ALLE ZEIT WACH
SJ
1842

J. Prieto J. Rodés D.A. Shafritz (Eds.)

# Hepatobiliary Diseases

With 215 Figures, Some in Color
and 114 Tables

Springer-Verlag
Berlin Heidelberg New York London Paris
Tokyo Hong Kong Barcelona Budapest

Jesús Prieto, M.D.
Professor of Medicine, Department of Medicine and Liver Unit,
Clinica Universitaria and School of Medicine
University of Navarra, Pamplona, Spain

Joan Rodés, M.D.
Professor of Medicine, Liver Unit, Hospital Clinic i Provincial,
University of Barcelona, Barcelona, Spain

David A. Shafritz, M.D.
Professor of Medicine and Cell Biology and Director Marion Bessin
Liver Research Center, Albert Einstein College of Medicine
Bronx, NY, USA

ISBN-13:978-3-642-76804-0 e-ISBN-13:978-3-642-76802-6
DOI: 10.1007/978-3-642-76802-6

Library of Congress Cataloging-in-Publication Data. Hepatobiliary diseases / J. Prieto, J. Rodés, D.A. Shafritz (eds.). p. cm. Includes bibliographical references and index. ISBN-13:978-3-642-76804-0 1. Liver—Diseases. 2. Biliary tract—Diseases. I. Prieto Valtüena, Jesús Ma. II. Rodës, Joan. III. Shafritz, D. A. (David A.) [DNLM: 1. Biliary Tract Diseases. 2. Liver Diseases. WI 700 H52885] RC845.H43 1992 616.3'6—dc20 DNLM/DLC for Library of Congress 91-5205


Softcover reprint of the hardcover 1st edition 1992



Typesetting: Best-set Typesetter Ltd., Hong Kong
10/3130-5 4 3 2 1 0 – Printed on acid-free paper

*"In salute corporis et in virtute animae, libertas"*

To all our teachers and students

# Preface

The last few years have witnessed major developments in molecular biology which have had a significant impact on biomedical knowledge. As a result new concepts in cell biology have emerged, new etiologic agents have been discovered, and new drugs have become available. Furthermore, the world of mediators, cytokines, and humoral factors has enlarged considerably in a relatively short period and this has modified our views of diverse physiopathologic processes as well as opened up new therapeutic prospects. In addition, recent technologic advances have revolutionized our diagnostic methodology and have greatly enhanced the power of our therapeutic resources. All these factors have contributed to a substantial remodeling of both liver science and clinical hepatology, and these changes have generated the motivation for the production of the present book, which attempts to give an account of well-known clinical facts in the light of current thinking. It is the fruit of the coordinated work of experts from different countries in three continents. In a sense, it is a manifestation of the fact that international cooperation is becoming increasingly important not only in the expansion of science but also in its exposition.

We hope that *Hepatobiliary Diseases* will be useful to both students and clinicians and that internists, gastroenterologists, and general practitioners will find in its contents a satifactory coverage of their field of interest.

We would like to thank our secretaries, and especially Maria Dolores Barrio, for their continual help and dedication, which have been so important for the completion of this book. We would also like to express our gratitude to all those institutions and foundations (among them Fundación Ramón Areces) that have provided generous help to liver research.

J. PRIETO · J. RODÉS · D.A. SHAFRITZ

# Contents

# List of Contributors

Vicente Arroyo, M.D.; Professor of Medicine, Liver Unit, Hospital Clinic i Provincial, University of Barcelona, Barcelona, Spain

Charles Balabaud M.D.; Professor of Hepatogastroenterology, Service des maladies de l'appareil digestif, hôpital St André, Bordeaux et Laboratoire des Interactions Cellulaires, Université de Bordeaux II, Bordeaux Cedex, France

Oscar Beloqui, M.D., Ph.D.; Consultant Physician, Department of Medicine and Liver Unit, Clinica Universitaria and School of Medicine, University of Navarra, Pamplona, Spain

José I. Bilbao, M.D.; Consultant Radiologist, Department of Radiology, Clinica Universitaria and School of Medicine, University of Navarra, Pamplona, Spain

Paulette Bioulac-Sage, M.D.; Professor of Pathology, Laboratoire d'Anatomie Pathologique, CHU Pellegrin, Bordeaux et Laboratoire des Interactions Cellulaires, Université de Bordeaux II, Bordeaux Cedex, France

Johannes Bircher, M.D.; Professor of Clinical Pharmacology and Internal Medicine, University of Witten/Herdecke, Beckweg 4, Herdecke, FRG

Jaime Bosch, M.D.; Professor of Medicine, Liver Unit, Hospital Clinic i Provincial, University of Barcelona, Barcelona, Spain

Daniel W. Bradley, M.D.; Hepatitis Branch, Division of Viral and Rickettsial Diseases, Center for Infectious Diseases, Centers for Disease Control, Atlanta, USA

Miguel Bruguera, M.D.; Professor of Medicine. Liver Unit, Hospital Clinic, University of Barcelona, Medical School, Barcelona, Spain

Patrizia Burra, M.D.; Liver Unit, Queen Elizabeth Hospital, Birmingham, U.K.

Andrew K. Burroughs, MB, ChB (Hons), MRCP; Senior Lecturer in Medicine and Honorary Consultant Physician, Hepatobiliary and Liver Transplantation Unit, Royal Free Hospital and School of Medicine, London, U.K.

Joan Camps, M.D.; Clinical Associate, Department of Medicine and Liver Unit, Clinica Universitaria and School of Medicine, University of Navarra, Pamplona, Spain

FLAIR JOSÉ CARRILHO, M.D.; Hepatology Branch, Discipline of Clinical Gastroenterology, University of Sao Paulo School of Medicine, Sao Paulo, SP. Brazil

ALBERTO CASTILLA, M.D.; Professor of Medicine, Department of Medicine and Liver Unit, Clinica Universitaria and School of Medicine, University of Navarra, Pamplona, Spain

PEDRO PAULO CHIEFFI, M.D.; Laboratory of Hepatology (LIM-47), Instituto de Medicina Tropical de Sao Paulo, Department of Preventive Medicine, University of Sao Paulo School of Medicine, Sao Paulo, SP. Brazil

MARÍA P. CIVEIRA, M.D.; Professor of Medicine, Department of Medicine and Liver Unit, Clinica Universitaria and School of Medicine, University of Navarre, Pamplona, Spain

MASSIMO COLOMBO, M.D.; Professor of Medicine, Institute of Internal Medicine University of Milan, Milan, Italy

FEDERICO CONCHILLO, M.D.; Associate Professor, Department of Medicine and Gastroenterological Unit, Clinica Universitaria and School of Medicine, University of Navarra, Pamplona, Spain

LUIZ CAETANO DA SILVA, M.D.; Hepatology Branch, Discipline of Clinical Gastroenterology, Laboratory of Hepatology (LIM-47), Instituto de Medicina Tropical de Sao Paulo, University of Sao Paulo School of Medicine, Sao Paulo, SP. Brazil

ROBERT J. DE KNEGT, M.D.; Department of Internal Medicine II, University Hospital Dijkzigt, Rotterdam, The Netherlands

VALEER DESMET, M.D., Ph.D.; Professor of Histology and Pathology, Head, Department of Pathology II, University Hospital St. Rafaël, Catholic University of Leuven, Leuven, Belgium

ELWYN ELIAS, M.D.; Liver Unit, Queen Elizabeth Hospital, Birmingham, U.K.

RAFAEL ESTEBAN, M.D.; Professor of Medicine, Chief, Liver Unit, Hospital General Universitario Vall d'Hebron, Universitat Autónoma de Barcelona, Barcelona, Spain

NELSON FAUSTO, M.D.; Professor and Chairman, Department of Pathology and Laboratory Medicine, Brown University, Providence, USA

FAUSTO FEU, M.D.; Research Associate Hepatic Haemodynamics Laboratory and Liver Unit, Hospital Clinic i Provincial, University of Barcelona, Barcelona, Spain

JOHAN FEVERY, M.D., Ph.D.; Professor of Medicine, Chief Division of Hepatobiliary and Pancreatic Diseases, University Hospital Gasthuisberg, Catholic University of Leuven, Leuven, Belgium

JUAN CARLOS GARCIA-PAGÁN, M.D.; Research Associate, Hepatic Haemodynamics Laboratory and Liver Unit, Hospital Clinic i Provincial, University of Barcelona, Barcelona, Spain

PERE GINÈS, M.D.; Staff member, Liver Unit, Hospital Clinic i Provincial, University of Barcelona, Barcelona, Spain

John L. Gollan, M.D., Ph.D., F.R.A.C.P., F.R.C.P.; Director, Gastroenterology Division, Brigham and Women's Hospital, Associate Professor of Medicine, Harvard Medical School Boston, USA

Javier Gonzalez-Gallego, M.D.; Professor and Director, Department of Physiology, Pharmacology and Toxicology, University of Leon, Leon, Spain

Jaime Guardia, M.D.; Professor of Medicine, Chief, Department of Medicine, Hospital General Universitario Vall d'Hebron, Universitat Autónoma de Barcelona, Barcelona, Spain

Sanjeev Gupta, M.B.B.S., M.D., M.R.C.P. (U.K.); Assistant Professor of Medicine, Department of Medicine and Marion Bessin Liver Research Center, Albert Einstein College of Medicine, Physician, Weiler Hospital of the Albert Einstein College of Medicine, Montefiore Medical Center and Bronx Municipal Hospital Center Bronx, New York, USA

June W. Halliday, B.Sc. (Hons.), Ph.D.; Senior Principal Research Fellow and Professor, Dept. of Medicine, Univ. of Queensland, Queensland Institute of Medical Research, Brisbane, Australia

Krzysztof Krawczynski, M.D.; Hepatitis Branch, Division of Viral and Rickettsial Diseases, Center for Infectious Diseases, Centers for Disease Control, Atlanta, USA

Brigitte Le Bail, M.D.; Pathologist, Laboratoire d'Anatomie Pathologique. CHU Pellegrin, Bordeaux et Laboratoire des Interactions Cellulaires, Université de Bordeaux II, Bordeaux Cedex, France

Francisco J. Lecumberri, M.D.; Consultant Radiologist, Department of Radiology, Clinica Universitaria and School of Medicine, University of Navarra, Pamplona, Spain

Stanley M. Lemon, M.D.; Professor of Medicine and Microbiology and Immunology, The University of North Carolina at Chapel Hill, Chapel Hill, North Carolina. USA

Jesús M. Longo, M.D.; Consultant Radiologist, Department of Radiology, Clinica Universitaria and School of Medicine, University of Navarra, Pamplona, Spain

Michael P. Manns, Professor Dr. med.; Medizinische Hochschule Hannover, Abt. Gastroenterologie und Hepatologie, Hannover, Germany

P. Aiden McCormick, M.B., M.R.C.P. (U.K.); Lecturer in Medicine and Honorary Senior Registrar, Hepatobiliary and Liver Transplantation Unit, Royal Free Hospital and School of Medicine, London, U.K.

Neil McIntyre, M.D.; Professor of Medicine, Head, Department of Medicine, Royal Free Hospital and School of Medicine, Pond Street, London, U.K.

Harold J. Metselaar, M.D., Ph.D.; Department of Internal Medicine II, University Hospital Dijkzigt, Rotterdam, The Netherlands

Karl-Herrmann Meyer zum Büschenfelde, Professor Dr. med.; Medizinische Klinik I, Johannes Gutenberg Universität, Mainz, Germany

Giordina Mieli-Vergani, King's College School of Medicine, Bessemer Road, London SE5 9PJ, England

Alberto Moreno, M.D.; Department of Pathology, Hospital Ramón y Cajal, Madrid, Spain

Alex P. Mowat, M.D.; Professor of Paediatric Hepatology, Department of Child Health, Variety Club Children's Hospital, King's College School of Medicine and Dentistry, Bessemer Road of King's College London, London SE5 9PJ, U.K.

Miguel Muñoz, M.D.; Consultant Physician and Chief of Endoscopy Unit, Department of Medicine, Clinica Universitaria and School of Medicine, University of Navarra, Pamplona, Spain

María T. Muñoz Yagüe, M.D.; Associate Professor of Medicine. Clinical Associate, Unit of Gastroenterology, Hospital Doce de Octubre School of Medicine, Universidad Complutense, Madrid, Spain

Albert Parés, M.D.; Clinical Assistant, Liver Unit, Hospital Clinic i Provincial, University of Barcelona, Barcelona, Spain

Dominique Pessayre, M.D.; Director of Research, INSERM U24, Hôpital Beaujon, Clichy, France

María P. Pizcueta, Ph.D. (Biol.), Ph.D. (Phar.); Research Associate, Hepatic Haemodynamics Laboratory and Liver Unit, Hospital Clinic i Provincial, University of Barcelona, Barcelona, Spain

Lawrie W. Powell, A.C., M.D., Ph.D., F.R.C.P. (Lond.), F.R.A.C.P.; Director, Queensland Institute of Medical Research and Professor of Medicine, University of Queensland, Brisbane, Australia

Jesús Prieto, M.D.; Professor of Medicine, Department of Medicine and Liver Unit, Clinica Universitaria and School of Medicine, University of Navarra, Pamplona, Spain

Jorge Quiroga, M.D.; Consultant Physician, Department of Medicine and Liver Unit, Clinica Universitaria and School of Medicine, University of Navarra, Pamplona, Spain

Joan Rodés, M.D.; Professor of Medicine, Director of Liver Unit, Hospital Clinic i Provincial, University of Barcelona, Barcelona, Spain

Sidney Rosalki, M.D.; Department of Chemical Pathology, Royal Free Hospital and School of Medicine, London, U.K.

Mikko Salaspuro, M.D., Ph.D.; Professor of Alcoholic Diseases, Research Unit of Alcohol Diseases, University of Helsinki, Helsinki, Finland

José M. Sánchez-Tapias, M.D.; Associate Professor of Medicine Liver Unit, Hospital Clinic, University of Barcelona, Barcelona, Spain

Bruno Sangro, M.D.; Clinical Associate, Department of Medicine and Liver Unit, Clinica Universitaria and School of Medicine, University of Navarra, Pamplona, Spain

Solko W. Schalm, M.D., Ph.D.; Professor of Medicine, Department of Internal Medicine II, University Hospital Dijkzigt, Rotterdam, The Netherlands

David A. Shafritz, M.D.; Professor of Medicine and Cell Biology and Director, Marion Bessin Liver Research Center, Albert Einstein College of Medicine, Morris Park Avenue, Bronx, New York. USA

José A. Solis Herruzo, M.D.; Professor of Medicine, Gastroenterology Unit. Hospital Doce de Octubre, School of Medicine, Universidad Complutense, Madrid, Spain

Waltraud Sommer, M.D.; University of Witten/Herdecke Beckweg 4, Herdecke, FRG

John A. Summerfield, M.D., F.R.C.P.; Reader in Medicine, Department of Medicine, St Mary's Hospital Medical School, London, U.K.

Kim M. Summers, B.Sc. (Hons.), Ph.D.; Senior Research Officer, Queensland Institute of Medical Research, Brisbane, Australia

Victor Vargas, M.D.; Professor of Medicine, Staff, Liver Unit, Hospital General Universitario Vall d'Hebron, Universitat Autónoma de Barcelona, Barcelona, Spain

J. Jaime Vázquez, M.D.; Professor of Pathology, Department of Pathology, Clinica Universitaria and School of Medicine, University of Navarra, Pamplona, Spain

Bart van den Berg, M.D., Ph.D.; Department of Internal Medicine II, University Hospital Dijkzigt, Rotterdam, The Netherlands

Peter Van Eyken, M.D., Ph.D.; Assistant, Department of Pathology II, University Hospital St. Rafaël, Catholic University of Leuven, Leuven, Belgium

Diego Vergani, M.D.; Department of Immunology, King's College School of Medicine, Bessemer Road, London SE5 9PJ, England

José M. Zozaya, M.D.; Consultant Physician, Department of Medicine and Liver Unit, Clinica Universitaria and School of Medicine, University of Navarra, Pamplona, Spain

Stephen D. Zucker, M.D.; Associate Physician, Gastroenterology Division, Brigham and Women's Hospital, Instructor in Medicine, Harvard Medical School, Boston, USA

# 1 Anatomy and Structure of the Liver and Biliary Tree*

B. LE BAIL, C. BALABAUD, and P. BIOULAC-SAGE

## 1 Introduction

The liver is a voluminous organ, interposed between the digestive tract and the rest of the organism, which functions both as an exocrine gland (bile secretion) and as a complex endocrine gland. It is richly vascularized and composed of different structural elements: hepatocytes, sinusoids, biliary system, and extracellular matrix. All these elements are closely associated in a well-defined pattern perfectly adapted for the various hepatic functions and mainly characterized by:

- A double blood supply, arterial and venous (oxygenation, hormone and nutrient supply)
- The arrangement of hepatocytes in unicellular plates separated by fenestrated capillaries with no basement membrane (blood–hepatocyte exchanges, cellular heterogeneity)
- The exposure of Kupffer, endothelial, and pit cells to different exogenous, immunogenic, or tumoral elements (immunologic functions)
- The presence of extracellular matrix in the Disse space, between sinusoidal cells and hepatocytes (intercellular regulation, communication, homeostasis)
- The specific intracellular organization of hepatocytes (exocrine and endocrine secretions, intercellular communications)

We shall first discuss the general anatomy of the liver and the biliary tree and then consider the main histologic and ultrastructural features, including liver organization, analysis of the different components, functional histologic models, and an outline of functional anatomy [for general reviews see 1–6].

---

* All micrographs shown in this chapter illustrate human material from control patients. For light microscopy, 3 μm thick paraffin-embedded sections from 10% formalin-fixed specimens and 1 μm thick epon-embedded sections from perfusion-fixed biopsy specimens (1.5% glutaraldehyde) were used. Ultrathin sections for transmission electron microscopy and blocks for scanning electron microscopy were from perfusion-fixed biopsy specimens (1.5% glutaraldehyde).

## 2 Gross Anatomy

### 2.1 Liver

The liver is a large pyramidal-shaped organ that weighs 1200–1500 g in adults and is situated in the right upper quadrant of the abdomen, under the diaphragm and sheltered by the ribs. It is red-brown and has a smooth surface due to the presence of a thin connective capsule (Glisson's capsule).

The liver has three main faces. The *upper face* is convex, tapering to a point on the left and linked to the right dome of the diaphragm by the falciform ligament. The *lower face* is positioned obliquely, inclined forward and turned to the left. It harbors three hollows: one is transversal and corresponds to the hilus of the organ (porta hepatis); the others are posteroanterior and correspond to the position of the gallbladder (right) or to a vestige of the Arantius canal (left). The *posterior face* is triangular, vertical, and close to the vena cava. The liver is held in place by the

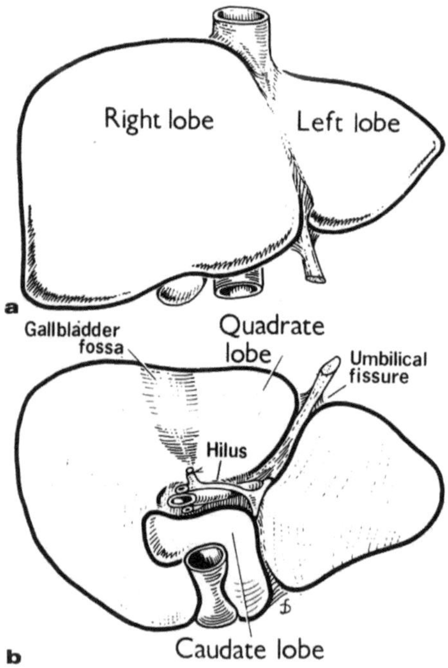


**Fig. 1a,b.** Morphologic aspect of the liver. The liver is divided into a right and a left lobe as seen from the front (**a**). From underneath (**b**), the back of the right lobe is delimited by the transverse or hilar fissure. The quadrate lobe is outlined on the left by the umbilical fissure, on the right by the gallbladder fossa. Behind the hilar fissure is the caudate (spigelian) lobe. [Reproduced with permission from Bismuth H (1988) In: Blumgart LH (ed) Surgery of the liver and biliary tract. Churchill Livingstone, Edinburgh, 1:1–9]

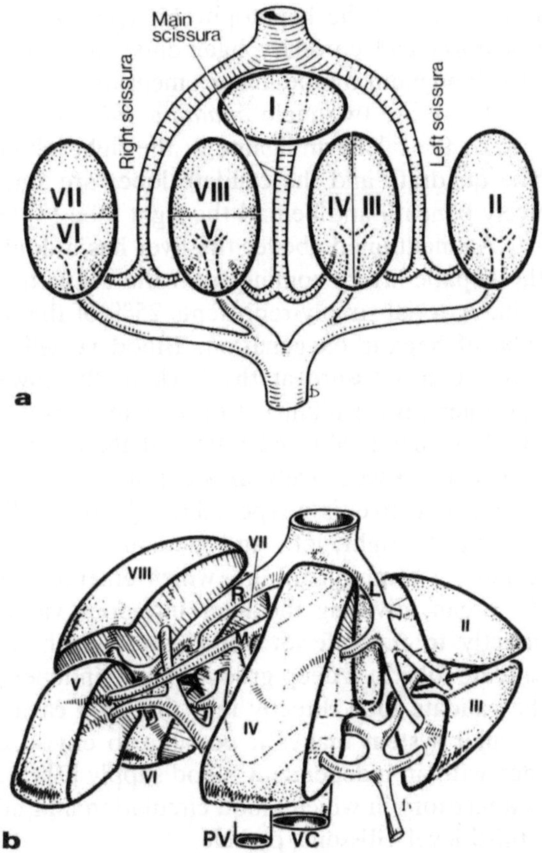


**Fig. 2. a** Schematic representation of the functional anatomy of the liver. There are three main hepatic veins lying within the liver scissurae and dividing the liver into four sectors, each receiving a portal pedicle. Hepatic veins and portal pedicles are intertwined as would be the fingers of two hands. **b** Segmentation of the liver according to Couinaud's nomenclature. The liver appears to be divided into two livers by the main hepatic scissura within which the middle hepatic vein (*M*) runs. The right liver is divided into two sectors by the right portal scissura within which runs the right hepatic vein (*R*). Each of these two sectors is divided into two segments: anterior sector – segments V and VIII, and posterior sector – segments VI and VII. The left liver is divided into two sectors by the left portal scissura in which the left hepatic vein runs (*L*). The anterior sector is divided by the umbilical fissure into two segments: a median segment IV (quadrate lobe) and a lateral segment III. The posterior sector comprises only one segment (II), which is the posterior part of the left lobe. The Spigel lobe (segment I) is an autonomous segment. It receives vessels not only from the left but also from the right branches of the portal vein (*PV*) and hepatic artery. Its hepatic veins are independent and drain directly into the inferior vena cava (*VC*). [Reproduced with permission from Bismuth H (1988) In: Blumgart LH (ed) Surgery of the liver and biliary tract. Churchill Livingstone, Edinburgh, 1:1–9]

vena cava and the hepatophrenic (posterior face) and peritoneal ligaments (falciform and coronary ligaments) and anchored to the stomach and the first duodenum by the lesser omentum.

There are two main *anatomic lobes* in the liver, separated on the front face by the falciform ligament; the right lobe is six times the size of the left. The quadrate and the caudate lobes are smaller segments situated respectively beneath and behind the right lobe [7] (Fig. 1).

As mentioned above, the liver has a double blood supply: arterial from the hepatic artery coming from the celiac trunk, and venous via the portal vein. Arterial supply represents 25% of the total blood supply but provides 50% of hepatic oxygenation. Blood vessels enter the liver and bile ducts leave it in a fissure at the back of the lower face of the right lobe, the porta hepatis (or hilum). At this point venous and arterial vessels divide into two branches (right and left) and then enter the parenchyma, where they branch out successively and continue in association with a bile duct and some connective tissue (portal or Glisson' pedicles). Venous blood leaves the liver by the right, left, and median hepatic veins (the left and the median forming a common trunk), which emerge at the back of the upper face of the organ, dividing the liver into four vascular sectors. These veins lead directly to the inferior vena cava, which furrows along the right of the caudate lobe in a deep groove. Small independent venules drain blood from the caudate lobe directly into the vena cava. Functional study of the liver vascular system makes it possible to envisage the liver as eight segments, each with an independent blood supply [7] (Fig. 2). Each segment is defined as a territory in which blood circulation and biliary drainage are provided by a third level Glisson's pedicle.

Lymphatic vessels drain mainly into the nodes around the porta hepatis and the celiac trunk; another group drains directly into the mediastinal nodes.

The hepatic nerve plexus runs close to biliary and vascular ramifications and contains fibers from sympathetic ganglia (T7–T10), the right and left vagus nerves, and the right phrenic nerves.

## 2.2 Gallbladder and Extrahepatic Bile Ducts

The extrahepatic biliary tract is composed of three parts. It is subject to many anatomic variations (such as size, position, and orientation), particularly at the different confluences; we shall concentrate on the most common features.

The main biliary tract comprises the two hepatic ducts (right and left) coming from the right and left hepatic lobes, the common hepatic duct, and the common bile duct [8]. The accessory biliary tract includes the gallbladder and the cystic duct and represents a diverticulum of the main tract.

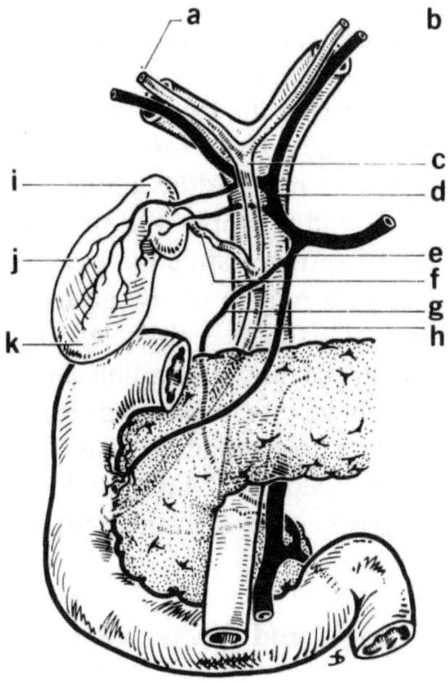


**Fig. 3.** Front view of the biliary tree. *a*, right hepatic duct; *b*, left hepatic duct; *c*, common hepatic duct; *d*, hepatic artery; *e*, gastroduodenal artery; *f*, cystic duct; *g*, retroduodenal artery; *h*, common bile duct; *i*, neck of the gallbladder; *j*, body of the gallbladder; *k*, fundus of the gallbladder. Note particularly the position of the hepatic bile duct confluence in front of the right branch of the portal vein, the cystic artery behind the common hepatic duct, and the proximity of the neck of the gallbladder to the right branch of the hepatic artery. [Reproduced with permission from SMADJA C and BLUMGART LH (1988) In: BLUMGART LH (ed) Surgery of the liver and biliary tract. Churchill Livingstone, Edinburgh, 1:11–22]

The terminal part of the common bile duct represents the zone of entry into the duodenal wall (Fig. 3).

The gallbladder is a pear-shaped bag 9–12 cm long and 2.5–5 cm wide that can contain 30–50 ml of bile. It lies in a fossa on the lower edge of the right lobe and extends to the right end of the porta hepatis. It is divided into four zones: the fundus (bottom), the body, the infundibulum, and the neck. This last segment forms an "S" that tapers into the cystic duct and comprises a small saccus called the Hartmann's pouch where stones can often be blocked.

The right and left hepatic ducts drain bile from the right and left hepatic lobes and meet at the porta hepatis to form the common hepatic duct (0.8–5 cm long). The cystic duct coming from the gallbladder (0.4–6.5 cm long) drains shortly afterwards into the common hepatic duct to form the common bile duct (1.5–9 cm long and 0.5–1.5 cm in diameter). This duct runs into and along the omentum, in front of the portal vein and to the right of the hepatic artery, and passes behind the first portion of the duodenum in a groove on the back of the head of the pancreas to enter the second part of the duodenum.

Once in the duodenum wall, the common bile duct joins with the main pancreatic duct to form the ampulla of Vater; this emerges in the duodenal lumen surrounded by a mucosal pad, the duodenal papilla.

Blood is supplied to the gallbladder by the cystic artery, a branch of the hepatic artery, while the common bile duct is supplied by the retroduodenal artery, a branch of the gastroduodenal artery. Venous blood coming from the gallbladder is collected in a network of small vessels connected to a similar plexus surrounding the extrahepatic bile ducts; this plexus drains into the cholecystic veins that enter directly into the liver, where they subdivide into capillaries. The lymphatic vessels of the gallbladder enter the pericholedochal lymph node situated near the origin of the cystic duct; lymph then flows to the peripancreatic nodes.

## 3 Light and Electron Microscopy

### 3.1 General Organization

On histologic sections, the liver appears as a homogenous and richly vascularized tissue. Hepatocytes represent 80%–90% of the parenchyma, composing unicellular plates forming a regular, radial pattern between vascular structures. Blood is supplied by branches of the portal vein and the hepatic artery. These vessels together with branches of the biliary tree, lymphatics, nerves, and a few lymphocytes are surrounded by loose connective tissue; these pedicles of varying size are called the portal tracts. Between the incoming vessels of the portal tracts and the central veins lies the network of hepatic sinusoids, which allows exchanges between blood and the unicellular sheets of hepatocytes (Figs. 4–7).

### 3.2 Hepatocytes

Hepatocytes are voluminous polygonal cells which make up approximately 80% of the liver cell population. They are arranged in unicellular plates or laminae of about 20 cells (Remak's plates) which branch and anastomose with one another to form a complicated walling system, the hepatic muralium, extending from portal tracts to the central veins [9–11] (Figs. 4–7).

Adjacent hepatic plates are separated by specialized capillaries: the hepatic sinuoids (Fig. 7). The rim of hepatocytes surrounding the portal tract (which constitutes an interface between the connective tissue of the tract and the parenchyma) forms the limiting plate. In each Remak's plate,

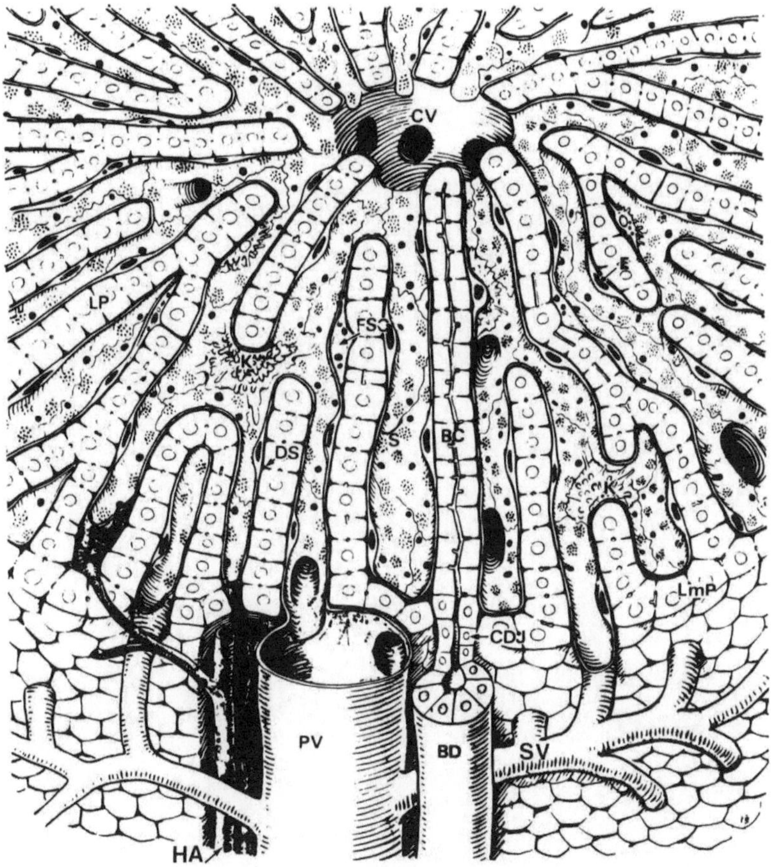


**Fig. 4.** Three-dimensional structure of the lobule according to MUTO. This schematic figure summarizes the three-dimensional structure of the hepatic lobule as revealed by scanning electron microscopy. *CV*, central vein; *K*, Kupffer cell; *FSC*, fat-storing cell (perisinusoidal cell, Ito cell); *BC*, bile canaliculus; *E*, endothelial cell; *S*, sinusoid; *DS*, Disse's space; *HA*, hepatic artery branch; *PV*, portal vein branch; *CDJ*, canaliculoductular junction (canal of Hering); *BD*, interlobular bile duct; *LmP*, limiting plate; *LP*, liver plates; *SV*, septal branch of the portal vein. [Reproduced with permission from MOTTA P et al. (1978) The liver: an atlas of scanning electron microscopy. Igaku-Shoin, Tokyo]

each hepatocyte is in contact with the adjacent hepatocyte and with the sinusoidal lumen through the Disse space (Figs. 7, 8).

Hepatocytes are polyhedral cells approximately 30 µm long and 20 µm wide, with a mean volume of 5000 $\mu m^3$. The nucleus is spherical and voluminous, occupying 5%–10% of the cell volume, with one or more prominent nucleoli and scattered chromatin (Figs. 8, 9). About 25% of the cells are binucleate. The adult liver has a very low mitotic index, with

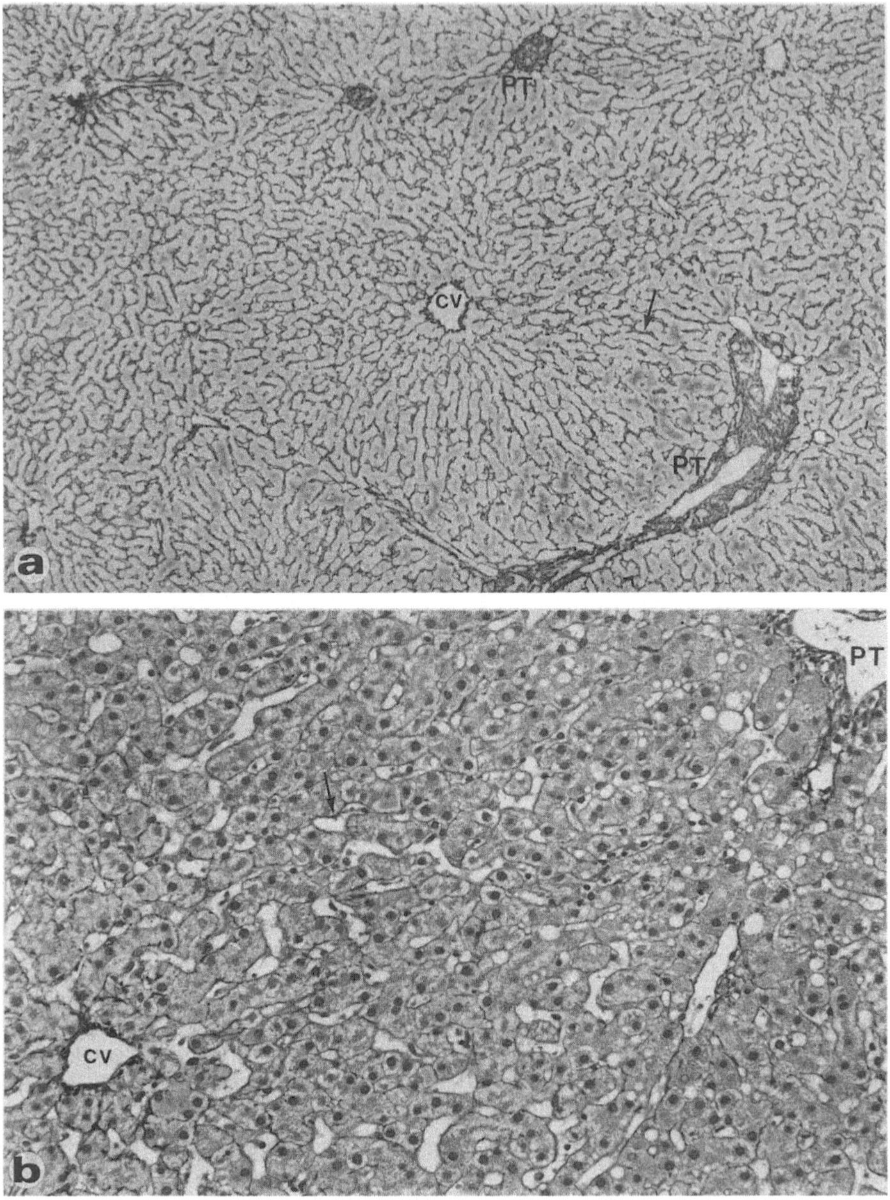


**Fig. 5a,b.** Hepatic parenchyma. Paraffin embedding (3 μm thick sections). **a** The classic polygonal lobule is seen with a centrolobular vein (*CV*) in the center and portal tracts (*PT*) at the periphery. Hepatocytic plates are separated by the reticulin network (*arrow*) surrounding sinusoids. Reticulin staining, ×63. **b** Sirius red staining allows identification of the thin perisinusoidal matrical network (*arrow*) and of the fibrous tissue around the centrolobular vein (*CV*) and the portal tract (*PT*). ×220

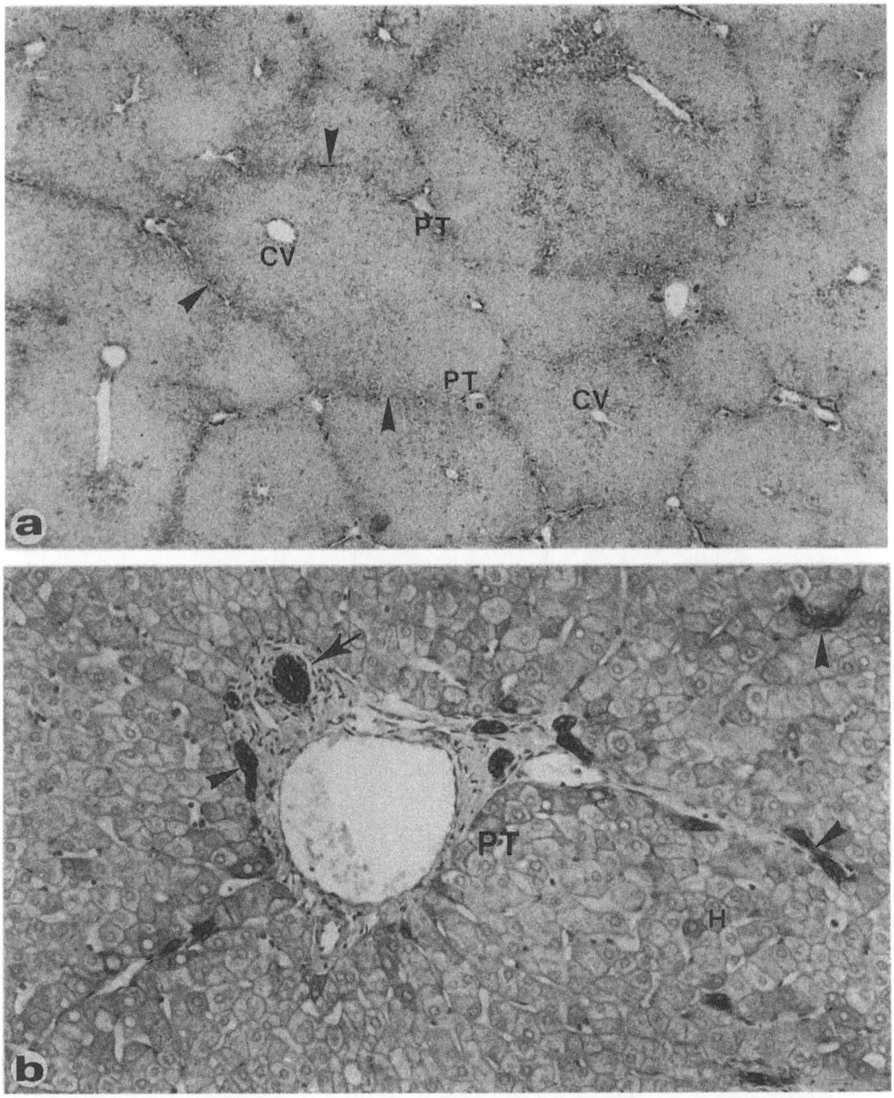


**Fig. 6a,b.** Hepatic parenchyma. Paraffin embedding (3 µm thick sections); peroxidase–antiperoxidase immunostaining for cytokeratin KL 1 (Immunotech). **a** The septa of the lobules can be clearly seen thanks to the staining of cholangioles (*arrowheads*) in the terminal branches of portal tracts (*PT*). *CV*, centrolobular veins. ×30. **b** In this portal tract (*PT*), interlobular bile ducts (*arrows*) and cholangioles (*arrowheads*) at the periphery show diffuse and dense cytoplasmic staining whereas hepatocytes (*H*) show only fine peripheral cytoplasmic staining. ×220

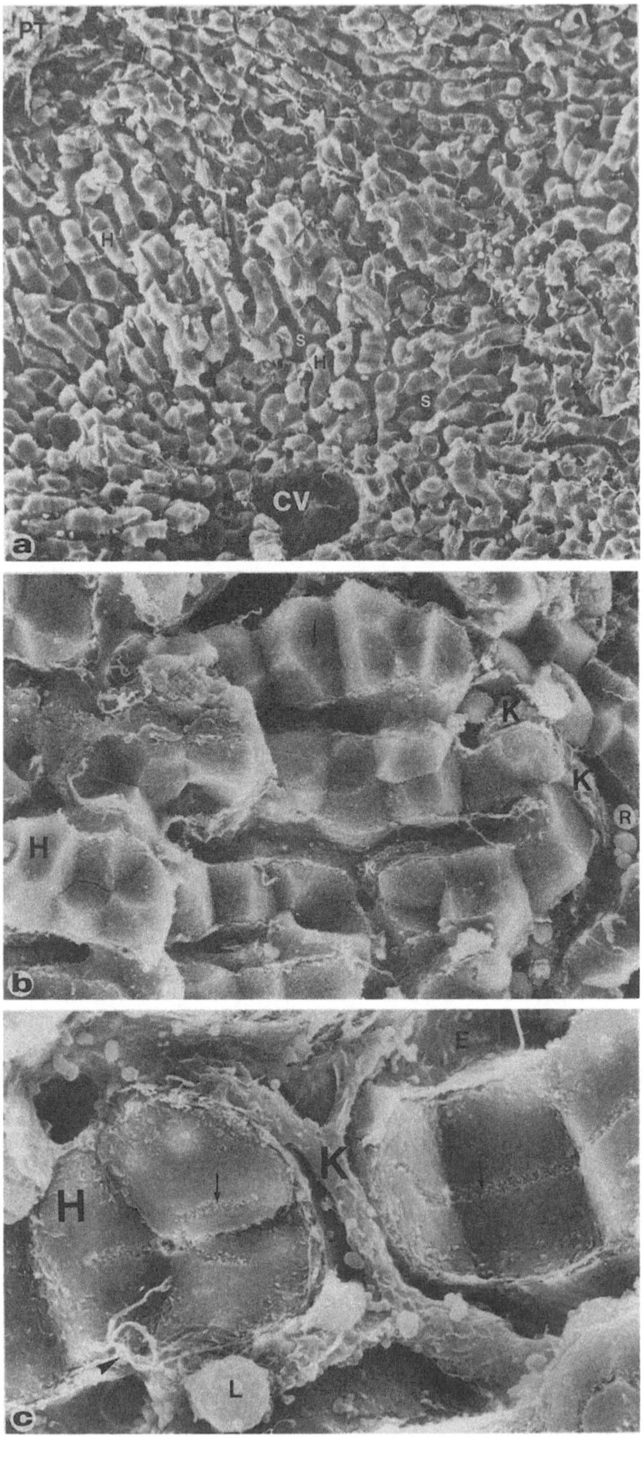


Fig. 7a–c

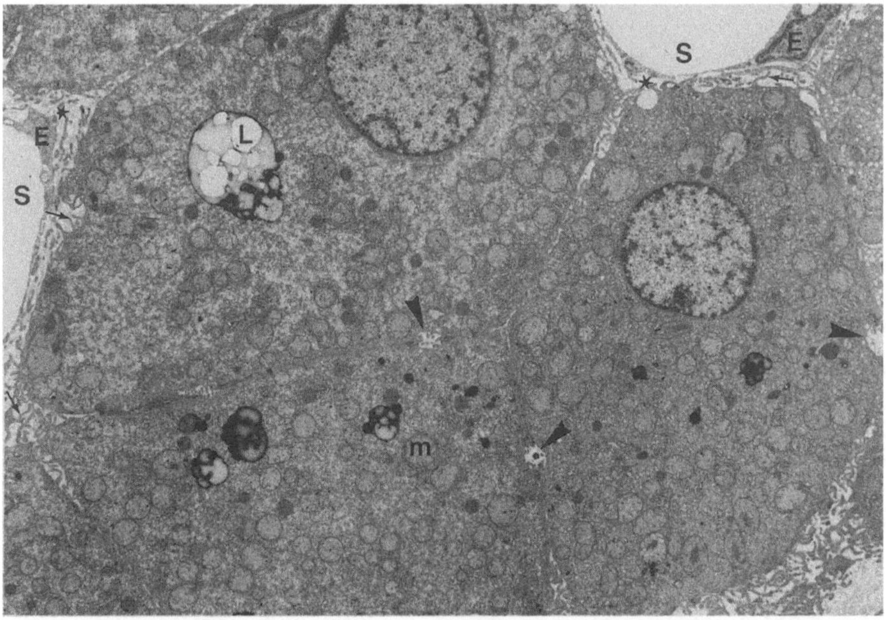


**Fig. 8.** Transmission electron microscopy. These three hepatocytes are limited by their sinusoidal membranes with microvilli (*arrows*) and lateral and canalicular (*arrowheads*) membranes. Mitochondria (*m*), other organelles, and lipofuscins (*L*) can be seen in the cytoplasm. Two round and regular nuclei are visible. *S*, sinusoid; *E*, endothelial wall; *star*, Disse space. ×2850

estimates ranging from 2 mitoses per 1000 cells to 1 per 10000 cells. Nuclear size seems to correlate to ploidy and increases with aging.

*Light microscopy* reveals the hepatocellular cytoplasm to be slightly eosinophilic, with granular clumps of basophilic material which correspond on electron microscopy to rough endoplasmic reticulum. Near the bile canaliculi, the cytoplasm frequently contains fine brown granules of lipofuscin pigment. These are more abundant with age, particularly in the centrolobular zone. A few hepatocytes may contain fat vacuoles. Histochemical procedures are essential to identify glycogen, hemosiderin, lipids, etc.

---

**Fig. 7a–c.** Scanning electron microscopy. **a** At this low magnification, the unicellular sheets of hepatocytes (*H*) separated by sinusoids (*S*) can be clearly seen with the centrolobular vein (*CV*) at the center of the lobule and a portal tract (*PT*) at the periphery. ×400. **b** It happens frequently that liver blocks are broken between the lateral surface of hepatocytes (*H*), which allows clear visualization of the biliary hemicanaliculi (*arrow*). Kupffer cells (*K*) protrude in the sinusoidal lumen. *R*, red blood cell. ×1300. **c** In between two hepatocytes (*H*), a Kupffer cell (*K*) protrudes at the confluence of two sinusoids, attached by filipodia to the endothelial wall (*E*). *Arrowhead*, collagen fibers; *L*, lymphocyte; *arrows*, biliary hemicanaliculi. ×3150

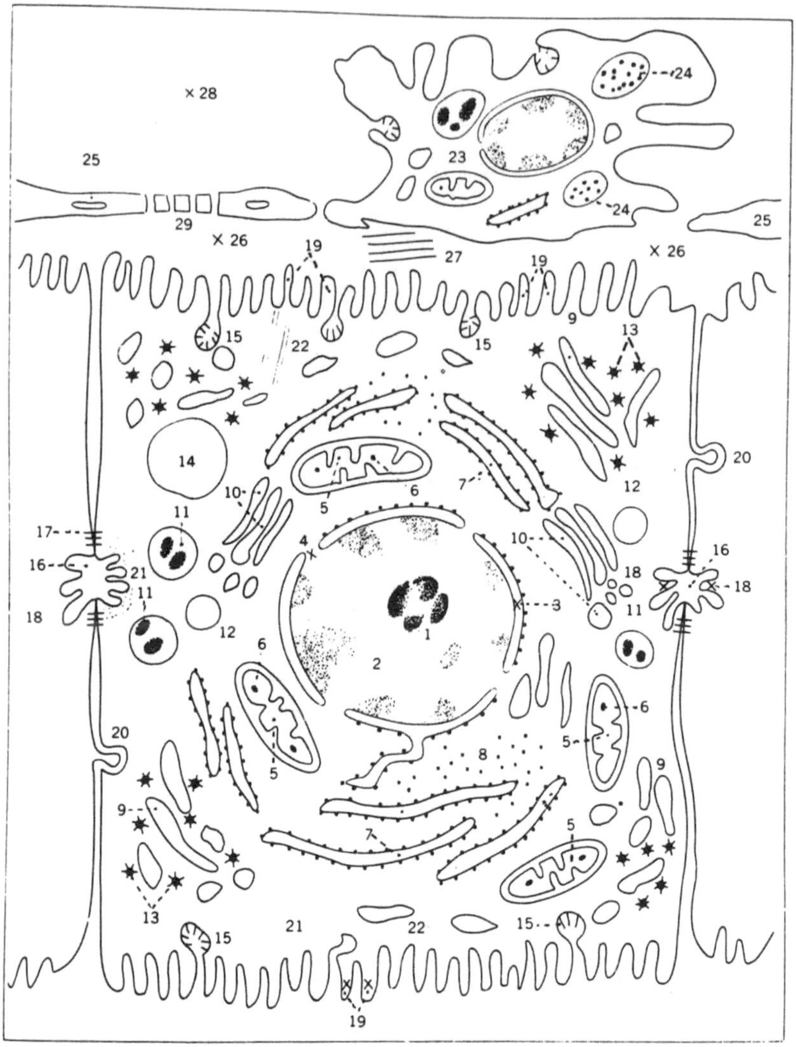


**Fig. 9.** Schematic view of hepatocyte ultrastructure and its position with regard to the sinusoid. *1*, nucleolus; *2*, nucleoplasm; *3*, nuclear envelope; *4*, nuclear pore; *5*, mitochondrion; *6*, mitochondrial granule; *7*, rough surfaced endoplasmic reticulum; *8*, free ribosomes; *9*, smooth surfaced endoplasmic reticulum; *10*, Golgi apparatus; *11*, lysosome; *12*, peroxisome; *13*, glycogen particles; *14*, fat droplet; *15*, pinocytic invagination; *16*, bile canaliculus; *17*, junctional complex; *18*, microvilli of the bile canaliculus; *19*, microvilli of the sinusoidal pole; *20*, a studlike projection of the cytoplasm; *21*, microfilaments; *22*, microtubules; *23*, Kupffer cell; *24*, phagocytosed material; *25*, endothelial cell; *26*, Disse space; *27*, fibers of the extracellular matrix; *28*, sinusoidal lumen; *29*, endothelial fenestrae forming a sieve plate. [Reproduced with permission from Bioulac-Sage P et al. (to be published) In: McIntyre N et al. (eds) Oxford textbook of clinical hepatology. Oxford University Press, Oxford]

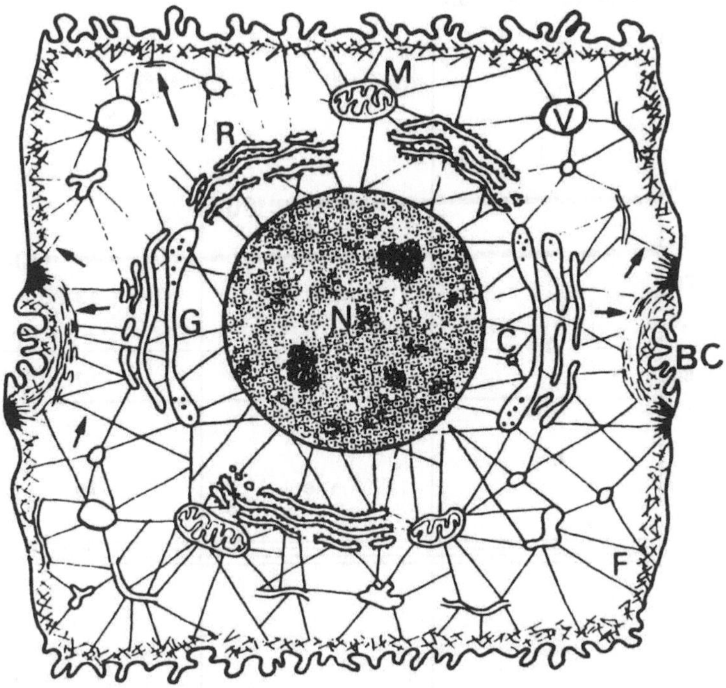


**Fig. 10.** Schematic representation of the cytoskeleton of the hepatocyte. *F*, microfilaments; *short arrows*, intermediate filaments; *long arrow*, microtubules; *BC*, bile canaliculus; *N*, nucleus; *G*, Golgi apparatus; *C*, centriole; *R*, rough endoplasmic reticulum; *M*, mitochondrion; *V*, vesicle. [Reproduced with permission from French SW et al. (1982) Hepatology 1:29–38]

*Electron microscopy* is necessary to visualize organelles (Figs. 8, 9). There is an abundant rough and smooth endoplasmic reticulum, a Golgi apparatus close to the biliary pole, and numerous mitochondria (1000–1500 per cell) and peroxisomes (about 200 per cell). The hepatocyte is rich in glycogen rosettes, the quantity depending on the time of food intake. The cytoskeleton of the cell comprises microfilaments, intermediate filaments, and microtubules which are shown by immunocytochemistry to correspond to actin, cytokeratin, and tubulin respectively; microfilaments are located mainly at the periphery of the cell and are connected to the plasma membrane whereas intermediate filaments and microtubules are scattered throughout the whole cytoplasm (Fig. 10) [12]. The main morphometric data concerning organelles are presented in Fig. 11.

The hepatocyte is limited by a plasma membrane in which three zones can be distinguished that represent morphologic and functional differentiation (Figs. 8, 9):

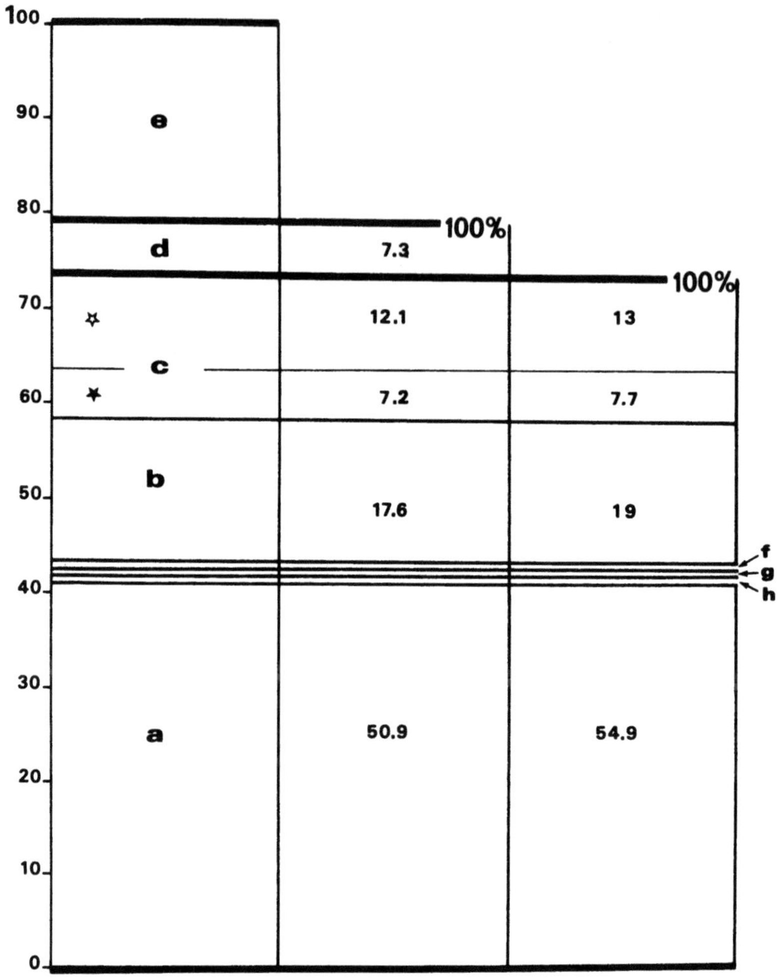


**Fig. 11.** Morphometric data: volumetric composition (expressed as a percentage) of the liver parenchyma (*left column*), an average hepatocyte (*middle column*), and hepatocytic cytoplasm (*right column*). *a*, hyaloplasm; *b*, mitochondria; *c*, endoplasmic reticulum: rough (*white star*), smooth (*black star*); *d*, nucleus; *e*, extrahepatocytic space (sinusoids and bile canaliculi); *f*, lysosomes; *g*, lipids; *h*, peroxisomes. Lysosome, lipid, and peroxisome volume density, expressed as % of the cytoplasm, are 2, 2.1, and 1.3 respectively

- The *sinusoidal membrane* is in contact with the Disse space and permits exchanges between blood and hepatocytes (exo- and endocytosis). It represents 70% of total cell surface owing to the presence of microvilli (0.5 μm long), which increase the surface area sixfold (Figs. 8, 12, 13c, 14c). At each extremity, the sinusoidal membrane burrows down, thus delimiting, with the sinusoidal membrane of the adjacent hepatocyte, the interhepatocytic space.

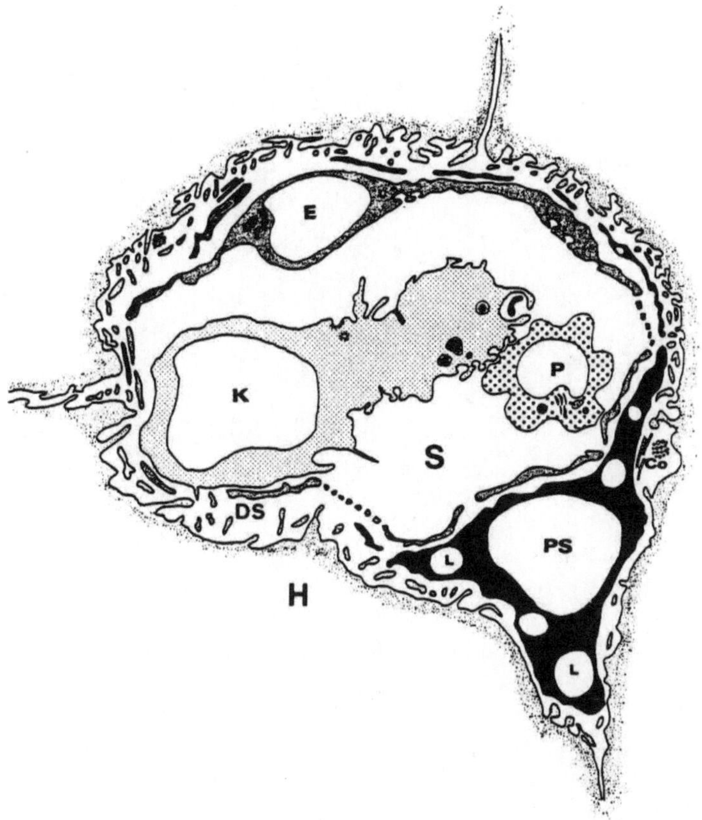


**Fig. 12.** Schematic representation of a sinusoid (*S*) and sinusoidal cells. *E*, endothelial cell; *K*, Kupffer cell; *PS*, perisinusoidal cell containing lipids (*L*); *P*, pit cell (large granular lymphocyte); *H*, hepatocyte; *DS*, Disse space; *Co*, collagen

- The *canalicular membrane* (15% of total cell surface area) is situated at the biliary pole of the hepatocyte and is formed by a depression in the plasma membrane, covered by microvilli; juxtaposition of the canalicular membranes of two neighboring hepatocytes delimits a groove-like space where bile is excreted: the biliary canaliculus (Fig. 7b,c). The canalicular lumen is isolated from the Disse space by tight junctions and is reinforced by numerous actin microfilaments (Fig. 15a).
- The *lateral membrane* (15% of the cell surface) is anchored to the lateral membrane of adjacent hepatocytes by various junctional complexes: desmosomes, gap junctions, intermediate junctions, and tight junctions (Fig. 15a). Between these points, hepatocytes are separated by an intercellular space of 15 nm (Figs. 8, 9).

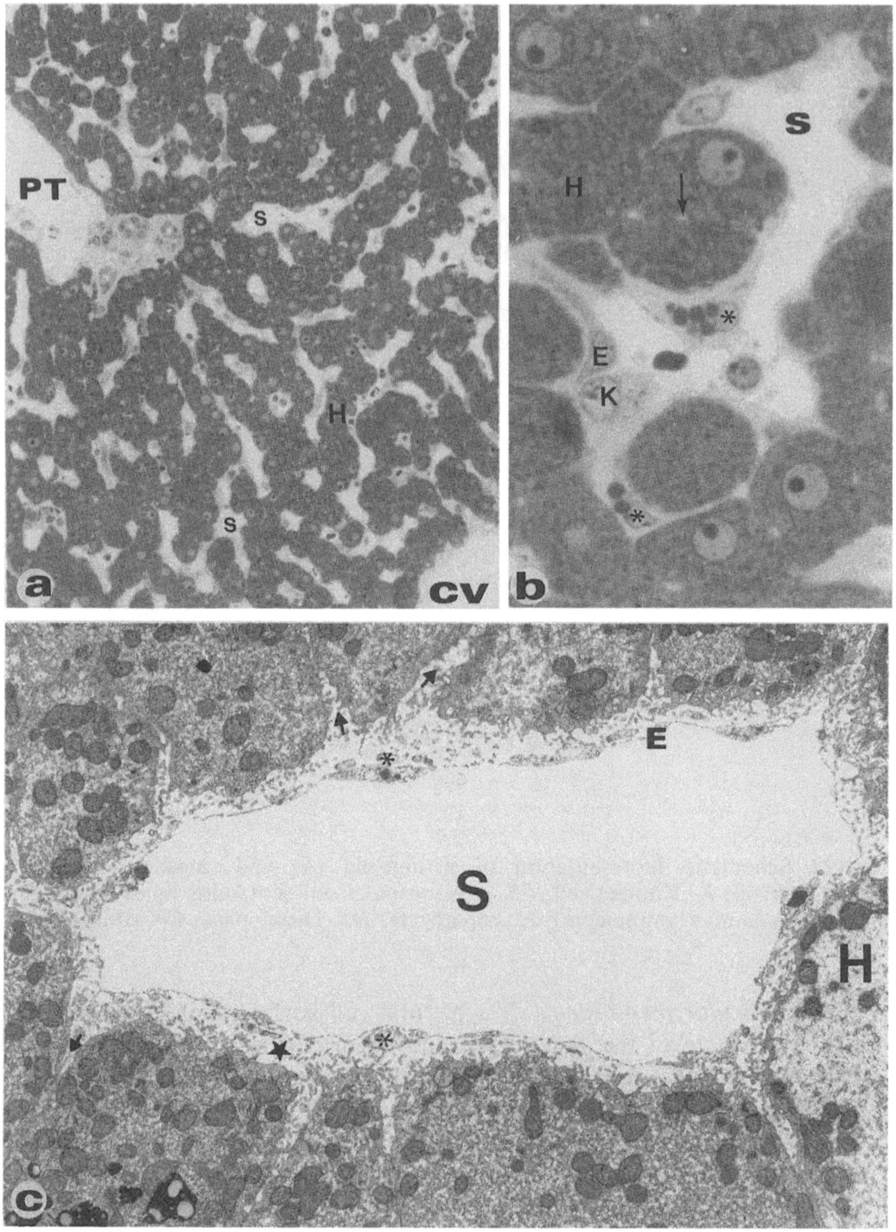


**Fig. 13a–c.** Epon embedding. **a,b** 1 μm thick section, toluidine blue; **c** transmission electron microscopy. **a** Sinusoids (*S*) are clearly visible, in between the unicellular sheets of hepatocytes (*H*), from the portal tract (*PT*) to the centrolobular vein (*CV*). ×220. **b** At higher magnification, sinusoidal cells can be identified: Kupffer (*K*), endothelial (*E*), and perisinusoidal (*asterisk*) cells. *Arrow*, bile canaliculus. ×1100. **c** This sinusoidal barrier is formed only by a thin fenestrated endothelial wall (*E*). Numerous cross-sections of hepatocyte (*H*) microvilli are visible in the Disse space (*star*) and the lateral recessus (*arrow*); *asterisk*, perisinusoidal cell processes. ×3500

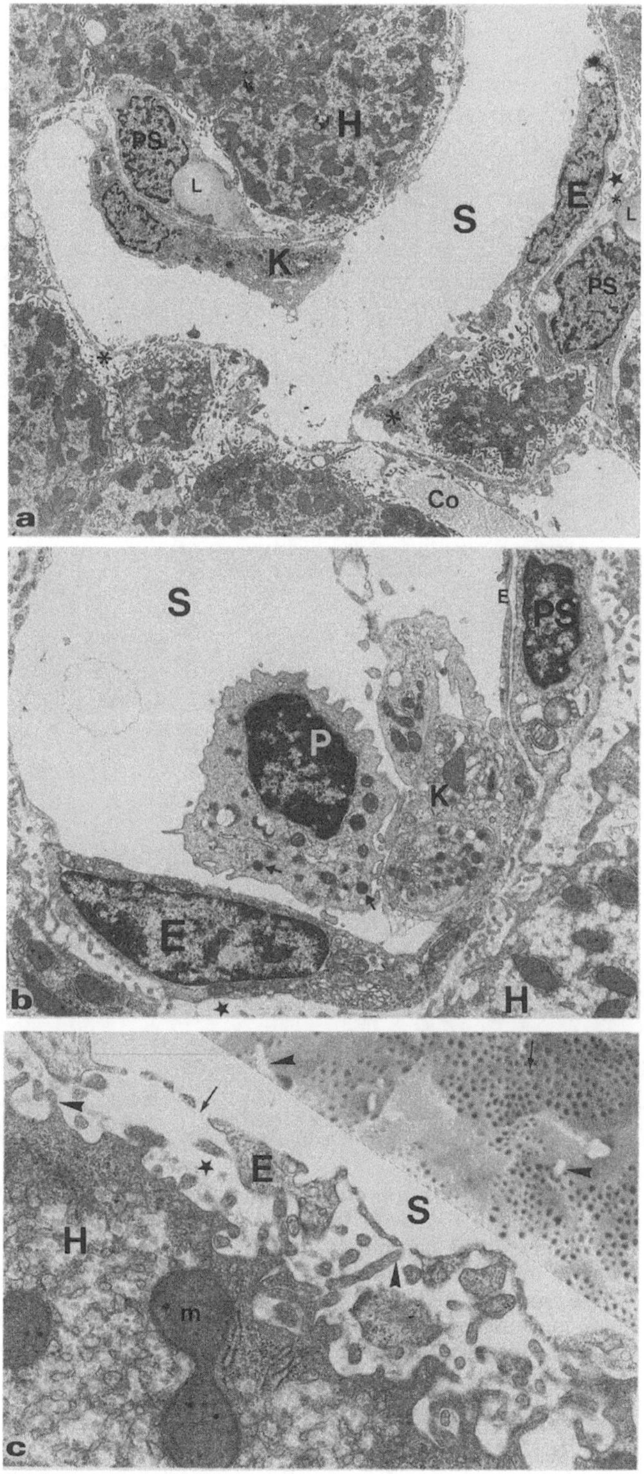


**Fig. 14a–c.** Transmission electron microscopy. **a** This wide sinusoid (*S*) is delimited by an endothelial cell with its cell body (*E*) and processes and by a Kupffer cell (*K*). Two perisinusoidal cells (*PS*) containing lipids (*L*) and their processes (*asterisk*) can be seen in the Disse space (*star*), next to collagen bundles (*Co*). *H*, hepatocytes. ×3300. **b** All four types of sinusoidal cells are seen in this sinusoid (*S*). The perisinusoidal cell (*PS*), devoid of lipids, lies under the endothelial cell (*E*); the pit cell (*P*) with two characteristic granules (*arrows*) is close to the Kupffer cell (*K*). *Star*, Disse space. ×7500. **c** This endothelial process shows open fenestrae (*arrow*). Microvilli (*arrowheads*) of the sinusoidal membrane of an hepatocyte (*H*) can be seen in the Disse space (*star*). In the visible part of its cytoplasm, rough and smooth endoplasmic reticulum, glycogen, and mitochondria (*m*) are clearly visible. ×22500. *Inset* (top right): scanning electron microscopy of endothelial fenestrae (*arrow*) grouped in sieve plates. *Arrowheads*: hepatocyte microvilli protruding in the lumen. ×21000

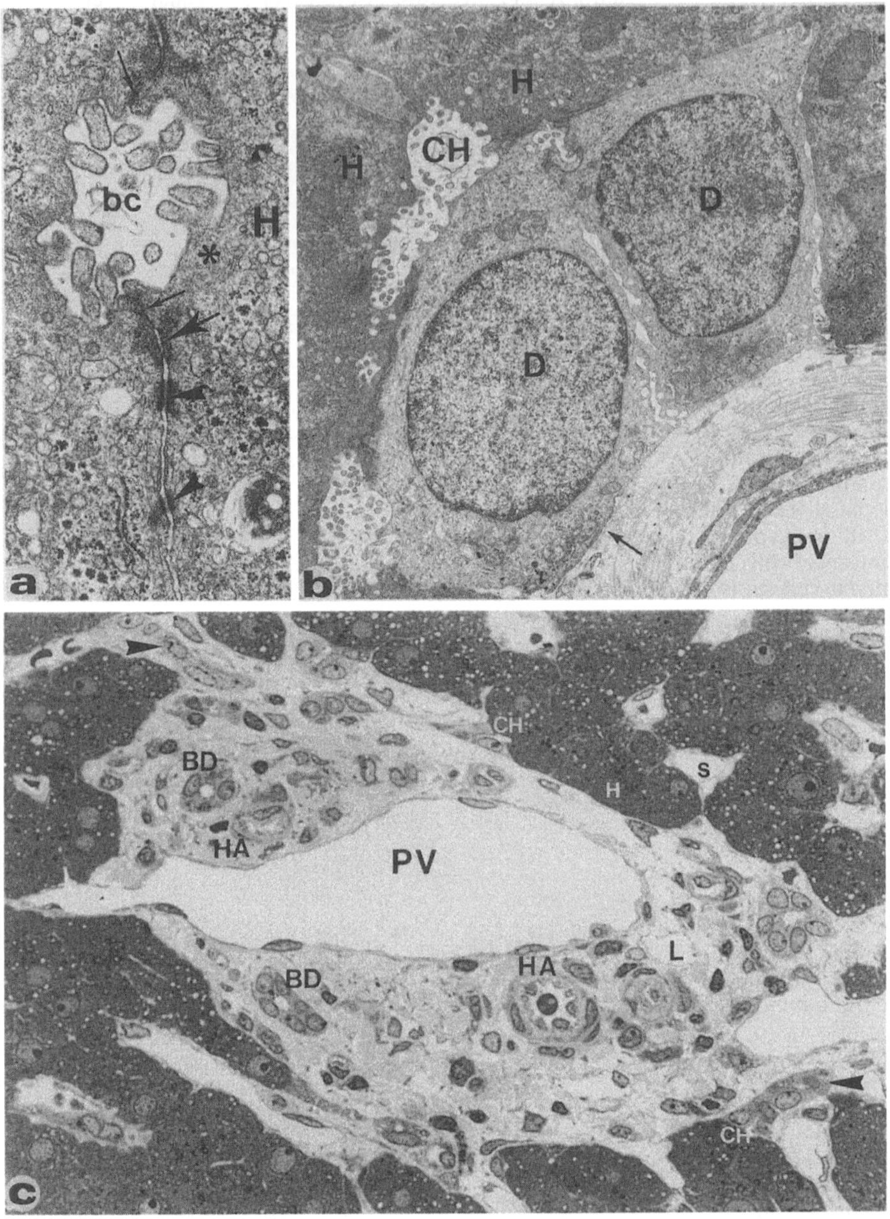


**Fig. 15a,b.** Transmission electron microscopy; **c** light microscopy. **a** Bile canaliculus (*bc*), with microvilli from the lining hepatocytes (*H*) protruding into the lumen. Junctional complexes on the edge of the lumen: tight junctions (*thin arrows*), intermediate junction (*thick arrow*), desmosomes (*arrowheads*). The narrow zone of hepatocytic cytoplasm (*asterisk*) surrounding the canalicular lumen appears to be denser and contains no organelles. ×20 000. **b** The lumen of a canalicular–ductular junction at the periphery of a portal tract (canal of Hering, *CH*) is lined by two hepatocytes (*H*) and two ductular epithelial cells (*D*) partially surrounded by a basement membrane (*arrow*). ×5500 **c** At the periphery of this portal tract, several canals of Hering (*CH*) and cholangioles (*arrowheads*) can be seen. Interlobular bile ducts (*BD*) are close to arterioles (*HA*). *PV*, portal vein; *H*, hepatocytes forming the periportal limiting plate; *S*, sinusoids; *L*, lymphatic vessel. ×560

### 3.3 Sinusoids and Sinusoidal Cells

The liver sinusoid is a fenestrated capillary lining the unicellular layers of hepatocytes on both lateral sides, from the terminal axis of the portal vein to the branches of the hepatic vein (Figs. 4, 7a). The sinusoidal barrier around the sinusoidal lumen is formed of endothelial cells surrounded by perisinusoidal cells (Figs. 12–14). Endothelial cells are separated from hepatocyte microvilli by the Disse space which contains the perisinusoidal cells and the extracellular matrix. This peculiar capillary is unique in that macrophages inside the lumen are anchored to the endothelial wall, the endothelium is fenestrated (Fig. 14c), perisinusoidal cells contain vitamin A lipid droplets, and there is no genuine basement membrane. Furthermore, as has been shown recently, sinusoids also harbor a population of large granular lymphocytes (pit cells) [13].

#### *Endothelial Cells*

Endothelial cells (ECs) are the most numerous of the sinusoidal cells, as they constitute the wall of the liver sinusoid [14, 15]. They occupy, in the rat, 2.8% of total liver volume and represent 44% of the volume of sinusoidal cells. Their main functions are filtration and endocytosis. These cells present two distinct zones, a perinuclear region that protrudes to varying degrees into the sinusoidal lumen, and a cytoplasm characterized by its extreme thinness, lining the sinusoidal wall and harboring characteristic and numerous fenestrae (best seen by scanning electron microscopy) (Figs. 12–14). These fenestrae are often arranged in clusters that have been given the name of "sieve plates" (Fig. 14c); 9% of the total endothelial lining is fenestrated. When cut perpendicular to the cell, these fenestrae look like small transcellular pores with no diaphragms; the mean diameter of fenestrae is in the 100 nm range. Larger fenestrae or gaps have been described but could correspond to fixation artifacts. The fenestrae allow direct communication between the sinusoidal lumen and the Disse space, which itself is in direct contact with hepatocytes, since ECs generally have no continuous basement membrane.

Recent results have shown lobular differences in the diameter and number of fenestrae and all studies confirm that the number of fenestrae, and hence porosity, are greater in zone 3 (perivenous or centrolobular) than in zone 1 (periportal). In normal liver, filtration capacity is thus greater in zone 3 than in zone 1, not only since the presence of more fenestrae guarantees higher porosity but also because periportal sinusoids are narrower than centrolobular sinusoids. The influence of different compounds or of tumor cells on the size and number of fenestrae has been investigated by several authors. Wisse et al., having found that blood cells, especially white cells, are often larger than periportal and, to a lesser extent, centrolobular sinusoids, introduced the concepts of "forced sieving" and "endothelial massage" for these mechanisms that could facilitate exchanges through fenestrae and cause movement of fluid in the Disse space [16]. ECs have been reported to be active in endocytosis. This is made possible by the presence of specific organelles such as micropinocytic vesicles, endosomes, and lysosomes. ECs are capable of more efficient endocytosis than Kupffer cells for certain substances (e.g., heparin, colloidal albumin).

***Kupffer Cells***

Kupffer cells (KCs), the macrophages of the liver, lie inside sinusoids in direct contact with the blood (Figs. 12, 14a,b), which they can clear of different types of material [14, 17]. They represent the most important population of resident macrophages in the body (range of $10-20 \cdot 10^6$ KCs per gram of liver). They are voluminous stellate cells easily visible by light microscopy (Fig. 13b). Using liver scanning electron microscopy (SEM), they can be seen bulging into the sinusoidal lumen and have numerous characteristic microvilli and filopodia (Fig. 7b,c).

The endocytic capacity of these cells is very high and is made possible by the development of numerous pinocytic and phagocytic structures and the presence of a large number of different kinds of lysosomes (Fig. 14). Two other structures have been said to be characteristic of KCs: worm-like structures and annulated lamellae.

Kupffer cells have been found predominantly in the periportal region, which may be the best location for endocytosis of the blood-borne material entering the liver. However, even if the periportal zone is the richest in KCs, it has been shown that these cells are far from absent elsewhere. Different studies have shown varying ratios for the three zones (periportal, midzone, and centrolobular) of approximately 4:3:2. Periportal KCs are also the largest and the most active in phagocytosis.

The functions of KCs are numerous. KCs can clear several types of pathogens, such as viruses, bacteria, fungi, and parasites. The liver has long been known to play an important role in the detoxification of circulating endotoxins. KCs can also clear the blood of immune complexes, tumor cells, liposomes, lipid microspheres, iron, and several other particulate or cellular elements. They have also been shown to make an important contribution to host-defense function through their complement receptors and to play a role in immune response. KCs respond to a great variety of immunomodulators, including oligopeptides (interferon, granulocyte-macrophage colony-stimulating factor, macrophage-activating factor), lipids (phorbol myristate acetate, lipopolysaccharides, platelet-activating factor, eicosanoids, glucocorticoids), and $Ca^{2+}$ ionophores. Under stimulation they can release mediators (tumor necrosis factor, interleukins 1 and 6, eicosanoids, interferon-α and -β) and agents (active oxygen species, cytolytic proteases, plasminogen activators, lytic enzymes, etc.) which may be harmful to hepatocytes.

***Perisinusoidal Cells***

Perisinusoidal cells (PSCs) originate from mesenchymal cells in the septum transversum and belong to the myofibroblast family [15, 18]. They are located in the Disse space beneath the endothelial barrier, often in the recesses delimited by two hepatocytes. Usually, PSCs are not visible on standard sections for light microscopy; their study requires semithin sections or electron microscopic examination (Figs. 12, 13b, 14a).

Under the electron microscope, one can see their stellate shape. The cell body is round or elongated with a high ratio of nucleus to cytoplasm. The nucleus is irregular and often indented by lipid droplets (Fig. 14a). Lipids are present in 75% of cells on tissue sections. The size and number of lipid droplets are highly variable from one cell to another and from one area to another. In general, lipid droplets are non-membrane-bound. Rough endoplasmic reticulum cisternae and free polysomes are easily visible. There are numerous smooth-surfaced and a few coated caveolae and vesicles, particularly along the plasma membrane.

The cytoskeleton is particularly well developed, with numerous microtubules, microfilaments, and intermediate filaments. Both the latter are clearly visible on tangential sections, running parallel to the plasma membrane. They are often concentrated in the ectoplasmic layer and occasionally condensed in small patches below the plasma membrane. Cytoskeleton proteins consist of tubulin, actin, vimentin, and desmin. The PSCs processes are thick near the cell body, and narrow further away. They run parallel to the endothelial wall. Short or long digitations often sprout from the processes, the longer ones occasionally partly, or completely, covering the cell body. Processes contain abundant cytoskeleton more or less parallel to the long axis of the process, numerous coated and smooth-surfaced caveolae and vesicles, occasional small lipid droplets, and some rough endoplasmic reticulum profiles.

According to some authors, the distribution of PSCs is homogeneous in the acinus; according to others, PSCs are predominantly located in the centrolobular zone. The number of PSCs is approximately 5–20 per 100 hepatocytes ($18 \pm 1.5/0.1\,mm^2$). Volume density represents 1.9% of the hepatic parenchyma. The volume and surface densities of PSCs processes represent 70% and 90% of total PSCs volume and surface densities, respectively. PSCs are involved in the storage of vitamin A and in fibrogenesis.

Immunocytochemical studies on isolated and cultured PSCs and on tissue sections have produced clear evidence for the secretion of different components of the extracellular matrix (intracellular localization): (1) collagen I, III, IV, fibronectin, laminin; (2) glycosaminoglycans (GAG): mainly dermatan and chondroitin sulfates (particularly abundant in fibrotic liver), but also heparan sulfate (which is the predominant GAG in normal liver, mainly secreted by hepatocytes). Perisinusoidal cells show the submicroscopic characteristics of fibroblasts (shape, organelles) and of myofibroblasts (desmin-positive intermediate filaments).

#### *Large Granular Lymphocytes ("Pit Cells")*

Pit cells are considered to be resident large granular lymphocytes (LGLs) with natural killer activity; they represent the largest population of LGLs in the organism. They are located in the sinusoidal lumen and adhere to the endothelial wall or KCs (Fig. 12) [13]. Far fewer in number (one for ten KCs) they can only be identified by electron microscopy. They are round lymphoid cells, 8–15 μm in diameter, with short pseudopodia, a large round nucleus, and a reduced cytoplasm containing two characteristic organelles: dense granules and rod-cored vesicles (Fig. 14b). They play a role in antiviral and antitumoral defense.

### 3.4 Extracellular Matrix

The extracellular matrix is located in the perisinusoidal Disse space and is composed of three components: collagens, proteoglycans, and glycoproteins (Fig. 14a). Although not normally discernible by light microscopy, part or all of the extracellular matrix can be visualized with special staining such as silver impregnation (Fig. 5a) or Sirius red (Fig. 5b). The stain forms a delicate network delimiting the shape of sinusoids.

Two main functions are classically attributed to the hepatic connective matrix: support and mediation between hepatocytes and sinusoidal cells. The knowledge we have at present of the functional properties of matrical proteins would suggest that:

1. The extreme flexibility of the Disse connective matrix could be due either to the predominance of type III collagen over type I, or to the simultaneous presence of these two collagens.
2. Fibronectin, known to be a molecule involved in cell–matrix interaction in the microvascular system, may be responsible for the cohesion of the heterogeneous cell–matrix edifice.
3. The presence of type IV collagen could explain the nonthrombogenic properties of the lining; in association with heparan sulfate proteoglycan, it would allow the selective filtration of blood signal substances for target cells, in this case hepatocytes.
4. The absence of a well-developed basement membrane could enable selected molecules to transit from the blood to hepatocytes and from hepatocytes to the bloodstream, across the Disse space.

The importance of cell–matrix interactions in modulation of the phenotypic expression of sinusoidal cells and hepatocytes has recently been underlined [19, 20].

## 3.5 Biliary Tree

### *The Intrahepatic Biliary Tree*

Bile secreted by hepatocytes flows through the canalicular network (0.4% of the lobular parenchyma) which forms a structurally and functionally coherent system (average diameter 0.5–1 μm in zone 3 and 1–1.25 μm in zone 1) (Figs. 7b,c, 8, 15a). Tone is provided by an encircling mesh of contractile microfilaments fixed on the zonula adherens which follow the outline of the microvilli. Bile flows in the opposite direction to plasma and enters small ductules or cholangioles. The junction between the last hepatocyte and the first of two spindle-shaped biliary cells is called the *canal of Hering* (Fig. 15b,c). A putative stem cell with a dual differentiation potentiality (hepatocellular, biliary) has been identified and described between the last hepatocyte and the first biliary cell.

Lined by three or four cells that become cuboidal, cholangioles are usually less than 15 μm in diameter and are situated in the vascular axis of Rappaport's acinus (Figs. 6, 15). On light microscopy they are at the periphery of the portal tract and are not accompanied by vessels. They drain bile into interlobular bile ducts located in portal tracts (Figs. 6b, 15c, 16b,c). Running close to these ducts (diameter <100 μm) lined by a cuboidal epithelium are arteries of similar diameter. The confluence of two or more interlobular bile ducts forms a septal duct (diameter >100 μm) lined by a cylindrical epithelium (Fig. 16d). Segmental ducts (diameter between 400 and 800 μm) as well as left and right bile ducts are histologically similar. The biliary columnar epithelium lined by a basement membrane (Fig. 16e) is surrounded by dense fibrous tissue containing many elastic fibers. A peribiliary vascular plexus (branches of the hepatic artery) supplies all the intrahepatic bile ducts. This plexus drains principally into hepatic sinusoids. The biliary tree plays a role not only in excreting bile but also in absorption and secretion. In addition to the enterohepatic cycle it has been suggested that a cholehepatic cycle may also exist.

### *The Extrahepatic Biliary Tree*

The gallbladder wall comprises four layers [21] (Fig. 17): a mucosa, a plexiform muscularis, perimuscular connective tissue, and a fold of the visceral peritoneum (or serosa). In the gallbladder, bile is concentrated and stored.

The mucosa is lined by a columnar single-layer epithelium separated by a basal membrane from a layer of loose connective tissue (lamina propria). It forms multiple primary and secondary folds that flatten as the gallbladder fills. The villosities are separated by epithelial crypts sometimes extending across the entire width of the muscular layer and communicating with the lumen: Rokitansky-Aschoff sinuses or crypts. The mucosa is mainly lined by

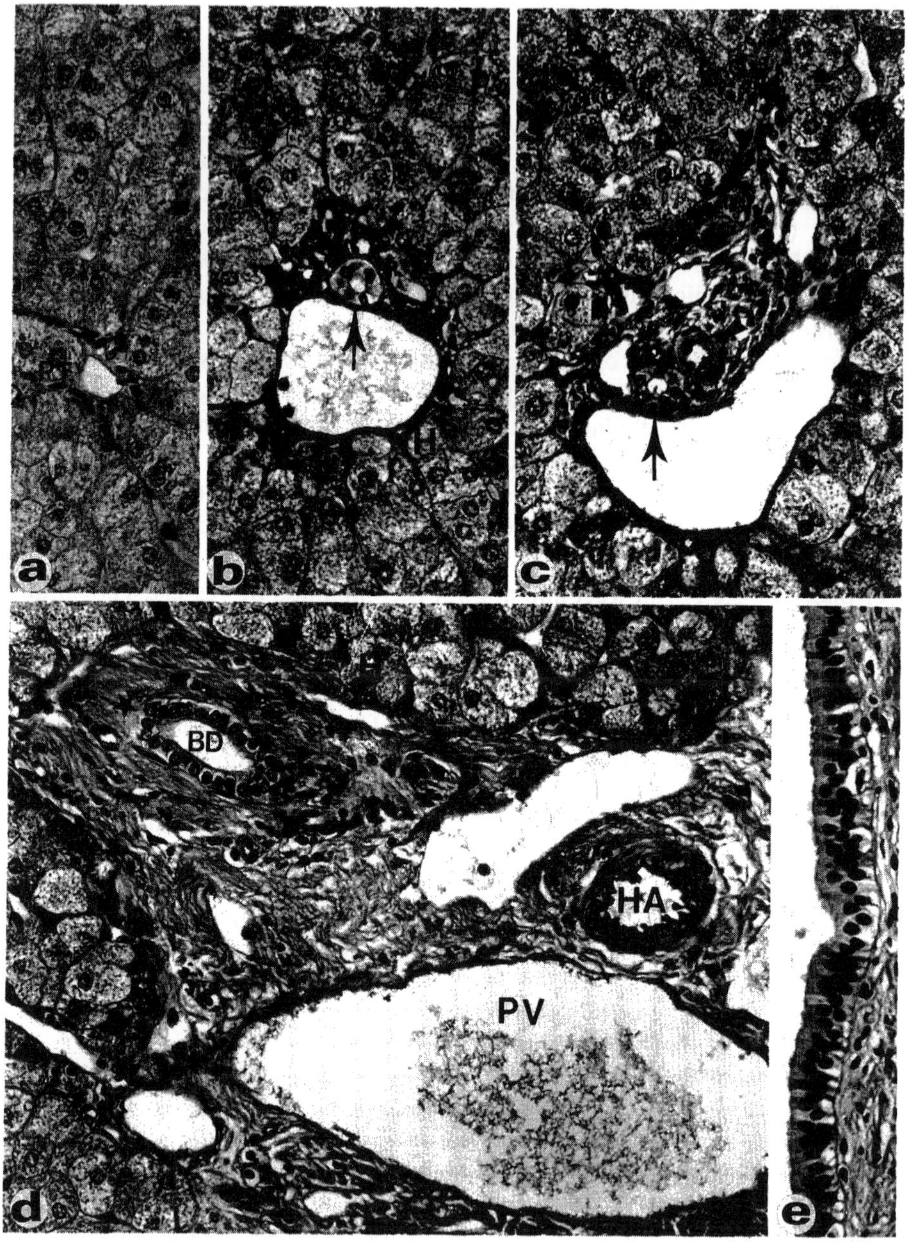


**Fig. 16a–e.** Paraffin embedding (3 μm thick sections). Different types of bile ducts (*arrows*) at the same magnification, in portal tracts (*PT*) of different sizes. At the periphery of the portal tracts, hepatocytes (*H*) form the periportal limiting plate. ×250. **a** In this very small portal tract, the bile duct is below the limit of visibility. **b,c** These interlobular bile ducts are formed by four or five cuboidal cells, around a narrow, round lumen; an artery (*arrowhead*) of the same size runs close to them. **d** In this larger portal tract, the septal bile duct (*BD*) is lined by a cubocylindrical epithelium, surrounded by a rim of dense fibrous tissue (*star*); the lumen is wider and elongated. Note the abundant connective tissue in the tract around the portal vein (*PV*) and artery (*HA*). **e** Cylindrical epithelium of a segmental bile duct in a large portal tract, near the porta hepatis

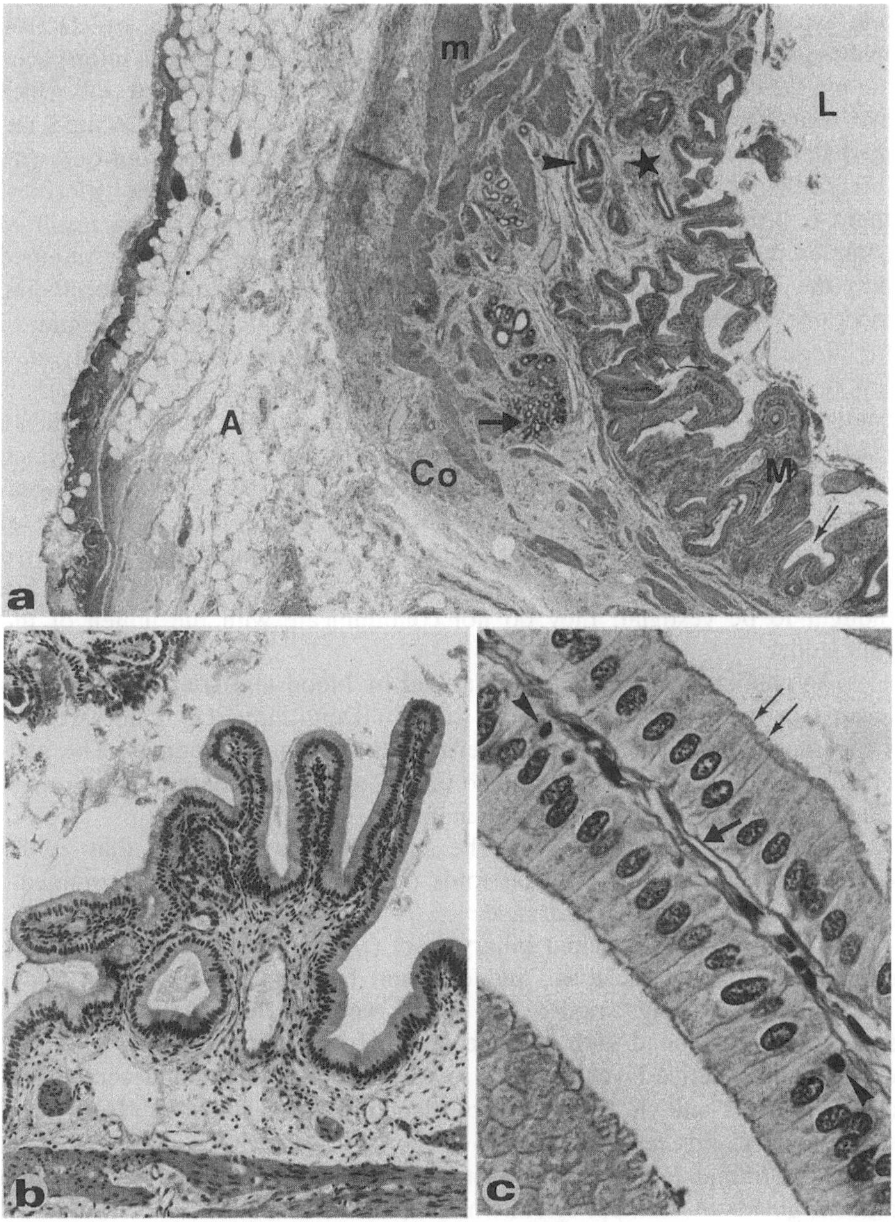


**Fig. 17a–c.** Normal gallbladder. Paraffin embedding (3 μm thick sections). **a** The whole gallbladder wall is shown. The mucosa (*M*) presents numerous villosities protruding in the lumen (*L*) and crypts (*thin arrow*) extending into the lamina propria (*star*), forming Aschoff-Rokitansky sinuses (*arrowhead*). Luschka's diverticula (*thick arrow*) can be seen in the smooth muscle layer (*m*) surrounded by perimuscular connective tissue (*Co*). The adventitia (*A*) is a thin fibroadipose tissue. ×30. **b** The mucosal folds are formed by columnar epithelium, covering a digitation of connective tissue which contains some inflammatory cells. ×110. **c** The epithelium consists of a single layer of tall uniform columnar cells with a striated apical pole (*thin arrows*) and ovoid basal nucleus; it is supported by a basement membrane (*thick arrow*). Some intraepithelial lymphocytes (*arrowheads*) are also seen. ×560

a single layer of tall columnar cells (95%) with an ovoid basal nucleus and a pale cytoplasm with microvilli at the apex (only visible by electron microscopy). Pencil-like cells are narrow and dark-staining cells interspaced among the columnar cells; their function is unknown. Some basal cells which are rounder and smaller than the other epithelial cells are located immediately above the basement membrane and should not be confused with intraepithelial lymphocytes, which are more common. Within the villosities, there is little connective tissue. Concentration of the bile is the result of complex mechanisms occurring in the mucosa. Sodium is actively pumped into the intercellular cleft between columnar cells, below the occluding junctions, creating a standing gradient that moves water from the lumen to the blood vessels in the wall of the gallbladder. In the neck of the organ, a few mucous glands can be found in the lamina propria. The muscularis is composed of circular, longitudinal, and oblique smooth muscle cells in an elastic connective tissue. The perimuscular layer is a connective tissue which contains blood vessels, lymphatic channels, nerves, adipocytes, and occasional paraganglions. Aberrant bile ducts with a cuboidal biliary type of epithelium can occasionally be seen in the perimuscular connective tissue adjacent to the liver. These ducts, called *Luschka's ducts*, are thought to be vestigial; they do not communicate with the lumen of the gallbladder.

The gallbladder is richly vascularized by blood and lymphatic plexuses located in the lamina propria and in the adventitium; it is innervated by sympathetic motor fibers and numerous sensitive nerve endings. The gallbladder is emptied by the combined action of cholecystokinin on the musculature and peristalsis in the duodenum.

The structure of the wall of the cystic duct is similar to that of the gallbladder, except that mucosal folds (valves of Heister) are prominent, giving the duct a spiral appearance.

The wall of the principal biliary tract (right and left extrahepatic bile ducts, common hepatic duct, and common bile duct) is 0.5–1 mm thick. The mucosa is fairly smooth but forms irregular longitudinal pleats or small folds. It is lined with a single layer of tall columnar cells. The subepithelial connective layer contains numerous elastic fibers and very sparse circular smooth muscle fibers, except near the Oddi's sphincter. Intramural seromucous glands can be seen.

The terminal common bile duct has a thick wall containing numerous mucous glands of vestigial origin which open into the ductal lumen in small pits, the Beale sacculi. The lumen is narrow and fairly villous. A muscular sphincter is formed by longitudinal and circular smooth muscle fibers, sometimes attached to the mucosa of the duodenum. The duct is anchored to the intestinal wall by thin muscular fibers. The ampulla of Vater is lined by long parallel villosities covered by a regular columnar epithelium which play an antireflux role. It is encircled by numerous smooth muscle fibers which penetrate into the axis of the villosities.

### 3.6 Nerves

Nerves enter at the porta hepatis. In humans, the liver receives both sympathetic and parasympathetic nerve fibers. Intrinsic innervation mainly consists of fibers within the vascular and biliary systems. Immunocytochemistry has revealed not only, as expected, the presence of adrenergic nerves in portal tracts and a few cholinergic bundles, but also neuropeptides (substance P, vasoactive intestinal peptides, neuropeptide Y) both in portal tracts and along sinusoids. Using electron microscopy [6], unmyelinated nerve bundles surrounded by Schwann cells and nerve endings have been observed close to the surface, without real synapses, of (a) fibroblasts surrounding the portal veins, bile ducts, hepatic arteries, and lymph vessels, (b) PSCs in the Disse space, (c) myofibroblasts around central veins, and (d) hepatocytes. Nerve endings contained many granular and agranular vesicles. Hepatic nerve functions are both efferent and sensory. Efferent nerves influence liver cell metabolism (glucose release) and play a role in the regulation of blood flow. The close contact between nerve endings and PSCs suggests that nerves may in part regulate the hemodynamic process at sinusoidal level.

### 3.7 Lymphatics

Lymph is first formed in the perisinusoidal Disse space. Fluid then enters the periportal tissue of the Mall space, which lies between portal connective tissue and the limiting plate, and from there the lymphatic capillaries. Lymph is then collected in lymphatics present in the portal tract, and conveyed by increasingly large lymphatic vessels which leave the liver at the porta hepatis to reach the thoracic duct. The liver capsule and stroma contain numerous lymphatic vessels which form loose plexuses that connect at intervals with underlying lymphatic vesssels.

## 4 Functional Anatomy

### 4.1 Functional Unit of the Liver

For the histologist and physiologist, the functional unit (vascular and biliary) is not the classic lobule. The functional unit could be better represented by Rappaport's acinus or Matsumoto's primary lobule.

#### *Kiernan's Lobule*

The portal tracts of the pig liver form a continuous network that, on section, divides the liver into polygonal units called lobules. In humans, these septa are less developed (Figs. 5a, 6a) and often even absent. Each lobule is a polygonal area of parenchyma, 0.7 mm in diagonal, delimited by its angles which correspond to portal tracts. The center of the lobule is occupied by a centrolobular venule (or hepatic venule). Plates of hepatocytes separated by sinusoids converge toward this venule.

### *Rappaport's Liver Acinus*

Rappaport's acinus is a diamond-shaped parenchymal mass lying between two centrolobular veins [22] (Fig. 18). The axis is the terminal branch of the portal vein in the septa (<40 μm in diameter) situated between two portal

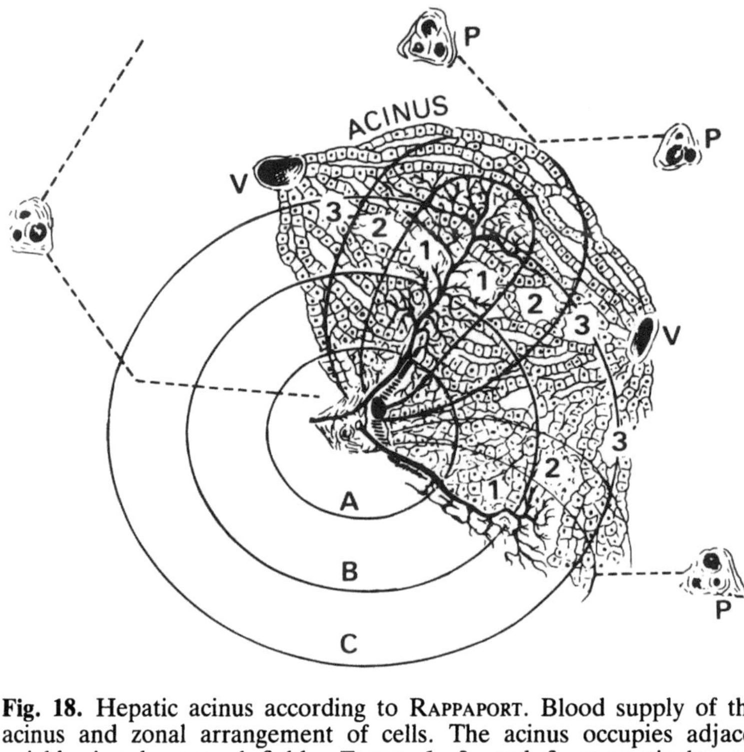


**Fig. 18.** Hepatic acinus according to Rappaport. Blood supply of the simple liver acinus and zonal arrangement of cells. The acinus occupies adjacent sectors of neighboring hexagonal fields. Zones *1*, *2*, and *3*, respectively, represent areas supplied with blood of first, second, and third quality in terms of substrate, oxygen, and nutrients. These zones are arranged around the terminal afferent vascular branches, terminal bile ductules, lymph vessels, and nerves and extend into the triangular portal field from which these branches originate. Zones *1'*, *2'*, and *3'* designate corresponding areas in a portion of an adjacent acinar unit. In zones *1* and *1'*, the afferent vascular twigs empty into the sinusoids. *Circles B* and *C* indicate peripheral circulatory areas as commonly described around a "periportal" area *A*. *P*, portal tract; *V*, terminal hepatic venules ("central veins"). [Reproduced with permission from Rappaport AM (1987) In: Schiff L and Schiff ER (eds) Diseases of the liver. J.B. Lippincott, Philadelphia, pp 1–46]

tracts. It is accompanied by an arteriole and a bile ductule. Blood flows into sinusoids, forming a right angle with the septa, and irrigates hepatocytes, from periportal to centrolobular, subdividing the acinus into three vascular zones (afferent: 1, intermediate: 2, efferent: 3). These three zones surround the parenchymal branches of the portal vessels like the layers of a bulb. However, this model, although nowadays widely accepted, does not in fact correspond to the physiologic reality (see below).

### *Matsumoto's Primary Lobule*

The study by MATSUMOTO and KAWAKAMI focused on the detailed description of human hepatic angioarchitecture [23]. Each "classic" lobule consists of six to eight primary lobules (Fig. 19). Each primary lobule is cone shaped, with its convex surface at the periphery of the classic lobule fed by the terminal branches of portal venules and hepatic arterioles and its apex at the center of the classic lobule drained by a central (terminal) hepatic venule. Terminal portal venules together with the sinusoids (which emerge between parallel terminal portal venules originating from the same distributing portal venule) form a "vascular septum."

In the periportal area, the sinusoids follow a tortuous course whereas in the pericentral area they straighten into a convergent pattern. It is possible that these tortuous sinusoids constitute a zone of high flux of blood, which then pours uniformly into radial sinusoids. Unfortunately MATSUMOTO's three-dimensional model presents the lobules as isolated entities with the ensuing artificial concept of portal blood passing from a single (distributing) vein to adjacent units.

### *Lamers's Concept of Lobular Metabolism*

Hepatocytes belong to different exocrine and endocrine units. Exocrine and endocrine units partially overlap, with their respective axes regularly spaced within the liver. The only shared parameters between these exocrine and endocrine units are therefore the distance between the portal and the central veins and the position of the hepatocytes along this line. Since both units play a role in hepatic metabolism, it seemed rational to develop a concept of liver architecture based on the metabolic properties of hepatocytes.

Taking into account the three-dimensional angioarchitecture and perfusion pattern of the liver, and the three-dimensional pattern of tissue oxygenation and the distribution of hepatocyte-specific enzymes, LAMERS et al. [24] proposed a concept (Fig. 20b) of lobular metabolism in which the pericentral zone is circular and discrete (rather than stellate and reticular as proposed by RAPPAPORT: Fig. 20a), whereas the periportal zone is reticular, i.e., contiguous between adjacent acini (rather than discrete). Seen three-dimensionally, the structure of the pericentral zone follows the branching pattern of the terminal hepatic vein, whereas that of the periportal zone envelops the pericentral compartment, forming an extensive network.

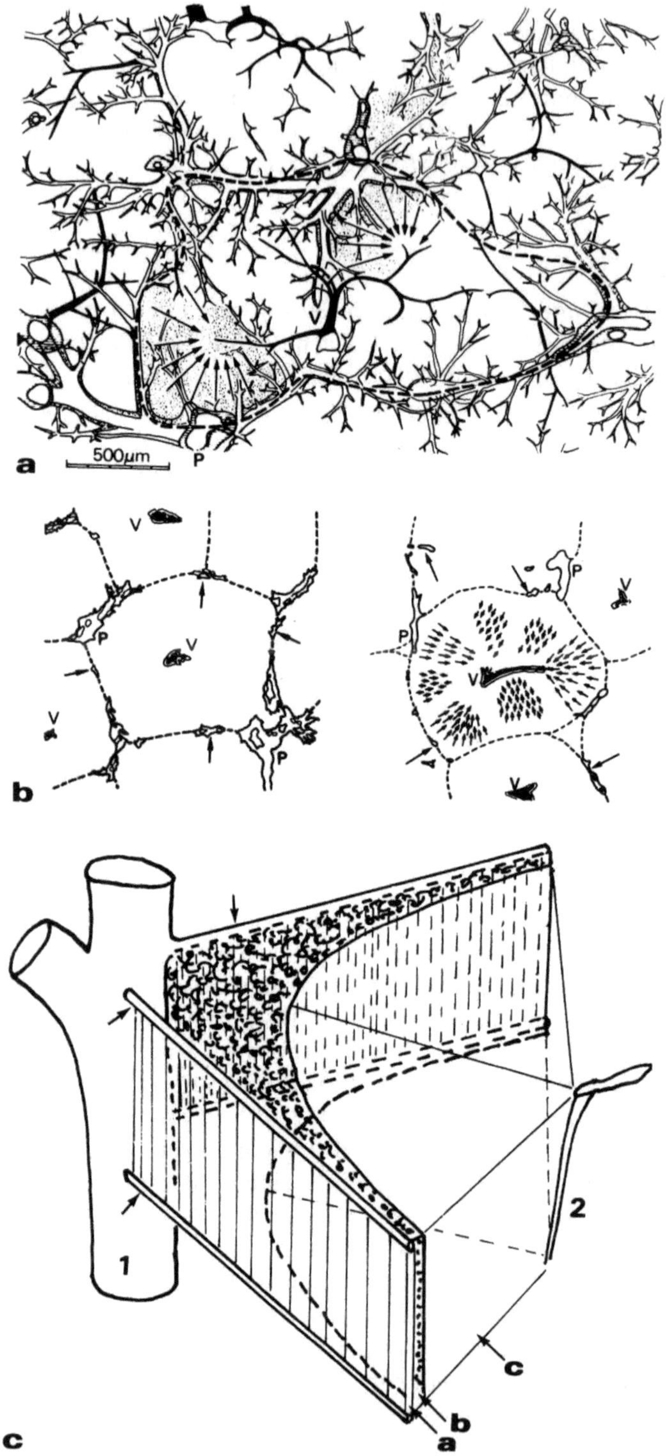


Fig. 19a–c

Only the parenchymal (terminal) branches of the portal vein and hepatic veins have a structural role in lobular architecture and therefore in hepatic microcirculation. There is regular interdigitation of the afferent and efferent vessels.

## 4.2 Microcirculation

Blood mainly enters sinusoids from portal venules. These inlets are usually guarded by sphincters made up of cells from the sinusoidal lining and termed "afferent" or "inlet" sphincters. Arterial blood enters sinusoids principally through branches of the hepatic arterioles. These vessels, arteriosinus twigs, terminate in sinusoids near where these emerge from portal venules. Occasional direct connections (arterioportal anastomoses), have also been observed with terminal portal venules. Since all these structures can contract independently, sinusoids receive a varying mixture of venous and hepatic blood from the portal vein and hepatic artery. The fraction of blood delivered to sinusoids by the hepatic artery seems to vary between the hilus and the periphery of the hepatic lobes.

Near their origins in portal venules, sinusoids are slightly narrower as well as being more tortuous and anastomotic than their straighter terminations in central venules. In the periportal area, the liver volume occupied by sinusoids is greater than that of sinusoids surrounding central venules. However, due to the smaller size and anastomotic nature of periportal sinusoids, the surface available for exchange in this area (surface/volume ratio) is greater than in centrolobular sinusoids. KCs are also more numerous in the periportal region. The size and pattern of distribution of endothelial fenestrae vary all along the sinusoid. At the portal end, fenestrae are

**Fig. 19a–c.** MATSUMOTO's model. **a** The secondary lobule is delimited by the *broken line*. It is composed of primary lobules, some of which are illustrated by *arrows* in the *shaded area*. The direction of the *arrows* indicates the direction of blood flow. The central vein (*V*) comprises six to eight draining poles arranged in such a way that each of these poles drains a primary lobule. *P*, Portal tract. **b** *Left side*: Secondary lobule (classical lobule). *Arrows*, septal branches; *broken line*, transverse section of vascular septa; *V*, central vein; *P*, portal tract. *Right side*: Primary lobules. Each primary lobule is represented by a *group of small arrows*. The secondary lobule is made up of six to eight primary lobules. **c** Primary lobule (three-dimensional view). The septal zone (*a*) lies between two parallel septal branches (*arrows*) emerging from the portal vein (*1*); it is constituted by a two-dimensional sinusoidal network. In the sickle-shaped portal zone (*b*, *shaded area*) sinusoids from the septal zone branch out three-dimensionally. At the apex, sinusoids converge in a radial pattern toward the branches of the hepatic vein (*2*). The septal zone (*a*) could correspond in the Rappaport model to the axis, the portal zone (*b*) to the periportal zone, and the radial zone (*c*) to zones 2 and 3. [**a** and **b** reproduced with permission from MATSUMOTO T and col. (1979) Jikeikai Med J 26:1–40]

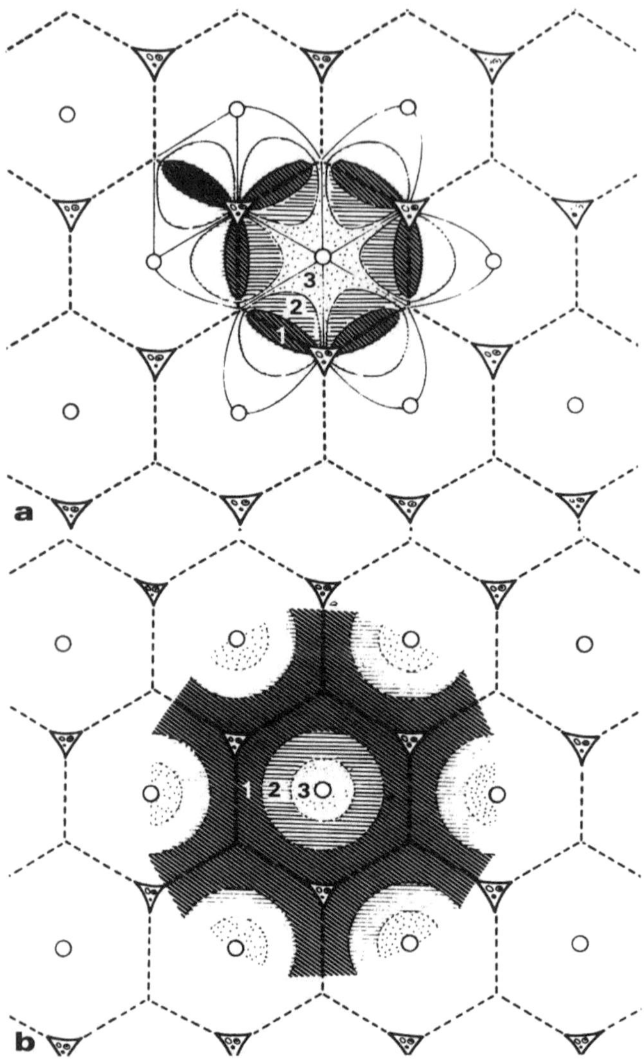


**Fig. 20a,b.** Diagram of Rappaport's model of acinar zonation (**a**) and Lamers's modification (**b**). These hypothetical sections are cut in the plane of the distributing portal vein and perpendicular to the central vein. Whereas Rappaport's zones surround the terminal afferent vessels like the layers of a bulb, Lamers's model stresses circular layers around perpendicularly orientated afferent and efferent vessels. Furthermore, in **a**, adjacent acini are characterized by discrete periportal zones and contiguous large pericentral zones, whereas in **b** adjacent acini are characterized by contiguous large periportal zones and discrete pericentral zones. *1*, zone 1 (periportal); *2*, zone 2 (intermediate); *3*, zone 3 (pericentral); *triangle*, portal tracts with conducting part of the portal vein, the hepatic artery, and the bile duct; *dashed line*, distributing part of the portal vein; *circle*, central (terminal hepatic) vein. [Reproduced with permission from LAMERS WH et al. (1989) Hepatology 10:72–76]

larger but account for less of the endothelial surface area than they do in the pericentral region. The functional significance of these differences is unclear, but it is tempting to relate them to the functional metabolic heterogeneity that has been demonstrated for hepatocytes in different regions of the lobule.

Portal venules and central veins contain limited amounts of smooth muscle in their walls in relation to the size of their lumens, but are nevertheless contractile and respond to pharmacologic agents; hepatic arterioles are more responsive, with a higher proportion of smooth muscle and relatively small lumens.

It is, however, within the sinusoid itself that blood flow is principally regulated and it is in the sinusoid that there is the greatest reduction in blood pressure [25]. Here the ECs and KCs are responsive to a wide variety of pharmacodynamic substances. By contracting (or swelling) they can selectively reduce the patency of the sinusoidal lumen, thereby altering the rate and distribution of blood flow. The relative role of KCs versus ECs in this process has not yet been resolved, but both appear to be involved. Whether PSCs are involved in the regulation of sinusoidal diameter has yet to be established. Slender processes of the cellular extensions of PSCs branch out at fairly regular intervals, encircling the sinusoid. The arrangement of these branches would suggest that these cells play an important role in regulating the size of the sinusoidal lumen inasmuch as nerves have been shown to be closely related to PSCs. In addition, it should be noted that all three cell types contain filaments, tubules, and contractile proteins that would suggest contractile activity. Because of these structures, blood flow through individual sinusoids is variable (Fig. 21). At sites where the lumen is narrowed by protrusion of the nuclear regions of sinusoidal lining cells, flow may be impeded by leukocytes, which transiently plug the vessel and obstruct flow. Transient leukocyte plugging is more frequent in periportal sinusoids, which are narrower and more tortuous than in the centrolobular region. The more plastic erythrocytes usually flow easily through such sites unless the lumen is reduced to near zero. Some sinusoids, however, may act as throughway channels and have relatively constant rates of blood flow, while others have more intermittent flow. This may depend not only on the distribution of intrasinusoidal sphincter cells but also on that of arteriosinus twigs and the contribution of arterial blood flowing to individual sinusoids. The average velocity of erythrocyte flow in sinusoids as measured in the rat ranges between 25 and 300 μm/s, with a volumetric rate of flow averaging 6.0 ml/s. The wide variations in flow are due to the structural features previously described for sinusoids and also to intermittent arterial inflow into sinusoids. While blood pressures in portal and central venules have been measured to be about 6–7 cm $H_2O$ and 1.5–3.0 cm $H_2O$, respectively, arterial blood enters the sinusoid at pressures ranging from 12 to 25 cm $H_2O$.

The neural and humoral mechanisms that regulate blood flow through hepatic sinusoids have yet to be completely elucidated.

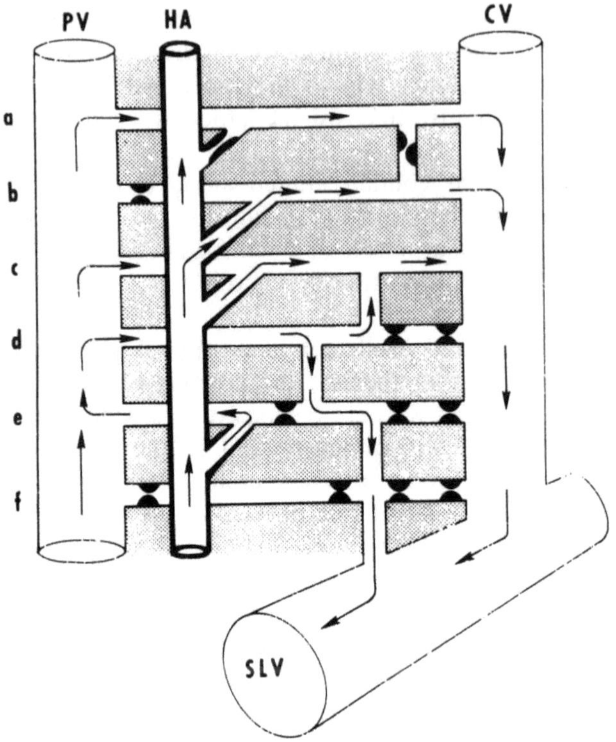


**Fig. 21.** Liver microcirculation patterns observed by in vivo microscopy. Closed sphincters are indicated by *black semicircles*. *a*, Sinusoid supplied only with portal venous blood due to constricted arteriosinus twig. *b*, Sinusoid supplied only with arterial blood due to closed inlet sphincter. *c*, Sinusoid supplied with a mixture of arterial and portal venous blood. There is no mixture of blood between *a* and *b* due to closed intersinusoidal sphincters. *d*, Sinusoid perfused only in peripheral part of lobule due to closed, centrally located sphincters. *e*, "Functional" arterioportal anastomosis formed by arteriosinus twig and initial segment of sinusoid whose remaining segment is closed by sphincters. *f*, Sinusoid in which there is no blood flow due to closed sphincters. *PV*, portal venule; *HA*, hepatic arteriole; *CV*, central venule; *SLV*, sublobular hepatic venule. *Arrows* indicate direction of flow. [Reproduced with permission from McCuskey RS (1988) In: Bioulac-Sage P and Balabaud C (eds) Sinusoids in human liver: health and disease. The Kupffer Cell Foundation, Rijswijk, pp 151–164]

### 4.3 Liver Heterogeneity

It has been shown in perfusion experiments that, when the direction of perfusion (anterograde or retrograde) changes, the areas of maximal oxygen consumption, gluconeogenesis, glycolysis, and ketogenesis vary immediately.

There is evidence that periportal hepatocytes (zone 1) differ from centrolobular hepatocytes (zone 3) both *structurally* (stereologic electron microscopy) and *functionally* (histochemistry, immunohistochemistry, microspectrophotometry, in situ hybridization). For example: (a) periportal hepatocytes contain approximately twice as many Golgi complexes as centrolobular hepatocytes, which conversely contain more lysosomes and smooth endoplasmic reticulum, and (b) carbonyl phosphate synthetase is predominantly located in periportal and midzonal hepatocytes whereas glutamine synthetase is located exclusively in one or two hepatocytes surrounding hepatic venules. Some examples of metabolic zonation are presented in Table 1.

There seem to be at least two elements commanding zonal responses. The first is the sequential delivery of substrates, as illustrated by carbohydrate metabolism. The unidirectional blood perfusion of the liver acinus results in the exposure of periportal hepatocytes to a high concentration of solutes. The importance of the direction of blood flow for metabolic compartmentation within the liver acinus has been clearly demonstrated. The second factor is the zonal pattern of gene expression. Some genes, such as albumin gene, are expressed by hepatocytes of the whole acinus. In contrast, other genes are expressed in a rather restricted manner, e.g., glutamine synthetase or $\alpha_2$-microglobulin, which are expressed only in the one or two hepatocytes surrounding hepatic venules. It has been proposed that these genes may be under the modulatory influence of mesothelial or endothelial cells in these vessels. It is also plausible that gene expression in hepatocytes of the portal limiting plate may be regulated differently. These hepatocytes may be the precursors of intrahepatic bile ducts. They are capable of multiplication under physiologic cell removal but show less regenerative capacity than hepatocytes which are two to three cells further from the portal venules during liver regeneration following partial hepatectomy. Their role in transport mechanisms is different from that of other periportal hepatocytes.

When all this is taken into account, the present division of the liver acinus into three functional zones may be inappropriate and restrictive. While it may be possible to characterize the various functional zones according to patterns of expression and types of regulation, it may be more realistic and useful to subdivide the acinus in terms of the function to be studied [26].

## 5 Conclusion

The liver is a voluminous organ implicated in numerous essential functions such as metabolism (nutrients, drugs, etc.), protein synthesis (inflammation, coagulation, etc.), and immune response. Homogeneous at the macroscopic level, at the microscopic level it presents a complex cellular and matrical organization which can be arbitrarily divided on the basis of structure and function into several sectors: vascular, biliary, metabolic, and immunologic.

**Table 1.** Metabolic zonation of liver parenchyma; predominant localization of major functions

| Predominantly periportal | Predominantly centrolobular | Equally distributed |
|---|---|---|
| Carbohydrate<br>– Glucose release<br>– Glycogen degradation to glucose<br>– Gluconeogenesis | Carbohydrate<br>– Glucose uptake<br>– Glycogen synthesis from glucose<br>– Glycolysis<br>– Ketogenesis<br>– Liponeogenesis | |
| Drug metabolism<br>– Sulfation | Drug metabolism<br>– Monooxygenation (phenobarbital treated)<br>– Glucuronidation (phenobarbital treated) | Drug metabolism<br>– Monooxygenation (normal) (methylcholanthrene treated)<br>– Glucuronidation (normal) (methylcholanthrene treated) |
| Oxidative energy metabolism<br>– Oxygen uptake<br>– Fatty acid oxidation<br>– Citrate cycle<br>– Respiratory chain | | |
| Amino acid metabolism<br>– Amino acid utilization<br>– Amino acid conversion to glucose<br>– Amino acid degradation<br>– Ureagenesis from amino acid nitrogen | Amino acid metabolism<br>– Ammonia detoxification<br>– Ureagenesis from ammonia nitrogen | |
| Bile secretion<br>– Bilirubin excretion<br>– Cholic acid excretion | Bile secretion<br>– Bile salt independent fraction | |
| Alcohol<br>– Oxidation (glutathione) | | |

Nevertheless, the liver is an entity and can be considered as a bioecological system, interconnected with other systems (digestive, immunologic, vascular, etc.) in which each cell interacts with other cell types and with the extracellular matrix. The functional capacity of each cell is constantly modified by the metabolic activity of others [27].

Thanks to new techniques (such as in situ hybridization, flow cytometry, and three-dimensional reconstruction of digital images) coupled with classical histologic techniques (light and ultrastructural immunocytochemistry, etc.), it is possible to go a step further in the morphologic approach to biologic processes. Investigation of processes such as cell differentiation (e.g., transdifferentiation of hepatocytes into biliary cells), cellular motility (e.g., migration of Kupffer cells), cell multiplication (e.g., liver regeneration), interactions between sinusoidal cells and matrix (e.g., fibrotic and cirrhotic processes), or the zonal expression of genes is essential for the comprehension and treatment of liver disease.

## References


1. Jones AL, Spring-Mills E (1984) The liver and gallbladder. In: Weiss L (ed) Modern concepts of gastrointestinal histology. Elsevier Science, New York, 20:707–747
2. MacSween RNM, Scothorne RJ (1987) Developmental anatomy and normal structure. In: MacSween RNM, Anthony PP, Scheuer PJ (eds) Pathology of the liver. Churchill Livingstone, Edinburgh, pp 1–45
3. Millward-Sadler GH, Jezequel AM (1985) Normal histology and ultrastructure. In: Wright R, Millward-Sadler GH, Alberti KGMM, Karran S (eds) Liver and biliary disease. Baillière Tindall, Eastbourne, pp 13–44
4. Miyai K (1988) Structure-function relationship of the liver in health disease. In: Gitnick G (ed) Principles and practice of gastroenterology and hepatology. Elsevier Science, New York, pp 1051–1068
5. Bloom W, Fawcett DW (1975) A textbook of histology. WB Saunders, Philadelphia, pp 688–725
6. Motta P, Muto M, Fujita T (1978) The liver: an atlas of scanning electron microscopy. Igaku-Shoin, Tokyo
7. Bismuth H (1988) Surgical anatomy and anatomical surgery of the liver. In: Blumgart LH (ed) Surgery of the liver and biliary tract. Churchill Livingstone, Edinburgh, 1:1–9
8. Smadja C, Blumgart LH (1988) The biliary tract and the anatomy of biliary exposure. In: Blumgart LH (ed) Surgery of the liver and biliary tract. Churchill Livingstone, Edinburgh, 1:11–21
9. Tanikawa K (1979) Ultrastructural aspects of the liver and its disorders, 2nd edn. Igaku-Shoin, Tokyo
10. Bioulac-Sage P, Le Bail B, Balabaud C (to be published) Liver and biliary tract histology. In: McIntyre N, Benhamou JP, Bircher J, Rizzetto M, Rodes J (eds) Oxford textbook of clinical hepatology. Oxford University Press Oxford
11. Phillips MJ, Poucell S, Patterson J, Valencia P (eds) The normal liver. In: The liver: an atlas and text of ultrastructural pathology. Raven, New York, pp 1–35
12. French SW, Kondo I, Irie T et al. (1982) Morphologic study of intermediate filaments in rat hepatocytes. Hepatology 1:29–38
13. Balabaud C, Boulard A, Quinton A et al. (1988) Light and transmission electron microscopy of sinusoids in human liver. In: Bioulac-Sage P, Balabaud C (eds) Sinusoids in human liver: health and disease. The Kupffer Cell Foundation, Rijswijk, pp 87–110
14. Gendrault JL, Steffan AM, Bingen A, et al. (1988) Kupffer and endothelial cells. In: Bioulac-Sage P, Balabaud C (eds) Sinusoids in human liver: health and disease. The Kupffer Cell Foundation, Rijswijk, pp 17–38
15. Brouwer A, Wisse E, Knook DL (1988) Sinusoidal endothelial cells and perisinusoidal fat-storing cells. In: Arias IM, Jakoby WB, Popper H, Schachter D, Shafritz DA, (eds) The liver. Biology and pathobiology. Raven, New York, pp 665–682

16. Wisse E, De Zanger RB, Charels K et al. (1985) The liver sieve: considerations concerning the structure and function of endothelial fenestrae, the sinusoidal wall and the space of Disse. Hepatology 5:683–692
17. Jones EA, Summerfield JA (1988) Kupffer cells. In: Arias IM, Jakoby WB, Popper H, Schachter D, Shafritz DA (eds) The liver. Biology and pathobiology. Raven, New York, pp 683–704
18. Bioulac-Sage P, Lafon ME, Le Bail B et al. (1988) Perisinusoidal and pit cells in liver sinusoids. In: Bioulac-Sage P, Balabaud C (eds) Sinusoids in Human liver: health and disease. The Kupffer Cell Foundation, Rijswijk, pp 39–62
19. Rojkind M (1988) Extracellular matrix. In: Arias IM, Jakoby WB, Poper H, Schachter D, Shafritz DA (eds) The liver. Biology and pathobiology. Raven, New York, pp 707–716
20. Peyrol S, Grimaud JA (1988) Perisinusoidal connective matrix. Immunohistochemical mapping of the major matricial components. In: Bioulac-Sage P, Balabaud C (eds) Sinusoids in human liver: health and disease. The Kupffer Cell Foundation, Rijswijk, pp 323–340
21. Albores-Saavedra J, Henson DE (1986) Normal anatomy. In: Tumors of the gallbladder and extrahepatic bile ducts. AFIP, Washington, 2nd series, pp 3–16
22. Rappaport AM (1987) Physioanatomic considerations. In: Schiff L, Schiff ER (eds) Diseases of the liver. J.B. Lippincott, Philadelphia, pp 1–46
23. Matsumoto T, Kawakami M (1982) The unit-concept of hepatic parenchyma: a reexamination based on angio-architectural studies. Acta Pathol Jpn 32:285–314
24. Lamers WH, Hilberts A, Furt E et al. (1989) Hepatic enzymic zonation: a reevaluation of the concept of the liver acinus. Hepatology 10:72–76
25. McCuskey RS (1988) Hepatic microcirculation. In: Bioulac-Sage P, Balabaud C (eds) Sinusoids in human liver: health and disease. The Kupffer Cell Foundation, Rijswijk, pp 151–164
26. Gumucio JJ (1989) Hepatocyte heterogeneity: the coming of age. From the description of a biological curiosity to a partial understanding of its physiological meaning and regulation. Hepatology 9:154–160
27. Rojkind M, Greenwel P (1988) The liver as a bioecological system. In: Arias IM, Jakoby WB, Popper H, Schachter D, Shafritz DA (eds) The liver. Biology and pathobiology. Raven, New York, pp 1269–1286

# 2 Biochemical Investigations in the Management of Liver Disease

N. McIntyre and S. Rosalki

Clinical laboratories use a small battery of biochemical tests for the detection and subsequent management of liver disease. Although called "liver function tests", they do not really assess liver function. Many such tests have been proposed (Table 1), but there is much overlap between them.

Most laboratories measure serum (or plasma) total bilirubin, aspartate and/or alanine aminotransferase, alkaline phosphatase, and serum albumin; some add serum $\gamma$-glutamyltransferase, and/or bile acids to the battery. Tests for urinary bilirubin and urobilinogen are usually done in the ward or clinic. Prothrombin and partial thromboplastin times, which are useful markers of the severity of liver disease, are usually measured in the haematology laboratory, and are not generally considered as "liver function tests".

These tests are not specific for liver disease; increased levels of plasma total bilirubin, aspartate and alanine aminotransferase, alkaline phosphatase and $\gamma$-glutamyltransferase, and low levels of albumin may all be caused by other disorders.

Specific aspects of hepatic function are assessed using various clearance tests, including galactose elimination, bile acid clearance, and aminopyrine breath tests, and by measuring the excretion of certain dyes. These tests are inconvenient to perform and are relatively expensive, but they help us to assess the functional effects of therapy. Other tests, e.g., of specific proteins in serum, may help define a specific disorder.

It is important to know how to interpret liver function tests, to appreciate when they are useful, and to understand their limitations.

## 1 Serum Bilirubin [1, 2, Table 2]

Several forms of bilirubin may be present in jaundiced sera. Bilirubin itself does not give a colour reaction with Ehrlich's diazo reagent except in the presence of ethanol or another "accelerator" and is therefore called "indirect" bilirubin. The bilirubin which does react directly with Ehrlich's diazo reagent ("direct" bilirubin) is a mixture of bilirubin mono- and diglucuronides (i.e., bilirubin esters). Bilirubin is esterified in the liver and normally the glucuronides are efficiently excreted in bile, little appearing in

**Table 1.** Some tests used as "liver function tests"

| | |
|---|---|
| A. Tests used as indices of uptake, conjugation and excretion of anionic compounds | |
| | Serum total bilirubin (and direct and indirect) |
| | Urinary bilirubin (and urobilinogen) |
| | Bile acids |
| B. Tests reflecting hepatocellular damage | |
| | Aspartate and/or alanine aminotransferase |
| | Glutathione-*S*-transferase |
| | Lactate dehydrogenase (isoenzyme 5) |
| | Clearance tests |
| | Serum ferritin |
| | Vitamin $B_{12}$ |
| C. Tests used to indicate obstruction to bile flow | |
| | Alkaline phosphatase |
| | γ-Glutamyltransferase |
| | 5′-Nucleotidase |
| | Lipoprotein-X |
| D. Tests of synthetic function | |
| | Serum albumin |
| | Prealbumin |
| | Cholinesterase |
| | Lecithin cholesterol acyltransferase |
| | Serum proteins – electrophoresis |
| | Prothrombin and partial thromboplastin times |
| E. Test suggesting increased hepatic collagen formation | |
| | Procollagen peptide |

blood. There is a disproportionate increase in bilirubin glucuronides in the blood in various types of liver disease, but not with haemolytic jaundice.

Bilirubin itself is insoluble in water and is bound to albumin; therefore it does not appear in the urine. Bilirubin glucuronides are water soluble and are excreted in urine when their plasma level rises. When there is an increase in plasma bilirubin glucuronides some become covalently bound to serum albumin and other proteins and this fraction (bili-alb or bili-protein) can be a major component of serum total bilirubin, particularly during recovery from jaundice. It is not filtered by the glomerulus, and thus a negative test for urinary bilirubin does not exclude the presence of conjugated hyperbilirubinaemia.

In most laboratories serum bilirubin is measured as total bilirubin; some also measure "direct" bilirubin; "indirect" bilirubin is the difference between total and "direct" measurements. This is not an accurate way of measuring bilirubin and bilirubin esters as some free bilirubin reacts directly with the reagent. "Direct" bilirubin underestimates bilirubin esters at high bilirubin concentrations and overestimates them at low bilirubin levels; this is unfortunate because it is important to measure bilirubin esters when there is only a small increase of total bilirubin, as this allows identification

**Table 2.** Causes of hyperbilirubinaemia

| |
|---|
| *Unconjugated (pre-microsomal)* |
| Excessive bilirubin production (haemolytic) |
| Ineffective haemopoiesis |
| Hemolytic disorders |
| Abnormal bilirubin metabolism (congenital) |
| Immaturity of enzyme systems |
| Physiological jaundice of newborn |
| Jaundice of prematurity |
| Inherited defects |
| Gilbert's syndrome |
| Crigler-Najjar syndrome |
| Drug effects |
| *Conjugated and unconjugated (post-microsomal)* |
| Hepatocellular abnormality (hepatocellular) |
| Primary hepatocyte disease (hepatitis, cirrhosis, neoplasm, drugs) |
| Intrahepatic cholestasis (drugs, pregnancy) |
| Benign postoperative jaundice |
| Congenital conjugated hyperbilirubinaemia |
| Dubin-Johnson syndrome |
| Rotor syndrome |
| Mechanical obstruction of bile ducts (obstructive) |
| Extrahepatic (calculus, neoplasm, stricture, atresia) |
| Intrahepatic (infantile obstructive cholangiopathy, sclerosing cholangitis, primary biliary cirrhosis) |

Based on ROSOFF L and ROSOFF L (1977) Surg Clin North Am 57:257–273

of "unconjugated hyperbilirubinaemia", as in Gilbert's syndrome and haemolysis.

There are now accurate methods for measuring bilirubin and its mono- and diconjugates, but they are rarely employed in routine laboratories. Conjugated bilirubins make up only about 4%–5% (<1 μmol/litre) of total bilirubin in normal subjects, but the upper limit for "direct reacting" bilirubin is usually taken as about 3 μmol/litre; levels above 5 μmol/litre, in patients with a normal total bilirubin, suggest hepatobiliary disease, if reliable measurement can be assured. Accurate measurement of bilirubin conjugates (e.g., by alkaline methanolysis and high performance liquid chromatography) is a sensitive marker of hepatobiliary disease, allowing the distinction between the "unconjugated hyperbilirubinaemia" of Gilbert's syndrome and that of haemolysis, as the proportion of bilirubin conjugates (as a % of total bilirubin) is normal in patients with haemolysis but low (<1.7%) in Gilbert's syndrome.

## 2 Interpretation of Bilirubin Levels

The reference interval ("normal" range) for total bilirubin concentration in serum or plasma is between about 3 and 17 μmol/litre. The mean total bilirubin level is about 3–4 µmol/litre higher in men than in women; as Gilbert's syndrome is often "diagnosed" when the plasma bilirubin is only just above the upper limit of 17 µmol/litre, this explains, in part, why the condition appears more prevalent in men.

Bilirubin levels between 17 and 70 µmol/litre are seen, without an increased conjugated bilirubin or other abnormal liver function tests, in patients with a benign unconjugated hyperbilirubinaemia, or with haemolysis. Haematological investigations usually indicate the presence of haemolysis and often the cause. When haemolysis occurs in the presence of liver damage, bilirubin levels tend to be much higher.

When other liver function tests are also abnormal, and bilirubin esters are elevated, bilirubin levels above 17 µmol/litre usually indicate liver disease. The actual level of total bilirubin is of little diagnostic value. An elevated serum total bilirubin reflects increased production, reduced hepatic uptake and/or conjugation, or decreased biliary excretion of the pigment.

Even with complete bile duct obstruction, the bilirubin tends to plateau between 170 and 500 µmol/litre; most of this bilirubin is removed by urinary excretion, but there is also breakdown of bilirubin to unidentified compounds. Extreme hyperbilirubinaemia (up to 1250 µmol/litre) is more likely to occur in severe parenchymal liver disease, usually in association with renal failure and/or haemolysis, or with blood transfusion.

In acute liver diseases the serum bilirubin level is of some prognostic value, but complete recovery usually occurs, even after deep jaundice, if the underlying condition can be treated (e.g., biliary obstruction) or improves spontaneously (e.g., acute viral hepatitis). With chronic liver diseases, however, an increasing serum bilirubin, without obvious cause (such as blood transfusion or certain drugs), is a bad sign.

## 3 Urinary Bilirubin

Bilirubin gives urine a dark brown colour. Other compounds also cause dark urine (Table 3) so the presence of bilirubin must be confirmed. Bilirubin test strips are easy to use and can detect 1–2 µmol of bilirubin per litre.

Bilirubinuria is an important pointer to liver damage, occurring with only small increases in plasma conjugated bilirubin (if it is not bound to protein) and usually preceding clinical jaundice; it is often found when the total plasma bilirubin is normal or only slightly elevated.

In jaundiced patients the absence of bilirubinuria is important, particularly if other liver function tests are normal, as it suggests an unconjugated hyperbilirubinaemia or haemolysis. However, it may be absent if conjugated pigment is present in plasma mainly as bili-alb. During recovery from acute viral hepatitis, bilirubin may be absent from the urine even at

**Table 3.** Causes of dark urine other than bilirubinuria

| Colour | Cause |
|---|---|
| Orange | Concentrated urine, urobilin, drugs |
| Orange-reddish brown | Drugs, rhubarb ingestion |
| Dark brown | Altered blood, myoglobin, porphyrins[a], phenolic drugs[a] |
| Red | Blood, beetroot or blackberry ingestion (acid urine), food dyes, drugs, urates |
| Purple-red | Phenolphthalein laxatives (alkaline urine) |
| Port-wine | Porphyrin[a], altered blood |
| Brown-black | Melanin[a], homogentisic acid, altered blood, phenolic drug poisoning[a] |

[a] Colour develops on standing

serum bilirubin levels as high as 170 μmol/litre; at the onset, bilirubinuria is usually present before jaundice appears.

## 4 Urinary Urobilinogen

Bilirubin esters entering the intestine in bile undergo bacterial hydrolysis and degradation in the ileum and colon with the production of "urobilinogen" (a term used for a mixture of isomers). Urobilinogen is excreted in the faeces, but some is absorbed and carried via the portal vein to the liver, where most is removed and excreted in bile. A little escapes hepatic uptake and is excreted in the urine.

A dipstick containing Ehrlich's aldehyde reagent allows rough and ready quantification of urinary urobilinogen. The test should be done on freshly voided urine. Although much emphasis is placed on urobilinogen metabolism in undergraduate texts, the detection and/or quantification of urinary urobilinogen is of little clinical value.

More urobilinogen is made when bilirubin is over-produced, as with haemolysis, and with constipation or bacterial contamination of the small bowel. With liver damage, more urobilinogen escapes hepatic uptake and biliary excretion, and more is excreted in urine. However, with biliary obstruction, urinary levels fall as less bilirubin enters the intestine for conversion to urobilinogen and less urobilinogen is absorbed. Urobilinogen production and urinary excretion also fall with diarrhoea and following treatment with antibiotics. Thus, changes in urinary urobilinogen can occur which are unrelated to changes in hepatic function.

Urinary excretion of urobilinogen depends on urine pH; tubular reabsorption increases with urinary acidity, which also renders urobilinogen unstable. Estimation of urinary urobilinogen in an acid urine is thus an unreliable index of plasma urinobilinogen.

## 5 Aspartate and Alanine Aminotransferases [3]

Elevations of serum aspartate aminotransferase (AST; glutamic-oxaloacetic transaminase; SGOT) and alanine aminotransferase (ALT; glutamic-pyruvate transaminase; SGPT) are found in patients with many types of hepatic damage. Although they are not specific for liver disease they are an index of liver cell injury, and can be used to identify or confirm liver disease.

### 5.1 Properties of the Aminotransferase Enzymes

Aspartate aminotransferase and ALT catalyse respectively the reversible transfer of an amino group from aspartate (or alanine) to α-oxoglutarate to yield oxaloacetate (or pyruvate) and glutamate.

Aspartate aminotransferase is found in high concentrations in liver, heart muscle, skeletal muscle, kidney, pancreas and red cells; with damage to these tissues AST is released into the blood, and the serum level rises. The organ source of serum AST cannot be identified, but it is possible to distinguish between two isoenzymes (one from cytoplasm, the other from mitochondria) which can be measured individually in serum.

Alanine aminotransferase is present in low concentration in tissues other than liver, where it is confined to the cytoplasm; high serum levels of ALT are therefore relatively specific for hepatic damage, although elevations also result from muscle diseases (such as Duchenne dystrophy or active polymyositis). ALT generally rises and falls in parallel with AST, but a small elevation of ALT often occurs without an increase of AST and may persist longer following hepatocellular injury.

Both enzymes are released from damaged cells, due to increased permeability of the cell membrane or to cell necrosis. Release of mitochondrial AST from hepatocytes is thought to imply more severe cellular damage than release of the cytoplasmic isoenzyme or of ALT. The ratio of the mitochondrial to cytoplasmic or total AST has been proposed as a "diagnostic" test, as it increases in severe cell necrosis and in alcoholic liver disease, but it is rarely used; few laboratories measure mitochondrial isoenzyme activity.

Haemolysis causes a small but definite increase in serum AST levels, and plasma or serum should be separated soon after blood collection to avoid release of erythrocyte enzyme.

Some laboratories measure both these enzymes, others only one. There is debate over their relative value. ALT is more specific for liver disease, but this is of little practical value as it is rarely difficult on clinical grounds to decide that an elevation of AST is due to hepatic damage. Measurement of ALT activity is of little value except for liver disease; for the laboratory which wishes to perform only one test, AST can also be used to detect damage to cardiac muscle. However, it has been suggested that the AST–ALT ratio may be of diagnostic value (see below).

The major value of aminotransferase measurements is in detecting hepatocellular damage, and in monitoring the patient's subsequent progress; return to normal suggests resolution of the factors causing hepatocellular damage.

Because they are increased in so many conditions, even quite marked elevations of aminotransferase levels are of limited value in differential diagnosis. They have been used to differentiate "hepatocellular" (when they are high) from "obstructive" jaundice (when they are low). This interpretation is often misleading, and the classification of jaundice into hepatocellular and obstructive causes on the basis of liver function test changes is undesirable (see later).

Very high aminotransferase levels are of diagnostic value. An aminotransferase level above 20x the upper reference limit (about 1000 units/litre at 37°C) is strongly suggestive of an acute hepatitis, due to viral hepatitis or to drugs. Normal or low aminotransferase levels early in an illness virtually exclude acute hepatitis as a cause; however, levels tend to drop rapidly, and if blood is not taken early in the illness, aminotransferase levels are of little diagnostic value. A striking elevation also occurs with a marked fall in blood pressure, as in shock, and with acute heart failure, but these diagnoses are usually obvious on clinical grounds. In viral hepatitis, and with most drugs, there is a gradual rise in aminotransferase levels for a week or two before the onset of jaundice. In shock and acute heart failure there is usually an abrupt rise, and a rapid fall with resolution of the circulatory problem.

Occasionally, striking elevations are seen with extrahepatic obstruction, with chronic active hepatitis, and with ascending cholangitis; an erroneous diagnosis of acute hepatitis may be made. Rare cases are described of marked elevation of serum AST due to complexing of the enzyme with high molecular weight immunoglobulin (usually IgG); this finding, analogous to macroamylasaemia, may cause diagnostic confusion.

In most patients with uncomplicated viral hepatitis, in which the initial levels are very high, aminotransferase levels return to normal within 8 weeks of the onset of illness. In hepatitis B, C and D infections more persistent elevations of ALT and AST suggest that chronic liver disease may be developing, but it is usual to wait for 6 months before reaching this conclusion. Even in hepatitis A infection, which has no long-term sequelae, aminotransferase levels may take many months to return to normal, and there may be increases suggesting exacerbation of the disease.

More modest aminotransferase increases, up to about eight times normal, are seen in many types of liver disease, e.g., chronic hepatocellular disease, cirrhosis, hepatic infiltration or neoplasia and cholestatic jaundice, and they are also found in the later stages of acute hepatitis. ALT is more frequently increased, except in alcoholic cirrhosis and infiltrative disease. A minor aminotransferase increase, generally below twice the upper reference limit, is occasionally found when there is little evidence of significant liver disease on liver biopsy. This is particularly true for ALT, which rises in many conditions, e.g., in patients with obesity, and for AST, which goes up after short periods of binge drinking in healthy subjects.

Not all liver diseases show aminotransferase elevation; levels may be normal with established but well-compensated cirrhosis and with chronic and incomplete biliary obstruction. While levels usually rise in acute liver diseases, relatively small increases are sometimes encountered, even in fulminant hepatitis. AST levels may appear disproportionately low in patients with Wilson's disease even when the disease presents as fulminant hepatitis or subacute hepatic necrosis.

Many have tried to use the AST–ALT ratio to distinguish between various types of liver disease. In general, ALT activity exceeds AST activity in toxic and viral hepatitis, chronic active hepatitis and cholestatic jaundice. AST is the higher of the two in alcoholic liver disease, in neoplastic and infiltrative liver disease and in non-biliary cirrhosis. It has been claimed [4] that an AST–ALT ratio >2 is evidence of alcoholic hepatitis and/or cirrhosis, distinguishing patients with these conditions from those with extra-hepatic obstruction and viral hepatitis, in which the ratio is normally <2. But this distinction is rarely difficult on clinical grounds and the sensitivity and specificity of this ratio are only about 70%; values >2 occur in many patients with post-necrotic cirrhosis and chronic hepatitis, with Wilson's disease and occasionally with viral hepatitis. A low hepatic ALT has been suggested as the reason for the high AST–ALT ratio seen in plasma in alcoholic liver disease.

It has recently been claimed that an increase in the AST–ALT ratio suggests the development of cirrhosis in patients with chronic viral hepatitis (B, delta and non-A, non-B) and "primary biliary cirrhosis" [5], but there is considerable overlap in individual cases.

Attempts to use the degree of abnormality, and change in AST relative to the change in bilirubin, alkaline phosphatase and other biochemical markers, in order to identify different hepatobiliary diseases have been disappointing [6]. The AST–bilirubin ratio is not of diagnostic value even in hepatitis. The AST–alkaline phosphatase ratio has been considered useful in distinguishing between acute hepatitis and obstructive jaundice, but about 5%–10% of patients show inappropriate results.

The serum AST increases in many other diseases, including myocardial infarction, myocarditis and pulmonary embolism. It goes up in skeletal myopathies and with trauma (even with intramuscular injections); measurement of serum creatine kinase helps to identify aminotransferase elevations due to muscle disease. Confusion may arise when these conditions coincide with liver disease; then ALT estimations may be helpful, although severe muscle disease also causes an increase in this enzyme.

## 6 Other Tests Indicating the Presence of Hepatocellular Damage or Necrosis

The plasma concentrations of other substances rise with hepatocellular damage (Table 1). Some are other enzymes, presumably released from damaged hepatocytes. The pattern of response does not necessarily mirror that of aminotransferases. Not surprisingly, many have been advocated as useful liver function tests in their own right, but they have not been widely used and have little advantage over aminotransferase estimations, though glutathione-*S*-transferase is more sensitive to acute hepatocellular injury.

Modest elevation of serum lactate dehydrogenase (LD) activity, generally averaging twice the upper reference limit, may be found early in the course of viral hepatitis; in most other liver diseases normal, or near normal, values are usual. With malignant liver disease LD values increase in up to 80% of patients, the frequency depending on the extent of metastatic disease, and high levels may be found. Many disorders raise the total serum LD, but only liver disease, malignancy and muscle disorders cause a preferential increase in the LD5 isoenzyme.

Plasma vitamin $B_{12}$ levels increase with various kinds of liver disease; it appears to be released from damaged hepatocytes. The amount bound to transcobalamin I (the major $B_{12}$ carrier in normal blood) increases, and there is a more striking rise in the amount bound to transcobalamin II. There is a rise in urinary $B_{12}$ excretion in association with a marked increase in dialysable serum $B_{12}$ levels. Serum $B_{12}$ binding proteins may increase with hepatocellular carcinoma, and there seems to be a particular association with the fibrolamellar form of the tumour [7].

Serum ferritin levels are elevated in patients with hepatocellular damage, from almost any cause, and they also rise in patients with various types of iron overload, including haemochromatosis.

## 7 Alkaline Phosphatases (Liver, Biliary, Tumour, Bone, Intestinal, Placental) [3, 8]

Alkaline phosphatases are zinc metallo-enzymes, with a serine at the active centre; they release inorganic phosphate from a variety of organic orthophosphates. They are present in nearly all tissues and there are several isoenzymes. The natural substrates are thought to include pyrophosphate, phosphoserine and phosphatidylethanolamine; intestinal alkaline phosphatase may act as a $Ca^{2+}$-dependent ATPase. In the liver, alkaline phosphatase can be found histochemically in the microvilli of the bile canaliculus and on the sinusoidal surface of hepatocytes. The genes for various alkaline phosphatases have been sequenced. Alkaline phosphatase isoforms from liver, bone and kidney are thought to be coded by the same gene, while the alkaline phosphatases from intestine and placenta are the product of separate genes and represent true isoenzymes.

Alkaline phosphatase activity in normal serum is due mainly to the presence of isoforms derived from bone and liver; an intestinal alkaline phosphatase is present in about 20% of normal subjects and may contribute up to 20% of total activity.

In most clinical laboratories the measurement of total serum alkaline phosphatase is a standard "liver function test", although it is well recognised that elevated serum alkaline phosphatase activity occurs in many clinical conditions in which the liver is not involved.

A number of methods have been used for the measurement of serum alkaline phosphatase activity. Heparinised plasma can be used, but the test should not be done on plasma if citrate, oxalate or EDTA have been used as anticoagulants as they form a complex with the zinc in the alkaline phosphatase, resulting in irreversible enzyme inactivation.

The reference range (and units) for total alkaline phosphatase activity varies with the method of determination, with the age and sex of the patient, and with a number of other factors. Serum alkaline phosphatase is above the normal adult range until about 20 years of age; there are two peaks, one in the neonatal period and the other in adolescence (i.e., during periods of increased bone growth). Alkaline phosphatase levels also tend to rise in older subjects, with increased contributions by liver alkaline phosphatase in elderly males and bone alkaline phosphatase in post-menopausal females (Table 4). A post-prandial increase in alkaline phosphatase, due to intestinal isoenzyme, may occur after a fatty meal in some normal subjects, usually those from blood groups B and O who also carry the ABH red cell antigen and are Lewis antigen negative.

In normal pregnancy the serum alkaline phosphatase increases during the 3rd month, rises up to three times the usual adult female level in late pregnancy, and may remain elevated for a few weeks after delivery. The main source of this increase is the placenta. It has been suggested that the serum level after delivery is higher in mothers who breast-feed their babies.

The various alkaline phosphatase isoenzymes in serum can be identified and measured by a number of methods, and sometimes one isoenzyme is found to be elevated even when the total alkaline phosphatase is normal.

For routine analysis of alkaline phosphatase isoenzymes, electrophoresis (on cellulose acetate, agarose or polyacrylamide gels) is the method of choice, separation depending mainly on charge. The liver ("slow" liver band) and bone isoenzymes in normal sera are found in similar proportions, but they may be difficult to distinguish from each other. The placental and intestinal isoenzymes are easily identified. The main clinical question is whether an increased alkaline phosphatase level is due to liver or bone isoenzyme. These can be easily distinguished, and quantified, using wheat-germ lectin affinity electrophoresis or non-electrophoretically by precipitation of the bone isoform with wheat-germ lectin [9]. Tumour isoenzymes, a

**Table 4.** Causes of "isolated" serum alkaline phosphatase increase

| |
|---|
| *Increased liver isoenzyme* |
| Hepatic metastases or infiltrative disease |
| Primary biliary cirrhosis |
| Cholelithiasis |
| (N.B. all usually accompanied by γ-glutamyltransferase increase) |
| Minor increase with age |
| *Increased bone isoenzyme* |
| Physiological – childhood, puberty, postmenopausal (minor) |
| Osteoblastic bone disease, e.g., Paget's, osteomalacia, metastases |
| *Increased intestinal isoenzyme* |
| Liver disease (cirrhosis) |
| Diabetes mellitus |
| Chronic renal failure |
| Intestinal disease (lymphoma, α-chain disease) |
| Physiological (minor) increase after fat ingestion, especially in H-substance secretors of blood groups O and B |
| *Placental isoenzyme* |
| Physiological – pregnancy |
| Malignant disease (minor activity increase) |
| Indian childhood cirrhosis |
| *Variant or unusual forms* |
| Immunoglobulin-bound – autoimmune disease, inflammatory bowel disease |
| Tumour-derived – ovarian, testicular, hepatocellular cancer (minor activity increase) |
| Liver-like + bone – benign transient hyperphosphatasaemia (massive increase) |
| *Genetically determined increase* |
| Any or all isoenzyme form(s) |

high molecular mass "biliary" (or fast liver) isoenzyme, and one or more unusual hepatic isoenzymes can also be identified by electrophoresis.

### 7.1 Alkaline Phosphatase and Liver Disease

In 1934, King and Armstrong described their classic method for measuring serum alkaline phosphatase. Levels greater than 30 King-Armstrong (KA) units were common in large bile duct obstruction; unfortunately this became a diagnostic criterion for extrahepatic obstruction, even though early workers cast doubt on the value of phosphatase measurements in the differential diagnosis of jaundice because values above 30 KA units were sometimes found in hepatitis and cirrhosis.

The serum alkaline phosphatase activity rises in many types of liver disease; the highest levels are seen with obstruction to the flow of bile, either intrahepatic or extrahepatic, or with intrahepatic space-occupying lesions such as primary or metastatic liver tumours. The elevated plasma alkaline phosphatase seen with liver disease is not due to failure of the liver to excrete the enzyme. The phosphatase accumulating is produced in the liver. There are at least two hepatic isoenzymes, one from hepatocytes ("slow" liver) and a high molecular mass biliary or "fast" liver alkaline phosphatase which originates from the plasma membrane. "Biliary" enzyme seems to be a better marker of biliary obstruction than total serum alkaline phosphatase activity.

In acute viral hepatitis, alkaline phosphatase is usually either normal or moderately raised, but up to 40% may have levels two and a half times the upper reference limit. Hepatitis A infection may cause a cholestatic picture with marked and prolonged itching and elevation of alkaline phosphatase; cholestatic features may also be seen with chronic hepatitis B infection. A very high alkaline phosphatase has been reported in Epstein-Barr virus infection ("glandular fever"), even with normal bilirubin levels.

The serum alkaline phosphatase is increased (a) by drugs which cause cholestatic liver disease, (b) in Hodgkin's disease, (c) in congestive heart failure, and (d) in infectious and inflammatory diseases not primarily involving the liver, such as polymyalgia rheumatica.

Although a high alkaline phosphatase is usually found in "cholestatic" liver diseases this is not always the case. Even with a confirmed extrahepatic block, due to tumour or stones, the alkaline phosphatase may be normal or only slightly raised in some cases. A normal alkaline phosphatase has also been seen in patients with primary biliary cirrhosis or primary sclerosing cholangitis; this may cause diagnostic confusion.

In about 25% of patients with cirrhosis an intestinal band is seen on electrophoresis and it may be the major alkaline phosphatase in serum (normally it does not exceed 20% of the total phosphatase activity). This may result from diminished hepatic uptake or diminished hepatic excretion or catabolism. In some jaundiced patients increased amounts of the bone isoenzyme can be detected (presumably as a result of secondary bone disease, e.g., hepatic osteodystrophy or osteomalacia complicating liver disease).

Alkaline phosphatase may be secreted into plasma by tumours. In some tumours specific isoenzymes are produced, e.g., the Regan and Kasahara isoenzymes. The Regan isoenzyme can be found with carcinoma of the bile duct, the Kasahara isoenzyme in about 30% of patients with primary liver cell carcinoma. Unfortunately, these isoenzymes are of relatively little diagnostic value in liver disease; they are present in few patients with tumours, and generally at a low level of activity, so that sensitive immunological methods are required for their identification. They may be of value for monitoring anti-tumour therapy; successful treatment is associated with a fall or with disappearance of the isoenzyme from the plasma.

Identification of alkaline phosphatase isoenzymes is of only limited value in distinguishing various kinds of liver disease. Isoenzyme studies can certainly help to decide whether an elevated alkaline phosphatase activity is due to liver disease or bone disease. Where alkaline phosphatase isoenzyme determinations are not available, it is usual to look at other markers of biliary obstruction (Table 1), such as γ-glutamyltransferase or sometimes 5′-nucleotidase, in order to confirm a hepatic origin for raised alkaline phosphatase levels. The measurement of γ-glutamyltransferase has 90% sensitivity and specificity for this purpose, as it is normal in bone disease.

Occasionally liver phosphatase in serum, like AST, is increased due to binding with serum immunoglobulins which interferes with the normal clearance of the enzyme from plasma. This occurs particularly in association with auto-immune disease and ulcerative colitis. Rarely a familial increase in liver alkaline phosphatase is found without other evidence of liver disease.

Alkaline phosphatase elevation occurs in many diseases other than those involving the liver. A list of causes of an isolated increase in serum alkaline phosphatase is given in Table 4 (and in [8]).

### 7.2 5′-Nucleotidase [3]

5′-Nucleotidase is an alkaline phosphatase which attacks nucleotides with a phosphate at the 5′ position of the pentose. It is present in all human tissues but only liver disease appears to cause significant elevation of serum 5′-nucleotidase activity. The normal range of activity in plasma is from 1–15 IU/litre (measured at 37°C).

The highest levels are found with either intrahepatic or extrahepatic obstruction to bile flow, but increases are also seen with chronic active hepatitis, cirrhosis, hepatitis and other hepatocellular disorders. In routine practice measurement of 5′-nucleotidase activity has been used to confirm that liver disease is indeed the cause of an elevated alkaline phosphatase but its use for this purpose has now been largely superseded by isoenzyme determinations or by measurement of γ-glutamyltransferase.

## 8 γ-Glutamyltransferase [10, 11]

γ-Glutamyltransferase (GGT) is a membrane-bound glycoprotein which catalyses the transfer of γ-glutamyl groups from γ-glutamyl peptides, particularly glutathione, to other peptides, to amino acids and to water. It is found mainly in the membranes of cells with a high rate of secretory or absorptive activity. Large amounts are found in the kidneys, pancreas, liver, intestine and prostate, and the enzyme is also found in many other tissues. GGT is present in bile, where the activity is approximately 100 times greater than in normal serum.

Several isoforms of GGT have been described, but there is no clear evidence of tissue specificity. The heterogeneity appears to be related to the number of sialic acid residues, to the degree of glycosylation and to binding to lipoproteins.

The reference interval for serum GGT is higher in men than in women. The level is very high in neonates and infants up to 1 year, and levels appear to increase above the age of 60. Levels exceeding the usually accepted upper reference limit (approximately 50 mU/litre at 37°C in men, 30 mU/litre in women) are so common that some laboratories have readjusted the upper limit to 80 in men, and 50 in women. Even then, about 6% of men have an abnormal level, and in 4% it is greater than 100 mU/litre. Reference levels are lower in lifelong abstainers from alcohol than in the general population.

Serum GGT levels rise in almost all kinds of liver disease and consequently the determination is of little differential diagnostic value. Abnormal levels are found in about 90% of patients suffering from hepatobiliary disease. GGT is a very sensitive indicator of the presence of liver disease (sensitivity 0.87–0.95), but specificity is limited by the many other conditions, not primarily hepatic, which cause an increase in GGT as a consequence of mild, clinically insignificant hepatic involvement. The highest levels of GGT (averaging 10–20 times the upper limit of normal) are found with intrahepatic biliary obstruction or with primary or secondary hepatic malignancies. However, a normal or low GGT may be seen occasionally in patients with intrahepatic cholestasis, even with a very high bilirubin and alkaline phosphatase. This does not appear to be due to an inhibitor in plasma. In infants with idiopathic cholestasis a normal GGT was found to be of poor prognostic significance [12].

In acute viral hepatitis, serum GGT levels rise to reach a peak in the 2nd or 3rd week of the illness, and in some patients the GGT level is still up at 6 weeks. Levels remain high with the development of chronic active hepatitis or cirrhosis.

γ-Glutamyltransferase levels are of definite, though limited, value in the management of alcoholic patients. Such patients may have high GGT levels, presumably due to enzyme induction, even when there is no significant underlying liver disease; but there is a poor correlation between alcohol intake and serum GGT activity. On cessation of drinking, GGT falls to normal over 2–5 weeks; if it does not return to normal continued alcohol intake is likely, liver damage may have occurred, or there may be another reason for the high GGT. Unfortunately, about a third to a half of heavy drinkers show no elevation of GGT in the absence of liver disease, so it is not a sensitive screening test for alcoholism. GGT levels do not rise as the result of an alcoholic binge in healthy subjects, but may do so in alcoholics and patients with other liver disorders.

An increase in GGT activity is seen in conditions other than liver disease and alcoholism. It increases in acute pancreatitis, and in 50%–70% of cases of acute myocardial infarction. The source of the increase with myocardial infarction is not clear, as there is no measurable activity in cardiac or skeletal muscle; it is probably due to secondary effects on the liver, as high levels are also found in congestive cardiac failure.

**Table 5.** Causes of "isolated" plasma GGT increase

| |
|---|
| Hepatobiliary disease |
| Pancreatic disease |
| Alcohol |
| Drugs (especially enzyme inducers) |
| Non-hepatobiliary disease with liver involvement (slight GGT increase) |
| Anorexia nervosa |
| Dystrophia myotonica |
| Guillain-Barré syndrome |
| Hyperthyroidism |
| Obesity-hyperlipidaemia/diabetes mellitus |
| Porphyria cutanea tarda |
| Postmyocardial infarction |
| Neurological disease (slight GGT increase) |
| Malignant disease/radiotherapy (GGT increase possibly from shedding of enzyme-containing plasma membrane fragments) |

Serum GGT activity increases with enzyme-inducing drugs. Moderate increases are seen with phenobarbitone, phenytoin and other anticonvulsant drugs, paracetamol, tricyclic antidepressants and glutethimide. Smaller increases occur with anticoagulants, oral contraceptives and antihyperlipidaemic drugs.

Elevated blood GGT activity is found in about 20% of patients with uncomplicated diabetes mellitus; levels are rarely more than twice the upper limit of normal. The liver is thought to be the source of the enzyme but other clinical or biochemical evidence of liver disease is not usually found. Some have disputed this association with diabetes mellitus, arguing that the raised GGT in diabetic patients is due to associated conditions.

Causes of an isolated increase in GGT are presented in Table 5. Sometimes very high levels of serum GGT are found (ca. 1000 u/litre) with no obvious cause.

## 9 Plasma Proteins

The liver is the source of many circulating plasma proteins. The effects of liver disease on their plasma concentration are complex, depending not only on changes in protein synthesis, but also on changes in the volume and distribution of extracellular fluids, in the half-life of the individual proteins and in their catabolism by various tissues. There may also be altered metabolism of proteins produced outside the liver. The estimation of "total plasma protein" alone is of relatively little value. It is often normal even when there are gross disturbances of the individual components. When the total level is either high or low its significance can only be interpreted by measurement of the major fractions. Measurement of total protein together with albumin is used for the calculation of globulin by difference;

serum protein electrophoresis is often performed in conjunction with these measurements.

Certain types of electrophoretic pattern are characteristic, but not diagnostic, of certain types of liver disease [13]. Patients with chronic active hepatitis often have a marked elevation of $\gamma$-globulin while patients with non-biliary cirrhosis have a low albumin and high $\gamma$-globulin concentration. With biliary obstruction there may be an excess of $\alpha_2$- and $\beta$-globulins due to the accumulation of abnormal lipoproteins. A low $\alpha_2$ band can occur with intravascular haemolysis (due to decreased haptoglobin concentration), while $\alpha_1$-antitrypsin deficiency may be suspected if the strip shows a poor $\alpha_1$ band.

Overall the electrophoretic strip is of little value in liver disease as the various abnormalities are also found in other conditions.

### 9.1 Serum or Plasma Albumin [14]

Albumin is the most abundant circulating protein. It is an important determinant of the colloid osmotic pressure of plasma, and has binding sites with great affinity for many naturally occurring compounds, including bilirubin, and for many drugs. The liver is the only site of synthesis, producing approximately 15 g/day in a normal 70-kg person; about 1 g is lost into the gastrointestinal tract, and most of the rest is degraded by a mechanism

**Table 6.** Causes of low plasma albumin concentration

| |
|---|
| *Impaired albumin synthesis* |
| Malnutrition |
| Malabsorption |
| Liver disease |
| Malignant disease |
| *Increased albumin loss* |
| Proteinuria, e.g., nephrotic syndrome |
| Protein-losing enteropathy – inflammatory bowel disease |
| Burns |
| Exudative skin disease |
| *Increased albumin catabolism* |
| Hypercatabolic states – injury, postoperation |
| *Altered distribution between intra-extravascular compartments from increased vascular permeability* |
| Inflammatory states – acute phase reaction |
| *Overhydration* |
| *Genetic variation* |
| Analbuminaemia |
| *Interrupted synthesis* |
| Acute (and chronic) inflammatory conditions |

which is under metabolic control. When synthesis is reduced, the fall in plasma albumin is minimised by a reduction in the fractional catabolic rate for albumin. The total exchangeable pool of albumin is normally about 3.5–5.0 g/kg body weight; about 40% is within the intravascular space. The plasma albumin concentration is normally between 35 and 50 g/litre.

The plasma albumin level has been used as a test of liver function, because it is affected by hepatic protein synthesis. However, synthesis is only one of several factors affecting plasma albumin; low values also result from increased gastrointestinal or renal loss, increased catabolism, altered vascular permeability or overhydration. Even when synthesis is markedly reduced it may take many days to see an effect on plasma albumin because of its long half-life (about 20 days). In patients without pre-existing liver disease who suffer fever or trauma, the albumin half-life may fall to about 7 days, and albumin levels fall rapidly to below 30 g/litre, indicating a marked increase in albumin removal as well as inhibition of albumin synthesis.

The low serum albumin level found in many patients with severe chronic liver disease is largely due to reduced albumin synthesis. But with ascites, levels may also be low because the plasma volume is large and, despite hypoalbuminaemia, there may be more albumin than normal in the extravascular space. The absolute rate of degradation, and synthesis, may be normal or even high but with a low fractional catabolic rate.

Alterations in the concentration of plasma albumin must be interpreted with caution because of the many conditions other than liver disease which may result in low plasma albumin levels. These are listed in Table 6.

## 9.2 Specific Protein Measurements

The changes in the plasma protein electrophoretic pattern outlined above result from changes in the specific proteins from which the globulin fraction is derived. $\alpha_1$-Globulin is principally composed of $\alpha_1$-antitrypsin and $\alpha_1$-acid glycoprotein (orosomucoid); both are acute phase proteins which increase in a variety of inflammatory disorders, the latter being especially responsive in liver disease. Within the $\alpha_2$-globulin complex, haptoglobin is also an acute phase protein. Increased clearance of haptoglobin–haemoglobin complexes reduces the haptoglobin level in intravascular or severe extravascular haemolysis. In non-biliary cirrhosis the $\beta$-globulin iron-binding protein, transferrin, may be reduced; it also falls in a variety of inflammatory disorders. Immunoglobulins (principally IgG, IgA and IgM) are located within the $\gamma$-globulin fraction and extend anodally therefrom; a diffuse (polyclonal) increase of staining in this region if often observed in chronic liver disease (especially chronic active hepatitis) as well as in chronic inflammatory and auto-immune disorders. In non-biliary cirrhosis (especially alcoholic) there may be an increase in IgA; this runs in the $\beta$–$\gamma$ region, causing the appearance known as $\beta$–$\gamma$ "fusion" or bridging.

Changes in the specific proteins considered above are better defined by quantitative immunological measurement. Of particular interest in relation to liver disease are prealbumin, $\alpha_1$-antitrypsin, $\alpha$-fetoprotein, caeruloplasmin and the immunoglobulins.

### ***Prealbumin*** *(Transthyretin [15])*

Prealbumin is a tetramer of four identical subunits which binds iodothyronines. It also binds one molecule of retinol-binding protein (RBP), thus helping to reduce urinary excretion of RBP. The plasma prealbumin concentration is 0.2–0.3 g/litre, that of RBP, 0.04–0.05 g/litre. Measurement of prealbumin has been proposed as a liver function test as its concentration tends to fall in liver disease, presumably from impaired synthesis. Because of its short half-life (1.9 days), changes precede alterations in serum albumin.

### ***Serum Caeruloplasmin*** *[16]*

Caeruloplasmin is a blue $\alpha_2$-globulin, normally present in plasma at a concentration of 0.2–0.4 g/litre. Its physiological function is unknown. It is synthesised in liver and is an acute phase protein. The plasma concentration (determined immunologically) rises in pregnancy and with oestrogens, with infections, with rheumatoid arthritis, with some malignancies, with active non-Wilson's liver disease and in obstructive jaundice.

Serum caeruloplasmin is an important diagnostic marker in Wilson's disease, in which the plasma level is usually reduced. A low caeruloplasmin is also seen in neonates, Menkes' disease, kwashiorkor and marasmus, protein-losing enteropathy, nephrotic syndrome, severe hepatic insufficiency, copper deficiency and hereditary hypocaeruloplasminaemia.

### ***$\alpha_1$-Antitrypsin*** *[17]*

$\alpha_1$-Antitrypsin, a glycoprotein of $M_r$ approximately 54000, acts as an inhibitor of serine proteinases, especially elastase. It is synthesised by the liver. It is present in serum at a concentration of 1–1.6 g/litre and is an acute phase protein, serum levels increasing with inflammatory disorders; they also increase in pregnancy and in women receiving oral contraceptives.

Liver disease occurs with $\alpha_1$-antitrypsin deficiency, an inherited disorder sometimes identifiable by a reduced $\alpha_1$ band on electrophoresis; deficiency should be confirmed by quantitative measurement. $\alpha_1$-Antitrypsin shows genetic polymorphism. Approximately 90% of Caucasian populations are homozygous for the M allele (i.e., MM phenotype); other alleles include F, S, Z and null forms. $\alpha_1$-Antitrypsin phenotype is best determined by isoelectric focussing; allelic variation may be associated with both low plasma concentration and deficient functional (inhibitory) capacity. Plasma levels of

$\alpha_1$-antitrypsin vary with phenotype; they are approximately 15% of normal with ZZ, 38% with SZ, and about 60% with MZ and FZ.

The presence of the Z allele, particularly in the homozygous form, is associated with defective processing of the protein in the liver. The precursor protein, deficient in sialic acid, is poorly secreted by the hepatocytes; its intrahepatic accumulation may be a factor in the genesis of liver damage. Neonatal hepatitis is seen in Pi ZZ homozygotes, and less frequently with MZ and SZ phenotypes. Cirrhosis in adults has been found with ZZ, MZ, SZ and FZ phenotypes.

***α-Fetoprotein** [18]*

α-Fetoprotein is the principal fetal protein in plasma in early gestation, but is later present at very low levels (reference limit 25 µg/litre or ng/ml). More than 90% of patients with hepatocellular carcinoma have increased serum levels. It also increases in up to 15% of cirrhotics without hepatocellular carcinoma, in chronic hepatitis, in the regeneration phase of viral hepatitis and with hepatic metastases; however, these elevations are generally minor compared with that observed in hepatocellular carcinoma, and they are frequently transient. To improve specificity (with some loss of sensitivity) high α-fetoprotein levels (above 400 µg/litre) are generally regarded as a diagnostic prerequisite; at such levels 70% or more patients with hepatocellular carcinoma will show abnormality with less than 5% false-positives. High α-fetoprotein levels are more often found in blacks and Chinese with hepatocellular carcinoma, and less often in white Europeans.

Serial determination of α-fetoprotein is valuable for monitoring patients with cirrhosis, as increasing levels should lead to a search for a hepatocellular carcinoma; it is also valuable in monitoring the treatment of hepatocellular carcinoma as its concentration should fall to low levels following successful therapy.

## 10 Other Tests Sometimes Used to Investigate Liver Function

### 10.1 Cholinesterase [19, 20]

Cholinesterase is a plasma enzyme which hydrolyses several choline esters. It is produced by the liver, and serum levels fall when there is decreased hepatic protein synthesis, generally in parallel with serum albumin. Low values are occasionally encountered due to genetic polymorphism.

In acute hepatitis, of infective or toxic origin, mildly reduced plasma cholinesterase levels are found within days of onset, returning gradually to normal with recovery. Chronic hepatitis, cirrhosis and neoplastic and other infiltrative diseases of the liver are also accompanied by low levels. In obstructive jaundice normal values are usually present, unless the obstruction is due to malignancy, when reduced values are found. Malignant disease, even when localised and not involving the liver, can give low enzyme levels as a consequence of impaired enzyme synthesis. In steatosis levels are normal or somewhat increased.

Cholinesterase has been used to assess liver function before and after hepatic transplantation. It is a useful prognostic tool when used serially; a sudden or marked fall to a quarter of the usual activity indicates ominous deterioration.

## 10.2 Serum Bile Acids *[21]*

Bile acids are derived from catabolism of cholesterol. The two main primary bile acids, cholic and chenodeoxycholic acids, are produced in the liver, conjugated with glycine or taurine, and excreted in bile. They play an important role in the digestion and absorption of fat and fat-soluble compounds. They are reabsorbed in the terminal ileum by a very efficient active transport mechanism, but some escape into the colon where bacteria cause deconjugation and/or dehydroxylation of the molecule at the 7-α-position. The latter reaction converts cholic acid to deoxycholic acid, and chenodeoxycholic to lithocholic acid. These secondary bile acids are absorbed from the colon and travel to the liver via the portal vein. The normal liver removes primary and secondary bile acids very efficiently and excretes them into bile, thus completing the enterohepatic circulation of bile acids (i.e., liver–bile–intestine–portal vein–liver).

With liver disease there may be a reduction in primary bile acid synthesis or a change in the relative proportions of cholic and deoxycholic acids (normally about twice as much cholic acid is produced); unusual bile acids may be produced. The amount of bile acid conjugated may alter or there may be a change in the taurine–glycine ratio. As less primary bile acid enters the intestine there is sometimes less secondary bile acid synthesis and reduced plasma levels of deoxycholate. Impaired liver function, or diversion of portal blood, impairs hepatic bile acid removal from portal blood, causing increased levels of plasma bile acids, particularly after meals. Biliary obstruction causes a rise in plasma bile acids, due to their regurgitation into the bloodstream. High plasma bile acid levels increase urinary excretion of bile acids.

Few of these effects are of value in the clinical assessment of patients. The simplest bile acid measurement is the total bile acid concentration, either in the fasting state or 2 h after a meal, but this test is rarely available in routine laboratories. The normal fasting serum bile acid level is up to about 15 µmol/litre (depending on the method used, which varies from laboratory to laboratory). The fasting serum bile acid level is elevated in only about two-thirds of patients with a variety of types of liver disease. It is therefore of relatively limited value in screening for patients who might have liver disease. Levels remain high after a meal in almost all patients with significant liver disease and the 2-h post-prandial bile acid level is a valuable screening test for liver disease. The finding of a high serum bile acid level has high specificity for the detection of liver disease (when compared with other individual tests), but its sensitivity is limited.

### 10.3 Ammonia

Arterial ammonia levels tend to be raised in patients with chronic liver disease, particularly if they have evidence of hepatic encephalopathy or if there is much portal systemic shunting; it also increases in severe acute hepatitis and with fulminant hepatic failure. There is a poor correlation between the ammonia level and the degree of encephalopathy. The measurement of blood ammonia is of relatively little clinical value in liver disease.

High blood ammonia levels are also seen in the hereditary deficiencies of urea cycle enzymes; in these conditions the blood ammonia is usually higher than in acquired liver diseases and other liver function tests tend to be normal.

## 11 Other Tests Which May Be Useful in Managing Patients with Liver Disease

### 11.1 Glucose

Blood glucose measurements are useful in patients with liver disease. Their frequent use is mandatory in patients with fulminant hepatic failure and in acute fatty liver of pregnancy, as symptomatic hypoglycaemia is common in these conditions. High glucose levels and frank diabetes mellitus are common in patients with cirrhosis, particularly when corticosteroids are used in the management of autoimmune chronic hepatitis.

### 11.2 Cholesterol, Triglyceride, Lipoproteins

The serum total cholesterol level often rises in biliary obstruction and may reach very high levels in some forms of chronic intrahepatic cholestasis, such as primary biliary cirrhosis. It tends to fall in severe parenchymal liver disease, whether acute or chronic, and in acute hepatitis there may be a rebound hypercholesterolaemia during the recovery phase. Serum triglyceride levels may be moderately elevated in patients with various types of liver disease, often showing reciprocal changes with the total serum cholesterol. In patients with either obstructive jaundice or severe parenchymal disease, lipoprotein electrophoresis may show an abnormal patterns, with loss of the α (HDL) and pre-β (VLDL) bands and a prominent β band.

An abnormal lipoprotein, LP-X, has been considered of diagnostic value in liver disease, because of its association with histological cholestasis [22]. It is, however, of little differential value, as "cholestasis" is sometimes found in hepatitis and cirrhosis and other causes of intrahepatic cholestasis as well as in extrahepatic obstruction. Furthermore LP-X may be undetectable in patients with clear evidence of surgical or other forms of obstruction to the biliary tree. This limits the value of LP-X even for screening.

### 11.3 Lecithin Cholesterol Acyltransferase

Lecithin cholesterol acyltransferase (LCAT) is a protein produced in the liver for secretion into plasma, where it catalyses the formation of cholesteryl ester. Reduced plasma LCAT activity is an important determinant of the plasma lipid and lipoprotein changes found in liver disease. It has a short half-life in plasma and some believe that, as a single test, it is the most sensitive index of hepatocellular dysfunction [23].

### 11.4 Urea and Creatinine

The blood or plasma urea is an important measurement in patients with liver disease. In severe liver disease plasma urea may be low because of reduced hepatic urea synthesis, and it is then an index of hepatocellular function. An increase in urea may occur due to vascular or extravascular volume depletion (particularly as a result of diuretic therapy for oedema and/or ascites), to renal failure secondary to liver disease (which may be exacerbated by drugs), and to gastro-intestinal bleeding, which increases urea production due to protein loading.

Measurement of plasma creatinine is a better indicator of impaired renal function than urea because it is not affected by protein catabolism or reduced hepatocellular function, but high levels of bilirubin interfere with some methods for determining creatinine causing spuriously low values.

## 12 Tests Used for Research [24, 25]

### 12.1 Galactose Elimination Capacity

Following absorption, galactose is removed from blood only by the liver and kidneys. At high plasma galactose levels there is a constant rate of removal of galactose by the liver consequent upon its hepatic conversion to galactose-1-phosphate.

Hepatic galactose uptake can be measured by intravenous injection of galactose 0.5 g/kg body weight over about 5 min, with measurement of plasma galactose levels at 5-min intervals for 60 min; urinary galactose elimination is also measured. From 20–40 min after injection the disappearance of galactose from the blood is linear with time and one can calculate the galactose elimination capacity. In normal subjects it is approximately 270 ± 40 (S.D.) mg/min per $m^2$ of body surface area or 6.7 ± 1.0 mg/min per kg body mass.

The galactose elimination capacity correlates well with other indices of hepatocellular function, e.g., prothrombin time, plasma albumin concentration and aminopyrine clearance, and has the advantage that it measures a single aspect of hepatocellular function. It is affected only by the number of individual hepatocytes and by their functional capacity, i.e., it provides a measure of functioning cell mass. There is considerable overlap between normal subjects and patients with several kinds of liver disease and the test is most useful for repeated studies done on individual subjects.

## 12.2 Aminopyrine Removal and Breath Test

Labelled aminopyrine ($^{14}C$-dimethyl amino-antipyrine) has been used to study hepatic drug metabolism. Its disappearance rate from plasma can be measured after intravenous injection, but the main attraction of this compound lies in its use in simple breath tests. If $^{14}C$-aminopyrine is given orally to non-ambulant subjects $CO_2$ can be collected from the breath. The specific activity of the breath $CO_2$ is measured and, assuming constant endogenous production of $CO_2$, the amount of labelled $^{14}CO_2$ produced by demethylation of aminopyrine can be calculated.

If the specific activity of $CO_2$ is plotted against time the disappearance curve over about 12 h is roughly exponential and a decay constant, $K_b$ can be estimated. This seems to be the best index which can be obtained from breath analyses and correlates well with bromosulphthalein disappearance (see below) and with the galactose elimination capacity. It is rather tedious to sample the breath over many hours. The breath test has been modified to obtain results after a period of 2 h, by taking the mean value for $CO_2$ specific activity during the first 2 h after the ingestion of the drug, or by sampling the breath at 2 h. Specific activity values obtained from normal subjects have been compared with those obtained from patients with various kinds of liver disease. Values for patients with hepatocellular dysfunction are generally lower than those found in normal subjects but normal values may be found in patients with biliary obstruction. Increased values may be found with hepatic enzyme induction from drugs or alcohol.

The aminopyrine 2-h breath test is not a useful diagnostic test but it does allow serial measurements of one aspect of hepatic function to be made in the same patient, the coefficient of variation of duplicate tests being about

6%. There is, of course, some reluctance to use radioactive material with a long half-life for repeated studies in man, but the radiation dosage of the test is small.

## 12.3 Hepatic Removal of Bromosulphthalein and Indocyanine Green

Bromosulphthalein (BSP) is removed from blood by hepatic parenchymal cells, bound by intracellular proteins such as ligandin and Z protein, and excreted in bile either unconjugated (approximately 30%) or following conjugation with glutathione. It is easy to measure in blood and bile. In the past a simple test of BSP excretion was widely used to detect hepatobiliary disease in non-jaundiced subjects. For this, 5 mg BSP per kg body weight is injected intravenously over 30 s. The plasma concentration of BSP is measured in a single blood specimen taken 45 min later, and the retention of BSP at 45 min calculated. In normal subjects this is up to 7% of the original dose. Higher values are found with many types of liver disease. In the familial conjugated hyperbilirubinaemia of Dubin-Johnson syndrome retention at 45 min is usually normal but a secondary rise at 90 min is usual. This contrasts with Rotor's syndrome, in which BSP retention is normal at 45 min, with no secondary rise.

The conventional BSP removal test has never been popular in Britain, because it provides very limited information and it is a potentially dangerous test. Local damage results if BSP extravasates at the site of injection: anaphylaxis has been reported, and if the BSP is not properly prepared for injection there may be neurological problems associated with the injection of microcrystals.

More complex studies of BSP removal may provide details about different aspects of the liver's handling of BSP. Following a single intravenous injection of BSP the plasma disappearance curve can be represented by two exponentials. If a two-compartment model (i.e., plasma and liver) is assumed, one can calculate the size of the plasma compartment, hepatic storage, the transfer of dye between the compartments, urinary excretion and the rate of biliary excretion, which has a theoretical maximum level, Tm. Unfortunately, such studies do not take into account the conjugation of BSP, and other problems affect interpretation. However, repeated measurements of BSP removal by this method do offer a useful method of evaluating changes in a defined function of the liver. Kinetic analysis of plasma disappearance curves has demonstrated abnormalities of hepatic BSP uptake in 30%–50% of patients with Gilbert's disease.

Indocyanine green (ICG) is rapidly removed by the liver, and is excreted into the bile without conjugation. It is much safer than BSP, is simple to measure, and can also be used to study hepatic uptake, storage and transport of an exogenous dye. ICG retention at 20 min can be measured and plasma disappearance curves can be analysed as for BSP disappearance curves. The major disadvantages of using ICG are its high cost relative to BSP and its instability in plasma, which means that plasma levels have to be measured soon after withdrawal of the sample.

Both BSP and ICG have been used to measure hepatic blood flow on the basis of the Fick principle. Plasma levels of either BSP or ICG are held constant during a continuous infusion of the dye; hepatic blood flow can then be calculated by dividing the rate of infusion by the difference in concentration of dye between arterial and hepatic venous plasma. The blood flow through the liver is clearly an important functional characteristic and it is unfortunate that its measurement involves hepatic venous catheterisation.

### 12.4 Dynamic Studies of Bilirubin Metabolism

Following injection of radioactive unconjugated bilirubin, the label is rapidly removed from the plasma, and its disappearance curve can be represented as the product of three exponentials. A number of estimates can be made directly from this curve, including the mass of unconjugated bilirubin in the initial pool, the initial distribution volume of the injected material, the quantity of unlabelled bilirubin which enters the plasma per unit of time, the hepatic clearance of bilirubin and the plasma bilirubin turnover rate. If it is assumed that the bilirubin enters three comparlments then it is also possible to derive various parameters which indicate the rate of transfer between these comparlments and the size of the comparlments, but the calculations depend on assumptions made in constructing the model. Such analyses have been useful for interpretation of disorders such as Gilbert's syndrome and the Crigler-Najjar syndrome, but the method, which is both expensive and time consuming, does not allow interpretation of findings in conjugated hyperbilirubinaemia. It is therefore of little value in patients with most types of liver disease.

### 12.5 Dynamic Studies of Bile Acid Metabolism

Theoretically one can measure the fractional disappearance of bile acids from plasma after injection of radiolabelled bile acids. They disappear very rapidly (within minutes) from plasma; interpretation of the data is complicated, as there may be considerable removal of label before adequate mixing. While it is possible to show differences in removal rate with impairment of hepatic function, there are problems in deciding the physiological meaning of the changes.

It is possible to follow the fate of a labelled bile acid through the various compartments of the total bile acid pool. Mathematical interpretation of the results is extremely complicated because of enterohepatic recirculation, the conversion of primary to secondary bile acids, and both conjugation and deconjugation with taurine and glycine. This method is of little value for repeated study of patients with liver disease.

### 12.6 Caffeine Clearance [26]

The clearance of caffeine provides a quantitative measure of cytochrome P-448-mediated hepatic microsomal demethylation, and measurement of caffeine levels in saliva after oral caffeine provides a simple non-invasive non-harmful means of investigating hepatocellular function. Clearance is markedly decreased in cirrhosis and mildly reduced in non-cirrhotic disease. Caffeine clearance correlates with other clearance tests (e.g., aminopyrine breath test and galactose capacity) but appears more sensitive.

### 12.7 Lignocaine Clearance [27]

In this test, the metabolite of lignocaine, monoethylglycine xylidide, formed by hepatic de-ethylation is measured in serum 15 min after intravenous lignocaine. A high level indicates good hepatocellular function. The procedure has been recommended as a rapid method of assessing liver function in potential liver transplant donors and in their recipients, and for post-transplant follow-up.

## 13 The Use of Liver Function Tests

Most standard liver function tests are simple to perform, are relatively inexpensive and, as they are easily automated, are included in the output of multichannel automatic analysers. Physicians may therefore receive the results of liver function tests even if they did not request them (or they may ask for them without apparent reason). Often, of course, liver function tests are requested because a doctor hopes that they will confirm a suspicion about the presence of liver disease and provide a clue to the diagnosis. If the results are normal, no further action results in most cases, and little harm will result. If the results are abnormal, problems may arise. The doctor may not notice the abnormal test results (if he did not request them); he may ignore them (if they do not fit within his clinical preconceptions); or he may be stung into action!

## 14 Applications of Liver Function Tests

Liver function tests can be used for:

1. Screening (or profiling), that is to detect the presence of unsuspected liver disease
2. Confirmation of the presence of liver disease in patients in whom it is suspected (with varying degrees of probability) on clinical grounds
3. Differential diagnosis
4. Prognosis
5. Monitoring the progress of a patient with liver disease and assessing the response to therapy
6. Clinical research

No investigation is equally useful for all of these purposes.

## 15 Screening and Profiling

"Screening" may be defined as the routine performance of investigations on an apparently healthy population; "profiling" as the routine use of tests on patients, regardless of the clinical presentation. Screening and profiling are done mainly to detect unsuspected conditions for which treatment would be beneficial. Profiling may also shed light on the cause of the patient's symptoms and, if the results are negative, it may allow confident exclusion of certain conditions. Profiling also provides background data that may be helpful later if new problems arise. For example, if jaundice occurs during treatment with a potentially hepatotoxic drug it is helpful to know that liver function tests were normal before the start of therapy.

For screening or profiling, the main concern is to detect unsuspected disease and we want to be confident that a negative test excludes the disease. False-positives are less important as the position can be clarified by further diagnostic tests; they are a major problem only if further diagnostic tests are costly or if they are potentially hazardous to the patient. For screening or profiling, therefore, a test must have high sensitivity (see Appendix).

Screening and profiling tests are done on very large numbers of patients. Such tests must therefore be cheap to perform, and they must not cause patients discomfort or inconvenience.

## 16 "Batteries" of Liver Function Tests

A single liver function test is of little value for screening because serious liver disease may be present with normal serum levels of either bilirubin, AST or ALT, alkaline phosphatase, albumin or GGT. With any one of these tests false-negatives would be unacceptably high. Furthermore, a positive result for only one of these tests has limited value, as many other diseases not involving the liver cause an increase in bilirubin, aspartate aminotransferase, alkaline phosphatase and GGT, or a reduction in albumin.

With a battery of liver function tests, however, the number of false-negatives is minimised. Only a small number of patients with significant liver disease have a completely normal set of results with the commonly used batteries of liver function tests (usually patients with well compensated cirrhosis); if their liver disease is missed on screening it is unlikely that there would be untoward clinical consequences as they would tolerate drugs, surgical procedures, and other treatments far better than those showing clear evidence of liver damage.

The use of a battery of liver function tests also gives high specificity; when more than one liver function test is abnormal, the probability of liver disease is very high. False-positives are uncommon; but they do occur (e.g., a patient with chronic malabsorption may have a high serum alkaline phosphatase of bone origin and a low serum albumin; a patient with myocardial infarction may have a high AST from cardiac muscle and an elevated bilirubin, due perhaps to a functional and relatively trivial hepatic disturbance).

We believe that a battery of liver function tests should be performed routinely on hospital in-patients and out-patients. In a hospital population about 4% have a raised AST and more have an increased ALT. Alcoholic liver disease (often just a fatty liver) is the major cause, and levels may fall with abstinence; obesity is also an important factor [28]. About 4%–5% have an increased alkaline phosphatase; bone disease, such as Paget's disease, is an important cause in the elderly. Only in a few patients does the finding of a high alkaline phosphatase lead to a new diagnosis of liver disease. Similar results have been found in "healthy" out-patient populations.

Most of these abnormalities (ca. 90%) will not have been previously recognised, but confirmatory action is taken in only 20%–25% of cases, and a new diagnosis is established in only about 10% of those with the abnormal results.

Although there is not a high diagnostic yield from profiling there are other advantages – reassurance for the patient, data that make other tests unnecessary, and baseline investigations against which to compare future test results. The last of these is particularly valuable in the hospital setting.

If an apparently healthy population is screened, unsuspected liver disease, usually due to excessive alcohol intake, is found in approximately 1% of the subjects in Britain. In some countries there might be a significant number of patients with previously unrecognised chronic viral hepatitis/cirrhosis. A plasma total bilirubin above 17 μmol/litre is found in about 5% of subjects; approximately 2% of men have a level >25 μmol/litre, but only 0.5% of women. This hyperbilirubinaemia is almost always due to Gilbert's syndrome, a completely benign condition. Finding this high bilirubin may sometimes prove deleterious, as the patient may be subjected to expensive and potentially hazardous medical or surgical intervention! However, knowing about the presence of Gilbert's syndrome may also be a help, as it may prevent unnecessary intervention if a patient with this condition becomes jaundiced, as often happens when they reduce their food intake (after surgery), or if they have abdominal pain or nausea or vomiting.

The value of GGT as a screening test is controversial. It is undoubtedly a very sensitive indicator of the presence of liver disease (0.87–0.95) but lacks specificity, since many conditions with only minimal liver disturbance cause an increase in GGT. Levels exceeding the usually accepted upper limit of normal (50 mU/litre in men, 30 mU/litre in women) have been found in about 15% of people screened.

## 17 Role of Liver Function Tests in Diagnosis

Standard liver function tests have only limited differential diagnostic value. They allow patients to be categorised as having simple unconjugated hyperbilirubinaemia (i.e., an elevation of serum total bilirubin with little or no increase in conjugated bilirubin, absence of bilirubinuria, and no abnormality of other liver function tests). Also, when the aminotransferases are very high (in the thousands) the patient is almost certainly suffering from an acute hepatitis, due to a virus or drugs, or an acute reduction in hepatic blood flow.

Liver function tests should not be used to classify jaundice for diagnostic purposes, e.g., as "*haemolytic jaundice*" when jaundice is acholuric (i.e., urinary bilirubin is absent) and the serum bilirubin is predominantly unconjugated; as "*hepatocellular jaundice*" when there is an increase in both unconjugated bilirubin and bilirubin esters, with a normal or only slightly increased alkaline phosphatase and a marked increase in aminotransferases; or as "*obstructive jaundice*" (or "cholestasis") when most of the serum bilirubin is conjugated (although this is rarely confirmed), aminotransferase levels are only moderately elevated, and there is a more marked increase in alkaline phosphatase (more than two and a half times the upper reference limit).

If used in this way, many conditions generally considered "hepatocellular", e.g., viral hepatitis, drug-induced hepatitis, alcoholic liver disease, chronic active hepatitis and cirrhosis, might be classified as obstructive or cholestatic jaundice since they may all present with biochemical (and clinical) features which are "typical" of extrahepatic biliary obstruction.

To assess the ability of any liver function test to effect diagnostic discrimination it is essential that a variety of hepatobiliary disorders with both typical and atypical clinical features be studied in adequate numbers of patients and that attention is paid to the degree of overlap in results between disease categories. Furthermore, it is essential to consider sensitivity, specificity, predictive accuracy and efficiency and the effect of disease prevalence when the diagnostic usefulness of any test or combination of tests is being assessed (see Appendix).

## 18 Diagnostic Classification of Liver Disease

A sound diagnostic strategy must be based on a sound diagnostic classification. The classes should not only be collectively exhaustive, but should, ideally, be mutually exclusive (i.e., all diagnostic possibilities should be included but they should not appear under more than one heading).

A more useful classification for diagnostic purposes, in which the groups are mutually exclusive (although more than one condition may be present in an individual patient), is to divide hepatobiliary diseases into:

1. Unconjugated hyperbilirubinaemia
2. Large bile duct disease (identifiable on cholangiography)
3. Diffuse parenchymal liver disease
4. Space-occupying lesions (and infiltrations)
5. Disorders of the hepatic circulation

This classification is applicable both for jaundiced patients and for patients with other types of presentation, and it takes into account that hepatobiliary diseases may present without hyperbilirubinaemia, even in patients with obstructive lesions of the main bile ducts such as gallstones, tumours or strictures (if the obstruction is incomplete or intermittent).

The familial unconjugated hyperbilirubinaemias have been frequently classified under "hepatocellular" jaundice (even though there is no increase in bilirubin esters), but they have few features in common with the other conditions in that group. It seems more logical to group them, based on the initial biochemical findings, under the heading "unconjugated hyperbilirubinaemia" together with haemolytic disorders.

It is clear that the other groups cannot usually be distinguished on the basis of liver function tests. Even though patients with large duct obstruction and space-occupying lesions tend to have "cholestatic" liver function tests and patients with parenchymal and vascular lesions tend to have "hepatocellular" test results, there are many exceptions; differential diagnosis must therefore depend on other evidence such as viral markers, autoantibodies, history of alcohol abuse or drug intake, indices of iron and copper metabolism, cholangiography, ultrasound or CT scanning or liver biopsy.

## 19 Monitoring

Much of the work of chemical pathology and haematology laboratories involves repetition of tests that are done to monitor progress, but there is little theoretical basis for deciding on the best way to use them. Tests for monitoring should be either quantitative (measures of a continuous variable) or semiquantitative (giving points on a scale with sufficient intervals to allow adequate documentation of change), and the methods should be sufficiently precise to ensure that observed changes are real and not the result of experimental error. When repeated measurements are done on a single patient, it may be possible to detect clinically significant trends, even if all results remain within the conventional normal range. Tests for monitoring are repeated on many occasions. They should, therefore, be cheap; expensive tests are justified only if they are used to make important clinical decisions.

Conventional liver function tests are satisfactory for monitoring progress. They are quantitative, precise and cheap. When results are abnormal due to liver disease, they tend to change only in one direction, i.e., increasing in the case of bilirubin, AST and ALT, alkaline phosphatase, and GGT, and decreasing in the case of albumin. The degree of change of aminotransferases and alkaline phosphatase may be of little prognostic significance, but high levels of bilirubin and low levels of albumin (or clotting factors) tend to indicate severe liver damage. Improvement in hepatic status is usually, but not invariably, accompanied by a return of all tests towards normal values. The results of individual tests often change in opposite directions; for example, in acute hepatitis the aminotransferase levels may fall from a very high level while the bilirubin level continues to rise.

## 20 Appendix: Sensitivity, Specificity and Predictive Accuracy

It can be assumed that in a large population some patients will have a particular disease. If a test for that disease is applied to the whole population, then a certain number of those with the disease will have a positive result (true-positives) and some will have a negative result (false-negatives). Of those without the disease, some will have a positive result (false-positives) and some, a negative result (true-negatives). The sensitivity of such a test is defined as the number of true-positive results divided by the total number of subjects who have the disease (that is, true-positives plus false-negatives). A test is therefore considered sensitive to the extent that it detects patients with the disease and excludes those without the disease.

Specificity is calculated by dividing the true-negatives by the number of subjects without the disease (that is, true-negatives plus false-positives). A test is specific to the extent that it identifies those who do not have the disease, particularly in that it minimises false-positives.

These indices are of relatively little value to the practising clinician, who does not need to know the sensitivity or the specificity of a test, but its predictive accuracy. In other words he needs to know the probability that a positive test indicates the presence of disease (that is, true-positives divided by true-positives plus false-positives) or that a negative test indicates the absence of disease (that is, true-negatives divided by true-negatives plus false-negatives). Unfortunately, the predictive accuracy of a test is markedly dependent on the type of population studied and the proportion of those who have the disease. When there are very few subjects with the disease, even a small percentage of false-positives in the large healthy subgroup would mean that a positive result would have little predictive value; this would be true even if the test was highly sensitive and highly specific. The predictive accuracy of a negative result would be very high under these circumstances. By contrast, a positive result of a test with a specificity and sensitivity no better than tossing a coin might have a high predictive accuracy if there was a very high prevalence of the disease.

These principles have been ignored in many of the studies done to evaluate tests for hepatobiliary disease. Often they have been done on selected groups of patients in whom the prevalence of various diseases is high. This is particularly unsatisfactory if the tests are then used in another population in which the prevalence is quite different (for example, if a test evaluated on in-patients is applied to a quite different out-patient population).

## References

1. Billing BH (1978) Twenty-five years of progress in bilirubin metabolism (1952–1977). Gut 19:481–491
2. Billing BH (1983) A 1983 assessment of the value of bile pigment determinations in the diagnosis of jaundice. Postgrad Med J 59:19–25
3. Rosalki SB (1976) Enzyme tests in disease of the liver and biliary tract. In: Wilkinson SH (ed) Principles and practice of diagnostic enzymology. Edward Arnold, London, Chap. 20
4. Cohen JA, Kaplan MM (1979) The SGOT/SGPT ratio – an indicator of alcoholic liver disease. Dig Dis Sci 24:835–838
5. Williams ALB, Hoofnagle JA (1988) Ratio of serum aspartate to alanine aminotransferase in chronic hepatitis: relationship to cirrhosis. Gastroenterology 95:734
6. Clermont RJ, Chalmers TC (1967) The transaminase tests in liver disease. Medicine 46:197–207
7. Paradinas FJ, Melia WM, Wilkinson ML, Portmann B, Johnson PJ, Murray-Lyon IM, Williams R (1982) High serum vitamin $B_{12}$ binding capacity as a marker of the fibrolamellar variant of hepatocellular carcinoma. Br Med J 285:840–842
8. Nemesanszky E (1986) Alkaline phosphatase. In: Lott JA, Wolf PL (eds) Clinical enzymology. Field Rich and Assoc., New York (distributed by Year Book Publishers), Chap. 3
9. Rosalki SB, Foo Ay (1984) Two methods for separating and quantifying bone and liver alkaline phosphatase isoenzymes in plasma. Clin Chem 30:1182–1186
10. Rosalki SB (1975) Gamma-glutamyl transpeptidase. Adv Clin Chem 17:53–107
11. Nemesanszky E (1986) Gammaglutamyltransferase (GGT). In: Lott JA, Wolf PL (eds) Clinical enzymology. Field Rich and Assoc., New York (distributed by Year Book Publishers), Chap. 9

12. Maggiore G, Bernard O, Riely CA, Hadchouel M, Lemonnier A, Alagille D (1987) Normal serum gamma-glutamyl-transpeptidase activity identifies groups of infants wth idiopathic cholestasis with poor prognosis. J Pediatr 111:251–255
13. Hobbs JR (1967) Serum proteins in liver disease. Proc R Soc Med 60:1250–1254
14. Rothschild MA, Oratz M, Schreiber SS (1988) Serum albumin. Hepatology 8:385–401
15. Hutchinson DR, Halliwell RP, Smith MG, Parke DV (1981) Serum "prealbumin" as an index of liver function in human hepatobiliary disease. Clin Chim Acta 114:69–74
16. Strickland GT, Leu ML (1975) Wilson's disease. Clinical and laboratory manifestations in 40 patients. Medicine 54:113–137
17. Feld RD (1989) Heterozygosity at alpha-1-antitrypsin: a health risk. Clin Lab Sci 27:461–481
18. Kew MC (1975) Alpha-fetoprotein. In: Read A (ed) Modern trends in gastroenterology, vol 5. Butterworth, London, pp 91–114
19. Brown SS, Kalow W, Pilz W et al. (1981) The plasma cholinesterases: a new perspective. Adv Clin Chem 22:1–123
20. Sawhney AK, Lott JA (1986) Acetylcholinesterase and cholinesterase. In: Lott JA, Wolf PL (eds) Clinical enzymology. Field Rich and Assoc., New York (distributed by Year Book Publishers), Chap. 1
21. Berry W, Reichen J (1983) Bile acid metabolism: its relation to chinical disease. Semin Liver Dis 3:330–340
22. Seidel D, Gretz H, Ruppert C (1973) Significance of the LP-X test in differential diagnosis of jaundice. Clin Chem 19:86–91
23. Simko V, Kelley RE, Dincsoy HP (1985) Predicting severity of liver disease: twelve laboratory tests evaluated by multiple regression. J Int Med Res 13:249–254
24. Larrey D, Branch RA (1983) Clearance by the liver: current concepts in understanding the hepatic disposition of drugs. Semin Liver Dis 3:285–297
25. Preisig R (1986) Clinical evaluation of liver function. Recent Adv Hepatol 1:1–12
26. Jost G, Wahllander A, von Mandach U, Preisig R (1987) Overnight salivary caffeine clearance: a liver function test suitable for routine use. Hepatology 7:338–344
27. Oellerich M, Burdelski M, Ringe B et al. (1989) Lignocaine metabolite formation as a measure of pre-transplant liver function. Lancet I:640–642
28. Friedman LS, Dienstag JL, Watkins E, Hinkle CA, Spiers JA, Rieder SV, Huggins CE (1987) Evaluation of blood donors with elevated serum alanine aminotransferase levels. Ann Intern Med 107:137–144
29. Rosoff L, Rosoff L (1977) Biochemical tests for hepatobiliary disease. Surg Clin North Am 57:257–273

# 3 Molecular Biology of the Liver

N. FAUSTO

Because of its physiologic importance, the predominance of a single cell type, its size, and its relative accessibility, the liver has become a focal point for studies of gene regulation. These studies have not only enhanced our knowledge about mechanisms of gene expression in general but also provided major insights on questions regarding normal and abnormal liver development, function, and growth. Major areas of research that heavily rely on molecular biology techniques include the analysis of transcriptional factors in developing and adult liver, studies on proto-oncogenes, growth factors and other growth-associated genes, the investigation of coordinated gene expression in the acute phase response, the expression of extracellular matrix genes in liver fibrosis, and the analysis of the structure and regulation of individual genes that may regulate hepatic function or structure. A more recent area of research, which should eventually lead to clinical applications, involves the replacement or inactivation of hepatic genes in vivo. This line of work became possible due to the successful development of methods to transfer genes into cultured liver cells.

Each liver cell contains approximately 100000 genes, but only 5%–10% of these are active [1]. Active genes may have multiple copies on the DNA; genes for ribosomal RNAs (rRNA) and transfer RNA (tRNA) are heavily repeated in the human genome (280 and 1300 gene copies, respectively [2, 3]). In contrast, other genes are present only once in the genome (unique sequences or single-copy genes). Among the single-copy genes there are those which may be active exclusively or predominantly in the liver ("liver-specific" genes such as albumin and α-fetoprotein) and those which are also transcribed in other tissues. Genes which code for proteins necessary for cell maintenance functions are known as "housekeeping" genes [2, 3].

One of the central issues regarding the regulation of gene expression in complex organisms is to understand how tissue-specific patterns of expression develop from common DNA sequences present in all tissues. To put it more directly, it is still not known how liver cells make albumin while muscle cells make myosin, despite the presence of both genes in the two types of cells. The problem is even more complex because in the liver, as in other tissues, tissue-specific, housekeeping genes, growth-associated genes, etc. may be expressed simultaneously. Questions regarding the developmental determination of tissue specificity are generally less relevant in the study of neoplastic transformation or fibrosis because growth-associated genes and those encoding extracellular matrix proteins are not liver specific but are expressed in other tissues as well. Nevertheless, α-fetoprotein, because of its oncodevelopmental pattern of expression, is an example of a "liver-specific" gene that is also of importance in hepatic tumorigenesis [4].

Not only is the coordination of gene expression enormously complicated in a single cell but another level of complexity is added at the tissue level as various cell types differ in their pattern of gene expression. For instance, Kupffer cells and endothelial cells produce growth factors not made by hepatocytes (TGFβ, platelet-derived growth factor, interleukins, etc.) but do not make albumin or α-fetoprotein, while lipocytes (Ito cells) are rich sources for extracellular matrix proteins [5–8]. Moreover, gene expression in hepatocytes may depend both qualitatively and quantitatively on interactions with nonparenchymal cells [9].

## 1 Gene Transcription

Active genes can be identified because they transcribe RNA, but even in the absence of a transcriptional product an active gene might be detectable by the presence of sites which are highly sensitive to deoxyribonuclease I (DNase I) digestion [3]. In these sites (generally comprising 100–400 base pairs) the DNA-protein structure (chromatin) is modified either by folding (secondary structure) or by altered spacing of the protein along the DNA chain. The weaker DNA-protein association in DNase-hypersensitive sites permits the interaction between DNA and cellular proteins that can bind to it. These proteins are capable of modulating gene transcription and are known as transcriptional factors or transactivators. The correlation between transcriptional activity and DNase-hypersensitive sites found in most genes is, however, not absolute, and DNase hypersensitivity may be present in inactive genes [3].

The synthesis of ribosomal RNA (rRNA), messenger RNA (mRNA), and transfer RNA (tRNA) is catalyzed by RNA polymerases I, II, and III respectively. Almost 90% of cellular RNA is constituted by rRNA. RNA polymerase II is the enzyme involved in the transcription of protein-encoding genes. Messenger RNA constitutes only 1%–2% of the total amount of cellular RNA.

The ends of DNA or RNA molecules are designated 5′ or 3′ depending on whether the terminal deoxyribose (DNA) or ribose (RNA) has a non-bonded 5′ or 3′ carbon. The primary transcript copied from the DNA template is not functional but requires modifications (processing) that consist of cleavage at the 3′ end, addition of polyadenylic acid sequences (poly A), and splicing (Fig. 1). Splicing is required because in most genes the transcriptional units encoding the sequence of a protein (exons) are separated by intervening sequences (introns). The introns do not generally

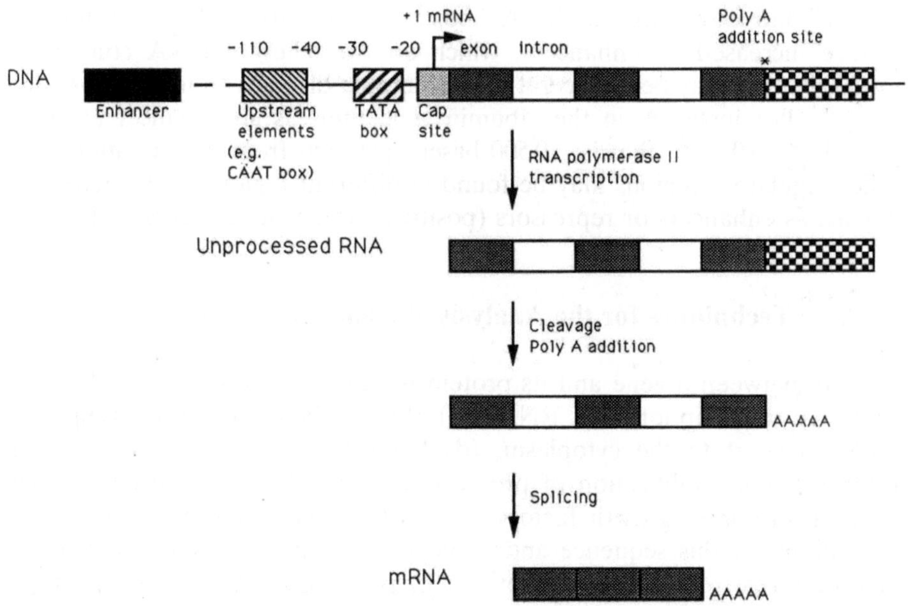


**Fig. 1.** Gene structure, mRNA transcription and processing. The diagram shows a hypothetical gene containing exons (coding sequences) interrupted by introns (generally noncoding). The cap site where mRNA transcription is initiated is indicated as +1. Several transcriptional regulatory sites are indicated: the TATA and CAAT boxes located in the promoter region (+1 to −110) and distant enhancer sequences located 5′ (upstream) from the promoter area. The unprocessed transcript contains all exons and introns. During processing 3′ noncoding regions are cleaved and poly A is added at the 3′ end. Splicing eliminates introns and places the coding exons in contiguous positions

encode protein sequences and are removed during processing of the primary RNA transcript. In the mature mRNA transported to the cytoplasm, the exons are spliced together, constituting a molecule that contains the uninterrupted code for the protein sequence (Fig. 1).

The site at which transcription is initiated is called a CAP, named because of the "capping" (addition of a 7-methylguanosine residue) that takes place in the 5′ end of nascent mRNA. By convention, the mRNA initiation site on the DNA is numbered +1. Active and correct initiation of RNA transcription depends on the promoter region, generally located within 200 base pairs (bp) in a 5′ direction (upstream) from the start site. In most genes this region contains common sequences (consensus sequences) that can specifically bind transcriptional factors that regulate promoter activity (Fig. 1). Two of these consensus elements have been particularly well studied: (a) a region rich in adenine and thymine known as "TATA box" located 20–30 bases upstream from the initiation site (−20 to −30), and (b) a region generally located at −70 to −90 containing the sequence

CCAAT and known as the "CAAT box". The activity of the promoter can also be increased by enhancers, which are stretches of DNA containing 50–300 bp that may be located at a considerable distance from the promoter (Fig. 1). For instance, in the albumin gene there is an enhancer element located at −10.5 kb, that is, 10500 bases upstream from the initiation site. Other regulatory regions may be found at different regions of the gene and may act as enhancers or repressors (positive and negative regulators).

## 2 Basic Techniques for the Analysis of Gene Expression

The link between a gene and its protein product includes a series of steps: (a) DNA transcription into RNA; (b) RNA splicing and processing; (c) RNA transport to the cytoplasm; (d) RNA translation into protein; (e) posttranslation modification of proteins (Fig. 2) [10]. External or internal stimuli (hormones, growth factors, metabolic changes, etc.) act at one or more points in this sequence and, depending on their site of action, their effects are referred to as transcriptional or posttranscriptional.

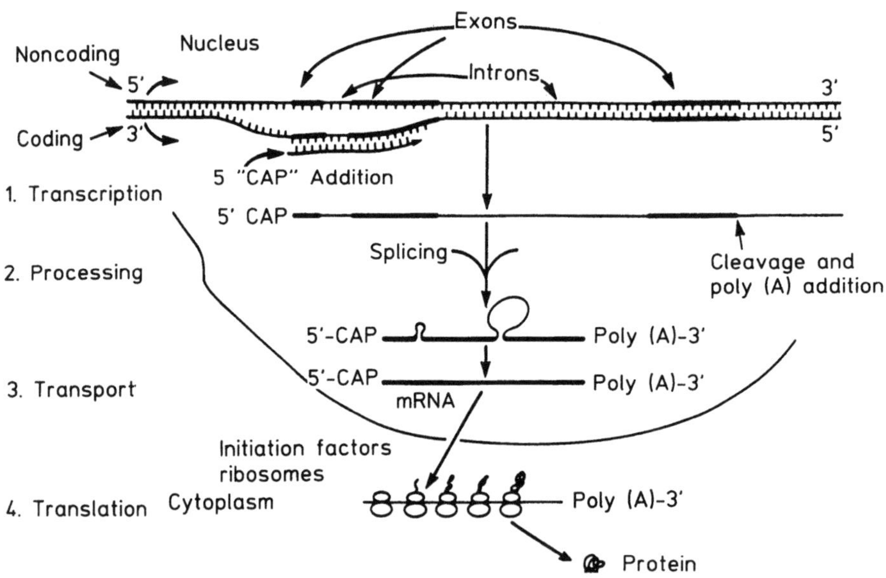


**Fig. 2.** Steps involved in gene expression. The diagram shows a gene with exons and introns and the 5′ and 3′ ends of each DNA strand. The steps illustrated are: *1*, transcription of the coding DNA strand and "capping" on the nascent transcript; *2*, processing of the transcript involving cleavage at the 3′ end, poly A addition, and splicing to remove introns; *3*, transport of mature mRNA to cytoplasm; and *4*, translation of mRNA into protein in ribosomes. [Reproduced with permission from Nienhuis AW and Maniatis T (1987) in: Stamatoyannopoulos G et al. (eds) The molecular basis of blood diseases. W.B. Saunders, Philadelphia, p 28]

The analysis of gene expression relies on a number of basic techniques, some of which have become routine and are used in both research and clinical laboratories. When combined with immunohistochemical or cytologic procedures, these techniques permit the analysis of the expression of individual genes in specific cells. Procedures for the analysis of gene expression continue to be actively developed and simplified for more general use. A detailed description of techniques is available in some excellent manuals [11, 12]. General features of gene expression are very well presented in references 2, 3, 10, and 11.

### 2.1 Northern, Southern, and Western Blots

Northern, Southern, and Western blots are used to detect specific DNA (Southern), RNA (Northern), or protein (Western) molecules in cellular extracts. Northern blot analysis is used to examine the expression of a specific gene in RNA preparations obtained from whole tissue, isolated cells, or subcellular compartments. Southern blot is used to determine the number of copies of a particular gene in the genome, gene amplification, deletions, gross mutations, viral integration sites, etc. It is also an essential technique for work involving gene cloning and transfer. The DNA technique was named after its inventor, E.M. Southern [12]. When the method was adapted to RNA analysis it received the name "Northern," an indication that molecular biologists are not completely lacking in humor. A further development was the "Western" blot used for the detection of specific proteins.

In the Southern, Northern, and Western techniques, DNA, RNA, or proteins (respectively) are first separated according to size by electrophoresis on a gel matrix of polyacrylamide, agarose, or a mixture of the two (Fig. 3). The blotting step consists of the transfer of fractionated DNA, RNA, or protein from the gel into a solid support (usually nitrocellulose or nylon filters). Specific DNA or RNA sequences become immobilized in the solid support and are detected using the following steps: (a) hybridization with a labeled complementary DNA or RNA sequence (Fig. 3A, preparation of labeled probes); (b) termination of the hybridization reaction, washing the filter and placing it in contact with x-ray film; (c) developing the film after variable exposure time to visualize the bands corresponding to the radioactive hybrids (Fig. 3B). In Western blots, individual immobilized proteins are detected by reaction with a specific antibody.

A variation of these techniques for DNA and RNA detection is known as dot blotting. In this case RNA or DNA extracted from tissues is directly bound to nitrocellulose or nylon filters (without previous electrophoretic fractionation) and hybridized to specific probes. This is a fast technique useful for screening multiple samples.

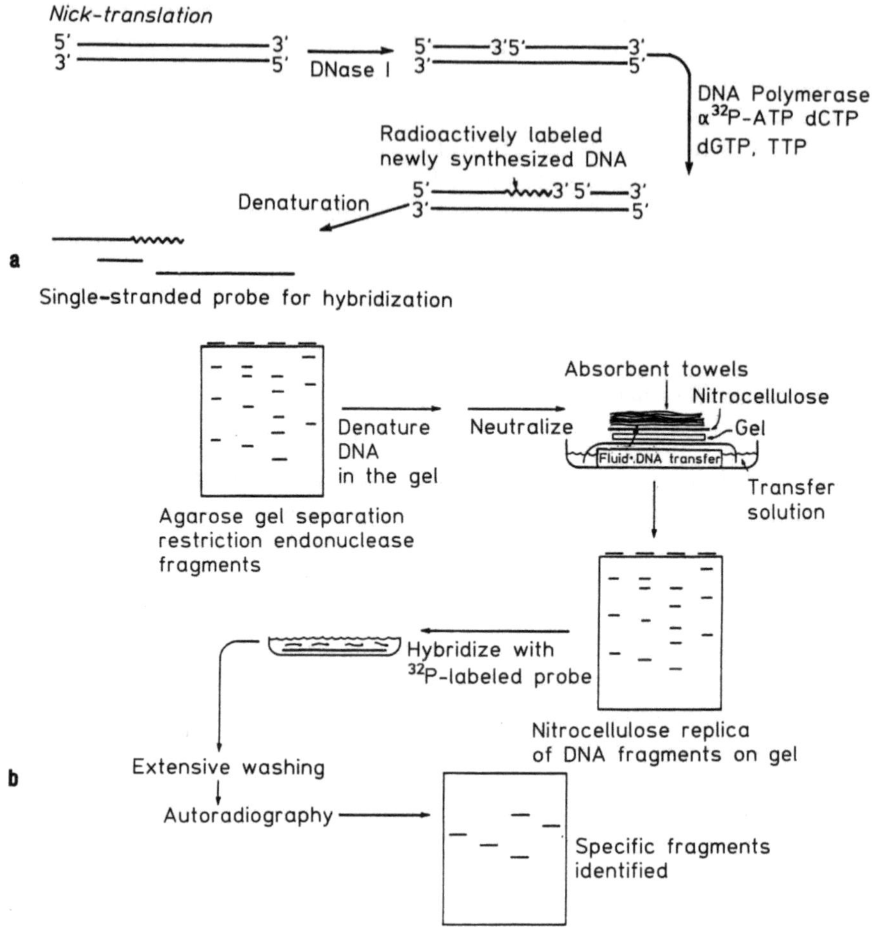


**Fig. 3. a** Preparation of labeled probes by "Nick-translation." Nick-translation is a method used to incorporate radioactive nucleotides into double-stranded DNA. Digestion of DNA with pancreatic deoxyribonuclease (DNase I) creates a cut (nick) in one of the DNA strands. The enzyme DNA polymerase I (*E. coli*) is then used to add labeled nucleotides to the 3′ end of the nicked strand. The nicks are created randomly by DNase I digestion. The strands are separated by denaturation and the labeled single-stranded material can be used as a probe for hybridization. **b** Southern/Northern blotting procedure. In the Southern procedure illustrated in the figure, DNA is first digested with restriction endonucleases and the fragments generated in the digestion are separated by electrophoresis in agarose gels. The DNA fragments in the gel are denatured by alkali treatment, neutralized, and transferred ("blotted") to nitrocellulose or nylon filters. In the Northern procedure, RNA is fractionated by gel electrophoresis and transferred directly to the filter. Northern or Southern blots are then hybridized with $^{32}$P-labeled probes, washed extensively, placed in contact with x-ray film, and developed (autoradiography). The specific bands corresponding to DNA (Southern) or RNA (Northern) molecules that hybridized with the labeled probe can then be visualized and quantitated by densitometric scanning. [Reproduced with permission from FRITSCH EF and MANIATIS T (1987) In: STAMATOYANNOPOULOS G et al. (eds) The molecular basis of blood diseases. W.B. Saunders, Philadelphia, p 1]

## 2.2 Ribonuclease Protection Assay

Specific RNA molecules in cellular or tissue RNA preparations can also be detected by a nuclease protection assay, a method that is more sensitive than Northern blotting. Nuclease protection assays consist of: (a) hybridization of an RNA probe made from a DNA template with the RNA preparation to be analyzed; (b) digestion with nucleases (ribonucleases A and T) that digest only single-stranded sequences (nonhybridized sequences), leaving intact the hybrid; (c) analysis of the hybrids by gel electrophoresis. Nuclease protection with S1 nuclease from Aspergillus oryzae can be utilized to both quantify and to "map" transcripts that is, determine the exact locations of 5′ and 3′ ends and intron/exon junctions. For S1 nuclease protection assays single-stranded DNA is used as a probe.

## 2.3 RNA Transcription by Isolated Nuclei

The amounts of specific mRNAs measured by Northern blot analysis may change in the cytoplasm in response to various stimuli (growth, metabolism, etc.). It is then important to determine whether the change in the amounts of mRNA (steady-state levels) depends on transcriptional or posttranscriptional regulation. The method known as "run-on transcription" can be used to directly determine the rate of transcription in isolated nuclei (Fig. 4). A good example of the use of this technique is for the analysis of the mechanisms that account for increased steady-state levels of mRNAs from several proto-oncogenes after partial hepatectomy. To determine whether the elevation in mRNA levels depends on transcriptional mechanisms the following strategy can be used: (a) isolation of nuclei from livers of partially hepatectomized animals; (b) incubation of nuclei in an appropriate medium containing at least one labeled nucleotide; (c) hybridization of the labeled RNA product with specific DNA probes (in this case from proto-oncogenes) previously immobilized into nitrocellulose or nylon filters; (d) film exposure and development as described above (Fig. 4). This assay measures the elongation of RNA molecules whose transcription had been initiated in vivo before the isolation of the nuclei. Little or no new initiation occurs in the isolated nuclei during the assay in vitro.

## 2.4 In Situ Hybridization – Analysis of Gene Expression at the Cellular Level

In *in situ* hybridization techniques the hybridization reaction with a labeled, specific, probe is performed on a tissue section (frozen or paraffin embedded) or cytologic preparation [13]. This method is often the most sensitive technique available for mRNA detection (for instance in cases where the mRNA

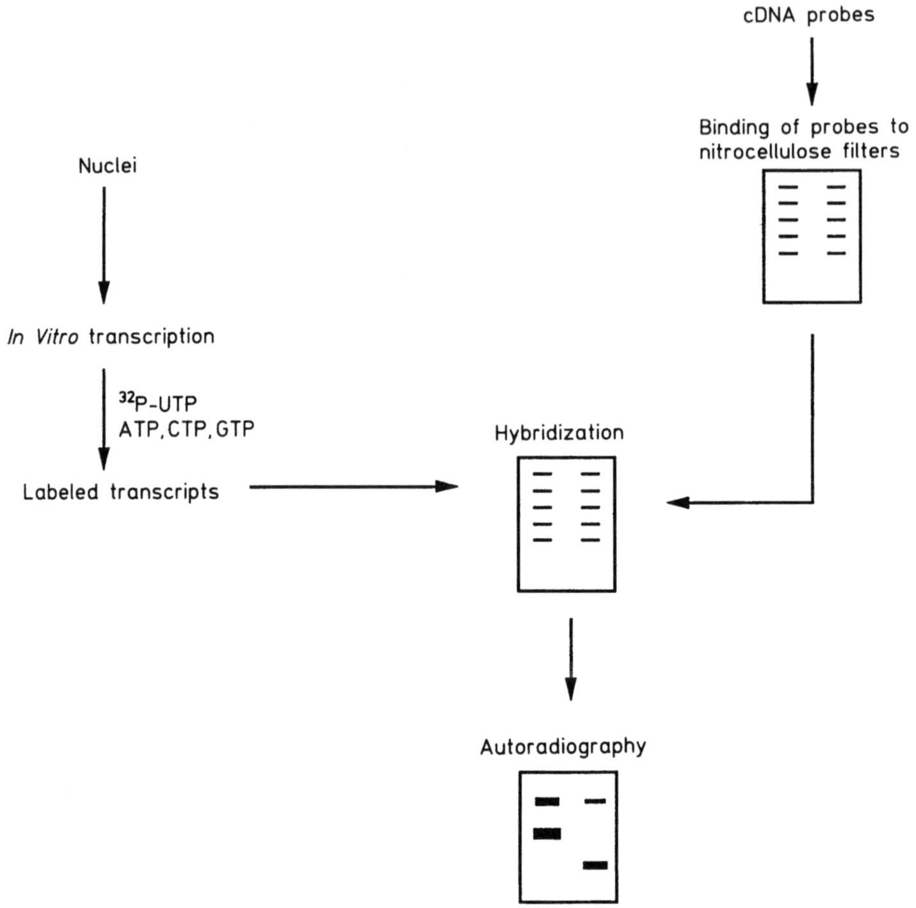


**Fig. 4.** Nuclear "run-on" transcription assay. For this assay nuclei are isolated from tissues or cells in culture and incubated in a reaction mixture containing the four nucleotides, at least one of which labeled with $^{32}P$. The labeled RNA formed in this reaction is hybridized to DNA probes which are complementary to the sequences of the gene to be detected. The probes are bound to cellulose or nylon filters before hybridization to the labeled RNA. After appropriate washing, the filters are placed in contact with x-ray film. The films are exposed and developed to detect labeled RNA transcripts which have hybridized with the complementary probes. In this technique DNA probes are pipetted into the filters in symmetrical rows with the help of a plastic template to form a series of parallel dots or slots

is not abundant or is expressed by only a few cells in the tissue) and provides both molecular and morphologic data. In this procedure, tissue fixation, slide preparation (free of nuclease), and prehybridization treatment of the sections are crucial steps that may determine the success of the method. Both DNA and RNA probes can be used for detection of mRNA transcripts in tissues but there are many advantages in utilizing RNA probes. RNA probes are synthesized to be complementary to the transcribed mRNA molecule being studied in the tissue (antisense RNA probe) and they hybridize with the specific cellular mRNA to form stable RNA-RNA duplexes. After digestion of the unhybridized probe, labeled duplexes can be visualized by conventional autoradiography techniques. When care is taken to minimize background and the proper controls are run (using 'sense" probes which have identical sequences to the cellular mRNA and thus cannot form complementary duplexes), in situ hybridization can detect the presence of a few molecules of a specific mRNA in the cell.

## 2.5 Polymerase Chain Reaction

Polymerase chain reaction (PCR), devised less than 10 years ago, has found wide application in research and clinical work. In this technique, which may be completed in less than 1 h, a short segment of DNA or RNA is amplified in a Thermocycler instrument. Each amplification cycle takes about 5 min and 30–40 cycles are generally run (Fig. 5) [14, 15]. The cycles consist of: (a) denaturation of the double-stranded DNA by heating at 90°C; (b) annealing to the DNA (at 55°C) of two single-stranded oligonucleotide primers that flank the sequences to be amplified; (c) extension of the

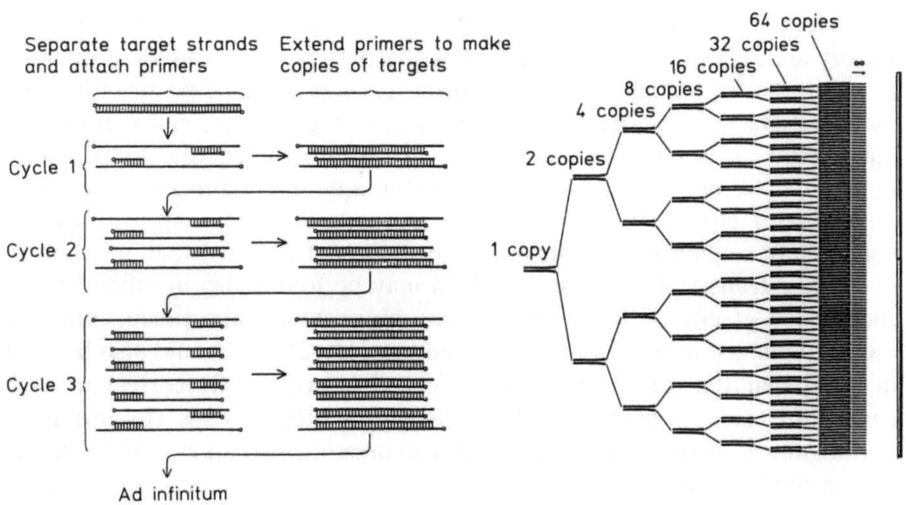


**Fig. 5.** Polymerase chain reaction. Each cycle consists of denaturation of DNA to separate the strands, hybridization of each strand to oligonucleotide primers, and extension of primers by DNA polymerase. The number of cycles can be repeated and, as the number of copies increases exponentially in each cycle, more than 100 million copies of the original RNA or DNA sequence can be obtained using 1–5 μg of starting material. For RNA amplification, complementary DNA (cDNA) to the target RNA molecule is first prepared. [Reproduced with permission from Mullis KB (1990) Sci Am 263:56–65]

primers by a DNA polymerase that synthesizes complementary DNA (at 72°C with Thermus aquaticus, "Taq," polymerase). By repeating this amplification cycle many times, it is possible to obtain 20–100 million-fold amplification of a short DNA or RNA fragment (Fig. 5). For use in the PCR technique, RNA is transcribed into complementary DNA by reverse transcriptase before the first amplification cycle. The procedure requires very small quantities of tissue (1–5 μg DNA or RNA), amounts available in biopsy specimens or paraffin blocks. PCR has a very broad range of applications, including detection of rare cellular transcripts (hepatitis virus transcripts, oncogenes, etc.), analysis of the structure of transcripts, detection of oncogene mutations in tissue specimens, and nucleic acid sequencing to detect genetic variability or insertion sites.

## 3 Regulation of Liver-Specific Genes; Albumin and α-Fetoprotein

The liver-specific genes that have been studied in considerable detail include albumin, α-fetoprotein (AFP), $\alpha_1$-antitrypsin, α and β fibrinogen, pro-albumin (transthyretin), aldolase B, and pyruvic kinase L [16]. The central hypothesis guiding the study of these genes was that their expression may be regulated at the transcriptional level by proteins (transcriptional factors) which are unique to or enriched in liver cells. These proteins act as transcriptional activators by virtue of their ability to bind specific DNA sequences in the target genes. However, as most "liver" transcriptional factors are also present in other tissues the preferential expression of some genes in the liver might be explained by: (a) liver-specific posttranslational modifications (phosphorylation for instance) of transcriptional factors that make them capable of binding to DNA, (b) specific chromatin conformation in hepatocytes allowing DNA binding; (c) unique interactions between transcriptional factors. Results of recent research indicate that liver-specific genes share sequences (and probably secondary structures) that are capable of binding transcriptional factors which may be found also in other tissues. Indeed few if any of these factors are unique to hepatic tissue, although their abundance in other organs may be low [16–24]. It should also be kept in mind that the term "liver-specific gene" is not strictly correct as such genes can also be expressed at low levels in other tissues (for instance, fibrinogen, $\alpha_1$-antitrypsin, and albumin expression in kidney; AFP expression in fetal intestine, etc.).

At least five transcriptional factors that may regulate the expression of liver-specific genes have been identified [16]. They are known by their abbreviations HNF-1, HNF-3, HNF-4 (hepatocyte nuclear factor 1, 3, and 4), C/EBP ("CAAT/enhancer binding protein"), and DBP ("D" site binding protein). The genes for HNF-1, HNF-3, and C/EBP have been cloned, making it possible to investigate the tissue distribution of their respective mRNAs [16–20]. HNF-1 transcripts are present in liver and kidney (although there is some disagreement about these observations) while C/EBP mRNA is very abundant in fat cells [17, 19]. HNF-3A transcripts have been, so far found only in liver [18]. The detection of these factors and their transcripts in liver tissue does not by itself provide information on how their synthesis and activity might be regulated and how transcriptional factors regulate the expression of liver-specific genes. The amount of each factor in hepatic tissue appears to be transcriptionally regulated although DBP expression may be controlled at a posttranscriptional level [21]. Whatever mechanism regulates their synthesis, the transcriptional factors can bind to a short DNA sequence present in most liver-specific genes. In each of these genes there are binding sites for the five liver-specific factors as well as for more ubiquitous transcriptional activator proteins and binding sites for a single factor may be found dispersed in different locations in the gene.

In the albumin gene, the best studied among liver-specific genes, there are at least three regulatory regions in 5′ upstream sequences [16, 22–24]. The promoter region extending approximately 100 bases upstream from the transcription initiation site, a region distant 3.5 kb 5′ from the start site, and an enhancer region located 10.5 kb upstream from the start site. In each of these three regions there are sequences that can be recognized by various transcriptional factors (for instance, HNF-1 binds to the promoter site; C/EBP binds to the three sites). Simultaneous occupation of various sites is apparently required for maximum transcriptional rates.

Analysis of the structure and expression of the AFP gene in mouse and rat liver revealed the presence of two binding sites for HNF-1 in the promoter region [25, 26] which are essential for transcription of the gene in the liver. Transcription may be increased by three distant enhancer elements located at 2.5, 5.0, and 6.5 kb upstream from the start site. The repression of liver AFP transcription that occurs after birth depends on a repressor element located 5′ to the promoter region which is believed to become active only after birth. Furthermore, in mice, repression of AFP transcription is also under the control of a transactivating locus known as RAF ("regulation of AFP"). In addition to the liver and the yolk sac, transcription of the AFP gene also occurs in the fetal intestine, but at levels that are at least 100-fold lower than those of fetal liver. It is not known what accounts for the differential transcription of the gene in fetal liver and intestine but in contrast to liver, the middle enhancer element is not active in the intestine [25, 26].

The identification of transcriptional factors and the analysis of the mechanisms that regulate their activity are the subject of very active research. The increased complexity of such studies has made it clear that transcription regulation is a complicated process and that the idea that a single factor might determine the expression of an individual gene is no longer tenable [27]. Instead, the recent work indicates that single regulatory sequences in DNA can interact with multiple proteins, that the proteins themselves may have differing function depending on their subunit composition, and that various combinations of transcriptional factors binding to regulatory sites in a gene may have different effects on the transcriptional activity and tissue specificity of the gene [27].

## 4 The Expression of Growth-Associated Genes: Proto-oncogenes, Oncogenes, Growth Factors, and Suppressor Genes

Oncogenes were first identified in acute transforming RNA tumor viruses (retroviruses) as the sequences coding for proteins responsible for tumorigenesis in vivo and cell transformation in culture [28, 29]. The transforming sequence, not found in nontransforming viruses, was called a viral oncogene (v-*onc*). Further studies revealed that V-ONCS are slightly modified cellular genes generated by the transduction of a normal cellular gene into a nontransforming virus during infection. The cellular genes which are homologous to V-ONCS became known as proto-oncogenes. Analysis of human and animal genomes showed that there are many proto-oncogenes in cellular DNA that do not have equivalents in viral DNA [28, 29]. The definition of proto-oncogenes was then broadened to include any gene whose modification could lead to tumorigenesis. By this definition, proto-oncogenes are normal genes, generally associated with cell growth and development, which are the normal counterparts of genes (oncogenes) which have transforming capacity. Proto-oncogenes can be converted to oncogenes by: (a) transduction into a virus (V-ONC); (b) mutation by single-base substitution or chromosomal rearrangement; (c) amplification in the genome; (d) overexpression caused by the insertion of a virus adjacent to the gene (insertional mutagenesis). The study of proto-oncogenes and oncogenes has become intimately connected to that of growth factors. These are peptides which bind to plasma membrane receptors and initiate a cascade of events (signal transduction) which results in gene activation. Growth factors themselves or their receptors may function as proto-oncogenes as in the following examples: (a) the identity between the B chain of platelet-derived growth factor (PDGF) and the v-*sis* oncogene; (b) the homology between the EGF receptor and the v-*erb* gene; (c) the homology between the CSF-1 (colony stimulating factor-1) and the c-*fms* gene [28, 29].

A further class of genes related to tumorigenesis act as suppressors, that is, they must be lost or inactivated for transformation to occur [30, 31]. Two of these genes, the retinoblastoma (Rb) and p53, have been the subject of much recent work. The Rb protein is not present in retinoblastomas or in some other tumors such as small cell lung carcinomas as a consequence of a delection or inactivation of the gene [32, 33]. This was first detected by the analysis of restriction fragment length polymorphisms in chromosome 13. Further studies revealed that the Rb gene encodes a DNA-binding protein that becomes inactivated by phosphorylation during the $G_1$/S phase of the cell cycle [34, 35]. p53 inactivation or its mutation into a transforming protein is associated with the development of colon cancers [36]. Apparently the normal function of the gene is to permit cell cycle progression in replicating cells [37]. Thus, it has become evident that tumor development requires the interplay between activating (oncogenes, growth factors) and suppressor genes.

## 5 Gene Expression During Liver Regeneration

### 5.1 Immediate Early Genes

The removal of 70% of the liver mass (partial hepatectomy) initiates a chain of events involving the expression of several proto-oncogenes that culminates in DNA replication in more than 90% of hepatocytes [38]. The expression of three proto-oncogenes (c-*fos*, c-*jun*, and c-*myc*) is markedly increased in the first 4 h after partial hepatectomy (Fig. 6) [39–45]. Because the response of these genes is also rapid in cells in culture stimulated to proliferate by the addition of growth factors or serum, they became known as "immediate early" genes. These three genes are certainly not the only ones that respond rapidly to partial hepatectomy. Indeed, they are prototypes for a class of genes that may include a dozen or more sequences which change in expres-

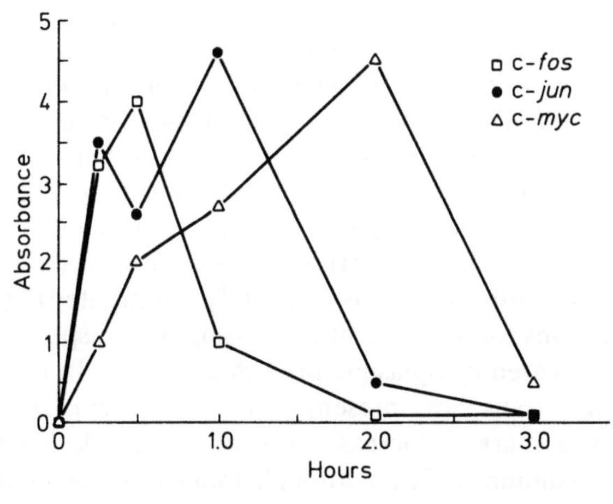


**Fig. 6.** Expression of c-fos, c-jun and c-myc in the early stages of liver regeneration. These three genes are prototypes for a category of genes known as "immediate early" genes because their expression changes rapidly after growth stimuli. The products of c-*fos* and c-*jun* form dimers which bind to DNA and function as transcriptional activators for other genes involved in the growth response. Myc protein can regulate the expression of other genes by acting both at the transcriptional and the posttranscriptional level. In the regenerating liver there is a sequential increase in the mRNA for the three genes: the increase is rapid for c-*fos* and c-*jun* and slower for c-*myc*. Steady-state levels of the mRNAs return to normal 3 h after partial hepatectomy

sion after growth stimulation both in liver and in cultured cells [46]. After partial hepatectomy, c-*fos* transcripts increase within 0.5 h, followed by a sequential accumulation of c-*jun* and c-*myc* RNA. The mRNAs for these proto-oncogenes return to normal by 3 h (Fig. 6).

The response of immediate early genes to partial hepatectomy appears to be one of the first events of the regenerative response. Although c-*fos*, c-*jun*, and c-*myc* expression is not directly linked to DNA synthesis (which starts 10–12 h later), these genes probably function as master switches that trigger the expression of other genes required for the progression of quiescent hepatocytes through the cell cycle. The proteins encoded by c-*fos* and c-*jun* serve as transcriptional activators of other genes (by convention c-*fos*, c-*jun*, and c-*myc* proteins are referred to as Fos, Jun, and Myc) by virtue of their capacity to form homo- (Jun-Jun) or heterodimers (Jun-Fos) that bind to DNA [47, 48]. The proteins dimerize through leucine-rich domains called leucine zippers and also contain a DNA-binding domain that recognizes the sequence TGACTCA (Jun/AP-1 recognition sequence or enhancer). This sequence is present in many different genes such as proto-oncogenes, genes for growth factors, and extracellular matrix components [49]. The transcription of sets of genes that contain the Jun/AP-1 site can thus be simultaneously activated as a consequence of the increased expression of c-*fos* and c-*jun* shortly after partial hepatectomy. Similarly, Myc also induces the expression of other genes, and acts at both the transcriptional and the posttranscriptional level of regulation.

It is important to understand the mechanisms that control the expression of immediate early genes in the regenerating liver because their activation may be closely linked to the triggering of the regenerative process. The regulation of c-*myc* has been studied in detail [39, 40, 45] and will be summarized below because it illustrates the various levels at which gene expression might be regulated. The regulation of c-*myc* expression is complex and may involve modulation of: (a) transcription initiation; (b) "pausing," that is, the completion of transcription once initiated (transcripts may "pause" after the first exon and be prematurely terminated); (c) posttranscriptional mechanisms (more efficient processing or transport of transcripts in the nucleus of increased cytoplasmic mRNA stability). In the normal liver there are few c-*myc* transcripts present in the cytoplasm. After partial hepatectomy there is a marked increase in c-*myc* mRNA (steady-state levels), reaching a maximum at 2 h. Although there is some increase in c-*myc* transcriptional initiation after partial hepatectomy, most of the elevation of c-*myc* mRNA in the cytoplasm depends on posttranscriptional events. Surprisingly, higher transcriptional initiation after partial hepatectomy is associated with an increase in the pausing process which prevents the completion of initiated transcripts. The net result is that there is only a small increase in the number of completed transcripts produced in the regenerating liver [39, 40] (Fig. 7). The reason for this apparently paradoxical phenomenon (increase in both initiation and pausing) is not known but pausing of the gene may serve to

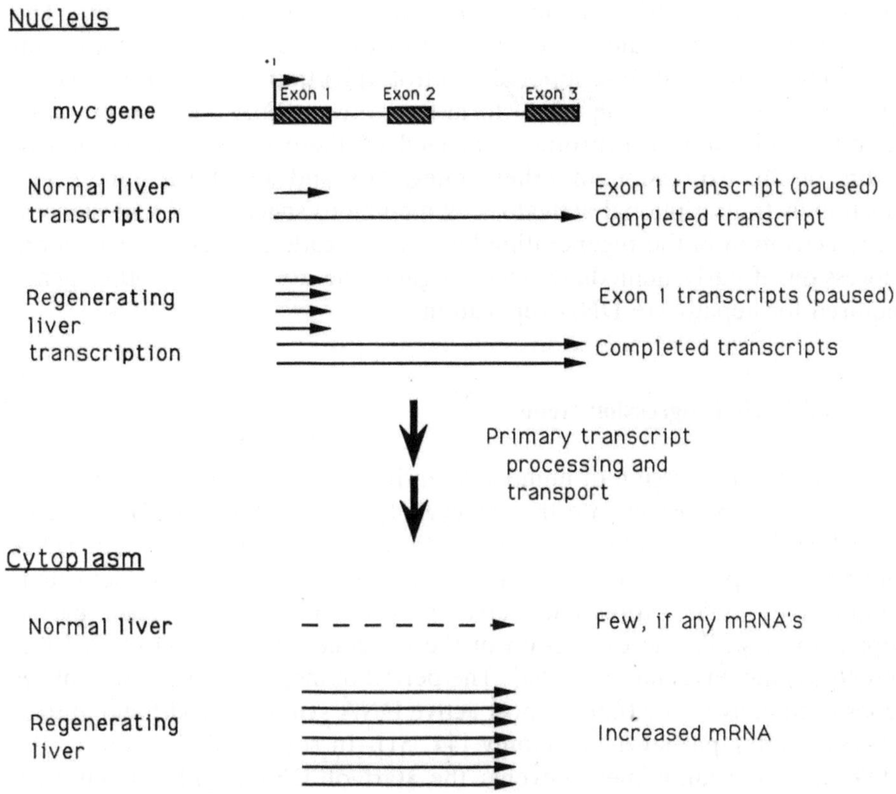


**Fig. 7.** Mechanisms of expression of c-myc during liver regeneration. The c-*myc* gene has three exons separated by introns. In the normal liver some transcripts are terminated prematurely ("pause") while others are completed. However, practically no mRNA accumulates in the cytoplasm. In the regenerating liver initiation of transcription increases almost tenfold but very few of the initiated transcripts are completed. mRNA accumulates in the cytoplasm probably because of more efficient transport of completed mRNA molecules from nucleus to cytoplasm. Cytoplasmic c-*myc* mRNA stability is apparently not significantly modified in the regenerating liver

prevent its overexpression. However, even if the increase in full length transcripts is relatively small in the regenerating liver, the amount of cytoplasmic c-*myc* in RNA increases markedly after partial hepatectomy probably as a consequence of more efficient processing and/or transport of nuclear transcripts [39]. The elevation of c-*fos* and c-*jun* expression during liver regeneration also depends, at least in part, on posttranscriptional mechanisms but it is not known whether the mechanism of posttranscriptional regulation of c-*fos* and c-*jun* is similar to that of c-*myc* [39, 40].

In summary, at least three immediate early genes (c-*fos*, c-*jun*, and c-*myc*) are activated rapidly in the regenerating liver, as indicated by an elevation of their mRNAs during the first 2h after the operation. The mechanisms that regulate the expression of these genes involve both transcriptional and posttranscriptional control; posttranscriptional regulation appears to be the most important form for c-*myc* mRNA and also probably for c-*fos* and c-*jun*. The proteins encoded by these genes can act as activators of the expression of other genes; Fos and Jun form dimers and function as transcriptional activators by binding to specific DNA sequences. Gene activation in the regenerating liver is a cascade of events in which the expression of early immediate genes triggers the activation of other genes required for hepatocyte DNA replication.

### 5.2 Cell Cycle Progression Genes

The increased expression of immediate early genes is a marker for the entry of quiescent hepatocytes into the cell cycle (passage from $G_0$ to $G_1$ phase of the cell cycle). As hepatocytes progress through the $G_1$ phase to start DNA replication (S phase) and mitosis (M) other proto-oncogenes are activated. Among these, p53 expression increases between 8 and 18h after partial hepatectomy while the expression of the *ras* gene family (c-Ha-*ras*, Ki-*ras*, and N-*ras*) increases later [44, 50]. The period of increased expression of *ras* genes encompasses the time of most active DNA synthesis (24h) and mitosis (30–36h) after partial hepatectomy [44, 51]. In some cells in culture, the addition of *ras* antibodies prevents the start of DNA synthesis but such experiments have so far not been performed with hepatocytes [52].

The increase in p53 expression during mid $G_1$ is a convenient marker for hepatocyte cell cycle progression but it is puzzling considering the tumor suppressor properties of p53 [53]. It is not known whether in the regenerating liver p53 activation directly causes cell cycle progression or is a shut-off signal for immediate early genes.

### 5.3 Growth Factor Genes

The pattern of proto-oncogene expression in the regenerating liver suggests that the process consists of sequential phases, each mediated by one or more growth factors [54]. These factors may be extrinsic or intrinsic and new research indicates that both types of factors exist [55]. Among the intrinsic factors, the transforming growth factors α and β1 (TGFα and β) and acidic fibroblast growth factor (aFGF) appear to play important roles. Among extrinsic factors (or factors that can be both extrinsic and intrinsic) the newly cloned hepatocyte growth factor (HGF) is of major interest [56, 57]. Both TGFα and β1 are made from longer precursor molecules [58]. TGFα is active as a secreted, processed, 50 amino acid peptide as well as a larger form that remains anchored in the plasma membrane [59]. TGFα is made by proliferating hepatocytes in vivo and in culture and stimulates hepatocyte DNA synthesis when added to primary cultures [60].

In most tissues and presumably also in the liver, TGFβ1 is made in a latent form that consists of the mature peptide bound to portions of the precursor and to a latency protein [61]. Although latent complexes can be activated in vitro by heat, acid, or protease digestion, the physiologic mechanisms that activate the growth factor in the liver or any other tissue remain unknown [62]. TGFβ1 is a potent inhibitor of hepatocyte DNA synthesis in vitro and in vivo and an inducer of liver fibrogenesis [63–71]. It is produced by nonparenchymal cells, and in fibrotic liver Ito cells appear to be a major site for TGFβ1 synthesis.

TGFα and β1 constitute good examples of factors which are produced in hepatic tissue during growth and act locally. TGFα is an autocrine stimulator of hepatocyte DNA synthesis (hepatocytes both produce and are stimulated by the factor) while TGFβ1 is a paracrine repressor of hepatocyte DNA synthesis (the factor is made in nonparenchymal cells but can act on hepatocytes). aFGF is another example of an intrinsic growth factor produced in the liver during growth [72]. It can function by both autocrine and paracrine mechanisms to regulate the balance between TGFα and β1 [60].

HGF has been cloned from human plasma, leukocytes, and rat platelets [56, 57, 73]. It has an approximate molecular weight of 85000 and is composed of two different peptide chains of 30000 and 60000 daltons [55]. The factor increases in the blood of patients with fulminant liver failure and in the serum of rats after partial hepatectomy and toxic liver injury [55–57]. The site(s) of synthesis of the peptide is not known but its mRNA can be found in various tissues as well as in the liver of rats shortly after toxic injury [56, 73]. In hepatic tissue HGF mRNA was detected in nonparenchymal cell but not in hepatocytes [74]. HGF is a very potent stimulator of DNA synthesis for cultured hepatocytes and might play an important role in liver regeneration in humans and experimental animals. At this time, its mechanism of action and potential interactions with intrinsic growth factors remain to be established.

### 5.4 Extracellular Matrix Genes

Another group of genes whose expression is increased after partial hepatectomy is that of genes encoding extracellular matrix proteins [75]. It has been shown that Col I, Col III, fibronectin, vitronectin, and laminin mRNAs as well as that of transin (an extracellular matrix degrading protease) increase after partial hepatectomy [41, 76]. The increase in Col I mRNA is prolonged, lasting for 3–4 days after the operation, while the messages for most other components increase only during the first 24 h. As liver regeneration after partial hepatectomy does not involve fibrosis or would healing, these changes probably reflect increased turnover and/or synthesis of new molecules needed to restore the ratio between cellular and extracellular components in the regenerating liver [77].

### 5.5 Heat Shock and Drug Resistance Genes

Besides growth regulatory and extracellular matrix genes it is to be expected that the expression of many individual genes encoding housekeeping functions or structural components may become elevated in hepatocytes as they prepare for replication. More difficult to explain is the finding that there is a significant elevation in the expression of heat shock genes and the multidrug response (MDR) gene [78, 79]. In mammals the MDR 1 gene encodes the 170-kd p-glycoprotein. The protein is located in the canalicular domain of the hepatocyte plasma membrane and functions as a multidrug transporter [80]. Although the multidrug resistance phenomenon can be induced by carcinogens or drugs in experimental animals, in cancer of the liver and intestine there may be "spontaneous" overexpression of the p-glycoprotein without previous exposure to anticancer drugs or chemicals. Increased expression of heat shock and MDR genes in the regenerating liver may represent a "stress-type" response and suggests that the replicative process is accompanied by the activation of metabolic functions not directly associated to cell proliferation.

*Acknowledgments.* I thank Mark Fitzgerald and Douglas Laird for ideas, lively discussions and the preparation of the figures.

### References

1. Fausto N, Schultz-Ellison G, Atryzek V et al. (1982) Distribution and specificity of sequences in polyadenylated nuclear RNA of normal, regenerating, and neoplastic liver. J Biol Chem 257:2200–2206
2. Darnell J, Lodish H, Baltimore D (1986) Molecular cell biology. Scientific American Books, New York
3. Lewin B (1987) Genes, 3rd edn. John Wiley, New York
4. Tamaoki T, Fausto N (1984) Expression of the alpha-fetoprotein gene during development, regeneration and carcinogenesis. In: Stein G, Stein J (eds) Recombinant DNA approaches to studying control of cell proliferation. Academic, New York, p 145
5. Braun L, Mead JE, Panzica M et al. (1988) Elevation of transforming growth factor-beta mRNA during liver regeneration: a possible paracrine mechanism of growth regulation. Proc Natl Acad Sci USA 85:1534–1538
6. Armendariz-Borunda J, Seyer JM, Kang AK et al. (1990) Regulation of TGFβ gene expression in rat liver intoxicated with carbon tetrachloride. FASEB J 4:215–221
7. Maher JJ, McGuire RF (1990) Extracellular matrix gene expression increases preferentially in rat lipocytes and sinusoidal endothelial cells during hepatic fibrosis in vivo. J Clin Invest 86:1641–1648

8. Milani S, Herbst H, Schuppan D et al. (1990) Cellular localization of type I, III, and IV procollagen gene transcripts in normal and fibrotic human liver. Am J Pathol 137:59–70
9. Guguen-Guillouzo C, Clement B, Baffet G et al. (1983) Maintenance and reversibility of active albumin secretion by adult rat hepatocytes co-cultured with another liver epithelial cell type. Exp Cell Res 143:47–54
10. Fritsch EF, Maniatis T (1987) Methods of molecular genetics. In: Stamatoyannopoulos G, Nienhus AW, Leder P, Majerus PW (eds) The molecular basis of blood diseases. W.B. Saunders, Philadelphia, p 1
11. Nienhuis AW, Maniatis T (1987) Structure and expression of globin genes in erythroid cells. In: Stamatoyannopoulos G, Nienhuis AW, Leder P, Majerus PW (eds) The molecular basis of blood diseases. W.B. Saunders, Philadelphia, p 28
12. Southern EM (1975) Detection of specific sequences among DNA fragments separated by gel electrophoresis. J Mol Biol 98:503–517
13. Bernuau D, Feldmann G (1990) In situ hybridization: application to the study of gene expression during experimental hepatocarcinogenesis and human hepatocellular carcinoma. Tumor Biol 11:173–180
14. Mullis KB (1990) The unusual origin of the polymerase chain reaction. Sci Am 263:56–65
15. Brechot C (1990) Polymerase chain reaction: a new tool for the study of viral infections in hepatology. J Hepatol 11:124–129
16. Johnson PF (1990) Transcriptional activators in hepatocytes. Cell Growth Diff 1:47–52
17. Kuo CJ, Conley PB, Hsieh C-L et al. (1990) Molecular cloning, functional expression, and chromosomal localization of mouse hepatocyte nuclear factor 1. Proc Natl Acad Sci USA 87:9838–9842
18. Lai E, Prezioso VR, Smith E et al. (1990) HNF-3A, a hepatocyte-enriched transcription factor of novel structure is regulated transcriptionally. Genes Dev 4:1427–1436
19. Monaci P, Nicosia A, Cortese R (1988) Two different liver-specific factors stimulate in vitro transcription from the human $\alpha_1$-antitrypsin promoter. EMBO J 7:2075–2087
20. Landschulz WH, Johnson PF, Adashi EY et al. (1988) Isolation of a recombinant copy of the gene encoding C/EBP. Genes Dev 2:786–800
21. Mueller CR, Maire P, Schibler U (1990) DBP, a liver-enriched transcriptional activator, is expressed late in ontogeny and its tissue specificity is determined posttranscriptionally. Cell 61:279–291
22. Liu J-K, Bergman Y, Zaret KS (1988) The mouse albumin promoter and a distal upstream site are simultaneously DNase I hypersensitive in liver chromatin and bind similar liver-abundant factors in vitro. Genes Dev 2:528–541
23. Lichtsteiner S, Schibler U (1989) A glycosylated liver-specific transcription factor stimulates transcription of the albumin gene. Cell 57:1179–1187
24. Cereghini S, Raymondjean M, Carranca AG et al. (1987) Factors involved in control of tissue-specific expression of albumin gene. Cell 50:627–638
25. Tyner AL, Godbout R, Compton RS et al. (1990) The ontogeny of α-fetoprotein gene expression in the mouse gastrointestinal tract. J Cell Biol 110:915–927
26. Vacher J, Tilghman SM (1990) Dominant negative regulation of the mouse α-fetoprotein gene in adult liver. Science 250:1732–1735
27. Berk AJ, Schmidt MC (1990) How do transcription factors work? Genes Dev 4:151–155
28. Varmus H (1987) Cellular and viral oncogenes. In: Stamatoyannopoulos G, Nienhuis AW, Leder P, Majerus PW (eds) The molecular basis of blood diseases. W.B. Saunders, Philadelphia, p 271
29. Bishop JM (1983) Cellular oncogenes and retroviruses. Annu Rev Biochem 52:301–354
30. Sager R (1989) Tumor suppressor genes: the puzzle and the promise. Science 246:1406–1412

31. Stanbridge EJ (1990) Identifying tumor suppressor genes in human colorectal cancer. Science 247:12–13
32. Lee W-H, Bookstein R, Hong F et al. (1987) Human retinoblastoma susceptibility gene: cloning, identification, and sequence. Science 235:1394–1399
33. Horowitz JM, Park S-H, Bogenmann E (1990) Frequent inactivation of the retinoblastoma anti-oncogene is restricted to a subset of human tumor cells. Proc Natl Acad Sci USA 87:2775–2779
34. Chen L-P, Scully P, Shew J-Y et al. (1989) Phosphorylation of the retinoblastoma gene product is modulated during the cell cycle and cellular differentiation. Cell 58:1193–1198
35. DeCaprio JA, Ludlow JW, Lynch D et al. (1989) The product of the retinoblastoma susceptibility gene has properties of a cell cycle regulatory element. Cell 58:1085–1095
36. Vogelstein B, Fearon ER, Hamilton SR et al. (1988) Genetic alterations during colorectal-tumor development. N Engl J Med 319:525–532
37. Deppert W, Buschhausen-Denker G, Patschinsky T et al. (1990) Cell cycle control of p53 in normal (3T3) and chemically transformed (Meth A) mouse cells. II. Requirement for cell cycle progression. Oncogene 5:1701–1706
38. Fausto N, Mead JE (1990) Role of protooncogenes and transforming growth factors in normal and neoplastic liver growth. In: Popper H, Schaffner F (eds) Progress in liver disease, vol IX. W.B. Saunders, Philadelphia, p 57
39. Morello D, Fitzgerald MJ, Babinet C et al. (1990) *C-myc*, *c-fos*, and *c-jun* regulation in the regenerating liver of normal and H-2K/*c-myc* transgenic mice. Mol Cell Biol 10:3185–3193
40. Morello D, Lavenu A, Babinet C (1990) Differential regulation and expression of *c-jun*, *c-fos* and *c-myc* proto-oncogenes during mouse liver regeneration and after inhibition of protein synthesis. Oncogene 5:1511–1519
41. Alcorn JA, Feitelberg SP, Brenner DA (1990) Transient induction of *c-jun* during hepatic regeneration. Hepatology 11:909–915
42. Mohn KL, Laz TM, Melby AE et al. (1990) Immediate-early gene expression differs between regenerating liver, insulin-stimulated H-35 cells, and mitogen-stimulated Balb/c 3T3 cells. J Biol Chem 265:21914–21921
43. Makino R, Hayashi K, Sugimura T (1984) *C-myc* transcript is induced in rat liver at a very early stage of regeneration or by cycloheximide treatment. Nature 310:697–698
44. Thompson NL, Mead JE, Braun L et al. (1986) Sequential proto-oncogene expression during liver regeneration. Cancer Res 46:3111–3117
45. Sobczak J, Mechti N, Tournier M-F et al. (1989) *C-myc* and *c-fos* gene regulation during mouse liver regeneration. Oncogene 4:1503–1508
46. DuBois RN (1990) Early changes in gene expression during liver regeneration: What do they mean? Hepatology 11:1079–1082
47. Landschulz WH, Johnson PF, McKnight SL (1989) The DNA binding domain of the rat liver nuclear protein C/EBP is bipartite. Science 243:1681–1688
48. Turner R, Tjian R (1989) Leucine repeats and an adjacent DNA binding domain mediate the formation of functional cFos-cJun heterodimers. Science 243:1689–1694
49. Kerr LD, Holt JT, Matrisian LM (1988) Growth factors regulate transin gene expression by *c-fos*-dependent and *c-fos*-independent pathways. Science 242:1424–1427
50. Mead JE, Braun L, Martin D et al. (1990) Induction of replicative competence ("priming") in the normal liver in vivo. Cancer Res 50:7023–7030
51. Goyette M, Petropoulos CJ, Shank PR et al. (1983) Expression of a cellular oncogene during liver regeneration. Science 219:510–512
52. Barbacid M (1987) *ras* genes. Annu Rev Biochem 56:779–827
53. Baker SJ, Markowitz S, Fearon ER et al. (1990) Suppression of human colorectal carcinoma cell growth by wild-type p53. Science 249:912–915

54. Fausto N, Mead JE (1989) Regulation of liver growth: protooncogenes and transforming growth factors. Lab Invest 60:4–13
55. Michalopoulos GK (1990) Liver regeneration: molecular mechanisms of growth control. FASEB 4:176–187
56. Tashiro K, Hagiya M, Nishizawa T et al. (1990) Deduced primary structure of rat hepatocyte growth factor and expression of the mRNA in rat tissues. Proc Natl Acad Sci USA 87:3200–3204
57. Miyazawa K, Tsubouchi H, Naka D et al. (1989) Molecular cloning and sequence analysis of cDNA for human hepatocyte growth factor. Biochem Biophys Res Commun 163:967–973
58. Roberts AB, Sporn MB (1990) The transforming growth factor-betas. In: Sporn MB, Roberts AB (eds) Peptide growth factors and their receptors. Springer Berlin Heidelberg New York, p 425
59. Massague J (1990) Transforming growth factor-α. J Biol Chem 265:21393–21396
60. Mead JE, Fausto N (1989) Transforming growth factor-α may be a physiological regulator of liver regeneration by means of an autocrine mechanism. Proc Natl Acad Sci USA 86:1558–1562
61. Wakefield LM, Smith DM, Flanders KC et al. (1988) Latent transforming growth factor-β from human platelets: a high molecular weight complex containing precursor sequences. J Biol Chem 263:7646–7654
62. Lyons RM, Gentry LE, Purchio AF et al. (1990) Mechanism of activation of latent recombinant transforming growth factor β1 by plasmin. J Cell Biol 110:1361–1367
63. Fausto N, Mead JE, Gruppuso PA et al. (1990) TGFβ in liver development, regeneration and carcinogenesis. Ann NY Acad Sci 592:231–242
64. McMahon JB, Richards WL, del Campo AA et al. (1986) Differential effects of transforming growth factor-β on proliferation of normal and malignant rat liver epithelial cells in culture. Cancer Res 46:4665–4671
65. Nakamura T, Tomita Y, Hirai R et al. (1985) Inhibitory effect of transforming growth factor-β on DNA synthesis of adult rat hepatocytes in primary culture. Biochem Biophys Res Commun 133:1042–1049
66. Carr BI, Hayashi I, Branum EL et al. (1986) Inhibition of DNA synthesis in rat hepatocytes by platelet-derived type transforming growth factor. Cancer Res 46:2330–2334
67. Russell WE, Coffey RJ, Ouellette AJ (1988) Type beta transforming growth factor reversibly inhibits the early proliferative response to partial hepatectomy in the rat. Proc Natl Acad Sci USA 85:5126–5130
68. Schackert HK, Fan D, Fidler IJ (1990) Transient inhibition of liver regeneration in mice by transforming growth factor-beta 1 encapsulated in liposomes. Cancer Commun 2:165–171
69. Weiner FR, Giambrone M-A, Czaja MJ et al. (1990) Ito-cell gene expression and collagen regulation. Hepatology 11:111–117
70. Nakatsukasa H, Nagy P, Evarts RP et al. (1990) Cellular distribution of transforming growth factor-β1 and procollagen types I, III, and IV transcripts in carbon tetrachloride-induced rat liver fibrosis. J Clin Invest 85:1833–1843
71. Matsuoka M, Tsukamoto H (1990) Stimulation of hepatic lipocyte collagen production by Kupffer cell-derived transforming growth factor β: implication for a pathogenetic role in alcoholic liver fibrogenesis. Hepatology 11:599–605
72. Kan M, Huang J, Masson PE et al. (1989) Heparin-binding growth factor type 1 (acidic fibroblast growth factor): a potential biphasic autocrine and paracrine regulator of hepatocyte regeneration. Proc Natl Acad Sci USA 86:7432–7436
73. Seki T, Ihara I, Sugimura A et al. (1990) Isolation and expression of cDNA for different forms of hepatocyte growth factor from human leukocyte. Biochem Biophys Res Commun 172:321–327
74. Kinoshita T, Tashiro K, Nakamura T (1989) Marked increase of HGF mRNA in nonparenchymal liver cells of rats treated with hepatotoxins. Biochem Biophys Res Commun 165:1229–1234

75. Nakatsukasa H, Evarts RP, Hsia C-C et al. (1990) Transforming growth factor-β1 and type I procollagen transcripts during regeneration and early fibrosis of rat liver. Lab Invest 63:171–180
76. Jakowlew SB, Mead JE, Danielpour D et al. (1991) Transforming growth factor-β (TGF-β) isoforms in rat liver regeneration: messenger RNA expression and activation of latent TGF-β. Cell Regul 2:535–548
77. Rojkind M, Greenwel P (1988) The liver as a bioecological system. In: Arias IM, Jakoby WB, Popper H, Schachter D, Shafritz DA (eds) The liver. Biology and pathobiology. Raven, New York, p 1269
78. Carr BI, Huang TH, Buzin CH et al. (1986) Induction of heat shock gene expression without heat shock by hepatocarcinogens and during hepatic regeneration in rat liver. Cancer Res 46:5106–5111
79. Thorgeirsson SS, Huber BE, Sorrell S et al. (1987) Expression of the multidrug-resistance gene in hepatocarcinogenesis and regenerating rat liver. Science 236:1120–1122
80. Arias IM (1990) Multidrug resistance genes, p-glycoprotein and the liver. Hepatology 12:159–165

# 4 Immunology and the Liver

G. Mieli-Vergani, M.P. Civeira, and D. Vergani

## 1 The Immune Response

The immune response is a cascade of events that follows the encounter, under appropriate conditions, of an immunocompetent cell with a foreign molecule, usually referred to as the antigen.

Both lymphocytes and accessory cells (monocytes and macrophages) participate in the immune response. Three lymphocyte populations have been recognised: B lymphocytes, T lymphocytes and null cells [natural killer (NK) cells].

T lymphocytes bear on their surface the T cell receptor (TCR) with specificity for the antigen. The TCR is a heterodimer with variable regions, which recognises peptides bound to molecules of the major histocompatibility complex (MHC). Two main groups of MHC molecules are known in man. HLA-A, HLA-B and HLA-C constitute the MHC class I, whereas HLA-DP, HLA-DQ and HLA-DR constitute the MHC class II.

T lymphocytes can be grouped into two main subpopulations: helper T cells and cytotoxic T cells (CTLs). The former bear the molecule CD4 on their surface and recognise antigenic peptides bound to MHC class II molecules while the latter express CD8 molecules on their membrane and bind peptides associated with MHC class I proteins.

Recognition of the antigen by CD4-positive T cells is the starting point of the immune response. In addition to TCR, the membrane-bound protein CD4 is required for the interaction of helper T cells with the antigen. CD4 has affinity for class II MHC molecules, thus increasing interactions between TCR and its ligand. Cell adhesion molecules (CAMs) of the integrin family, like LFA-1 on T cells, are also important. These molecules bind to receptors on antigen-presenting cells (I-CAM-1 for LFA-1), promoting cell–cell contact and cell activation (Fig. 1). After activation, helper T cells proliferate and secrete lymphokines, such as interleukin-2 (IL-2) and interferon-$\gamma$, which promote growth and differentiation of other lymphoid cells. CD4-positive T cells represent 60% of circulating lymphocytes.

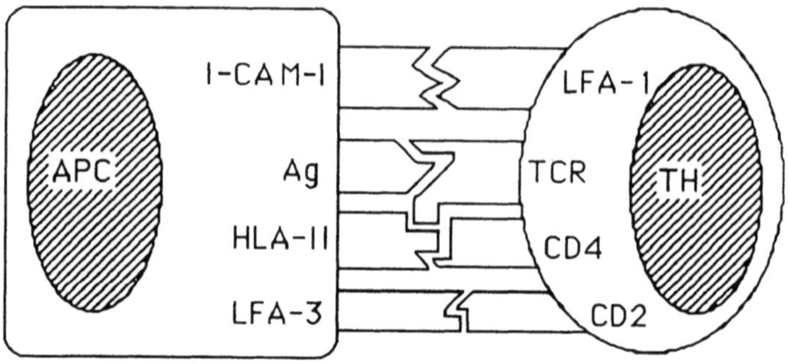


**Fig. 1.** Interactions between antigen-presenting cells (*APC*) and T helper (*TH*) cells for antigen recognition. T cell receptor (*TCR*) binds the antigen (*Ag*). CD4 molecule binds HLA class II molecules. CD2 molecule binds LFA-3 and LFA-1 binds I-CAM-1

### 1.1 Antigen Presentation

T cells recognise antigens after their processing by another cell. This process converts complex antigens into smaller fragments, some of which are presented on the cell surface. Macrophages, dendritic cells and B lymphocytes express MHC class II molecules as components of their membrane. These are the predominant antigen-processing and -presenting cells. In the liver, 75% of class II MHC positive cells are macrophages. Many cell types may express MHC class II molecules following interferon stimulation and, thus, behave as antigen-presenting cells (APCs). This "ectopic" MHC-II expression has been described in various cells including hepatocytes and biliary epithelial cells.

Macrophages internalise and process exogenous antigens via endosome formation. Small fragments of antigen are displayed on the cell surface in association with class II MHC molecules, where they are recognised by helper T cells (Fig. 2).

Unlike T cells, which bind a processed form of the antigen, B lymphocytes are able to interact directly with the antigen via their immunoglobulin receptors. Once this interaction has occurred, B cells internalise the antigen and process it. Following antigen processing, small peptides may be displayed in association with class II MHC molecules at the surface of the B cell. Recognition of the complex MHC class II peptide by the TCR will result in proliferation of this B cell, which in turn will elicit antibodies specific for the region (epitope) of the antigen which had interacted with the surface immunoglobulin. B cells with the specificity for the antigen, acting as APCs, ensure the T cell help required for their own differentiation and proliferation.

Antigen-presenting cells are involved in the activation of helper T cells by supplying costimulating factors. The best-known of these costimulators is interleukin-1 (IL-1), which has broad effects on lymphokine release and on increasing the number of growth factor receptors on T cells.

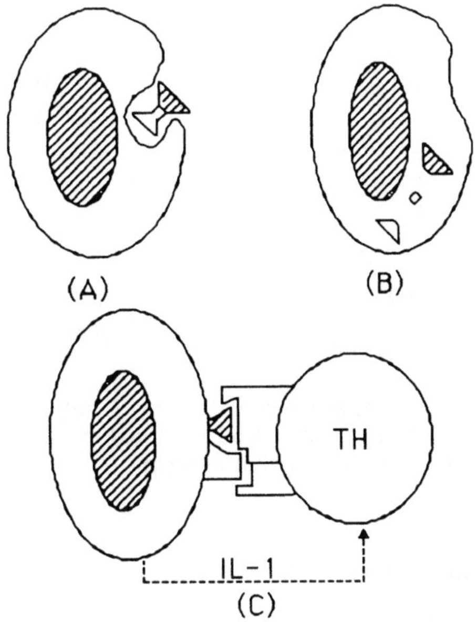


**Fig. 2.** Macrophages internalise (*A*) and process (*B*) exogenous antigens which are then displayed on the cell surface in association with class II MHC molecules (*C*). After TH cell recognition, macrophages become activated and secrete costimulator factors (e.g. IL-1)

## 1.2 Interleukin Production

Antigen recognition is followed by several events: (a) activation of antigen-presenting and -recognising cells, (b) secretion of soluble factors (cytokines) and (c) expression on the cell surface of growth factor receptors that allow clonal expansion of specific effector cells. Depending on the soluble factors released, probably by two groups of helper T cells (clearly characterised only in mice), two types of immune response are elicited. When interleukin-4 (IL-4) and interleukin-5 are the main cytokines released, B cell differentiation and proliferation occur. This results in antibody production. On the other hand when IL-2 and interferon-γ are produced, cytolytic T cells proliferate, and thus specific cytolytic clones are expanded (Fig. 3).

Interleukin-2 is the most important factor regulating T cell growth. IL-4, formerly thought to be only a B cell growth and differentiation factor, can also function as T cell growth factor, restricted to certain subsets of T cells.

Similar to other members of the interferon family, interferon-γ has antiviral activity. It activates cytotoxic macrophages and NK cells and enhances class II gene expression, which facilitates antigen presentation.

Macrophage activation is followed by the release of IL-1, interleukin-6 (IL-6) and tumour necrosis factor (TNF). These cytokines have a broad spectrum of biological activity on multiple target cells.

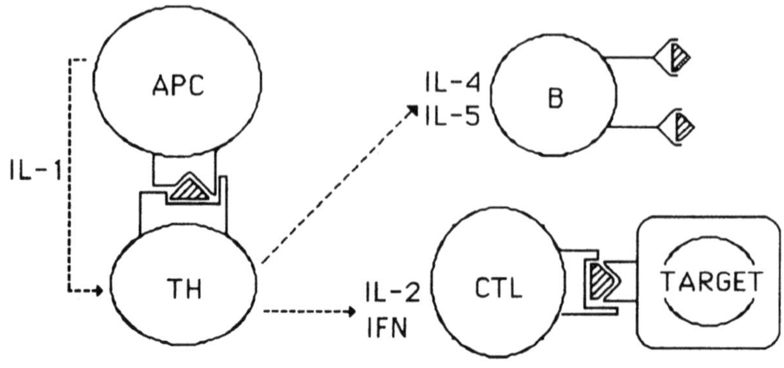


**Fig. 3.** Antigen recognition by T helper (*TH*) cells is followed by the secretion of soluble factors that lead to clonal expansion of B cells and cytotoxic T lymphocytes (*CTL*) specific for that antigen

## 1.3 Effector Mechanisms

Soluble antigens are bound by specific antibodies. Formation of immune complexes facilitates removal of circulating antigens and promotes different biological activities via their immunoglobulin Fc fragment.

Endogenous antigens, such as virally encoded proteins produced within infected cells, are subjected to cytoplasmic processing. If the processed fragments are recognised by MHC-I molecules, they are transported and expressed on the cell surface in association with these molecules. Once on the cell surface, the antigen–MHC molecule is recognised by CTLs.

Cytotoxic T cells are mostly CD8-bearing T lymphocytes that recognise antigen in the context of self class I MHC molecules and exert a lytic effect on target cells. The CD8 molecule has affinity for MHC-I molecules and helps cell–cell interactions. Once CTLs have seen the antigen, they are stimulated to proliferate (clonal expansion). IL-2, produced by helper T cells, induces growth and differentiation of CTLs. Other cells, phenotypically different from T lymphocytes, also possess cytolytic activity. The so-called NK cells have the ability to destroy malignant or virally infected cells, irrespective of MHC display and without involvement of specific antigen recognition. Interferon-$\gamma$ is a potent inducer of NK activity.

## 1.4 Immune Regulation

Once the immune reaction is initiated, different mechanisms control the magnitude and duration of the response. The existence of a specific subpopulation of suppressor T cells that inhibit T cell activation has been postulated. However, neither the antigen specificity of these cells nor the suppressive mechanisms involved are clear. On the other hand it has been shown that immune responses against the variable regions of immunoglobulin chains or of TCR (anti-idiotipic reaction) can also limit the intensity of the immune response.

### 1.5 Immune-Mediated Tissue Damage

Although in many cases the immune response is protective, in certain circumstances the immune reaction can in itself produce cell damage. Five major mechanisms of immune-mediated tissue injury (leaving aside IgE-mediated reactions) can be distinguished:

1. Antibodies may cause disturbances in cell function by blocking or stimulating cell surface receptors without destroying cells. They may also opsonise cells, facilitating phagocytosis, or may induce complement-dependent lysis of the target cell. On the other hand, antigen–antibody complexes may be deposited in tissues, resulting in complement activation, inflammation and tissue injury. Antibodies may also bind antigens on the surface of a cell, inducing antibody-dependent cell-mediated cytotoxicity (ADCC). NK cells, which have on their membrane receptors for the Fc fragment of IgG, can destroy cells through this mechanism. ADCC is a more efficient lytic mechanism than complement-mediated cytotoxicity.
2. Macrophages can mediate ADCC and generate pro-inflammatory monokines, such as tumour necrosis factor.
3. CD8+ cytolytic T lymphocytes directly lyse target cells bearing class I MHC-associated viral (or other foreign) antigens without the participation of macrophages or any other effector mechanisms.
4. NK cells may lyse virus-infected or tumoral cells through cytotoxic mechanisms that do not involve specific antigen recognition.
5. Cytokines released by helper T cells can activate macrophages and initiate an inflammatory reaction characterised by dense mononuclear infiltrate (delayed hypersensitivity).

### 1.6 Autoimmunity

Autoimmunity occurs when an immune response is directed against "self" antigens. Susceptibility to the development of autoimmune diseases is genetically controlled by genes within the MHC complex. Other unidentified genes also play a role.

Autoreactive T cell clones are deleted in the thymus. Inactivation of T cell clones directed against self antigens can also occur in extrathymic sites. The acquisition of self-tolerance by T cells seems to depend on the display of autoantigens at a critical step in ontogeny. Although autoreactive T cells are eliminated or inactivated, B cells able to produce autoantibodies are found in the normal immune system.

Several mechanisms may explain loss of self-tolerance and development of autoimmunity:

1. It has been proposed that one of these mechanisms might be autoantigen presentation to T cells through ectopic expression of MHC molecules. This can take place when interferon-γ is produced locally as a result of viral infections and induces expression of class II molecules by neighbouring cells.
2. A foreign antigen that cross-reacts with self-constituents might elicit T cell help which stimulates an autoimmune response.
3. Defective T cell immunoregulation including excessive T cell help or loss of antigen-specific suppressor T cells can also lead to autoimmunity.
4. Idiotypic networks may influence autoimmunisation. If an idiotype imitates the structure of an autoantigen, the anti-idiotypic response could provoke autoantibody formation. The idiotypic network could also influence helper and suppressor cell function.

## 2 Role of the Immune System in Liver Disease

It is widely accepted that the immune system plays a central or a contributory role in the pathogenesis of a variety of liver diseases. In addition, liver diseases may be characterised by distinctive immune reactions, which, though not responsible for liver damage, are of great diagnostic importance.

### 2.1 Autoimmune Chronic Liver Diseases

Autoimmune chronic active hepatitis, a form of juvenile primary sclerosing cholangitis and conceivably primary biliary cirrhosis are examples of organ-specific autoimmune diseases in which the immune system targets the liver.

#### *Autoimmune Chronic Active Hepatitis*

Autoimmune chronic active hepatitis (aCAH) is characterised by the histological picture of chronic aggressive hepatitis and elevated levels of serum immunoglobulins and non-organ- and liver-specific autoantibodies in the absence of a known cause of liver disease. The involvement of the immune system in the pathogenesis of CAH was suspected shortly after its first description in 1947 [1]. Several authors [2–4] drew attention to the fact that the affected patients, mainly females, have high serum γ-globulin levels and that the inflammatory cells characteristically present in portal and periportal areas are mainly lymphocytes and plasma cells. These patients were subsequently shown to have high titres of circulating autoantibodies reacting against nuclear components [5], the actin of smooth muscle [6], liver/kidney microsomes [7] or a liver cell cytoplasmic protein called soluble liver antigen (SLA) [8]. Recently, aCAH has been divided into subgroups according to the type of autoantibodies detected [9], type I being aCAH associated with smooth muscle antibody (SMA) with or without antinuclear antibody (ANA) and type II aCAH associated with anti-liver/kidney microsomal (LKM) antibody. The latter type is often associated with IgA deficiency and usually has a more severe course, with rapid progression to cirrhosis despite immunosuppressive treatment. The LKM antibody found in type II aCAH is directed to cytochrome P-450 db1 [10], a drug-metabolising enzyme with a known genetic polymorphism, and is known as LKM-1. A third subgroup of aCAH would be characterised by the presence of anti-SLA antibody, which is usually present in isolation. Although most of these autoantibodies are non-organ-specific and may be found in other diseases [7, 11], when present at high titres they are important diagnostic markers of aCAH.

*Autoantibodies Against Liver-Specific Membrane Antigens*

Autoantibodies directed against liver-specific antigens in patients with aCAH were first described by Meyer zum Büschenfelde et al. in 1968 [12]. These antibodies react with a macromolecular antigenic complex called "liver-specific lipoprotein" or LSP on the hepatocyte cell membrane [13]. Only a few of the LSP antigenic determinants are liver specific, while the others are not organ specific, and within both categories there are antigens which are species specific and some which have species cross-reactive components [14]. Early animal experimental work showed that the antibodies to the LSP complex were rapidly cleared during perfusion through isolated liver preparations and that this was associated with complement consumption [15], suggesting that LSP was derived from a superficial layer of the liver cell membrane and could be readily accessible to circulating antibodies in vivo. Later, the development of a radio-immunoassay for anti-LSP [16] allowed the demonstration that patients with aCAH had high serum concentrations of anti-LSP and that there was a close relationship between the serum anti-LSP titre and the extent of histologically assessed liver damage [17]. More recently, McFarlane et al. have demonstrated that patients with aCAH have circulating antibodies against the human asialoglycoprotein receptor (ASGPR) and that anti-ASGPR titres are correlated with disease activity [18]. The ASGPR is a well-characterised component of LSP expressed on the surface of the plasma membrane of the hepatocytes [19] and therefore likely to be a target for the immune attack.

Studies using fluorescein-conjugated anti-immunoglobulin G (IgG) show that hepatocytes isolated from diagnostic liver biopsies of patients with aCAH are coated in vivo with antibodies [20], suggesting a direct role for autoantibodies in producing damage to the liver cell.

*Mechanism of Liver Damage* (Fig. 4)

Liver damage in aCAH is likely to be orchestrated by CD4-positive (helper/inducer) T lymphocytes recognising as foreign a self antigenic peptide, possibly derived from ASGPR. To trigger an autoimmune response, the peptide must be embraced by HLA molecules, since T lymphocytes recognise as antigenic only peptides encased within the cleft which is found on the external aspect of the HLA molecule. The peptide is presented to the helper/inducer T cells by either a professional APC such as a macrophage or by the hepatocyte itself. The T helper cell becomes activated and can initiate a cascade of immune reactions by producing cytokines, activating cytotoxic T cells and inducing autoantibody production by B lymphocytes. This model is supported by a number of observations: (a) hepatocytes from patients

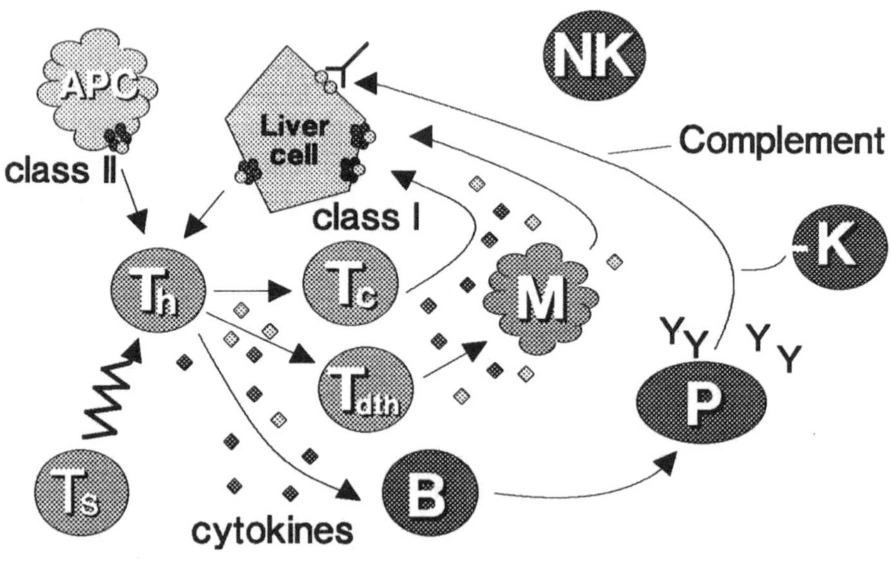


**Fig. 4.** Liver cell autoimmune attack. A normal component of the liver cell membrane is presented to T helper (*Th*) lymphocytes either directly on the hepatocyte or by an antigen-presenting cell (*APC*), in the context of class II HLA antigens. If there is no opposition from T suppressor (*Ts*) lymphocytes, then a variety of effector mechanisms are triggered. Liver cell destruction could derive from the action of: (a) T cytotoxic (*Tc*) lymphocytes which react with the self antigen(s) in the context of class I HLA antigens; (b) cytokines produced by T helper, T delayed type hypersensitivity (*Tdth*) lymphocytes and recruited macrophages; or (c) autoantibody production by B lymphocytes with activation of complement and/or engagement of killer (*K*) lymphocytes, *NK*, natural killer cell; *B*, blymphocyte; *M*, macrophage; *P*, plasma cell

with active aCAH express class II HLA antigens not normally expressed on liver cells [21] and can therefore present autoantigenic peptides; (b) CD4-positive and activated lymphocytes are present in areas of piecemeal necrosis [22, 23]; (c) a high proportion of circulating helper T lymphocytes express the activation marker IL-2 receptor (IL-2R) [24]; and (d) high titre liver-specific autoantibodies are present in the circulation of these patients, as mentioned above.

Once the autoimmune reaction is initiated, hepatocytes can be destroyed through various mechanisms. These include direct T cell cytotoxicity, the cytolytic action of cytokines or autoantibody-directed complement- or killer (K) cell-mediated lysis.

In vitro microcytotoxicity assays, in which lymphocytes and hepatocytes prepared from the same patient are co-cultured to ensure histocompatibility between the effector and target cells, have shown increased cytotoxicity in aCAH patients with active disease [25]. Experiments using subpopulations of T and non-T lymphocytes indicated that cytotoxicity was mediated by non-T lymphocytes [25]. This observation and the blocking effect of aggregated IgG suggest that cytotoxicity, in aCAH, is an antibody-dependent cell-mediated mechanism. Thus the non-T cells are K cells which become attached, through their Fc receptor, to the hepatocyte membrane by an antibody reacting with a plasma membrane antigen. Since the reaction can be blocked by LSP, the antigen is most probably within the LSP complex, on the liver cell surface. Further evidence for this mechanism was obtained by experiments in which hepatocytes from patients with aCAH carrying surface IgG, as detected by immunofluorescence, proved to be susceptible to damage by lymphocytes (K cells) prepared from healthy subjects [20].

Studies to investigate the possible role of complement in generating liver cell damage have failed to demonstrate any association between complement activation and biochemical evidence of hepatocyte injury in aCAH [26].

Although the study of cytokines has started only recently, the involvement of these soluble mediators in the pathogenesis of aCAH is suggested by the finding that circulating levels of IL-1 and IL-6, TNF and interferon-$\gamma$ are increased in patients with active disease [27].

### *T Cell Cloning*

Cloning in vitro activated T lymphocytes from the peripheral blood and the liver tissue of patients with aCAH has enhanced our capacity to understand the mechanisms leading to autoimmune liver damage and to design novel therapeutic approaches. Cloning, i.e. the generation of millions of daughter cells from a single progenitor, has been successfully achieved in aCAH by exploiting the ability of activated T lymphocytes expressing the IL-2 receptor to proliferate in the presence of IL-2.

Liver-specific CD4-positive T cell clones have been obtained both from the peripheral blood and from liver biopsies of aCAH patients [28, 29]. Such clones have been shown to stimulate autologous B lymphocytes to produce liver membrane-specific autoantibodies and antibody to the ASGPR [28]. Recently, T cell clones obtained from the liver biopsy of patients with aCAH and expressing the $\gamma\delta$ receptor have been shown to be cytotoxic to a variety of targets, but to exert preferential killing of liver-derived cells as opposed to target cells derived from other organs [29], suggesting that they may contribute to hepatocyte damage.

Manoeuvres designed to inhibit or remove the offending clones, such as anticlonotypic antibodies [30], peptide immunotherapy [31], or "lymphocyte vaccination" [32], have been able to prevent or cure experimentally induced autoimmune diseases in animals. The demonstration that circulating activated T helper cells in autoimmune CAH are sensitised to liver membrane antigens and are of potential pathogenic importance may provide a basis for similar approaches to therapy.

### *T-Suppressor Function*

The finding of a variety of non-organ- and liver-specific autoantibodies, as well as evidence of unrestrained autoimmune liver cell damage, has led to the hypothesis of a defect in the immunoregulatory control mechanisms in patients with aCAH [33]. Using various in vitro assays, impaired non-antigen-specific T cell suppressor function has been demonstrated in both adults [34, 35] and children [36] with aCAH and in their first-degree relatives. This defect was shown to segregate with the possession of the HLA haplotype B8/DR3 [37]. In addition, it has been shown that patients with aCAH have a specific defect in a subpopulation of suppressor T cells controlling the immune response to liver-specific membrane antigens [38]. Impaired immunoregulation due to the decreased T cell suppressor function could play an important pathogenic role in CAH by leading to the persistence of autoimmune reactions. In one study [35], a suppressor T cell defect in patients with aCAH was uniformly improved by incubation of the lymphocytes with concentrations of prednisolone akin to those present in plasma during maintenance treatment of CAH, thus suggesting that a direct influence on T cell suppressor function might be an important mechanism of action of steroids in this condition.

### *Genetic Predisposition*

Patients with aCAH have an increased frequency of the histocompatibility antigens HLA A1/B8/DR3, a haplotype characteristically associated with other autoimmune conditions, such as sicca syndrome, autoimmune thyroiditis, systemic lupus erythematosus and insulin-dependent diabetes [39], in which there is excessive production of antibody to extrinsic antigens and autoantigens. As early as 1974 [33], it was postulated that HLA B8 is a marker of defective T cell function and that individuals possessing this antigen would be inefficient at switching off immune and autoimmune reactions triggered by environmental factors, which could include viruses. Indirect confirmation of this hypothesis is provided by the results of family studies showing high titres of autoantibodies in B8-positive patients and their first-degree relatives [40]. Curiously, although possession of HLA A1/B8/DR3 augments susceptibility not only to aCAH but also to a wide range of other autoimmune disorders, very little overlap exists amongst them, implying that HLA A1/B8/DR3 is a phenotypic marker of weak immunoregulatory activity but that other genetic and/or environmental factors must determine which organs or tissues are affected. In a reported family with multiple occurrence of aCAH, female sex and possession of DR3 were more important than B8 in conferring susceptibility to the disease [41], suggesting that defective antigen recognition by T cells in the context of class II HLA molecules plays a central role in generating autoimmunity, in association with gender-determined factors (genes and hormones). Recently, it has been shown that susceptibility to aCAH is conferred independently by two genes within the MHC linked to the DR3 and DR4 genes [42]. When compared with the DR4-positive patients, those with A1/B8/DR3 have been shown to present at an earlier age, to relapse more frequently and to be more frequently referred for liver transplantation. Haplotypes conferring susceptibility to the juvenile or mature form of aCAH have been further characterised. The DR3 haplotype predisposing to the juvenile form is DRB1*0301--DRB3*0101--DQA1*0501--DQB1*0201, with the individual alleles DRB3*0101 and DQA1*0501 exerting the greatest predisposing effect, while the DR4 haplotype associated with the mature form is DRB1*0401--DRB4*0101--DQA1*0301--DQB1*0301 [43].

Patients with aCAH have an isolated partial deficiency of the complement component C4, which is not due to impaired hepatic synthesis or immune consumption, but is genetically determined and is associated with the possession of a silent gene at the C4A locus, C4AQ0 [44]. C4AQ0, either in linkage with A1/B8/DR3 or on its own, has been reported in association with other autoimmune disorders [45] and could represent the true disease susceptibility gene. The genetically determined partial C4 deficiency resulting from the possession of null C4 genes may be a predisposing factor to autoimmunity. C4 has a key role in virus neutralisation [46] and failure to eliminate viruses might lead to the development of immune and autoimmune reactions directed against antigens on the persistently infected cells. The specificity of the autoimmune reaction would possibly derive from the tropism of the virus. An additional genetic factor which might contribute to the development of aCAH is the immunoglobulin Gm allotype Gm ax. The presence of both HLA B8 and Gm ax in the same individual confers a 40-fold risk for the disease [47]. All the above data suggest that aCAH conforms to a multifactorial model [48]. It is proposed that a disease develops when a threshold is exceeded by a number of different combinations or interactions of multiple genetic and environmental factors.

### *Autoimmune Primary Sclerosing Cholangitis*

Primary sclerosing cholangitis (PSC) is an uncommon disorder of unknown aetiology, characterised by chronic inflammation and fibrosis of the intrahepatic or extrahepatic bile ducts or both, with obliteration of interlobular bile ducts and narrowing and dilatation of all or part of the major bile ducts. The condition is well recognised in adults, being associated in one-half to two-thirds of cases with chronic inflammatory bowel disease, particularly ulcerative colitis. For a long time PSC has been thought to be extremely rare in children.

Recently, a retrospective study on 13 children with PSC [49] showed that such patients may present with clinical, biochemical, immunological and histological features indistinguishable from those of aCAH and can therefore be erroneously diagnosed. In both conditions there was an increase in the levels of IgG and circulating non-organ-specific autoantibodies, in particular ANA and SMA. Histological features common to both conditions were portal tract infiltrate and piecemeal necrosis. In some cases, the correct diagnosis could be made only by demonstrating the characteristic bile duct abnormalities by endoscopic retrograde cholangiopancreatography.

#### *Mechanism of Liver Damage*

As in aCAH, liver-specific autoantibodies, including antibodies to LSP and ASGPR, are found in the juvenile autoimmune form of PSC [50]. Autologous microcytotoxicity assays have shown that in PSC, too, liver cell damage is likely to be mediated by K cells [50]. Increased levels of circulating activated T lymphocytes are also found in PSC. Unlike in aCAH, T suppressor cell number and non-antigen-specific suppressor function tend to be normal in patients with PSC [50]. It therefore appears that although liver-damaging effector mechanisms are similar in the two conditions, there are differences in the behaviour of immunomodulatory cells.

#### *Genetic Predisposition*

Similarly to patients with aCAH, children and adults with PSC tend to possess the HLA haplotype A1/B8/DR3 [51].

Whether the juvenile autoimmune form of PSC and aCAH are two distinct entities or different manifestations of the same disease remains to be elucidated.

### *Primary Biliary Cirrhosis*

Primary biliary cirrhosis is a chronic liver disease of unknown aetiology characterised by slowly progressive intrahepatic cholestasis due to an inflammatory destruction of small intrahepatic bile ducts. The clinical course of PBC is variable, ranging from a few years in rapidly progressive cases to a normal life expectancy in a proportion of asymptomatic cases. It has long been recognised that the disease is characterised by the presence of high titre antimitochondrial antibodies (AMA) and elevated serum IgM [52–54]. This, in addition to the observation that these patients often have associated autoimmune disorders (rheumatoid arthritis, sicca syndrome, thyroiditis, scleroderma), has led to the concept that PBC is an autoimmune disease. The role of the HLA system in predisposing to this disease has not been fully clarified, although an association with HLA-DRw8 [55] has been reported.

#### *Antimitochondrial Antibodies and Mitochondrial Autoantigens*

Primary biliary cirrhosis is characterised by disease-specific subtypes of AMA, including M2, M4, M8 and M9. Anti-M2 is the diagnostic marker for PBC, while anti-M4, anti-M8 and anti-M9 identify either particular subsets or stages of PBC. For example, anti-M4 (with anti-M2) identifies the chronic active hepatitis–PBC overlap syndrome, and anti-M9 may identify cases with a benign clinical course. Gel electrophoresis and Western immunoblotting, using human placental mitochondria, disclosed that anti-M2 sera reacted to very high titres with two major mitochondrial polypeptides of molecular sizes initially estimated as 70 and 45 kd [56]. Molecular cloning has been successfully applied to characterise the main 70-kd mitochondrial antigen [57]. The M2 autoantigens have been identified as mitochondrial 2-oxo-acid dehydrogenase enzymes. These include pyruvate dehydrogenase (PDH) (70–74 kd antigen) and branched chain 2-oxo-acid dehydrogenase and 2-oxo-acid glutaric dehydrogenase (45–52 kd antigens). Each of these enzymes has three subunits, E1 to E3. For PDH, an autoepitope has been identified as a decapeptide containing the attachment site of lipoic acid, an essential cofactor for enzyme activity. Current questions include the degree to which antibodies to PDH, and related enzymes, account for the mitochondrial reactivity defined by immunofluorescence or other procedures, the cell surface expression of M2 autoantigens, and the significance of the occurrence of non-mitochondrial (such as centromeric) autoantibodies in PBC [57]. The reasons for the localisation of the lesions of PBC to intrahepatic biliary ductules is unclear since mitochondrial autoantigen is not tissue specific. It has been speculated that there are allelic forms of PDH specific to the hepatobiliary cells [58], that bile favours penetrance of immune effector agents such as antibodies or T cells [58], and that the biliary tract is colonised by a micro-organism with a particular capacity to display the appropriate epitopes, since homology between the bacterial and mammalian forms of the dehydrogenase enzymes has been described [59].

*Mechanisms of Liver Damage*

The few available histochemical studies agree that in PBC, among the portal lymphoid infiltrate, T lymphocytes greatly outnumber other lymphoid cells [60–62], and these T cells exhibit markers of activation. CD4 helper T cells predominate overall but are localised more in the portal infiltrates, whereas the T cells around and in the walls of bile ducts, which may be the actual effectors, are of the cytotoxic (CD8-positive) phenotype [62]. Immunohistochemistry also has been applied to the identification of MHC-encoded molecules on hepatocytes and bile duct cells [63]. Bile duct epithelium normally expresses MHC class I molecules. In PBC, MHC class II molecules also become expressed on biliary epithelial cells, presumably under the influence of lymphokines, including interferon-γ. Such expression may be relevant to the pathogenesis of PBC, since biliary epithelial cells that express MHC class II molecules could act as APCs for CD4 helper T cells. Bile duct damage may derive from different effector mechanisms. Given that MHC class I molecules are constitutively expressed on biliary epithelial cells and that CD8-positive cytotoxic T cells are identifiable histochemically at sites of damage, a cytotoxic T cell response to a mitochondrial peptide, associated with a class I MHC molecule, on the biliary epithelial surface is one possibility. An alternative (or coexisting) process would be an induction of CD4-positive helper T lymphocytes, with release by activated cells of lymphokines with tissue-damaging potential. The role of lymphocytes in causing damage is suggested by the ability to induce characteristic histological lesions in severe combined immunodeficiency (SCID) mice [64], i.e. in animals that cannot mount their own immune response, injected with PBC patients' peripheral blood lymphocytes. Our ability to dissect the pathogenic mechanisms leading to PBC has greatly improved in recent years. Thus, the identification of mitochondrial autoantigens and their encoding DNA and the possibility of establishing B and T cell clones from peripheral blood and liver tissue of patients with PBC should enable the reconstruction of the pathogenic events leading to bile duct damage. This in turn should lead to the establishment of new specific immunotherapy (see Sect. 2.1.1.3).

## 2.2 Viral Hepatitis

***Hepatitis B***

The liver damage caused by the hepatitis B virus (HBV) varies greatly in severity: it can be mild and transient, severe and prolonged, or fulminant.

The mechanisms responsible for determining the course and outcome of hepatitis B are not known. However, many investigations have suggested that HBV is not directly cytopathic, and that liver damage derives from the host immune response to the virus-infected hepatocytes [65]. A normal immune response would lead to self-limiting acute hepatitis, a decreased immune response to chronic hepatitis, and a hyperactive response to fulminant hepatic failure. Immune surveillance against viral infections begins with the recognition by T lymphocytes of the viral antigens on the surface of the infected cell in association with HLA molecules [66]. During intracellular viral replication, viral peptides can bind to HLA class I molecules, which carry the viral antigens to the cell surface, where the complex becomes a target for CD8-positive (cytotoxic) T lymphocytes [66]. Recently, HLA class I restricted cytotoxic T cells reacting with the amino-terminal end of the HBV core molecule have been demonstrated in the peripheral blood of patients with acute hepatitis B [67]. CD4-positive (helper/inducer) T lymphocytes also play a key role in virus elimination by recognising viral antigens ingested and processed by APCs and expressed on the surface of the APC within the groove of HLA class II molecules [68]. Thus, HLA class II restricted CD4-positive T lymphocytes recognising an immunodominant 20 amino acid sequence located within the amino-terminal half of the core molecule have been identified in the peripheral blood of patients with self-limiting acute hepatitis B [69]. Moreover, this interaction between the HLA-restricted T cell receptors and the MHC viral antigenic complex is believed to activate the T lymphocyte to proliferate and/or to produce specific lymphokines necessary in the elaboration of the immune response. Thus CD4-positive lymphocytes, obtained from liver biopsies and cloned in vitro, are capable of providing help to B cells for anti-HBc production [70]. A high percentage of CD8- and CD4-positive activated T lymphocytes expressing HLA DR have been described in children with chronic HBV infection and evidence of ongoing viral replication [71]. Such cells may play a central role in engendering persistent liver injury. Experimental work suggests that the direct damage to the HBV-infected liver cells in chronic hepatitis is mediated by two different mechanisms. On the one hand, cytotoxic T lymphocytes react with viral antigenic determinants (mainly HBcAg and HBeAg) expressed on the hepatocyte membrane [72, 73]. On the other hand, patients produce autoantibodies directed against the "liver-specific protein" (LSP) (see above) [16], which induce damage through an antibody-dependent non-T cell-mediated cytotoxic reaction [74].

It is not clear why certain patients progress to chronic infection while others clear HBV after acute infection. Persistence of infection probably derives from complex virus–host interactions. HLA molecules or viral determinants on the infected cells may be hidden by excessive production of antiviral antibody and escape immune clearance [72]. Lymphocytes infected and functionally impaired by the HBV [75] may be unable to mount a normal immune response. Another possibility is a genetic or acquired deficiency in interferon production [76, 77]. It has also been suggested that HBsAg-specific T suppressor cells play a role in the maintenance of non-responsiveness to HBsAg in chronic HBV carriers [78]. A further mechanism for viral persistence is alteration in viral replication and viral antigen production by a change in transcription and translation of the viral genes. This mechanism underlies persistence of viruses that produce defective interfering particles or generate a great number of mutants. In chronic hepatitis B, defective viral particles are produced in great numbers [79], and recent data indicate that spontaneous mutations in the genome are associated with the development of particularly aggressive forms of chronic hepatitis [80, 81] or fulminant hepatic failure [82–84].

### *Hepatitis A*

The liver damage in acute hepatitis A has long been thought to derive from a direct cytopathic effect of the virus. It is now believed that a T cell-mediated immune attack in response to virus-infected cells plays a major additional pathogenic role [85–87], similarly to what happens in hepatitis B (see above). HAV infection, however, does not become chronic, suggesting that the interaction between virus and host is different from that observed in HBV infection, and that the immune system is generally very efficient in eliminating HAV.

### *Hepatitis C*

Akin to hepatitis B, hepatitis caused by the recently described C virus can be acute and self-limiting, run a fulminant course or progress to chronic liver damage. The mechanisms leading to hepatocyte injury remain to be elucidated. Early studies showed that a high proportion of patients defined as having aCAH were positive for anti-HCV antibodies detected by first generation assays [88, 89]. However, a further study showed that anti-HCV positivity was confined to patients with high IgG levels, suggesting that seropositivity could be non-specific [90]. A convincing association between anti-HCV positivity with second generation assays and LKM-positive CAH has been reported recently [91]. Such an association appears to divide LKM-positive CAH into two subgroups: young patients, usually females with high levels of anti-LKM and negative for anti-HCV, in whom liver damage may be due to a direct autoimmune attack, and older patients, frequently males, with low titres of anti-LKM and positive anti-HCV, in whom the autoimmune process may be a consequence of the viral disease.

Antibodies reacting against host-encoded sequences (anti-GOR) have been described in a high proportion of patients with chronic HCV infection, as detected by polymerase chain reaction, emphasising the possible connection between viral infection and autoimmunity [92].

## 2.3 Drug-Induced Hepatitis

The best-documented example of drug-induced liver damage with an immune pathogenesis is severe hepatitis after halothane exposure.

***Halothane-Induced Hepatitis***

The spectrum of liver damage that may follow halothane exposure varies from minor increases in the concentration of serum aminotransferases to the rarer instances of fulminant hepatic failure [93]. It is not clear whether they represent two different forms of liver damage or extreme ends of a spectrum. The severe form of halothane hepatitis is very uncommon and more frequent in patients exposed to halothane on more than one occasion. Many of the clinical and serological features of patients who develop halothane hepatitis suggest that the severe form of liver damage is an immune-mediated adverse reaction. Thus, the disease is rare, affects mainly females and is often associated with features of immunological disturbance, such as circulating immune complexes, peripheral eosinophilia and non-organ-specific autoantibodies (particularly anti-LKM). Studies have shown that such patients also have a high incidence of antibodies to both normal liver cell components and specifically to halothane-related antigens [94]. These antigens, which have not yet been fully defined, are associated with metabolism of halothane by the oxidative route [95], and occur in both laboratory animals and in man. It remains to be established whether these halothane antibodies are involved in the pathogenesis of halothane hepatitis. In vitro studies showing that lymphocytes from patients with severe halothane hepatitis are cytotoxic to hepatocytes prepared from rabbits following halothane anaesthesia, but not from normal rabbits [96], and that halothane antibody-coated liver cells become susceptible to damage by lymphocytes prepared from normal individuals [94], suggest that these antibodies are likely to be involved in the pathogenesis of the disease.

## References

1. Kelsall AR, Stewart A, Witts LJ (1947) Subacute and chronic hepatitis. Lancet II:195–198
2. Waldenström J (1950) Leber, Blutprotein und Nahrungseiweiss – Stoffwechsel. Report of session. Bad Kissingen, special vol 15:8–10
3. Kunkel HG, Ahrens EH, Eisenmenger WJ, Bongiovanni AM, Slater RJ (1951) Extreme hypergammaglobulinemia in young women with liver disease of unknown aetiology. J Clin Invest 30:654
4. Saint EG, King WE, Joske RA, Finckh ES (1953) The course of infectious hepatitis with special reference to prognosis and to the chronic stage. Australas Ann Med 2:113–127
5. Bouchier IAD, Rhodes K, Sherlock S (1964) Serological abnormalities in patients with liver disease. Br Med J I:592–594

6. Johnson GD, Holborow EJ, Glynn LE (1965) Antibody to smooth muscle in patients with liver disease. Lancet II:878–879
7. Rizzetto M, Swana G, Doniach D (1973) Microsomal antibodies in active chronic hepatitis and other disorders. Clin Exp Immunol 15:331–344
8. Manns M, Gerken G, Kyriatsoulis A, Staritz M, Meyer zum Büschenfelde KH (1987) Characterization of a new subgroup of autoimmune chronic active hepatitis by autoantibodies against a soluble liver antigen. Lancet I:292–294
9. Homberg JC, Abuaf N, Bernard O, et al. (1987) Chronic active hepatitis associated with anti liver/kidney microsome antibody type 1: a second type of "autoimmune" hepatitis. Hepatology 7:1333–1339
10. Manns MP, Johnson EF, Griffin KJ, Tan EM, Sullivan KF (1989) The major antigen of liver kidney microsomal autoantibodies in idiopathic autoimmune hepatitis is cytochrome P450 db1. J Clin Invest 83:1066–1072
11. Whitehouse JM, Holborow EJ (1971) Smooth muscle antibody in malignant disease. Br Med J IV:511–513
12. Meyer zum Büschenfelde KH (1968) Untersuchungen über die immunobiologische Bedeutung löslicher Leberproteine. Z Gesamte Exp Med 148: 131–135
13. Meyer zum Büschenfelde KH, Miescher PA (1972) Liver specific antigens, purification and characterization. Clin Exp Immunol 10:89–102
14. McFarlane IG (1984) Editorial review – autoimmunity in liver disease. Clin Sci 67:569–578
15. Meyer zum Büschenfelde KH, Kossling FK (1971) Characterization and isolation of liver-specific protein in different species: their importance for experimental models and in diagnosis of chronic active hepatits. In: Smith A, Williams R (eds) Immunology of the liver. Heinemann, London, pp 169–185
16. Jensen DM, McFarlane IG, Nicholson A, Eddleston ALWF, Williams R (1978) The development of a radioimmunoassay for the detection of antibodies to a liver specific membrane lipoprotein (LSP). J Clin Immunol 1:31–35
17. Jensen DM, McFarlane IG, Portmann B, Eddleston ALWF, Williams R (1978) Detection of antibodies directed against a liver-specific lipoprotein in patients with acute and chronic active hepatitis. N Engl J Med 299:1–7
18. McFarlane BM, McSorley CG, Vergani D, McFarlane IG, Williams R (1986) Serum antibodies reacting with the hepatic asialoglycoprotein receptor (hepatic lectin) in acute and chronic liver disorders. J Hepatol vol 3:196–205
19. McFarlane IG, McFarlane BM, Major GN, Tolley P, Williams R (1984) Identification of the hepatic asialoglycoprotein receptor (hepatic lectin) as a component of liver specific membrane lipoprotein (LSP). Clin Exp Immunol 55:347–354
20. Vergani D, Mieli-Vergani G, Mondelli M, Portmann B, Eddleston ALWF (1987) Immunoglobulin on the surface of isolated hepatocytes is associated with antibody-dependent cell-mediated cytotoxicity and liver damage. Liver 7:307–315
21. Lobo Yeo A, Senaldi G, Portmann B, Mowat AP, Mieli-Vergani G, Vergani D (1990) Class I and class II major histocompatibility complex antigen expression on hepatocytes. A study in children with liver disease. Hepatology 12:224–232
22. Colucci G, Colombo M, Del Ninno E, Paronetto F (1983) In situ characterization by monoclonal antibodies of the mononuclear cell infiltrate in chronic active hepatitis. Gastroenterology 85:1138–1145
23. Senaldi G (1990) Mononuclear cell infiltrate characterisation and hepatocyte expression analysis of class I and II major histocompatibility complex molecules in liver biopsies from children with hepatic disorders. PhD thesis, University of London, pp 132–152
24. Lobo Yeo A, Alviggi L, Mieli-Vergani G, Portmann B, Mowat AP, Vergani D (1987) Preferential activation of helper/inducer T lymphocytes in children with autoimmune chronic active hepatitis. Clin Exp Immunol 67:95–104

25. Mieli-Vergani G, Vergani D, Jenkins PJ, Portmann B, Mowat AP, Eddleston ALWF, Williams R (1979) Lymphocyte cytotoxicity to autologous hepatocytes in HBsAg negative chronic active hepatitis. Clin Exp Immunol 38:16–21
26. Vergani D, Wells L, Larcher VF, Nasarruddin BA, Davies ET, Mieli-Vergani G, Mowat AP (1985) Genetically determined low C4: a predisposing factor to autoimmune chronic active hepatitis. Lancet 2:294–298
27. Hussain MJ, Mowat AP, Mieli-Vergani G, Vergani D (1991) Interleukin-1 (IL-1), soluble interleukin-2 receptor (SIL2R), tumour necrosis factor (TNF) and interferon $\gamma$ (IFN $\gamma$) in children with chronic liver disease (CLD) (abstr). J Pediatr Gastroenterol Nutr (in press)
28. Wen L, Peakman M, Lobo-Yeo A, McFarlane BM, Mowat AP, Mieli-Vergani G, Vergani D (1990) T-cell-directed hepatocyte damage in autoimmune chronic active hepatitis. Lancet 336:1527–1530
29. Wen L, Peakman M, Mowat AP, Mieli-Vergani G, Vergani D (1991) $\gamma\delta^+$ T cell clones from liver biopsies of children with autoimmune chronic active hepatitis (aCAH) and primary sclerosing cholangitis (aPSC) are cytotoxic to human liver target cells (abstr). J Hepatol 13:580
30. Acha-Orbea H, Mitchell DJ, Timmermann L et al. (1988) Limited heterogeneity of T cell receptors from lymphocytes mediating autoimmune encephalomyelitis allows specific immune intervention. Cell 54:263–273
31. Wraith DC, McDevitt HO, Steinman L, Acha-Orbea H (1989) T cell recognition as the target for immune intervention in autoimmune disease. Cell 57:709–715
32. Lider O, Karin N, Shinitzky M, Cohen IR (1987) Therapeutic vaccination against adjuvant arthritis using autoimmune T cells treated with hydrostatic pressure. Proc Natl Acad Sci USA 84:4577–4580
33. Eddleston ALWF, Williams R (1974) Inadequate antibody response to HBAg or suppressor T-cell defect in development of active chronic hepatitis. Lancet II:1543–1545
34. Kashio T, Motta R, Kakumu S (1981) Lymphocyte suppressor cell activity in acute and chronic liver disease. Clin Exp Immunol 44:459–466
35. Nouri Aria KT, Hegarty JE, Alexander GJ, Eddleston ALWF, Williams R (1982) Effect of corticosteroids in suppressor cell activity in "autoimmune" and viral chronic active hepatitis. N Engl J Med 307:1301–1304
36. Nouri Aria K, Lobo Yeo A, Vergani D, Mieli-Vergani G, Eddleston ALWF, Mowat AP (1985) T suppressor cell function and number in children with liver disease. Clin Exp Immunol 61:283–289
37. Nouri Aria KT, Donaldson PT, Hegarty JE, Eddleston ALWF, Williams R (1985) HLA A1-B8-DR3 and suppressor cell function in first degree relatives of patients with autoimmune chronic active hepatitis. J Hepatol 1:235–241
38. Vento S, Hegarty JE, Bottazzo G, Macchia E, Williams R, Eddleston ALWF (1984) Antigen specific suppressor cell function in autoimmune chronic active hepatitis. Lancet I:1200–1204
39. Stastny P, Ball EJ, Dry PJ, Nunez G (1983) The human immune response region (HLA-D) and disease susceptibility. Immunol Rev 70:113–153
40. Galbraith RM, Eddleston ALWF, Williams R et al. (1976) Enhanced antibody response in active chronic hepatitis. Relationship to HLAB8 and HLAB12 and portosystemic shunting. Lancet I:930–934
41. Hodges S, Lobo-Yeo A, Donaldson P, Tanner MS, Vergani D (1991) Autoimmune chronic active hepatitis in a family. Gut 32:299–302
42. Donaldson PT, Doherty DG, Hayllar KM, McFarlane IG, Johnson PJ, Williams R (1990) Susceptibility to autoimmune chronic active hepatitis: human leukocyte antigens DR4 and A1-B8-DR3 are independent risk factors. Hepatology 13: 701–706
43. Doherty DJ, Donaldson PT, Farrant JM et al. (1991) Strong association between HLA-DQA, DQB and DRB3 alleles and autoimmune chronic active hepatitis demonstrated by PCR oligonucleotide analysis (abstr). J Hepatol 13:S25

44. Vergani D, Wells L, Larcher VF, Nassarruddin BA, Davies ET, Mieli-Vergani G, Mowat P (1985) Genetically determined low C4: a predisposing factor to autoimmune chronic active hepatitis. Lancet II:294–298
45. Lachmann PJ, Peters DK (1982) Complement. In: Lachmann PJ, Peters DK (eds) Clinical aspects of immunology. Blackwell, Oxford, pp 18–49
46. Daniels CA, Borsos T, Rapp HJ, Shyderman R, Notkins AL (1969) Neutralisation of sensitised virus by the fourth component of complement. Science 165:508–509
47. Whittingham S, Mathews JD, Schanfield MS, Tait BD, Mackay IR (1981) Interaction of HLA and GM in autoimmune chronic active hepatitis. Clin Exp Immunol 43:80–86
48. Falconer DS (1965) The inheritance of liability of certain diseases estimated from the incidence among relatives. Ann Hum Genet 29:51–76
49. El-Shabrawi M, Wilkinson M, Portmann B, Mieli-Vergani G, Chong SKF, Williams R, Mowat AP (1987) Primary sclerosing cholangitis in childhood. Gastroenterology 92:1226–1235
50. Mieli-Vergani G, Lobo-Yeo A, McFarlane BM, McFarlane IG, Mowat AP, Vergani D (1989) Different immune mechanisms leading to autoimmunity in primary sclerosing cholangitis and autoimmune chronic active hepatitis of childhood. Hepatology 9:198–203
51. Donaldson PT, Farrant JM, Wilkinson ML, Hayllar K, Portmann BC, Williams R (1991) Dual association of HLA DR2 and DR3 with primary sclerosing cholangitis. Hepatology 13:129–133
52. Mackay IR (1958) Primary biliary cirrhosis showing a high titer of autoantibody. N Engl J Med 258:185–187
53. Walker JG, Doniach D, Roitt IM, Sherlock S (1965) Serological tests in diagnosis of primary biliary cirrhosis. Lancet I:827–829
54. Berg PA, Doniach D, Roitt IM (1967) Mitochondrial antibodies in primary biliary cirrhosis. I. Localization of the antigen to mitochondrial membranes. J Exp Med 126:277–290
55. Gores GJ, Moore SB, Fisher LD et al. (1987) Primary biliary cirrhosis: association with class II major histocompatibility complex antigens. Hepatology 7:889–892
56. Frazer IH, Mackay IR, Jordan TW et al. (1985) Reactivity of mitochondrial autoantibodies in primary biliary cirrhosis: definition of two novel mitochondrial polypeptide autoantignes. J Immunol 135:1739–1745
57. Gershwin ME, Mackay IR (1991) Primary biliary cirrhosis: paradigm or paradox for autoimmunity. Gastroenterology 100:822–833
58. Mackay IR, Gershwin ME (1990) Primary biliary cirrhosis: current knowledge, perspectives, and future directions. Semin Liver Dis 9:149–157
59. Baum H (1989) Nature of the mitochondrial antigens of primary biliary cirrhosis and their possible relationship to the etiology of the disease. Semin Liver Dis 9:117–123
60. Si L, Whiteside TL, Shade RR, et al. (1981) T lymphocyte subsets in liver tissues of patients with primary biliary cirrhosis (PBC), patients with primary sclerosing cholangitis (PSC) and normal controls. J Clin Immunol 4:262–272
61. Colucci G, Shaffner F, Paronetto F (1986) In Situ characterization of the cell surface antigens of the mononuclear cell infiltrate and bile duct epithelium in primary biliary cirrhosis. Clin Immunol Immunopathol 41:35–42
62. Shimizu M, Yuh K, Aoyama S et al. (1986) Immunohistochemical characterization of infilammatory of infilammatory infiltrates at the side of bile duct injury in primary biliary cirrhosis. Liver 6:1–6
63. Ballardini G, Mirakian R, Bianchi FB, Pisi, E, Doniach F, Salmon C (1984) Aberrant expression of HLA-DR antigens on bile duct epithelium in primary biliary cirrhosis: relevance to pathogenesis. Lancet II:1009–1013

64. Krams SM, Dorshikind K, Gershwin ME (1989) Generation of biliary lesions following transfer of human lymphocytes into SCID mice. J Exp Med 170: 1919–1930
65. Mondelli M, Eddleston ALWF (1984) Mechanisms of liver injury in acute and chronic hepatitis B. Semin Liver Dis 4:47–57
66. Unanue ER, Cerottini JC (1990) Antigen presenattion. FSEB J 3:2496–2502
67. Bertoletti A, Ferrari C, Penna A et al. (1991) HLA class I restricted cytotoxic T cells in acute viral hepatitis B (abstr). J Hepatol 13:S11
68. Unanue ER, Allen PM (1987) The basis for the immunoregulatory role of macrophages and other accessory cells. Science 236:551–554
69. Ferrari C, Bertoletti A, Penna A et al. (1991) Identification of immunodominant T cell epitopes of the hepatitis B virus nucleocapsid antigen. J Clin Invest 88:214–222
70. Ferrari C, Chisari FV, Ribera E, Penna A, Mondelli MU (1988) Functional modulation of hepatitis B core antigen-specific T lymphocytes by an autoreactive T cell clone. J Immunol 141:1155–1160
71. Vegnente A, Guida S, Lobo-Yeo A et al. (1991) T lymphocyte activation is associated with viral replication in chronic hepatitis B virus infection of childhood. Clin Exp Immunol 84:190–194
72. Mondelli M, Mieli-Vergani G, Alberti A, Vergani D, Portmann B, Eddleston ALWF, Williams R (1982) Specificity of T-lymphocyte cytotoxicity to autologous hepatocytes in chronic hepatitis B virus infection: evidence that T-cells are directed against HBV core antigen expressed on hepatocytes. J Immunol 129: 2773–2778
73. Pignatelli M, Waters J, Lever AML, Iwarson S, Gerety R, Thomas HC (1987) Cytotoxic T cell responses to the nucleocapsid proteins of HBV in chronic hepatitis. J Hepatol 4:15–21
74. Mondelli M, Mieli-Vergani G, Bortolotti F et al. (1985) Different mechanisms responsible for in vitro cell-mediated cytotoxicity to autologous hepatocytes in children with autoimmune and HBsAg positive chronic liver disease. J Pediatr 106:899–906
75. Lamelin JP, Trepo C (1990) The hepatitis B virus and the peripheral blood mononuclear cells: a brief review. J Hepatol 10:120–124
76. Abb J, Zachoval R, Eisenburg J, Pape GR, Zachoval U, Deinhardt F (1985) Production of interferon alpha and interferon gamma by peripheral blood leucocytes from patients with chronic hepatitis B virus infection. J Med Virol 16:171–176
77. Twu JS, Lee CH, Lin MP, Schloemer RH (1988) Hepatitis B virus suppresses expression of human β-interferon. Proc Natl Acad Sci 85:252–256
78. Vento S, Hegarty JE, Alberti A et al. (1985) T lymphocyte sensitization to HBcAg in hepatitis B virus mediated unresponsiveness to HBsAg in hepatitis B virus related chronic liver disease. Hepatology 5:192–197
79. Ganem D, Varmus HE (1987) The molecular biology of the hepatitis B viruses. Annu Rev Biochem 56:651–693
80. Carman WF, Jacyna MR, Hadziyannis S, Karayiannis P, McGarvey MJ, Makris A, Monias HC (1989) Mutation preventing formation of hepatitis B e antigen in patients with chronic hepatitis B virus infection. Lancet II:588–590
81. Brunetto MR, Stemler M, Bonino F et al. (1990) A new hepatitis B virus strain in patients with severe anti-HBe positive chronic hepatitis B. J Hepatol 10:258–261
82. Liang TJ, Hasegawa K, Rimon N, Wands JR, Ben-Porath E (1991) A hepatitis B virus mutant associated with an epidemic of fulminant hepatitis. N Engl J Med 324:1705–1709
83. Omata M, Ehata T, Yokosuka O, Hosoda K, Ohto M (1991) Mutations in the precore region of hepatitis B virus DNA in patients with fulminant and severe hepatitis. N Engl J Med 324:1699–1704

84. Kosaka Y, Takase K, Kojima M et al. (1991) Fulminant hepatitis B: induction by hepatitis B virus mutants defective in the precore region and incapable of encoding e antigen. Gastroenterology 100:1087–1094
85. Vallbracht A, Gabriel P, Maier K et al. (1986) Cell-mediated cytotoxicity in hepatitis A virus infection. Hepatology 6:1308–1314
86. Kurane I, Binn LN, Bancroft WH, Ennis FA (1985) Human lymphocyte responses to hepatitis A virus-infected cells: interferon production and lysis of infected cells. J Immunol 135:2140–2144
87. Fasel-Felley J, Overby LR, Frei PC (1986) A specific immune response to purified HA antigen (HAAg) demonstrated by leukocyte migration inhibition in patients recovering from viral hepatitis A. J Hepatol 2:237–244
88. Esteban JI, Esteban R, Viladomiu L et al. (1989) Hepatitis C virus antibodies among risk groups in Spain. Lancet II:294–297
89. Lenzi M, Ballardini G, Gusconi M et al. (1990) Type 2 autoimmune hepatitis and hepatitis C virus infection. Lancet 335:258–259
90. McFarlane IG, Smith HM, Johnson PJ et al. (1990) Hepatitis C Virus antibodies in chronic active hepatitis: pathogenetic factor or false positive result? Lancet 335:754–757
91. Lunel F, Homberg JC, Grippon P et al. (1991) Type 2 autoimmune hepatitis and hepatitis C virus: a study group of 83 patients (abstr). J Hepatol 13:S47
92. Mishiro S, Hoshi Y, Takeda K et al (1990) Non-A, non-B hepatitis specific antibodies directed to host-derived epitope: implications for an autoimmune process. Lancet 336:1400–1403
93. Neuberger JM, Williams R (1984) Halothane anaesthesia and liver damage. Br Med J 289:1136–1139
94. Vergani D, Mieli-Vergani G, Alberti A et al. (1980) Antibodies to the surface of halothane-altered rabbit hepatocytes in patients with severe halothane-associated hepatitis. N Engl J Med 303:66–71
95. Neuberger J, Mieli-Vergani G, Tredger JM, Davis M, Williams R (1981) Oxidative metabolism of halothane in the production of altered hepatocyte membrane antigens in acute halothane-induced hepatic necrosis. Gut 22:669–672
96. Mieli-Vergani G, Vergani D, Tredger JM, Eddleston ALWF, Davis M, Williams R (1980) Lymphocyte cytotoxicity to halothane altered hepatocytes in patients with severe hepatic necrosis following halothane anaesthesia. J Clin Lab Immunol 4:49–51

# 5 Diagnostic Imaging of the Hepatobiliary System

F.J. LECUMBERRI, J.I. BILBAO, J.M. LONGO, and M. MUÑOZ

## 1 Introduction

The study of liver diseases by means of imaging methods has changed substantially in the last decade owing to advances in ultrasound (US), angiography, computed tomography (CT), and radionuclide studies. In recent years, we have witnessed important developments in the selection of diagnostic methods. In the 1960s, selective hepatic arteriography was the "gold standard" in the diagnosis of numerous hepatic lesions (hepatocellular carcinoma, hemangioma, metastasis, etc.). However, since then the role of arteriography in diagnosis has become less important and it is now used mainly as an exploratory procedure prior to surgery. In its place, other methods, such as scintigraphy, US, CT, and magnetic resonance imaging (MRI), are used. Each of these procedures is useful, but a specific radiologic diagnosis is most often reached with a combination of investigations rather than with a single modality. In addition, percutaneous fine-needle aspiration biopsy (PFNAB) under US or CT guidance may be performed without significant complications, contributing to histopathologic diagnosis in a large number of cases.

## 2 Plain Radiographs

The diagnostic information provided by plain films is limited. Nonopaque gallstones (composed of cholesterol) cannot be visualized by this method. Calcified gallstones, however, are identified. Similarly, milk of calcium bile and calcium in the gallbladder wall (porcelain gallbladder) can be confidently diagnosed.

Aerobilia constitutes a frequent event in cholecystectomized patients and also after choledochal stone passage and sphincterotomy. Gas in the gallbladder wall indicates emphysematous cholecystitis. Bubbles in the hepatic parenchyma can be seen in hepatic abscesses.

## 3 Oral Cholecystography

Oral cholecystography (OCG) was the standard procedure in gallbladder imaging until the advent of cross-sectional imaging techniques. Nowadays,

US has largely replaced OCG in gallbladder evaluation [1]. However, OCG is as effective as US in the diagnosis of gallstones [2], and some authors have claimed that it is more accurate in evaluating hyperplastic cholecystopathy and gallbladder polyps.

Iopanoic acid (Telepaque) is given orally and is readily absorbed into the bloodstream. The hepatic microsomes conjugate the iopanoic acid with glucuronic acid and it is excreted in this form into bile. Thus, both failure of absorption from the gut and liver insufficiency can lead to poor visualization of the gallbladder. Opacification of the gallbladder also requires a patent cystic duct. Maximal opacification usually occurs 17 h after ingestion of iopanoic acid [3].

Stones, polyps, and masses arising in the gallbladder wall are clearly outlined by the opacified bile. OCG is accurate in determining the number and size of stones and also provides information regarding the patency of the cystic duct. It is regaining popularity as a means of evaluating the exact number of stones and the emptying of the gallbladder when biliary lithotripsy is warranted [2].

## 4 Intravenous Cholangiography

With the advent of US and the widespread use of more accurate direct opacification techniques, such as endoscopic retrograde cholangiopancreatography and percutaneous transhepatic cholangiography, intravenous cholangiography (IVC) is now of limited use.

The contrast agent (methylglucamine iodipamide, Cholografin) is concentrated by the liver and excreted into the bile ducts. Visualization of the hepatic and common bile ducts precedes gallbladder opacification. Plain films and tomograms are taken at 20-min intervals to detect common bile duct opacification.

In the presence of jaundice, biliary visualization is markedly impaired. IVC is useless when the level of serum conjugated bilirubin exceeds 2 mg/100 ml.

Morbidity related to IVC contrast agents can represent a significant risk, as the prevalence of hypersensitivity reactions is around 1%.

## 5 Hepatic Radionuclide Imaging

Radionuclide imaging studies of the liver are based on their ability to analyze the functional status of this organ. Functional studies performed with radiolabeled tracers may be directed toward analyzing the reticuloendothelial system, hepatic blood flow, or production of bile.

Technetium-99 m ($^{99m}Tc$) is the radionuclide of choice for various purposes. Many intrahepatic lesions can be detected and differentiated

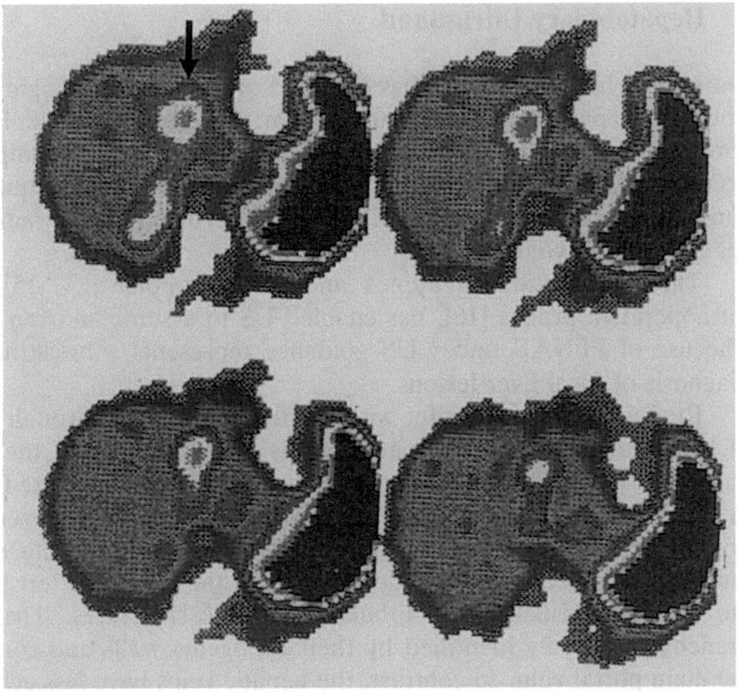

**Fig. 1.** Cavernous hepatic hemangioma. SPECT scan shows persistence of activity in the left lobe of the liver (*arrow*). Incidentially, splenomegaly is also evident

(colloidal liver scans) [4]. Iminodiacetic acid derivatives labeled with $^{99m}$Tc-pertechnetate allow the possibility of studying the biliary transport system and detecting the presence or absence of cystic duct obstruction and post-surgical bile leakage [5–7].

Gallium citrate ($^{67}$Ga) is a good tracer for obtaining specific images in tumoral or inflammatory lesions [8, 9]. $^{99m}$Tc-labeled red blood cell imaging is one of the methods of choice for the diagnosis of hepatic cavernous hemangiomas when other noninvasive radiologic methods have failed to yield a definite diagnosis of this entity [10, 11].

Conventional radionuclide studies are performed with the intravenous injection of a radiotracer and the detection of the emitted radiation with a gamma camera. This safe and simple technique has recently been rendered more sophisticated and efficient by the introduction of single photon emission computed tomography (SPECT) [12, 13] (Fig. 1), which enables transaxial tomographic images to be acquired with conventional nuclear imaging equipment and conventional radiotracers. The signal intensity needed for imaging is lower and more precise information can be obtained; for this reason, some radiotracers (like labeled antibodies), less active but more specific, can be used for diagnostic purposes.

## 6 Hepatobiliary Ultrasound

During the last decade, US has emerged as the primary imaging modality in both the hepatic and the biliary system. Several factors explain its widespread use: its availability, noninvasiveness, low cost, and high diagnostic accuracy. Furthermore, it can be used at the bedside and sequential studies can be performed. Finally, as US does not involve ionizing radiation, harmful effects are avoided.

The introduction of duplex and color Doppler [14, 15], as well as intraoperative probes [16], has enabled US to assume an even greater role. The use of PFNAB under US guidance represents a breakthrough in the diagnosis of focal liver lesions.

Real-time machines offer within a few minutes a thorough visualization of liver parenchyma and hepatic vessels. The gallbladder, the head of the pancreas, and most surrounding structures are clearly depicted. Alterations in the size and shape of the liver are easily seen. The parenchyma of a normal liver appears as a uniformly reflective structure, with evenly distributed midlevel echoes. Hepatic vessels and the right and left hepatic ducts are regularly visualized as tubular, anechoic structures. The portal vein branches are easily identified by their echogenic walls and continuity from the main portal vein. In contrast, the hepatic veins have less echogenic walls and are directed posteriorly, toward the inferior vena cava.

An echogenic liver is most often caused by fatty infiltration. Focal fatty changes are frequent. They can mimic hepatic masses by leaving other zones unaffected [17].

Ultrasound-based diagnosis of diffuse liver diseases is difficult unless there is gross distortion of the normal echogenicity. US is unreliable in assessing the severity of histologic changes. Increased echogenicity, scattered high amplitude echoes (a "coarsened" echo pattern), and increased attenuation of the beam are frequently found in chronic hepatopathies. Cirrhosis, fatty infiltration, chronic active hepatitis, and hemochromatosis can all alter the normal echo pattern. However, specific diagnosis is not possible in most cases.

Gross morphologic changes present in advanced cirrhosis can easily be seen by means of US [18]. Right lobe shrinkage, caudate lobe enlargement, and rounded nodular contours are frequent findings. Ascites, even minimal, is easily detected.

Morphologic vascular changes associated with portal hypertension are usually evident in US examination. The normal diameter of the main portal vein is less than 1.3 cm in most patients. Increases in the portal diameter, splenomegaly, and collateral circulation are highly suggestive of portal hypertension. Portal venous collaterals are commonly seen by US.

Doppler US allows measurements of the portal vein flow. However, its accuracy has not yet been proven.

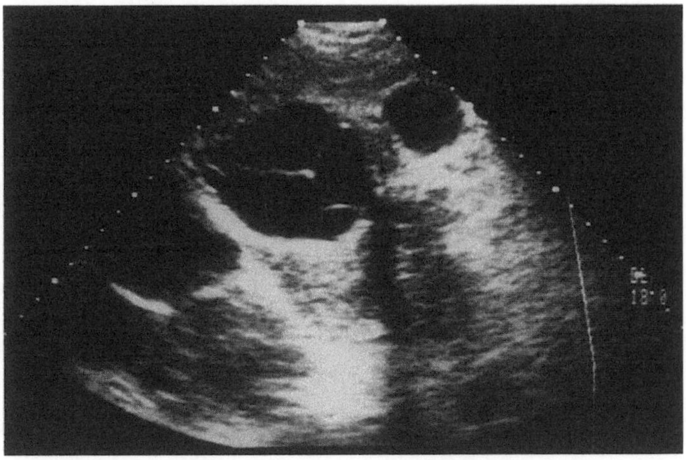

**Fig. 2.** Echinococcal cyst. Well-marginated cystic lesion with multiple septa

Hepatic masses disrupting the normal echo pattern are easily detected. US can detect lesions as small as 1 cm in diameter and can accurately differentiate between solid and cystic lesions. Cysts exhibit a well-defined wall and no internal echoes [19]. Increased sound transmission through the lesion results in acoustic enhancement. Simple cysts are a frequent finding in US examinations of the liver. They have a thin, well-defined wall. Echinococcal cysts (hydatid disease) usually exhibit a thicker wall. Daughter cysts, membrane detachment, and wall calcification can be demonstrated [20] (Fig. 2).

Although the detection rate of focal liver lesions by US is high (80%–90%), a specific diagnosis based on US findings alone is frequently not achievable. In this setting, PFNAB under US guidance provides a safe and reliable method of obtaining a definitive diagnosis. Over the last decade, US-guided PFNAB of liver lesions has become a routine procedure in most radiologic departments.

With the widespread use of US, cavernous hemangiomas are often incidentally discovered. Most of them appear as a hyperechoic, well-defined lesion less than 3 cm in diameter (Fig. 3). However, atypical forms are not infrequent (occurring in up to 15% of cases) and can pose a diagnostic challenge. The complementary role of the different imaging techniques is well shown in these cases.

Solid lesions can appear as hyper- or hypoechoic. Involvement of neighboring structures and hepatic hilar adenopathies can be evaluated.

A hepatic abscess usually appears as a fluid or mixed pattern mass. Percutaneous drainage using small-bore catheters under imaging guidance, either US or CT, has largely supplanted open surgery over the last 5 years

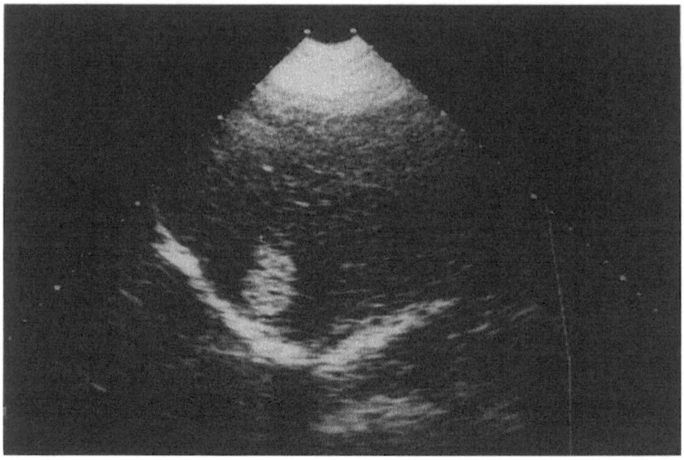

**Fig. 3.** Cavernous hemangioma. Well-defined echogenic mass with slightly lobulated contours

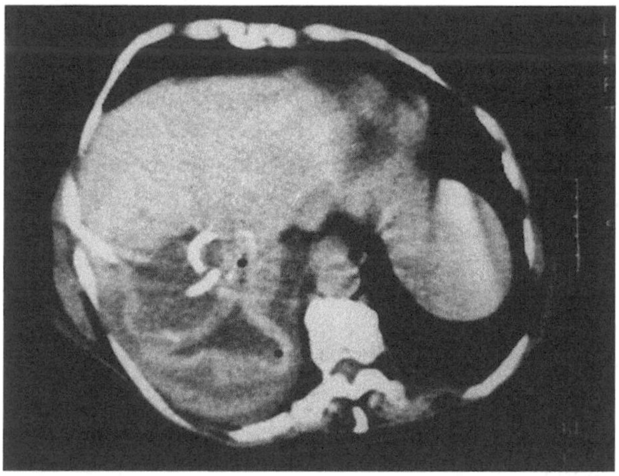

**Fig. 4.** Liver abscess. CT imaging allows safe insertion of a pigtail catheter for drainage

(Fig. 4). In addition, bilomas, hematomas, and perihepatic fluid collections can be both detected and drained.

Ultrasound is the first imaging technique to be used in patients with cholestasis. The normal intrahepatic biliary ducts are too small to be visualized by US. When dilated, the biliary ducts become easily visible as tubular structures parallel to the portal vein branches, producing the typical "double channel" appearance. The proximal main bile duct is regularly

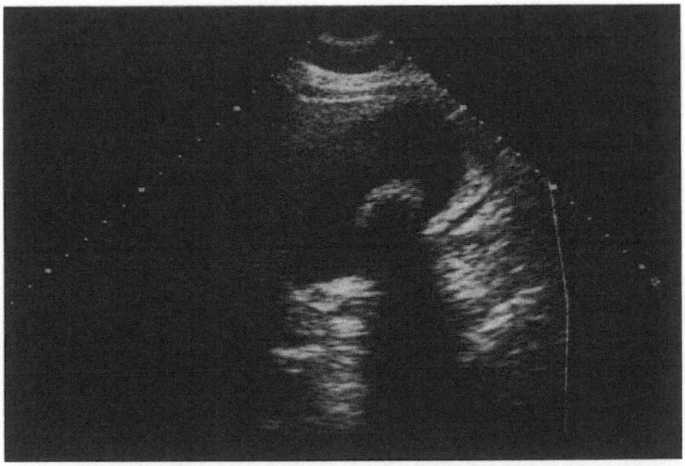

**Fig. 5.** Gallstone. Echodense stone is seen in the dependent portion of the gallbladder, with associated acoustic shadowing

visualized at the hepatic hilum where it crosses the portal vein. However, evaluation of its distal portion can be hindered by overlying gas in the duodenum. For this reason, US is not as accurate as CT in visualizing the cause of the dilatation.

Segmental dilatation of the hepatic ducts (Caroli's disease) can be detected by US. Congenital abnormalities, such as choledochal cyst and choledochocele, can also be demonstrated.

The normal gallbladder appears as a pear-shaped, anechoic cystic structure lying below the inferior edge of the right hepatic lobe. Examination in the fasting state results in a distended gallbladder in which both the walls and the content can be thoroughly scanned.

Ultrasound has become the ideal procedure in evaluating cholelithiasis [21]. Stones typically appear as brightly echogenic structures with associated acoustic shadowing (Fig. 5). With current equipment, stones as small as 3 mm can be detected. US plays a key role in biliary lithotripsy. Both the targeting of the shock wave and monitoring of the fragmentation are carried out under continuous US evaluation.

Masses arising from the gallbladder wall are readily visualised [1]. The invasion of surrounding organs by a cholangioarcinoma can be evaluated by US.

*Acute* cholecystitis typically appears as a distended gallbladder with thick, irregular walls [1]. Gallstones are usually present. At times, a gallstone obstructing the neck of the gallbladder can be seen. Selective pain on compression with the transducer (the sonographic Murphy's sign) can aid in the diagnosis. Pericholecystic fluid collections usually indicate wall necrosis and gallbladder perforation [22]. In *chronic* cholecystitis, a contracted gall-

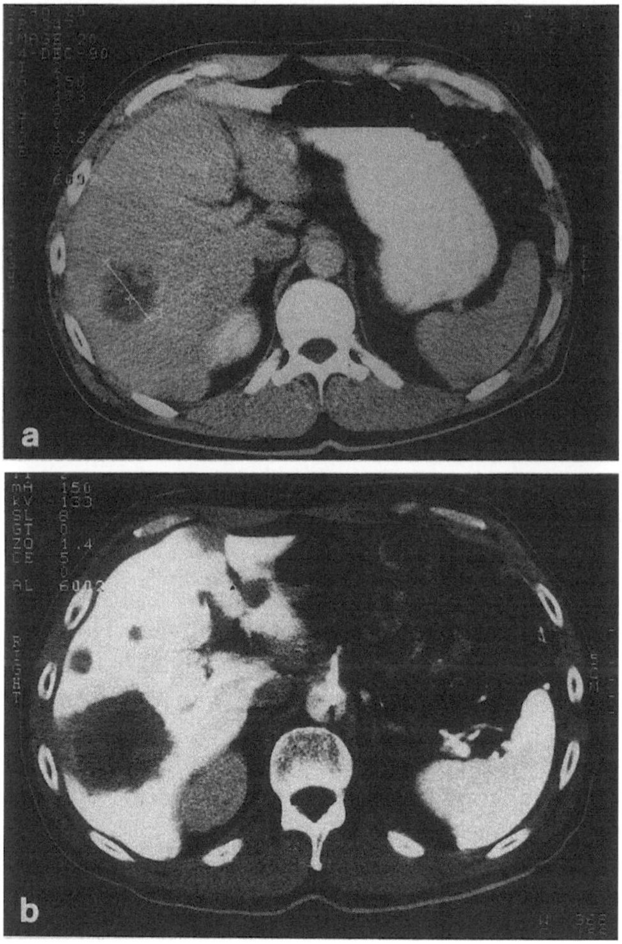

**Fig. 6a,b.** Liver metastases in carcinoma of the colon. **a** Bolus CT scan shows a single metastatic lesion in the right lobe of the liver. **b** CTAP scan at the same level as **a**. The true extent of the lesion is shown. In addition, four smaller metastases ranging down to 8 mm in diameter were also detected. (The tip of the infusion catheter is positioned in the splenic artery.)

bladder can be difficult to depict. The "WES triad" (wall, echo, shadow) usually indicates multiple lithiasis in a contracted gallbladder [23].

## 7 Hepatobiliary Computed Tomography

Hepatic lesions are revealed on CT scans by alterations in the density. The administration of iodinated contrast is used to augment the differences in density between healthy tissue and hepatic lesions. There are numerous methods for administering the contrast:

- Using modern equipment, the ideal technique is the administration of iodinated contrast material by intravenous bolus injection with dynamic sequential scans. During and after the injection, contiguous scans are made through the liver within 3 min. As a screening procedure for hepatic tumors, it has a sensitivity of about 85%–90% [24].
- A more sensitive method for the evaluation of hepatic tumors is CT during arterial portography (CTAP) [25, 26], with injection of contrast in the splenic or superior mesenteric artery. Nevertheless, it is an invasive technique which is reserved as a step prior to surgery in order to ascertain the number of lesions and their location (Fig. 6).

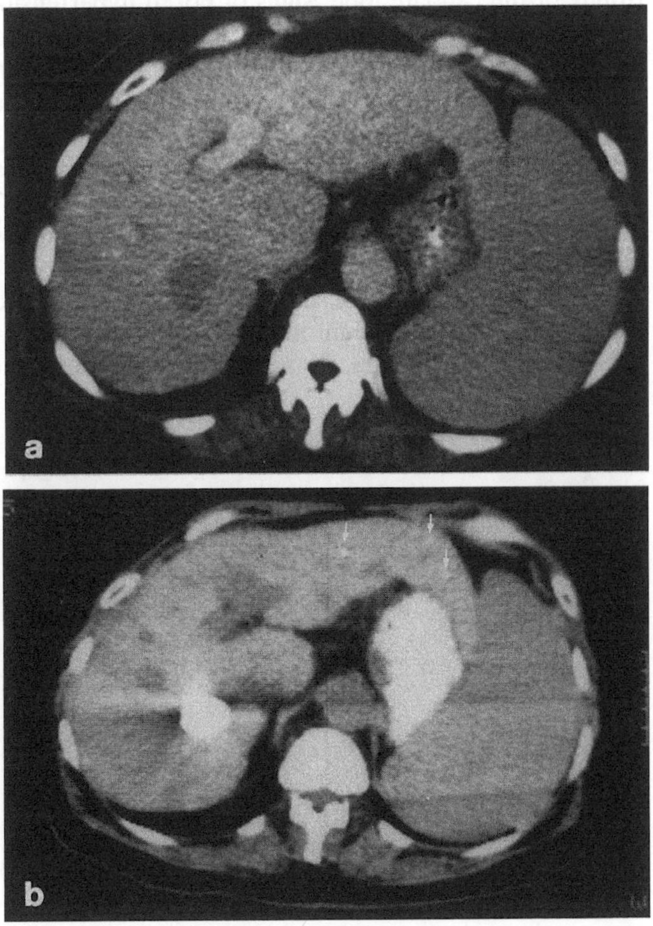


**Fig. 7a,b.** Hepatocellular carcinoma in a cirrhotic patient. **a** CT after bolus enhancement. A solitary hypodense lesion is observed in the right lobe of the liver. **b** Fifteen days after the intraarterial injection of Lipiodol. Three more satellite lesions, ranging from 2 to 5 mm in diameter, are also observed in the left lobe of the liver (*arrows*); curative resection is not possible

- When massive doses of contrast medium are used (60–80 g iodine), its excretion (about 1%–2%) by the hepatocytes results in an increase in the density of normal tissue. CT study is carried out 4–6 h later (delayed CT), allowing better tumor detection [27].
- Finally, Lipiodol injected intraarterially is retained in abnormal sinusoids of hepatic tumors [28]. In the appraisal of hepatocellular carcinoma, CT is performed 10–15 days later, allowing the representation of the exact shape of the lesion and the detection of possible multiple nodules (Fig. 7).

Even though the fundamental use of CT resides in the evaluation of focal lesions, there are several diffuse lesions that can be readily diagnosed by CT: steatosis (diffuse diminution in hepatic density), hemochromatosis (increase in density), and hepatic cirrhosis (lobulations of contours, hypertrophy of the caudate lobe, signs of portal hypertension, etc.) [29] (Fig. 8).

Computed tomography and MRI have become the primary diagnostic imaging modalities for focal hepatic lesions. The accuracy of each is dependent on the technique used, the equipment available, and the experience of the examiner. When focal lesions are cystic, there is no difficulty in their diagnosis because of the difference between their CT attenuation value and that of healthy liver. Hydatid cysts (Fig. 9) present CT aspects that permit their differentiation from other cystic lesions and allow the identification of complications [30].

One inconvenience of modern imaging techniques is that they make benign tumors more evident than they used to be, and their further exploration increases health care costs and may give rise to iatrogenic problems.

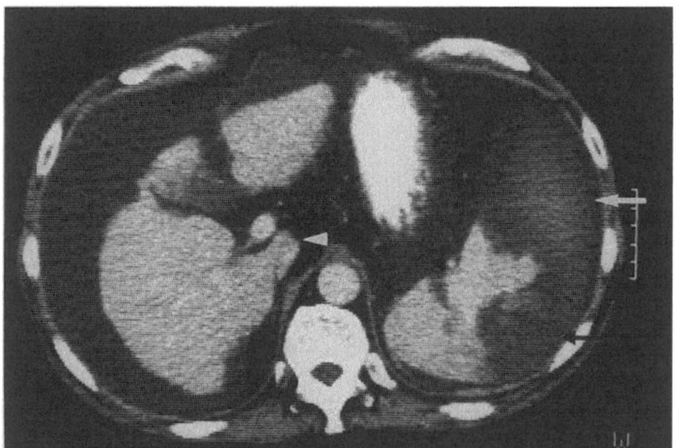

**Fig. 8.** Liver cirrhosis. Several radiologic signs are observed: lobulation of contours, caudate lobe enlargement (*arrowhead*), and ascites. Splenomegaly is evident; hypodense areas due to previous therapeutic splenic embolization are clearly depicted (*arrows*)

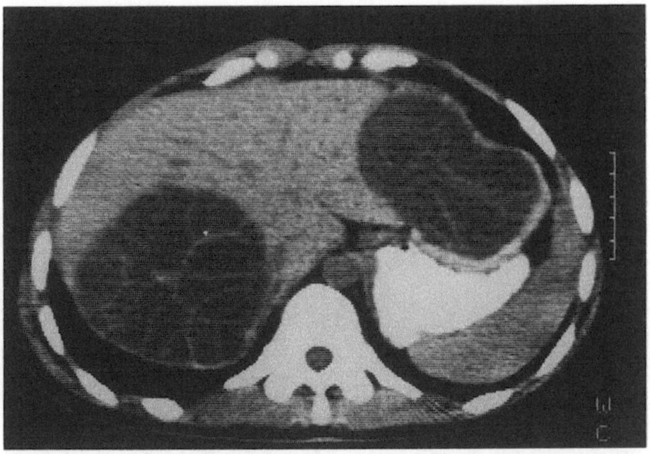

**Fig. 9.** Multiple hydatid cysts. Unilocular cyst in the left lobe shows membrane detachment; the lesion observed in the right lobe presents the typical appearance of a multivesicular cyst. Both lesions are clearly delineated from the surrounding normal liver

Hemangioma is the most common benign hepatic tumor. Dynamic CT studies allow its characterization in 56%–85% of cases (hypodense mass with contrast enhancement from the periphery to the center, with isodense filling compared to the rest of the liver in delayed phases) [31–33] (Fig. 10). Atypical cases should be studied by means of MRI or $^{99m}$Tc red blood cell scintigraphy.

Focal nodular hyperplasia and hepatic cell adenomas may have a similar appearance on CT scans. On occasion, the central scar in focal nodular hyperplasia and the capsule in adenomas may be appreciated. Adenomas may be multiple and tend to bleed. Unenhanced CT may demonstrate areas of increased density within a hypodense lesion corresponding to recent intratumoral hemorrhage; this is a characteristic finding in adenoma (Fig. 11). Most of these lesions are hypervascular. Hepatic adenomas and focal nodular hyperplasia typically present as a discrete mass or masses that show homogeneous rapid, transient enhancement on dynamic CT, except in areas with acute or remote hemorrhage. For the diagnosis of these lesions, the utilization of diverse procedures is required (scintigraphy, US, CT, angiography, etc.) [34, 35]. Nevertheless, on many occasions exact diagnosis is not obtained even by PFNAB (larger gauge needles carry a high risk of hemorrhage) and therefore surgery may be needed.

Hepatocellular carcinoma is the most frequent malignant primary hepatic tumor. In our environment, it appears as a complication of cirrhosis of any etiology (alcoholic, viral, hemochromatosis, etc.). Studies using CT and US have a sensitivity close to 90% in different series. The CT scan demonstrates the localization of the tumor, venous invasion, and extra-

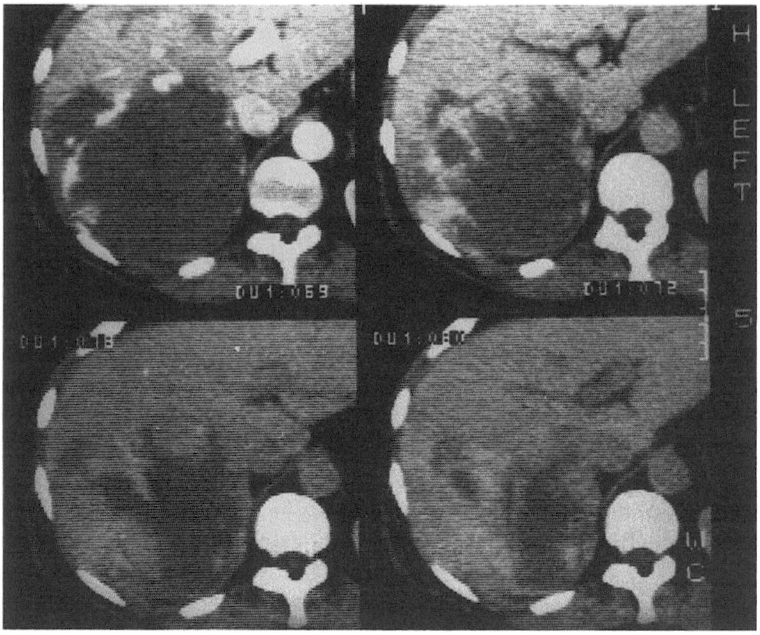

**Fig. 10.** Hepatic cavernous hemangioma. Sequential liver CT scan after bolus injection of contrast. There is a hypodense area in the right lobe which enhances peripherally. Progressive centripetal filling of the lesion is seen 10 min later

hepatic metastasis. At the same time, it serves as a guide to percutaneous biopsy. Usually, the tumor is seen as a unifocal or multifocal mass with decreased attenuation and heterogeneous contrast enhancement [25, 28, 36] (Fig. 12). The diffuse, infiltrating form can be difficult to detect but can be recognized after a bolus of contrast material.

Fibrolamellar hepatocellular carcinoma is a variant of hepatocellular carcinoma that has a better prognosis and, generally, appears in young patients with no underlying liver disease. Using CT, we can better appreciate its delineation, compartmentalization, and central scar and the possible presence of calcification [37].

Metastases are the most common malignant tumors of the liver. They may be solitary or multifocal (Fig. 6). Generally, in CT they appear as solid lesions with diminished attenuation relative to the normal hepatic parenchyma [26, 27, 31, 38]. Nevertheless, some hypervascular metastases (hypernephroma, carcinoid tumors, melanoma, etc.) may show contrast enhancement and become isodense with respect to the rest of the liver. Metastases of primary mucinous tumors with necrosis can develop calcifications.

Gallbladder disorders may be studied using CT but usually they are diagnosed by US. Both US and CT have been advocated as the initial

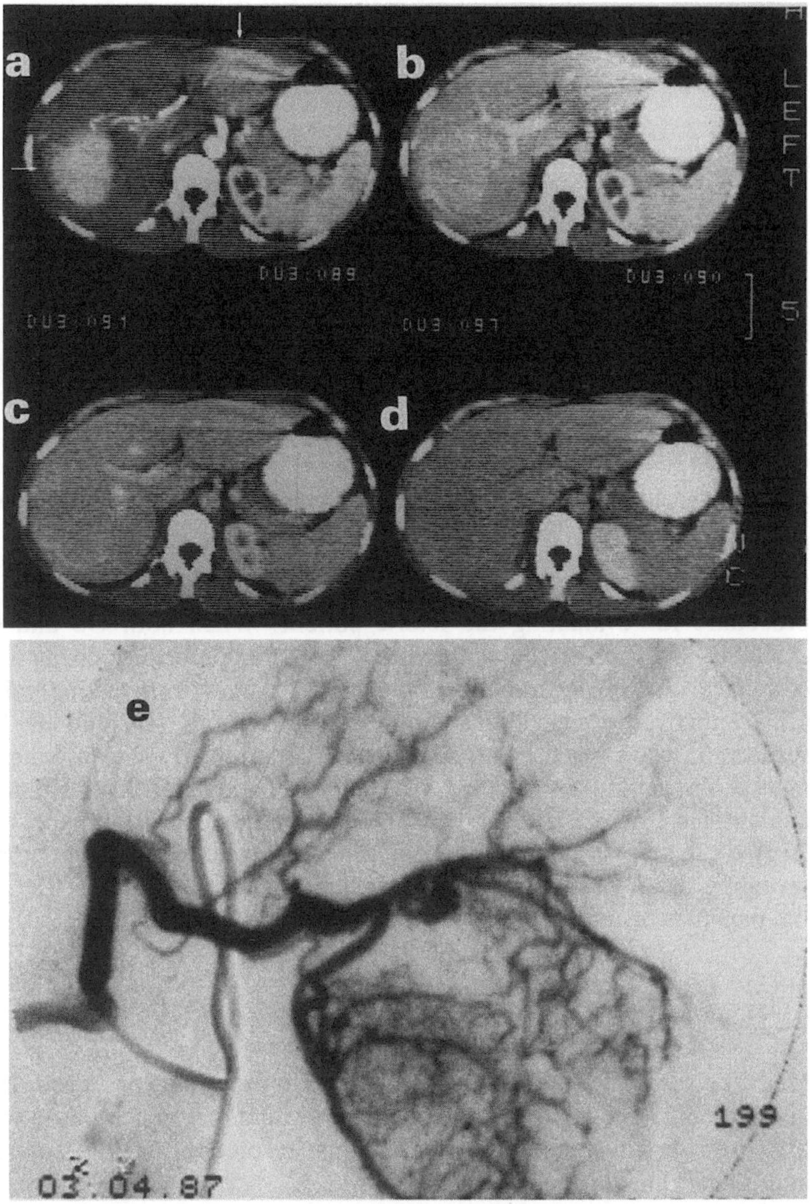


**Fig. 11a–e.** Hepatic adenomas (dynamic CT scan). **a** Early arterial phase. Marked hypervascularization of lesions located in both lobes (*arrows*). **b** Thirty seconds later (portal phase) the lesions are becoming isodense with the normal liver. **c,d** One and two minutes later both lesions are hypodense. **e** Left hepatic arteriography: well-delineated hypervascular lesion with tumoral vessels entering the lesion from the periphery

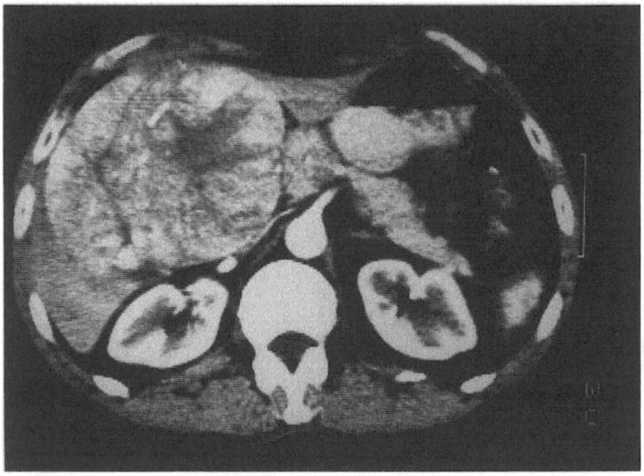

**Fig. 12.** Hepatocellular carcinoma (bolus CT scan in arterial phase). Well-delineated mass with intense and heterogeneous enhancement

procedure for evaluating the icteric patient. When both US and CT are available, US is preferred as the initial screening procedure owing to its low cost, lack of ionizing radiation, and high accuracy in detecting gallstones. CT is employed whenever US findings are ambiguous, when a mass lesion is suspected, when the distal common duct is not clearly shown, when a segmental obstruction is suspected, or when a hepatic parenchymal abnormality is identified [39]. CT shows whether the jaundice is obstructive or not, the level of the obstruction, and sometimes the etiology. CT is superior in revealing distal obstructions (choledocholithiasis, neoplasia of the head of the pancreas or ampulla, etc.).

## 8 Hepatic Magnetic Resonance Imaging

Magnetic resonance imaging is a technique in development, whose final role in hepatobiliary diagnosis remains to be evaluated. As compared with CT, MRI has the advantage of better contrast resolution and the possibility of multiplanar imaging.

Magnetic resonance imaging of the liver is performed to detect primary or metastatic neoplastic lesions, to document patency of intrahepatic veins, to define the extent of disease for preoperative planning, to differentiate hemangiomas from malignant neoplasms, and to demonstrate vascular and portosystemic shunt patency. Given the high dependence of CT on contrast media for its efficacy and the fact that MRI is comparable to contrast-aided CT, MRI should be the imaging modality of choice in any patient with a contraindication to contrast media [40].

Magnetic resonance imaging is the most sensitive imaging method in the detection of hepatic masses. The increase in sensitivity impinges especially on surgical indications. With the introduction of more aggressive procedures, more patients benefit from segmental resections in attempts to cure hepatic malignancy. Therefore, in addition to showing the existence or not of metastases, it is necessary to define the extension (number and location of metastatic foci) with precision [41]. MRI has a greater potential for characterizing hepatic lesions than any other tomographic technique.

Hepatic cysts and hemangiomas are hypointense on T1-weighted images and extremely hyperintense on T2-weighted images. Generally, hemangiomas are well delimited; they present smooth contours or, more frequently, lobulated as well as central heterogeneous zones (fibrosis, thrombosis or calcifications) [42, 43].

MRI allows distinction between FNH and adenomas owing to the former's isointensity on all pulse sequences, the central scar being hypointense on T1-weighted images and hyperintense on T2-weighted images [44].

Nodular hepatocellular carcinomas and their satellite nodules are usually hyperintense on T2-weighted images, while on T1-weighted images they are either isointense or slightly hyperintense owing to fatty metamorphosis (Fig. 13) [45]. A peripheral rim, hypointense on T1-weighted images and hyperintense on T2-weighted images, is sometimes present. Vascular invasion (portal thrombosis), hyperintensity of the liver, and focal atrophy are additional characteristics.

Metastasic lesions are heterogeneous and can present a central zone of necrosis, badly delimited margins, and peritumoral edema. These features are more evident on T2-weighted images, where they do not appear as

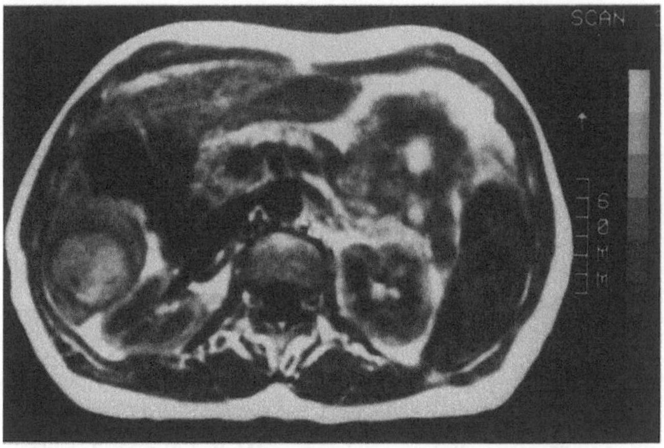


**Fig. 13.** Nodular hepatocellular carcinoma (T1-weighted image). Slightly hyperintense lesion due to fatty metamorphosis, with hypointense peripheral rim

hyperintense as hemangiomas (except in the case of certain hypervascular metastases like pancreatic insulinoma, pheochromocytoma, and soft tissue sarcomas) [42, 43].

Spectroscopic studies by MRI are currently still at the experimental stage.

## 9 Hepatic Angiographic Studies

Until the arrival of sectional techniques (US and CT), hepatic arteriography and other vascular studies were the most accurate method for analysis of a liver mass [46–48]. The indications for a vascular study have now changed dramatically. The role of hepatic vascular studies for diagnostic purposes is confined to aiding sectional studies (CTAP) [49–51] (Fig. 6b) or to confirming the presence of or analyzing a suspected liver mass when other, nonaggressive, methods have failed [52]. However, the role of vascular studies in therapeutic intervention is expanding.

In hepatic arteriography, sequential films are obtained during the injection of contrast into the vascular pedicle of the liver (mainly the common hepatic artery). Contrast is injected by means of a catheter placed percutaneously via a peripheral vascular approach (usually the common femoral artery).

Vascular displacements, amputations, areas of hypervascularization, and arteriovenous shunts are signs that must be looked for on the sequential films. Recently, the introduction of computerized techniques (digital sub-

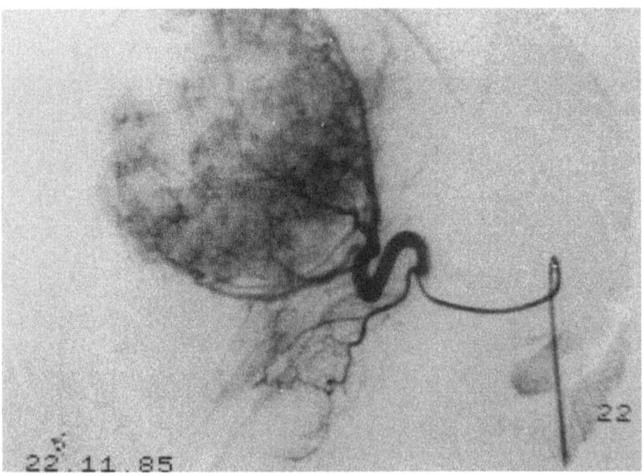


**Fig. 14.** Hepatocellular carcinoma. Well-delineated lesion with arterial branches entering from the periphery. Several areas of neovascularization and necrosis are observed within the lesion

traction angiography) [53] has permitted better definition and enabled additional data to be obtained (quantification of parenchymal contrast uptake in different areas, etc.).

As already pointed out, hepatic arteriography is now scarcely performed for diagnostic purposes [46–48]. Hepatic adenoma, focal nodular hyperplasia, and hepatocellular carcinoma (Figs. 11e, 14) can be detected and differentiated with angiography but today this can be achieved with other nonaggressive methods like dynamic CT or radionuclide studies or even by PFNAB and cytologic study. In some specific situations, e.g., atypical cavernous hemangiomas, arteriography is still needed.

A few years ago, several Japanese authors observed the persistence of Lipiodol in the tumor mass and peritumoral neovascular vessels. This observation suggested the possibility of treating tumoral masses (mainly hepatocellular carcinomas) with selective injection of Lipiodol-antitumoral drugs and subsequent embolization of the tumoral vessels (liver chemoembolization) [54–56]. With this therapeutic approach, tumor necrosis and increased life expectancy have been observed. Other interventional procedures can be performed for therapeutic purposes: intraarterial chemotherapy for inoperable tumors, superselective embolization in liver parenchymal bleeding and hemobilia, etc. [57–61].

Portographic studies have maintained or even gained actuality. In spite of sectional studies, portography is still often needed in order to analyze portosystemic collaterals in portal hypertension or to detect vascular tumoral infiltrations in presurgical planning. Portal interventional procedures are performed in different circumstances, but mainly in the control of variceal bleeding in portal hypertension [62]. A percutaneous transhepatic approach to the portal vein with superselective catheterization of the bleeding vessel and its subsequent occlusion has been used as a therapeutic modality. Other percutaneous interventional procedures, e.g., the creation of a stable portocaval shunt using a transjugular approach and the insertion of an expandable endoprosthesis, have recently been added to the therapeutic armamentarium for portal hypertension, and initial results have been promising [63].

## 10 Biliary Invasive Studies

There are basically two invasive techniques for study of the biliary system: percutaneous transhepatic cholangiography (PTC) and endoscopic retrograde cholangiopancreatography (ERCP). Both provide radiologic images of high quality for diagnostic purposes [64, 65].

Percutaneous transhepatic cholangiography is an old and well-known technique that involves percutaneous insertion of a fine needle (Chiba needle) into a biliary radicle. Needle insertion is performed under local anesthesia at the level of the middle axillary line. Once a biliary radicle is

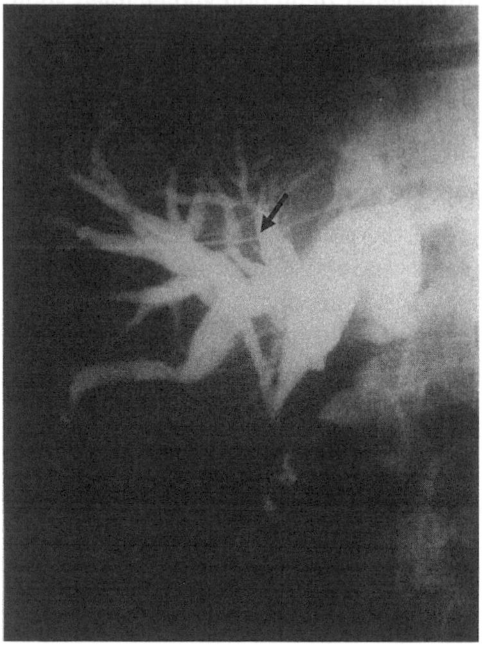

**Fig. 15.** Cholangiocarcinoma (technique: PTC). Severe dilatation of bile radicles in both lobes due to a common hepatic duct obstruction (*arrow*: fine needle entering a left lobe radicle)

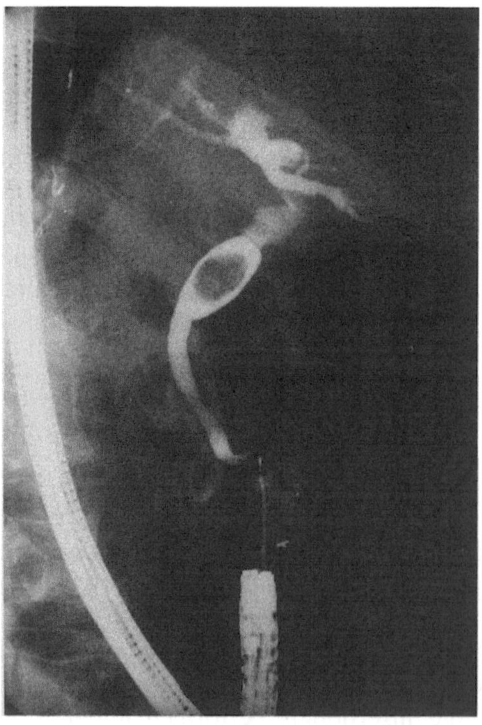

**Fig. 16.** Bile duct stone (technique: ERCP)

punctured, bile is extracted for cytologic and microbiologic purposes and contrast is introduced in order to detect and delineate the cause of the biliary obstruction [66] (Fig. 15)

In spite of the use of fine needles and even if the operator is highly skilled, PTC is not free of complications such as pneumothorax, massive bleeding, and septicemia [67]. For this reason, ERCP has recently gained great popularity. This technique is performed with the aid of an endoscope placed in the duodenum and a small catheter traversing the sphincter of Oddi for the injection of contrast medium (Fig. 16). Although this technique is safer than PTC, more skill is needed on the part of the operator, and some complications have been reported [68, 69].

Both techniques not only yield high-quality images but also permit, under fluoroscopic guidance, interventional techniques in order to palliate cholestasis, retrieve retained biliary stones, dilate postsurgical stenosis, etc. This new therapeutic approach (catheter biliary intervention), percutaneously or endoscopically performed, is now an important indication for PTC or ERCP [70, 71].

## References


1. Cooperberg PL, Gibney RG (1987) Imaging of the gallbladder, 1987. Radiology 163:605–613
2. Maglinte DDT, Torres WE, Laufer I (1991) Oral cholecystography in contemporary gallstone imaging: a review. Radiology 178:49–58
3. Whalen JP, Rizzuti RJ, Evans JA (1972) Time of optimal gallbladder opacification with Telepaque (iopanoic acid). Radiology 105:523–524
4. Drum DF (1982) Current status of radiocolloid hepatic scintiphotography for space-occupying disease. Semin Nucl Mde 12:64–74
5. Rosenthall L, Shaffer EA, Lisbona R, Parc P (1978) Diagnosis of hepatobiliary disease by $^{99m}$Tc-HIDA cholescintigraphy. Radiology 126:467–747
6. Lieberman DA, Krishnamurthy GT (1986) Intrahepatic versus extrahepatic cholestasis discrimination with biliary scintigraphy combined with ultrasound. Gastroenterology 90:734–743
7. Lee AW, Ram MD, Shih W-J et al. (1986) Technetium 99m HIDA biliary scintigrapy in the evaluation of the jaundiced patient. J Nucl Med 12:1407–1412
8. Tsan MF, Scheffel U (1986) Mechanism of gallium-67 accumulation in tumors. Nucl Med 27:1215–1219
9. Tsan MF (1985) Mechanism of gallium-67 accumulation in inflammatory lesions. J Nucl Med 26:88–92
10. Rabinowitz SA, McKusick KA, Strauss HW (1984) 99m Tc red blood cell scintigraphy in evaluating focal liver lesions. AJR 143:63–68
11. Moinuddin M, Allison JR, Montgomery JH et al. (1985) Scintigraphic diagnosis of hepatic hemangioma: its role in the management of hepatic mass lesions. AJR 145:223–228
12. Jaszczak RS, Whitehead FR, Lim CB, Coleman RE (1982) Lesion detection with single-photon emission computed tomography (SPECT) compared with conventional imaging. J Nucl Med 23:97–102
13. Deland FH, Shih WJ (1984) The status of SPECT in tumor diagnosis. J Nucl Med 25:1375–1379

14. Ralls PW (1990) Color Doppler sonography of the hepatic artery and portal venous system. AJR 155:517–525
15. Patriquin H, Lafortune M, Burns PN, Dauzat M (1987) Duplex Doppler examination in portal hypertension: technique and anatomy. AJR 149:71–76
16. Rifkin ND, Rosato FE, Branch M et al. (1987) Intraoperative ultrasound of the liver: an important adjunctive tool for decision making in the operating room. Ann Surg 205:446–471
17. Kawashima A, Suehiro S, Murayama S, Russell WJ (1986) Focal fatty infiltration of the liver mimicking a tumor: sonographic and CT features. J Comput Assist Tomogr 10:329–331
18. Richard PH, Bouniaud P, Barthelemy C et al. (1985) Valeur de l'ultrasonographie dans le diagnostic des cirrhoses: étude prospective de 128 patients. J Radiol 66:503–506
19. Gaines PA, Sampson MA (1989) Prevalence and characterization of simple hepatic cysts by ultrasound examination. Br J Radiol 62:335–337
20. Lewall DB, McCorkell SJ (1985) Hepatic echinococcal cysts: sonographic appearance and classification. Radiology 155:773–775
21. Cooperberg PL, Burhenne HS (1980) Real-time ultrasonography. Diagnostic technique of choice in calculous gallbladder disease. N Engl J Med 302:1277–1279
22. Madrazo BL, Francis I, Hricak H, Sandler MA, Hudak S, Gitschlag K (1982) Sonographic findings in perforation of the gallbladder. AJR 139:491–496
23. MacDonald FR, Cooperberg PL, Cohen MM (1981) The WES triad: a specific sonographic sign of gallstones in the contracted gallbladder. Gastrointest Radiol 6:39–41
24. Platt JF, Glazer GM (1988) IV contrast material for abdominal CT. Comparison of three methods of administration. AJR 151:275–277
25. Matsui O, Takashima T, Kadoya M et al. (1985) Dynamic computed tomography during arterial portography: the most sensitive examination for small hepatocellular carcinoma. J Comput Assist Tomogr 9:19–24
26. Matsui O, Takashima T, Kadoya M et al. (1987) Liver metastases from colorectal cancers: detection with CT during arterial portography. Radiology 165:65–69
27. Bernardino ME, Erwing BC, Steinberg HV et al. (1986) Delayed hepatic CT scanning: increased confidence and improved detection of hepatic metastases. Radiology 159:71–74
28. Yumoto Y, Jinno K, Tokuyama K et al. (1985) Hepatocellular carcinoma detected by iodized oil. Radiology 154:19–24
29. Torres WE, Whitmire LF, Geddaudas-McKleesk, Bernardino ME (1986) Computed tomography of hepatic morphologic changes in cirrhosis of the liver. J Comput Assist Tomogr 10:47–50
30. De Diego J, Lecumberri FJ, Franquet T, Ostiz S (1982) Computed tomography in hepatic echinococcosis. AJR 139:699–702
31. Freeny PC, Marks WM (1986) Patterns of contrast enhancement of benign and malignant hepatic neoplasms during bolus dynamic and delayed CT. Radiology 160:613–618
32. Freeny PC, Marks WM (1986) Hepatic hemangioma: dynamic bolus CT. AJR 147:711–719
33. Ashida CH, Fishman EK, Zerhouni EA, Herlog FH, Siegelman SS (1987) Computed tomography of hepatic cavernous hemangioma. J Comput Assist Tomogr 11:455–460
34. Welch TJ, Sheedy PF, Johnson CM et al. (1985) Focal nodular hyperplasia and hepatic adenoma: comparison of angiography, CT, US and scintigraphy. Radiology 156:593–595
35. Mathieu D, Brunneton JN, Drouillard J, Pointreau CC, Vasile N (1986) Hepatic adenomas and focal nodular hyperplasia: dynamic CT study. Radiology 160:53–58

36. Itay Y, Araki T, Furni S et al. (1981) Differential diagnosis of hepatic mass on computed tomography with particular reference to hepatocellular carcinoma. J Comput Assist Tomogr 5:834–842
37. Adam A, Gibson RN, Soreide O et al. (1986) The radiology of fibrolamellar hepatoma. Clin Radiol 37:355–358
38. Miller DL, Simmons JT, Chang R et al. (1987) Hepatic metastases detection. Comparison of three CT contrast enhancement methods. Radiology 165:785–790
39. Moss AA (1983) Computed tomography of the hepatobiliary system. In: Moss AA, Gamsu G, Genant HK (eds) Computed tomography of the body. W.B. Saunders, Philadelphia, p 676
40. Mattrey R, Trambat M, Edelman RR (1990) MR imaging of the upper abdomen and adrenal glands. In: Edelman RR, Hesselink JR (eds) MRI clinical magnetic resonance imaging. W.B. Saunders, Philadelphia, p 854
41. Ferrucci JT, Freeny PC, Stark DD et al. (1988) Advances in hepatobiliary radiology. Radiology 168:319–338
42. Wittemberg J, Stark DD, Forman BH et al. (1988) Differentiation of hepatic metastases from hepatic hemangiomas and cysts by using MR imaging. AJR 151:79–84
43. Ferrucci JT (1986) MR imaging of the liver. AJR 147:1103–1116
44. Mattison GR, Glazer GM, Quint LE et al. (1987) MR imaging of hepatic focal nodular hyperplasia: characterization and distinction from primary malignant hepatic tumors. AJR 148:711–715
45. Rummeny E, Weissleder R, Stark DD et al. (1989) Primary liver tumors: diagnosis by MR imaging. AJR 152:63–72
46. Reuter SR, Redman HC, Siders DB (1970) The spectrum of angiographic findings in hepatoma. Radiology 94:89–94
47. Okuda K, Obatta H, Jinnouchi S et al. (1977) Angiographic assessment of gross anatomy of hepatocellular carcinoma: comparison of celiac angiograms and liver pathology in 100 cases. Radiology 123:21–29
48. Goldstein HM, Heiman HL, Mena E et al. (1974) Angiographic findings in benign liver cell tumors. Radiology 119:339–343
49. Heiken JP, Weyman PJ, Lee JKT et al. (1989) Detection of focal hepatic masses: prospective evaluation with CT. Delayed CT, CT during arterial portography and MR imaging. Radiology 171:47–51
50. Passariello R (1985) Angio-CT. Techniques. Eur J Radiol 5:193–198
51. Vlachos L, Trakadas S, Gouliamas A, Lazarou S, Moorikes D, Ioannu R (1990) Comparative study between ultrasound, computed tomography, intra-arterial digital subtraction angiography, and magnetic resonance imaging in the differentiation of tumors of the liver. Gastrointest Radiol 15:102–106
52. Okuda K, Musha H, Yoshida T et al. (1975) Demonstration of growing casts of hepatocellular carcinoma in the portal vein by celiac angiography: the thread and streaks sign. Radiology 117:303–309
53. Takahashi K, Furuse M, Saito K et al. (1989) Intra-arterial digital subtraction angiography in the detection of hepatocellular carcinoma. Cardiovasc Intervent Radiol 12:61–65
54. Inoue H, Kobayashi H, Itoh Y, Shinohara S (1989) Treatment of liver metastases by arterial injection of adriamycin/mitomycin C Lipiodol suspension. Acta Radiol 30:603–608
55. Guo S, Yen D, Huang B, Hu G, Liv P (1989) Transcatheter arterial chemoembolization with anticancer drug in iodized oil for primary hepatic carcinoma. Cardiovasc Intervent Radiol 12:181–187
56. Raby N, Karani J, Michell M, Gimson A, Nunnerly H, Williams R (1989) Lipiodol enhanced CT scanning in assessment of hepatocellular carcinoma. Clin Radiol 40:480–485
57. Cho KJ, Andrews JC, Williams DM, Doenz F, Guy GE (1989) Hepatic arterial chemotherapy. Role of angiography. Radiology 173:783–791

58. Charnsangavej CH, Carrasco CH, Wallace S, Richli W, Haynie TP (1987) Hepatic arterial flow distribution with hepatic neoplasms: significance in infusion chemotherapy. Radiology 165:71–73
59. Patt YZ, Charnsangavej CH, Boddie A et al. (1989) Treatment of hepatocellular carcinoma with hepatic arterial fluoxuridine, doxorubicin and mitomycin C (FUDRAM) with or without hepatic artery embolization: factors associated with longer survivals. Reg Cancer Treat 2:98–104
60. Kuroda CH, Sakurai M, Monden M et al. (1989) Transcatheter arterial embolization for metastatic liver tumors: a study in resected cases. Cardiovasc Intervent Radiol 12:72–75
61. Coldwell DM (1990) Hepatic arterial embolization utilizing a coaxial catheter system: technical note. Cardiovasc Intervent Radiol 13:53–54
62. Okuda K, Kimura K, Takayasu K (1982) Percutaneous transhepatic portography and sclerotheraphy. Semin Liver Dis 2:57–66
63. Richter GM, Noeldge G, Palmaz JC, Roessle M (1990) The transjugular intrahepatic portosystemic stent-shunt (TISS): results of a pilot study. Cardiovasc Intervent Radiol 13:200–207
64. Scharschmidt BF, Goldberg HI, Schmidt R (1983) Approach to the patient with cholestatic jaundice. N Engl J Med 308:1515–1519
65. Richter JM, Silverstein MD, Schapiro R (1983) Suspected obstructive jaundice: a decision analysis of diagnostic strategies. Ann Intern Med 99:46–51
66. Ferrucci JT, Freeny PC, Stark DD et al. (1988) Symposium: advances in hepatobiliary radiology. Radiology 168:319–338.
67. Hoevels S, Nilsson U (1980) Intrahepatic vascular lesions following nonsurgical percutaneous transhepatic bile duct intubation. Gastrointest Radiol 5:127–135
68. Summerfield JA (1988) Biliary obstruction is best managed by endoscopists. Gut 29:741–745
69. Zimmon DS, Breslaw J, Kessler RE (1975) Endoscopy with endocopic cholangiopancreatography. The combination as a primary diagnostic procedure. JAMA 233:447–449
70. Zimmon DS, Falkenstein DB, Kessler RE (1976) Management of biliary calculi by retrograde endoscopic instrumentation (lithocenosis). Gastrointest Endoscopy 23:82–86
71. Coons HG, Carey PH (1983) Large-bore, long biliary endoprostheses (biliary stents) for improved drainage. Radiology 148:89–94

## Suggested Reading

Berk PD (ed). Hepatic imaging. Semin Liver Dis 9

Castañeda-Zúñiga WR, Tadavarthy SM (1988) Interventional radiology. Williams and Wilkins, Baltimore.

Dondelinger RF, Rossi P, Kurdziel JC, Wallace S (1990) Interventional radiology. Thieme, Stuttgart.

Edelman RR, Hesselink JR (1990) Clinical magnetic resonance imaging. W.B. Saunders, Philadelphia

Freeny PC (1990) Radiologic diagnosis of hepatic neoplasm. Postgrad Radiol 10:265–284

Friedman AC (1987) Radiology of the liver, biliary tract, pancreas and spleen. Williams and Wilkins, Baltimore

Johnsrude IS, Jackson DC, Dunnick MR (1987) A practical approach to angiography, 2nd edn. Little, Brown & Co., Boston

Lee JKT (1989) Computed body tomography with MRI correlation, 2nd edn. Raven, New York

Mittelstaedt CA (1987) Abdominal ultrasound. Churchill-Li-vingstone, New York
Zeman RK, Burrell MI (1987) Gallbladder and bile duct imaging. A clinical radiologic approach. Churchill-Li-vingstone, New York

# 6 The Role of Direct Morphologic Methods

## A. Liver Biopsy and Elementary Hepatic Lesions

J.J. VÁZQUEZ and A. MORENO

### 1 Introduction

Classification of liver diseases relies mainly upon morphologic alterations. Therefore, liver biopsy is mandatory for the correct diagnosis of most liver diseases and plays a central role in the prognosis and treatment of patients.

Needle biopsy is the technique usually employed. The specimen must be handled with care, avoiding unnecessary handling. After its fixation, usually in 10% buffered formalin, it is embedded in paraffin. A small piece may be taken for electron microscopy, which requires a special procedure. When hepatic porphyria is suspected, the observation of the unfixed specimen under Wood's light is mandatory. The stains routinely applied are: hematoxylin and eosin, reticulin, periodic acid-Schiff, trichrome, Perl's Prussian blue, and Shikata's stain for HBsAg and elastic fibers.

In the presentation of this chapter, we have followed the steps a pathologist undertakes when analyzing a hepatic biopsy. After considering the macroscopic description, the initial approach to the microscopic examination is to assess the lobular architecture as a whole. Then, the examination proceeds from the general aspects to particular details. For instance, when dealing with the hepatic parenchyma, attention is paid first to the liver cell plates, then to the entire hepatocyte, and finally to the cellular parts (i.e., cytoplasm and nucleus).

### 2 Hepatic Architecture and Its Alterations

Here we will only deal with histologic features of particular interest for biopsy interpretation.

Obviously, the architecture may be normal, altered without cirrhosis, or cirrhotic. It may be assumed that the *normal* liver structure is preserved when the conventional units, the acini, have a normal appearance, i.e., when there are interconnecting liver cell plates, usually one cell thick, separated from each other by the sinusoids. Liver cell plates appear to radiate from the hepatic venule. Portal tracts and hepatic venules are regularly and alternately arranged, being 500 (±200) μm apart from each other. This kind of regular alternation allows us to speak of preserved

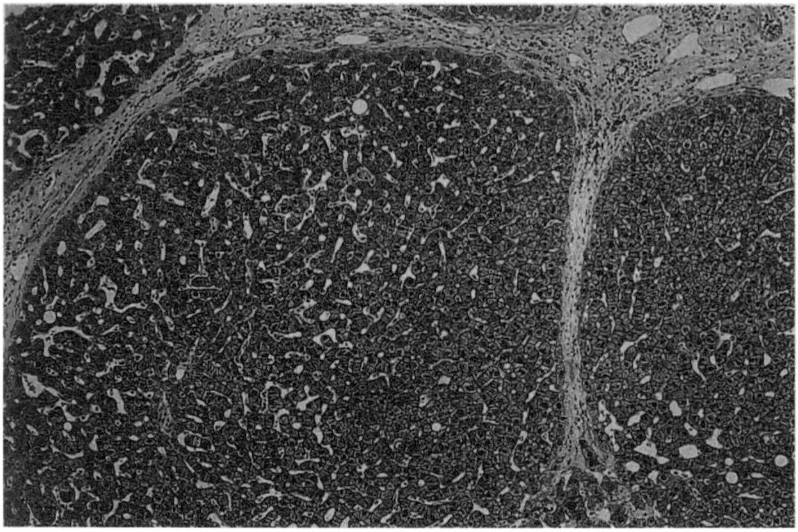

**Fig. 1.** Macronodular cirrhosis, incomplete septal variant. Well-differentiated nodules demarcated by often incomplete, slender septa. Trichrome, ×80

structural relationships between portal tracts and central veins, which is the most relevant feature of architectural integrity. Normal alternation is lost in some diseases, particularly in the case of cirrhosis. When the specimen includes only tissue from a cirrhotic macronodule, this may be the single diagnostic feature [1].

In other cases, the architecture may be *abnormal*, but without evidence of cirrhosis. Usually the abnormal structure is recognized by fibrosis which is manifested as a confluent septal fibrosis, to be discussed below. This is observed (a) in different chronic liver diseases before the development of cirrhosis; (b) as residual change after severe liver injury, for instance, after severe acute hepatitis with confluent necrosis; and (c) in chronic venous congestion. In addition to fibrosis, structural changes without cirrhosis may be found in cases of focal hyperplasia and nodule formation, which will be considered when dealing with the liver cell plates.

In still other cases, there is a *cirrhotic* architecture, characterized by the replacement of the normal acinar structure by nodules separated by fibrous septa. This is easily recognized in the case of micronodular cirrhosis when there is an adequate sample. In contrast, it may be very difficult to recognize in macronodular cirrhosis unless large samples are available (Fig. 1). In this case, it is necessary to apply criteria of "high confidence," such as the presence of round fragments (nodules), demarcated by connective tissue, or criteria of "probability," such as the finding of slender fibrous septa which intersect the parenchyma and the presence of hepatic venules in excess, placed very close to each other and to broad fibrous bands. In addition to these changes, regenerative activity produces distortion of the architecture due to focal expansion of the liver cell plates, which in some fields are two or more cells thick. This growth at different rates leads to the development of nodules within nodules. In the absence of obvious fibrosis, when these subtle features are present, the diagnosis of macronodular cirrhosis must be considered as very probable [1].

When the biopsy sample is not fully representative, the clinical features become more important than the histologic findings.

## 3 Portal Tracts

Portal tracts, located at the periphery of the classic lobule, are the intrahepatic branches of the connective tissue which enters the liver through the hilum. In these portal tracts, connective tissue branches of portal vein, hepatic artery, and bile ducts, together with efferent lymph vessels, are embedded. In a biopsy sample, three categories of portal tract can be observed according to their size: the larger ones are referred to as septal or trabecular and they have an irregular stellate shape; the middle-sized tracts are interlobular, having a triangular shape; and the smaller ones are referred to as terminal portal tracts, being round.

In portal tracts attention should be paid to the inflammatory infiltrate, alterations of the connective tissue, bile ducts, and vascular disorders.

### 3.1 Inflammatory Infiltrate

The degree, cell type, and location of the inflammatory infiltrate is very useful for accurate diagnosis. In a normal liver few lymphocytes may be found. The inflammatory infiltrate usually consists of different cell types, although a particular type commonly prevails.

#### *Predominant Lymphocytic Infiltrate*

Predominant lymphocytic infiltrate comprises lymphocytes and sometimes plasma cells and some macrophages. According to the location, two different types of infiltrate may be distinguished.

1. *Infiltrate limited to portal stroma*. This takes the form of infiltration with lymphocytes which is heavier in the center of the portal tracts. This type of infiltrate is found in chronic persistent hepatitis (Fig. 2), acute hepatitis (there are then associated liver cell changes), reactive hepatitis, and primary biliary cirrhosis. In chronic hepatitis, the infiltrates usually are heavy and most or all tracts are affected. In contrast, in reactive hepatitis there is an irregular distribution, with sparing of some portal tracts.

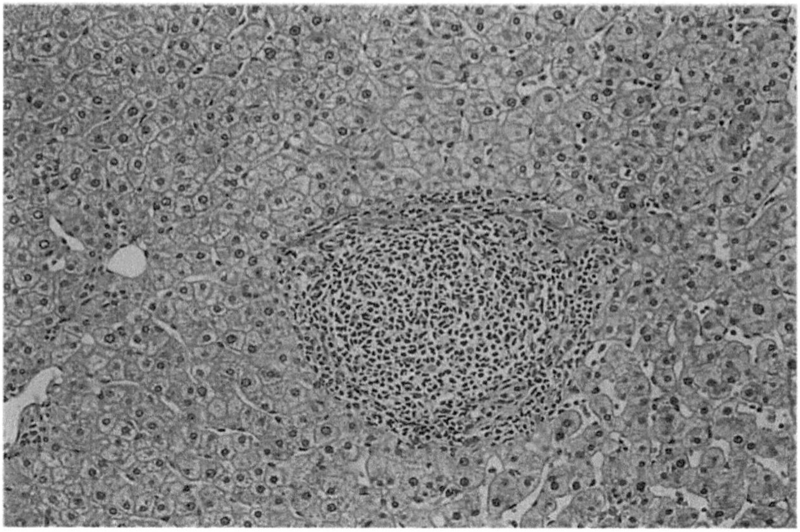

**Fig. 2.** Chronic persistent hepatitis. The portal tract is heavily infiltrated with lymphoid cells. H&E, ×150

2. *Periportal infiltrate with piecemeal necrosis*. The infiltration is predominantly located at the periphery of the portal tract and extends to the adjacent periportal parenchyma, accompanying a process of erosion of the hepatocytic limiting plate (Fig. 3) that is known as "piecemeal" necrosis or erosive parcellar necrosis (see below). This is characteristic of chronic active hepatitis. In very severe cases, plasma cells may predominate.

Focal dense infiltrates made up of lymphocytes, often tightly aggregated, taking a follicular appearance, and located in portal tracts, are more often found in non-A, non-B hepatitis than in other types of hepatitis [2]. The macrophages which usually accompany the lymphocytes and plasma cells in these infiltrates may contain granules of different material in their cytoplasm, which may help diagnosis.

Diffuse or discrete atypical cell infiltrate of the liver is common in both myeloid and lymphocytic proliferative disorders. Its differential diagnosis from inflammatory infiltrates rests on the cytologic features and the more extensive, diffuse, and intense nature of the malignant infiltrate.

A polymorphous infiltrate, containing immunoblastic cells, is found in infectious mononucleosis and cytomegalovirus infection.

### *Predominant Neutrophilic Infiltrate*

In a normal liver, the portal tracts do not contain neutrophils; therefore, their presence, even in small numbers, must be considered abnormal. They are usually found together with edema of the connective tissue in different entities:

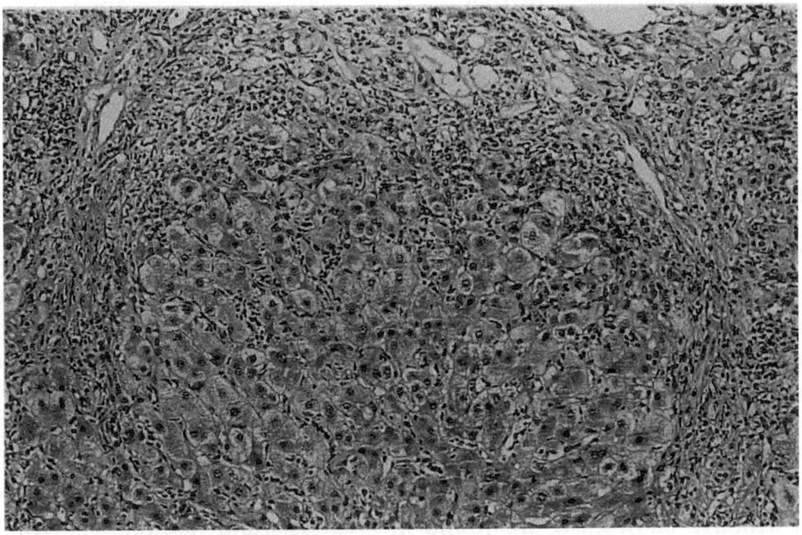

**Fig. 3.** Chronic active hepatitis. The interface between parenchyma and connective tissue is irregular due to liver cell necrosis (piecemeal necrosis). There are numerous lymphoid cells in this area. H&E, ×150

1. *In acute cholangitis*. The inflammatory infiltrate is located not only around the bile ducts but also in their walls and lumens. When an intermittent or partial *obstruction* is present (ascending cholangitis), there is a dense neutrophil infiltrate associated with parenchymatous cholestasis and ductular proliferation. Cholestasis may be absent, particularly when the inflammation is heavy. Bile ducts in small portal tracts are preferentially affected. In the case of prolonged obstruction, the infiltrate contains, in addition to neutrophils, increased numbers of plasma cells.

In 75% of cases of acute cholecystitis, portal tracts are acutely inflamed. In septicemia, the inflammation principally affects the canals of Hering, which contain inspissated bile, and larger ducts. Other causes of inflammation include acute cholangitis associated with congenital abnormalities of bile ducts (Caroli's disease, polycystic disease) and the peculiar oriental recurrent pyogenic cholangitis.

2. *In large bile duct obstruction*. The neutrophilic infiltrate is mild and located around ductules. The cholestasis is usually heavy.

3. *In other situations*. Neutrophils in portal tracts also may be found in intrahepatic cholestasis induced by drugs and other substances, in cholestatic viral hepatitis, in polyarteritis nodosa, and in alcoholic hepatitis, the latter suggesting concomitant pancreatitis.

Diffuse edema very often accompanies the neutrophilic infiltrate. It is more pronounced in the smaller terminal ramifications and is observed in acute large bile duct obstruction. The small portal tracts appear round and pale stained.

### *Predominant Eosinophilic Infiltrate*

Occasionally, scarce eosinophils may be found in the portal tract in normal liver. Their presence in rather large numbers may be related to systemic eosinophilia, to eosinophilic gastroenteritis, or to a primary liver disorder. Eosinophilic infiltrate without other changes has been described in systemic eosinophilia, in the paraneoplastic syndrome [particularly in cases of lymphoproliferative diseases and carcinomatosis (lung, ovary, and rectal carcinoma, mesothelioma)], associated with collagen or parasitic diseases (hydatid), and in toxic reactions.

The presence of an eosinophilic infiltrate associated with intrahepatic cholestasis and cholangitis or cytolytic changes points to a drug effect or to a viral infection. On the other hand, eosinophils in association with obstructive cholestasis are found in ascariasis and fascioliasis. Granulomas are present in Hodgkins's disease, parasitic infestation, particularly by *Toxocara*, and eosinophilic gastroenteritis. In polyarteritis nodosa, arterial lesions and infarctions may be found. Venous lesions are usually present in some parasitic diseases, such as schistosomiasis, and in the toxic oil syndrome [3].

### *Macrophages in Portal Tracts; Granulomas*

Macrophages loaded with hemosiderin granules are common in posttransfusional siderosis. Clumped macrophages containing ceroid pigment, which may also be iron-positive, are very often found in the late stage of acute viral hepatitis. PAS-positive granular macrophages may be found in widespread systemic involvement of Whipple's disease and other metabolic diseases.

Portal tract granulomas are observed in many conditions [4]: primary biliary cirrhosis, sarcoidosis, tuberculosis, Hodgkin's disease, schistosomiasis, chronic inflammatory bowel diseases (ulcerative colitis and Crohn's disease) and some gastrointestinal neoplasias, drug reactions (phenylbutazone, halothane, sulfonamide, steroids, allopurinol), and exposure to foreign material (contrast media, mineral oil as a food additive, narcotics). In many of these entities, granulomas are also found within the acinus.

## 3.2 Connective Tissue

### *Edema*

Edema, in addition to occurring in large bile duct obstruction (see above), is usually present in cholestatic acute hepatitis and in the second stage of primary biliary cirrhosis when ductular proliferation and neutrophil infiltrates are predominant features. Edema is also found in the vicinity of tumoral nodules. A particular type is periseptal lamellar edema (halo effect), which is found in precirrhotic and cirrhotic livers in which there is a prominent biliary obstructive component. It is recognized as parallel lamellae of very loose connective tissue arranged around the parenchymal nodules. When the lamellar edema fades, it leaves broad bands of connective tissue with parallel fibers.

### *Fibrosis*

Fibrosis may be *diffuse* or *periductal*. Diffuse fibrosis may be found in alcoholic liver disease, congenital hepatic fibrosis, and cirrhosis. Periductal fibrosis is found in patients with bile duct obstruction and particularly in primary and secondary sclerosing cholangitis. An "onion-skin" type of fibrosis develops around the bile ducts. In addition, in sclerosing cholangitis some ducts may disappear completely, being replaced by fibrous scars.

## 3.3 Bile Ducts

The bile ducts are usually centrally located in the portal tract near the artery and the vein. The smaller ducts, called terminal ducts, have a basement membrane and are lined by three to five cuboidal cells. They are found throughout the limiting plate and within the terminal portal tracts, forming the interlobular bile ducts, which anastomose and increase in size to form larger septal or trabecular ducts located in large portal tracts, lined by columnar cells.

When observing a biopsy, it is important to assess the number, caliber, and shape of the bile ducts, inflammatory lesions, and epithelial changes [5]. In normal liver, arteries are regularly accompanied by bile ducts.

### *Changes in Number, Caliber, and Shape*

Several entities are characterized by an absence of or a decrease in the number of bile ducts. In intrahepatic biliary atresia or paucity of bile ducts in childhood, the ducts progressively disappear. This is the hallmark of Alagille's syndrome. It must be taken into account that the paucity of bile ducts as the only histologic feature is not specific to any entity or syndrome and may be observed in other cholestatic conditions, among them $\alpha_1$-antitrypsin deficiency, coprostanic acidemia, some viral infections, and rare cases of intrahepatic familial cholestasis.

A decrease in bile duct number in adults is observed in primary biliary cirrhosis, primary sclerosing cholangitis, sarcoidosis, some drug-induced liver diseases, graft-versus-host disease, hepatic allograft rejection, and other chronic hepatic diseases [6].

An idiopathic adulthood ductopenia has recently been described in which the age of onset may be the only distinguishing feature from neonatal or infantile nonsyndromic intrahepatic bile duct paucity [7].

An increase in the number of bile ducts occurs particularly in obstructive cholestasis. Several causes of extrahepatic cholestasis may be considered, such as choledocholithiasis, "benign" stenosis (after surgery) and fistulas, chronic pancreatitis, extrahepatic biliary atresia, and cystic fibrosis. A quite different picture is the cholangiolar increase observed in intra- and extrahapatic cholestasis.

Bile ducts appear dilated in cases of obstruction, tumors, and notably in Caroli's disease (congenital dilatation of the intrahepatic bile ducts).

Finally, malformed ducts are found in polycystic disease, congenital hepatic fibrosis, and microhamartomatosis (Meyenburg's complexes). Histologically, there is an increase in the number of biliary channels, which appear to anastomose and are lined by a cuboidal, very regular epithelium. They are immersed in a dense fibrous stroma.

The bile ducts may contain bile thrombi (obstruction, cholestatic hepatitis, severe hemolysis, dehydration, sepsis, congenital hepatic fibrosis, microhamartoma), leukocytes (acute cholangitis), parasitic ova (ascariasis, schistosomiasis), blood, hemoglobin, and mucous plugs.

### *Inflammation*

Bile duct inflammation may be acute or chronic. In acute cholangitis, edema and neutrophilic infiltrate are found in and around the ducts (see above). A similar picture may be found in septicemia.

Some neutrophils may be found in large bile duct obstruction accompanying the edema.

In *primary biliary cirrhosis*, a chronic nonsuppurative destructive cholangitis leading to progressive fibrosis, the medium-sized (interlobular) bile ducts are affected. Four overlapping histologic stages have been described, reflecting the progression of the lesion.

The early lesions are focal and the bile ducts are segmentally affected. The bile duct epithelium becomes swollen and irregular. Some epithelial cells become vacuolated and more eosinophilic than normal. The basement membrane is focally disrupted and lymphocytes may extend into the epithelium. The damage to bile ducts may lead to rupture of the wall. Around the affected bile ducts there is an inflammatory infiltrate made up predominantly of lymphocytes which may form aggregates. Plasma cells may be numerous and a variable number of macrophages and eosinophils are also found. In relation to the ruptured ducts, granulomas develop (Fig. 4). They may be well-formed lesions, resembling those observed in sarcoidosis, or ill-defined collections of macrophages. The destruction of the bile ducts leads to a sharp reduction in their number. Similar lesions very occasionally occur

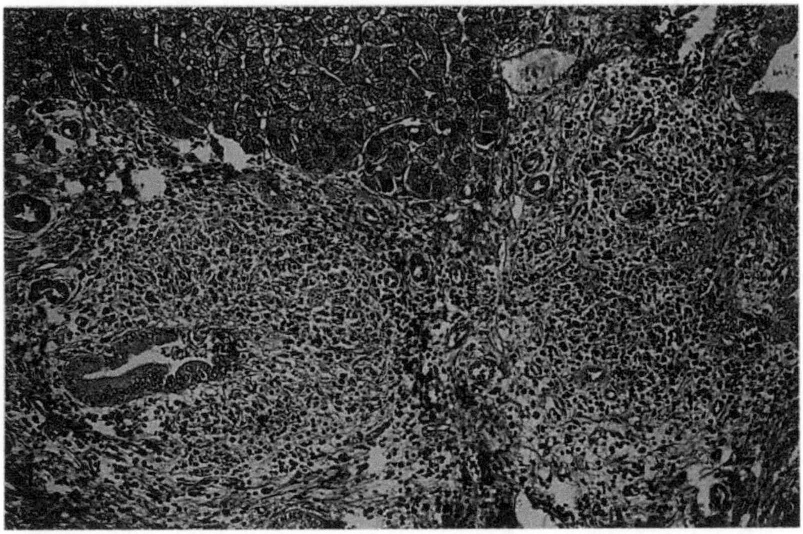

**Fig. 4.** Primary biliary cirrhosis. Epithelioid granulomas lie close to damaged interlobular bile ducts. The wall of the duct on the left has a focal rupture. Trichrome, ×150

in sarcoidosis and portal hypertension and may also be induced by some drugs. When disease progresses, histologic features of cholestasis become evident and the lesion extends beyond the portal tracts. The periportal inflammatory infiltrate, usually rich in neutrophils, together with the ductular transformation, produces a blurred appearance of the parenchyma–connective tissue interface (biliary piecemeal necrosis).

Bile ducts lesions consisting of marked plasma cell infiltration and occasional periductal granulomas have been observed in incomplete septal cirrhosis and idiopathic portal hypertension [6].

A dense concentric fibrosis may develop around the ducts (periductal fibrosis) in *sclerosing cholangitis* (Fig. 5), strictures of the biliary tree, ulcerative colitis, and chronic duct obstruction.

Bile duct injury is an essential part of the histologic changes of acute *liver allograft rejection*. The changes graded according to severity are: (a) mononuclear inflammatory infiltrate involving the bile duct epithelium, (b) pleomorphism of the epithelial cells with nuclear and cytoplasmic alterations, and (c) inflammatory disruption of the ductular walls, which may lead to complete disappearance of the duct [8, 9].

### 3.4 Portal Tract Vessels

Portal tracts contain branches of the hepatic artery, branches of the portal vein, and lymphatic vessels.

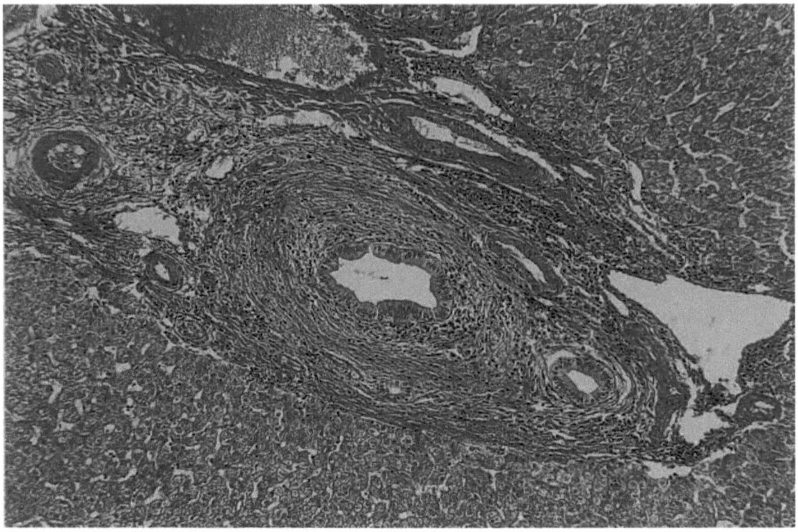

**Fig. 5.** Primary sclerosing cholangitis. Dense concentric fibrosis and inflammation are observed around a large bile duct. H&E, ×80

The branches of the hepatic arteries may be involved in the same diseases as other systemic arteries [10]. The wall may be thickened because of hyalinization, as occurs in systemic hypertension, diabetes mellitus, senility, amyloid deposits, and congenital hepatis fibrosis.

Intimal hyperplasia is a common complication of the chronic use of oral contraceptives [11].

In liver grafts, a subintimal accumulation of foamy lipid-laden macrophages is quite characteristic of chronic rejection, which usually is also accompanied by accumulation of such cells in the sinusoids [12, 13]. The narrowing of the lumen causes parenchymal atrophy. Necrotizing angiitis, with deposits of fibrinoid material, is found in polyarteritis nodosa and after treatment with some drugs (sulfonamides, penicillin, diphenylhydantoin, allopurinol).

Other changes include the presence of fibrin thrombi (disseminated intravascular coagulation, sepsis, paroxysmal nocturnal hemoglobinuria), aneurysmatic dilatation (hemangiomatosis, Rendu-Osler-Weber disease), and arteriovenous fistulas.

Portal vein branches may present intimal thickening which may be eccentric as in obliterative portal venopathy and schistosomiasis, pylephlebitis produced by a diffuse bacterial infection from areas drained by the portal vein system (appendicitis, diverticulitis, typhoid fever, ulcerative colitis, Crohn's disease), and thrombosis.

The lymphatic vessels are dilated in cases of severe venous congestion and outflow obstruction, a change often associated with ascites.

## 4 The Hepatic Acinus

The classical lobule is represented as a hexagonal structure bearing a venule at its center (centrolobular vein) which represents a terminal tributary of the hepatic vein. The hepatic unit that now receives general acceptance is the Rappaport acinus, which is defined as the parenchymal mass arranged around a terminal portal vein and its accompanying arteriole and bile duct. The acinus sinusoids drain into efferent venules. The acinus is functionally divided into zones 1, 2, and 3, zone 1 being the nearest to the terminal portal vein and zone 3 the farthest away, which is in continuity with zone 3 of adjacent acini.

Within the acinus, hepatocytes are arranged in plates or laminae, one cell in thickness in the adult. The hepatic laminae branch and anastomose together, forming a complicated system, the hepatic muralium. The labyrinth of pathways between the laminae is occupied by the sinusoids, which interconnect with each other. The term "periportal" designates the parenchyma adjacent to the portal tract. The hepatocytic layer immediately adjacent to the portal connective tissue forms the limiting plate.

### 4.1 Changes in the Liver Cell Plates

The normal laminar structure of the acinus may be modified in different ways.

#### *Hyperplasia*

The thickness increases because of the increase in the liver cell number. The liver cell plates appear arranged in a rather compact structure producing a cobblestone pattern [14], with the sinusoids spaced out and having narrow lumens. The parenchyma is paler than normal and liver cells display regeneration signs: nuclear polyploidy, frequent binucleation, and prominent nucleoli. Liver cell regeneration is a very common, nonspecific event, occurring as a reparative process after many injuries.

Hyperplasia may be simple or nodular. *Simple hyperplasia* is usually mild or moderate and may have a zonal, diffuse, or irregular distribution. *Focal nodular hyperplasia* consists of well-demarcated nodules ranging from 1 to several centimeters in diameter with a quite extensive central fibrous scar (Fig. 6). Histologically, the parenchyma appears dissected by dense fibrous septa which contain large thick-walled arteries and bile duct-like structures. Occasionally prominent cholestatic features are observed.

In *nodular regenerative hyperplasia*, multiple hyperplastic parenchymal foci with thickened liver cell plates, without significant fibrosis, are observed. Nodular regenerative hyperplasia is associated with a wide range of disorders: chronic venous congestion; rheumatoid arthritis, particularly when

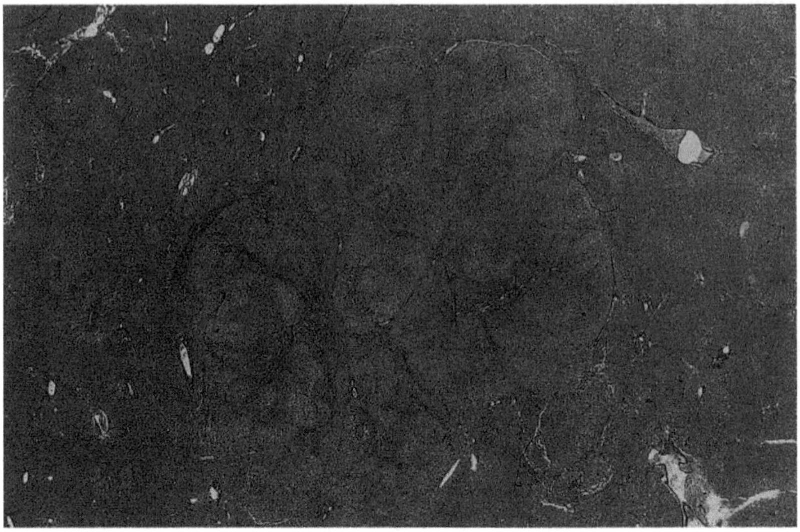

**Fig. 6.** Focal nodular hyperplasia. The nodule is lobulated and well demarcated from the normal parenchyma. Photograph taken from the histologic section. Trichrome, ×6

associated with leukopenia and splenomegaly (Felty's syndrome); myeloproliferative disorders; prolonged treatment with anabolic steroids and gold salts [15], and in Spain the toxic oil syndrome [16]. An extensive review of the associated conditions has recently been published by Wanless [17].

The regeneration of liver cells does not always result in hyperplasia. After acute and heavy loss of hepatocytes, particularly after an ischemic process, many mitotic figures may be seen leading to a normal regeneration. On the other hand, when hyperplasia develops mitoses are observed very rarely or not at all.

### *Atrophy*

There is a decrease in thickness of the liver cell plates because of the reduction in the size of hepatocytic cytoplasm, which becomes denser than normal. The sinusoids are usually dilated. The atrophy may be dependent on hypoxemic conditions and compression. A very common type of atrophy is that due to chronic venous congestion, in which both factors play a role. In this condition, the atrophy is zonal, being localized in zone 3 of the acinus. Granulomas and tumour nodules cause local atrophy by compression.

### *Pleomorphism*

The laminar structure is blurred owing to severe changes in the form, size, and stain affinity of liver cells (Fig. 7). This is caused by the simultaneous

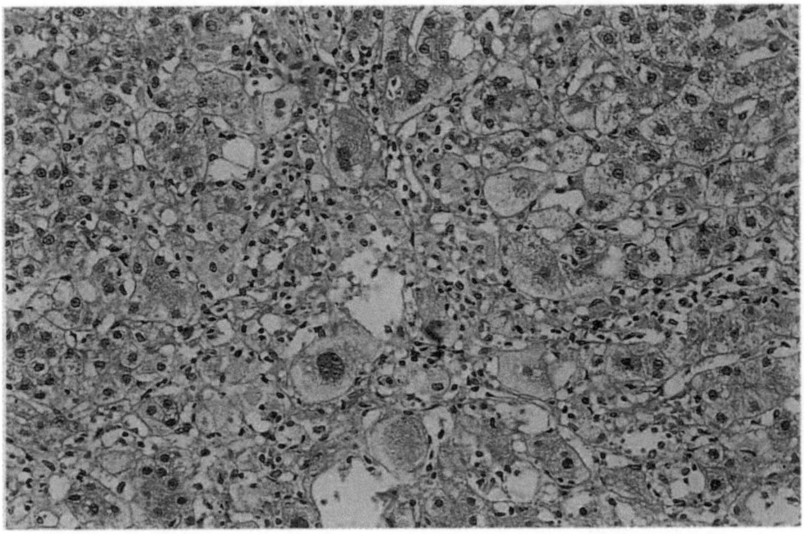

**Fig. 7.** Acute viral hepatitis. Many hepatocytes have undergone ballooning degeneration. An outstanding pleomorphism is also observed. H&E, ×150

appearance of degenerative changes, necrosis, and regeneration. It may be diffuse throughout the acinar parenchyma, although the hepatocytic changes are usually more severe in zone 3, particularly in many toxic injuries. Pleomorphism is very characteristic of overt acute hepatitis (Fig. 7), either viral or toxic. In these cases, hepatocytic changes are accompanied by inflammatory infiltrate. Pleomorphism is also seen when in the course of chronic active hepatitis a reactivation, with lobular cytolysis, takes place; for instance, in a superimposed delta virus infection.

### *Rosettoid Rearrangement*

In long-standing canalicular cholestasis, liver cell laminae often acquire a tubular arrangement, which in cross-sections appears as rosettes formed by more than two cells around a dilated canaliculus [18].

In some circumstances, such as in chronic active hepatitis, the surviving liver cells at the periphery of the lobule undergo rearrangement to pseudorosettes, which appear as round solid structures composed of several hepatocytes (Fig. 8). Together with these pseudorosettes, true rosettes bearing a small lumen may be seen. Fibrosis and inflammation usually accompany this change.

### *Necrosis*

Another lesion to be observed in the liver cell plates is necrosis. As it takes place in hepatocytes, we will deal with it below, in the section concerning liver cells.

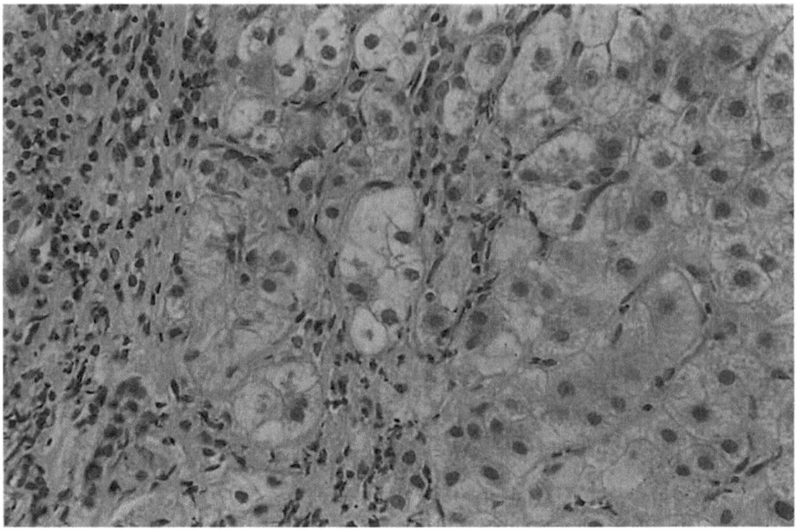

**Fig. 8.** Chronic active hepatitis. The surviving liver cells at the periphery have formed pseudorosettes. H&E, ×400

## 4.2 Liver Cells

Hepatocytes are roughly polyhedral cells, and each cell contains at least a spherical nucleus with one or more prominent nucleoli and abundant euchromatin. Some cells are binucleated, an event which together with polyploidy increases with age. The cytoplasm contains clumps of rough endoplasmic reticulum profiles which are continuous with smooth endoplasmic reticulum tubules. Mitochondria are numerous, particularly in zone 3, in which they are smaller than in zone 1. Glycogen is usually abundant and disposed in alpha granules. Lysosomes are usually polarized at the bile canalicular pole.

Hepatocytes have three types of surface: sinusoidal, facing the space of Disse, which bears microvilli; canalicular, which takes part in forming the bile canaliculus; and intercellular, facing other hepatocytes.

Hepatocytes may undergo different changes, some of which are adaptive; others are degenerative, which may lead to necrosis.

### *Liver Cell Damage and Cell Death*

Several types of cell damage and cell death can be identified in biopsy specimens.

1. *Acidophil degeneration and necrosis*. The liver cell undergoes shrinkage, becoming deeply eosinophilic with an irregular rhomboid outline.

These cells are thought to be precursors of acidophilic (Councilman) bodies, which represent a particular form of apoptosis. The cell as a whole or its fragments become rounded, deeply eosinophilic, and refractile, and detach from neighboring hepatocytes [19].

A few acidophilic bodies may be found in a great variety of conditions. However, their presence in large number points to overt liver lobular damage and is characteristically found in acute hepatitis (viral or toxic), chronic lobular hepatitis, and active cirrhosis.

A mild perivenular acidophilia, without nuclear changes but with frequent mitoses, occasional bile intracanalicular thrombi, and erythrophagocytosis are characteristically found in leptospirosis.

2. *Coagulation necrosis*. A special pattern of coagulation necrosis occurs in hypoperfusion (shock, severe hypotension, heart failure). In such circumstances, the general architecture may be preserved for some time and there is no inflammation.

Liver cells may undergo coagulation necrosis, as in acute hepatitis, or liquefaction necrosis, as caused by many toxic agents, among them alcohol and carbon tetrachloride. Necrosis may occur in individual cells or in groups of cells. It may be roughly classified according to its distribution in different types, although more than one type may be seen in different parts of the same liver.

*Spotty* or *focal necroses* are small areas, not always sharply demarcated, in which single hepatocytes or small groups of cells undergo necrosis. An inflammatory reaction takes place in relation to necrotic cells. When the necrotic hepatocytes vanish, the infiltrate remains as clumps of macrophagic cells which may represent the sole stigma of the lesion. Spotty necrosis represents an important lesion of acute viral hepatitis although it is not in itself specific, being often observed as a nonspecific reaction to diseases located elsewhere in the body [10].

*Confluent necrosis* refers to the death of larger groups of adjacent liver cells. They are often perivenular in location or form bridges between vascular structures, particularly between terminal hepatic venules and between terminal hepatic venules and portal tract vessels (bridging necrosis). They may be observed in acute hepatitis, either viral or drug-induced (being then accompanied by inflammatory reaction), in ischemia (left ventricular failure, shock), and as a consequence of a variety of chemical poisons, chloroform and carbon tetrachloride among them. Confluent necrosis of the acinus is called *panacinar necrosis*, while the necrosis of two or more adjacent acini is referred to as *multiacinar necrosis* [20].

*Piecemeal necrosis*, or *erosive necrosis*, may be defined as a process of erosion of the hepatocytic limiting plate due to the death of single or small groups of hepatocytes at the interface of parenchyma and connective tissue, accompanied by chronic inflammation and fibrosis. Piecemeal necrosis is the defining feature of chronic active hepatitis, although it also may be present

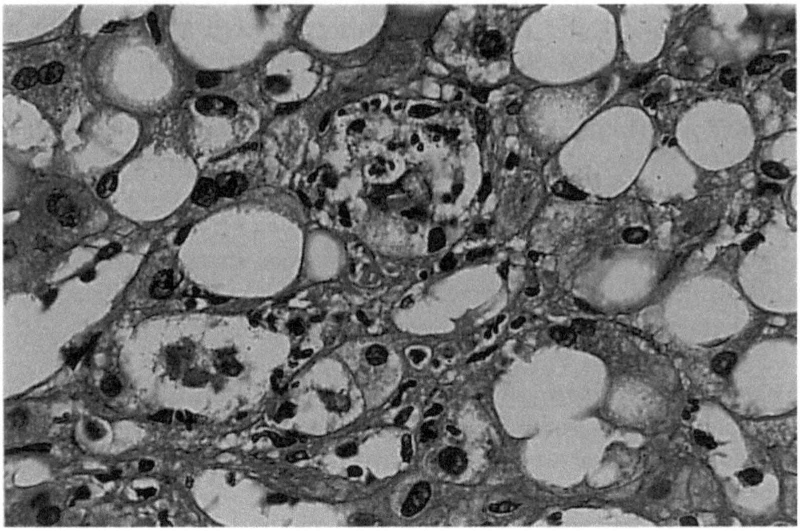

**Fig. 9.** Alcoholic hepatitis. A ballooned liver cell contains Mallory bodies. A clump of neutrophil leukocytes is observed within a damaged hepatocyte which also contains Mallory bodies. In addition, many other hepatocytes show fatty change. H&E, ×400

in acute hepatitis. Without piecemeal necrosis a histologic diagnosis of chronic active hepatitis is difficult to establish. In livers with a normal structure, the piecemeal necrosis is limited to the periportal zone (a simple form of chronic active hepatitis). Piecemeal necrosis is not always easy to distinguish from periportal hepatitis seen in type A hepatitis, in which a sleeve of necrosis surrounds the portal tract [20].

3. *Hydropic or ballooning degeneration*. This is a swelling and rounding of hepatocytes, which become pale-stained as a result of intracellular edema. Two different types are observed in acute viral hepatitis and alcoholic liver disease (Fig. 9). Ultrastructurally, an intense swelling of rough endoplasmic reticulum is observed. Ballooning degeneration associated with pleomorphism of liver cell plates and acidophil necrosis is characteristic of acute viral hepatitis (Fig. 7).

Alcoholic hepatitis is often accompanied by Mallory bodies (alcoholic hyalin), which are accumulations of disarranged intermediate filaments of the cytoskeleton. On light microscopy, Mallory bodies appear as strands or clumps of an amphophilic material, arranged around the nucleus.

4. *Feathery degeneration*. This is usually observed in single cells or in small groups. The cells appear swollen with a thread-like reticular appearance of the cytoplasm. Feathery degeneration is characteristic of cholestasis and is probably due to the toxic effect of bile components, resulting in lytic necrosis.

A list of other possible changes of the whole hepatocyte include atrophy and regeneration (as pointed out above), dysplasia, neoplastic transformation, and hypertrophy.

### *Cytoplasmic Changes*

1. *Fatty change*. This is very common. It may be microvesicular (alcoholism, Reye's syndrome, fatty liver of pregnancy, and that induced by some drugs) or macrovesicular (alcohol excess, among many other possible causes).

2. *Ground-glass hepatocytes*. A variety of histologic patterns merging imperceptibly with each other have been observed. Although they look alike on routine examination, they can be caused by diverse conditions. The hepatocytic change consists basically of homogeneous areas which are weakly eosinophilic in hematoxylin and eosin-stained sections. They are frequently referred to as "inclusion" bodies, even though they are not true inclusions.

The best-known type of ground-glass hepatocytes are those observed in HBsAg carriers. They can be stained with orcein or Victoria blue and display strong reactivity when treated with antibodies raised against HBsAg. In addition, they give a PAS-positive reaction. On electron microscopy the ground-glass areas show hyperplasia of the smooth endoplasmic reticulum, containing long filaments similar to the HBsAg filaments found in the serum of these patients.

A peculiar type of ground-glass change is the cyanamide-induced "inclusion" bodies described in alcoholic patients treated to discourage them from drinking alcohol [21–23]. They consist of round or kidney-shaped, homogeneous or partly granular areas and often displace the nucleus to the cell periphery. In PAS-stained sections, the "inclusions" give a strongly positive reaction which disappears after incubation with saliva, although total digestion of the glycogen requires longer time. (Fig. 10). On electron microscopy, the "inclusions" contain a large amount of glycogen disposed in beta granules, secondary lysosomes, and residues of degenerating organelles. The distribution of "inclusion" bodies through the lobule varies according to the duration of treatment. The lesion starts at the periportal area and progresses toward the center. The development of these "inclusion" bodies may result in progressive fibrosis [24].

Other drugs produce liver cell changes which resemble ground-glass hepatocytes, e.g., the adaptive changes observed in long-term treatment with anticonvulsant drugs, phenobarbital or phenytoin, rifampicin, etc. Ultrastructurally, a pronounced increase in smooth endoplasmic reticulum is observed.

"Inclusion" bodies described in the liver tissue in cases of myoclonic epilepsy (Lafora's disease) appear quite similar to the cyanamide-induced "inclusions" on observation by light microscopy. They are also periportal in location.

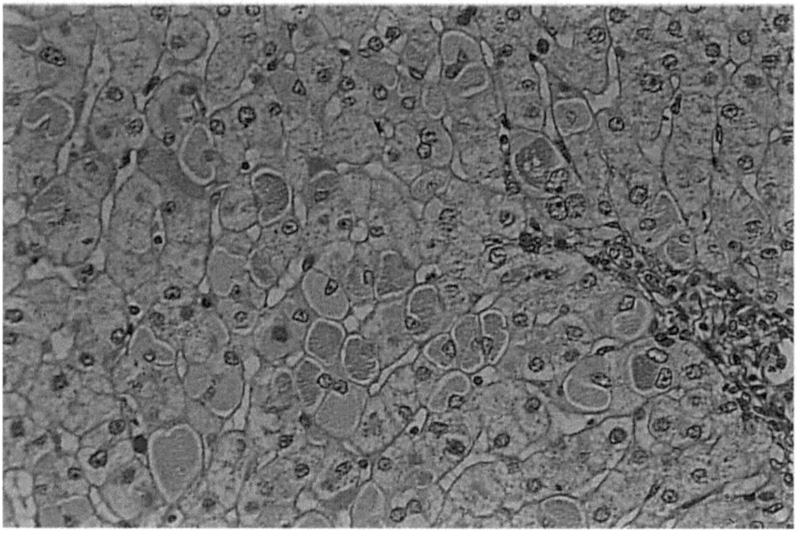

**Fig. 10.** Biopsy taken from a patient on cyanamide. Many liver cells bear "inclusion" bodies. PAS stain after saliva incubation for a short time. The "inclusions" still contain a little glycogen. ×400

Very similar to the previously described bodies are the "inclusions" observed in type IV glycogenosis, which is due to branching enzyme deficiency [25]. This lesion, like that produced by cyanamide, is followed by a progressive fibrosis which eventually progresses to cirrhosis.

Another change also giving a rather vague ground-glass appearance to the cytoplasm is that resulting from intracytoplasmic accumulation of fibrinogen, observed in neoplastic and nonneoplastic hepatocytes. The resulting inclusions give a negative reaction with PAS staining and immunocytochemically react strongly for fibrinogen. Ultrastructurally, they are bounded by a membrane which bears ribosomes.

Coexistence of different types of ground-glass hepatocytes in a liver biopsy, due to different causes, has been described [26].

3. *Cytoplasmic inclusions*. Needle-shaped birefringent porphyrin crystals have been described in biopsy specimens from patients with porphyria cutanea tarda. They are water-soluble, which makes it very difficult to observe them in routinely prepared paraffin sections. The crystals are best seen in unstained sections [27].

In $\alpha_1$-antitrypsin deficiency, characteristic PAS-positive, diastase-resistant globules of different size are found predominantly in periportal hepatocytes. They can be specifically demonstrated by immunocytochemical staining and ultrastructurally the material is found in the endoplasmic reticulum. Granules of copper binding protein which accumulate in chronic cholestasis, particularly in primary biliary cirrhosis and Wilson's disease, have a similar distribution but are orcein positive.

4. *Changes in mitochondria*. Giant mitochondria are seen as round eosinophilic bodies, often reaching the size of the nucleus. They are frequently found in alcoholic liver diseases [28] and may be considered as a good indicator of chronic alcoholism. Megamitochondria have more often been described in association with mild than with severe alcoholic hepatitis [29].

In patients with cirrhosis or severe chronic autoimmune hepatitis, an oncocytic change is sometimes observed in single hepatocytes or more often in small groups of hepatocytes. Their cytoplasm has a granular appearance and stains intensively with eosin and acid fucsin because of the large amount of mitochondria.

5. *Pigments and abnormal lysosome*. Different types of pigments may be seen in the cytoplasm of liver cells. Brown-yellow bile pigment is observed particularly in cholestasis, usually associated with bile thrombi in dilated canaliculi.

Lipofuscin is present in a normal liver from the second decade onward and increases with age. It is seen as fine, diastase-resistant, acid-fast small granules which are located at the canalicular pole of the cell. It is predominant in the perivenular area. Lipofuscin granules themselves are secondary lysosomes (wear and tear pigment). Large amounts of lipofuscin are found in Gilbert's disease, after treatment with many drugs which increase autophagocytotic events, and in ceroidolipofuscinosis. In Dubin-Johnson syndrome, hepatocytes contain large amounts of a diagnostic dark-brown pigment which resembles lipofuscin granules. Like lipofuscin pigment, it occupies the canalicular pole and predominates in the perivenular zone.

Lysosomes accumulate iron pigment in various iron metabolic disorders, particularly in hemochromatosis, in which the periportal hepatocytes are especially overloaded.

In many inborn errors of metabolism, lysosomes increase in size and number and accumulate large amounts of undigested material (Niemann-Pick disease, type II glycogenosis, mucopolysaccharidosis, oligosaccharidosis, mucolipidosis).

### *Nuclear Changes*

Binucleation and anisokaryosis are normal findings which increase with age and after many lesions. Anisokaryosis is due to endomitosis which leads to polyploidy. Mitotic divisions are rare in normal liver.

Mitotic figures may be numerous after different pathologic conditions and reflect the parenchymal regeneration after necrosis of a large number of hepatocytes.

Glycogen nuclear inclusions are quite common and are seen as eosinophilic vacuoles which displace the chromatin to the nuclear membrane. Nuclear glycogenation is a prominent finding in diabetes mellitus and venous congestion, affecting predominantly the periportal hepatocytes.

Characteristic viral inclusions may be found in some viral infections (cytomegalovirus, herpesvirus, adenovirus). In patients with hepatitis D, eosinophilic inclusions, giving the nucleus a "sandy" appearance ("sanded" nuclei), were described by Moreno et al. [30]. This type of nuclear inclusion had been previously related to HBcAg.

### 4.3 Sinusoids

Hepatic sinusoids are fairly straight in the perivenular area and tortuous in the periportal space. The lining consists of endothelial cells and Kupffer cells. Endothelial cells are extremely thin and perforated by small fenestrae arranged in groups forming "sieve plates." There is no basement membrane; therefore, the plasma can flow through into the space of Disse, into which the microvilli of the liver cells project.

Kupffer cells have an irregular stellate shape and are located within the sinusoidal lumen. They belong to the mononuclear phagocytic system. They undergo hyperplasia when stimulated by liver injury.

#### *Changes in the Lumen Size*

Sinusoidal dilatation in zone 3 with extension to zone 2 is typically observed in Budd-Chiari syndrome, veno-occlusive disease, and congestive heart

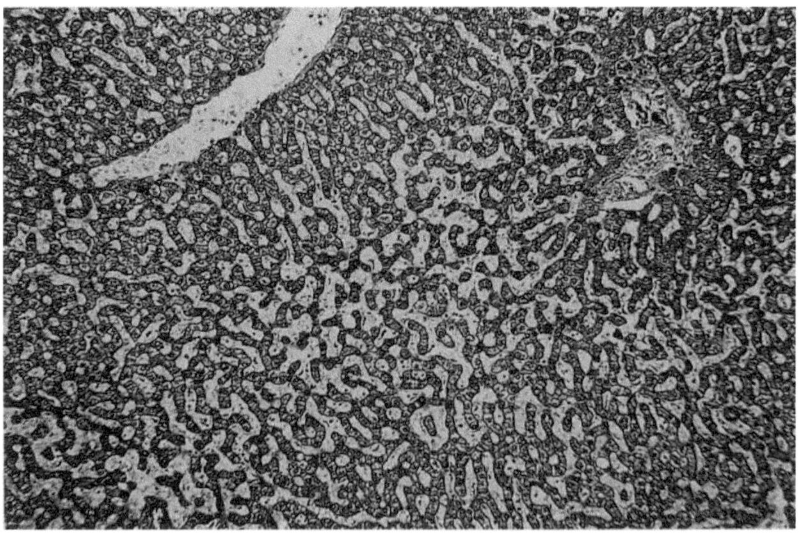

**Fig. 11.** Sinusoidal dilatation in a patient with Hodgkin's disease. Trichrome, ×80

failure. In chronic stages, atrophy of liver cell plates and perisinusoidal fibrosis are seen. When they are severe, intervenular linkage (reverse lobulation) is observed.

Patchy or diffuse sinusoidal dilatation has been described in several conditions (Fig. 11), especially in patients with granulomas or tumors, even when these do not involve the liver [31]. Sinusoidal dilatation is quite common in Hodgkin's disease [32], renal cell carcinoma [33], and rheumatoid arthritis [34]. Dilatation of periportal sinusoids occurs in patients taking anabolic and oral contraceptive steroids, being periportal in the latter [35, 36].

*Peliosis hepatis* is a particular form of sinusoidal dilatation, with small cysts filled with blood which communicate with sinusoids. This lesion sometimes complicates steroid hormone therapy [37, 38] and treatment with other drugs (e.g., tamoxifen, danazol), and also may occur in patients with hypervitaminosis A [39].

Peliosis has been described in association with nodular regenerative hyperplasia [40]. A combination of peliosis and cirrhosis has also been observed after long-term use of oral contraceptives [41].

### *Granulomas*

Granulomas may be defined as distinct aggregates of mature cells of the phagocytic mononuclear system. They are found in 5%–10% of hepatic biopsies performed for a variety of disorders. Fever and elevation of alkaline phosphatase are commonly associated findings when the basic process is infectious in nature. When aminotransferases are also high, the picture is referred to as *granulomatous hepatitis*, in which focal necrosis of liver cells and clumps of macrophages bearing ceroid pigment are usually present.

The list of causes of granulomas is very long and includes many bacteria, mycobacteria, viruses, rickettsiae, spirochetes, fungi, parasites, hypersensitivity reactions, immunodeficiency diseases, drugs, neoplasms, and foreign materials [4]. A peculiar type of granuloma with a fibrin ring has been described in Q fever and in other conditions [42].

### *Space of Disse*

The space of Disse in a normal liver contains occasional bundles of type III collagen fibers, which constitute the reticulin framework, and some lipocytes (synonyms: perisinusoidal cells, Ito cells) which may transform into fibroblast-like cells involved in the process of fibrosis.

The space of Disse may be enlarged because of edema or when containing abnormal material: collagen (fibrosis), amyloid substance, immunoglobulin light chain, acidophilic bodies (see above), hemopoietic cells.

Sinusoidal fibrosis may be focal, zonal, or diffuse. Focal fibrosis develops as a result of inflammatory infiltrates, the presence of clumps of macrophages, and granulomas.

Zonal fibrosis may be perivenular or periportal. Perivenular fibrosis is observed in chronic alcoholic disease, congestive cardiac failure, narrowing or occlusion of hepatic veins or the inferior vena cava (Budd-Chiari syndrome), and hypervitaminosis A. Periportal fibrosis occurs in chronic active hepatitis and severe, long-standing cholestasis (lamellar fibrosis). In alcoholic hepatitis, pericellular fibrosis and capillarization of sinusoids are observed in association with perivenular fibrosis. Deposition of collagen and development of basement membrane around the sinusoids take place as in normal capillaries. The capillarization interferes with the normal exchange between the blood and hepatocytes.

Diffuse fibrosis takes place after multiacinar necrosis (viral or toxic hepatitis, alcoholic hepatitis), after protracted methotrexate treatment, and in patients with congenital syphilis.

The liver is commonly involved in systemic amyloidosis. Amyloid substance is deposited in the space of Disse or in the arterial walls. The perisinusoidal deposits compress the sinusoids and the liver cell plates, leading to atrophy.

Hemopoiesis may be seen in the lumen of sinusoids and the space of Disse, in both physiologic (fetal, neonatal) and pathologic (myeloproliferative disorders, severe anemias) conditions.

## 4.4 Hepatic Veins

After perfusing the acinus via the sinusoids, the blood enters the efferent venule whose wall consists only of a thin endothelium, with fenestrae which communicate with sinusoids, and some delicate bundles of collagen fibers. The efferent venules unite to form intercalated veins which flow into larger hepatic veins.

Four main alterations may be found in efferent venules: dilatation, endothelialitis, endosclerosis/thrombosis, and perivenular fibrosis.

Hepatic vein *dilatation* is typically observed in congestive cardiac failure.

*Endothelialitis* consists in attachment of lymphocytes to the vein endothelium with or without subendothelial inflammation [13]. It may also affect the portal tract vein. It is a characteristic feature of liver allograft rejection, although a similar lesion has been described in alcoholic liver disease in precirrhotic and cirrhotic stages affecting terminal venules and intercalated veins [43].

*Endosclerosis* with partial or complete luminal occlusion by subintimal proliferation of connective tissue is observed in veno-occlusive disease (Fig. 12). The lesion is observed in efferent venules and intercalated veins.

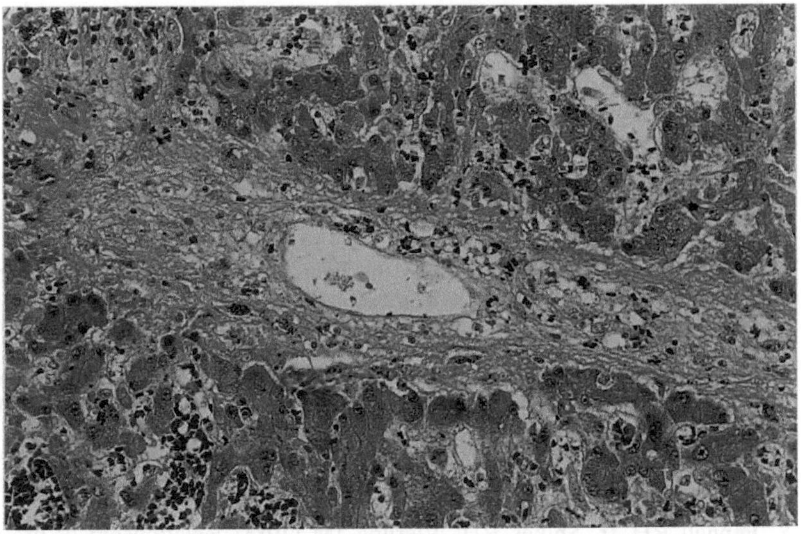

**Fig. 12.** Chronic veno-occlusive disease in alcoholic liver. Partial luminal occlusion is observed. Trichrome, ×150

Endosclerosis may run an acute or a chronic course. Acute veno-occlusive disease may follow chemotherapy for cancer or immunosuppressive therapy after transplantation. Azathioprine has been considered as the culprit in renal transplant patients [44, 45]. Chronic veno-occlusive disease is very common in alcoholic liver disease in both precirrhotic and cirrhotic stages [43]. A similar lesion follows the administration of pyrrolizidine alkaloids from *Crotalaria* and *Senecio* species [46], which may also produce an acute course.

*Thrombosis* of the main hepatic vein branches constitutes the Budd-Chiari syndrome.

*Perivenular fibrosis* is a very common feature of alcoholic hepatitis and probably represents an intermediate stage in the transition to cirrhosis. Fibrosis starts around the efferent venule in association with liver cell necrosis, and progresses to pericellular fibrosis. In trichromic-stained preparations, thin bands of collagen are observed in the space of Disse surrounding enlarged hepatocytes.

A mixed form of perivenular fibrosis and endosclerosis has been described by Edmonson et al. [47] under the name of "sclerosing hyaline necrosis." It consists of extensive perivenular necrosis which is followed by the development of a large scar.

After severe confluent necrosis (see above), fibrous bridges connect the perivenular fibrosis with portal tracts or adjacent perivenular areas.

## References


1. Sciot R, Staessen D, Van Damme B et al. (1988) Incomplete septal cirrhosis: histopathological aspects. Histopathology 13:593–603
2. Underwood JCE (1990) Hepatitis C virus and transfusion transmitted liver disease: review. J Clin Pathol 43:445–447
3. Solís-Herruzo JA, Castellano G, Colina F et al. (1984) Hepatic injury in the toxic epidemic syndrome caused by ingestion of adulterated cooking oil (Spain, 1981). Hepatology 4:131–139
4. Ishak KG (1983) Cranulomas of the liver. In: Joachim HL (ed) Pathology of granulomas. Raven, New York, pp 307–369
5. Baptista A, Bianchi L, De Groote J et al. (1983) Histopathology of the intrahepatic biliary tree. Liver 3:161–175
6. Nakanuma Y, Ohta G, Takeshita H et al. (1983) Florid duct lesions and extensive bile duct loss of the intrahepatic biliary tree in chronic liver diseases other than primary biliary cirrhosis. Acta Pathol Jpn 33:1095–1104
7. Ludwig J, Weisner RH, LaRusso NF (1988) Idiopathic adulthood ductopenia. A cause of chronic cholestatic liver disease and biliary cirrhosis. J Hepatol 7:193–199
8. Fennell RH Jr, Shikes RH, Vierling JM (1983) Relationship of pretransplant hepatobiliary disease to bile duct damage occurring in the liver allograft. Hepatology 3:84–89
9. Kemnitz J, Ringe B, Cohnert TR et al. (1989) Bile duct injury as a part of diagnostic criteria for liver allograft rejection. Hum Pathol 20:132–143
10. Scheuer PJ (1988) Liver biopsy interpretation; 4th edn. Baillière Tindall, London
11. Irey NS, Norris HJ (1973) Intimal vascular lesions associated with female reproductive steroid. Arch Pathol 96:227–234
12. Demetris AJ, Lasky S, Van Thiel DH et al. (1985) Pathology of hepatic transplantation. A review of 62 adult allograft recipients immunosuppressed with a cyclosporine/steroid regimen. Am J Pathol 118:151–161
13. Snover DC, Sibley RK, Freese DK et al. (1984) Orthotopic liver transplantation: a pathological study of 63 serial liver biopsies from 17 patients with special reference to the diagnostic features and natural history of rejection. Hepatology 4:1212–1222
14. Peters RL, Craig JR (1986) Liver pathology. Churchill Livingstone, New York
15. Stromeyer FW, Ishak KG (1981) Nodular transformation (nodular "regenerative" hyperplasia) of the liver. A clinicopathologic study of 30 cases. Hum Pathol 12:60–71
16. Solís-Herruzo JA, Vidal JV, Colina F et al. (1986) Nodular regenerative hyperplasia of the liver associated with the toxic oil syndrome: report of the five cases. Hepatology 6:687–693
17. Wanless IR (1990) Micronodular transformation (nodular regenerative hyperplasia) of the liver: a report of 64 cases among 2,500 autopsies and a new classification of benign hepatocellular nodules. Hepatology 11:787–797
18. Nagore N, Howe S, Boxer L et al. (1989) Liver cell rosettes: structural differences in cholestasis and hepatitis. Liver 9:43–51
19. Bianchi L (1983) Liver biopsy interpretation in hepatitis. Part I. Presentation of critical morphologic features used in diagnosis (Glossary). Pathol Res Pract 178:2–19
20. Baptista A, Bianchi L, De Groote J et al. (1988) The diagnostic significance of periportal hepatic necrosis and inflammation. Histopathology 12:569–579
21. Vázquez JJ, Pardo-Mindán J (1979) Liver cell injury (bodies similar to Lafora's) in alcoholics treated with disulfiram (Antabuse). Histopathology 3:377–384
22. Vázquez JJ, Cervera S (1980) Cyanamide-induced liver injury in alcoholics Lancet I:361–362

23. Vázquez JJ, Guillén FJ, Zozaya J et al. (1983) Cyanamide-induced liver injury. A predictable lesion. Liver 3:225–230
24. Moreno A, Vázquez JJ, Ruíz del Arbol L et al. (1984) Structural hepatic changes associated with cyanamide treatment: cholangiolar proliferation, fibrosis and cirrhosis. Liver 4:15–21
25. Santonja C, Moreno A, Suárez L et al. (1990) Liver biopsy diagnosis of Andersen's disease. J Pediatr Gastroenterol Nutr 10:274
26. Alonso-Martí C, Moreno A, Barat A et al. (1990) Co-existence of hepatocyte ground-glass inclusions from several causes. Histopathology 16:304–307
27. Cortés JM, Oliva H, Paradinas FJ et al. (1980) The pathology of the liver in porphyria cutanea tarda. Histopathology 4:471–485
28. Iseri OA, Gottlied LS (1971) Alcoholic hyalin and megamitochondria as separate and distinct entities in liver disease associated with alcoholism. Gastroenterology 60:1027–1035
29. Chedid A, Mendenhall CL, Tosch T et al. (1986) Significance of megamitochondria in alcoholic liver disease. Gastroenterology 90:1858–1864
30. Moreno A, Ramón y Cajal S, Marazuela M et al. (1989) Sanded nuclei in delta hepatitis. Liver 9:367–371
31. Bruguera M, Aranguibel F, Ros E et al. (1978) Incidence and clinical significance of sinusoidal dilatation in liver biopsy. Gastroenterology 75:474–478
32. Bruguera M, Caballero T, Carreras E et al. (1987) Hepatic sinusoidal dilatation in Hodgkin's disease. Liver 7:76–80
33. Aoyagi T, Mori I, Ueyama Y et al. (1989) Sinusoidal dilatation of the liver as a paraneoplastic manifestation of renal cell carcinoma. Hum Pathol 20:1193–1197
34. Laffon A, Moreno A, Gutierrez-Bucero A et al. (1989) Hepatic sinusoidal dilatation in rheumatoid arthritis. J Clin Gastroenterol 11:653–657
35. Winkler K, Poulsen H (1975) Liver disease with periportal sinusoidal dilatation. A possible complication to contraceptive steroids. Scand J Gastroenterol 10: 699–704
36. MacSween RNM, Anthony PP, Scheuer PJ (1987) Pathology of the liver, 2nd edn. Churchill Livingstone, Edinburgh
37. Bagheri SA, Boyer JL (1974) Peliosis hepatis associated with androgenic-anabolic steroid therapy. A severe form of hepatic injury. Ann Intern Med 81:610–618
38. Karasawa T, Shikata T, Smith RD (1979) Peliosis hepatis. Report of nine cases. Acta Pathol Jpn 29:457–469
39. Ishak KG, Schiff ER, Schiff L (1987) Needle biopsy of the liver. In: Schiff L, Schiff ER (eds) Disease of the liver, 6th edn. Lippincott, Philadelphia, pp 399–441
40. Voinchet O, Degott C, Scoazec J-Y et al. (1988) Peliosis hepatis, nodular regenerative hyperplasia of the liver, and light-chain deposition in a patient with Waldenström's macroglobulinemia. Gastroenterology 95:482–486
41. van Erpecum KJ, Janssens AR, Kreuning J et al. (1988) Generalized peliosis hepatitis and cirrhosis after long-term use of oral contraceptives. Am J Gastroenterol 83:572–575
42. Marazuela M, Moreno A, Yebra M et al. (1991) Hepatic fibrin-ring granulomas: a clinicopathological study of 23 patients. Hum Pathol 22:607–613
43. Goodman ZD, Ishak KG (1982) Occlusive venous lesions in alcoholic liver disease. A study of 200 cases. Gastroenterology 83:786–796
44. Marubbio AT, Danielson B (1975) Hepatic veno-occlusive disease in a renal transplant patient receiving azathioprine. Gastroenterology 69:739–743
45. Liaño F, Moreno A, Matesanz R et al. (1989) Veno-occlusive hepatic disease of the liver in renal transplanation: Is azathioprine the cause? Nephron 51:509–516
46. Tandon BN, Tandon RK, Tandon HD et al. (1976) An epidemic of veno-occlusive disease of liver in central India. Lancet II:271–272
47. Edmonson HA, Peters RL, Reynolds TB et al. (1963) Sclerosing hyaline necrosis of the liver in the chronic alcoholic. A recognizable clinical syndrome. Ann Intern Med 59:646–673

## B. Laparoscopy

J.A. Solis Herruzo and M.T. Muñoz Yagüe

Laparoscopy is an endoscopic procedure that allows direct visualization of many of the intra-abdominal organs. Selective liver and peritoneal biopsies, cholangiography, splenoportography, ultrasonography, and some therapeutic operations [1–3] are feasible with the aid of laparoscopy.

For decades, laparoscopy has been a major diagnostic technique in the evaluation of patients with liver, gallbladder, and peritoneal diseases, at least in many European countries. In the United Kingdom and the United States, laparoscopy was practically abandoned during and following World War II.

Between the 1920s and 1960s, a large number of reports showed the potential of laparoscopy as a diagnostic tool. The improvement of optic systems and methods of illumination was important in promoting the widespread use of laparoscopy during the 1960s and 1970s. Critical evaluations of its diagnostic usefulness, risks, complication rate, etc. were published during these years. The widespread use of diagnostic imaging techniques (ultrasonography, computed tomography, etc.) during the 1980s has had a serious impact on the use of laparoscopy in gastroenterology, and accordingly a critical evaluation of its indications in this field is now needed.

### 1 Indications

Table 1 shows the indications for laparoscopy prior to and since the routine use of ultrasonography in our hospital.

#### 1.1 Peritoneal Diseases

Laparoscopy allows direct examination of a great part of the peritoneal surface; therefore, this procedure – with the aid of guided biopsy – is the most accurate method in the diagnosis of peritoneal diseases as well as in the evaluation of ascites of unknown origin [4]. Cirrhosis of the liver, as a cause of ascites, is easily identified, and peritoneal implants of tumor, as

**Table 1.** Indications for laparoscopy in the authors' hospital in the years 1976 and 1983 (i.e., prior to and after the routine use of ultrasonography)

| | 1976 | 1983 |
|---|---|---|
| *Diffuse liver diseases* | 208 (66.2%) | 336 (84.6%) |
| Chronic persistent hepatitis | 24 | 46* |
| Chronic active hepatitis | 31 | 65* |
| Cirrhosis of the liver | 67 | 80 |
| Alcoholic liver disease | 18 | 44* |
| Acute hepatitis | 7 | 1 |
| Fatty liver | 18 | 11 |
| Granulomatosis | 10 | 7 |
| Nodular regenerative hyperplasia | – | 3 |
| Hepatic porphyria | 11 | 13 |
| Hepatomegaly | 22 | 52* |
| Toxic oil syndrome | – | 14* |
| *Focal liver diseases* | 53 (16.8%) | 32 (8.1%)** |
| Primary liver cancer | 12 | 9 |
| Secondary liver cancer | 18 | 13 |
| Lymphoma | 4 | 6 |
| Hydatid cyst | 14 | 3* |
| Renal polycystic disease | 2 | – |
| Polyarteritis nodosa | 2 | – |
| Hemangioma | 1 | 1 |
| *Cholestasis* | 37 (11.8%) | 15 (3.8%)* |
| Extrahepatic cholestasis | 30 | 8* |
| Distal obstruction | 12 | 3* |
| Proximal obstruction | 1 | 1 |
| Gallbladder diseases | 6 | 1* |
| Chronic cholecystitis | 11 | 3* |
| Intrahepatic cholestasis | 7 | 7 |
| Primary biliary cirrhosis | 5 | 5 |
| Cirrhosis | 2 | 2 |
| *Nonhepatobiliary diseases* | 16 (5.1%) | 14 (3.5%) |
| Gastric cancer | 4 | 0 |
| Carcinoma of the colon | 1 | 1 |
| Pancreatic carcinoma | 1 | 1 |
| Retroperitoneal tumor | 3 | 1 |
| Splenomegaly | 2 | 5 |
| Ovaric tumor | 2 | 2 |
| Peritoneal tumor | 2 | 4 |
| Crohn's disease | 1 | 0 |
| *Total no. of laparoscopies* | 314 | 397 |

* $P < 0.05$; ** $P < 0.01$ between 1976 and 1983

well as granuloma, can be seen and biopsied. Likewise, laparoscopy may reveal characteristic features in malignant diseases of the liver or ovary, lymphomas, eosinophilic gastroenteritis [5], familial paroxysmal polyserositis, ovarian cystadenocarcinoma, and *Chlamydia trachomatis* [6] infection.

## 1.2 Diseases of the Gastrointestinal Tract and Intra-abdominal Masses

The serosal side of a part of the gastrointestinal tract is visible under laparoscopy, and hyperemia, local efflorescences, wall infiltrations, and tumoral masses or adhesions can be seen in patients with malignant tumors or inflammatory processes of the gastrointestinal tract. Nevertheless, laparoscopy is not the diagnostic procedure of choice in these diseases of the gastrointestinal tract. Rather, it should be considered only in selected cases in which other methods (endoscopy, roentgenology, etc.) have failed to clarify the diagnosis. The same holds true in respect of intra-abdominal masses, since the diagnostic imaging techniques usually provide useful information on the nature of these conditions. Although laparoscopy is able to visualize the pancreas in 60% of cases [7], it has never been included among the diagnostic procedures for pancreatic disease.

## 1.3 Diffuse Liver Diseases

Imaging techniques can occasionally detect changes suggesting diffuse liver diseases; however, the diagnostic efficiency of these new procedures is too low in this group of diseases, and evaluation of suspected liver disease by direct morphologic methods such as laparoscopy and histology is necessary.

Liver biopsy can be performed percutaneously. This procedure is easier, less time consuming, and cheaper than laparoscopy; nevertheless, in various respects percutaneous blind liver biopsy is less satisfactory. The criteria for diffuse parenchymal liver diseases are essentially histologic; therefore, diagnosis of these diseases can be established if adequate liver specimens are obtained. However, diagnosis of cirrhosis on blind biopsy has a rate of false-negative results of up to 20%, and inter- and intraobserver variability is too high. By contrast, assessment of cirrhosis or of its absence is achieved in 100% of cases when laparoscopic and histologic data are combined. Moreover, liver biopsy with laparoscopic guidance is safer than the percutaneous approach. Finally, laparoscopy may reveal associated conditions, such as small focal lesions, primary hepatocellular carcinoma, hemangioma, tuberculous peritonitis, and portal hypertension.

## 1.4 Focal Liver Lesions

There is no doubt that liver biopsy performed under laparoscopic guidance is superior to percutaneous blind liver biopsy in the diagnosis of focal liver lesions. The likelihood of a percutaneous liver biopsy being positive is 60% [8], while the sensitivity and specificity of laparoscopy and guided liver biopsy in these patients are 92% and 100%, respectively [9, 10]. Evaluation of focal lesions can now be achieved by means of ultrasonography and other diagnostic imaging methods, and it has also become possible to perform fine-needle cytology and aspiration biopsies under the guidance of such methods. The accuracy of ultrasonography is approximately 80%–90% and the new diagnostic imaging methods can display areas not routinely identified at laparoscopy. In the absence of adhesions, laparoscopy visually detects approximately 70%–80% of the surface of the liver, but deep-seated lesions within the hepatic parenchyma may go undetected even if the liver surface is visualized. Accordingly, it might be considered doubtful whether laparoscopy is indicated. However, ultrasonography and other diagnostic imaging methods also have their limitations. Not all patients have an optimal body habitus, and the value of ultrasonography is limited in respect of certain lesions (small masses, regenerative nodules, hyperplasia of the liver, or areas of fatty infiltration). In spite of this, when a focal lesion is suspected, ultrasonography, possibly with guided liver biopsy, should be performed first. If biopsy is negative or if the filling defect is confined to the left lobe, then laparoscopy with liver biopsy is mandatory. Laparoscopy is specifically indicated when primary hepatocellular carcinoma is suspected, not only because it is able to determine the presence and location of the tumor, but also because the presence or absence of cirrhosis can be established with certainty and the spread of the tumor into other lobes of the liver or the involvement of other organs is easily detected. Moreover, liver biopsy can be directed to the less vascularized areas or nodules and incidental bleeding can be treated early.

Cystic lesions, such as hydatid cysts and polycystic disease of the liver, have virtually ceased to be an indication for laparoscopy, since these lesions are easily diagnosed by imaging methods.

### 1.5 Other Indications

Laparoscopy is a useful procedure for staging intra-abdominal lymphomas, including Hodgkin's disease, since the demonstration of liver involvement by laparoscopy and guided liver biopsy may make a staging laparotomy unnecessary [11, 12]. Laparoscopy has also been used for the evaluation of necrotizing angiitis [13], fever of unknown origin [14], splenomegaly [15], granulomatous hepatitis [16], and metabolic disorders such as porphyria [17, 18], Wilson's disease, or amyloidosis [19]. Although laparoscopy allows the diagnosis of acute cholecystitis, appendicitis, mesenteric infarction, tubal pregnancy, rupture of the spleen and liver, endometriosis, torsion of ovarian cysts, etc., *emergency endoscopy* has been used only by a few groups of gastroenterologists [20]. In these conditions, clinical evaluation and simple laboratory tests are usually enough for planning therapeutic strategy. Laparoscopy has replaced culdoscopy as the preferred method of diagnostic pelvic endoscopy, and several surgical interventions under laparoscopic control have become very common in gynecology [21, 22] and surgery (cholecystectomy).

**Table 2.** Complications of laparoscopy in 46364 examinations

| Complications | Surgery | Deaths |
|---|---|---|
| *Complications of laparoscopy* | | |
| Bleeding from the abdominal wall | 10 | 8 |
| Bleeding from mesenteric veins | 1 | 0 |
| Bleeding of unknown origin | 1 | 0 |
| Splenic injuries | 4 | 0 |
| Injury to the iliac artery | 1 | 0 |
| Perforation of the gallbladder | 1 | 0 |
| Intestinal perforations | 7 | 0 |
| *Complications of liver biopsy guided by laparoscopy* | | |
| Bleeding | 4 | 7 |
| Cholerrhagic flow | 6 | 0 |
| Biliary peritonitis | 6 | 10 |
| Biliary abscess | 1 | 0 |
| Puncture of a gallbladder empyema | 1 | 0 |
| Splenic bleeding | 1 | 0 |

Reproduced from HENNING H and LOOK D (1985) Laparoskopie, Atlas und Lehrbuch. Thieme, Stuttgart

## 2 Contraindications

Laparoscopy is usually a safe procedure; nevertheless, there are a few situations in which it may be hazardous. Congestive heart failure, acute or recent myocardial infarction, severe chronic obstructive lung disease, respiratory failure, severe hemorrhagic dyscrasias (prothrombin activity less than 50%, platelet count less than 70000/mm$^3$), acute sepsis, and some particular local conditions (excessive collateral circulation in the abdominal wall, extensive intra-abdominal masses, multiple abdominal scars, advanced pregnancy) are contraindications to laparoscopy, although in some of the aforementioned circumstances the appropriateness of laparoscopy should be evaluated on an individual basis. This should also be the policy in patients who have previously undergone abdominal surgery [23]. Most recently, abdominal hernias, acute abdomen, obesity, and massive ascites are no longer considered contraindications to laparoscopy; these conditions may cause some limitations or technical difficulties but these can be overcome by certain changes in technique.

## 3 **Complications** (Table 2)

The frequency of major complications is low, particularly when contraindications to and anatomic limitations upon laparoscopy are taken into account and the procedure is performed by an experienced operator. In BRÜHL's large review of 63845 laparoscopies performed by 67 physicians the overall complication rate was found to be 2.5% and the mortality, 0.029% [24]. Henning and Look reviewed the 46364 laparoscopies reported by 17 groups of workers and found a complication rate of 0.149% and a mortality of 0.054% [25]. Moreover, most of the reported morbidity and mortality associated with laparoscopy is in fact due to the liver biopsy, and not to the laparoscopic procedure per se.

## 4 Technique

The technique of laparoscopy is not described in this chapter. The reader is referred to textbooks of laparoscopy where this procedure is described in every detail [12, 25–27].

## 5 Diagnostic Value of Changes Detected by Laparoscopy

### 5.1 Peritoneum

Normal peritoneum is smooth, shining, and transparent, allowing distinction of the color of the organs and tissues of the abdominal cavity (fat tissue under the parietal peritoneum or greater omentum, liver, gallbladder, abdominal musculature, etc.). By contrast, the peritoneum is *thickened* and there is reduced light reflection in the presence of primary (pneumococcal, gonococcal, streptococcal, recurrent polyserositis, eosinophilic gastroenteritis) and secondary peritonitis (tuberculosis, starch, talcum, peritoneal catheters) and peritoneal tumors (mesothelioma, pseudomyxoma peritonei, secondary peritoneal carcinoma). Peritoneum is usually hyperemic, edematous, and with adhesions in primary and secondary peritonitis; however, the formation of fibrotic bands is a particular response of the peritoneum to any possible aggression. Thus, adhesions can be seen not only after peritonitis, but also following abdominal trauma and surgery and occasionally in peritoneal malignancy.

Particularly striking is the presence of *nodules* distributed throughout the peritoneal surface. This finding can be seen in peritonitis (tuberculosis [28, 29], sarcoidosis, eosinophilic gastroenteritis [5]) and peritoneal malignancies (carcinomatosis, mesothelioma [30], pseudomyxoma peritonei). Although nodules may appear similar in all these conditions at laparoscopy, those of tuberculous origin are described as multiple, small, homogeneous, miliary, disseminated over the entire peritoneal cavity, and with a whitish or pale-yellowish color and translucent contour. By contrast, typical nodules in peritoneal malignancies are more prominent, projecting from the peritoneal surface, vary in size, and may be confluent or infiltrate the peritoneum superficially. In some cases, malignant tumors may mimic peritoneal tuberculosis or may appear as a single, isolated nodule of uncertain origin.

Therefore, guided biopsy is mandatory in any patient with peritoneal nodules.

Peritoneum is an organ rich in vessels; however, the normal vascular pattern is delicate and difficult to recognize. *Vasculature of the peritoneum* is increased in all types of peritonitis, in recurrent polyserositis [31], and also sometimes in peritoneal carcinomatosis. When hyperemia is confined to an area of the abdominal cavity, it may suggest the origin of the peritonitis. Portal hypertension is a common cause of vascular congestion of the peritoneal serosa, and its vascular pattern is characteristic. In this condition, veins are swollen, tortuous, and cyanotic.

## 5.2 Liver

The normal liver has a smooth and glistening surface covered by a transparent Glisson's capsule.

In patients with abnormal liver function tests and a smooth liver surface at laparoscopy, liver biopsy usually shows acute hepatitis or chronic persistent hepatitis; nevertheless, chronic active hepatitis cannot be ruled out (Table 3). When laparoscopy shows a *granular or undulate liver surface*, biopsy will probably demonstrate chronic active hepatitis and occasionally

**Table 3.** Findings of laparoscopy and liver biopsy in patients with abnormal liver function tests

| | No. of patients | % |
|---|---|---|
| *Liver with smooth surface* | 92 | 100 |
| Acute hepatitis | 48 | 52.1 |
| Chronic persistent hepatitis | 16 | 17.4 |
| Chronic active hepatitis | 6 | 6.5 |
| Fibrosis | 22 | 24.0 |
| Cirrhosis of the liver | 0 | 0 |
| *Liver with undulated surface* | 74 | |
| Chronic active hepatitis | 32 | 43.2 |
| Chronic persistent hepatitis | 3 | 4.0 |
| Liver fibrosis | 3 | 4.0 |
| Cirrhosis of the liver | 29 | 39.1 |
| Normal liver | 1 | 1.3 |
| Others | 6 | 8.1 |
| *Liver with nodular surface* | 239 | |
| Regenerative nodules | 209 | 87.4 |
| Cirrhosis of the liver | 207 | 86.6 |
| Nodular regenerative hyperplasia | 2 | 0.8 |
| Normal liver architecture | 24 | 10.0 |
| Normal liver | 12 | 5.0 |
| Chronic active hepatitis | 11 | 4.6 |
| Amyloidosis | 1 | 0.4 |
| Nonevaluable biopsies | 6 | 2.5 |

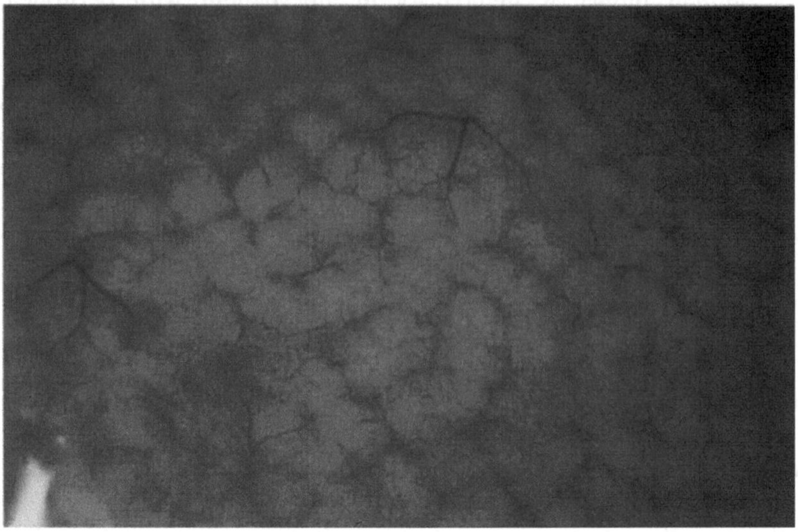

**Fig. 1.** Fatty liver

liver cirrhosis. Although the most characteristic feature of cirrhosis is the presence of regenerative nodules, discrimination between an undulate and a nodular surface may be troublesome and a matter of subjective interpretation. Histologic cirrhosis in the absence of a nodular surface is particularly found in alcoholic cirrhosis with high-grade fatty changes. Differentiation between advanced active chronic hepatitis and liver cirrhosis when the liver surface is not clearly nodular may be feasible if signs of portal hypertension are present.

The presence of a liver surface distorted by *nodules* has to be regarded as strongly indicative of liver cirrhosis, even in the absence of histologic proof. On the other hand, a similar laparoscopic picture can be found in nodular regenerative hyperplasia of the liver [32]. Normal consistency of the liver parenchyma upon palpation is then to be considered suggestive of the latter condition [32, 33].

The *color* of the normal liver parenchyma varies from person to person between light red or pink and reddish-brown. These variations are related to the blood perfusion and the amount of lipofuscin deposited in the liver. Significant deviations from this normal color may have diagnostic implications. A yellowish liver parenchyma should always suggest a fatty liver. Depending on the severity of fatty infiltration, the color may vary from orange-red to marked yellow. In cases of zonal fatty changes, the lobular pattern appears exaggerated by a honeycomb-like marking in which the yellow areas are enclosed in a meshlike tissue of brownish-red color (Fig. 1). A grayish or bluish color can be found in some types of hepatic porphyria (porphyria cutanea tarda, porphyria variegata), erythropoietic proto-

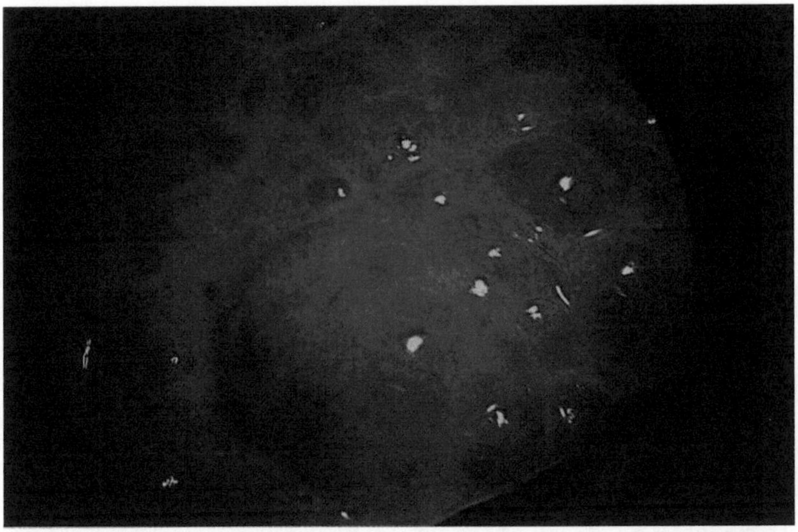

**Fig. 2.** Wilson's disease. The liver surface is distorted by large nodules with the characteristic metallic blue color

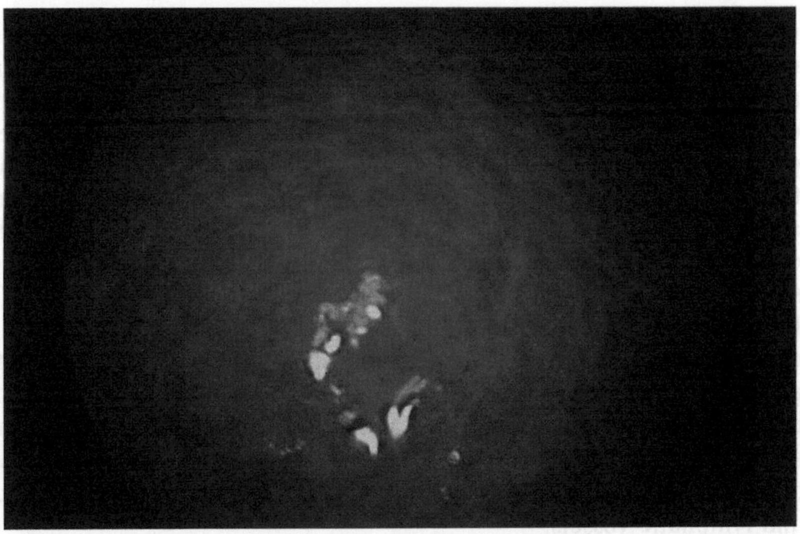

**Fig. 3.** Porphyria cutanea tarda and hemochromatosis. The liver shows a granular surface and the parenchyma displays a dark-brown discoloration (siderosis) and multiple grayish spots scattered throughout the liver

porphyria, and Wilson's disease (Figs. 2, 3) [17–19]. The pattern of distribution in the porphyrias ranges from diffuse to geographic or lobular stippling. In porphyria cutanea tarda, liver biopsy specimens show a characteristic red fluorescence under a Wood's lamp. In Wilson's disease, the more

**Fig. 4.** Peliosis hepatis. Networks and stellate formations of a reddish-violet color, which tend to enhance the normal lobular pattern

metallic blue color is particularly marked in the apical zones of cirrhotic nodules. A dark grayish to black liver suggests Dubin-Johnson syndrome, although this color has also been described when there are deposits of ceroid or malarial pigment in the liver [27]. Cyanotic discoloration can be seen in passive congestion of the liver (Budd-Chiari syndrome, right-sided cardiac failure), systemic cyanosis (respiratory failure), intrahepatic masses (metastases, primary liver cancer, lymphoma, hydatid cyst, abscess), and peliosis of the liver. In the last-mentioned condition, liver parenchyma reveals a spotty or meshlike bluish-red formation or cyanotic marks [34] (Fig. 4). Dark brown discoloration suggests iron deposition (siderosis, hemochromatosis) or lipofuscin pigmentation (Fig. 3). A green color of the liver parenchyma indicates cholestasis, although this finding does not allow differentiation between the intra- and extrahepatic forms. A bright red liver suggests inflammatory activity (acute viral hepatitis) and is usually associated with other signs of inflammation, such as increased markings of blood and lymphatic vessels.

On close examination, the color of the liver parenchyma is not uniform but shows a fine honeycomb pattern that has been named a "lobular or surface pattern" (Fig. 5). Although this pattern is not always easily recognizable in the normal liver, its increase or effacement may have diagnostic implications. The surface pattern disappears in acute hepatitis (95%), active chronic hepatitis (94%), liver cirrhosis (100%), and frequently also chronic persistent hepatitis (53%). On the other hand, it is increased when hepatic lobules are partially infiltrated by cells (lymphomas, granulomas), iron

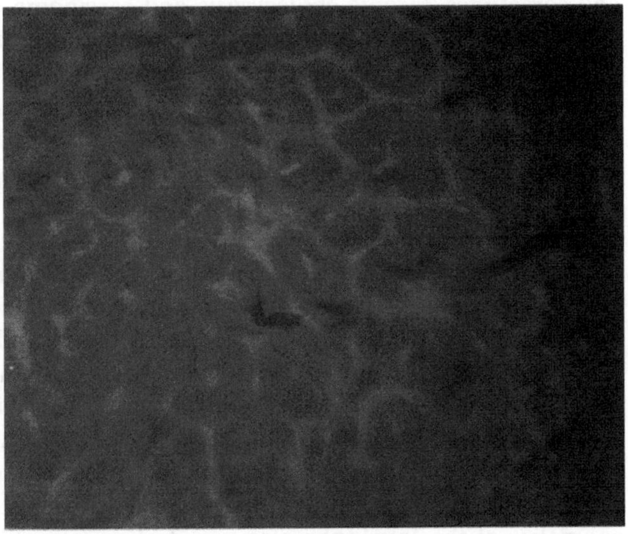

**Fig. 5.** Normal lobular or surface pattern

(siderosis). bile (cholestasis), fat, amyloid, or lipofuscin, or when there is fibrosis restricted to some areas of the lobule.

Whether liver parenchyma is normal or pathologic, laparoscopy may reveal a variety of focal lesions. When these are greater than 1–2 cm in diameter, it is likely that they will have been previously identified and perhaps biopsied employing some other diagnostic imaging method. This is the case for hydatid cysts, hemangiomas, and abscesses. Occasionally, the size of these lesions does not allow detection by the imaging methods, but they may be visible during laparoscopy. Some of these lesions appear as single or multiple nodules (metastases, primary carcinoma of the liver, lymphoma, liver cell adenoma, etc.) or maculae of white (granulomatosis, lymphoma, Meyenburg's complexes), yellowish (focal fatty liver degeneration), or cyanotic color (peliosis) [27, 34]. Guided biopsy, taken with forceps, for histologic and/or microbiologic studies will usually allow diagnosis of the causal disease.

### 5.3 Gallbladder

Although the gallbladder is easily visible during laparoscopy and most of its anomalies and diseases can be diagnosed by means of laparoscopy, nowadays these diseases rarely constitute an indication for this procedure. Sometimes, palpation reveals the gallbladder to be enlarged and tense. This is the case with biliary obstruction below the cystic duct, acute cholecystitis, and sometimes chronic cholecystitis and carcinoma of the gallbladder. The organ can also be distended after several hours of fasting, as well as in cirrhotic patients. However, the gallbladder wall can be depressed with the palpation probe in these conditions. Occasionally, laparoscopy shows a small and contracted or atrophic gallbladder with a thickened wall and adhesions to surrounding tissues (chronic cholecystitis) or a small or totally collapsed gallbladder associated with a cholestatic liver (proximal extrahepatic biliary duct obstruction, severe intrahepatic cholestasis). Sometimes, the normal gallbladder appears empty; generally this is the result of easy evacuation when the liver is fixed to the abdominal wall.

The wall of the normal gallbladder is bluish and translucent; nevertheless, it may appear whitish when it is thickened (edema, chronic cholecystitis, carcinoma) or when the gallbladder contains little bile. Finally, the normal gallbladder has a globular or ovoid shape, but this shape can be lost in a number of conditions, including chronic cholecystitis, malignancies, cholelithiasis, adenomyomatosis, vesical diverticulum, and congenital anomalies of the form (phrygian cap, trabecular gallbladder).

## 5.4 Spleen

The spleen can almost always be seen by laparoscopy and this procedure has been shown to be useful in the differential diagnosis of splenomegaly in 75% of cases. In spite of this, laparoscopy is seldom indicated in diseases of the spleen. This organ can display a number of changes (shape, color, appearance of its surface, etc.); however, only in a few instances are they semispecific ("dark brown spleen" [27], "sugar-icing spleen," granules, nodules) [15]. If laparoscopy has proved useful in the diagnosis of splenomegaly, this has to be ascribed not to the features of the spleen but to the laparoscopic appearance of the remaining abdominal organs (liver, collateral circulation, etc.).

## References

1. Semm K (1983) Endoscopic appendectomy. Endoscopy 15:59–64
2. Gangai HT, Gangai MH (1987) Laparoscopic appendicectomy. Endoscopy 19: 127–129
3. Cuschieri A, Abd El Ghany AA, Holley MP (1989) Successful chemical cholecystectomy: a laparoscopic guided technique. Gut 30:1786–1794
4. Nafeh MA, Shahwan MM, Mohammed SS, Rashvan NM (1983) Endoscopic diagnosis of ascites in Assint Province, Upper Egypt. Endoscopy 15:347–349
5. Solis Herruzo JA, Cuenca B, Muñoz Yague MT (1988) Laparoscopic findings in serosal eosinophilic gastroenteritis. Endoscopy 20:152–153
6. Poynard T, Mazeron C, Florent C et al. (1982) La périhépatite a chlamydia trachomatis n'est pas une urgence chirurgicale. Gastroenterol Clin Biol 6:2–3

7. Meyer-Burg J (1972) The inspection, palpation and biopsy of the pancreas by peritoneoscopy. Endoscopy 4:99–101
8. Jori GP, Peschle C (1972) Combined peritoneoscopy and liver biopsy in the diagnosis of hepatic neoplasm. Gastroenterology 63:1016–1019
9. Ishida H, Dohrono T, Furukawa Y, Kobayashi M, Tsuneoko K (1984) Laparoscopy and biopsy in the diagnosis of malignant intraabdominal tumors. Endoscopy 16:140–142
10. Lightdale CJ, Winawer SJ, Kurtz RC, Knapper WH (1979) Laparoscopic diagnosis of suspected liver neoplasms; value of prior liver scans. Dig Dis Sci 24:588–593
11. Solis Herruzo JA (1978) Contribución de la laparoscopia al estudio de los linfomas malignos. Gastrenterol Hepatol 1:253–259
12. Dagnini G (1978) "La laparoscopia nella diagnostica clinica". Piccin Editore, Padova
13. Solis Herruzo JA, Muñoz Yague MT, Colina F (1981) Laparoscopic findings in polyarteritis nodosa. Endoscopy 13:9–13
14. Solis Herruzo JA, Benita V, Morillas JD (1981) Laparoscopy in fever of unknown origin. Study of seventy cases. Endoscopy 13:207–210
15. Garcia Molinero MJ, Solis Herruzo JA, Muñoz Yague MT (1981) La laparoscopia en el estudio de las esplenomegalias. Gastroenterol Hepatol 4:515–519
16. Moreto M, Restillano M, Zaballa M, Suarez M, Ibañez S (1988) Diagnostic yield and endoscopic pattern of laparoscopy in the diagnosis of granulomatosis hepatitis. Endoscopy 20:294–297
17. Solis Herruzo JA, Muñoz Yagüe MT, Enriquez de Salamanca R (1978) Laparoskopische Befunde bei der chronischen hepatischen Porphyrie: Graufleckung der Leberoberfläche. Leber Magen Darm 8:101–103
18. Solis Herruzo JA, Perez Peña F (1974) Laparoskopische Befunde bei erythropoetischer Protoporphyrie. Z Gastroenterol 12:335–340
19. Solis Herruzo JA (1982) La laparoscopia en las enfermedades metabólicas. Gastrum April:40–52
20. Llanio R (1977) Laparoscopia en urgencias. Editorial Científico-Técnica, La Habana
21. Hulka JF (1985) Textbook of laparoscopy. Grune & Stratton, Orlando
22. Cibils LA (1975) Gynecologic laparoscopy. Diagnostic and operatory. Lea & Febiger, Philadelphia
23. Orlando R, Lirussi F, Okoliesanyi L (1977) Validity of laparoscopy after abdominal surgery. Endoscopy 19:150–152
24. Brühl W (1966) Zwischenfälle und komplikationen bei der Laparoskopie und gezielten Leberpunktion. Dtsch Med Wochenschr 51:2297–2299
25. Henning H, Look D (1985) Laparoskopie. Atlas und Lehrbuch. Thieme, Stuttgart
26. Solis Herruzo JA (1975) Atlas de diagnóstico diferencial laparoscópico. Editorial Paz Montalvo, Madrid
27. Beck K (1984) Color atlas of laparoscopy, 2nd edn. W.B. Saunders, Philadelphia
28. Jorge AD (1984) Peritoneal tuberculosis. Endoscopy 16:10–12
29. Rodriguez de Lopez C, San Miguel Joglar G, Pons Romero F (1982) Laparoscopic diagnosis of tuberculous ascites. Endoscopy 14:178–179
30. McCallum RW, Maceri DR, Hensen D, Berci G (1979) Laparoscopic diagnosis of peritoneal mesothelioma. Dig Dis Sci 24:170–174
31. Sarles H, Bernard P (1956) Maladie périodique. Constatation par laparoscopie d'une intense vasodilatacion peritonéale au cours des crises. Arch Mal App Digest 45:183
32. Solis Herruzo JA, Duran A, Colina F et al. (1985) Laparoscopic and histological problems in the diagnosis of nodular regenerative hyperplasia of the liver. Endoscopy 17:91–126

33. Cano Ruiz A, Martin Scapa MA, Larraona JL, Gonzalez Martin JA, Moreno Caparros A, Garcia Plaza A (1985) Laparoscopic findings in seven patients with nodular regenerative hyperplasia of the liver. Am J Gastroenterol 80:796–800
34. Solis Herruzo JA, Colina F, Muñoz Yagüe MT, Castellano G, Morillas JD (1983) Reddish-purple areas on the liver surface. The laparoscopic picture of peliosis hepatis. Endoscopy 15:95–100

# 7 Bilirubin Metabolism and Hyperbilirubinemia

J. FEVERY and J. GONZALEZ-GALLEGO

## 1 Introduction

It has long been recognized that the appearance of jaundice indicates the existence of hematologic or hepatobiliary alterations. Determination of serum bilirubin is nowadays a widely used test for evaluation of liver function. The understanding of various aspects of bilirubin chemistry, transport, and metabolism is therefore of great importance for correct interpretation of serum bilirubin levels and for adequate treatment of clinical conditions characterized by the presence of jaundice.

Bilirubin is derived from hemoglobin and other hemoproteins and is carried in the blood circulation by binding to albumin. After being taken up by the hepatocytes, it is esterified at the endoplasmic reticulum with a variety of UDP-sugars. Bilirubin mono- and diester conjugates are then excreted into bile and eliminated via the feces after conversion to bilinoids [1].

High plasma levels of bilirubin may induce toxic effects in different tissues, particularly in the neonatal nervous system, leading to the development of kernicterus or bilirubin-induced encephalopathy. For this reason bilirubin has been regarded for years as a waste product that must be eliminated from the organism. Recent data indicate, however, that circulating bilirubin could function as an antioxidant of physiologic value and protect against deleterious effects of free radical formation and lipid peroxidation [2].

## 2 Chemistry of Bilirubin

Bilirubin-IXα, the most abundant isomer of bilirubin in the body, is a linear tetrapyrrole derived from oxidation of the α-meso bridge in protoporphyrin-IX (Fig. 1). The pigment is characterized by a low water solubility due to the presence of six intramolecular hydrogen bonds that yield a configuration like a two-bladed propeller [3]. At alkaline pH the solubility of bilirubin-IXα is increased by disruption of the intramolecular bonds. The pigment is solubilized in plasma by binding to albumin. Intrahepatocytic conjugation

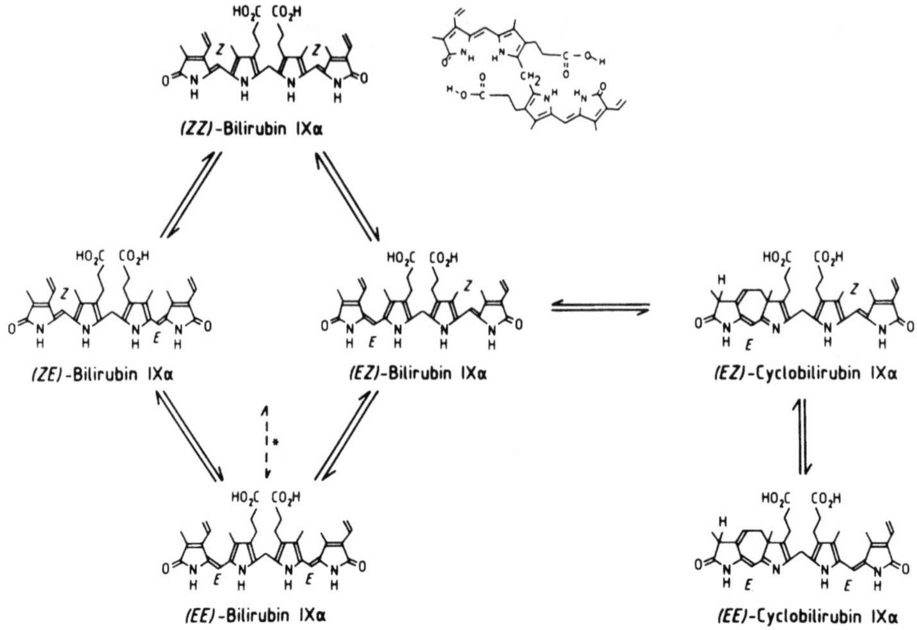


**Fig. 1.** Structure of bilirubin. [Reproduced with permission from Fevery J et al. (1989) Clin Gastroenterol 3:2]

introduces polar glycosyl residues in the molecule at one or both of the carboxylic groups, which prevents the formation of hydrogen bonds.

When exposed to light, the intramolecular bonds of the natural bilirubin isomer (bilirubin-IXα Z-Z) are disrupted, with formation of Z-E configurational photoisomers and cyclization to form the structural isomer cyclobilirubin or lumirubin [4]. These isomers are much more polar than bilirubin and therefore can be excreted in bile or urine without prior esterification. For this reason, phototherapy has proved to be an extraordinarily useful treatment of neonatal jaundice and protects against the potential neurologic damage that bilirubin can cause. It reduces the need for exchange transfusions. Commercial and laboratory bilirubin preparations can also contain a significant proportion of nonphysiologic IIIα and IXα isomers formed by disproportionation of the asymmetric bilirubin-IXα.

## 3 Bilirubin Formation and Plasma Transport

Bilirubin is mainly derived from hemoglobin breakdown of senescent red cells in the reticuloendothelial system. In addition, 10%–20% arises from prematurely destroyed erythrocyte precursors in the bone marrow or from the turnover of cytochrome P-450 and other hepatic hemoproteins.

Formation of bilirubin involves two enzymatic steps (Fig. 2). The heme molecule is first converted to biliverdin by microsomal heme oxygenase in

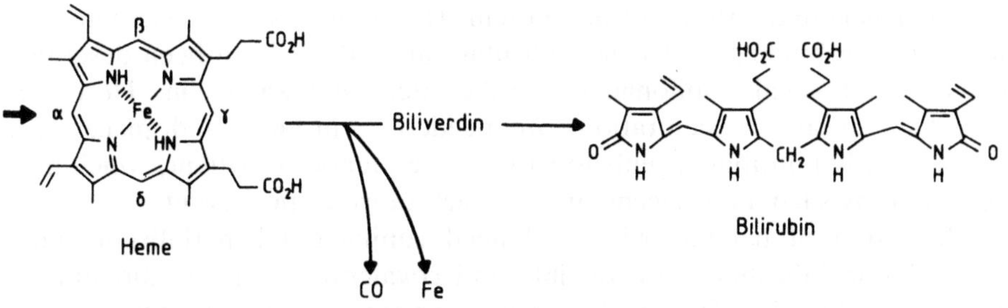


**Fig. 2.** Formation of bilirubin

a reaction requiring oxygen and the concerted action of the microsomal NADPH-cytochrome c reductase [5]. Heme oxygenase is localized in the endoplasmic reticulum of spleen and other tissues and shows a high specificity for the α-meso bridge of the heme substrate. This seems to explain the predominance of the IXα-isomers of biliverdin and bilirubin. The initial reaction of oxygen with the α-bridge carbons gives α-oxyheme, which is rapidly cleaved to bilirubin with release of CO and iron. Microsomal heme oxygenase exhibits a relatively high degree of substrate specificity. However, its catalytic site recognizes some metalloporphyrins, such as Sn-protoporphyrin and other related molecules, that act as competitive inhibitors of heme oxygenase. These compounds are becoming of therapeutic use by virtue of their ability to suppress bilirubin production.

Biliverdin is then reduced by cytosolic biliverdin reductase. This enzyme shows a high activity in liver, spleen, and kidney and catalyzes the formation of bilirubin in a reaction that requires NAD or NADPH. Biliverdin reductase activity is not present in birds, reptiles, or amphibia, so that in lower animals biliverdin is excreted directly into bile as the end product of heme degradation. The reduction of biliverdin to bilirubin and the subsequent hepatic conjugation of bilirubin in humans and most mammals is an intriguing subject, considering that these are expensive energy reactions and that bilirubin is a toxic compound when it accumulates in high concentrations. The prevalent hypothesis is that the physiologic requirement for bilirubin formation could have evolved to facilitate placental transfer from fetus to mother of bilirubin, which can cross biologic membranes more easily than biliverdin owing to its higher lipophilicity.

Daily production rate of bilirubin can be estimated by plasma turnover studies with radiolabeled bilirubin or by measuring endogenous CO production. Values obtained in normal adults average 4.4 ± 0.7 mg/kg per day and 3.89 ± 0.67 mg/kg per day respectively. The slightly higher values obtained with the labelled method are probably more accurate, because they take into account the fraction of bilirubin produced in the liver and directly excreted without entering the plasma compartment.

Unconjugated bilirubin in plasma is transported bound to albumin. Binding is critically dependent on lysine groups and secondarily on serine and phenylalanine residues of the protein. Different substances can interfere with albumin binding to displace bilirubin, and effects have been described for free fatty acids, sulfonamides, salicylates, and ampicillin. However, very high plasma concentrations are needed to produce a displacement. Consequently bilirubin encephalopathy in the jaundiced patient, which may be caused by such a displacement, is in fact a rare clinical event.

In serum of patients with prolonged conjugated hyperbilirubinemia, most plasma bilirubin is irreversibly and covalently bound to albumin (δ bilirubin or bil-alb). This fraction cannot undergo glomerular filtration, in contrast to the unbound conjugated pigment. It is thus responsible for the persistence of high plasma bilirubin levels that is observed during the resolution phase of various liver diseases [6].

## 4 Hepatocyte Uptake and Intracellular Storage

Bilirubin is almost exclusively cleared from plasma by the liver. Most studies concerning bilirubin uptake have been carried out using more polar and soluble organic anions, such as sulfobromophthalein, that apparently share common hepatic transport mechanisms. It has been demonstrated that carrier-mediated uptake of sulfobromophthalein is electrogenic and that only charged species are translocated by carrier(s) into the hepatocyte against electrogenic gradients [7]. Chloride ions seem to be linked to the uptake of sulfobromophthalein, because an inwardly directed gradient stimulates this process.

Bilirubin dissociates from albumin before being taken up by the liver cells and the traditional view has been that the unbound pigment is immediately available for uptake. More recently, a specific albumin receptor has been proposed to exist in the membrane of the hepatocyte that interacts with the albumin–bilirubin complex. However, different experimental results, such as the efficient uptake of bilirubin and other organic anions by analbuminemic rats and the fact that uptake kinetics do not change with binding proteins other than albumin, make the existence of such a receptor unlikely. Although albumin binding may prevent bilirubin from nonspecific diffusion into tissues, it is not necessary for hepatocytic uptake of the pigment.

Some proteins of the basolateral membrane of the hepatocyte have been postulated to the putative carriers for hepatic uptake of bilirubin and other organic anions [8]. At least three different proteins have been studied. Two of them are 54- to 55-kd molecules that have different PI values, amino acid sequences, and DNA coding. The third (bilitranslocase) is a 37-kd bilirubin and sulfobromophthalein binding protein that could also be involved in the transport of fatty acids. The relative role of these proteins in the hepatocellular uptake of bilirubin probably depends on different factors.

The carrier system responsible for the uptake of bilirubin, sulfobromo phthalein, and other dyės such as disulfobromophthalein or indocyanine green seems to be different from that involved in the hapatic uptake of bile acids. However, some data do not support such a concept and indicate that bilirubin or sulfobromophthalein may compete for hepatic uptake with certain bile acids. It has been proposed that bile acid and bilirubin binding proteins could be different forms of the same carrier system, having preferential specificities but being able to transport other anions at lower rates.

Once bilirubin is transferred across the cell membrane into the hepatocyte, it is reversibly bound to the intracellular proteins ligandin and fatty acid binding protein. The most important binding protein is ligandin (or Y protein), which constitutes 2% of total protein in the cytosol of human liver. This protein is able to bind not only bilirubin but also different organic anions, steroids, and carcinogens. In rat liver it is apparently identical to some glutathione-*S*-transferase isoenzymes, and at least two different ligandins with identical or nonidentical subunits have been identified. The site for bilirubin binding is not shared by glutathione acceptor substrates.

The role of bilirubin binding to cytosolic proteins would be to prevent reflux of the pigment back to the circulation and to limit nonspecific diffusion into compartments of the hepatocyte.

## 5 Conjugation

Although bilirubin is assumed to be shuttled from sinusoidal to intracellular membranes by binding to cytosolic proteins, some evidence suggests that it could be transported in part by membrane to membrane transfer and diffusion within the lateral plane of membranes to the site of conjugation [9]. The amount of bilirubin partitioned into intracellular membranes may be relatively small under physiologic conditions, but membrane-bound pigment appears to be delivered more efficiently to the microsomal membrane.

Bilirubin is conjugated in the endoplasmic reticulum with different UDP-sugars (glucuronic acid, glucose, or xylose), giving monoesterified or diesterified derivatives [10]. Glucuronide conjugates are the predominant pigment in human bile, with about 80% in the form of bilirubin diglucuronide. Conjugation is catalyzed by bilirubin UDP-glucuronyltransferase, probably a tetramer with a molecular weight of 209 kd. In rat and human liver, bilirubin is sequentially converted to the monoglucuronide and the diglucuronide in UDP-glucuronic acid-dependent reactions catalyzed by this enzyme. The previously postulated enzymic formation of diglucuronides by dismutation from two different monoglucuronide molecules has been demonstrated to be the consequence of nonenzymic artifactual dipyrrole exchange.

Under physiologic conditions the microsomal membrane is poorly permeable to cofactors and polar substrates and exhibits a considerable latency. Activity is enhanced when microsomes are permeabilized by detergents, sonication, freeze-thawing, or phospholipase treatment. Enzyme activation has been explained by two different models. The compartment model proposes that there is a compartmented arrangement in the microsomal membrane. The enzyme would be in the cisternal (internal) side of the endoplasmic reticulum and a carrier system (permease) would allow access of UDP-sugars through the membrane carrier to the luminal compartment [11]. Permeabilizing agents would bypass the translocation step, allowing full expression of the enzyme. An alternative hypothesis, the constraining model, suggests that the increase in enzyme activity brought about by permeabilizing agents is due to indirect effects related to altered organization of the microenvironment in the native microsomal membrane that induces conformational changes of the transferase [12]. The relative roles of membrane conformation and permeability and putative transporters of UDP-sugars still remain to be fully elucidated.

UDP-glucuronyltransferase shows functional heterogeneity, catalyzing the transfer of glucuronic acid to a variety of endogenous compounds and xenobiotics. In the rat, activity toward phenolic substrates develops in late fetal life, while transferases catalyzing the glucuronidation of bilirubin and sex hormones develop in early neonatal life. Enzyme activity toward bilirubin also increases in human liver after birth, attaining adult levels by 14 weeks of age. Evidence suggests that conjugation of bilirubin is mainly catalyzed by a UDP-glucuronyltransferase isoform that presents a common site for the different UDP-sugars. In homozygous Gunn rats with a functionally defective form of this enzyme, esterification of bilirubin is completely impaired while conjugation of other acceptor substrates is normal or only partially reduced.

The cytosolic nucleotide UDP-*N*-acetylglucosamine appears to play a regulatory role in UDP-glucuronyltransferase activity. This cofactor functions as an allosteric effector and facilitates the transport of UDP-glucuronic acid from the cytosol to the enzyme. Enzyme activity can also be modulated by a variety of hormonal factors. It has been reported that in the rat UDP-glucuronyltransferase activity is decreased by oophorectomy or *L*-thyroxine administration and is increased by orchiectomy, thyroidectomy, or pretreatment with secretin or glucagon and a series of enzyme inducing agents such as phenobarbitone, clofibrate, glutethimide, and spironolactone [13, 14]. The exact physiologic relevance of these effects is still unknown. Nutrition may be another regulatory factor in UDP-glucuronyltransferase activity, acting by altering membrane composition or UDP-glucuronic acid synthesis.

At least in the Gunn rat, evidence supports an alternative pathway of bilirubin metabolism involving cytochrome P-448-dependent monooxygenases, although oxidation of bilirubin by microsomal system has still not been demonstrated in vitro. In rat intestine, kidney, and liver, oxidation of bilirubin may be catalyzed by a mitochondrial bilirubin oxidase [15]. Its activity is not increased in homozygous Gunn rats and probably has no physiologic relevance for bilirubin metabolism in these animals, although it might play a role in some disease states.

## 6 Secretion and Intestinal Fate

The mono- and diester conjugates of bilirubin formed in the endoplasmic reticulum are secreted by an apparently energy-dependent process that transports the pigment against concentration gradients and operates at a lower capacity than that of the hepatic uptake. Changes in UDP-glucuronyl-transferase activity result in parallel changes in the maximal bilirubin secretion [13, 14, 16] and in the proportion of diconjugates as compared to monoconjugates in bile, which suggests a rate-limiting role for conjugation on the overall hepatobiliary transport of the pigment. Bile flow per se does not influence the maximal bilirubin secretion but delays the hepatic transport of bilirubin conjugates (bilirubinostasis or cholestasis) and results in a longer time available for conversion of mono- to diconjugates; this results in an increase in the bilirubin diconjugate–monoconjugate ratio in bile [17]. Although a small proportion of unconjugated bilirubin can be found in bile, it most probably derives from cleavage from monoester conjugates of the pigment because a close relation exists between the amount of unconjugated and monoconjugated pigment in bile.

Analysis of the hepatic transport of injected radiolabeled bilirubin suggests that bilirubin mono- and diconjugates traverse the hepatocyte via a transcellular pathway that appears to be different from that of the unconjugated pigment and from that of endogenously formed conjugates. Different studies have shown that a small fraction of newly formed bilirubin conjugates normally reflux into plasma, and a compartment model in which there is bidirectional transfer across the sinusoidal membrane for both unconjugated bilirubin and bilirubin glucuronides has been proposed [18].

The canalicular transport system of bilirubin is shared by different organic anions but not by bile acids. This conclusion is sustained by the observation of normal bile acid secretion in patients in whom biliary secretion of several organic anions is impaired, as e.g. in Dubin-Johnson syndrome, in mutant Corriedale sheep, and in transport-deficient rats. The latter mutant rats exhibit defective canalicular secretion not only for bilirubin and sulfobromophthalein but also for ouabain, cysteinyl leukotrienes, disulfobromophthalein, and glutathione [19], suggesting that the involved transport mechanism has a broad substrate specificity.

Despite their separate secretory carriers, bile acids are able to influence the excretion of bilirubin and other organic anions. Increases in bilirubin transport maximum have been found following infusions of bile acids [20, 21], although results obtained vary with doses of bile acid and species of animal. At this moment a clear explanation for this interaction is still lacking. A recent paper suggests that following bile acid infusion a microtubule-dependent system able to increase the transhepatic transport of bilirubin is recruited [22].

A relationship of bilirubin secretion with that of phospholipid and cholesterol has also been reported. Like other organic anions such as ampicillin, sulfobromophthalein or iodipamide, bilirubin, when presented to the liver, reduces biliary cholesterol and phospholipid secretion without affecting that of bile acids. A generalized mechanism has not yet been proposed, although uncoupling effects are most probably exerted at the level of the canalicular membrane or intracellular transport.

Conjugated bilirubin is not absorbed in the intestine or gallbladder. Colonic bacteria degrade bilirubin conjugates to a series of tetrapyrroles collectively termed urobilinogens. Although urobilinogens may undergo enterohepatic circulation, only a small fraction is reabsorbed from the intestine and more than 90% of this is then reexcreted into bile. In neonates or in cases of intestinal stasis, deconjugation of bilirubin conjugates may occur and absorption of unconjugated bilirubin may contribute to the development of unconjugated hyperbilirubinemia.

## 7 Hyperbilirubinemia

Disorders of the bilirubin metabolism mainly become apparent by the clinical appearance of jaundice or by the detection of unconjugated or conjugated hyperbilirubinemia. Values of plasma total bilirubin are between 0.2 and 1.0 mg/dl in 95% of a healthy population. Usually, 1.0 mg/dl or 17 μmol/liter is accepted as the upper limit of normal. Levels of conjugated bilirubin are usually approximated by a direct-diazo reaction. This procedure does not represent an exact reproduction of the amount of conjugates present; the result may vary widely according to the method used [23, 24] but can yield clinically useful information [25]. In our hands the upper limit of the 10-min direct-reacting bilirubin in normals was 0.4 mg/dl. The development of the alkaline methanolysis procedure [26] allowed a specific and sensitive assay of esterified bilirubins. Using alkaline methanolysis and reverse phase high-performance liquid chromatography (HPLC), the upper limit of normal was 0.40 μmol/liter [18]. By means of this method, one can subdivide hyperbilirubinemia into various categories (Table 1). Increased levels of conjugated pigments can be demonstrated in patients with liver disease even at normal levels of total bilirubin [27]. It was further demonstrated that unlike in Gilbert's syndrome or Crigler-Najjar disease, patients with hyperbilirubinemia due to bilirubin overproduction display a parallel increase in both unconjugated and conjugated bilirubins [18, 28, 29]. Clinical differential diagnosis is outlined in Table 2.

**Table 1.** Causes of hyperbilirubinemia

1. Increased unconjugated bilirubin
    - Decreased hepatic uptake
        - Drugs (such as flavaspidic acid, rifamycin, contrast media)
        - Fasting
        - Cardiac decompensation
        - Gilbert's syndrome
    - Decreased bilirubin conjugation
        - Gilbert's syndrome
        - Crigler-Najjar syndrome
        - Neonatal jaundice
        - Acquired conjugation defect?
            - Drug inhibition (such as pregnanediol, chloramphenicol)
            - Hepatocellular disease (chronic hepatitis, Wilson's disease)
2. Increased in unconjugated and conjugated bilirubins with a predominantly unconjugated hyperbilirubinemia
    - Overproduction
        - Hemolysis (sometimes present in septicemia)
        - Ineffective erythropoiesis
        - Fasting
3. Predominantly conjugated hyperbilirunbinemia
    - Intrahepatic biliary obstruction
        - Hepatocellular disease (viral or drug induced)
        - Drug-induced cholestasis (such as steroids)
        - Sepsis
        - Recurrent (benign) intrahepatic cholestasis
        - Cholestatic jaundice of pregnancy
        - Dubin-Johnson syndrome
        - Rotor's syndrome
    - Extrahepatic biliary obstruction (such as stones, tumors, strictures)

Three fundamental alterations of bilirubin metabolism are reflected by three different patterns of serum bilirubins, which can be differentiated by alkaline methanolysis–HPLC or thin-layer chromatography (TLC).

1. Purely unconjugated hyperbilirubinemia is associated with deficient hepatic conjugation (Gilbert's syndrome, Crigler-Najjar disease) that is characterized by a selective increase in unconjugated bilirubin with normal or decreased absolute concentrations of the ester conjugates, resulting in a decreased percentage of esterified versus total bilirubin.
2. A parallel increase in both unconjugated and esterified bilirubins with a normal ratio of esterified to total pigment is characteristic of increased pigment production.
3. A normal or a moderately increased unconjugated bilirubin with a markedly increased concentration of esterified bilirubin resulting in an increased percentage of esterified to total pigment is found in hepatobiliary disease.

**Table 2.** Differential diagnosis of hyperbilirubinemia

| | Hyperbilirubinemia | | | | |
|---|---|---|---|---|---|
| | increased indirect-reacting bilirubin, no bilirubinuria | | | increased direct-reacting bilirubin, bilirubinuria | increased indirect + direct-react. bil. |
| reticulocyte count: | ↑ | nl | nl | ↓ | ↓ |
| serum haptoglobin: | ↓ | low or nl | nl | | |
| hemoglobin: | nl or ↓ | nl or low | nl | | |
| urobilinuria: | ↑ | urobilinuria | nl | | |
| red cell survival (*Cr): | ↓ | nl | nl to slightly ↓ (in 50%) | △△ hepatitis, cirrhosis, obstructive jaundice | mixed pathology, e.g. cirrhosis + hemolysis, Zieve syndrome, Overloading, Rifamycine therapy |
| | ↓ | ↓ | ↓ | | |
| | hemolytic jaundice | possibly dys-erythropoiesis; to test with "Fe kinetics | usually Gilbert's syndrome to be confirmed by<br>• fasting, nicotinic acid<br>• glucuronyltransferase assay in liver<br>• serum or bile analysis (bilirubin conjugates)<br>• trial with phenobarbitone or glutethimide<br>P.S. Storage disease to be excluded by<br>• BSP Tm and S<br>• Ligandin determination on liver | | |

**Table 3.** Hemolysis

I . Intracorpuscular defects
- A. Abnormalities of the red cell membrane
  1. Hereditary spherocytosis
  2. Hereditary elliptocytosis
  3. Acanthocytosis
  4. Stomatocytosis
  5. Abnormalities of lipid
- B. Paroxysmal nocturnal hemoglobinuria
- C. Abnormalities of red cell enzymes
  1. Defects of the Embden-Meyerhof pathway
  2. Defects of the pentose phosphate pathway
  3. ATPase deficiency
- D. Inherited abnormalities of hemoglobin
  1. Abnormalities of globin due to amino acid substitutions and delections: the unstable hemoglobins
  2. Sickle cell disease
  3. The thalassemias

II. Extracorpuscular defects
- A. The autoimmune hemolytic anemias
- B. Hemolysis due to infections and to the direct action of drugs and chemical agents: the Heinz body anemias.
- C. Hemolysis due to direct trauma or to physical agents (microangiopathic hemolytic anemia)

## 7.1 Overproduction of Bilirubin

Overproduction of bilirubin can result from hemolysis (Table 3) or dyserythropoiesis and rarely from breakdown of extravasated erythrocytes (e.g., in a hematoma) or enhanced turnover of hemoproteins. In most hemolytic disorders, destruction of defective or injured red cells occurs in mononuclear phagocytic cells of the spleen, liver, and bone marrow. In intravascular hemolysis erythrocytes are destroyed within the circulation and hemoglobin is released directly into plasma. Hemoglobin is bound to haptoglobin and this complex is taken up and degraded principally by hepatic parenchymal cells [30]. If large amounts of hemoglobin are released (in excess of 1–2 mg/ml plasma), haptoglobin may be depleted and unbound hemoglobin will appear in plasma, where it is rapidly oxidized to methemoglobin. Oxidized heme (ferric heme or hemin), which dissociates more readily from globin that does its reduced form, binds to hemopexin and albumin. The heme–hemopexin complex also enters the parenchymal liver cell, where it is degraded to bilirubin. In addition, a major portion of circulating unbound hemoglobin or methemoglobin is cleared by the kidneys. After dissociation of the tetrametric hemoglobin or methemoglobin into globin pairs, each containing an $\alpha$ and a $\beta$ subunit, the dimers undergo glomerular filtration to be largely reabsorbed by the proximal tubular cells, where heme is degraded to bilirubin. Thus during intravascular hemolysis, parenchymal cells of both liver and kidney are important sites of bilirubin production.

Megaloblastic anemia, sideroblastic anemia, erythroleukemia, and lead poisoning, in addition to a hereditary syndrome of unknown pathogenesis called "primary shunt hyperbilirubinemia" or "idiopathic dyserythropoietic jaundice," are associated with ineffective erythropoiesis. The erythropoietic early labeled bile pigment fractions have been estimated to range from 30% to 80% of all bile pigments formed. A marked erythroid hyperplasia of the bone marrow occurs with active erythrophagocytosis on occasions, a greatly accelerated plasma iron turnover, and a relatively low reticulocytosis when compared to the degree of anemia.

Bilirubin overproduction leads to enchanced serum levels of both unconjugated and conjugated pigments [18] but the hyperbilirubinemia remains predominantly unconjugated. With increasing rates of pigment production the plasma bilirubin concentration will rise linearly until a new steady state is reached in which hepatic bilirubin removal equals pigment production. Since erythropoiesis can be increased maximally by eight- to tenfold, the highest plasma bilirubin concentrations in severe chronic hemolysis do not exceed 40 mg/liter provided hepatic bilirubin clearance is normal; higher concentrations indicate that hepatic bilirubin removal is (also) defective [31]. In acute hemolytic crises plasma bilirubin levels in excess of 40 mg/liter are encountered, regardless of the prevailing hepatic bilirubin clearance.

The increased production rate remains far below the maximal conjugating and secretory capacity. The increased bilirubin load will thus lead to an enhanced excretion of bilirubin conjugates in bile and this will augment the fecal and urinary urobilinogen excretion.

## 7.2 Decreased Conjugation of Bilirubin

A decreased conjugation will result in unconjugated hyperbilirubinemia. According to the degree of deficiency one can recognize three major types (Table 4).

Crigler-Najjar disease is rare. It is subdivided into two types mainly on the basis of the response of serum bilirubin levels to treatment with phenobarbital. Type I, the more serious disease, is characterized by a pronounced unconjugated hyperbilirubinemia which does not decrease by more than 20% under phenobarbital (10 mg/kg). Bile of these patients contains low concentrations of bile pigments; they are composed of unconjugated (≥75%) and monoconjugated (5%–25%) bilirubin whereas diconjugates are absent or only present in trace amounts. Children with Crigler-Najjar disease run a severe risk of dying from kernicterus. Phototherapy is the only way of keeping them alive until hepatic transplantation can be carried out safely.

**Table 4.** Inherited unconjugated hyperbilirubinemias

| | Crigler-Najjar disease, type I | Crigler-Najjar Disease, type II | Gilbert's syndrome |
|---|---|---|---|
| Incidence | Rare | Rare | 5%–7% of adult population |
| Jaundice | Severe, beginning 3–4 days after birth | Usually beginning shortly after birth | Mild, fluctuating, recognized in early adulthood; many instances remain undetected |
| Bilirubin encephalopathy | Developing within 18 months but occasionally delayed until early adulthood | Very rare | None |
| Plasma bilirubin | 17–50 mg/dl; usually >20 mg/dl | 6–22 mg/dl; usually <20 mg/dl | <6 mg/dl; usually <3 mg/dl and fluctuating |
| Plasma bilirubin turnover | Normal | Normal | Normal or moderately increased in a significant proportion of individuals |
| Plasma bilirubin clearance | <50% of normal | <50% of normal | Approximately 30% of normal |
| Response to phenobarbital | Absent | Marked improvement (to <50%) of plasma bilirubin levels | Virtual normalization of plasma bilirubin clearance and concentration |
| Bile | Yellow: contains unconjugated bilirubin and bilirubin mono-glucuronides | Yellow: contains mostly bilirubin mono-glucuronides | Yellow: decreased proportion of bilirubin diconjugates |
| Hepatic bilirubin UDP-glucuronosyltransferase activity | Absent or near zero | Absent or near zero | Reduced to about a third of normal |

Type II is the more benign condition, where phenobarbital therapy usually can keep the bilirubin levels at safe concentrations below 150 μmol/liter. Kernicterus can develop when serum bilirubin levels rise during infections or fasting.

Gilbert's syndrome is a far more common abnormality, said to occur in approximately 5%–7% of the adult male population. The incidence in females is, however, underestimated as the upper limit of normal serum bilirubin levels is lower in postpubertal females than in males [32]. The syndrome is characterized by a mild chronic unconjugated hyperbilirubinemia in the absence of overt hemolysis or liver disease [33]. It constitutes a totally benign mild jaundice, observed mostly at or after puberty. This seems to be attributable to changes in plasma bilirubin levels occurring at puberty and due presumably to alterations in bilirubin UDP-glucuronyltransferase activity. Indeed, testosterone decreases and estro-progesterone enhances transferase activity [34]. The syndrome is inherited as an autosomal-dominant trait.

Individuals with Gilbert's syndrome are asymptomatic or present with vague symptoms of fatigue or abdominal discomfort not caused by the jaundice but frequently representing the reason for seeking medical advice, at which occasion the jaundice is recognized. Indeed, caloric deprivation occurring during any illness will enhance the jaundice. Studies by Gollan et al. [35] demonstrated that the lipid compound of the food was important besides the total amount of calories. The diagnosis is based upon the finding of a chronic unconjugated hyperbilirubinemia in the absence of hemolysis, dyserythropoiesis, or liver disease. Serum bile acids, haptoglobin, and the reticulocyte count are normal. Development of sensitive methods has allowed documentation of a sole increase in unconjugated bilirubin concentrations with an enhanced ratio of mono- to diconjugates [18, 28]. If necessary, caloric restriction to 400 kcal/day for 48 h [36] or an intravenous load of nicotinic acid [37] can be used to elicit a pronounced and diagnostic rise in serum unconjugated bilirubin. Bilirubin levels normalize with phenobarbitone, glutethimide, or clofibrate [38], all inducers of bilirubin UDP-glucuronyltransferase [14], but the disorder does not need treatment besides confirmation of its benign, innocent nature.

### 7.3 Bilirubinostasis and Cholestasis

The hepatocyte secretory mechanism is very susceptible to many kinds of agents and situations, and biliary secretion is disturbed in all hepatic diseases. This becomes apparent through the increase in bilirubin conjugates in plasma [27] or in covalently linked bilirubin–albumin conjugates [6, 39]. Bilirubinostasis points to a sole disturbance of bilirubin secretion (see, e.g., also Sect. 7.4) whereas cholestasis represents a more frequent and more generally disturbed biliary secretion. Its intensity can vary markedly. Cholestasis can be due to functional alterations of the canalicular secretory apparatus or to mechanical obstructions of bile duct or ductules, or be associated with hepatocellular necrosis (Table 5). Characteristically, serum concentrations of bile acids, bilirubin conjugates, alkaline phosphatase, γ-glutamyltranspeptidase, 5′-nucleotidase, etc. are increased.

The plasma levels of esterified bilirubins are enhanced and when the cholestasis is prolonged, non-C-1 isomers are demonstrated in serum. Furthermore it recently became clear that an additional pigment fraction is present which is direct-diazo reacting and strongly protein bound, pre-

**Table 5.** Conditions associated with hampered biliary secretion of bilirubin conjugates

| | |
|---|---|
| 1. *Only disturbed bilirubin secretion* | |
| Postoperative jaundice due to overload with anoxia | |
| Dubin-Johnson syndrome | |
| 2. *Cholestasis* | |
| a) Functional disturbances | |
| – ranging from pure cholestasis | Anabolic steroids<br>Drugs such as chlorpromazine<br>$\alpha_1$-Antitrypsin deficiency |
| – to hepatocellular necrosis | Hepatitis cirrhosis |
| b) Mechanical disorders | |
| – of small bile ducts | Primary biliary cirrhosis<br>Sclerosing cholangitis |
| – of large bile ducts | Cholangiocarcinoma<br>Common duct stones<br>Ampulloma<br>Pancreatic carcinoma |

sumably by covalent binding with albumin [39–42]. It is responsible for the discrepancy between the diazo reaction and the lower concentrations obtained by the alkaline methanolysis procedure; indeed the latter procedure is carried out after deproteinization, whereby the protein-bound pigment is not extracted and thus not revealed in the TLC or HPLC analysis. These bilirubin–protein conjugates can be produced in vitro by incubation of glucuronides with serum albumin. Bilirubin β-D-1-*O* mono- and/or diglucuronide during stasis is known to undergo intramolecular base-catalyzed dearrangement or so-called acyl shift to 2-*O*-, 3-*O*-, and 4-*O*-acylglucuronides via ortho-acid intermediates [43, 44]. Studies in vitro sustained by observations in vivo led McDonagh et al. [41] to propose that a similar acyl shift occurs but via O → N migration of a bilirubin acyl group from glucuronide acid to a reactive -$NH_2$ group of albumin. Some hydrolysis to unconjugated bilirubin appears to occur at the same time, especially at pH values above 7.4. It should be noted that the covalent interaction of *O*-acylglucuronides with albumin is not limited to bilirubin as this was recently also described for zomepirac, an anti-inflammatory agent [45], and for glucuronides of other drugs [46].

It will be clear from the mechanism discussed above that protein conjugates are only formed from ester glucuronides. They are thus only present in chronic conjugated hyperbilirubinemias. The protein linkage renders these pigments nondialyzable; they are not taken up by the liver and thus not excreted in bile. They remain in plasma and appear to have a plasma half-life comparable to that of serum albumin. Bile duct ligation in the rat results in a bilirubin–protein conjugate fraction of approximately 17% of total serum bilirubin after 48 h; this fraction increases with time. In patients with cholestasis it can amount to 50% or more [6, 27]. When a mechanical obstruction is removed, the glucuronide ester conjugates rapidly decrease whereas the protein conjugates have a very slow plasma clearance; as a result their proportion increases to 85%–90% of total pigment. Bilirubinuria is present during and shortly after relief of obstruction but not later, despite the persistence of conjugated hyperbilirubinemia; this is due to the fact that the protein conjugates are not dialyzable. They can now be measured directly in plasma.

Acute obstruction of the bile ducts results initially in increased transaminases; some hours later bilirubin conjugates are elevated in plasma and only later still are higher levels of alkaline phosphatases observed. Indeed, the latter are newly synthesized by the hepatocytes [47] and this requires some time. Acute cholestasis leads to a predominance of diconjugates [48]. This is presumably secondary to retention of monoconjugates within the hepatocytes whereby a more efficient transformation to diconjugates is possible. Indeed, similar events have been observed when the biliary secretion of bilirubin conjugates was hampered by infusion of ioglycamide [17] and also in mutant rats with defective biliary secretion [19].

## 8 Dubin-Johnson Syndrome and Rotor's Syndrome [49, 50]

The Dubin-Johnson syndrome presents an inherited defect of the biliary transport of conjugated bilirubin and sulfobromophthalein and an unexplained abnormality in coproporphyrin metabolism. The liver has a black appearance due to retention of a melanine-like pigment. Most patients are asymptomatic and the plasma bilirubin levels range between 20 and 50 mg/liter (35–85 µmol/liter). It is a direct-reacting hyperbilirubinemia with bilirubinuria. Non-C-1-bilirubin glucuronides are present as well as bilirubin–protein conjugates. The kinetics of injected sulfobromophthalein are highly characteristic: initial plasma disappearance rate is normal but a secondary rise due to reflux of conjugated sulfobromophthalein is observed after 45–90 min. This secondary rise is not noted with disulfobromophthalein or indocyanine green, two substances which can be secreted without conjugation. The computed hepatic uptake and storage capacity are (near) normal, the secretory maximum ($T_m$) is grossly impaired. In this syndrome urinary excretion of coproporphyrins is normal, but isomer III excretion is reduced whereas that of the I isomer is enhanced to approximately 80% of total coproporphyrins (in normal individuals it is <45%).

Rotor's syndrome seems to be identical with hepatic storage disease. This rare disorder is characterized by fluctuating direct-reacting hyperbilirubinemia. In contrast to Dubin-Johnson syndrome, coproporphyrin excretion in urine is enhanced and the ratio of I to III isomers only mildly increased. Plasma sulfobromophthalein kinetics show a decreased disappearance rate resulting in increased retention at 45 min. Autosomal-recessive inheritance has been suggested.

Analysis of bilirubin conjugates in serum revealed a predominance of the diester conjugates in Dubin-Johnson syndrome, in agreement with data obtained in bilirubinostasis in the rat [17], and a predominance of the C-12 monoconjugate in Rotor's syndrome [51].

## References


1. Crawford JM, Hauser SC, Gollan JL (1988) Formation, hepatic metabolism and transport of bile pigments: a status report. Semin Liver Dis 8:105–118
2. Stocker R, Glaze AN, Ames BN (1987) Antioxidant activity of albumin-bound bilirubin. Proc Natl Acad Sci USA 84:5918–5922
3. Lightner DA, Wijekoon WMD, Zhang MH (1988) Understanding bilirubin conformation and binding. J Biol Chem 263:16669–16676
4. Tiribelli C, Ostrow DJ (1989) New concepts on bilirubin chemistry, transport and metabolism: report of the International Bilirubin Workshop, 6–8 April, 1989, Trieste, Italy. Hepatology 11:303–313
5. Schacter B (1988) Heme catabolism by heme oxygenase: physiology, regulation and mechanism of action. Semin Hematol 25:349–369
6. Weiss JS, Gautam A, Lauff JJ, Sundberg MW, Jatlow P, Boyer JL, Seligson D (1983) The clinical importance of a protein-bound fraction of serum bilirubin in patients with hyperbilirubinemia. N Engl J Med 309:147–150
7. Sorrentino D, Berk PD (1988) Mechanistic aspects of hepatic bilirubin uptake. Semin Liver Dis 8:119–136
8. Tiribelli C, Ballentani S, Lunazzi GC, Sottocasa GL (1988) Role and nature of plasma membrane carrier proteins in the hepatic transport of organic anions. J Gastroenterol Hepatol 4:215–225
9. Whitmer ID, Russell PE, Gollan JL (1987) Membrane-membrane interactions associated with rapid transfer of bilirubin to microsomal UDP-glucuronyl transferase: releveance for hepatocellular transport and biotransformation of hydrophobic substrates. Biochem J 244:41–47
10. Fevery J, Van de Vijer M, Michiels R, Heirwegh KPM (1977) Comparison in different species of bilirubin-IXα conjugates with the activities of hepatic and renal bilirubin-IXα UDP-glycosyltransferases. Biochem J 164:737–746
11. Vanstapel F, Blanckaert N (1988) Topology and regulation of bilirubin UDP-glucuronosyl transferase in sealed native microsomes from rat liver. Arch Biochem Biophys 263:216–225
12. Zakim D, Vessey DA (1982) The role of microsomal membrane in modulating the activity of UDP-glucuronyl transferase. In: Marroussi A (ed) Membranes and transport. Plenum, New York, pp 269–273
13. Van Steenbergen W, Fevery J, De Vos R, Leyten R, Heirwegh KPM, De Groote J (1989) Thyroid hormones and the hepatic handling of bilirubin. I. Hepatic transport of bilirubin mono- and diconjugates in the Wistar rat. Hepatology 9:314–321
14. Van Steenbergen W, Fevery J (1990) Effects of uridine diphosphate glucuronosyltransferase activity on the maximal secretion rate of bilirubin conjugates in the rat. Gastroenterology 99:488–499
15. Yokosuka O, Billing BH (1987) Enzymatic oxidation of bilirubin by intestinal mucosa. Biochem Biophys Acta 923:268–274
16. Muñoz ME, Esteller A, Gonzalez J (1987) Substrate induction of bilirubin conjugation and biliary excretion in the rat. Clin Sci 73:371–375
17. Mesa AM, Fevery J, Heirwegh KPM, De Groote J (1985) Effects of ioglycamide on the hepatic transport of bilirubin and its mono- and diconjugates in the rat. Hepatology 5:600–606

18. Muraca M, Fevery J, Blanckaert N (1987) Relationship between serum bilirubins and production and conjugation of bilirubin: studies in Gilbert's syndrome, Crigler-Najjar disease, hemolytic disorders and rat models. Gastroenterology 92:309–317
19. Jansen PLM, Peters WH, Lamers WH (1985) Hereditary chronic unconjugated hyperbilirubinemia in mutant rats caused by defective hepatic anion transport. Hepatology 5:573–579
20. Ricci GL, Cornelis M, Fevery J, De Groote J (1983) Maximal hepatic bilirubin transport in the rat during somatostatin-induced cholestasis and taurocholate-induced cholestasis and taurocholate-choleresis. J Lab Clin Med 101:835–846
21. Galan AI, Jimenez R, Muñoz ME, Gonzalez J (1990) Effects of ursodeoxycholate on maximal biliary secretion of bilirubin in the rat. Biochem Pharmacol 39: 1175–1180
22. Crawford JM, Gollan JL (1988) Hepatocyte cotransport of bilirubin glucuronides: role of microtubules. Am J Physiol 255:G121–G131
23. Nosslin B (1960) The direct diazo reaction of bile pigments in serum. Experimental and clinical studies. Scand J Clin Lab Invest 12[Suppl 49]
24. Killenberg PG, Stevens RD, Wildermann RF et al. (1980) The laboratory method as a variable in the interpretation of serum bilirubin fractionation. Gastroenterology 78:1011–1015
25. Fevery J, Claes J, Heirwegh K, De Groote J (1967) Hyperbilirubinemia: significance of the ratio between direct-reacting and total bilirubin. Clin Chim Acta 17:73–79
26. Blanckaert N (1980) Analysis of bilirubin and bilirubin mono- and diconjugates. Determination of their relative amounts in biological fluids. Biochem J 185: 115–128
27. Van Hootegem P, Fevery J, Blanckaert N (1985) Serum bilirubins in hepatobiliary disease: comparison with other liver function tests and changes in the post obstructive period. Hepatology 5:112–117
28. Sieg A, Stiehl A, Raedsch R, Ullrich D, Messmer B, Kommerell B (1986) Gilbert's syndrome: diagnosis by typical serum bilirubin pattern. Clin Chim Acta 154:41–48
29. Sieg A, König R, Ullrich D, Fevery J (1990) Subfractionation of serum bilirubins by alkaline methanolysis and thin-layer chromatography. An aid in the differential diagnosis of icteric disease. J Hepatol 11:159–164
30. Bissell DM (1986) Heme catabolism and bilirubin formation. In: Ostrow JD (ed) Bile pigments and jaundice. Marcel Dekker, New York, pp 133–156
31. Berk PD, Isola LM, Jones EA (1986) Specific defects in hepatic storage and clearance of bilirubin. In: Ostrow JD (ed) Bile pigments and jaundice. Marcel Dekker, New York, pp 270–316
32. Werner M, Tolls RE, Hultin JV et al. (1970) Influence of sex and age on the normal range of eleven serum constituents. Z Klin Chem Klin Biochem 8:105–115
33. Okolicsanyi L, Fevery J, Billing B, Berthelot P, Thompson RPH, Schmid R, Berk PD (1983) How should mild isolated unconjugated hyperbilirubinemia be investigated? Semin Liver Dis 3:36–41
34. Muraca M, Fevery J (1984) Influence of sex and sex steroids on bilirubin uridine diphosphate-glucuronosyltransferase activity of rat liver. Gastroenterology 87:308–313
35. Gollan JL, Bateman C, Billing BH (1976) Effect of dietary composition on the unconjugated hyperbilirubinaemia of Gilbert's syndrome. Gut 17:335–340
36. Barrett PVD (1975) Effects of caloric and non-caloric materials in fasting hyperbilirubinemia. Gastroenterology 68:361–369
37. Gentile S, Orzes N, Persico M, Marmo R, Bronzino P, Tiribelli C (1985) Comparison of nicotinic-acid and caloric restriction-induced hyperbilirubinemia in the diagnosis of Gilbert's syndrome. J Hepatol 1:537–543

38. Kutz K, Kandler H, Gugler R, Fevery J (1984) Effect of clofibrate on the metabolism of bilirubin; bromosulphophthalein and indocyanine green and on the biliary lipid composition in Gilbert's syndrome. Clin Sci 66:389–397
39. Wu TW (1984) Bilirubin analysis – the state of the art and future prospects. Clin Biochem 17:221–229
40. Lauff JJ, Kasper HE, Ambrose RT (1981) Separation of bilirubin species in serum and bile by high performance liquid chromatography. J Chromatogr 226:391–402
41. McDonagh AF, Palma LA, Lauff JL, Wu TW (1984) Origin of mammalian biliprotein and rearrangement of bilirubin glucuronides in vivo in the rat. J Clin Invest 74:763–770
42. Blanckaert N, Servaes R, Leroy P (1986) Measurements of bilirubin-protein conjugates in serum and application to human and rat sera. J Lab Clin Med 108:77–87
43. Compernolle F, Van Hees GP, Blanckaert N et al. (1978) Glucuronic acid conjugates of bilirubin-IXα glucuronide in cholestasis and during storage in vitro. Intramolecular rearrangement to positional isomers of glucuronic acid. Biochem J 171:185–201
44. Compernolle F, Van Hees GP, Heirwegh KPM (1978) Rearranged glucuronic acid conjugates of bilirubin-IXα in post-obstructive bile. Structure elucidation of azopigments β and γ as ethyl anthranilate *N*-glycosides derived from 2-, 3- and 4-*O*-acyl glucuronides. Biomed Mass Spectrom 5:453–459
45. Smith PC, McDonagh AF, Benet LZ (1986) Irreversible binding of zomepirac to plasma protein in vitro and in vivo. J Clin Invest 77:934–939
46. Wells DS, Janssen FW, Ruelius HW (1987) Interactions between oxaprozin glucuronide and albumin. Xenobiotica 17:1437–1449
47. Kaplan MM, Okhubo A, Quaroni EG, Sze-Tu D (1983) Increased synthesis of rat liver alkaline phosphatase by bile duct ligation. Hepatology 3:368–376
48. Mesa VA, De Vos R, De Groote J, Fevery J (1987) Increase in the ratio of bilirubin di- to monoconjugates (BDC:BMC) in bile and serum constitutes a sensitive marker of cholestasis in rats. J Hepatol 15:S168
49. Wolkoff AW, Cohen LE, Arias IM (1973) Inheritance of the Dubin-Johnson syndrome. N Engl J Med 288:113–117
50. Wolkoff AW, Wolpert E, Fascasio FM et al. (1976) Rotor's syndrome: a distinct pathophysiologic entity. Am J Med 60:173–179
51. Rosenthal P, Blanckaert N (1984) Differentiation of Rotor syndrome from Dubin-Johnson syndrome by fractionation of serum bilirubins (abstr). Hepatology 4:1026

# 8 Bile Salts, Bile Flow, and Cholestasis*

J. Quiroga

## 1 Bile Salts and the Enterohepatic Circulation: Physiology and Pathophysiology

### 1.1 Bile Composition

Bile is a solution of organic and inorganic compounds in water. It is produced by hepatocytes and secreted into the bile canaliculi (canalicular bile). It is then modified as it passes through intrahepatic bile ductules and ducts (ductular bile). Most of the bile entering the extrahepatic biliary tree enters the gallbladder, where it is concentrated and stored between periods of digestion (gallbladder bile). Finally, meals stimulate gallbladder emptying which projects bile through the common bile duct into the duodenum, where bile facilitates digestion.

Figure 1 shows the components of human hepatic bile. The exact composition of primary hepatocytic bile is unknown, since its direct sampling is not possible owing to the canalicular diameter (1 µm). Unlike other biologic fluids, bile contains substantial amounts of lipidic compounds. This reflects the key role of the liver both in regulation of lipoprotein metabolism and in clearance of lipophilic metabolites from the body.

Organic bile solutes comprise about 30 g/liter. Of these, 67% are bile salts, 22% phospholipids, 4% unesterified cholesterol, 4.5% proteins, and less than 0.5% bilirubin. Bile also contains derivatives of several metabolic pathways, such as uro- and coproporphyrins, various kinds of steroid hormones, vitamin $D_2$, cysteinyl leukotrienes, prostaglandins, and many other compounds that are subjected to hepatic excretion. Most xenobiotics, especially lipophilic substances, are eliminated in bile, including opioids,

---

* *Abbreviations used in this chapter*: AIDS, acquired immunodeficiency syndrome; BADF, bile acid-dependent bile flow; BAIF, bile acid-independent bile flow; BPOC, benign postoperative cholestasis; CMC, critical micellar concentration (of bile acids); EHC, enterohepatic circulation (of bile acids); ERCP, endoscopic retrograde cholangiopancreatography; GGT, γ-glutamyltranspeptidase; GVHD, graft versus host disease; $Na^+,K^+$-ATPase, sodium and potassium-dependent adenosine triphosphatase; OLTx, orthotopic liver transplantation; PTHC, percutaneous transhepatic cholangiography SAMe, *S*-adenosylmethionine; UDCA, ursodeoxycholate.

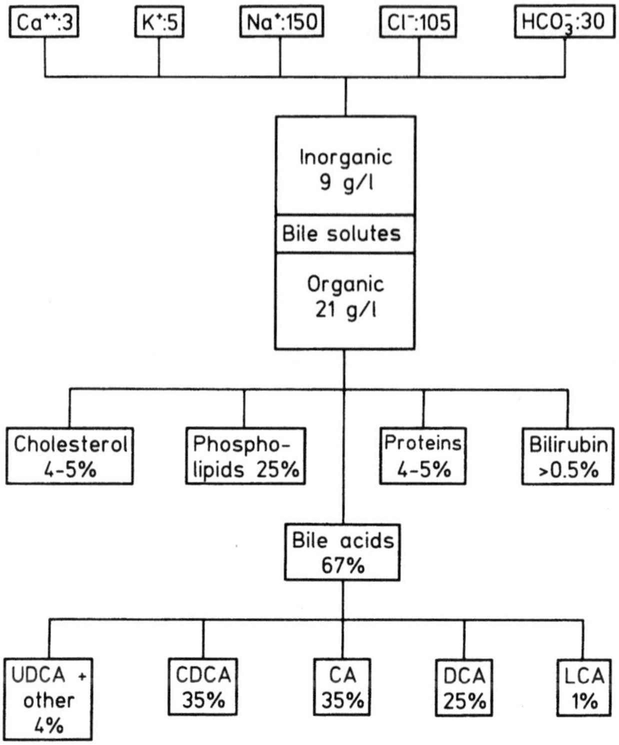


**Fig. 1.** Composition of human hepatic bile. Total solute concentration in hepatic bile is 30 g/liter. Values in the figure are averages from data in references 1–4. Bile electrolyte values are expressed as mmol/liter. Values of individual organic compounds are expressed as the percentage of total organic compounds. *CA*, cholic acid; *CDCA*, chenodeoxycholic acid; *DCA*, deoxycholic acid; *LCA* lithocholic acid; *UDCA*, ursodeoxycholic acid. More than 99% of the bile acids are conjugated with taurine (24%) or glycine (75%)

digitalis, ampicillin, and cephalosporins among many other drugs. Bile proteins include lysosomal and canalicular enzymes, specific bile proteins with the ability to bind copper and other substances, IgA coupled to the secretory piece, and albumin and other serum proteins in minimal quantities. Of the organic bile compounds, bile salts are the essential biological element accounting for most, if not all, of the physiologic functions of bile [1–4].

The concentrations of inorganic ions in ductal bile and in plasma are similar (Fig. 1). The anion gap is greater in bile than in plasma, the difference being accounted for by the presence of bile acids and other organic anions. Bile osmolality measured by freezing point depression is about 300 mosm/kg, whereas its value obtained by calculation from ionic bile composition is higher. This difference is due to the presence in bile of polymolecular bile salt aggregates. Bile osmolality tends to equilibrate rapidly with plasma osmolality. In gallbladder bile, organic materials are concentrated up to 100 g/liter by reabsorption of electrolytes and water [1–4].

### 1.2 Bile Salts: Chemistry, Biosynthesis, and Structure–Activity Relationships

Bile salts are organic substances with unique physicochemical properties. They recirculate in a restricted circuit where they exert their physiologic functions.

Bile salts (or bile acids when non ionized, see legend to Fig. 2) are a family of steroid substances synthesized from cholesterol by liver cells. This conversion involves several enzyme-mediated changes both in the sterol nucleus and in the side chain of the cholesterol molecule. The key intermediate reaction in this process is the 7α-hydroxylation of cholesterol (to 7α-hydroxycholesterol), which is catalyzed by a microsomal 7α-hydroxylase, the activity of which constitutes the rate-limiting step in bile acid synthesis. The size of the total bile acid pool regulates the activity of this enzyme through a negative feedback mechanism. Physiologic bile acids contain 24 carbon atoms and are amphiphilic molecules which exhibit a hydrophilic (polar; α-side) and a hydrophobic (nonpolar; β-side) domain. This structure confers upon bile acids the ability to perform some of their specific functions but also contributes to their toxic potential [5–8].

Bile acids are able to solubilize lipid compounds. This property is directly related to the hydrophobicity of each particular bile acid molecule and is referred to as their detergent-like activity. An additional characteristic of bile acids is their ability to form self-aggregates called simple micelles. Micelle formation requires a certain level, or threshold, of bile acid concentration which is unique for each bile acid and is known as the "critical micellar concentration" (CMC). Above the CMC, bile acids form mixed micelles with phospholipids (lecithin) and cholesterol. This is a crucial function of bile acids that allows completely hydrophobic molecules such as cholesterol and lecithin to be maintained in solution. The amphiphilic nature of bile acids permits the hydrophilic side of the molecule to be directed to the aqueous external milieu, while the hydrophobic pole is in contact with the micellar core, containing cholesterol and lecithin. Hence, bile acids may be present in bile as single molecules, simple micelles, or mixed micelles [9–12].

The basic structure common to all physiologic bile acids is that of 5β-cholanic acid (see Fig. 2). The polarity, solubility, detergent potency, and capacity for micelle formation of each particular bile salt are basically dependent upon four factors: the number of hydroxyl groups added to the basic molecule of cholanic acid, the orientation of these hydroxyl groups in space, the ionization of the terminal COOH ($COO^-$) radical, and conjugation with either taurine or glycine. Bile salts may be mono-, di-, or trihydroxylated. Hydroxyl groups are inserted in the α position in one or

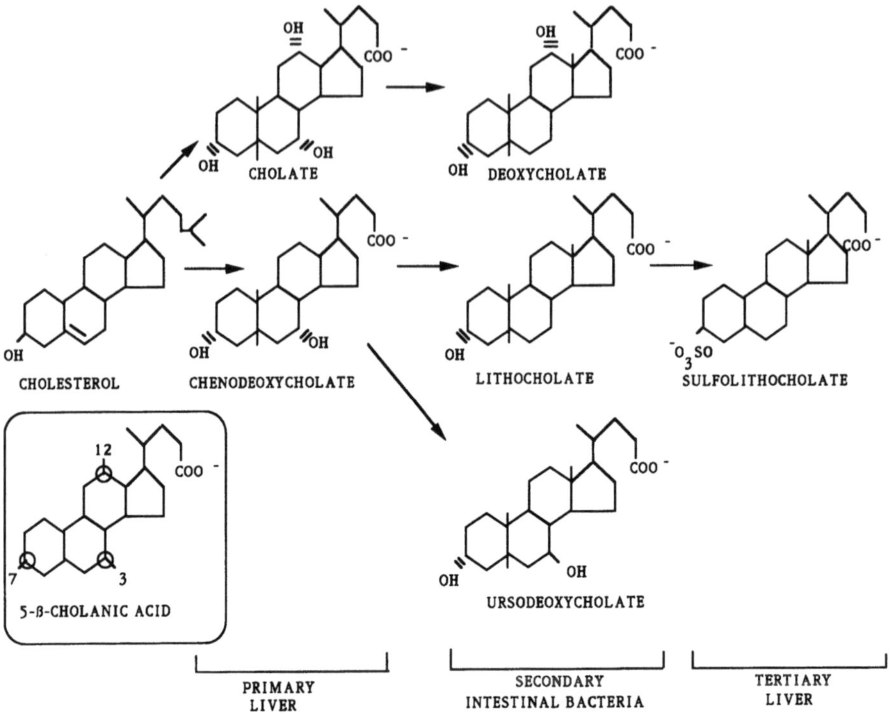


**Fig. 2.** Synthesis and chemistry of primary, secondary, and tertiary bile acids. *Left*: Basic molecule of 5β-cholanic acid. Normal sites for hydroxylation of physiologic bile acids are indicated. *Right*: Formulas in the figure correspond to the unconjugated forms of bile acids. In vivo, virtually all bile acids are ionized, forming taurine- or glycine-conjugated bile salts

more of carbons 3, 7, and 12 (see Fig. 2). In man, hydroxylations at positions other than those indicated above are unusual. Under pathologic conditions, minor amounts of bile acids hydroxylated at position 6 may be detected. β-Hydroxylations are also unusual but are functionally important, since they imply the positioning of a hydrophilic radical in the hydrophobic face of the molecule. Hydroxylations take place in the liver, whereas bile acids are dehydroxylated by the gut flora during their colonic transit. At physiologic pH, virtually all bile acids are ionized and form sodium and potassium salts. Bile acids are conjugated with either taurine or glycine as *N*-acyl amidates in the liver and are deconjugated by the colonic bacteria. At the time of their secretion by the liver, more than 99% of bile acids are conjugated. Additional conjugations with glucuronic acid or sulfate may also occur in the liver. As a general rule, ionization, conjugation, hydroxylation, and especially β-hydroxylation make a bile salt molecule less hydrophobic, less detergent active, less able to form micelles, and less toxic. Therefore, among bile acids, monohydroxy and nonconjugated species will be the most lipophilic and detergent, but also those with the greatest toxic potential. Amidation lowers the pKa of bile acids, avoiding their precipitation in the intestine over a wide range of pH variation. Specific amidations with taurine or glycine, but not with other amino acids, are resistant to the action of pancreatic enzymes, so bile acids remain conjugated in the intestinal lumen. Glucuronidation and sulfation increase the water solubility of bile acids, which in this form may be eliminated in urine [1–10].

### 1.3 The Enterohepatic Circulation

The crucial functions of bile salts are accomplished in the liver and in the lumen of the small bowel. Bile salts are not all lost in the feces but are efficiently reabsorbed in the intestine to be conveyed to the liver by the portal system. In the liver, bile salts are taken up by hepatocytes and resecreted into bile. Thus, bile salts are subjected to a continuous recycling through the liver, biliary tree, intestine, portal blood, and to the liver again. This is known as the enterohepatic circulation (EHC). EHC enhances the functional effectiveness and minimizes the toxic potential of bile acids. There are some specific points to be emphasized [1–4]:

1. Recovery of virtually all bile acids from the intestine allows the bile salt pool to be constant in size with daily synthesis of only minimal amounts of bile acids to match daily fecal loss.
2. The very efficient first-pass extraction of bile acids from portal blood by the liver confines the vast majority of the bile acid pool to the EHC, thus avoiding systemic toxic effects of these compounds.
3. Recirculation of the total bile acid pool several times a day amplifies the biologic activity of bile acids inside the EHC.
4. Pumping of bile salts into the duodenum by the gallbladder to coincide with meals makes possible the digestion of large amounts of dietary fat with a relatively small bile acid pool.
5. In addition to bile salts, many other compounds undergo enterohepatic circulation and may be recovered for reutilization.

A scheme of the EHC is presented in Fig. 3.

#### *Fate of Bile Salts in the Enterohepatic Circulation: Functions and Biotransformation*

*Liver and Biliary Tree.* The liver synthesizes the so-called primary bile salts, cholate and chenodeoxycholate, which are tri- and dihydroxylated respectively. Conjugation with taurine or glycine is carried out in the liver before bile salts are secreted to the canaliculus. Glycocholate is the most abundant bile salt in man. Under normal conditions, bile is continuously produced by hepatocytes and delivered to the biliary tree, where it is stored in the gallbladder between meals. Periodic contractions of the sphincter of

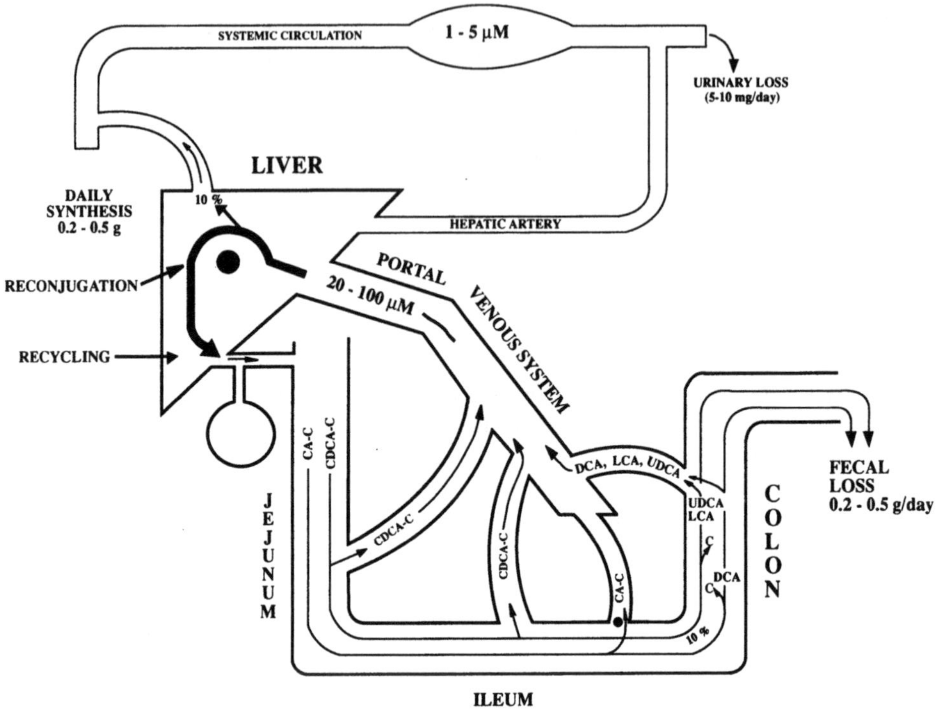


**Fig. 3.** Schematic representation of the EHC of bile salts. *CA*, cholic acid; *DCA*, deoxycholic acid; *CDCA*, chenodeoxycholic acid; *LCA*, lithocholic acid; *UDCA*, ursodeoxycholic acid. "*Bile acid-C*" indicates the conjugated form. *Thick lines* delimit the ECH. *Arrows* indicate the direction of the traffic of substances inside the EHC. *Black dots* indicate the sites where bile salts are transported by specific and energy-dependent systems

Oddi facilitate the entry of bile into the gallbladder. The stimulatory effect of cholecystokinin during the digestive period causes the emptying of this reservoir and the projection of bile into the duodenum.

Bile formation requires the active secretion of bile acids by the liver. The presence of bile acids in the canaliculi is the main driving force for bile formation. Secretion into the canaliculi of bilirubin, cholesterol, and phospholipids is dependent on bile acid secretion. Hence, the chief function of bile acids in the liver is stimulation of bile formation [1–6].

*Small Bowel.* Bile salts reach the intestine where they perform important physiologic functions, and in addition they undergo biotransformation and enterohepatic circulation. The bulk of the primary bile salts are reabsorbed in the small bowel. A specific carrier-mediated, sodium-coupled, active transport system is active in the distal ileum, translocating bile salts from intestinal lumen to the enterocytes which then release the bile salts into the portal venous system. This specific transport system is very efficient in the reabsorption of trihydroxy bile salts (tauro- and glycocholate). A large proportion of tauro- and glycochenodeoxycholate, which are more lipophilic than cholates, gains entry into the portal circulation by passive diffusion across the jejunal mucosa. Minor amounts (less than 10%) of the bile salts entering the duodenum escape intestinal reabsorption and reach the colon [11–15].

*Colon.* In the large bowel, bile salts are metabolized by bacterial anaerobic flora, mainly of the genera *Eubacterium* and *Clostridium*. Bile acids undergo deconjugation and then 7α-dehydroxylation. Taurine and glycine are reabsorbed. Cholate and chenodeoxycholate are converted to deoxycholate and lithocholate, which are di- and monohydroxy compounds, respectively, and are known as secondary bile salts. About 50% of deoxycholate and 20%–25% of lithocholate formed in the colon is reabsorbed and enters the portal system. The rest is lost in the stool and constitutes the only daily loss of bile acids [1–4, 17].

*Portal Venous System.* All bile salts recovered from the small and large bowel return to the liver through the portal circulation. Hepatocytes very efficiently take up bile salts from sinusoidal blood. First-pass clearance is as high as 90% for trihydroxy bile salts and 50%–70% for the remaining compounds. Bile salts which escape liver uptake reach the systemic circulation. Thus, under normal conditions the concentrations of bile acids in the portal blood (20–30 μM in the fasting state and probably as high as 100 μM after meals) far exceed systemic blood levels (1–5 μM). In blood, bile salts are tightly bound to albumin and to lipoproteins, especially to high density lipoproteins and to a lesser extent to low density and very low density lipoproteins [1–4].

*Liver Reuptake and Recycling of Bile Salts.* Once bile salts are taken up by the liver, they are subjected to further metabolism. Basically, all secondary bile acids are conjugated but not rehydroxylated. Lithocholic conjugates, which are poorly water soluble, are conjugated again with sulfate. The resulting sulfoglycolithocholate and sulfotaurolithocholate are excreted into bile. Finally, 7-oxolithocholate may be reduced in the liver to yield ursodeoxycholate, which in some individuals is the fourth most common bile acid in bile, although in general it does not exceed 2%–3% of total bile acids. The cycle of the EHC is reinitiated by the transfer of bile salts from sinusoidal blood to bile canaliculi. This is a very complex process that will be considered in detail below.

### *Regulation of the Enterohepatic Circulation and the Bile Salt Pool*

Fecal loss of bile salts is about 200–400 mg/day. It is equilibrated by hepatic synthesis, so that the total bile salt pool remains relatively constant under normal conditions. Total bile salt pool size is the main factor regulating the rate of bile acid synthesis. When bile salt losses are increased, there is a compensatory stimulation of their synthesis by the liver. This is accomplished by enhanced cholesterol production and its eventual metabolism to bile acids. A decreased bile acid pool size stimulates HMG-CoA reductase and 7α-hydroxylase. The EHC does not occur at a uniform rate throughout the day; rather it reaches a maximum during digestion, when bile acid flow to the intestine is promoted by gallbladder contraction. Cholecystokinin and to a lesser extent gastrin and neural cholinergic stimuli are the principal stimuli for gallbladder emptying. In man, the bile salt pool size is about 3 g. It recirculates 12 times per day on average; thus, a total of 36 g of bile salts is secreted and taken up by the liver daily [1–4, 18].

### *Summary of Bile Salt Functions*

Bile salts are the most important substances in bile and display the following functions [1–6]:

1. Bile salts are the principal osmotic force for the generation of bile flow.
2. In addition to water flow, bile salts stimulate the canalicular secretion of bilirubin and other organic anions.
3. Bile salts stimulate the canalicular secretion of cholesterol and phospholipids and solubilize these substances by forming stable aggregates in the form of simple or mixed micelles. This function requires that a critical micellar concentration of bile salts is achieved. The CMC is ~2 mM, ranging from 0.6 to 10 mM for different physiologic bile acids. The proportions in bile of bile salts, cholesterol and lecithin which permit all biliary cholesterol to be in soluble form vary within a narrow range. When this equilibrium is altered, usually by relative cholesterol excess or deficiency of bile salts, cholesterol precipitation in bile occurs and bile becomes "lithogenic."
4. In the intestine, bile salts emulsify dietary neutral lipids, making possible their digestion by pancreatic lipase and colipase. The products of fat digestion, monoglycerides and fatty acids, form micelles with bile salts in the intestinal lumen. In this way, these hydrophobic fat compounds can gain access to the absorptive surface of the enterocyte, which is covered with an unstirred water layer.
5. The size of the bile acid pool regulates cholesterol synthesis by the liver, modulating the activity of the key enzyme (HMG-CoA reductase) in cholesterol formation.
6. The size of bile salt pool exerts a negative feedback on the activity of 7α-hydroxylase, the enzyme which controls the rate-limiting step in bile acid synthesis from cholesterol. At the same time, self-regulation of bile salt synthesis influences cholesterol levels.
7. The size of the bile salt pool also controls the cycling rate in the EHC, so that changes in the pool size may be compensated by increased or

decreased cycling. It has been demonstrated that the cycling rate and size of the bile salt pool are inversely and closely correlated.

8. Transport of bile salts from sinusoids to canaliculi and from intestine to portal blood provides chemical pumping for the EHC and complements the mechanical pumping exerted by gallbladder contraction and intestinal peristalsis.

Thus, bile salts are crucial for bile flow generation, maintenance of cholesterol solubility in bile, digestion and subsequent absorption of dietary fat in the intestine, regulation of cholesterol metabolism, maintenance of the EHC, and self-regulation of their synthesis.

## 1.4 Pathophysiology of the Enterohepatic Circulation of Bile Salts

Alterations in the physiology of bile salts may originate at any level within the EHC.

Clinical manifestations may be derived either from deficiency of bile salts inside the EHC or from their abnormal presence outside the boundaries of the EHC, where they may be damaging. A detailed description of diseases related to the pathophysiology of the EHC is beyond the scope of this chapter. However, the main mechanisms responsible for "dysfunction" of the EHC will be briefly considered.

### *Congenital Abnormalities of Bile Acid Synthesis*

Examples of congenital abnormalities of bile acid synthesis include: benign recurrent intrahepatic cholestasis (Summerskill and Walshe), progressive intrahepatic cholestasis (Byler's disease), hereditary lymphedema with recurrent cholestasis (Aagenaes's sydrome, Norwegian cholestasis), cerebrohepatorenal syndrome (Zellweger syndrome), the tetrahydrocoprostanic acid syndrome, and cerebrotendinous xanthomatosis. These entities are extremely infrequent. The cause of these diseases is a proven, or in some cases suspected, aberration in the synthesis of bile acids by the liver [2, 4, 20].

### *Acquired Abnormalities of Bile Acid Synthesis or Metabolism*

*Liver Cirrhosis.* Liver cirrhosis is characterized by diminished functional hepatocellular mass and by the presence of portal hypertension. Liver parenchymal failure leads to reduced synthesis of primary bile acids, especially cholic acid. The bile salt pool may be reduced to 50% of normal. The hydrophobicity index of the bile salt acid pool is increased. Sulfation of bile acids is enhanced and their urinary elimination is increased. Recently, it has been demonstrated that patients with liver cirrhosis synthesize abnormal amounts of the so-called unusual trihydroxy bile acids [21], which are very hydrophilic. On the other hand, in cirrhotic patients, the uptake of bile acids by the liver is reduced which together with portasystemic shunting leads to an increase in bile acid concentration in systemic blood. In the presence of a reduced bile salt pool, this spillover of bile acids outside the EHC may induce a deficiency of bile salts in the intestine. This may cause mild steatorrhea, which in general is of minor degree and lacks clinical relevance. On the other hand, secretion of bile acids and phospholipids by the liver is reduced and cholesterol synthesis and secretion are markedly impaired. As a result bile is undersaturated with cholesterol. For reasons which are unclear, in liver cirrhosis there is an increased prevalence of gallstones composed of bilirubinate [2, 4, 22].

*Cholestasis.* Cholestasis produces an interruption of the EHC because of either the failure of the liver to make bile or the existence of an obstruction to the flow of bile from the liver to the duodenum. This issue is addressed later in this chapter.

*Cholesterol Gallstone Disease.* (see Chap. 34). In this condition, bile salt secretion by the liver is generally reduced because of the existence of a decreased bile salt pool size. The ratio of cholesterol to lecithin and bile salts in bile is shifted toward cholesterol excess. This results in the formation of cholesterol microcrystals which subsequently precipitate in bile, and finally cholesterol stones are formed. The process of cholesterol gallstone formation is, however, very complex and factors other than a reduction in bile acid pool size are involved [1–4].

***Ileal Disease Interfering with the Normal Absorption of Bile Acids***

*Cholerheic Diarrhea (Cholerheic Enteropathy).* Dysfunction of the ileal mucosa (i.e., Crohn's disease) or surgical resection of the terminal ileum may lead to bile acid malabsorption. The liver maintains the size of the bile acid pool by a compensatory increase in bile acid synthesis by the liver. However, the passage of excessive amounts of bile acids into the colon induces secretory diarrhea by increasing cAMP levels in the cells of colonic mucosa. The diarrheogenic effect is produced by hydrophobic bile acids, such as deoxycholate and chenodeoxycholate, but not by equimolar amounts of taurocholate or ursodeoxycholate. Treatment with cholestyramine is effective [23].

Idiopathic bile acid diarrhea is a variant of this syndrome in which no lesion is detected in the ileum despite the occurrence of bile acid malabsorption. It has been postulated that a deficiency in the number of ileal mucosal receptors for bile acids may be the cause of this condition [24, 25].

*Steatorrhea.* Ileal resection of more than 100 cm or severe diffuse mucosal damage will produce malabsorption of bile acids which cannot be compensated by increasing their synthesis in the liver. As a result, jejunal concentrations of bile acids are insufficient for micelle formation and fat malabsorption ensues. Intraluminal long chain fatty acids stimulate colonic secretion, thus augmenting fecal fluid loss. Reduction of dietary fat and administration of medium chain triglycerides, which are absorbed in the absence of bile acids, constitute the appropriate treatment [2, 4, 26].

*Abnormal Deconjugation of Bile Acids in the Small Bowel by Bacteria (Blind Loop Syndrome or Small Bowel Bacterial Overgrowth).* In this condition there is abnormal presence of colonic bacteria in the lumen of the jejunum and ileum. Anaerobic bacteria deconjugate bile acids which in this form are more easily absorbed by passive diffusion across the jejunal mucosa. This deprivation of bile acids in the intestinal lumen reduces their concentration to levels insufficient for adequate micellation of dietary fat. A toxic effect of the high concentrations of unconjugated bile acids on the jejunal mucosa is likely to contribute to fat malabosorption. Bacterial overgrowth of the small bowel may be secondary to jejunal diverticula, enterocolonic fistulae, strictures (in Crohn's disease), and alterations in the intestinal motility (in diabetes mellitus, scleroderma, idiopathic intestinal pseudo-obstruction, and often without clear cause in the elderly). If surgical correction is not undertaken, treatment with antibiotics can be effective [27].

### *Miscellaneous Rare Conditions*

*Cholecystocolonic Fistulae.* This rare complication is responsible for direct loss of bile salts from the gallbladder to the colon, thus bypassing the small bowel. Steatorrhea and cholerheic diarrhea are the main clinical manifestations [28].

*Zollinger-Ellison Syndrome.* In gastrinomas, the gastric content is still extremely acid when it enters the jejunum after meals (pH values: 1 and 3.8 at the entrance and at the end of the jejunum, respectively). This low pH reduces the ionization of conjugated bile salts, which may precipitate in the jejunal lumen. Micelle formation is therefore impaired and steatorrhea may occur. An important contributing factor in the production of steatorrhea in this syndrome is the deleterious effect of acid on the activity of pancreatic lipases [29].

*Retrograde Transit of Bile Acids in the Digestive Tract.* It has been proposed that retrograde transport of bile to the stomach because of the existence of duodenogastric reflux may induce damage to the gastric mucosa. However, the possible role of bile acids and specifically of deoxycholic acid in the pathogenesis of gastric ulcer is still a matter of debate [30].

## 2 Anatomic and Physiologic Bases of Bile Formation

### 2.1 Anatomic Basis

Hepatocytes produce primary, canalicular, or hepatocytic bile. Within the liver, bile flows successively through canaliculi, Hering canals, ductules, interlobular bile ducts, septal ducts, and lobar ducts (left and right) which join outside the liver and form the common hepatic duct, which is the beginning of the extrahepatic biliary tree.

Hepatocytes are highly polarized secretory cells showing in their plasma membrane three morphologically and functionally differentiated domains (Fig. 4). The anatomy of the liver is described in a previous chapter of

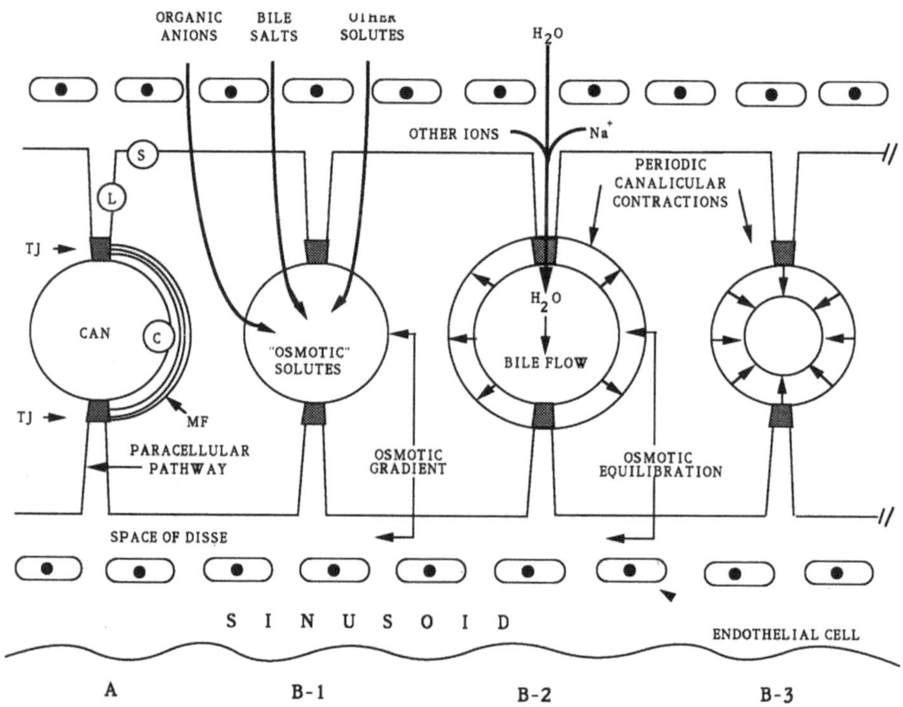


**Fig. 4.** Anatomic and physiologic basis of bile formation. *A*, Basic anatomic structures involved in bile formation. *CAN*, canaliculus; *encircled C, L, and S* identify, respectively, the canalicular, lateral, and sinusoidal domains of the plasma membrane. *TJ*, tight junctions; *MF*, microfilaments. B-1 to B-3, Basic steps in bile formation. *B-1*, Concentrative transport of bile salts and other solutes from sinusoidal blood to the canalicular lumen, generating an osmoic gradient which (*B-2*) determines the passage of water to the canaliculus through the paracellular pathway (transcellular transport of water may also exist – see text). The permselectivity of the tight junctions for small cations allows the entry of sodium by solvent drag. *B-3*, Propelling of bile toward cholangioles is accomplished by periodic microfilament-dependent contractions of the bile canliculus

this book. However, some important points concerning the structure of hepatocytes specifically related to bile flow formation are emphasized below [for reviews: 31–40].

### *Plasma Membrane*

*The sinusoidal domain* borders the space of Disse and is in direct contact with sinusoidal blood. Circulating substances which are to be secreted in bile are taken up by hepatocytes across the sinusoidal plasma membrane. The sinusoidal domain is endowed with specific membrane carriers and transport systems for the uptake of bile acids, organic anions, and other substances. The sodium- and potassium-dependent adenosine triphosphatase ($Na^+,K^+$-ATPase), the so-called sodium pump, is located in the sinusoidal and lateral membrane domains, while it is absent from the canalicular domain [41]. The activity of this enzyme maintains the transmembrane sodium gradient between the extracellular and intracellular fluids. This enzyme largely controls the membrane potential in hepatocytes and so it could influence several cell parameters and functions, such as intracellular pH and free calcium, cytoskeletal activity, and transport systems [42].

*The lateral domain* lies between the sinusoidal and the canalicular domains and faces the homologous membrane portion of an adjacent hepatocyte. The intercellular space between two adjacent cells corresponds functionally to the paracellular pathway [43]. The specific functions of the lateral membrane domain are cell-to-cell communication and adhesion. Junctional complexes between hepatocytes are constituted by the tight junction, belt desmosome, and spot desmosome (zonula occludens, zonula adherens, and macula adherens, respectively). An additional intercellular structure, the gap junction, may be associated with the tight junction or may be an independent element on the extracellular side of the plasma membrane.

Of these structures, the only one which provides continuous and strong cell-to-cell contact is the tight junction. It is, therefore, the only barrier between blood and bile at the intercellular level. The structure of tight junctions in the liver is similar to that found in other epithelia. They are composed of anastomosing and branching sealing strands. Each strand contains two rows of integral membrane proteins which make head-to-tail contact. This completely occludes the intercellular space to the transit of molecules. Trans-epithelial resistance to passage of ions is markedly influenced by the number of strands in the tight junctions. The urinary bladder of amphibia, which has up to 14 strands, exhibits high resistance to ions; however, the proximal renal tubule, having only one or two strands, is extremely permissive for the passage of ions. The liver, which has three to five strands, occupies an intermediate position. This allows rapid equilibration of osmolality between plasma and bile. The tight junctions prevent reflux of organic anions from canaliculi into the intercellular space, owing to their selectivity for cations [44]. Water and small cations, such as $Na^+$, may enter the canaliculi to achieve osmotic equilibration. In addition, tight junctions avoid lateral movement of lipids and proteins in the outer membrane layer from the canalicular to the basolateral domain, thus maintaining differences in chemical composition between canalicular and lateral plasma membranes. Belt desomosomes or intermediate junctions lie parallel to the tight junctions along the canaliculus. They can be considered as being an insertion line for actin filaments. These microfilaments are, in turn, the sealing strands of the tight junctions. In this area, plasma membranes of two adjacent hepatocytes are separated by a thin space of about 200 A. Spot desmosomes are points of contact for cell-to-cell attachment. At this level, the intercellular space is about 300 Å across. In both cases, the intercellular spaces are filled by filamentous material. Gap junctions are free communications between cells allowing cell-to-cell passage of molecules such as ions, sugars, and amino acids [31, 37, 38, 44].

Functionally, disruption of the tight junctions or an increase in their permeability will lead to free communication between the bile canaliculus and sinusoids.

*The canalicular domain* of the plasma membrane is the secretory pole of the hepatocyte and constitutes a hemicanaliculus. The canalicular membrane portions of two (often three) adjacent hepatocytes form the canaliculus, which is sealed off by the tight junctions. This membrane portion exhibits microvilli and has carriers and transport systems for bile salts, organic anions, glutathione, and bicarbonate and other compounds undergoing canalicular secretion. The canalicular membrane contains more cholesterol than basolateral domains: this makes the canalicular pole resistant to the toxic effect of bile acids which accumulate in this region of hepatocytes prior to secretion. The canaliculi show periodic contractions which facilitate the flow of bile. Canalicular contractions are mediated by microfilaments. The canalicular membrane is endowed with several enzymes specific to this location, such as $Mg^{2+}$-ATPase, which may be related to canalicular contraction, and alkaline phosphatase, $\gamma$-glutamyltranspeptidase (GGT), 5′-nucleotidase and leucine aminopeptidase, the functions of which are poorly understood [39, 40].

### *Golgi Complex*

Since a bile acid uptake system was detected in intracellular vesicles, it has been proposed that bile acids might be transported by the Golgi complex. However, it seems likely that only a minor part of total bile acid transport is carried out by this system, while the bulk of this function is accomplished by cytosolic proteins which bind bile acids. Vesicles mediate transport of lipids, IgA, and other substances into bile. Vesicular transport is intimately linked to microtubules. Recently, two types of vesicular transport system have been identified [45]: a fast, microtubule-independent and low capacity system (substances take 2 min to reach bile) and a slow, microtubule-dependent and high capacity system (substances taking 20–25 min to reach the bile).

### *Cytoskeleton*

The cytoskeleton of hepatocytes is composed of microfilaments, microtubules, and intermediate filaments. The microfilament network extends widely inside the hepatocytes. Microfilaments are located predominantly around the canaliculus, where they form the pericanalicular web. These thin actin filaments form the axis of microvilli and also insert on the inner side of the plasma membrane and in the tight junctions, where they are firmly attached. Microfilaments are responsible for canalicular contractions, modulate the structure and the tightness of tight junctions, and together with microtubules control the topography of membrane-associated proteins and cell shape. Microtubules are tubulin-containing structures, which, in addition to their coordinated actions with microfilaments, are essential for transcellular vectorial vesicular transport in the sinusoidal or canalicular direction. Secretory processes like canalicular secretion of lipids and IgA are dependent on microtubules. These two cytoskeletal components are dynamic structures subjected to rapid modulation through polymerization and depolymerization of their protein units under the influence of calcium and other lesser known mediators. Loss of function of these structures impairs bile flow (see below) [46].

## 2.2 Physiology

### *Basic Mechanisms*

Unlike urine formation, which results from hydrostatic filtration of the plasma, the genesis of bile is relatively independent of sinusoidal hydrostatic pressure. Bile formation depends on the concentrative transport of osmotically active compounds from sinusoidal blood to the canalicular lumen. The resultant osmotic gradient determines the passage of water into the canaliculus, generating bile flow [31–40]. This process, known as osmotic filtration, is carried out by hepatocytes. Physiologically, bile salts are the chief compounds generating this osmotic gradient. There are other solutes that contribute to bile formation (see below).

Biliary solutes are taken up at the sinusoidal pole of hepatocytes, transported transcellularly, and secreted across the canalicular portion of the plasma membrane. Additionally, cations may reach the canalicular lumen through the paracellular pathway, mainly accompanying water by the solvent drag effect.

Water movements in the liver are not fully understood. At present, there is evidence supporting passage of water to the canaliculus from the paracellular pathway across the tight junctions and from hepatocytes across the canalicular plasma membrane. This second system represents the last step of a transcytotic process [47]. The proportion of fluid transported by each system in unknown.

### *Fractions of Canalicular Bile Flow*

In all species studied so far, canalicular bile volume has been found to be linearly correlated with bile salt output. The calculation by extrapolation of the canalicular bile volume corresponding to zero (absent) bile salt output consistently gives a positive value in all species. Canalicular bile flow is therefore thought to have two fractions, known as "bile acid-dependent flow" (BADF) and "bile acid-independent flow" (BAIF), respectively [31–40]. This theory has not been definitively proven, since it is likely that bile salts, at very low concentrations, have a greater choleretic potency per molecule unit that at concentrations at which polymolecular aggregates do occur. In this case, values of BAIF obtained by extrapolation would be overestimated. In humans, total canalicular bile production is about 500 ml/day, with a 250 ml contribution of BAIF and BADF, although a markedly smaller contribution of BAIF is suggested by some other studies [31–40, 48]. The principal ionic pumps and transport systems thought to be involved in BADF and BAIF are represented in Fig. 5.

#### *Bile Acid-Dependent Bile Flow*

Bile acid concentration is at least 100-fold higher in bile than in portal blood. In fact, bile acids are transported against a concentration gradient from sinusoidal blood to hepatocytes and from hepatocytes to the canalicular lumen. Sinusoid-to-hepatocyte transport also takes place against an electric gradient. In other words, transport of bile acids is an active process requiring energy. The transport of bile acids by the liver is limited by a maximal secretory rate. The limiting step is canalicular secretion. The uptake capacity, although saturable, by far exceeds secretory Tm.

*Uptake of Bile Acids by Hepatocytes.* Conjugated, trihydroxy bile acids are taken up by a specific, carrier-mediated, sodium-coupled system. There is a mutual competitive inhibition for this system between different bile acids. The carrier is a 49-kd glycoprotein which binds distinct bile acids with different affinities and binds no other compounds. The internalization of bile acid molecules against both a concentration and an electric gradient is carried out through secondary active transport. Bile acids enter hepatocyte cotransported with sodium. A similar sodium-coupled transport is operative in hepatocytes for amino acid uptake, and perhaps for some organic anions,

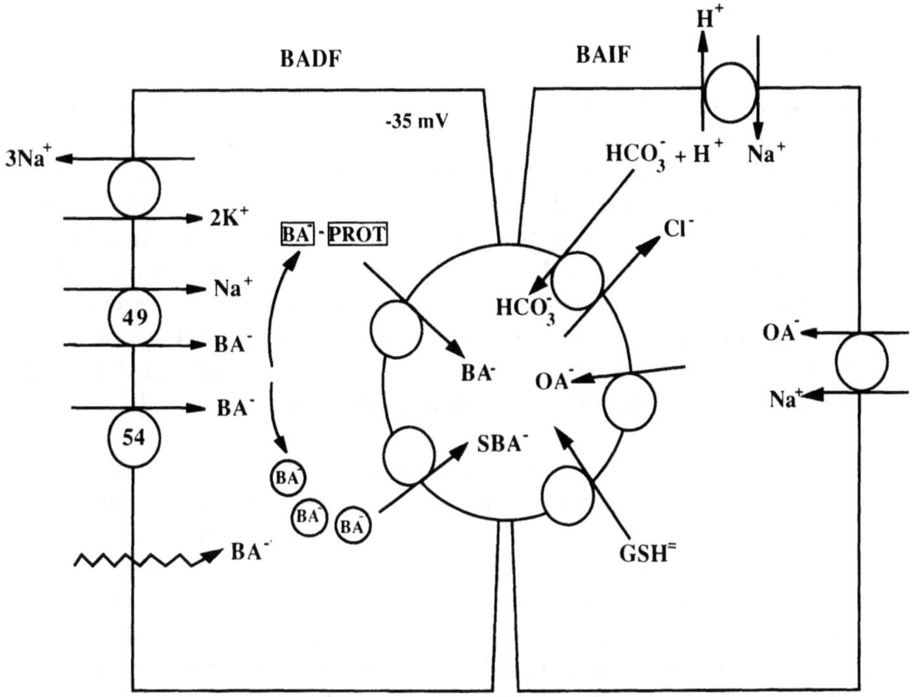


**Fig. 5.** Basic transport processes involved in the generation of the bile acid-dependent (BADF) and the bile acid-independent (BAIF) fractions of canalicular bile flow. *Left*: BADF. $Na^+$,$Ka^+$-ATPase maintains the transmembrane sodium gradient by the energy-dependent $3Na^+/2K^+$ exchange at the basolateral membrane domain. The basolateral uptake of bile salts by hepatocytes involves (a) carrier-mediated and $Na^+$-coupled bile salt transport, (b) bile salt transport mediated by a multispecific anion carrier, and (c) bile salt diffusion across the plasma membrane. The intracellular transport of bile salts is mediated by cytosolic carrier proteins and vesicles. Canalicular secretion: (a) carrier-mediated and electric potential-driven transport of taurocholate; (b) multispecific anion carrier-mediated transport of sulfated bile acids ($SBA^-$). *Right*: BAIF. Possible mechanisms involved in BAIF formation: (a) transport of sodium to the canaliculus; (b) $HCO_3^-/Cl^-$ canalicular exchanger, dependent on, and coupled to, basolateral $Na^+/H^+$ countertransport; (c) glutathione transport; (d) undefined organic anion transport

and is also similar to that which mediates bile acid reabsorption in the ileum. The entry of sodium into hepatocytes is favored by the transmembrane sodium gradient generated by the activity of the $Na^+$,$K^+$-ATPase, which continuously exchanges sodium for potassium across the basolateral plasma membrane. Thus, bile acids use the energy generated by the $Na^+$,$K^+$-ATPase to enter hepatocytes. A second system for bile acid uptake in hepatocytes involves a 54-kd carrier with affinity for cholate but also for oxalate, acetate, lactate, and other anions. A multispecific anion exchanger might, therefore, mediate part of the bile acid uptake. This mechanism has been suggested but remains to be proven. Less hydrophilic bile acids, such as deoxycholate, may diffuse across the lipid bilayer of the plasma membrane [31–40, 49–51].

*Transcellular Transport.* The transcellular transport of bile salts is incompletely understood. Binding of bile salts to cytosolic proteins having glutathione-*S*-transferase or 3α-hydroxysteroid dehydrogenase activities has been demonstrated. Some of these proteins, of 14, 33, and 45 kd, show overlapping specificity for bile acids and other organic anions. In addition, a minor fraction of bile acids is likely to be transported transcellularly in microtubule-dependent vesicles, a system which may be important in situations of bile acid overload. Both binding proteins and vesicles contribute to maintaining a low intracellular concentration of free bile acids which reduces their potential toxic effects in hepatocytes [51–55].

*Canalicular Secretion.* The canalicular secretion of bile salts takes place against a concentration gradient. This process is saturable and sodium independent. It seems to be energized by the electric gradient of about −40 mV established between the cell interior and the canalicular lumen and is mediated by a 100-kd glycoprotein carrier distinct from the sinusoidal carriers. This system is operative for taurocholate. Its contribution to the secretion of other bile acids is unknown. Another transport system seems to drive the secretion of sulfated and glucuronidated bile salts as well as of certain organic anions, such as bilirubin and sulfobromophthalein. In addition, vectorial vesicular transport followed by exocytosis seems to account for a fraction of bile acid secretion. A clear relationship between this vesicular system and the canalicular carriers has not been established. Canalicular secretion of bile salts with secondary generation of BADF requires the functional integrity of microtubules, microfilaments, vesicular systems, canalicular plasma membrane, and tight junctions, in addition to calcium availability. Effective sealing of canaliculi and their contractile activity are microfilament and calcium dependent [56–59].

*Choleresis Induced by Bile Salts.* Canalicular bile salts exert the main osmotic force contributing to the generation of bile flow. The amount of water entering the canaliculi in response to this osmotic force will depend on the intracanalicular concentration of bile acids and on the amount of water associated with the type of bile acid molecule. This is termed "apparent choleretic activity" and it is expressed in μl/μmol. Values of the apparent choleretic activity for physiologic bile acids vary between 7 and 10 μl/μmol and reach 20–25 μl/μmol for sulfated divalent bile acids [40].

Some bile acids exhibit a particularly high apparent choleretic activity. Ursodeoxycholate (UDCA), hyocholate, norursodeoxycholate, norchenodeoxycholate, and others share this property, with values ranging from 30 to more than 200 μl/μmol. In addition, hypercholeresis is associated with production of a bicarbonate-rich bile and it is induced only by the presence in bile of the unconjugated form of the bile salt [40].

Ursodeoxycholate, a dihydroxy bile acid, is a focus of special interest due to its therapeutic use. It produces a bicarbonate-rich choleresis, but in addition UDCA prevents the cholestatic effects of taurolithocholate or other monohydroxy bile acids. Its hypercholeretic properties are abolished by amiloride and amiloride analogs, which specifically inhibit the $Na^+/H^+$ countertransport [60]. Different hypotheses have been proposed to explain the hypercholeresis and the bicarbonate secretion induced by UDCA. These hypotheses are represented in Fig. 6.

In contrast, some bile acids, especially those which are monohydroxylated, may be cholestatic if administered at sufficient doses. The

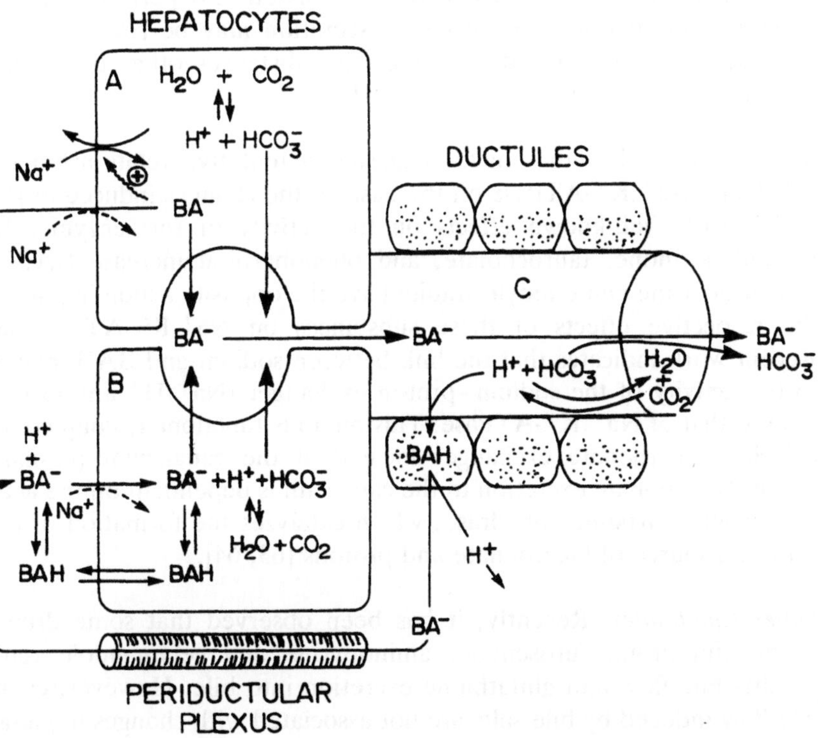


**Fig. 6.** Proposed mechanisms of the bicarbonate-rich hypercholeresis induced by ursodeoxycholate (UDCA). *A*, Stimulation of canalicular $HCO_3^-$ secretion via stimulation of apical $HCO_3^-$ transport or basolateral $Na^+/H^+$ exchange. *B*, $H^+/HCO_3^-$ transport mediated by cycling of UDCA at the level of the hepatocyte at either the canalicular or the sinusoidal lateral membrane. *C*, Cholehepatic recycling of unconjugated UDCA: Following secretion of UDCA as an anion, UDCA is taken up via ductular cells as protonated UDCA. UDCA is returned to the hepatocyte via the peribiliary plexus. The net effect is generation of biliary $HCO_3^-$. [Reproduced with permission from Lake JR et al. (1988) Gastroenterology 95:454–463]

classic representative is lithocholic acid. This effect is related to the detergent-like activity of these compounds, as previously mentioned.

*Bile Acid-Independent Bile Flow*

It is established that any osmotically active compound secreted into the canaliculus may generate bile flow. Physiologically, the agent or agents responsible for BAIF remain to be identified. However, some data suggest that inorganic ions are responsible, at least in part, for this fraction of canalicular bile [61].

*Bicarbonate.* A role for bicarbonate in BAIF generation is supported by the reduction of this fraction of bile flow which is observed after removal of bicarbonate from the perfusate of the isolated and perfused rat liver. In addition, stimulation of bicarbonate secretion may be responsible for the increase in BAIF induced by choleretic substances other than bile acids, such as aspirin and other salicylates [62, 63].

*Sodium.* Several studies have suggested a tentative relationship between BAIF and $Na^+$,$K^+$-ATPase on the basis of the changes induced in BAIF by agents with well-known effects on the activity of this enzyme. In fact, thyroid hormone, taurocholate, and phenobarbital increase BAIF, while chlorpromazine and ethinylestradiol have the opposite action in parallel with the respective effects of these substances on $Na^+$,$K^+$-ATPase activity. Recent work indicates that the link between sodium and BAIF may be due to the activity of the sodium–proton exchanger ($Na^+/H^+$ antiport), rather than to that of $Na^+$,$K^+$-ATPase. This pump is functionally coupled with the chloride–bicarbonate exchanger located at the canalicular plasma membrane. Bicarbonate excretion to the canaliculi is dependent on the activity of the enzyme carbonic anhydrase, which catalyzes the formation of carbonic acid as a source of bicarbonate and protons [63, 64].

*Other Candidates.* Recently, it has been observed that some drugs, such as nitrofurantoin, furosemide, aminopyrine and cefamandole reduce in parallel bile flow and glutathione excretion into bile. However, changes in bile flow induced by bile salts are not associated with changes in glutathione excretion. This suggests that glutathione excretion may be specifically related to BAIF, raising the possibility that glutathione would be a driving force for a fraction of BAIF [65].

In addition, some evidence in rats with hereditary hyperbilirubinemia and defective anion excretion supports a role for organic anions in the generation of BAIF [58]. These rats show impaired excretion of some organic anions, such as bilirubin, glutathione, sulfobromophthalein and cysteinyl leukotrienes, and exhibit normal bile acid excretion but reduced

BAIF. These findings suggest that the canalicular secretion of organic anions stimulates the formation of BAIF.

### *Biliary Secretion of Other Substances*

Cholesterol and phospholipids are integrated into vesicles, the formation of which is mediated by bile acids. Canalicular secretion of both compounds is dependent on bile acid secretion. Bile acid stimulation of phospholipid secretion occurs over a wide range of values of bile salt output into bile (0–2000 μmol/h) and determines a phospholipid output of 0–500 μmol/h. Cholesterol secretion is also stimulated in proportion to bile salt output but to a lesser extent than phospholipid secretion. Cholesterol secretion is 80–100 μmol/h for 500 μmol/h of bile salt output but only 125–150 μmol/h for 2000 μmol/h of secreted bile salts. This is a relationship that is important in avoiding supersaturation of cholesterol in bile.

Bilirubin and other organic anions, such as sulfobromophthalein or indocyanine green, share common characteristics with regard to their secretion by the liver. Canalicular secretion of these compounds is a saturable process, having a maximal secretory rate which is less than the maximal uptake capacity. Thus, the rate-limiting step in the clearance of these compounds from blood to bile is canalicular secretion. Competition exists between different organic anions for excretion, suggesting that they share a common transport system at the canalicular level. The infusion of bile acids in humans increases the Tm for bilirubin and other organic anions. However, choleresis induced by means other than bile acid infusion does not modify Tm for these substances. Although the exact mechanism responsible for this stimulation is still unknown, this points to the influence of bile acid secretion on many other secretory processes taking place at the canalicular level.

### *Modifications of the Hepatic Bile in Bile Ducts and Gallbladder*

Hepatocytic bile is modified in ductules and ducts by the secretion of a bicarbonate-rich fluid under secretin stimulation. The calculated bicarbonate concentration in the fluid secreted by ductules and ducts is 124 mmol/liter On the other hand, it is likely that ducts and ductules also have a reabsorptive capacity, but the physiologic role of this process seems to be irrelevant. Besides secretin, gastrin and cholinergic inputs seem to stimulate secretion by ducts and ductules, whereas somatostatin and vasoactive intestinal polypeptide stimulate reabsorption. In humans, total bile production is 600–560 ml/24 h, of which about one-third is of ductular and ductal origin.

The gallbladder concentrates and stores bile. Its capacity is 40 ml. The gallbladder reabsorbs 90% of bile water isosmotically. Organic compounds are not reabsorbed. Final concentrations of bile acids in gallbladder bile may be higher than 200 mmol/liter Some electrolytes are concentrated with respect to plasma and sodium may reach 200 mmol/liter [2, 4].

## 3 Cholestasis

### 3.1 Definition

The term "cholestasis" may be considered from different points of view. For the morphologist, cholestasis means the presence of stainable bile in the liver biopsy. For the physiologist, cholestasis is a reduction in the secretion of bile by the liver. The clinician defines cholestasis as a syndrome characterized by the abnormal presence of bile compounds in the blood and by the absence of these substances in the intestine. Summarizing these concepts, in the presence of normal synthesis of bile constituents, cholestasis may be defined as the failure of normal amounts of bile to reach the intestine.

### 3.2 Classification and Causes

Cholestasis can be classified as extrahepatic or intrahepatic. Extrahepatic cholestasis results from mechanical obstruction of the biliary tree outside the liver or within the porta hepatis. In intrahepatic cholestasis, the primary defect lies in the hepatocyte or the canaliculi (nonobstructive intrahepatic cholestasis) or in bile conduits within the liver (obstructive intrahepatic cholestasis), whereas the extrahepatic biliary tree remains patent. A list of causes of both types of cholestasis is provided in Table 1.

A second classification categorizes cholestasis according to its duration as acute or chronic, taking 3 months as the cut-off point. Since chronic cholestasis causes metabolic and nutritional derangements and may lead to secondary liver cirrhosis, this type of classification has prognostic and therapeutic implications.

### 3.3 Pathogenesis

#### *Initiation of Cholestasis*

Cholestasis may result from lesions localized at any point between the plasma membrane of the hepatocytes and the sphincter of Oddi. Lesions involving hepatocytes or canaliculi impair the formation of primary hepatocytic bile. Lesions beyond this point interfere with the normal flow of hepatocytic bile, leading to an obstructive form of intra- or extrahepatic cholestasis.

**Table 1.** Classification of the causes of cholestasis in adults

*Extrahepatic cholestasis*
Lithiasis
Pancreatic carcinoma (head)
Sclerosing cholangitis (primary or secondary)
Postsurgical stenosis
Neoplasms (primary: cholangiocarcinoma and others)
Neoplasms (secondary: lymphoma, metastatic melanoma)
Hemobilia
Parasites: hydatidosis, fascioliasis, ascariasis, Amebic abscess
Choledochal cyst
Duodenal ulcer (perforated)
Duodenal diverticula
Pancreatitis (acute and chronic)
Pancreatic pseudocyst

*Intrahepatic cholestasis*
*a) With intrahepatic mechanical obstruction*
Primary biliary cirrhosis (chronic nonsuppurative destructive cholangitis)
Chronic suppurative cholangitis
Primary sclerosing cholangitis
Cholangiocarcinoma
Hepatocellular carcinoma and other primary neoplasms of the liver
Metastases
Polycystic hepatic disease
Nonneoplastic space-occupying lesions
Cystic fibrosis
Granulomatosis
Caroli's disease
Syndromatic paucity of intrahepatic bile ducts (Alagille's disease)
Nonsyndromatic paucity of intrahepatic bile ducts
Benign recurrent familial cholestasis

*Intrahepatic cholestasis*
*b) Without demonstrable mechanical obstruction*
Drug-induced[a]
Hepatitis (viral, alcoholic, bacterial)
Hemolysis (sickle cell disease)
Bacterial sepsis
Benign postoperative cholestasis
Benign recurrent cholestasis of pregnancy
Total parenteral nutrition
Lymphoma (Hodgkin's), histiocytic medullary reticulosis
Congestive cholestasis
Sarcoidosis
Amyloidosis
Protoporphyrin cholestasis
Nonmetastatic hypernephroma (nephrogenic hepatic dysfunction syndrome)
Graft versus host disease
Hereditary lymphedema with recurrent cholestasis (Aagenaes's syndrome)[b]
$\alpha_1$-Antitrypsin deficiency[c]
Benign recurrent intrahepatic cholestasis[b]
Toxin-induced cholestasis
  The Epping jaundice (methylenedianiline)
  The toxic oil syndrome (Spain)

[a] See Table 3 and 4 for specific drugs
[b] Cholestasis is initiated in infancy but recurrent episodes may occur in adult life
[c] Common cause of cholestasis in the newborn: very rare in adults

## *Morphology of Cholestasis*

### *Light Microscopy*

The essential morphologic features of cholestasis are the same regardless of etiology: inspissated bile plugs are present in canaliculi, particularly in the centrilobular zone, where bile flow is lowest. Bile pigment is visible in hepatocytes and later in Kupffer cells. Feathery degeneration of hepatocytes is the morphologic consequence of cholestasis seen on light microscopy. The cell is swollen and consists of wisps of brownish cytoplasm separated by clear areas. Death of individual cells occurs in prolonged cholestasis and a local inflammatory response may develop. Proliferation of bile ductules and fibrosis take place in severe cholestasis [66, 67].

### *Ultrastructural Changes in the Hepatocytes*

In cholestasis, either intra- or extrahepatic, hepatocytes show a characteristic pattern of morphologic changes which predominate at the canalicular pole of the cell. The canaliculus is dilated and microvilli are lost from the outer aspect of the canalicular membrane. Golgi vesicles are distended and filled with opaque material. Their number is increased around the canalicular area at the onset of cholestasis, but later some transport vesicles are seen near the basolateral membrane. Both smooth and rough endoplasmic reticulum are reduced throughout the cell. Mitochondrial cristae are elongated. Thickening of the pericanalicular ectoplasm secondary to an increase in the number and disarray of microfilaments is prominent. Decreased number and density of strands in the tight junctions may be seen and in some cases these structures are anatomically disrupted [33, 37–39, 66, 67].

### *Specific Features in Extrahepatic Cholestasis*

Although morphologic changes are similar in intra- and extrahepatic cholestasis, large duct obstruction adds additional features to the morphology of cholestasis. Two diagnostic features are important. One is the extravasation of bile from bile ducts, which cannot be seen in intrahepatic cholestasis. The second is the presence of an area of necrosis in the lobule near the portal tract caused by bile leakage, which is called a bile infarct [66].

## ***Mechanisms of Extrahepatic Cholestasis***

The primary mechanism of extrahepatic cholestasis is physical obstruction. Obstruction of the biliary tree causes an increase in bile pressure upstream from the obstructed level and dilation of ducts ensues. Under normal conditions, bile duct pressure is about 10–15 $cmH_2O$. When obstruction begins, hepatocytes continue to make bile, thus producing a progressive increase in the pressure of the biliary system. Above 15 $cmH_2O$ bile flow begins to fall. Biliary system pressures above 30 $cmH_2O$ stop bile flow. For many years the concept persisted that the passage of bile compounds from an obstructed biliary tree to the blood occurred across ruptured ductules and distorted and unsealed canaliculi. Recent studies have demonstrated that in early extrahepatic cholestasis most of the biliary constituents present in plasma reach sinusoidal blood by transcellular transport. Vesicles travel from the canalicular to the basolateral areas of hepatocytes, where exocytosis occurs. Thus, inversion of hepatocellular polarity seems to represent a compensatory mechanism preventing excessive accumulation of material in the cell. The sinusoidal and basolateral portions of the hepatocyte's plasma membrane are in some way "canalicularized." For example, specific markers of the canalicular plasma membrane such as canalicular (100-kd) bile salt carriers or alkaline phosphatase activity have been isolated from basolateral fractions of the plasma membrane in this situation. An undefined fraction of the "returning materials" also pass to the sinusoids through tight junctions that are partially disrupted or the permeability of which is abnormally increased. This may be viewed as regurgitation [37, 67].

### *Mechanisms of Intrahepatic Cholestasis*

#### *Background*

Extensive efforts have been made in recent years to clarify whether there is a common primary mechanism for initiation of intrahepatic cholestasis. Available data suggest that a variety of primary lesions may produce a final common morphofunctional situation which may be thought of as "the palsy of the bile secretory apparatus." Knowledge about mechanisms of cholestasis has been gained largely from evaluation of experimentally induced cholestasis in animal models. The principal cholestatic agents used in these studies are monohydroxy bile acids (taurolithocholate or lithocholate), estrogens (ethinylestradiol), androgenic steroids (norethandrolone), antimicrofilament agents (phalloidin and cytochalasin B), antimicrotubular agents (colchicine), and chlorpromazine [36–39, 66–71].

#### *General Mechanisms*

Accordance with the previously described mechanisms of bile formation, the following factors, alone or in combination, should be expected to induce cholestasis:

1. Primary failure in establishing an osmotic gradient between the canalicular lumen and sinusoids. This may be due to alterations in the transport of bile acids or of substances generating BAIF, because of impairment in sinusoidal uptake, transcytotic transport, and/or canalicular secretion.
2. Failure of water to flow into canaliculi in response to the osmotic gradient. This situation may result from decreased permeability for water at the canalicular plasma membrane or junctional complex.
3. Dissipation of the osmotic gradient. This may occur because of increased permeability of the canalicular membrane or of the tight junctions or in

the presence of junctional disruption. These alterations cause retrograde diffusion or direct escape of canalicular content to the cells or to the paracellular pathway. An alternative mechanism may be the reduction of intracanalicular osmotic forces due to precipitation or aggregation of solutes in polymolecular structures (other than physiologic micelles).

4. Overriding of the expected osmotic gradient because of extracanalicular hyperosmolality (i.e., extreme hyperglycemia).
5. Failure of formed bile to flow because of a lack of mechanical canalicular pumping or intracanalicular obstruction.

*Mechanisms Supported by Clinical or Experimental Data*

*Alterations in the Plasma Membrane of Hepatocytes.* The lipidic composition of the plasma membrane, and specifically its cholesterol–phospholipid ratio, critically influences the functions of the plasma membrane and membrane-associated structures. Several cholestatic agents may modify this ratio, mainly by increasing the proportion of cholesterol. This results in changes in both the permeability and the fluidity of the plasma membrane [72–74]. Monohydroxy bile acids (lithocholate) characteristically decrease the permeability of the canalicular membrane, also affecting the tight junctions [75, 76]. This hampers the canalicular secretion of organic and inorganic compounds, including bile acids, and, in addition, the passage of water from the paracellular pathway to the canaliculus is reduced (see Sect. 3.4 for other effects of toxic bile acids). On the other hand, an increase in the permeability of the canalicular membrane may result in retrograde diffusion of solutes from the canalicular lumen to the hepatocytes. Great interest has been focused in recent years on the possible cholestatic role of changes in plasma membrane fluidity. This term refers to the diffusional freedom of membrane lipids. Membrane fluidity markedly influences the activity of membrane-associated enzymes, such as $Na^+$,$K^+$-ATPase, 5′-nucleotidase, or adenylate cyclase. Moreover, both the activity of membrane transport systems (i.e., $Na^+/H^+$ antiport, $Na^+$-coupled taurocholate uptake) and the mobility of membrane-associated carriers may be affected by changes in the membrane microenvironment [72–74]. Ethinylestradiol and chlorpromazine, which are two characteristic cholestatic agents, decrease the plasma membrane fluidity of hepatocytes. At least initially, this effect is restricted to the basolateral domain and is associated with decreased activity of the $Na^+$,$K^+$-ATPase and the $Na^+/H^+$ antiport, and also with a reduced uptake of bile acids by hepatocytes. However, whether these changes are responsible for the initiation of cholestasis or are secondary events has not been established. Indeed, the idea that decreased membrane fluidity might be one of the primary mechanisms of intrahepatic cholestasis is at odds with the effects of spironolactone, which decreases membrane fluidity and $Na^+$,$K^+$-ATPase activity while increasing bile flow [79]. Other studies demonstrating coupled changes in $Na^+$,$K^+$-ATPase activity and membrane fluidity failed to demonstrate consistently parallel variations in bile flow. Therefore, further studies are needed to define the true relevance of changes in plasma membrane fluidity in the development of cholestasis. In general, however, a role for structural and/or functional alterations of the plasma membrane and membrane-associated structures in the pathogenesis of cholestasis is widely accepted.

*Alterations in the Tight Junctions and Microfilament Dysfunction.* Loss of the anatomic integrity of the tight junctions results in direct communication between the canalicular lumen and sinusoidal space with consequent loss of the osmotic gradient. An increase in the permeability of the tight junctions is sufficient to make possible a retrograde diffusion of fluid [67–71]. Anatomic or functional alterations of the tight junctions have been detected in several experimental models of intrahepatic cholestasis [80–85]. In some cases, this modification results from changes in the lipidic composition of the membrane, as previously noted. In others, microfilament dysfunction leads to a true anatomic disruption of the tight junctions. The concept that changes in tight junctions may be a primary mechanism of cholestasis is supported by some data. Agents that specifically alter the polymerization–depolymerization equilibrium of the thin actin filaments, disorganizing tight junctions, cause cholestasis. Elias and Boyer studied cholestasis in phalloidin-treated rats and showed that the structural damage to the tight junctions was responsible for solute escape from the canaliculi and dissipation of the osmotic gradient [68, 81]. In addition, Phillips et al. demonstrated that the periodic contractile activity of canaliculi is impaired by the antimicrofilament agent cytochalasin B. Norethandrolone, another cholestatic agent, has also been reported to cause junctional complex dysfunction [83, 85]. Indian childhood cholestasis is the example of human cholestasis characterized by an altered function of microfilaments [84]. In summary, although the loss of activity of the pericanalicular microfilament network with secondary canalicular paralytic dilation occurs as a nonspecific event in cholestasis irrespective of etiology, microfilament dysfunction might play a primary role in some specific situations of intrahepatic cholestasis.

*Alterations in the Synthesis or Transport of Bile Acids.* Inhibition of bile acid transport reduces BADF. Canalicular bile acid secretion is the rate-limiting step in the overall process of transport of bile acids from the sinusoids to canaliculi. However, if the inhibition of bile acid uptake is intense, this can reduce canalicular secretion. Congenital aberrations in the synthesis of bile acids associated with cholestasis are described elsewhere in this chapter. These diseases are infrequent but they emphasize the importance of a normal bile acid metabolism in the genesis of bile flow. As previously stated, alterations in the transport of bile salts may occur secondarily to the dysfunction of several cell structures or functions. However, a primary role for this alteration in the initiation of cholestasis cannot be discounted in some situations. Uptake of bile salts may be inhibited by agents that modify the orientation or the mobility of bile salt carriers in the plasma membrane or by substances that lead to a dissipation of the transmembrane sodium gradient [35, 37, 67–71]. The principal cholestatic agents able to reduce bile acid uptake are chlorpromazine, ethinylestradiol, and cyclosporin A. It is likely that these substances act through more than one mechanism to impair bile acid uptake [67–71]. It has been suggested that amino acids entering hepatocytes by sodium cotransport may contribute to the cholestasis induced by total parenteral nutrition. Impairment of the intracellular transport of bile acids within hepatocytes may be involved in cholestasis but little is known on this subject. At the canalicular level, agents that modify the transport properties of the membrane (monohydroxy bile acids, antimicrofilament agents) or those interacting with canalicular carriers (phalloidin) inhibit canalicular secretion of bile acids. Finally, cholestasis, irrespective of the cause, impairs bile acid secretion by changing the functional polarity of hepatocytes, including the 100-kd bile acid carrier, which may be translocated to the basolateral membrane in cholestasis [37, 67].

*Impairment in Organic Anion Transport.* Definitive evidence that organic anions other than bile acids stimulate bile flow was provided by the study of a strain of rats with hereditary conjugated hyperbilirubinemia. These animals exhibit deficient secretion of several organic anions in association with reduced BAIF [58]. A similar phenomenon occurs in situations where glutathione secretion is impaired [65]. There is no evidence that impaired organic anion uptake may lead to cholestasis.

*Other Cell Systems* [67–71, 79]. Despite the fact that bile formation is energy dependent, there is no evidence that failure of hepatocytes to produce ATP in normal amounts specifically induces cholestasis. Changes in mitochondria, smooth and rough endoplasmic reticulum, lysosomes, and Golgi vesicles that have been observed in cholestatic livers seem to be secondary to cholestasis rather than initiating factors. However, impairment of vesicular transport may contribute to some forms of cholestasis, as recently demonstrated in rats receiving the immunosuppressant drug cyclosporin A. Functionally, vesicular transport is dependent on microtubules. Although antimicrotubular agents (colchicine and vinblastine) exert little effect on basal bile flow, they blunt the choleresis induced by bile acid overload. Thus, microtubular dysfunction cannot be ruled out as a possible cause of cholestasis as a primary or contributing event. Very recently, it has been demonstrated that the acute infusion of hypertonic glucose produces cholestasis in the rat. Although this reinforces the role of an osmotic force in the generation of bile flow, serum hyperosmolarity cannot be considered as a primary general mechanism of cholestasis.

*Intracanalicular Precipitates* [67–71, 86, 87]. Some drugs or drug metabolites may bind calcium, form polyaggregates with other bile solutes, or react with them. This may give rise to water-insoluble compounds precipitating in bile that may act as intracanalicular mechanical obstacles interfering with the normal flow of bile. Characteristically, lithocholate and chlorpromazine produce this alteration. Recently, benoxaprofen, and to a lesser extent ceftriaxone, have been found to produce bile precipitates, though not at the canalicular but rather at the cholangiolar or more distal levels in the biliary tree.

### *The Initiation of Cholestasis in Small or Large Bile Ducts Within the Liver*

In addition to the cholestasis initiated by hepatocyte dysfunction, a number of cholestatic conditions are due to an intrahepatic obstruction of the biliary tree. Diseases such as primary biliary cirrhosis, graft versus host disease, sarcoidosis and other liver granulomatoses, the intrahepatic forms of primary sclerosing cholangitis, and the chronic forms of drug-induced cholestasis are due to damage and obstruction of the small intrahepatic bile ducts. Whether, in some of these conditions, there is a primary defect in hepatocytes is unknown, but when cholestasis is established the most relevant lesions are located beyond the hepatic cells. It is of interest that a large majority of these conditions are attributed to immunologic mechanisms.

Compression or infiltration of the hepatic ducts within the liver is best considered as a large duct obstruction since it is clinically and pathologically indistinguishable from more distal obstructions of the biliary tree.

### *The Pericentral Occurrence of Cholestasis*

Morphologically, cholestasis predominates in the pericentral area of the liver lobule (zone 3) irrespective of its specific cause. This finding has been attributed by ELIAS and BOYER to the existence of a lobular gradient for bile formation from the periportal to the pericentral area [68]. In the hepatic lobule, the formed bile moves from perivenous to periportal areas, whereas blood flows in the opposite direction. Thus, a progressive fall in the blood content of bile salts occurs from periportal to perivenous zones. Accordingly, the amounts of bile salts taken up by hepatocytes will be far greater in zone 1 than in zone 3. As a result, bile produced by periportal hepatocytes largely corresponds to BADF, whereas that produced in zone 3 corresponds to BAIF. Under cholestatic conditions, a fall in the secretion of bile acids by zone 3 hepatocytes is very likely to lead to a situation in which the CMC of bile salts is not achieved, thus leading to the intracanalicular precipitation of water-insoluble materials. In addition, the activity of the enzyme systems responsible for drug metabolism is greater in zone 3 hepatocytes than in the rest of the liver. Therefore, drugs which cause cholestasis acting through

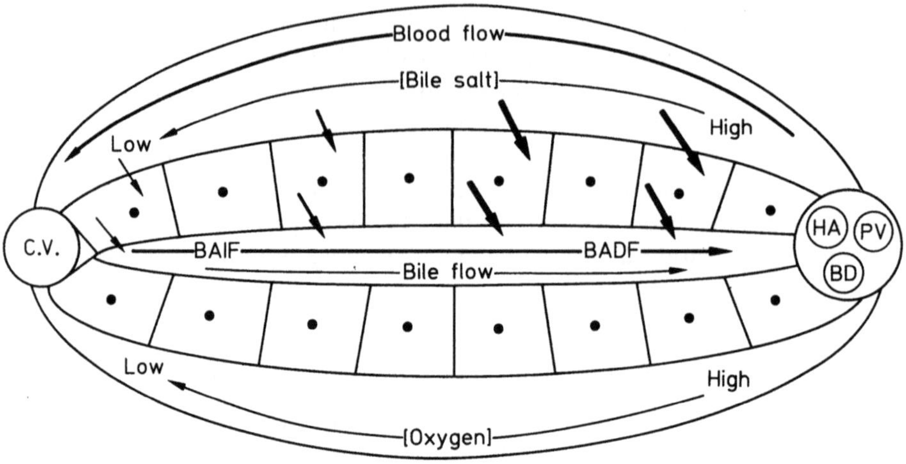


**Fig. 7.** Lobular gradient for bile formation. The *size of the arrows* in hepatocytes is in direct proportion to the amounts of bile salts taken up from sinusoidal blood and secreted to the canaliculus by these cells in the different areas of the hepatic lobule. *CV*, central vein. In the portal triad: *HA*, hepatic artery; *PV*, portal vein; *BD*, bile duct. (See text)

toxic metabolites will damage especially this area. The existence of a gradient for oxygen in the liver lobule implies that zone 3 is continuously perfused with relatively poorly oxygenated blood, another factor which may contribute to the predominant centrizonal localization of cholestatic features (Fig. 7).

### 3.4 Pathophysiology

Cholestasis results in the retention of bile solutes in the liver, in the presence of increased concentrations of these substances in serum, and in a deficiency of bile constituents in the intestinal lumen. In addition, liver function is altered as a result of both the primary lesion that induces cholestasis and the cholestasis itself [88–90].

#### *Liver Function Changes in Cholestasis*

##### *Retention of Bile Constituents in the Liver*

Failure of bile secretion leads to modifications of liver morphology and function. When cholestasis is transient, bile secretion returns to normal and liver function recovers without residual damage. However, in persistent forms of cholestasis, irreversible structural lesions resulting in secondary biliary cirrhosis may ensue. In cholestasis, changes in liver function may be "adaptive" or may be secondary to liver cell damage. The following alterations may take place:

*Liver Transport Processes.* Uptake processes are preserved since most substances appear in plasma in conjugated from, e.g., bile salts or bilirubin. Canalicular secretory processes, however, are blocked. Secretion of substances normally delivered to sinusoidal blood, like albumin or clotting factors, remains normal. In addition, a partial inversion of the functional polarity of hepatocytes allows some materials normally eliminated into bile to be released through the sinusoidal aspect of the plasma membrane. Conjugated bilirubin, bile acids, and lipid-containing vesicles are the most relevant of these materials [66].

*Transformation and Conjugation of Drugs and Endogenous Substrates.* Phase I reactions are partially impaired. In chronic cholestasis, the detergent activity of bile acids retained in the liver causes cytochrome P-450 dysfunction of variable degree. As a result, drug metabolism may be affected. Mixed oxidase function is still inducible by barbiturates until late stages of the disease. On the other hand, microsomal phase II reactions are preserved and shifted to glucuronidation and sulfation, whereas taurine and glycine conjugations are decreased. This modification renders water soluble some hydrophobic compounds, allowing their elimination in urine [91].

*Protein Synthesis by the Liver.* Protein synthesis is preserved in cholestasis. The synthesis of some canalicular enzymes, such as alkaline phosphatase and GGT, is accelerated. In the case of alkaline phosphatase, the stimulated synthesis is attributed to the high concentrations of intracellular bile acids. Increased biosynthesis of GGT seems to occur in biliary epithelial cells rather than in hepatocytes [94]. Circulating proteins of hepatic origin are normal in acute cholestasis. However, serum proteins may be decreased in patients with long-term cholestasis and secondary biliary cirrhosis or in those with protein–calorie malnutrition due to severe steatorrhea [92, 93].

*Bile Acid and Cholesterol Metabolism.* The bile acid concentration in hepatocytes increases several-fold. Changes in bile acid metabolism are directed toward minimizing the effects of the "detergent overload." Most bile acids are sulfated or glucuronidated [92]. These conjugations facilitate their urinary excretion. Thus, renal excretion of bile acids becomes important in cholestasis, increasing from 10 to 400 μmol/day. Minor amounts are hydroxylated in position 6, yielding hyocholic acid, a hydrophilic and non-toxic metabolite. In cholestatic diseases, the synthesis of bile acids and cholesterol in the liver is substantially inhibited, because bile acid overload inhibits HMG-CoA reductase and 7α-hydroxylase activities. This reduction in primary bile salt synthesis leads to a decrease in the trihydroxy to di-hydroxy bile acid ratio. As a result, the hydrophobicity of the bile acid pool increases. Serum cholesterol is high despite its diminished synthesis because of reduction in both degradation and elimination in feces. Bile salt pool size is decreased but its distribution is so profoundly altered that bile acid levels in serum and hepatocytes may increase greatly; because the supply of bile acids to the intestine is abolished or markedly reduced [2, 4, 70].

*Changes in Copper Metabolism.* Metals, especially copper, accumulate in cholestatic livers due to the lack of biliary excretion. In long-lasting cholestasis, liver copper stores may equal those seen in Wilson's disease. However, overt copper-induced liver damage does not occur, owing to the storage of the metal in a nontoxic form. S-Cu-S bonds augment the polymerization of metallothionein and prevent copper toxicity in liver cells. Serum copper is high, ceruloplasmin is normal, and, rarely, patients with chronic cholestasis may exhibit extrahepatic copper deposition. No neurologic manifestations of copper toxicity are seen. Occasionally, Kayser-Fleischer ring formation may be observed [94].

*Other Metabolic Changes in the Liver.* Impaired excretion of porphyrins into bile increases the urinary excretion of coproporphyrin and uroporphyrin. Less polar porphyrin derivatives cannot be excreted in urine owing to their poor solubility [95].

The liver takes up from blood, metabolizes, and eliminates in bile cysteinyl leukotrienes of systemic origin, a family of compounds with proinflammatory and vasoactive properties. In cholestasis, these compounds, still biologically active, accumulate in the liver and return to the systemic circulation. The effects of high amounts of cysteinyl leukotrienes in the liver may include edema, vasoconstriction, and progression of cholestasis. These agents, which are eliminated in urine in increased proportions, may be involved in the development of renal vasoconstriction, which often complicates cholestasis [96].

### *Mechanisms of Secondary Liver Damage*

Long-term cholestasis is associated with a progressive functional and structural deterioration of the liver which may lead, ultimately, to the development of secondary biliary cirrhosis. The following mechanisms contribute to cholestatic liver cell damage.

*Physical and Chemical Factors.* Bile salts are thought to be the agents responsible for cholestatic liver damage. Toxicity of bile acids is a function of their detergent potency. Lithocholate, the most toxic compound, is generated in very small amounts in cholestasis owing to the interruption of the EHC. However, the hydrophobicity index of the bile acid pool is increased. Bile acids at high concentrations solubilize cholesterol and phospholipids of the membrane systems, promoting detachment and loss of integral membrane proteins and changes in membrane lipid composition. Lipid composition determines the microviscosity (fluidity) of the plasma membranes, which, in turn, critically influences the functions of membrane-associated structures. Thus, the activities of $Na^+$,$K^+$-ATPase, $Mg^{2+}$-ATPase, or other membrane-associated enzymes, the orientation and mobility of membrane carriers, or the functions of transport membrane systems may be altered. Bile acids may directly affect the lipid bilayer of membrane systems, modifying their permeability. As a result, transmembrane traffic of water and solutes is disturbed and the transmembrane electric potential may be altered [72–74]. Bile acids may modify calcium transport in cells. In red blood cells, bile acids increase calcium entry across the plasma membrane [97]. In fact, their ability to induce hemolysis is directly related to their detergent potency. Similarly, hepatotoxic bile acids increase cytosolic calcium in hepatocytes, suggesting that this alteration may be responsible for the initiation of liver cell damage [98]. In addition, increased cytosolic calcium may modify many cell functions and constitutes a universal mechanism of cell death [98, 99]. It should be remembered that monohydroxy bile acids can induce not only cholestasis but also hepatocyte death in experimental studies. Therefore, altered bile acid metabolism and bile acid accumulation in hepatocytes may perpetuate cholestasis and cause cell damage. A vicious circle leading to irreversible liver injury may occur. Secondary biliary cirrhosis may develop after a variable period of months to years, depending on the severity of cholestasis.

Whether substances other than bile acids contribute to liver damage in cholestasis is unknown. Bilirubin, at high concentrations, may uncouple oxidative phosphorylation in mitochondria [100]. However, at high levels, bilirubin is likely to act also as a powerful antioxidant, an action that, at least theoretically, should be cytoprotective. The possible role of copper and peptidyl-leukotrienes has already been mentioned. At present, bile acids are considered the leading damaging agents in cholestasis.

*Immunologic Events.* Recently, it has been shown in cholestatic livers that class I molecules of the HLA system are abnormally displayed in hepatocytes, while the expression of both class I and class II molecules is abnormal in biliary epithelial cells [101]. On theoretical grounds, these abnormalities could trigger an immune response directed against both types of liver cells. It has been suggested that the predominant ductular and ductal damage observed in primary biliary cirrhosis or in the rare cases of drug-induced chronic cholestasis might be related, at least in part, to these immunologic events.

### *Bile Constituents in Serum*

Serum levels of conjugated bilirubin, bile salts, cholesterol, and phospholipids are abnormally elevated in cholestasis. Lipoprotein-X, a mixture of cholesterol, phospholipids, albumin, and fragments of the hepatocellular membrane, is found in serum in cholestatic patients [102]. These changes are caused by regurgitation from the liver.

Serum levels of alkaline phosphatase, GGT, leucine aminopeptidase, and 5′-nucleotidase, the so-called enzymes of cholestasis or canalicular enzymes, increase several-fold. This reflects increased synthesis rather than simple regurgitation, at least in the case of alkaline phosphatase and GGT [71, 88–90].

### *Pathophysiologic Consequences*

*Bilirubin* will return to plasma in conjugated form either from the hepatocyte across the sinusoidal plasma membrane or by regurgitation from disrupted canaliculi. This causes jaundice and bilirubin loss in urine (coluria), since glucuronidation renders bilirubin water soluble. Serum bilirubin does not increase much above 30 mg/100 ml, since at these levels urine elimination matches bilirubin production. Renal failure or increased substrate availability (i.e., in hemolysis) shifts the equilibrium and serum conjugated bilirubin will increase again. However, a few weeks after the onset of severe jaundice there is a progressive reduction in bilirubinuria. This is due to the formation of bilirubin–albumin conjugates. Up to 80% of serum bilirubin may be "sequestered" in this form of irreversible binding. Since this complex cannot be filtered in the glomeruli, the amount of bilirubin cleared daily by the kidneys decreases [103, 104].

Unlike the unconjugated compound, conjugated bilirubin does not cross the hematoencephalic barrier and, therefore, CNS toxicity is not seen in cholestasis.

In severe hyperbilirubinemia, marked deposition of bilirubin in renal tubuli does not occur, except in oliguric patients, in whom bilirubin casts are seen. Bilirubin is the most significant isolated risk factor for the development of renal failure in patients with obstructive jaundice. Levels above 20 mg/dl are critical for patients undergoing surgery. Whether this reflects a direct effect of bilirubin on renal function or merely represents a marker of the severity of cholestasis, or of a poor general condition, is not established [105].

*Serum bile acids* are always increased in cholestasis. Bile salts are thought to be responsible for the pruritus of cholestasis. However, the substance(s) causing pruritus remain to be defined. Retained bile salts were incriminated on the grounds that oral administration of cholestyramine (a bile salt chelating agent which prevents reabsorption of these substances in the intestine) improves pruritus in cholestatic patients. However, cholestyramine may bind substances other than bile acids. In addition, pruritus does not correlate with the concentration of any specific bile acid present in plasma or deposited in skin. Moreover, bile acid levels remain elevated after the spontaneous relief of pruritus in late stages of chronic cholestasis [71, 88–90]. A pruritogenic role for histamine has been suggested, since serum histamine is increased in cholestasis [106]. However, the extremely poor efficacy of histamine antagonists in relieving pruritus is against this theory. Recently, endogenous opiates have been proposed to play a role in the genesis of cholestatic pruritus [107]. This concept is based on the fact that pruritus is a frequent side-effect of opiate drugs, and the levels of endogenous opiates (at least, leuenkephalins) are increased in patients with liver disease. This increased opiatergic tone appears to be biologically relevant, since some clinical manifestations in cholestatic patients undergoing therapy with opioid antagonists correspond closely with an opioid withdrawal syndrome.

An additional pathophysiologic consequence of increased serum bile acid concentration is the induction of hemolysis and decreased osmotic resistance of red blood cells because of the detergent effect of these compounds on the erythrocyte membrane [97]. Similarly, alteration in the lipid composition of the erythrocyte membrane is responsible for changes in the shape and formation of target cells. Bile salts may also contribute to decrease vascular reactivity and to lower blood pressure in cholestatic patients. Bradycardia is a classic sign of obstructive jaundice attributed to bile salts. Finally, some studies suggest that the dysfunction of the reticuloendothelial system, and specifically the decreased phagocytic activity of Kupffer cells observed in cholestatic disorders, is caused by high serum levels of bile salts [108, 109].

In cholestatic diseases *hypercholesterolemia* is likely to accelerate atheromatosis. In addition, cholesterol deposition in the skin causes xanthomas and xanthelasma.

### *Endotoxemia in Cholestasis*

Endotoxemia is an abnormal finding observed repeatedly in patients with cholestasis, especially in those with obstructive jaundice [110]. It has been proposed that the lack of bile salts in the colon allows endotoxin to escape from the colonic lumen into portal blood [108]. Kupffer cell dysfunction is a contributing factor to the spillover of endotoxin. Circulating endotoxin has been suggested to be directly or indirectly responsible for the development of the systemic hyperkinetic circulation, the high frequency of acute renal failure and the rare occurrence of disseminated intravascular coagulation which may be observed in patients with obstructive jaundice.

### ***Lack of Bile Constituents in the Intestine***

*All bile compounds are absent or present in low concentrations in the intestine of patients with cholestasis. However, only the deficiency of bile salts is of pathophysiologic relevance [88–90].*

Neutral dietary fat is not emulsified in the intestine in the absence of bile acids. As a consequence, neutral fat resists the enzymatic attack of lipase and colipase. Even if partial fat digestion is possible, in the absence of bile salts the resultant monoglycerides and fatty acids cannot move across the unstirred water layer covering the microvilli of enterocytes. Therefore, fat malabsorption, often severe, does occur in this situation. Its magnitude is proportional to the intensity of bile acid deficiency in the intestine. If maintained and severe, fat malabsorption may lead to calorie–protein malnutrition.

Steatorrhea is associated with malabsorption of lipid-soluble vitamins (A, K, D, E) and calcium. The earliest clinical manifestations (occurring at 1 month or less) are due to vitamin K deficiency.

As previously noted, several studies suggest that the absence of bile acids in the colon is a permissive factor for the escape of endotoxin to the portal blood.

The lack of bilirubin in the intestine prevents urobilinogen and stercobilinogen from being formed. As a consequence the feces are colorless.

### 3.5 Clinical Features

The association of jaundice, pruritus, choluric urine, and pale stools constitutes the clinical hallmark of cholestasis.

*Jaundice, Choluria, and Alterations in Stools.* Jaundice develops slowly and becomes apparent when plasma bilirubin is above 2.5 mg/dl. In severe cholestasis, jaundice is marked and the skin is greenish. Choluric urine may be observed a day or a few days before jaundice is visible. As jaundice progresses, the feces become progressively discolored and pale. Fecal fat may be increased. Steatorrhea is easily recognizable because the feces are voluminous, soft, shiny, floating, and foul-smelling. In patients with choledochal stones, jaundice increases, in general up to moderate levels, and tends to fluctuate, since stones rarely produce complete obliteration of the bile duct lumen. In contrast, in patients with a tumor of the pancreatic head, jaundice progresses continuously until serum bilirubin levels reach 25–30 mg/dl. Pain in the upper right quadrant at the onset of jaundice may be present in patients with bile duct stones but it is nonspecific. A high, rapidly ascending, fever (septic fever), occurring in repeated episodes, suggests bile duct obstruction but also lacks specificity. In intrahepatic cholestasis, the course and the intensity of jaundice depend on its specific etiology. Drugs usually induce acute jaundice that declines slowly over several weeks or a few months after the offending agent is withdrawn. Cholestatic alcoholic hepatitis may follow a similar pattern, although severe jaundice maintained over weeks is not uncommon. Jaundice is slowly progressive, often evolving over several years in chronic cholestatic diseases, such as sclerosing cholangitis and primary biliary cirrhosis. In some cases of intrahepatic cholestasis, such as in liver granulomatosis or in the early stages of primary biliary cirrhosis, jaundice may be absent. In these cases pruritus, if present, and biochemical markers are the only diagnostic clues. In incomplete obstruction of the extrahepatic biliary tree, jaundice may be absent. Intermittent jaundice can be observed in cases of extrahepatic cholestasis in which spontaneous relief of the obstruction is followed in days or weeks by reobstruction, as occurs in ball valve-acting stones which move up and down in the common bile duct. Tumors of the papilla of Vater can have a typical, although infrequent, clinical presentation, with spontaneous improvement of jaundice following an episode of melena only to manifest jaundice again weeks later. Bleeding is due to tumor necrosis which leads to a transient relief of the papillary obstruction.

When urinary daily losses of bilirubin match bilirubin production, the intensity of jaundice stabilizes (at a level of about 30 mg/dl). Changes in the severity of jaundice and choluria as well as in the pigmentation of feces tend to run in parallel and are good indicators of the clinical evolution of cholestasis.

*Pruritus.* In most cases, pruritus is the earliest manifestation of cholestasis. Pruritus is a very disturbing symptom for the patient's quality of life. In fact, the presence of severe, intractable pruritus warrants liver transplantation in patients with chronic cholestatic liver diseases. Pruritus of cholestasis is perceived initially in the palms and soles and then tends to become generalized. It is more intense at night. Sleep may be markedly disturbed. Skin lesions due to scratching are frequent and may serve as an index of the intensity of pruritus. Hyperpigmentation of the skin is frequent in scratched areas. In chronic forms of cholestasis, pruritus fluctuates in intensity, often without a clear explanation. In late stages of these diseases, it tends to disappear as hepatic function abates.

*Xanthelasma and Xanthomas.* In chronic cholestasis, increased serum cholesterol may be deposited in the skin, leading to formation of xanthelasma and xanthomas. Xanthelasma are flat yellow lesions localized in the eyelids and less frequently in the neck and below the breasts. Chronologically, these lesions precede xanthomas, which are tuberous, prominent nodular formations predominantly located on the extensor surfaces of the limbs, in pressure areas, like the buttocks, and in scars. At least 3 months of plasma cholesterol levels above 450 mg/dl are required for xanthoma formation. If cholesterol levels fall, these lipid deposits may disappear.

*Other Physical Findings.* In most cases, a mild to moderate increase in liver size is found. Hepatomegaly is firm and nontender and there is no splenomegaly unless cirrhosis with portal hypertension develops in chronic cholestatic diseases. Overall, the general condition of patients is rather well preserved, except in those with neoplastic diseases or protein–calorie malnutrition.

*Bone Disease.* Cholestasis is associated with a particular form of bone disease known as osteopenia of cholestasis. About 50% of patients with chronic cholestatic diseases, such as primary biliary cirrhosis, show clinical manifestations of osteopenia, with great variations in intensity from patient to patient. In adults, clinical expression of osteopenia takes the form of bone pain, mainly back pain, vertebral crush fractures, hyperkyphosis, and hip fractures. In some patients back pain is extremely disabling. Incapacitation often ensues, especially in postmenopausal women owing to concomitant estrogen deprivation. Patients with long-lasting primary biliary cirrhosis constitute the paradigm of cholestatic osteopenia. On physical examination the only diagnostic sign of osteopenia is height loss as a consequence of crush fractures in the spine.

Bone loss may be assessed with poor sensitivity by lumbar spine and forearm x-ray studies. Assessment of bone mineral density by dual photon absorptiometry constitutes the best available method. It is useful for patient follow-up and provides an objective parameter for evaluation of the efficacy of new drugs in therapeutic trials. The disease is progressive. In patients with primary biliary cirrhosis, later stages are associated with a more intense osteopenia [111–114].

The frequent occurrence of steatorrhea in cholestasis supported the belief that osteomalacia is a chief element in cholestatic osteopenia. However, it is now established that osteoporosis rather than osteomalacia is the essential feature. Variable degrees of vitamin D deficiency, mild hypocalcemia, and hypophosphatemia have been reported in some studies, while others have failed to demonstrate these alterations [111–113]. Low levels of parathormone have been reported [114]. Probably, vitamin D deficiency is important in subsets of patients with severe long-term steatorrhea and is crucial for the development of rickets in children with chronic cholestatic diseases. Osteocalcin, a noncollagen bone protein, which is considered a useful index of bone turnover, has been found to be moderately decreased in plasma from patients with primary biliary cirrhosis in most but not all studies. This points to the existence of a low turnover osteoporosis. To be biologically active, osteocalcin has to be carboxylated, a function accomplished by vitamin K. Whether vitamin K deficiency contributes in this way to osteopenia of cholestasis remains to be established. Combination therapy with calcium, vitamin D, and calcitonin has been reported to be effective in controlling bone resorption in patients with primary biliary cirrhosis [114]. A preliminary report from the Mayo Clinic claims that liver transplantation not only stops but actually reverses bone damage in patients with primary biliary cirrhosis [115].

*Vitamin K Deficiency and Coagulation Disorders.* Vitamin K represents a family of liposoluble compounds contained in vegetable foods or synthesized by the colonic flora. Vitamin K carboxylates clotting factors II, VII, IX, and X and in addition, protein S and protein C, which have anticoagulant

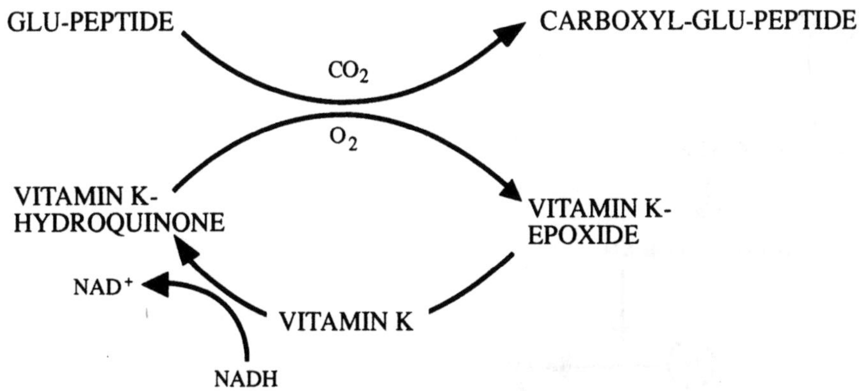


**Fig. 8.** Vitamin K-dependent protein carboxylation. The active form of vitamin K is the reduced vitamin K hydroquinone, which in the presence of $O_2$, $CO_2$, and a microsomal carboxylase is converted to its 2,3 epoxide at the same time as T-carboxylation takes place. The hydroquinone form of vitamin K is regenerated from the 2,3 epoxide by a coumarin-sensitive epoxide reductase. Vitamin K acts as essential cofactor for a microsomal enzyme system that activates peptide precursors by the conversion of glutamic acid residues (*GLU*) to T-carboxyglutamyl residues

properties, and osteocalcin [116] (Fig. 8). In the absence of vitamin K, these factors, all of them synthesized in the liver, remain inactive and a severe coagulopathy results. Deficiency of vitamin K is frequent in chronic cholestasis because of fat malabsorption. Easy bruising and petechial hemorrhages are frequently the first manifestations of vitamin K deficiency, but cerebral hemorrhages and gastrointetinal bleeding are also possible consequences. *Prothrombin time* is prolonged. A deficient synthesis of clotting factors by the liver may be ruled out by measuring prothrombin time before and 24 h after the parenteral administration of vitamin K (10 mg). Recovery of prothrombin time to normal values after a test dose of vitamin K indicates normal liver function and warrants substitution therapy with parenteral vitamin K. *Partial thromboplastin time* is also prolonged by vitamin K deficiency but it becomes altered later than prothrombin time and is not usually measured in cholestatic patients. The short half-life (5 hours) of factor VII is the cause of this difference, since deterioration of the extrinsic pathway of the clotting cascade occurs earlier than that of the intrinsic pathway (Fig. 9). Deficiency of activation of protein S and protein C, which under normal conditions will result in a tendency to hypercoagulability, is probably masked in cholestasis by deficiencies in clotting factors [116, 117].

*Vitamin A Deficiency.* Vitamin A deficiency may cause xerophthalmia and night blindness. It is lost in feces due to fat malabsorption. Serum carotene levels are low. Substitution therapy is indicated [118].

*Vitamin E Deficiency.* Vitamin E deficiency has no known clinical picture in adults. The relevance of its deficiency is unknown. It seems to be especially

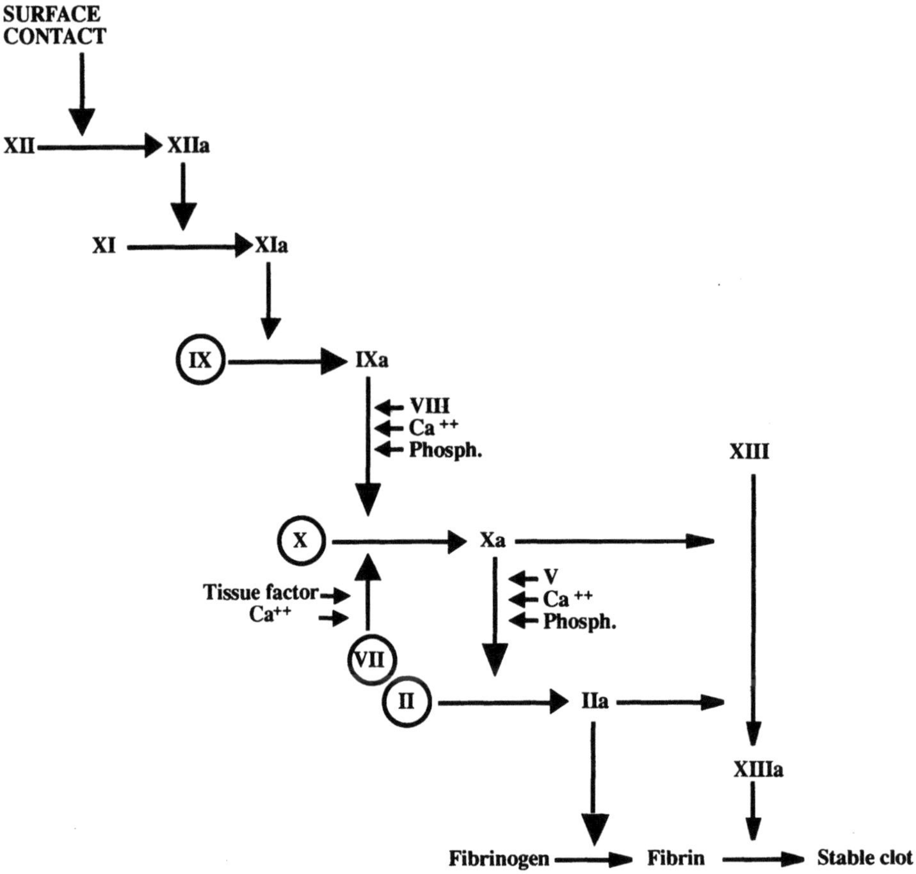


**Fig. 9.** Vitamin K-dependent clotting factors and their role in the clotting cascade. Vitamin K-dependent factors are encircled

important in children with chronic cholestasis who may develop severe neurologic alterations attributed to lack of vitamin E [118].

*Hemodynamic Alterations.* Hemodynamically, patients with cholestasis develop a hyperkinetic circulation of mild to moderate intensity which resembles the disturbed systemic hemodynamics of liver cirrhosis. A decrease in total peripheral vascular resistance seems to be the initial factor. A compensatory increase in cardiac output and overactivity of the pressor neurohumoral systems are observed. Arterial pressure tends to be slightly below normal, and there is a characteristic hemodynamic instability which is fully expressed at surgery. Increased serum bile acids and endotoxemia have been suggested to mediate these changes. A moderate bradycardia is frequently observed in obstructive jaundice. Myocardial contractility may be reduced [119, 120].

*Renal Function Disorders.* As previously noted, renal failure constitutes a frequent complication in obstructive cholestasis at the time of surgery [105]. Under normal conditions these patients show a mild renal vasoconstriction or at least renal blood flow redistribution with vasoconstriction of the renal cortex. Renal blood flow and glomerular filtration rate are maintained by an increased synthesis of renal vasodilatory prostaglandins which counteract the vasopressor effect of the increased levels of angiotensin II and norepinephrine present in these patients. This picture closely mimics renal function changes observed in cirrhotics with ascites. Alterations of systemic hemodynamics are, at least in part, responsible for this situation. Recent findings indicate that, initially, cholestasis causes a tubular dysfunction leading to renal sodium loss and defective ability to concentrate urine. Sodium retention occurs later in association with a fall in serum albumin concentration [105, 121].

*Infections.* Susceptibility to infections is increased in cholestatic patients, especially in those with obstructive jaundice. Cholangitis, cholecystitis, and gallbladder empyema may develop because of local obstructive factors. Sepsis associated with hepatobiliary diseases is commonly produced by *E. coli* and *Klebsiella*, *Enterobacter*, and *Serratia* species. The development of septic shock is a frequent and overwhelming complication in these patients, especially after biliary tract surgery [88–90].

### 3.6 Biochemical Findings

Biochemical findings are useful for the initial diagnosis and for monitoring the course of cholestasis. However, in most cases they are unreliable as a basis for distinguishing between extra- and intrahepatic cholestasis or between the different etiologic forms of the syndrome.

*Bile Acids.* Fasting serum total bile acids are markedly increased in cholestasis. However, this test is not routinely used in clinical practice, since it is not essential for the diagnosis and lacks specificity. Total bile acids and even differential quantitation of bile acid species might be useful for diagnosis of patients in whom a primary alteration in bile acid synthesis or metabolism is suspected or of patients still undiagnosed after the standard diagnostic workup has been completed. Techniques for the identification and differential quantitation of bile acids in serum or urine are complex, require skilled personnel, and are not available in most centers [122].

*Serum Bilirubin.* Conjugated hyperbilirubinemia is present in most but not all patients with cholestasis. A significant contribution from unconjugated hyperbilirubinemia should raise the suspicion of generalized hepatocellular damage, hemolysis, or congenital alterations in the uptake or conjugation of bilirubin. In recent years, newer laboratory methods have allowed the direct and accurate determination of unconjugated bilirubin, mono- and di-bilirubin glucuronides, and bilirubin–albumin conjugates [123]. Some interesting considerations emerged from comparison of these data with results obtained with the conventional diazo method still in use worldwide. Virtually all serum bilirubin is unconjugated in healthy people, while it is almost exclusively conjugated in cholestasis. As previously noted, in long-term cholestasis most serum bilirubin is incorporated in albumin–bilirubin conjugates. The marked persistence of conjugated hyperbilirubinemia in patients with recently relieved long-lasting obstructive jaundice may be explained by this fact. These conjugates have a half-life similar to that of albumin (2–3 weeks) and the components are bound irreversibly, thereby preventing glomerular filtration and urine elimination of this bilirubin fraction [104]. On the other hand, bilirubinuria is present while urobilinogenuria is absent in patients with complete biliary obstruction.

*Serum Alkaline Phosphatase and Other Canalicular Enzymes.* Serum alkaline phosphatase is always increased in cholestasis. It is a sensitive marker of cholestasis but is not specific since alkaline phosphatase isoenzymes are present in bone, kidney, intestine, and placenta, in addition to the liver [124]. Moderately raised levels of alkaline phosphatase may be found either in pregnant women (placenta) or in children (accelerated osteoblastic activity). In clinical practice, only cholestasic liver disease and some bone diseases may lead to significant elevations of serum alkaline phosphatase. The simultaneous determination of GGT, leucine aminopeptidase, or 5′-nucleotidase enables the clinician to establish the origin of this elevation, since none of them is present in bone whereas all are increased in cholestasis in parallel with alkaline phosphatase. This makes unnecessary the determination of alkaline phosphatase isoenzymes, although standardized methods are available. GGT is present in liver, kidney, pancreas, spleen, brain, heart, and seminal vesicles [125]. Increased GGT levels are due predominantly to liver, biliary tract, and pancreatic diseases. Its major clinical value is the confirmation of the hepatic origin of a coupled elevation in serum alkaline phosphatase. Isolated increases in GGT may be seen secondary to induction, such as in alcohol abuse or intake of drugs, especially barbiturates and phenytoin. Leucine aminopeptidase and 5′-nucleotidase are located in the canalicular plasma membrane. All these enzymes indicate impaired bile flow and are especially sensitive for the detection of compression of the microbiliary channels within the liver produced by disseminated space-occupying lesions, such as granulomas or diffuse tumoral infiltration.

*Serum Lipids.* Serum cholesterol levels are markedly elevated in cholestasis. Although lipoprotein-X is present almost exclusively in plasma from cholestatic patients, its determination is not routinely used for diagnosis.

*Serum Aminotransferases (AST and ALT).* These enzymes are minimally elevated in pure cholestasis. Their increase reflects the degree of hepatocellular necrosis.

*Prothrombin Time.* Prothrombin time may be prolonged as a result of vitamin K deficiency. If abnormal, a second determination must be performed 24 h after parenteral vitamin K (10 mg) has been given. Return to normal levels indicates vitamin K malabsorption secondary to cholestasis, whereas failure of correction points to defective synthesis of clotting factors by the liver. Determination of specific clotting factors is unnecessary for clinical purposes.

*Other Analytic Parameters.* Plasma proteins are normal. Hypergammaglobulinemia and hypoalbuminemia are present in long-lasting cholestasis with secondary biliary cirrhosis. Marked elevation of IgM is characteristic of primary biliary cirrhosis. Peripheral blood films do not show any alteration. Eosinophilia suggests parasitosis or drug-induced cholestasis. In chronic cholestasis, cholesterol accumulates in the membrane of red blood cells, leading to altered osmotic fragility and target cell formation. Anemia suggests complicated cholestasis. Infection, neoplasia, gastrointestinal bleeding, or associated hemolysis should be suspected in anemic patients. Leukocytosis with increased neutrophils is suggestive of infection.

### 3.7 Diagnosis

Cholestasis must be distinguished from conditions sharing some of its features. Jaundice due to hemolysis, shunt hyperbilirubinemia, or impaired uptake or conjugation of bilirubin by hepatocytes is associated with unconjugated hyperbilirubinemia. Jaundice in Dubin-Johnson and Rotor's syndromes is due to conjugated bilirubin, but serum bile salts and serum levels of alkaline phosphatase and other canalicular enzymes are normal in these conditions. Jaundice due to generalized hepatocellular injury, as in acute hepatitis, is associated with increased aminotransferase levels and mixed conjugated and unconjugated hyperbilirubinemia. Conversely, cholestasis may be anicteric in some situations, such as in partial obstruction of the main bile duct (i.e., stones, strictures), complete obstruction of one hepatic duct with patency of the other (i.e., early Klatskin tumor), space-occupying lesions without massive involvement of the intrahepatic biliary tree (i.e., metastases), disseminated microscopic lesions within the liver (i.e., granulomatosis, microabscesses), and the early stages of chronic progressive cholestatic liver diseases (i.e., primary biliary cirrhosis, sclerosing cholangitis). In these cases, cholestasis is recognized because serum levels of alkaline phosphatase, GGT, 5′-nucleotidase, or leucine aminopeptidase are increased.

The diagnosis of cholestasis must be completed by the investigation of etiologic factors and the location (intra- or extrahepatic) of the responsible lesion.

### *History and Clinical Examination*

Differentiation between intra- and extrahepatic cholestasis on clinical and biochemical grounds is often difficult. However, a careful clinical history and a detailed physical examination are essential steps in determining the diagnostic approach.

Gender and age of the patient, history of familial or personal episodes of jaundice, hemolysis, abdominal pain or hepatobiliary diseases, travel, environmental factors and profession, contact with animals, alcohol intake, and a careful revision of drug intake are important data. With regard to drugs, emphasis should be placed on over-the-counter drugs since some patients routinely taking analgesics, tranquilizers, sedatives, or contraceptive steroids may consider these drugs unimportant. Obtaining accurate data regarding the time when the symptoms began may distinguish acute cholestatic episodes from exacerbations of a preexistent liver disease or chronic cholestatic conditions. A detailed history of the rate of progression of jaundice, the existence of pruritus or other associated symptoms, and any change in the general condition of the patient is mandatory. In addition, symptoms or signs accompanying acute jaundice at the onset, and especially abdominal pain or fever, should be taken into account.

In patients with cholestasis developing on preexisting liver disease, the physical examination may reveal signs of liver failure or portal hypertension. On the other hand, relevant physical signs may be found in patients with cholestasis due to systemic conditions such as neoplasia, granulomatosis, cardiac disease, amyloidosis, or sarcoidosis.

### *Diagnostic Protocol*

There are no major differences between the diagnostic protocols for cholestasis proposed by several authors. Figure 10 presents a flow chart of diagnostic procedures. Changes should be introduced depending on the presentation of the patient. It must be remembered that diagnostic schedules are designed as an aid for the physician but never as a jail for clinical reasoning. In other words, diagnostic programs must always be subordinated to the physician's judgment.

Differentiation between intra- and extrahepatic cholestasis is attempted by means of hepatobiliary diagnostic imaging. The key finding is the dilation of intrahepatic bile ducts, which indicates the existence of a more distal mechanical obstruction. If this dilation is restricted to only one hepatic lobe, usually only the homolateral hepatic duct is obstructed. If bile duct dilation

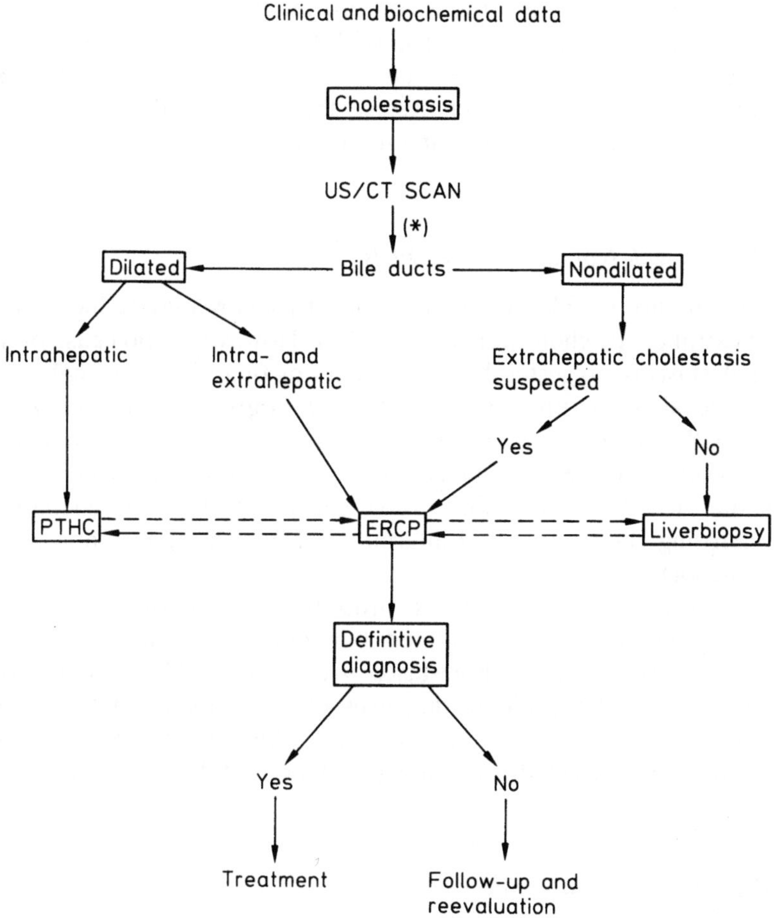


**Fig. 10.** Diagnosis of cholestasis. *US*, ultrasonography; *CT*, computed tomography; *PTHC*, percutaneous transhepatic cholangiography; *ERCP*, endoscopic retrograde cholangiopancreatography.
(*) Radionuclide scans (HIDA, DISIDA) may be useful in distinguishing between intra- and extrahepatic cholestasis.

is present in both hepatic lobes, the existence of dilation of the extrahepatic biliary tree and the level of its obstruction should be investigated.

*Abdominal ultrasonography* is the procedure of choice for the initial approach. Its success rate in diagnosing intra- versus extrahepatic cholestasis reaches 85% [126]. *Abdominal computed tomography* (CT) may substitute for ultrasonography with similar effectiveness in defining the existence of dilation of the biliary tree and with higher resolution in defining specific lesions. Disadvantages of CT compared with ultrasonography are patient irradiation and higher cost. CT offers better resolution for retroperitoneal structures and for the diagnosis of hepatic mass lesions and hilar processes

[126]. The use of intravenous contrast media enhances the resolution of CT scans for some types of lesions. With both techniques, a normal size of the biliary tree is not a reliable marker of intrahepatic cholestasis, since there are cases of extrahepatic cholestasis that cause no dilation of the bile ducts (i.e., stones in a nondilated main bile duct, sclerosing cholangitis).

### *Patients with Nondilated Bile Ducts*

The absence of bile duct dilation at ultrasonography reduces the likelihood of extrahepatic cholestasis to 5%–10%. However, if no cause of intrahepatic cholestasis is suggested by clinical data or there is a reasonable suspicion of an extrahepatic process, *endoscopic retrograde cholangiopancreatography* (ERCP) should be performed. This technique may provide the diagnosis of lesions in the bile ducts producing no dilation, such as choledochal stones, extrinsic infiltrations or malformations of the extrahepatic bile ducts, sclerosing cholangitis, and alterations in the intrapancreatic portion of the choledochal duct or even its parasitic invasion. If results of ERCP are normal, liver biopsy is the next procedure to be performed.

In patients with nondilated bile ducts and with no suspicion of an extrahepatic cause of cholestasis, *liver biopsy* will follow ultrasonography and/or CT. The etiologic diagnosis of intrahepatic cholestasis usually requires laboratory determinations in addition to histopathologic study. Laparoscopy-directed liver biopsy may be useful in some cases.

### *Patients with Dilated Bile Ducts*

Direct visualization of the biliary tree by means of *ERCP* or *percutaneous transhepatic cholangiography* (PTHC) is warranted when bile ducts are dilated. The choice between ERCP and PTHC depends in most cases on the particular conditions of a given hospital and specifically on the availability of personnel skilled in these techniques [127, 128]. The success rate for ERCP is markedly influenced by the skill and experience of the endoscopist. Table 2 summarizes the clinical indications, contraindications, success rate, and complications of these procedures.

Some patients with intrahepatic cholestasis remain undiagnosed after completion of the initial evaluation. This situation is more frequent in patients with mild jaundice or in those without hyperbilirubinemia but with isolated elevation of the serum alkaline phosphatase and related enzymes. The decision to stop or continue clinical diagnostic procedures depends on careful reevaluation of the case. A very important issue is whether the general condition of the patient is deteriorating or not. No invasive exploration should be undertaken in these patients until the clinical history and physical examination are again reviewed.

**Table 2.** Diagnostic procedures for direct visualization of bile ducts

| | Endoscopic retrograde cholangiography | Transparietal hepatic cholangiography |
|---|---|---|
| Indications[a] | 1. Suspected biliary tract obstruction with nondilated bile ducts<br>2. Intra- and extrahepatic bile duct dilation<br>3. Intrahepatic bile duct dilation | 1. Unilateral or bilateral intrahepatic bile duct dilation<br>2. Intra- and extrahepatic bile duct dilation<br>3. Suspected biliary tract obstruction with nondilated bile ducts |
| Success rate[b] | 75%–80% (very influenced by examiner's skills) | 95%–100% with dilated intrahepatic bile ducts; up to 70% with nondilated intrahepatic bile ducts |
| Contraindications | Pancreatitis<br>Anatomic alterations in the duodenum, especially after previous surgery<br>General of upper endoscopy | Massive ascites<br>Coagulopathy and/or thrombocytopenia<br>Parasitic cysts in the liver |
| Complications | 1%–2% (death rate <0.05%)<br>Pancreatitis<br>Cholangitis | 3.4%–10.1%[c] (death rate: 0.2%)<br>Hemoperitoneum (0.35%)<br>Bile leakage (1.45%)<br>Sepsis (1.4%) |
| Therapeutic usefulness | Sphincterectomy<br>Removal of stones | Placement of external or internal stents for biliary drainage |

[a] The two procedures are complementary for the same indications
[b] The success rate of TPHC increases with the number of passes

***Other Exploratory Procedures in Cholestasis***

*Radionuclide scans*: Hepatobiliary scintigraphy with technetium-99m, dimethyl acetanilide iminodiacetic acid (HIDA), or related compounds (DISIDA) may be used for the diagnosis of cholestasis in selected cases. This radionuclide is taken up by hepatocytes and eliminated into bile even in patients with moderately increased serum bilirubin levels. HIDA scans may be useful in patients with a suspicion of obstructive cholestasis but negative ultrasonographic and CT examinations [129]. It has been reported that the combined use of ultrasonography and scintigraphy yields up to an 85%–90% success rate in distinguishing between intra- and extrahepatic cholestasis [130]. This combined exploration is especially useful in extrahepatic cholestasis without bile duct dilation. However imaging with HIDA is not successful in patients with deep jaundice.

*Intravenous cholangiography* and *oral cholecystography* have virtually no indication at present for the diagnosis of cholestasis, since neither compares advantageously with modern imaging techniques.

## 3.8 Management

Management of cholestasis must be directed to the elimination of its cause when possible. With few exceptions diseases causing extrahepatic (obstructive) cholestasis are amenable to surgery, interventional endoscopy, interventional radiology, or extracorporeal shock-wave lithotripsy (see specific chapters). Exceptions are parasitic diseases which may be treated with drugs.

***Preoperative Care in Patients with Obstructive Jaundice***

Surgery for extrahepatic cholestasis is associated with high morbidity and mortality. Recently, Wait and Kahng [105] reevaluated data from 12 previously published hospital series comprising a total of 2007 patients who underwent surgery for extrahepatic cholestasis. The overall operative mortality was 16%. Acute renal failure occurred in 9% of patients, of whom 76% died. These data become even more impressive when one considers that no improvement in mortality was observed over the 25-year period encompassed by these studies.

Before surgery is undertaken, risk factors should be identified and, if possible, corrected. Deep jaundice, infection, and acute renal failure are the leading conditions worsening prognosis [105]. In other studies, discriminant evaluation of a series of independent parameters associated with poor outcome disclosed that serum creatinine >1.3 mg/dl, serum bilirubin >10 mg/dl, and serum albumin <3 g/liter were parameters with independent significance for poor prognosis [131]. Deep jaundice is associated, in turn, with an increased risk of renal failure. Indeed, several studies have shown that serum bilirubin above 20 mg/dl is associated with a high rate of acute renal failure with a fatal outcome. Such a serum bilirubin level matches the concentration of this compound that uncouples mitochondrial oxidative phosphorylation in vitro [103]. The possibility that bilirubin-induced mitochondrial dysfunction in the kidney might lead to renal failure remains to be evaluated. On the other hand, it is likely that the increased risk associated with very high bilirubin levels is related to the deterioration in the general condition of the patient in this situation.

Patients with obstructive jaundice tend to be hypotensive despite the fact that they show increased cardiac output and activation of the pressor neurohormonal systems. It seems that a decreased total peripheral vascular resistance is the primary hemodynamic alteration in these patients [119, 120]. During surgery, they are hemodynamically unstable and extremely sensitive to volume fluid loss. Recovery from hypotensive episodes as a rule, requires greater fluid replacement than in nonjaundiced patients. Indeed, in patients with obstructive jaundice, responsiveness to pressor agents is impaired and the ability of the kidneys to recover from transient hypoperfusion is poor. Overall, acute renal failure secondary to tubular necrosis, either intra- or postoperatively, is 30 times more frequent in these subjects than in nonjaundiced patients undergoing similar surgical procedures [132]. Surgical bleeding, often intense in jaundiced patients, constitutes an additional risk. Thus, low hematocrit values must be corrected before surgery. In addition, it has been shown that administration of 10% mannitol (500 ml) 2 h preoperatively protects renal function [133]. Nonsteroidal anti-inflammatory drugs and nephrotoxic antibiotics should be avoided.

As previously noted, it is thought that circulating endotoxin of intestinal origin may underlie some of these alterations. The occurrence of endotoxemia in patients with obstructive jaundice has been repeatedly verified [105, 108]. A recent study in normal subjects undergoing intravenous administration of endotoxin (4 ng/kg body wt.) showed a 46% decrease in systemic vascular resistance and a 56% increase in cardiac index 3 h after endotoxin challenge [134]. These findings, which mimic the hemodynamic behavior of patients with obstructive jaundice, reinforce the view that endotoxemia is involved in the pathogenesis of complications associated with surgery.

The "escape" of endotoxin from the intestinal lumen to portal blood in patients with obstructive cholestasis seems to be due to the lack of bile acids in the colon [109]. In normal subjects, this circulating endotoxin should be cleared by Kupffer cells in the liver, but in obstructive jaundice there is a spillover of endotoxin into the systemic circulation. Recently, it has been proposed that high serum bile acids are responsible for the reduced phagocytic activity observed in patients with obstructive jaundice [110]. Moreover, Kupffer cell dysfunction in rats was experimentally induced by high concentrations of lithocholic and taurolithocholic acid. Interestingly, tauroursodeoxycholate, which was very effective in preventing endotoxin absorption, did not impair Kupffer cell phagocytic activity [110].

It seems clear that bile acids prevent the absorption of free endotoxin from the intestinal lumen or participate in its inactivation. Complete or marked biliary obstruction eliminates this defense mechanism. Chronic cholestyramine administration may have a similar effect. Positioning of external biliary drainage in these situations ameliorates pruritus and decreases jaundice but does not restore the supply of bile acids to the intestine. Internal rather than external drainage should be placed when possible. In patients with external bile diversion, two studies have demonstrated that oral deoxycholate (500 mg, tid) given 2 days preoperatively prevents endotoxemia and postoperative renal dysfunction [135]. An additional study in the rat showed blockade of endotoxin absorption by tauroursodeoxycholate. If, in fact, endotoxin is relevant in determining perioperative complications, there is a rational basis for oral administration of bile acids and selective intestinal decontamination. Recently, oral norfloxacin (400 mg/day) has been found to be very effective in preventing Gram-negative spontaneous bacterial peritonitis in cirrhotic patients with ascites [136]. Gram-negative sepsis has been dramatically reduced in liver transplant patients by intestinal decontamination starting several days before surgery [137]. Thus, while controlled studies in patients with obstructive jaundice are not available, selective bacterial decontamination of the bowel seems to be justified in cholestatic patients undergoing biliary surgery, or at least in those with interrupted EHC. Elimination of endotoxemia would also improve the depressed cellular immunity and the hyperkinetic systemic circulation present in subjects with obstructive jaundice [110, 134].

*Therefore, the specific preoperative goals in patients with obstructive jaundice are the following: adequate nutritional support, amelioration of jaundice, prevention of endotoxemia and infection, protection of renal function, correction of anemia, and stabilization of hemodynamic status with adequate fluid supply.*

There is no place for surgery in intrahepatic cholestasis unless liver transplantation is indicated. Treatment for specific disease entities is included in the corresponding sections of this chapter or in other chapters in this book.

### *General Medical Management*

A series of general guidelines are useful for all forms of cholestasis, irrespective of specific etiologies. In acute, self-limited cholestasis, most of the measures indicated below are unnecessary.

#### *Nutritional Measures*

In patients with chronic cholestasis supplements should be given to avoid protein–calorie malnutrition and specific nutritional deficiencies.

*General Measures.* Lack of bile salts in the intestine makes neutral dietary fat indigestible and leads to steatorrhea. Fat intake should be restricted to 30–40 g/day. Supplementary fat in the form of medium chain triglycerides, which are easily absorbed in the absence of bile salts, may be administered in amounts covering 30%–40% of daily calorie intake. Total calorie intake should be adjusted on an individual basis, taking into consideration conditions that modify standard energy requirements (basal nutritional status, preexistent or associated metabolic diseases, severity of steatorrhea, etc.). Special attention must be given to conditions that increase the catabolic rate, such as infection or fever. Carbohydrates should be given in quantities sufficient to compensate fuel needs and prevent muscle wasting. Adequate protein intake should be secured. Protein restriction or administration of specific amino acid formulas is indicated only in patients with associated renal insufficiency or hepatic encephalopathy. Since appetite and tolerance to meals are quite variable among these patients, intravenous supplements in the form of glucose solutions may be advisable in some cases. Total parenteral nutrition is used only when the oral and enteral routes are contraindicated or clearly insufficient. Frequent monitoring of liver function tests is advisable in these patients.

*Lipid-Solube Vitamins.* Patients with chronic cholestatic diseases require supplements of lipid-soluble vitamins and calcium. These deficiencies are related to the degree of steatorrhea. In general, adequate substitution is achieved with the following schedule [138]:

- Vitamin A: 100000 IU i.m. (monthly)
- Vitamin D: 100000 IU i.m. (monthly)
- Vitamin K: 10 mg i.m. (weekly)
- Vitamin E: 50–200 IU p.o. (daily) or 1–2 mg/kg body wt. i.m. (daily)
- Calcium: in the form of gluconate, or carbonate in doses equivalent to 0.5–2 g of elemental calcium p.o. (daily)

Vitamins A and D are toxic in overdose. Since in most patients vitamins ingested with meals may be partially absorbed, patients should be watched for toxicity. Periodic determinations of serum retinol and serum and urinary calcium are desirable.

In addition, exposure to sunlight is recommended in patients with chronic cholestasis.

*Treatment of Pruritus and Unspecific Medical Treatment*

Treatment of pruritus is a priority in cholestasis because pruritus may have a devastating effect on the quality of life of patients. Since the substance responsible for pruritus is still unknown, no universally effective therapy is available. Classic therapy with cholestyramine remains the most extensively used. In recent years, several drugs have been tried with beneficial effect either for pruritus or in the cholestatic process. These are discussed below.

*Chelating Resins: Cholestyramine and Colestipol.* Cholestyramine is effective in controlling pruritus in most but not all patients. It takes several days before relief of pruritus is achieved. The drug is nonabsorbable and binds to bile acids in the intestinal lumen, preventing reabsorption. As a result, serum bile acid levels fall. This is thought to be the basis for relief of pruritus. Bile acid losses are initially compensated by increasing cholesterol and bile acid synthesis in the liver, but continuous treatment leads to a decrease in bile acid pool size and plasma cholesterol levels. Cholesterol absorption is also impaired by cholestyramine. If bile acids do not reach the intestine (i.e., there is total biliary tract obstruction), chelating agents are ineffective. Cholestyramine may induce malabsorption of fat and fat-soluble vitamins and worsening of preexistent steatorrhea. Digestive intolerance, flatulence, and abdominal discomfort are frequent complaints with this drug. Cholestyramine contains chloride (in fact it is a chloride exchanger). If it is given at very high doses per kilogram body weight, it may induce hyperchloremic acidosis. Simultaneous administration of cholestyramine with other drugs may result in their chelation and malabsorption. Cholestyramine (12–20 g/day) is given in doses of 4 g 30 min before meals. At breakfast, 8 g may be given. Avoidance of the evening dose may be needed for administration of other drugs at that time [139, 140].

The mechanism of action and effects of colestipol are the same as those of cholestyramine. Its advantages are a better (less bad) taste and digestive tolerance than the parent compound. Colestipol is scheduled as indicated for cholestyramine [140].

*Phenobarbital.* When intolerance to or ineffectiveness of cholestyramine precludes its use, phenobarbital may be employed. Phenobarbital is given at bedtime so that daytime somnolence is avoided. Doses of 2–5 mg/kg day are effective in some patients [141].

*Histamine Antagonists.* Histamine $H_1$ receptor antagonists, diphenhydramine (25–50 mg qid) or hydroxyzine (25 mg tid), may be useful for inducing sedation and improving night sleep, but their effectiveness in reducing pruritus is very poor. Drowsiness and diurnal somnolence are possible mild side-effects. Histamine $H_2$ receptor antagonists, like cimetidine or ranitidine, seem to be ineffective. Anti-$H_2$ drugs may produce antiandrogen effects and obtundation and may influence liver metabolism of other drugs [142].

*Opioid Antagonists.* The hypothesis that increased levels of endogenous opioids might be the cause of pruritus in cholestasis [107] prompted trials to evaluate opioid antagonists. Preliminary results are encouraging [107]. Both naloxone and nalmefene reduce pruritus in patients with primary biliary cirrhosis and other cholestatic disorders. However, administration of opioid antagonists in cholestasis cannot be recommended to physicians not enrolled in specific trials with these drugs, since reactions mimicking opioid withdrawal syndrome are not infrequent.

*Rifampin.* Rifampin, an antibiotic which induces cytochrome P-450, has been found to ameliorate pruritus in adult patients with primary biliary cirrhosis [143] and in children with chronic intrahepatic cholestasis [144]. Rifampin was given orally at a total daily dose of 10 mg/kg body wt. divided into two doses. Rifampin did not modify biochemical parameters of liver function. No side-effects were seen. The mechanism for pruritus relief is unknown. The long-term safety of rifampin administration in cholestasis needs to be evaluated.

*S-Adenosylmethionine* (SAMe). Besides its demonstrated effectiveness on estrogen-induced cholestasis, SAMe may be useful in other cholestatic conditions. In a recent study [145] involving 220 patients with cirrhosis, chronic active hepatitis, or primary biliary cirrhosis, all with some degree of cholestasis, SAMe (800 mg bid., p.o., 2 weeks) or placebo was given. The effect of SAMe on pruritus and fatigue was significant as compared with placebo. After discontinuation of the drug, both biochemical abnormalities and clinical complaints returned. Only a few minor side-effects were reported and with similar frequency as observed in the placebo group. Although its effects were limited, this is a safe drug which can be used as adjuvant therapy. Mechanisms of SAMe effects may include methylation of hepatocyte plasma membrane phospholipids, resulting in increased membrane fluidity, and sulfation of hepatotoxic endogenous bile acids.

*Ursodeoxycholate* (UDCA). Of the newer drugs recently assayed in the treatment of cholestasis, UDCA, a dihydroxylated hydrophilic bile acid initially introduced for the treatment of gallstones, is the most relevant. After the encouraging results of the initial study by Poupon et al. [146] in patients with primary biliary cirrhosis, several authors confirmed a marked improvement in pruritus and in biochemical parameters using UDCA. Trials with UDCA have extended to other diseases, such as primary sclerosing cholangitis, chronic active hepatitis, biliary atresia, cystic fibrosis with cholestasis and malabsorption, and undefined cases of intrahepatic cholestasis. In all cases, beneficial effects were reported [147].

Ursodeoxycholate seems to act in different ways:

1. It lowers the hydrophobicity index of the bile acid pool by replacing, at least in part, other more hydrophobic bile acids. With the current schedules for chronic treatment with UDCA, this compound reaches 30%–40% of the bile acid pool. The inhibition that UDCA exerts on the

intestinal absorption of physiologic bile acids contributes to this effect [148].
2. UDCA produces a bicarbonate-rich choleresis [40], the implication of which in the improvement of the biochemical markers of cholestasis is unknown.
3. UDCA seems to have "hepatoprotective" properties that do not depend on previously cited mechanisms. In experimental studies UDCA prevented cholestasis and hepatocellular necrosis induced by hydrophobic bile salts in both the in vivo rat and in isolated hepatocytes through mechanisms not yet defined [149]. It is of interest that hepatoprotection is exerted by both UDCA and its conjugates, while the induction of bicarbonate-rich choleresis requires the secretion of unconjugated UDCA into the canaliculi [40]. Hence, these properties of UDCA are likely to be independent.
4. UDCA reverses the abnormal class I HLA antigen display on hepatocytes that seems to be a consequence of cholestasis [150]. This action would have a beneficial long-term effect if the abnormal HLA display is triggering an immune attack against liver cells. The abnormal class II HLA antigen display on biliary epithelial cells, which is also present in cholestasis, is not affected by UDCA.
5. UDCA prevents endotoxin escape from the intestinal lumen to portal blood and does not affect the phagocytic activity of Kupffer cells, as previously noted.

Although these results have offered new insights into the treatment of cholestasis, evidence is still lacking that UDCA can modify the course of chronic cholestatic diseases. While waiting for the results of trials, UDCA may be considered as an apparently safe, effective, easy to follow, and moderately expensive form of therapy for cholestatic disorders. UDCA is administered orally at a total daily dose of 10 mg/kg body wt., divided into three doses.

## 3.9 Diseases Causing Cholestasis

### *Extrahepatic Cholestasis*

The most common causes of extrahepatic cholestasis are stones, pancreatic tumors, and tumors and strictures of the extrahepatic biliary tree. More infrequently, biliary obstruction may be due to blood (hemobilia), parasites, common bile cysts, and duodenal diverticula. Stones may obstruct the common hepatic duct and the common bile duct, and, rarely, a stone retained in the cystic duct may obstruct the lumen of the main bile duct (Mirrizzi's syndrome). A stone in the common bile duct may have a ball valve effect, in which case clinical manifestations may be intermittent. Cholangiocarcinomas arising from one hepatic duct near the bifurcation may compress the contralateral hepatic duct (Klatskin tumor) and produce obstructive jaundice clinically indistinguishable from that of extrahepatic origin. Dilation of intrahepatic bile ducts with an extrahepatic biliary tree of normal size on ultrasonographic examination is a characteristic finding of these cases.

Tumors of the head of pancreas are the most frequent nonhepatobiliary neoplasms leading to cholestasis. Progression of jaundice is rapid and may be painless. Palpation of a distended, nontender gallbladder (Curvoisier-Terrier sign) is virtually diagnostic of pancreatic head masses. Acute and chronic pancreatitis may also be associated with cholestasis, although such an association is rare.

Hydatid vesicles entering the bile ducts from a ruptured hepatic hydatid cyst may produce cholestasis if they are retained in the biliary tree. Right upper quadrant pain is frequent. Hypersensitivity reactions and marked eosinophilia are commonly observed due to massive release of parasitic antigens. Adult forms of *Fasciola hepatica* and *Ascaris lumbricoides* located intraluminally in extrahepatic bile ducts constitute unusual causes of obstructive jaundice. Extremely infrequent are instances of cholestasis due to the compression of the extrahepatic biliary tree as a result of infected duodenal diverticula or peritoneal reactions secondary to perforation of duodenal ulcers.

### *Intrahepatic Cholestasis*

#### *Cholestasis in Inborn Errors of Bile Salt Metabolism*

*Idiopathic Benign Recurrent Intrahepatic Cholestasis.* This disease was described by Summerskill and Walshe in 1959 [151]. Bouts of jaundice and pruritus lasting for up to 3 months start in childhood or in early adult life. Attacks frequently follow a prodromal period of anorexia, malaise, and weight loss. Hepatomegaly is absent. Serum levels of bile acids and alkaline phosphatase are markedly increased, aminotransferase levels are minimally raised, and hyperbilirubinemia may reach 20 mg/dl. Sulfobromophthalein transport is impaired. The underlying metabolic disorder is unknown. The disease is autosomal recessive with poor penetrance. The prognosis is good, although jaundice attacks cannot be prevented. In some patients, more than 25 attacks have been documented. Cholestyramine and phenobarbital are useful in controlling pruritus. There is no specific treatment [151, 152].

*Progressive Intrahepatic Cholestasis (Byler's Disease).* This disease was described in, and takes its name from, several members of an Amish community descended from a man called Jacob Byler. The defect underlying this disorder has yet to be determined. Available data suggest a deficient excretion of bile acids across the canalicular plasma membrane of the hepatocyte. Serum lithocholate has been found to be elevated in some but not all patients. Severe pruritus, jaundice, choluria and steatorrhea associated with hepatomegaly and in some cases splenomegaly occur between the 1st and the 10th month of life. Hypercholesterolemia and xanthomatosis are absent in these patients. Spontaneous remissions are followed by recurrent cholestatic episodes often triggered by upper respiratory tract infections. Growth retardation, rickets, and bleeding episodes are frequent complications. Bile acid levels are increased in serum and markedly decreased in the duodenum. Serum bilirubin may be increased to as high as 50 mg/dl and serum transaminases are elevated. Secondary biliary cirrhosis develops in patients with Byler's disease, generally leading to death at an age between 2 and 15 years although one patient has survived until 25 years. Medical treatments are ineffective in stopping the progression of the disease. In some cases, pruritus may be controlled with phenobarbital. Cholecystojejunostomy has been reported to ameliorate cholestasis in some patients [153–155].

*Hereditary Lymphedema with Recurrent Cholestasis (Aagenaes's Syndrome, Norwegian Cholestasis).* In this syndrome, cholestasis manifested by jaundice, pruritus, and steatorrhea develops in the 1st month of life and continues until the age of 1–6 years. Lymphedema of the lower extremities, early or late, occurs in all patients and becomes chronic. Growth retardation, bleeding, and rickets occur as complications. However, patients may have normal height in adult life, at which time transient episodes of recurrent cholestasis have been observed. Cirrhosis may develop and some patients have died from liver failure. In the cholestatic period, patients show hyperbilirubinemia and increased serum levels of bile acids, alkaline phosphatase, and transaminases. The cause of the disorder is unknown, although the existence of an abnormal lymphatic system both in the liver and in the lower limbs is supported by some data. No effective therapy is available [154, 156, 157].

*The Tetrahydrocoprostanic Acid Syndrome (THCA Syndrome).* Only four patients with the THCA syndrome have been described in two independent reports. In the report of EYSSEN et al. [158], THCA levels were elevated in the duodenal fluid and serum; cholestasis developed at 2–3 months of age and remitted 2 months later. The two reported infants had other congenital abnormalities, which were absent in the two patients described by HANSON et al. [159], who showed an otherwise similar cholestatic condition. Histopathologically, this syndrome was characterized by paucity of intrahepatic ductules with progression to portal fibrosis and cirrhosis. All four patients developed liver cirrhosis and died before the age of 2 years. Available data indicate that a deficiency of 24-hydroxylase is the cause of this disorder. This enzyme converts THCA to varanic acid, which is a precursor of cholic acid. THCA is absent in serum and bile in normal people.

*Arteriohepatic Dysplasia (Alagille's Disease).* See Chap. 28

*Cerebrohepatorenal Syndrome (Zellweger Syndrome).* See Chap. 27

*Cholestasis Associated with Bacterial Sepsis*

Jaundice may be associated with several infectious diseases, even though the liver is not directly invaded by the infectious agent. This association has been recognized in 6%–60% of children but only 1% of adults with Gram-negative bacterial infections. The incidence of cholestasis increases with the severity of infection. Thus, cholestasis occurs in 50%–60% of patients with septic shock. Infective agents involved in this complication are almost invariably Gram-negative bacteria. *E. coli*, *Klebsiella pneumoniae*, *Haemophilus influenzae*, *Pseudomonas aeruginosa* and *Salmonella* species are the most frequently cultured pathogens, although *Bacteroides* and *Proteus* species have also been implicated. As regards Gram-positive agents, jaundice may be seen in pneumococcal pneumonia (3%–67% of patients) and in 50% of patients with the staphylococcal toxic shock syndrome. Urinary tract infections, pyelonephritis, pneumonia, soft tissue infections, and intra-abdominal abscesses are the primary infections most frequently associated with cholestasis. Conjugated hyperbilirubinemia may reach 30 mg/dl or more, although usually it does not exceed 10 mg/dl. Serum alkaline phosphastase is increased in most cases and no or mild increases in transaminase levels are observed. Liver biopsy shows cholestasis, predominantly in zone 3, Kupffer cell hyperplasia, and a mild portal inflammation. Patients who develop septic shock with sustained arterial hypotension present with markedly elevated transaminase values due to centrizonal hepatocellular necrosis. Bacterial endotoxin is thought to be responsible for the development of cholestasis in bacterial Gram-negative sepsis. It has been proposed that an exotoxin may have a role in staphylococcal toxic shock syndrome. Large amounts of peptide-leukotrienes released in the course of sepsis might contribute to the development of cholestasis. Prognosis depends on the evolution of the primary infection. Mortality is high, with some series reporting up to 90%. This stresses the importance of an early diagnosis, especially in children in whom cholestasis may be the only sign of infection. Patients with increased serum alkaline phosphatase but without jaundice have a better prognosis. Cholestasis does not worsen prognosis by itself, but reflects the severity of the primary process. Liver function recovers rapidly if control of infection is achieved [96, 160–164].

*Cholestasis Associated with Total Parenteral Nutrition.* See Chap. 29

*Cholestasis Associated with Severe Hemolysis*

The rate-limiting step in the hepatic clearance of bilirubin is canalicular secretion. An acute bilirubin overload may saturate the canalicular transport system for conjugated bilirubin. Bilirubin itself might exert a cholestatic effect. However, an overt cholestatic jaundice as a result of severe hemolysis is likely to occur when cholestasis, even subclinical, is previously present. In this situation, bilirubin rapidly attains serum levels higher than those in obstructive jaundice. Massive blood transfusions in patients with mild liver dysfunction may have the same effect.

Sickle cell anemia is the hemolytic condition associated with the most severe hepatic involvement. Sickle cell crises present with acute episodes of fever, intense right upper quadrant pain, tender hepatomegaly, jaundice, and leukocytosis. Jaundice is predominantly due to conjugated bilirubin. Total bilirubin oscillates from near normal values to more than 50 mg/dl, although values above 20 mg/dl are infrequent. Serum alkaline phosphatase is moderately increased and aminotransferase levels display mild to severe elevation. Liver biopsy shows sinusoids which are occupied by Kupffer cells loaded with erythrocytes. Acidophil bodies and coagulative necrosis are seen. Lesions are predominantly in centrilobular areas. Improvement of the patients after a sickle cell crisis is rapid in cases with a favorable outcome. High bilirubin levels may be associated with poor prognosis, at least in adults. Sickle cell disease is also associated with instances of acute hepatic failure of unknown origin which present with transaminase levels only moderately elevated but with severe hyperbilirubinemia and coagulopathy. This complication is infrequent and has a very poor prognosis. Additionally, these patients may present with obstructive cholestasis due to bilirubin stones whose formation is increased in sickle cell anemia [165, 166].

*Recurrent Cholestasis of Pregnancy*. See Chap. 18

*Benign Postoperative Cholestasis*

Benign postoperative cholestasis (BPOC) is, in itself, the least threatening of the conditions which may lead to postoperative cholestasis. Thus, the diagnosis of BPOC is one of exclusion. Postoperative jaundice is seen in less than 1% of patients undergoing major surgery and constitutes a diagnostic challenge. In patients who have undergone hepatobiliary surgery, surgical complications of the biliary tract must be ruled out. Other frequent causes of postoperative cholestasis, such as halothane or viral hepatitis, drug toxicity and bacterial infection should be considered. In a majority of jaundiced patients, clinical, biochemical and ultrasonographic evaluation of the liver does not disclose any condition requiring specific therapeutic measures. In this situation, BPOC may be tentatively diagnosed. Patients with BPOC present with jaundice from the 1st or 2nd postoperative day. Moderate conjugated hyperbilirubinemia, moderately increased serum alkaline phosphatase, and minimally raised aminotransferase values are characteristic findings. This particular type of cholestasis is thought to be multifactorial in origin. Endotoxemia, transient liver hypoxia, hemolysis and total parenteral nutrition are factors probably contributing to the genesis of cholestasis in these patients. Pathologic findings are nonspecific. The hepatic architecture is preserved. Cholestasis of the canalicular type, with intracanalicular bile plugs and stainable bile pigments in centrizonal hepatocytes, is a frequent finding. Parenchymal necrosis is absent. Although hepatic disease is mild, the outcome of these patients depends on the severity of the associated illness. Mortality as high as 50% has been reported. Nevertheless, this type of cholestasis does not constitute, in itself, an additional risk factor. If the primary process resolves, no residual liver damage remains. There is no specific treatment [167–169].

*Alcoholic Cholestatic Hepatitis*. See also Chap. 20

Ethanol-induced liver damage may present as alcoholic cholestatic hepatitis. Although alcoholic hepatitis is a subacute or even chronic disease, the clinical presentation may have an abrupt onset. Jaundice and biochemical features of cholestasis may be associated with nausea and vomiting, abdominal discomfort, right upper quadrant pain and tenderness, fever, and leukocytosis. The risk of a wrong diagnosis of acute biliary tract disease is real and unfortunately such an incorrect diagnosis is not infrequently made. Jaundice is present in 50% of patients with alcoholic hepatitis. Serum bilirubin is one of the most important prognostic factors together with prothrombin time and encephalopathy. In fact, hyperbilirubinemia correlates directly with patient survival. Alcoholic hepatitis may occur when ethanol intake is above 80 g/day for at least 5 (men) or 2 (women) years and the patient is drinking actively at the time the disease develops. An enlarged liver is found in 90% of patients. The absence of hepatomegaly makes the diagnosis of alcoholic hepatitis unlikely. Characteristic biochemical findings are a prolonged prothrombin time and aspartate aminotransferase levels higher than those of alanine aminotransferase, with the values of these enzymes not exceeding 500 and 300 IU, respectively. Serum alkaline phosphatase is three times normal in 70% of patients and serum GGT may be disproportionately high in relation to alkaline phosphatase because of induction. Nevertheless, definite diagnosis of alcoholic hepatitis depends upon histopathologic findings, and liver biopsy is mandatory before the diagnosis is made. No effective specific treatment is available [170, 171].

*Viral Cholestatic Hepatitis*

Less than 10% of cases of acute viral hepatitis have a clinical course dominated by cholestatic features. Characteristically, deep jaundice with predominantly conjugated bilirubin and intense pruritus may be present for 10 or more weeks. Spontaneous resolution generally follows. Aminotransferase levels may normalize weeks before the jaundice begins to decline. The prognosis of the hepatitis is not influenced by its cholestatic evolution.

Symptomatic relief of pruritus and reassuring the patient with regard to the favorable final outcome are the only therapeutic measures required. In prolonged cases, vitamin K may be needed [172].

*Cholestasis in Congestive Heart Failure (Congestive Cholestasis)*

Liver damage is frequent in patients with congestive cardiac failure. In general, symptoms and signs of cardiac failure dominate the clinical picture but in some cases congestive heart failure may mimic acute hepatitis. Hyperbilirubinemia occurs in 25%–75% of patients with congestive heart failure and jaundice is clinically evident in 10%–20%. However, jaundice is rarely cholestatic, since more often 50%–60% of serum bilirubin is unconjugated. Furthermore, a serum level of alkaline phosphatase that is either normal or disproportionately low in relation to the degree of hyperbilirubinemia supports the diagnosis of congestive jaundice. Dramatic increases in serum bilirubin are seen in patients with acute decompensation of chronic right-sided cardiac failure. Aminotransferase levels manifest great variations. Biochemical findings show a poor correlation with right atrial pressure. The mechanism most likely to be responsible for liver dysfunction in cardiac failure is hypoxia. Increased hydrostatic pressure may play a contributory role. Histopathologically, lesions predominate in the pericentral area. Liver recovery depends on resolution of the cardiac failure. However, a prolonged prothrombin time unresponsive to vitamin K may persist for several weeks after cardiac compensation has been achieved [154, 173, 174].

*Neoplastic Cholestasis*

Primary and, more frequently, metastatic liver tumors may present with cholestatic jaundice. Jaundice rarely constitutes the first sign of hepatocellular carcinoma. If present when the patient is seen for the first time, it is mild or moderate. Subsequently, jaundice may progress as tumor size increases. In patients with previous liver cirrhosis the development of jaundice may herald the presence of neoplasia. Excluding lymph nodes, the liver is the organ most vulnerable to metastasis. Apart from primary brain tumors, all neoplasms may metastasize to the liver. The most frequent sources of liver metastases are tumors of the gastrointestinal tract, lung, and breast and melanomas. Although jaundice may be absent, increased serum levels of alkaline phosphatase may be an early indicator of neoplastic invasion. It has been reported that determination of 5′-nucleotidase activity is the most sensitive test in the detection of liver metastases [175]. In late stages, with extensive liver invasion, jaundice is frequent. In neoplastic jaundice, the mechanism of cholestasis is the compressive or infiltrative obstruction of either multiple intrahepatic bile ducts by generalized widespread liver metastases or the hepatic ducts by strategically localized mass lesions near the hilum. In addition to the treatment of the neoplasms, in some cases biliary drainage may be required for relief of pruritus [176, 177]. Massive infiltration of the liver leading to cholestasis may occur in Hodgkin's and non-Hodgkin's lymphomas and in histiocytic medullary reticulosis [178].

*Cholestasis in Hodgkin's Disease.* See Chap. 18

*Cholestasis Associated with Nonmetastatic Hypernephroma (The Nephrogenic Hepatic Dysfunction Syndrome)*

The nephrogenic hepatic dysfunction syndrome is very uncommon. It is characterized by systemic and hepatic manifestations occurring in patients with nonmetastatic hypernephroma. It was first described in 1961 [179]. Fever, weight loss, and enlarged liver and spleen occur in more than 50% of patients. Analytic abnormalities include marked elevations of serum alkaline phosphatase, GGT, and 5′-nucleotidase levels in about 90% of the patients; anemia and thrombocytosis are present in more than half. Abnormal sulfobromophthalein retention occurs in 100% of cases. Liver biopsy is nonspecific, showing proliferation of Kupffer cells and increased centrilobular expression of alkaline phosphatase. The diagnosis requires the demonstration that no metastases are present in the liver by means of imaging and histopathologic studies. The syndrome may disappear some weeks after successful surgery of the kidney tumor. The mechanisms of the hepatic dysfunction are unknown [154, 179, 180].

*Cholestasis in Sarcoidosis.* See also Chap. 18

Sarcoidosis is a systemic disease of unknown etiology which may affect virtually any organ in the body. Sarcoidosis may present as an acute disease or it may develop slowly in subacute or chronic form. Histopathologically, liver involvement is present in 60%–90% of patients, but signs or symptoms attributable to liver disease are present in only 20%–30%. The most frequent manifestations are liver enlargement, increased serum alkaline phosphatase and mild elevations of bilirubin and transaminase levels. Clinically, liver involvement is quite variable, ranging from asymptomatic patients to others who develop liver cirrhosis with portal hypertension [181]. Recently, a preliminary report including 97 patients with definitively proven hepatic sarcoidosis identified four major histopathologic patterns [182]: chronic cholestatic syndrome (57%), nonsuppurative destructive cholangitis similar to primary biliary cirrhosis (10%), periductal fibrosis similar to that seen in primary sclerosing cholangitis (12%), and acute suppurative cholangitis (12%). Typical noncaseating inflammatory granulomas were observed in 100% of liver biopsies. A reduced number of bile ducts is seen in 35% of the patients, hepatitis-like features in 39%, and sinusoidal dilation or nodular regenerative hyperplasia in 20%. Occasionally, differential diagnosis of primary biliary cirrhosis from sarcoidosis may be difficult. In sarcoidosis, antimitochondrial antibody is negative, angiotensin II converting enzyme is increased in 50%–70% of patients, and the chest x-ray film is abnormal in 90%. Administration of corticosteroids results in long-term improvement in biochemical parameters. The practical conclusion is that sarcoidosis must be included routinely in the differential diagnosis of cholestasis [182].

*Cholestasis in Amyloidosis.* See Chap. 18

*Cholestasis in Graft Versus Host Disease*

Graft versus host disease (GVHD) may occur when genetically foreign, immunologically active lymphocytes are transferred into an immunosuppressed patient incapable of rejecting these lymphocytes [183]. GVHD following allogeneic bone marrow transplantation develops in up to 70% of patients with successful grafts.

Skin and gut involvement is often the initial manifestation of GVHD, usually before liver function tests, especially bilirubin and alkaline phosphatase, become abnormal. Recorded cases with well-documented liver damage show that GVHD may induce several types of lesion, such as periportal fibrosis, nonspecific cholestatic hepatitis, bile duct degeneration, and a sclerosing cholangitis-like syndrome [184]. Progression to secondary liver cirrhosis is rare, although some cases with a fatal outcome have been reported recently [185]. Diagnosis of GVHD after bone marrow transplantation may be difficult, since the liver is exposed to several potentially damaging factors [183].

*Cholestasis in the Liver Transplant Patient* (see also Chap. 33)

Cholestasis is frequently observed postoperatively in patients undergoing orthotopic liver transplantation (OLTx). The causes of cholestasis are quite different in the early postoperative period and in later periods. The immediate weeks after OLTx are critical, because the risk of morbidity and mortality is higher in this period than at any other postoperative time. Patients may be exposed to hypoxia, hypothermia, hypotension, hepatotoxic drugs, general anesthesia, blood transfusions (often massive), infection, and primary graft malfunction due to preservation injury. In addition, this is the time of high risk for acute rejection, biliary tract complications, and Gram-negative sepsis, all of which are capable of inducing cholestasis. There are in addition a number of patients who present with cholestasis in the 1st post-transplant week and in whom none of the conditions cited above may be identified. This idiopathic posttransplant cholestasis evolves to spontaneous healing without residual damage. Jaundice appears within the first 3 post-operative days, peaks 10–12 days later, and may last for 30 or more days. Levels of serum bilirubin of 30 mg/dl or more (largely conjugated) are frequent, whereas serum alkaline phosphatase increases mildly. Both the intensity and the duration of jaundice are directly related to peak levels of transaminases in the 2 days following OLTx. Differentiation of idiopathic jaundice from jaundice due to other causes, and especially due to acute rejection, cannot be made with certainty on clinical grounds. Repeated liver biopsies are mandatory. As a rule, a delay in the diagnosis of acute rejection or of another major complication in the postoperative period of OLTx carries a much greater risk than that inherent to liver biopsy or other invasive diagnostic procedures. From the 2nd-3rd postoperative months, cytomegalovirus hepatitis and early cases of chronic rejection have to be included in the differential diagnosis of cholestasis [186–188].

Beyond 6 months after the operation, jaundice is unusual in OLTx patients in whom the immediate postoperative period has been relatively uneventful. When cholestasis occurs in this setting, chronic rejection, late bile duct complications or sequelae, recurrence of the primary liver disease in the graft, and drug toxicity are the most likely diagnoses [188, 189].

*Cholestasis in the Patient with AIDS*. See also Chap. 16

Liver disease is known to occur frequently in patients with AIDS, with several autopsy studies reporting the presence of intrahepatic opportunistic infections or malignancies in 33%–78% of postmortem examinations. SCHNEIDERMAN et al. evaluated 85 consecutive patients having liver biopsy or whose livers were evaluated at autopsy, to define the spectrum of hepatic disease in AIDS [190]. Overall, a normal liver histology was found in only 10 of 85 patients. Specific AIDS-related diseases involving the liver were found in 42.4% of the patients with the following distribution: 16.5% had *Mycobacterium avium–intracellulare* infections, 12.9% Kaposi sarcomas, 9.4% cytomegalovirus hepatitis, 4.7% lymphomas, and 4.7% fungal infections [190]. Cholestasis occurred frequently in patients with lymphoma or mycobacterial infection and was consistently associated with marked increases in serum alkaline phosphatase. Jaundice was infrequent except in the presence of lymphoma. It is noteworthy that in only two patients (one with lymphoma and one with mycobacterial infection) did these diseases involve exclusively the liver. In a vast majority of AIDS patients, hepatic involvement is a manifestation of systemic infection or neoplasia, and liver biopsy will seldom influence therapy. On the other hand, the biliary tract is also a target organ for AIDS-related diseases. AIDS cholangiopathy includes sclerosing lesions of the biliary tree that may have different specific etiologies [191]. Evaluation of AIDS patients by means of ERCP because of suspected biliary tract disease yields abnormal cholangiograms in more than 70% of cases. The most frequent lesion is the combination of papillary stenosis with sclerosing cholangitis, which accounts for about 50% of the abnormal examinations, followed by sclerosing cholangitis or papillary stenosis not associated with each other and the isolated presence of extrahepatic bile duct strictures. In most cases these alterations are secondary to infection with *Cryptosporidium*, *Cytomegalovirus*, or *Mycobacteria* or to infiltration by Kaposi's sarcoma or lymphoma. Ampullary biopsy and culture may identify the responsible process [191]. In AIDS patients with acute right upper quadrant abdominal pain and fever often associated with cholestatic liver tests, the possibility of acalculous cholecystitis should be considered because it has a significant mortality [192]. As a rule, in patients with AIDS and cholestasis, the diagnostic workup follows the same schedule as in non-AIDS patients, with noninvasive imaging studies preceding ERCP. Even liver biopsy, in spite of its limited utility, should precede ERCP in the absence of bile duct dilation [193].

### *Cholestasis Induced by 4,4-Diaminodiphenylmethane (the Epping Jaundice)*

Flour contaminated with 4,4-diaminodiphenylmethane (methylenedianiline) was the cause of an outbreak of jaundice which affected 84 people purchasing bread from a single baker in Epping, England, in 1965. This substance is an aromatic amine which is used in the manufacture of epoxy resin. The clinical picture included fever, abdominal and limb pain, rigors, cutaneous rash and moderate jaundice. Elevation of serum alkaline phosphatase and hyperbilirubinemia were commonly found. Markedly increased serum levels of aminotransferases were observed in some patients. A portal infiltrate of eosinophils and nonspecific cholestatic features were seen at liver biopsy in these patients. All those affected recovered without residual damage, although nonspecific symptoms were present in some patients for 2 years after the toxic insult. Subsequently, some additional isolated cases of toxicity due to this substance have been reported in workers handling epoxy resin [194, 195].

### *Cholestasis in the Toxic Oil Syndrome (Spain)*

The so-called toxic oil syndrome affected thousands of Spanish citizens in 1981. It was due to the fraudulent sale of a mixture of olive oil and denaturated rapeseed oil for home use. One year after the onset of this intoxication, 315 deaths among 19 828 affected patients had been reported [196]. The syndrome manifested initially as an interstitial pneumonitis associated with fever, arthralgia, myalgia, skin rash, and nonspecific digestive symptoms. Most patients showed high serum levels of transaminases, alkaline phosphatase, and GGT in association with eosinophilia and increased serum IgE. This first phase was attributed to the direct effects of an unidentified toxin. In the months following this acute episode, about a third of patients developed a multisystem disease with predominant neuromuscular manifestations, often with a dermatomyositis–scleroderma syndrome, pulmonary hypertension, and respiratory failure. This second stage of the disease was considered to be a manifestation of autoimmunity. Liver involvement was observed in about 25% of cases. Hepatomegaly and elevated serum levels of GGT (constant), alkaline phosphatase, and transaminases (frequent) were the most common findings, with some patients developing jaundice. Histopathology of the liver showed degenerative lesions in the bile duct, phlebitis in branches of the portal vein, sinusoidal eosinophilia, unicellular hepatocytic degeneration, and cholestasis. Liver disease was the cause of death in only one patient, who developed a Budd-Chiari syndrome. Patients who presented with jaundice in the initial phase of the disease were prone to develop a chronic cholestasis with paucity of septal ducts. This subgroup had a high incidence of HLA-DR3 and HLA-DR4. Five patients were reported as having developed focal nodular hyperplasia of the liver [197,198].

### 3.10 Drug-Induced Cholestasis (see also Chap. 19)

Drug toxicity is the leading cause of intrahepatic cholestasis in adults. Many drugs are reported to be cholestatic. Two main forms of acute drug-induced cholestasis are recognized [199]:

1. Pure or canalicular (bland) cholestasis: In this form hepatocellular damage and inflammation is minimal or absent. Biochemical features of cholestasis are accompanied by only a small rise in aminotransferase levels. Clinical presentation does not include systemic signs of hypersensitivity. Eosinophilia is absent (Table 3).
2. Hepatocanalicular cholestasis: In this type of drug-induced cholestasis there is associated liver cell damage of moderate to severe intensity together with mononuclear cell and eosinophilic infiltrate especially prominent in the portal triads. Transaminase levels are clearly increased but usually below the values found in acute hepatitis. Fever, rash, arthralgia, and peripheral blood eosinophilia are common clinical findings (Table 3). There are intermediate forms, and in general it should be considered that drugs able to produce hypersensitivity reactions may induce only pure cholestasis.

In some cases patients do not recover after an acute episode of drug-induced cholestasis. Rather, these patients develop a chronic liver disease which may persist for 2 or 3 years. On occasions, chronic irreversible cholestasis mimicking primary biliary cirrhosis ensues [199, 200]. A list of the drugs most commonly responsible for chronic cholestasis is provided in Table 4.

The clinical presentation of drug-induced cholestasis is frequently preceded by a prodromal period of malaise, fatigue, abdominal discomfort, loss of appetite and nausea. In some cases, and especially in the cholestasis induced by erythromycin estolate [201], the clinical presentation may be abrupt, with severe abdominal pain localized to the right upper quadrant,

**Table 3.** Drugs that may induce cholestasis

| Canalicular type (Pure or bland cholestasis) | Hepatocellular/hepatocanalicular type |
|---|---|
| Estrogens | Chlorpromazine |
| Anabolic steroids (17 substituted) | Desipramine |
| Organic arsenicals[a] | Haloperidol |
| Nitrofurantoin[a] | Amitriptyline |
| Ajmaline | Amineptine |
| Chlorpropamide | Imipramine |
| Tolbutamide | Propoxifen |
| Warfarin | Phenytoin |
| Cyclosporin A | Carbamazepine |
| Benoxaprofen | Allopurinol |
| | Indomethacin |
| | Isoniazid |
| | Rifampin |
| | Oxacillin |
| | Chloramphenicol |
| | Erythromycin (estolate and other salts) |
| | Oleandomycin |
| | *p*-Aminosalicylic acid |
| | Sulfonamides |
| | Busulfan |
| | Cimetidine |
| | Piperacillin |
| | Griseofulvin |
| | Captopril/enalapril |
| | Amoxicillin–clavulanic acid |

[a] Frequently produce hepatocanalicular cholestasis

**Table 4.** Drugs that may induce chronic cholestasis

| |
|---|
| Chlorpromazine |
| Imipramine |
| Amitriptyline |
| Carbamazepine |
| Cyproheptidine |
| Thiabendazole |
| Haloperidol |
| Phenytoin |
| Methyltestosterone |
| Ajmaline |
| Tolbutamide |
| Barbiturates |

nausea, vomiting and fever, mimicking an episode of acute cholecystitis. This may lead to a delay in the diagnosis.

*Mechanisms.* Estrogens decrease the fluidity of the basolateral plasma membrane by increasing its cholesterol–phospholipid ratio. In addition, $Na^+$,$K^+$-ATPase activity, $Na^+/H^+$ antiport, the uptake and secretion of bile salts and the secretory Tm of organic anions are also reduced in the liver of rats pretreated with ethinylestradiol. The primary mechanism of estrogen-induced cholestasis is unknown [202]. Norethandrolone-induced cholestasis has been less investigated. It has been suggested that this drug might impair microfilament function. Substitution at C-17 is essential in rendering these steroids cholestatic [203].

Chlorpromazine-induced cholestasis is due to the generation of toxic metabolites of this drug in the liver. Hydroxylated metabolites are toxic, whereas sulfoxide metabolites are not. The ability to form chlorpromazine sulfoxides has been found to be reduced in patients developing cholestasis as an effect of this drug. Cholestasis is multifactorial, since these toxic intermediates may damage membranes, microfilaments, and other structures. This drug reduces $Na^+$,$K^+$-ATPase and $Mg^{2+}$-ATPase activities, impairs bile acid synthesis and transport and produces intracanalicular precipitates [204, 205]. A chlorpromazine-induced abnormal gelation of actin filaments may be important in the development of cholestasis. Other phenothiazine drugs may have similar effects.

Erythromycin salts, especially erythromycin estolate, cause a dose-dependent decrease in bile salt secretion with a parallel fall in bile flow. The activity of both $Na^+$,$K^+$-ATPase and $Mg^{2+}$-ATPase is reduced by this drug. The primary mechanism of cholestasis is unknown but it is produced only by erythromycin salts and not by the base form of this antibiotic [201, 206]. Cholestasis induced by amitriptyline, imipramine, amineptine, and, in general, tricyclic antidepressants, seems to be due to the generation in the liver of oxidized metabolites of these drugs. These reactive compounds may bind covalently to proteins in liver cells. Some studies suggest that secondary immune mechanisms may contribute to the development of the cholestasis induced by these drugs [207].

Among drugs recently identified as cholestatic, benoxaprofen and cyclosporin A deserve comment. Benoxaprofen, a nonsteroidal anti-inflammatory drug which inhibits both the cyclo- and the lipoxygenase branch of the arachidonic acid cascade, was withdrawn from clinical use after it caused 31 fatalities due to induction of cholestasis and renal failure, mainly in elderly patients. In spite of the fact that patients showed a moderate increase in serum levels of transaminases, the cholestasis induced by benoxaprofen was predominantly of canalicular type. Its primary damaging mechanism is unknown. This drug produced a unique lesion: the accumulation of large laminated precipitates filling proliferated ductules [208]. Cyclosporin A, the most effective immunosuppressant available for regular use in organ transplantation, competitively inhibits bile salt uptake. In the rat, cyclosporin A impairs bile flow and bile salt and bilirubin secretion and interferes with vesicle-mediated transport processes without causing structural lesions. In clinical practice, recognition of cyclosporin A-induced cholestasis is often difficult, since transplant patients are exposed to a variety of cholestatic hazards. Cyclosporin A-induced cholestasis is of canalicular type, dose dependent, and reversible [209, 210].

## 3.11 Neonatal Cholestasis

Unconjugated hyperbilirubinemia immediately after birth and during the next few days is usually physiologic and benign. Conjugated hyperbilirubinemia is never physiologic or benign and it always deserves careful attention. It must be suspected in any neonate in whom the urine deepens in color. It occurs in about 1/500 infants. There are a host of diseases which may be responsible for neonatal cholestasis. This syndrome constitutes a frequent diagnostic problem in the neonatal period and in early childhood. Severe cholestasis in neonates or children has devastating consequences for nutritional status and growth. In addition, when cholestasis is susceptible to surgical correction, long-term results depend on the age of the infant at operation. Thus, early diagnosis is of great relevance in the management of this condition [211–214].

### *Approach to Infants with Neonatal Cholestasis*

Table 5 shows disease categories which may lead to neonatal cholestasis. In a series of 731 patients with conjugated hyperbilirubinemia referred to King's College Hospital and published in 1985, the definitive diagnoses were: extrahepatic biliary atresia (249 cases), idiopathic hepatitis of infancy (220 cases), $\alpha_1$-antitrypsin deficiency, PiZZ phenotype (128 cases), bile duct hypoplasia (41 cases), choledochal cyst (17 cases), and other diseases (76 cases) [215].

Clinical parameters are nonspecific. The diagnostic workup should be directed toward recognizing treatable causes of cholestasis, including sepsis, urinary tract infection, toxoplasmosis, tuberculosis, syphilis, listeriosis, malaria, hypothyroidism, panhypopituitarism, nutritional liver toxicity due to specific metabolic illnesses like galactosemia, and other rare metabolic disorders such as tyrosinemia. Cystic fibrosis and $\alpha_1$-antitrypsin deficiency should also be considered as potential causes of the syndrome [214]. If no specific diagnosis has been obtained, distinction should be made between extrahepatic biliary atresia (as the main cause of extrahepatic cholestasis) and intrahepatic diseases (neonatal hepatitis). Clinical differences are in most cases subtle, but may help to distinguish between them. Patients with extrahepatic cholestasis show normal weight at birth, may have firm hepatomegaly, and generally display earlier onset and higher frequency of acholic stools than children with intrahepatic cholestasis. In contrast, low birth weight, signs of generalized disease, and splenomegaly are more frequent in patients with neonatal hepatitis. Biochemical findings (excluding those associated with the specific diseases indicated above) are of no help in the differential diagnosis between intra- and extrahepatic cholestasis. Ultrasonography may reveal dilations or cysts in the biliary tree; ERCP and PTHC, extremely useful in adults, have very poor resolution in neonatal cholestasis. Often, scintigraphy with HIDA or DISIDA is helpful since in

**Table 5.** Causes of cholestasis in infancy and childhood

*A. Extrahepatic*
Biliary atresia
Biliary hypoplasia
Bile duct stenosis
Anomalies of choledochopancreaticoductal junction
Spontaneous perforation of the bile duct
Mass (neoplasm, stone)
Bile mucous plug

*B. Intrahepatic*
*I. Idiopathic*
Idiopathic neonatal hepatitis
Intrahepatic cholestasis, persistent
- Arteriohepatic dysplasia (Alagille's disease)
- Byler's disease
- Trihydroxycoprostanic acidemia (THCA syndrome)
- Zellweger syndrome
- Nonsyndromatic paucity of intrahepatic bile ducts

Intrahepatic cholestasis, recurrent
- Familial benign recurrent cholestasis
- Hereditary cholestasis with lymphedema (Aagenaes's syndrome)

*II. Anatomic*
Congenital hepatic fibrosis
Caroli's disease
*III. Metabolic diseases*
a) Primary alteration defined
- Tyrosinemia
- Wolman's disease
- Niemann-Pick disease
- Gaucher's disease
- Galactosemia
- Fructosemia
- Glycogenosis type IV

b) Primary alteration undefined
- $\alpha_1$-Antitrypsin deficiency
- Cystic fibrosis
- Idiopathic hypopituitarism
- Hypothyroidism
- Neonatal iron storage disease
- Infantile copper overload
- Multiple acyl-CoA dehydrogenation deficiency
- Familial erythrophagocytic lymphohistiocytosis

*IV. Hepatitis*
a) Infectious
- Cytomegalovirus
- Hepatitis B virus
- Hepatitis C virus
- Rubella virus
- Reovirus type 3
- Herpesvirus
- Varicella virus
- Coxsackie virus
- ECHO virus
- Toxoplasmosis
- Syphilis
- Tuberculosis
- Listeriosis

b) Toxic
- Cholestasis associated with total parenteral nutrition
- Cholestasis associated with bacterial sepsis

*V. Genetic*
Trisomy E
Down's syndrome
Donahue's syndrome (leprechaunism)
*VI. Miscellaneous*
Histiocytosis X
Shock or hypoperfusion
Intestinal obstruction
Polysplenia syndrome

Reproduced with permission from Balistreri WF (1987) Semin Liver Dis 7:2

**Table 6.** Differential histopathologic diagnosis between extrahepatic biliary atresia and neonatal hepatitis

| Histopathologic feature | Extrahepatic biliary atresia | Neonatal hepatitis |
|---|---|---|
| Lobular arrangement | Preserved | Diffusely disturbed |
| Portal tracts | Enlarged, fibrotic, with lymphedema | Normal |
| Bile ductules/ducts | Proliferated | Normal |
| Inflammatory infiltrate | Polymorphonuclear, restricted to portal tracts | Mononuclear, diffuse, intense |
| Bile plugs | Present | Absent |
| Hepatocellular necrosis | Absent | Present, focal |
| Fatty changes in hepatocytes | Absent | Present |
| Giant cells | Present | Present |
| Extramedullary erythropoiesis | Present | Present |

extrahepatic biliary atresia the uptake phase is unimpaired, whereas the intestinal excretion of the isotope cannot be detected. The reverse situation may be seen in neonatal hepatitis [211–215]. Liver biopsy is most helpful in differential diagnosis; characteristic findings are summarized in Table 6.

## References


1. Small DM, Dowling RH, Redinger RN (1972) The enterohepatic circulation of bile salts. Arch Intern Med 130:552–573
2. Carey MC, Cahalane MJ (1988) The enterohepatic circulation. In: Arias I, Jakoby BW, Popper H, Schachter D, Shafritz DA (eds) The liver biology and pathobiology. Raven, New York, pp 573–616
3. Hofmann AF (1989) The enterohepatic circulation of bile acids in health and disease. In Sleisenger MH, Fordtran JS (eds) Gastrointestinal disease, 4th edn. W.B. Saunders, Philadelphia, pp 144–161
4. Vlahcevic ZR, Heuman DM, Hylemon PB (1990) Physiology and pathophysiology of enterohepatic circulation of bile acids. In: Zakim D, Boyer TD (eds) Hepatology, a textbook of liver disease. W.B. Saunders, Philadelphia, pp 341–377
5. Danielsson H, Sjovall J (1975) Bile acid metabolism. Ann Rev Biochem 44:221–242
6. Hofmann AF (1988) Bile acids. In: Arias I, Jakoby BW, Popper H, Schachter D, Shafritz DA (eds) The liver biology and pathobiology. Raven, New York, pp 553–572
7. Shefer S, Hauser S, Mosbach EH (1968) 7α-Hydroxylation of cholestanol by rat liver microsomes. J Lipid Res 9:328–335
8. Bjorkhem I (1985) Mechanisms of bile acid biosynthesis in mammalian liver. In: Danielsson H, Sjoevall J (eds) Sterols and bile acids. Elsevier, Amsterdam, pp 231–278
9. Hofmann AF, Roda A (1984) Physicochemical properties of bile acids and their relationship to biological properties: an overview of the problem. J Lipid Res 25:1477–1489

10. Carey M (1985) Physico-chemical properties of bile acids and their salts. In: Danielsson H, Sjovall J (eds) Sterols and bile acids. Elsevier, Amsterdam, pp 345–403
11. Pattinson NR (1985) Solubilisation of cholesterol in human bile. FEBS Lett 181:339–342
12. Carey MC, Small DM (1972) Micelle formation by bile salts. Arch Intern Med 130:506–527
13. Carey MC, Small DM, Bliss CM (1983) Lipid digestion and absorption. Ann Rev Physiol 45:651–677
14. Van Dyke RW (1989) Mechanisms of digestion and absorption of food. In: Sleisinger MH, Fordtran JS (eds) Gastrointestinal disease, 4th edn. W.B. Saunders, Philadelphia, pp 1062–1083
15. Marcus SN, Schteingart CD, Marquez ML et al. (1991) Active absorption of conjugated bile acids in vivo. Gastroenterology 100:212–221
16. La Russo NF, Korman MG, Hoffman NE, Hofmann AF (1974) Dynamics of the enterohepatic circulation of bile acids. N Engl J Med 291:689–692
17. McDonald IA, Bokkenheuser VD, Winter J, McLernon AM, Mosbach EH (1983) Degradation of steroids in the human gut. J Lipid Res 24:675–700
18. Stiehl A, Ast E, Czygan P et al. (1978) Pool size, synthesis and turnover of sulfated and unsulfated cholic and chenodeoxycholic acid in patients with cirrhosis of the liver. Gastroenterology 74:572–577
19. Setchell KDR, Street JM (1987) Inborn errors of bile acid synthesis. Semin Liver Dis 7:85–96
20. Matern S, Gerok W (1979) Pathophysiology of the enterohepatic circulation. Rev Physiol Biochem Pharmacol 85:126–204
21. Nakashima T, Sano A, Seto Y et al. (1990) Unusual trihydroxy bile acids in the urine of patients treated with chenodeoxycholate, ursodeoxycholate or rifampicin and those with cirrhosis. Hepatology 11:255–260
22. Patterson TE, Vlahcevic ZR, Schwartz CC, Gustafsson J, Danielsson H, Swell L (1980) Bile acid metabolism in cirrhosis. VI. Sites of blockage in the bile acid pathways to primary bile acids. Gastroenterology 79:620–628
23. Binder HJ, Filburn C, Volpe BT (1975) Bile salt alteration of colonic electrolyte transport: role of cyclic adenosine monophosphate. Gastroenterology 68:503–509
24. Thaysen EH, Pedersen L (1976) Idiopathic bile acid catharsis. Gut 17:965–970
25. Popovic OS, Kostic KM, Milovic VB et al. (1987) Primary bile acid malabsorption: histologic and immunologic study in three patients. Gastroenterology 92:1851–1858
26. Hofmann AF, Poley JR (1972) Role of bile acid malabsorption in pathogenesis of diarrhea and steatorrhea in patients with ileal resection. I. Response to cholestyramine or replacement of long chain triglyceride by medium chain triglyceride. Gastroenterology 62:918–925
27. Tabaqchali S, Harzioannou J, Booth CC (1968) Bile salt deconjugation and steatorrhea in patients with the stagnant loop syndrome. Lancet II:12–16
28. Haff RC, Wise L, Ballinger WF (1971) Biliary-enteric fistulas. Surg Gynecol Obstet 133:84–89
29. McGuigan JE (1989) The Zollinger-Ellison syndrome. In: Sleisenger MH, Fordtran JS (eds) Gastrointestinal disease 4th edn. W.B. Saunders, Philadelphia, pp 909–923
30. Boyle JM, Neiderhiser DH, Dworken HJ (1984) Duodenogastric reflux in patients with gastric ulcer disease. J Lab Clin Med 103:14–21
31. Boyer JL (1980) New concepts of mechanisms of hepatocyte bile formation. Physiol Rev 60:303–326
32. Boyer JL, Gautam A, Graf J (1988) Mechanisms of bile secretion: insights from the isolated hepatocyte couplet. Semin Liver Dis 8:308–316

33. Erlinger S (1983) Hepatic Bile flow: facts and hypothesis. In: Berk PD, Chalmers TC (eds) Frontiers in liver disease. Neueherberg, pp 1–10
34. Erlinger S (1988) Bile flow. In: Arias I, Jakoby BW, Popper H, Schachter D, Shafritz DA (eds) The liver biology and pathobiology. Raven, New York, pp 643–662
35. Klaassen CD, Watkins JB (1984) Mechanisms of bile formation, hepatic uptake and biliary excretion. Pharmacol Rev 36:1–67
36. Moseley RH (1986) Mechanisms of bile formation and cholestasis: clinical significance of recent experimental work. Am J Gastroenterol 81:731–734
37. Sellinger M, Boyer JL (1990) Physiology of bile secretion and cholestasis. In: Popper H, Schaffner F (eds) Progress in liver diseases, vol IX. W.B. Saunders, Philadelphia, pp 237–259
38. Scharschmidt BF (1990) Bile formation and cholestasis. In: Zakim D, Boyer TD (eds) Hepatology, a textbook of liver diseases. W.B. Saunders, Philadelphia, pp 303–340
39. Desmet VJ (1983) Cholestasis: a problem. In: Csomos G, Thaler H (eds) Clinical hepatology. Springer, Berlin Heidelberg New York, pp 299–320
40. Scharschmidt BF, Lake JR (1989) Hepatocellular bile acid transport and ursodeoxycholic acid hypercholeresis. Dig Dis Sci 34 [Suppl]:5S–15S
41. Sellinger M, Barrett C, Malle P, Gordon ER, Boyer JL (1990) Cryptic $Na^+,K^+$-ATPase activity in rat liver canalicular plasma membranes: evidence for its basolateral origin. Hepatology 11:223–229
42. Sweadner KJ, Goldin SM (1980) Active transport of sodium and potassium ions: mechanisms, function and regulation. N Engl J Med 302:777–787
43. Layden TJ, Elias E, Boyer JL (1978) Bile formation in the rat. The role of the paracellular shunt pathway. J Clin Invest 62:1375–1385
44. Martínez-Palomo A, Erlij D (1975) Structure of tight junctions in epithelia with different permeability. Proc Natl Acad Sci USA 72:4487–4491
45. Hayakawa T, Cheng OI, Ma A, Boyer JL (1990) Taurocholate stimulates transcytotic vesicular pathways labeled by horseradish peroxidase in the isolated perfused rat liver. Gastroenterology 99:216–228
46. Phillips MJ, Satir P (1988) The cytoskeleton of the hepatocyte: organization, relationships and pathology. In: Arias I, Jakoby BW, Popper H, Schachter D, Shafritz DA (eds) The liver biology and pathobiology. Raven, New York, pp 11–27
47. LeSage GD, Robertson WE, Baumgart MA (1990) Demonstration of vesicular-dependent bile flow in the sucrose-loaded rat. Gastroenterology 99:478–487
48. Paumgartner G (1977) Physiology of bile secretion: bile acid-dependent bile flow. In: Bianchi L, Gerok W (eds) Liver and bile. University Park Press, Baltimore, pp 45–43
49. Kramer W, Bickel U, Buscher HG, Gerok W, Kurz G (1982) Bile salt binding polypeptides in plasma membranes of hepatocytes revealed by photoaffinity labelling. Eur J Biochem 129:13–24
50. Van Dyke RW, Stephens JE, Scharschmidt BF (1982) Bile acid transport in cultured rat hepatocytes. Am J Physiol 243:G484–G492
51. Ananthanarayanan M, von Dippe P, Levy D (1988) Identification of the hepatocyte $Na^+$-dependent bile acid transport protein using monoclonal antibodies. J Biol Chem 263:8338–8343
52. Stolz A, Sugiyama Y, Kuhlenkamp J, Kaplowitz N (1984) Identification and purification of a 36 kDa bile acid binder in human hepatic cytosol. FEBS Lett 177:31–35
53. Takikawa H, Stolz A, Kaplowitz N (1987) Cyclical oxidation-reduction of the C3 position on bile acids catalyzed by rat hepatic 3-α-hydroxysteroid dehydrogenase. I. Studies with the purified enzyme, isolated rat hepatocytes, and inhibition by indomethacin. J Clin Invest 80:852–860

54. Sugiyama U, Yamada T, Kaplowitz N (1983) Newly identified bile acid binders in rat liver cytosol: purification and comparison with glutathione-*S*-transferases. J Biol Chem 258:3602–3607
55. Kitamura T, Gatmaitan Z, Arias IM (1990) Serial quantitative image analysis and confocal microscopy of hepatic uptake, intracellular distribution and biliary secretion of fluorescent bile acid analog in rat hepatocyte doublets. Hepatology 12:1358–1364
56. Weinman SA, Graf J, Boyer JL (1989) Voltage-driven taurocholate-dependent secretion in isolated hepatocyte couplets. Am J Physiol 256:G826–G832
57. Ruetz ST, Fricker G, Hugentobler G, Winterhalter K, Kurz G, Meier PJ (1987) Isolation and characterization of the putative canalicular bile salt transport system of rat liver. J Biol Chem 262:11324–11330
58. Jansen PLM, Groothuis GMM, Peters WHM, Meijer DFM (1987) Selective hepatobiliary transport defect for organic anions and neutral steroids in mutant rats with hereditary conjugated hyperbilirubinemia. Hepatology 7:71–76
59. Oshio C, Phillips MJ (1981) Contractility of bile canaliculi: implications for liver function. Science 212:1041–1042
60. Lake JR, Van Dyke RW, Scharschmidt BF (1987) Effects of $Na^+$ replacement and amiloride on ursodeoxycholic acid-stimulated choleresis and biliary bicarbonate secretion. Am J Physiol 252:G163–G169
61. Anwer M, Hegner D (1983) Role of inorganic electrolytes in bile acid-independent canalicular bile formation. Am J Physiol 244:G116–G124
62. Van Dyke RW, Stephens JE, Scharschmidt BF (1982) Effect of ion substitution on bile acid-dependent and bile acid-independent bile formation by the isolated perfused rat liver. J Clin Invest 70:
63. Meier PJ, Knickelbein R, Moseley RH, Dobbins JW, Boyer JL (1985) Evidence for carrier-mediated/bicarbonate exchange in canalicular rat liver plasma membrane vesicles. J Clin Invest 75:1256–1263
64. Moseley RH, Meier PJ, Aronson PS, Boyer JL (1986) $Na^+$-$H^+$ exchange in rat liver basolateral but not canalicular plasma membrane vesicles. Am J Physiol 250:G35–G43
65. Ballatori N, Truong AT (1989) Relation between glutathione excretion and bile acid-independent bile flow. Am J Physiol 256:G22–G30
66. O'Brien M, Gottlieb LS (1979) The liver and biliary tract. In: Robbins SL, Cotran RS (eds) Pathologic basis of disease. W.B. Saunders, Philadelphia, pp 1009–1089
67. Phillips MJ, Poucell S (1987) Cholestasis: surgical pathology, mechanisms, and new concepts. In: Farber E, Phillips MJ, Kaufman N (eds) Pathogenesis of liver diseases. Williams & Wilkins, Baltimore, pp 65–94
68. Elias E, Boyer JL (1979) Mechanisms of intrahepatic cholestasis. In: Popper H, Schaffner F (eds) Progress in liver diseases, vol VI. Grune Stratton, New York, pp 457–470
69. Zimmerman HJ (1979) Intrahepatic cholestasis. Arch Intern Med 139:1038–1045
70. Reichen J, Simon FR. Cholestasis. In: Arias IM, Jakoby WB, Popper H, Schachter D, Shafritz DA (eds) The liver: biology and pathobiology. Raven, New York, pp 1105–1124
71. Popper H (1985) Cholestasis. In: Berk JE, Haubrich WS, Kalser MH, Roth JLA, Schaffner F (eds) Bockus, gastroenterology, vol 5. W.B. Saunders, Philadelphia, pp 2697–2731
72. Spector AA, Yorek MA (1985) Membrane lipid composition and cellular function. J Lipid Res 26:1015–1035
73. Smith DJ, Gordon ER (1987) Membrane fluidity and cholestasis. J Hepatol 5:362–365
74. Schachter D (1984) Fluidity and function of hepatocyte plasma membranes. Hepatology 4:146–151

75. Scharschmidt BF, Keefe EB, Vessey DA. Blankenship MN, Ockner RK (1981) In vitro effects of bile salts on rat liver plasma membrane, lipid fluidity and ATPase activity. Hepatology 1:137–145
76. Kakis G, Phillips MJ, Yousef IM (1980) The respective roles of membrane cholesterol and of sodium potassium adenosine triphosphatase in the pathogenesis of lithocholate-induced cholestasis. Lab Invest 43:73–81
77. Davis RA, Kern F, Showalter R et al. (1978) Alterations of hepatic $Na^+$,$K^+$-ATPase and bile flow by estrogen: effects of liver surface membrane structure and function. Proc Natl Acad Sci USA 75:4130–4134
78. Layden TJ, Boyer JL (1976) The effect of thyroid hormone on bile salt independent bile flow and $Na^+$,$K^+$-ATPase activity in liver plasma membranes enriched in bile canaliculi. J Clin Invest 57:1009–1018
79. Rutishauser SCB, Millward SE (1990) The effects of hypertonic glucose solutions on hepatic bile formation. J Hepatol 11:22–28
80. Elias E, Boyer JL (1980) Chlorpromazine and its metabolites alter polymerization and gelation of actin. Science 206:1404–1406
81. Elias E, Hruban Z, Wade J, Boyer JL (1980) Phalloidin-induced cholestasis: a microfilament-mediated change in junctional complex permeability. Proc Natl Acad Sci USA 77:2229–2233
82. Dubin M, Maurice M, Felman G, Erlinger S (1978) Phalloidin-induced cholestasis in the rat: relation to changes in microfilaments. Gastroenterology 75:450–455
83. Phillips MJ, Oda M, Fumatsu K (1978) Evidence for microfilament involvement in norethandrolone-induced intrahepatic cholestasis. Am J Pathol 93:729–739
84. Weber AM, Tuchweber B, Yousef IM et al. (1981) Severe familial cholestasis in North American Indian children: a clinical model of microfilament dysfunction?. Gastroenterology 81:653–662
85. Phillips MJ, Oshio C, Miyairi M, Smith CR (1983) Intrahepatic cholestasis as a canalicular motility disorder: evidence using cytochalasin. Lab Invest 48:205–211
86. Xia Y, Lambert KJ, Schteingart CD, Gu JJ, Hofmann (1990) Concentrative biliary secretion of ceftriaxone. Inhibition of lipid secretion and precipitation of calcium ceftriaxone in bile. Gastroenterology 99:454–465
87. Taggart HMcA, Alderdice JM (1982) Fatal cholestatic jaundice in elderly patients taking benoxaprofen. Br Med J 284:1372
88. Sherlock S (1989) Diseases of the liver and biliary system. Blackwell Scientific, Oxford, pp 248–272
89. Scharschmidt BF (1989) Jaundice. In: Sleisenger MH, Fordtran JS (eds) Gastrointestinal disease, 4th edn. W.B. Saunders, Philadelphia, pp 454–465
90. Scharschmidt BF (1983) Approach to the patient with cholestatic jaundice. N Engl J Med 308:1515–1519
91. Kawata S, Imai Y, Inada M et al. (1987) Selective reduction of hepatic cytochrome P-450 content in patients with intrahepatic cholestasis. A mechanism for impairment of microsomal drug oxidation. Gastroenterology 92:299–303
92. Hatoff DE, Hardison WGM (1979) Induced synthesis of alkaline phosphatase by bile acids in rat liver cell culture. Gastroenterology 77:1062–1067
93. Bulle F, Mavier P, Zafrani ES et al. (1990) Mechanism of γ-glutamyltranspeptidase release in serum during intrahepatic and extrahepatic cholestasis in the rat: a histochemical, biochemical and molecular approach. Hepatology 11:545–550
94. Janssens AR, Bosman FT, Ruiter DJ, van den Hamer CJA (1984) Immunohistochemical demonstration of the cytoplasmic copper-associated protein in the liver in primary biliary cirrhosis: its identification as metallothionein. Liver 4:139–147

95. Aziz MA, Schwartz S, Watson CJ (1964) Studies of coproporphyrin. VI. Reinvestigation of the isomer distribution in jaundice and liver disease. J Lab Clin Med 63:596–604
96. Keppler D, Hagmann W, Rapp S, Denzlinger C, Koch H (1985) The relation of leukotrienes to liver injury. Hepatology 5:883–891
97. Oelberg DG, Dubinsky WP, Sackman JW et al. (1987) Bile salts induced calcium uptake in vitro by human erythrocytes. Hepatology 7:245–252
98. Anwer MS, Engelking LR, Nolan K, Sullivan D, Zimniak P, Lester R (1988) Hepatotoxic bile acids increase cytosolic $CA^{2+}$ activity of isolated rat hepatocytes. Hepatology 8:887–891
99. Schanne FAX, Kane AB, Young EE et al. (1979) Calcium dependence of toxic cell death. A final common pathway. Science 206:700–702
100. Odell GB (1966) The distribution of bilirubin between albumin and mitochondria. J Pediatr 68:165–180
101. Innes GK, Nagafuchi Y, Fuller BJ, Hobbs KEF (1988) Increased expression of major histocompatibility antigens in the liver as a result of cholestasis. Transplantation 45:749–752
102. Narayanan S (1984) Biochemistry and clinical relevance of lipoprotein X. Ann Clin Lab Sci 14:371–376
103. Billing B (1987) Bilirubin metabolism. In: Schiff L, Schiff ER (eds) Diseases of the liver. J.B. Lippincott, Philadelphia, pp 103–127
104. Gautam A, Seligson H, Gordon DR, Seligson D, Boyer JL (1984) Irreversible binding of conjugated bilirubin to albumin in cholestatic rats. J Clin Invest 73:873–878
105. Wait RB, Kahng KU (1989) Renal failure complicating obstructive jaundice. Am J Surg 157:256–263
106. Gittlen SD, Schulman ES, Maddrey WC (1990) Raised histamine concentrations in chronic cholestatic liver disease. Gut 31:96–99
107. Jones EA, Bergasa NV (1990) The pruritus of cholestasis: from bile acids to opiate agonists. Hepatology 11:884–887
108. Pain JA, Bailey ME (1987) Measurement of operative plasma endotoxin levels in jaundiced and nonjaundiced patients. Eur J Surg Res 19:207–216
109. Van Bossuyt H, Desmaretz C, Gaeta GB, Wisse E (1990) The role of bile acids in the development of endotoxemia during obstructive jaundice in the rat. J Hepatol 10:274–279
110. Greve JW, Gouma DJ, Soeters PB, Buurman WA (1990) Suppression of cellular immunity in obstructive jaundice is caused by endotoxins: a study with germ-free rats. Gastroenterology 98:478–485
111. Van Berkum FNR, Beukers R, Birkenhäger JC, Kooij PPM, Schalm SW, Pols HAP (1990) Bone mass in women with primary biliary cirrhosis: the relation with histological stage and use of glucocorticoids. Gastroenterology 99:1134–1139
112. Diamond T, Stiel D, Lunzer M, Wilkinson M, Roche J, Posen S (1990) Osteoporosis and skeletal fractures in chronic liver disease. Gut 31:82–87
113. Watson RGP, Coulton L, Kanis JA et al. (1990) Circulating osteocalcin in primary biliary cirrhosis following liver transplantation and during treatment with cyclosporine. J Hepatol 11:354–358
114. Floreani A, Chiaramonte M, Giannini S et al. (1991) Longitudinal study on osteodystrophy in primary biliary cirrhosis and a pilot study on calcitonin treatment. J Hepatol 12:224–229
115. Hay JE, Dickson ER, Wiesner RH, Krom RAF (1990) Long-term effect of orthotopic liver transplantation on the osteopenia of primary biliary cirrhosis (abstr). Hepatology 12:838
116. Suttie JW (1987) Recent advances in hepatic vitamin K metabolism and function. Hepatology 7:367–376

117. Jorgensen MJ, Furie BC, Furie B (1988) Vitamin K-dependent blood coagulation proteins. In: Arias I, Jakoby BW, Popper H, Schachter D, Shafritz DA (eds) The liver biology and pathobiology. Raven, New York, pp 495–504
118. Jeffrey GP, Muller DPR, Burroughs AK et al. (1987) Vitamin E deficiency and its clinical significance in adults with primary biliary cirrhosis and other forms of cholestatic liver disease. J Hepatol 4:307–314
119. Bomzom A, Weinbroum A, Kamanetz L (1990) Systemic hypotension and pressor responsiveness in cholestasis. J Hepatol 11:70–76
120. Bina O, Bomzom A, Blendis LM et al. (1985) Obstructive jaundice blunts myocardial contractile response to isoprenaline in the dog: a clue to the susceptibility of jaundiced patients to shock?. Clin Sci 69:647–653
121. Sitprija V, Kashemsant U, Sriratanaban A, Arthachinta S, Poshyachinda V (1990) Renal function in obstructive jaundice in man: cholangiocarcinoma model. Kidney Int 38:948–955
122. Makino I, Hashimoto H, Shinozaki K, Yoshino K, Nakagava S (1975) Sulfated and nonsulfated bile acids in urine, serum and bile in patients with hepatobiliary diseases. Gastroenterology 68:545–553
123. Blanckaert N (1979) Analysis of bilirubin and bilirubin mono- and diconjugates. Determination of their relative amounts in biological samples. Biochem J 183:115–123
124. Stolz A, Kaplowitz N (1990) Biochemical test for liver disease. In: Zakim D, Boyer TD (eds) Hepatology, a textbook of liver disease. W.B. Saunders, Philadelphia, pp 637–666
125. Rosalki SB, Trlow D, Rau D (1971) Plasma γ-glutamyl-transpeptidase elevation in patients receiving enzyme-inducing drugs. Lancet II:376–377
126. Campbell WL (1989) Medical versus surgical jaundice. In: Straub WH (ed) Manual of diagnostic imaging. Little, Brown and Company, Boston, pp 152–155
127. Matzen P, Malcow-Moller A, Brun B et al. (1983) Ultrasonography, computed tomography and cholescintigraphy in suspected obstructive jaundice – a prospective comparative study. Gastroenterology 84:1492–1497
128. Ritcher JM, Silverstein MD, Shapiro R (1983) Suspected obstructive jaundice: a decision analysis of diagnostic strategies. Ann Intern Med 99:46–51
129. Thoeni RF, Goldberg HI (1990) Radiologic evaluation of disorders of the liver and biliary system. In: Zakim D, Boyer TD (eds) Hepatology, a textbook of liver disease. W.B. Saunders, Philadelphia, pp 667–686
130. Lieberman DA, Krishnamurthy GT (1986) Intrahepatic versus extrahepatic cholestasis. Discrimination with biliary scintigraphy combined with ultrasound. Gastroenterology 90:734–743
131. Blamey SL, Fearon KCH, Gilmour VH et al. (1983) Prediction of risk in biliary surgery. Br J Surg 70:535–538
132. Glenn F, McSherry CK (1963) Etiological factors in fatal complications following operations upon the biliary tract. Ann Surg 157:695–696
133. Dawson JL (1964) Jaundice and anoxic renal damage: protective effect of mannitol. Br Med J 1:810–811
134. Suffredini AF, Fromm RE, Parker MM et al. (1989) The cardiovascular response of normal humans to the administration of endotoxin. N Engl J Med 321:280–287
135. Cahill CJ, Pain JA, Bailey ME (1987) Bile salts, endotoxin and renal function in obstructive jaundice. Surg Gynecol Obstet 165:519–522
136. Ginés P, Rimola A, Planas R et al. (1990) Norfloxacin prevents spontaneous bacterial peritonitis recurrence in cirrhosis: results of a double-blind, placebo-controlled trial. Hepatology 12:716–724
137. Wiesner RH, Hermans PE, Rakela J et al. (1988) Selective bowel decontamination to decrease gram-negative aerobic bacterial and *Candida*

colonization and prevent infection after orthotopic liver transplantation. Transplantation 45:570–574
138. Marcus R, Coulston AM (1990) The vitamins. In: Goodman Gilman A, Rall TW, Nies AS, Taylor P (eds) The pharmacological basis of therapeutic. Pergamon, New York, pp 1523–1571
139. Datta DV, Sherlock S (1966) Cholestyramine for long term relief of the pruritus complicating intrahepatic cholestasis. Gastroenterology 50:323–332
140. Brown MS, Goldstein JL (1990) Drugs used in the treatment of hyperlipoproteinemias. In: Goodman Gilman A, Rall TW, Nies AS, Taylor P (eds) The pharmacological basis of therapeutics. Pergamon, New York, pp 874–896
141. Bloomer JR, Boyer JL (1975) Phenobarbital effects in cholestatic liver disease. Ann Intern Med 82:310–317
142. Duncan JS, Kennedy TH, Trigor DR (1984) Treatment of pruritus due to chronic obstructive liver disease. Br Med J 289:22–25
143. Ghent CN, Carrhuters SG (1988) Treatment of pruritus in primary biliary cirrhosis with rifampin. Gastroenterology 94:488–493
144. Cynamon HA, Andres JM, Iafrate RP (1990) Rifampin relieves pruritus in children with cholestatic liver disease. Gastroenterology 1013–1016
145. Frezza M, Surrenti C, Manzillo G, Fiaccadori F, Bortolini M, Di Padova C (1990) Oral *S*-adenosylmethionine in the symptomatic treatment of intrahepatic cholestasis. Gastroenterology 99:211–215
146. Poupon R, Chretien Y, Poupon Re, Ballet F, Calmus Y, Damis F (1986) Is ursodeoxycholic acid an effective treatment for primary biliary cirrhosis? Lancet I:834–836
147. James OFW (1990) Ursodeoxycholic acid treatment for chronic cholestatic liver disease. J Hepatol 11:5–8
148. Stiehl A, Rudolph G, Raedsch et al. (1990) Ursodeoxycholic acid-induced changes of plasma and urinary bile acids in patients with primary biliary cirrhosis. Hepatology 12:492–497
149. Stiehl A, Raedsch R, Rudolph G (1990) Acute effects of ursodeoxycholic and chenodeoxycholic acid on the small intestinal absorption of bile acids. Gastroenterology 98:424–428
150. Borum M, Fromm H (1990) Expression of HLA molecules on hepatocytes: Does ursodeoxycholic acid prevent immunologic injury? Gastroenterology 99:561–562
151. Summerskill WHJ, Walshe JM (1959) Benign recurrent intrahepatic "obstructive" jaundice. Lancet II:686–690
152. Tygstrup N (1960) Intermittent possibly familial intrahepatic cholestatic jaundice. Lancet I:1171
153. Clayton RJ, Iber FL, Ruebner BH et al. (1965) Byler's disease: fatal familiar intrahepatic cholestasis in an Amish kindred (abstr). J Pedriat 67:1025
154. Ghishan FK, Greene HL (1990) Inborn errors of metabolism that lead to permanent liver injury. In: Zakim D, Boyer TD (eds) Hepatology, a textbook of liver disease. W.B. Saunders, Philadelphia, pp 1300–1349
155. Mowat AP (1987) Hepatitis and cholestasis in infancy: intrahepatic disorders. In: Mowat AP (ed) Liver disorders in childhood. Butterworths, London, pp 37–71
156. Aagenaes O, Van Der Hagen CB, Refsum S (1968) Hereditary recurrent intrahepatic cholestasis from birth. Arch Dis Child 43:646–649
157. Aagenaes O, Cudeman B, Sigstad H et al. (1970) Clinical and experimental relationships between cholestasis and abnormal hepatic lymphatics. Pediatr Res 4:377–384
158. Eyssen H, Parmentier G, Compernolle F et al. (1972) Trihydroxycoprostanic acid in the duodenal fluid of two children with intrahepatic bile duct anomalies. Biochim Biophys Acta 273:212–218

159. Hanson RF, Isenberg JN, Williams GC et al. (1975) The metabolism of 3α,7α,12α-trihydroxy-5β-cholestan-26-oic acid in two siblings with cholestasis due to intrahepatic bile duct anomalies. J Clin Invest 56:226–233
160. Miller DJ, Keeton GR, Webber BL, Saunders SJ (1976) Jaundice in severe bacterial infection. Gastroenterology 71:94–97
161. Abernathy CO, Stocker JT, Utili R, Seeff LB (1989) Jaundice of systemic infection. In: Seeff LB, Lewis JH (eds) Current perspectives in hepatology. Plenum, New York, pp 337–356
162. Zimmerman HJ, Fang R, Utili R (1979) Jaundice due to bacterial infection. Gastroenterology 77:362–374
163. Shands KN, Schmid GP, Dan BB et al. (1980) Toxic-shock syndrome in menstruating women. Association with tampon use and *Staphylococcus aureus* and clinical features in 52 cases. N Engl J Med 303:1429–1435
164. Franson TR, Hierholzer WJ, LaBrecque DR (1985) Frequency and characteristics of hyperbilirubinemia associated with bacteremia. Rev Infect Dis 7:1–10
165. Cello JP, Grendell JH (1990) The liver in systemic conditions. In: Zakim D, Boyer TD (eds) Hepatology, a textbook of liver disease. W.B. Saunders, Philadelphia, pp 1411–1437
166. Bunn HF, Forget BG (1986) Sickle cell disease – clinical and epidemiological aspects; and molecular basis of sickle cell disease. In: Platt O, Nathan DG (eds) Hemoglobin: molecular, genetic and clinical aspects. W.B. Saunders, Philadelphia, pp 502–554
167. Koff RS (1975) Postoperative jaundice. Med Clin North Am 59:823
168. LaMont JT, Isselbacher KJ (1973) Postoperative jaundice. N Engl J Med 288:305–311
169. Farell GC (1990) Postoperative hepatic dysfunction. In: Zakim D, Boyer TD (eds) Hepatology, a textbook of liver disease. W.B. Saunders, Philadelphia, pp 869–890
170. Galambos JT (1985) Alcoholic liver disease: fatty liver, hepatitis and cirrhosis. In: Berk JE, Haubrich W, Kalser MH, Roth JL, Schaffner F (eds) Bockus gastroenterology, vol 5. W.B. Saunders, Philadelphia, pp 2985–3048
171. Zakim D, Boyer TD, Montgomery C (1990) Alcoholic liver disease. In: Zakim D, Boyer TD (eds) Hepatology, a textbook of liver disease. W.B. Saunders, Philadelphia, pp 821–868
172. Hoofnagle JH (1985) Acute viral hepatitis: clinical features, laboratory findings and treatment. In: Berk JE, Haubrich W, Kalser MH, Roth JL, Schaffner F (eds) Bockus gastroenterology, vol 5. W.B. Saunders, Philadelphia, pp 2856–2901
173. Dunn GD, Hayes P Breen KS (1973) The liver in congestive heart failure: a review. Am J Med Sci 265:174–185
174. Logan RG, Mowry FM, Judge RD (1962) Cardiac failure simulating viral hepatitis. Ann Intern Med 56:784–788
175. Huguier M, Lacaine F (1981) Hepatic metastases in gastrointestinal cancer. Diagnostic value of biochemical investigations. Arch Surg 399–401
176. Foster JH, Lundy J (1981) Liver metastases. Curr Probl Surg 18:160–282
177. Juniper K Jr. (1979) Prolonged severe obstructive jaundice in Hodgkin's disease. Gastroenterology 77:375–388
178. Gupta SM, Kranwickel RW, Herrera NE (1980) Pathogenesis of jaundice in histiocytic medullary reticulosis. A correlative scintigraphic, histologic and biochemical study. Am J Gastroenterol 73:500–502
179. Stauffer MH (1961) Nephrogenic hepatosplenomegaly (abstr). Gastroenterology 40:694
180. Strickland RC, Schenker S (1977) The nephrogenic hepatic dysfunction syndrome: a review. Dig Dis Sci 22:49–55
181. Bascom R, Johns CJ (1986) The natural history and management of sarcoidosis. Adv Intern Med 31:213

182. Epstein MS, Devaney KO, Goodman ZD, Zimmerman HJ, Ishak KG (1990) Liver disease in sarcoidosis (abstr). Hepatology 12:839
183. Ferrara JLM, Deeg HJ (1991) Graft-versus-host disease. N Engl J Med 324:667–674
184. Sullivan KM, Shulman HM, Storb R et al. (1981) Chronic graft-versus-host disease in 52 patients: adverse natural course and successful treatment with combination immunosuppression. Blood 7267–7276
185. Rhodes DF, Lee WM, Wingard JR et al. (1990) Orthotopic liver transplantation for graft versus host disease following bone marrow transplantation. Gastroenterology 99:536–538
186. Wight DGD (1986) Differential diagnosis of cholestasis in liver allografts. Transplant Proc XVIII [Suppl 4]:152–156
187. Williams JW, Vera S, Peters TG et al. (1986) Cholestatic jaundice after hepatic transplantation. Am J Surgery 151:65–70
188. Van Thiel DH, Dindzans VJ, Gavaler JS, Tarter RE (1990) The postoperative problems and management of the liver transplant recipient. In: Popper H, Schaffner F (eds) Progress in liver disease, vol IX. W.B. Saunders, Philadelphia, pp 657–685
189. Demetris AJ, Jaffe R, Starzl TE (1987) A review of adult and pediatric post-transplant liver pathology. Pathol Annu II:347
190. Schneiderman DJ, Arenson DM, Cello JP, Margaretten W, Weber TE (1987) Hepatic disease in patients with the acquired immune deficiency syndrome (AIDS). Hepatology 7:925–930
191. Cello J (1989) Acquired immunodeficiency syndrome cholangiopathy: spectrum of disease. Am J Med 86:539–546
192. LaRaja R, Rotherberg R, Odom J, Mueller S (1989) The incidence of intra-abdominal surgery in acquired immunodeficiency syndrome: a statistical review of 904 patients. Surgery 105:175–179
193. Simon D, Brandt LJ (1990) Biliary tract disease in AIDS: AIDS vs. NONAIDS. Hepatology 12:618–619
194. Kopelman H, Robertson MH, Saunders PG (1966) The Epping jaundice. Br Med J I:214–222
195. Kopelman H (1968) The Epping jaundice after two years. Postgrad Med J 44:78–85
196. Rodriguez-Noriega A, Gomez-Reino J, Lopez-Encuentra A et al. (1982) Toxic epidemic syndrome, Spain, 1981. Description of a new systemic disease. Lancet II:697–702
197. Solís-Herruzo JA, Castellano G, Colina F et al. (1984) Hepatic injury in the toxic epidemic syndrome caused by ingestion of adulterated cooking oil (Spain, 1981). Hepatology 4:131–139
198. Solís-Herruzo JA, Vidal JV, Colina F, Santalla F, Castellano G (1986) Nodular regenerative hyperplasia of the liver associated with the toxic oil syndrome: report of five cases. Hepatology 6:687–693
199. King PD, Blitzer BL (1990) Drug-induced cholestasis: pathogenesis and clinical features. Semin Liver Dis 10:316–321
200. Zimmerman HJ (1978) Indirect hepatotoxins – cholestatic. In: Zimmerman HJ (ed) Hepatotoxicity: the adverse effects of drugs and other chemicals on the liver. Appleton-Century-Crofts, New York, pp 259–276
201. Bachman BA, Boyd WP Jr., Brady PG (1982) Erythromycin ethylsuccinate-induced cholestasis. Am J Gastroenterol 77:397–400
202. Ishak KG (1981) Hepatic lesions caused by anabolic and contraceptive steroids. Semin Liver Dis 1:116–128
203. Bass NM, Ockner RK (1990) Drug-induced liver disease. In: Zakim D, Boyer TD (eds) Hepatology, a textbook of liver disease. W.B. Saunders, Philadelphia, pp 754–790
204. Ros E, Small DM, Carey MC (1980) Effects of chlorpromazine hydrochloride on bile flow, bile salt synthesis and biliary lipid secretion in the primate. In:

Paumgartner G, Gerok W (eds) Bile salt metabolism in health and disease. University Park Press, Baltimore, pp 219–227
205. Tavoloni N, Boyer JL (1980) Relationship between hepatic metabolism of chlorpromazine and cholestatic effects in the isolated perfused rat liver. J Pharmacol Exp Ther 214:269–274
206. Gaeta GB, Utili R, Adinolfi LE et al. (1985) Characterization of the effects of erythromycin estolate and erythromycin base on the excretory function of the isolated rat liver. Toxicol Appl Pharmacol 80:185–192
207. Kappus H, Remmer H (1975) Irreversible protein binding of 14-C-imipramine with rat and human liver microsomes. Biochem Pharmacol 24:1079–1084
208. Glanfield P, Nicholls A, Freeth M, Moorhead P, Triger D (1982) Fatal cholestatic jaundice in elderly patients taking benoxaprofen. Br Med J 285:62 (letter)
209. Román ID, Monte MJ, González-Buitrago JM, Esteller A, Jiménez R (1990) Inhibition of hepatocitary vesicular transport by cyclosporin A in the rat: relationship with cholestasis and hyperbilirubinemia. Hepatology 12:83–91
210. Stacey N, Kotecka B (1988) Inhibition of taurocholate and ouabain transport in isolated rat hepatocytes by cyclosporin A. Gastroenterology 95:780–786
211. Mowat AP (1987) Extrahepatic biliary atresia and other disorders of the extrahepatic bile ducts presenting in infancy. In: Mowat AP (ed) Liver disorders in childhood. Butterworths, London, pp 72–88
212. Desmet VJ, Callea F (1990) Cholestatic syndromes of infancy and childhood. In: Zakim D, Boyer TD (eds) Hepatology, a textbook of liver disease. W.B. Saunders, Philadelphia, pp 1355–1395
213. Balistreri WF, Stocker JT (1989) α-1-Antitrypsin deficiency and neonatal cholestasis. In: Seeff LB, Lewis JH (eds) Current perspectives in hepatology. Plenum Medical, New York, pp 271–286
214. Balistreri WF, Schubert WK (1986) Liver disease in infancy and childhood. In: Schiff L, Schiff E (eds) Diseases of the liver. Lippincott, Philadelphia, pp 1337–1426
215. Dick MC, Mowat AP (1985) Hepatitis syndrome in infancy, an epidemiological survey with 10-year follow-up. Arch Dis Child 60:512–519

# 9 Chronic Hepatitis and Cirrhosis

## A. Chronic Hepatitis

J. CAMPS, M.P. CIVEIRA, and J. PRIETO

Chronic hepatitis is defined as a persistent inflammatory reaction in the liver lasting for more than 6 months [1, 2]. Different agents can act as triggers of the inflammatory process. The cellular infiltrate is mainly composed of lymphocytes [3]. Neither the target antigens nor the pathogenic mechanisms are known in many cases.

Needle liver biopsy is required for diagnosis. The presence of elevated aminotransferase levels for longer than 6 months in an asymptomatic patient suggests the diagnosis of chronic hepatitis. However, liver biopsy is needed to ascertain the nature of the process since other entities such as hemochromatosis or non-alcoholic steatosis may have the same clinical presentation [4].

### 1 Pathology

In spite of a broad spectrum of causative agents [5], chronic hepatitis has the same basic liver histology. It has been typically divided into two histologic forms: chronic persistent (CPH) and chronic active hepatitis (CAH) [1]. A third type, chronic lobular hepatitis, has been described in patients during acute exacerbation of their disease [6].

In *chronic persistent hepatitis* the inflammatory process is restricted to the portal tracts, which are expanded by the presence of a mononuclear cell infiltrate and some fibrosis. The limiting plate of liver cells that surrounds the portal zones remains intact. Piecemeal necrosis is not observed (Fig. 1).

In *chronic active hepatitis* the inflammatory infiltrate expands the portal areas and invades the liver lobule, destroying the hepatocytes that surround the portal tracts. This is the so-called piecemeal necrosis [7] (Fig. 2). Areas of intralobular necrosis are frequently found. If necrosis is more conspicuous, fibrous septa extend between portal tracts or between portal tracts and central veins. This is called bridging necrosis. When present, it is a sign of a bad prognosis, with frequent progression to cirrhosis [8, 9]. In the severe form of CAH, cirrhosis may already be present, coexisting with the CAH.

In *chronic lobular hepatitis*, inflammation and necrosis are mainly intralobular, without piecemeal or bridging necrosis [6] (Fig. 3).

The histopathologic classification has previously established for autoimmune-type chronic hepatitis. It was originally thought that only CAH

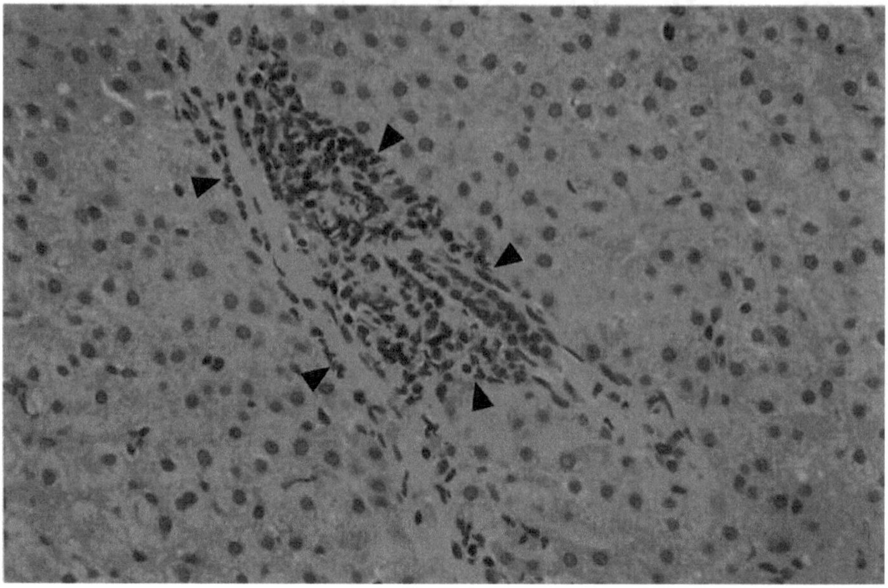

**Fig. 1.** Chronic persistent hepatitis. The inflammatory infiltrate is limited to portal tracts. The limiting plate remains intact (*arrowheads*). (By courtesy of Dr. E. de Alava and J. Vázquez, Department of Pathology, Clínica Universitaria de Navarra, Pamplona, Spain) H&E, ×100

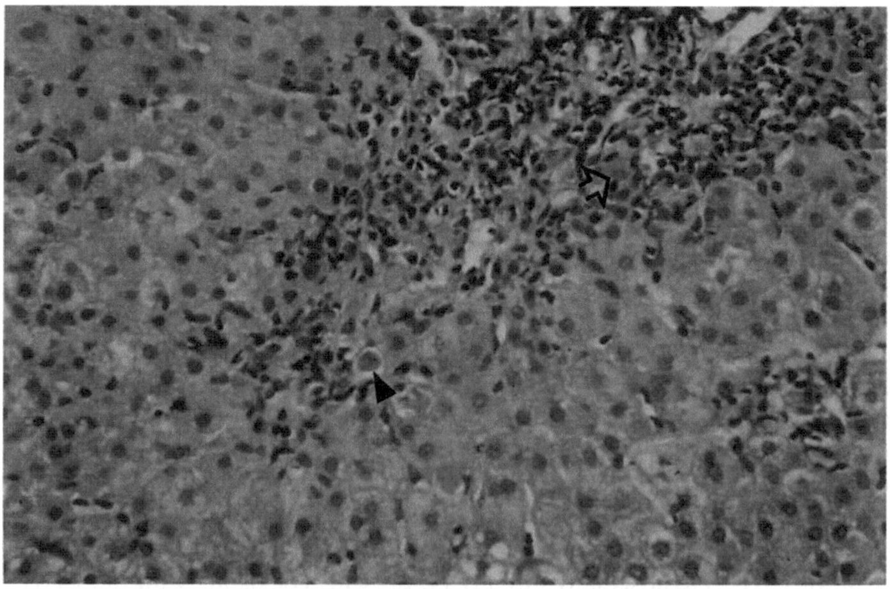

**Fig. 2.** Chronic active hepatitis. In this case piecemeal necrosis involves the complete perimeter of the portal tract. Some hepatocytes have been surrounded by inflammatory cells and are being destroyed (*arrow*). An eosinophilic body can be seen (*arrowhead*). (By courtesy of Dr. E. de Alava and J. Vázquez, Department of Pathology, Clínica Universitaria de Navarra, Pamplona, Spain) H&E, ×100

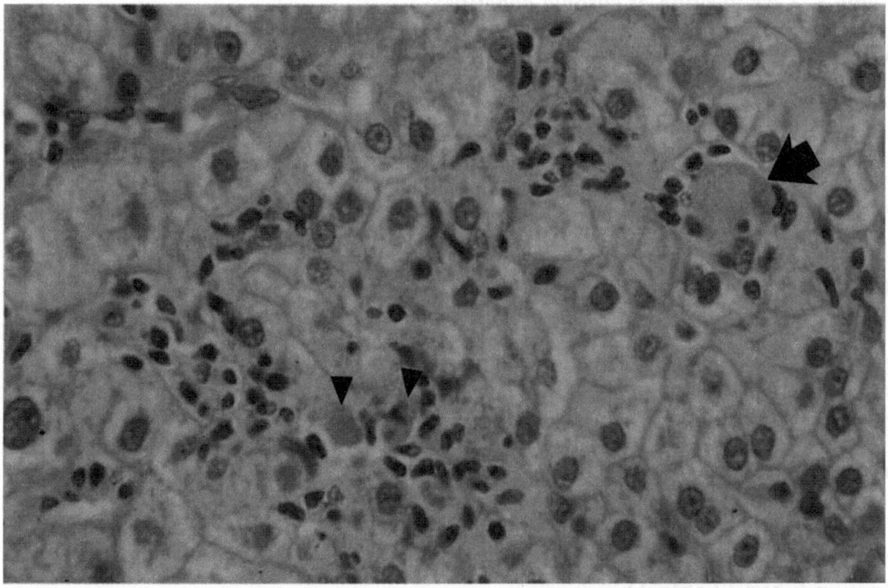

**Fig. 3.** Chronic lobular hepatitis. Inflammatory cells are present in the lobule, associated with scattered foci of hepatocyte necrosis. Two eosinophilic bodies can be seen (*arrowheads*) and another hepatocyte is beginning its process of necrosis (*arrow*). Hepatocyte ballooning is conspicuous. (By courtesy of Dr. E. de Alava and J. Vázquez, Department of Pathology, Clínica Universitaria de Navarra, Pamplona, Spain) H&E, ×400

would progress to cirrhosis. This concept is being modified by recent findings regarding the course and outcome of chronic hepatitis. In long-term follow-up studies, progression to cirrhosis has been observed in patients with CPH. However, this form of the disease entails in general a better prognosis. CAH with bridging necrosis or with cirrhosis has a relatively bad prognosis. Nevertheless, CAH can reverse to CPH or even to normal liver. This may happen in chronic hepatitis B after seroconversion to anti-HBe, in autoimmune hepatitis after steroid therapy, and in chronic hepatitis C after successful interferon therapy. Thus, the liver biopsy not only allows the diagnosis of chronic hepatitis to be made but also permits assessment of the evolution of the inflammatory process and the response to treatment. A numerical scoring system has been developed to estimate the histologic activity in chronic hepatitis [10]. This system is very useful in comparing serial liver biopsies in patients under treatment.

## 2 Etiologic Forms of Chronic Hepatitis

In chronic hepatitis, etiology is the main determinant of the clinical course, prognosis, and treatment. Based on etiology, chronic hepatitis can be

**Table 1.** Classification of chronic hepatitis[a]

| | | |
|---|---|---|
| *Viral* | Hepatitis B | High replication |
| | | Low replication |
| | | Undetectable replication |
| | Hepatitis D | |
| | Hepatitis C | |
| | Cytomegalovirus and Epstein-Barr virus | |
| *Autoimmune* | Classical autoimmune hepatitis: ANA-SMA (type I) | |
| | Anti-LKM1 autoimmune hepatitis (type II) | |
| | Anti-SLA autoimmune hepatitis (type III) | |
| *Metabolic* | Wilson's disease | |
| | α1-Antitrypsin deficiency | |
| | Porphyria cutanea tarda | |
| *Drug induced* | | |
| *Associated with inflammatory bowel disease* | | |

[a] Sometimes the histologic picture of primary biliary cirrhosis and alcoholic liver injury may resemble that of chronic hepatitis

categorized into four main groups: viral, autoimmune, metabolic, and drug-induced (Table 1).

### 2.1 Viral Chronic Hepatitis

Viruses are by far the most frequent cause of chronic hepatitis, accounting for more than 90% of cases [11]. Chronic viral infections represent the main cause of death due to liver failure or hepatocellular carcinoma.

#### *2.1.1 Chronic Hepatitis B* (see also Chap. 14)

The hepatitis B virus (HBV) is the main cause of chronic hepatitis in some areas of the world such as China and Southeast Asia, where 15%–20% of the population are carriers of HBV. Because of this, hepatitis B is the ninth major cause of death worldwide [12]. With the expanded programs of vaccination of newly born, it is conceivable that this disease will regress and even be eradicated in the near future [13].

Chronic hepatitis B is defined by the persistence of the hepatitis B surface antigen (HBsAg) in serum for more than 6 months, with liver biopsy revealing some degree of chronic hepatitis. The basic diagnostic serologic marker of this condition is the presence of HBsAg. Chronic hepatitis B may be the consequence of acute hepatitis followed by persistent viral replication; however, most often the acute episode goes unnoticed. The spectrum of clinical presentation in chronic hepatitis B is broad, ranging from elevation of aminotransferases in an asymptomatic subject at one end, to the clinical signs of advanced cirrhosis at the other. The level of aminotransferases does not consistently predict the outcome since patients with persistently low aminotransferase levels may have liver disease that progresses to cirrhosis while high aminotransferase levels in a chronic carrier of HBV may herald viral clearance and subsequent remission of necro-inflammatory activity [14, 15].

Liver injury in chronic hepatitis B is the result of two factors: the intensity of viral replication and the ability of the host to mount an immune response against the infected hepatocytes. HBV does not appear to be cytopathic by itself. It is currently believed that the viral nucleocapsid protein, HBcAg, expressed by the infected liver cells is the target antigen recognized by T lymphocytes [16]. This cellular immune response, which causes hepatocellular damage, is at the same time an important viral clearance mechanism. This explains why children who have acquired tolerance to HBV antigens in the perinatal period typically develop chronic hepatitis with low aminotransferase levels, scant hepatocellular injury, and high viral replication [17]. The same occurs in immunosuppressed patients with AIDS or during treatment with immunosuppressive drugs [14].

The level of viral replication has been used as a parameter to categorize chronic HBV infections [12, 14, 18]. The four markers of viral replication are: circulating viral DNA (serum HBV DNA), serum DNA-polymerase, serum HBeAg (a secreted protein structurally related to HBcAg), and HBcAg expressed in hepatocytes (detectable in liver biopsy by immunocytochemistry techniques). These four markers are usually coincident [19]. However, although HBeAg is closely associated with viral replication in North Europe, in Mediterranean countries serum HBV DNA is found in a variable proportion of HBeAg-negative patients due to the endemicity in this area of a virus mutant unable to produce HBe protein [20, 21].

Serum HBV DNA is detected and measured by molecular hybridization analysis. Slot or dot blot hybridization cannot detect less than 0.1 pg [22]. The polymerase chain reaction (PCR), a technique for amplifying nucleic acids, provides a greater than 100-fold increase in sensitivity over the conventional hybridization assay [23, 24].

According to the level of viral replication, chronic hepatitis B can be classified into three categories (Table 2):

1. Chronic hepatitis with high viral replication
2. Chronic hepatitis with low viral replication
3. Chronic hepatitis with viral replication undetectable by conventional techniques

Patients with *high viral replication* represent 20%–30% of chronic hepatitis B cases. In this group aminotransferase levels are variable according to the immunoreactivity of the patient. Although progression to cirrhosis is the rule [14, 25] – and in some cases may occur within months –, a minority of patients exhibit little liver damage. In these cases serum aminotransferase levels are low and there appears to exist a state of relative tolerance to the virus, which may last for years [14]. After a variable period of time and

**Table 2.** Serum markers in HBV infection

| Replication | HBsAg | Anti-HBs | HBeAg | Anti-HBe | Anti-HBcIgM | HBV DNA | HBcAg in hepatocytes |
|---|---|---|---|---|---|---|---|
| High | + | − | +[a] | −[a] | +/− | +++ | ++ |
| Low | + | − | +/− | −/+ | − | +/−[b] | + |
| Undetectable | + | − | − | + | − | −[c] | − |

[a] In precore mutants high replication coexists with anti-HBe(+)/HBeAg(−)
[b] HBV DNA may be only transiently detected by dot blot
[c] HBV DNA still may be positive by PCR

for unknown reasons, aminotransferase levels may increase while viral replication lessens. In patients with high viral replication, serum HBV DNA is always present at a high concentration (>200 pg/ml), HBcAg is found in the liver (Fig. 4), and serum HBeAg is positive. There are cases that, in spite of being HBeAg negative and anti-HBe positive, exhibit active viral replication (positive serum HBV DNA). In these instances the Mediterranean virus mutant referred to above is frequently found [20, 21]. In general in subjects with high viral replication the response to antiviral treatment is poor [26].

*Low viral replication* is present in about one-third of patients with chronic hepatitis B. In this group of patients aminotransferase levels are moderately to highly elevated. Episodes of reactivation of the disease may take place, and progression to cirrhosis may occur. Serum HBV DNA is detected at low levels and in many cases HBV DNA fluctuates with periods of nondetection [27]. In the liver biopsy HBcAg may be found in scattered hepatocytes. Serum HBeAg is usually positive but anti-HBe positive patients can also be found in this group. A significant proportion of patients with low viral replication respond to antiviral therapy with clearance of circulating HBV DNA [26]. On the other hand spontaneous seroconversion from HBeAg positive status to anti-HBe positive status occurs in 15%–20% per year, with a preference for those cases with high aminotransferase levels [28]. Seroconversion is preceded by clearance of serum HBV DNA and is associated with an improvement in the evolution of the disease and with a better prognosis [29].

In around 40% of subjects with chronic hepatitis, *viral replication is not detectable by conventional techniques*. In these individuals slot or dot blot molecular hybridization fails to demonstrate HBV DNA in serum and other markers of viral replication, such as HBcAg in the liver and HBeAg in the serum, are not detected either. However, in a significant proportion of these patients serum HBV DNA is positive using PCR [30]. Thus it appears that complete clearance of HBV DNA from the blood occurs only with difficulty in the patients with chronic disease. This explains the reactivation events that are sometimes observed in subjects with inactive disease [27, 31]. In

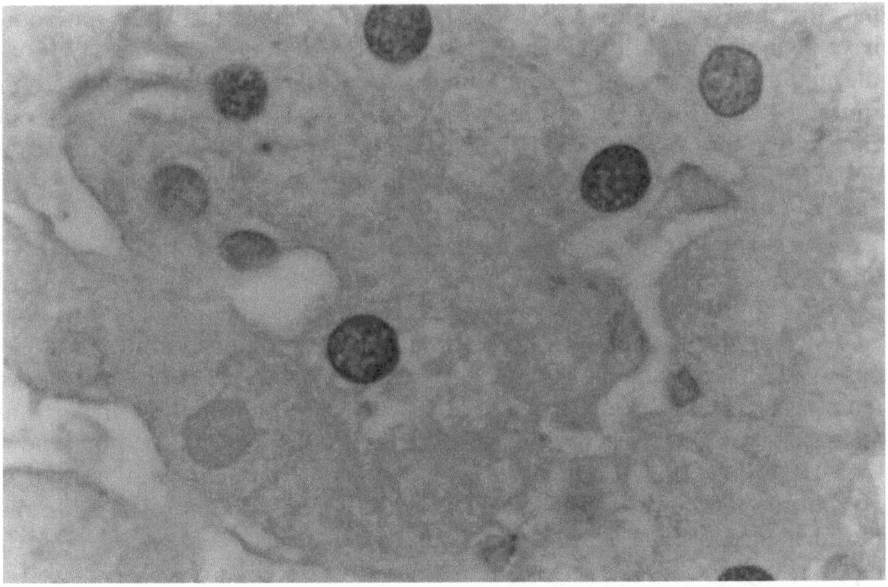

**Fig. 4.** HBcAg peroxidase staining. Positive cells are hepatocytes with viral replication in which HBcAg is expressed in the nucleus. (By courtesy of Dr. E. de Alava and J. Vázquez, Department of Pathology, Clínica Universitaria de Navarra, Pamplona, Spain) H&E, ×400

patients with undetectable viral replication, HBsAg, anti-HBe, and anti-HBc are present in serum and HBsAg can also be found in hepatocytes. Aminotransferases are usually normal.

HBV DNA can occasionally be detected by PCR in patients with chronic hepatitis in whom HBsAg is not detectable in serum. Anti-HBe, anti-HBc, and anti-HBs are generally present in these patients [23]. Moreover hepatitis B has been reported to have been transmitted from hepatitis-B-seronegative subjects [32]. The existence of a mutation on the surface region of the HBV genome has been proposed to explain these findings [33].

Integration of HBV DNA in the host genome may occur and this may open the way for the development of hepatocellular carcinoma [34]. Viral integration may take place in any of the forms of chronic hepatitis B and the chances that this may happen increase with the duration of the disease [35]. Cells with integrated HBV DNA may continue to produce HBsAg but do not express HBcAg.

### *2.1.2 Chronic Hepatitis C* (see also Chap. 15)

Hepatitis C virus (HCV), a single-stranded RNA virus of approximately 10 kb in size, has recently been identified and recognized as the agent of the parenteral form of non-A, non-B hepatitis [36]. Recombinant HCV antigens have become available and ELISA methods to detect anti-HCV antibodies have been developed [37]. Anti-HCV testing has demonstrated that HCV is the major cause, if not the only one, of both parenterally transmitted and sporadic non-A, non-B hepatitis worldwide [38] (leaving aside the enterally transmitted non-A, non-B hepatitis of developing countries caused by hepatitis E virus that is *not* associated with chronic liver disease or persistent viremia [39]).

Persistent infection and chronic hepatitis are the hallmarks of HCV infection [40]. After an acute episode of posttransfusional non-A, non-B hepatitis approximately 50% of patients develop biochemical and histologic evidence of chronic hepatitis [41], and a similar chronification rate has been observed in sporadic non-A, non-B hepatitis [42]. These estimates are mainly based on the occurrence of sustained or intermittent hypertransaminasemia after an acute episode of hepatitis. However, it is now known that HCV infection can evolve in a fluctuating manner with periods of normotransaminasemia that can be long [40]. It is therefore possible that the incidence of chronic infection after HCV exposure is higher than the reported figures.

Chronic hepatitis C is the most common form of chronic hepatitis in the Western world. This disease is found worldwide and appears to have a similar prevalence in developed and underdeveloped countries [43]. Using second generation assays, which incorporate recombinant structural and nonstructural viral proteins, anti-HCV antibodies are found in 97% of patients with chronic non-A, non-B hepatitis. Anti-HCV is also highly prevalent in patients with cryptogenic chronic hepatitis or cirrhosis [44, 45] and in patients with alcoholic liver disease and features of CAH [46, 47]. False-positive anti-HCV reactions have, however, been observed (mainly with the first generation test based on recombinant yeast fusion protein containing non-structural viral epitopes) in patients with chronic liver disease and in healthy blood donors [48, 49].

Serologic tests for HCV infection are evolving rapidly [43]. Second generation ELISA tests to detect antibodies against HCV are now commercially available. In addition, two new markers, HCV antigen and HCV RNA, have been found to possess diagnostic utility although at the present time they are only used for research purposes [43]. HCV antigen can be found by fluorescence microscopy in the cytoplasm of hepatocytes in acute and chronic hepatitis. Its sensitivity and specificity is under study. HCV RNA can be detected in serum or in the liver using PCR. With this technique serum HCV RNA is found in over 80% of patients with chronic hepatitis C. Detection and quantitation of HCV RNA may well be the most direct demonstration of HCV infection and the best means of assessing antiviral therapy in patients with chronic hepatitis C [50]. With these refinements in the detection of HCV it is becoming increasingly clear that, in spite of past claims on the existence of more than one agent of non-A, non-B hepatitis, the probability that a second agent might exist is very low.

Chronic hepatitis C is a disease of only moderate severity. In sporadic chronic non-A, non-B hepatitis liver biopsies demonstrate CPH in 60%, CAH in 35%, and severe CAH with signs of early cirrhosis in 5% [51, 52]. Histopathologic studies in cases of posttransfusional non-A, non-B hepatitis have shown that 50% have CAH and 10% cirrhosis when first biopsed [53].

#### *2.1.3 Chronic Hepatitis D* (see also Chap. 14)

Hepatitis D virus (HDV) is a defective RNA virus that requires HBsAg for its persistence and replication in the host. Simultaneous HDV and HBV infection (coinfection) induces an acute hepatitis that usually resolves. HDV superinfection of HBsAg carriers usually progress to chronicity. In 15% of patients, the disease is rapidly progressive, with cirrhosis developing within 2 years of onset [54]. HDV infection is found worldwide. In countries with low endemicity of HBsAg carriers, it prevails in high-risk groups such as intravenous drug abusers and hemophiliacs [55].

#### *2.1.4 Other Viruses*

In the newly born, and occasionally in the immunosuppressed patient, cytomegalovirus infection may lead to chronic hepatitis [56]. Paramyxoviral infection has been implicated in severe sporadic forms of chronic hepatitis. The finding of large syncytial giant hepatocytes is the distinctive histopathologic feature [57].

### 2.2 Autoimmune Chronic Hepatitis

The etiology of autoimmune chronic active hepatitis (Ai-CAH) is unknown. Altered immune regulation appears to be the basic mechanism. The presence of circulating autoantibodies is the serologic marker of this group of diseases. Female sex predominance, response to immunosuppressive therapy, and hypergammaglobulinemia are characteristic features. The most classical form of Ai-CAH is the "lupoid" variety (Ai-CAH type I), which is characterized by high titers of antinuclear antibodies (ANA). The prevalence of HLA-B8 in this disease is higher than 60%. It may be associated with a wide variety of immunopathogenetic disorders in other organs (skin rashes and vasculitis, arthritis, Coombs-positive hemolytic anemia, thrombocytopenia, thyrotoxicosis. Hashimoto's disease, pericarditis, pleurisy, fibrosing alveolitis, sicca syndrome, renal tubular acidosis, nephrotic syndrome, peripheral neuritis) [58]. Liver histology usually shows significant inflammatory activity [59] and progression to cirrhosis may take place within a few years after diagnosis. The "lupoid" form of CAH is the most common and the most easily recognized type of Ai-CAH, but it only represents 2%–3% of all forms of chronic hepatitis, although this percentage could be higher in areas with a low prevalence of viral hepatitis.

During the last few years new types of Ai-CAH have been defined (Chap. 21). Ai-CAH type II is characterized by the presence of anti liver-kidney microsomal antibodies class 1 (anti-LKM1) and Ai-CAH type III by the finding of antibodies against soluble liver antigen (anti-SLA). It has been suggested that patients with high titers of smooth muscle antibodies (SMA) but without ANA might represent a fourth type of Ai-CAH (Ai-CAH type IV). The real frequency of these forms of Ai-CAH has not been established. These studies are obscured by the fact that antibodies against HCV have been found in a substantial proportion of adult patients with Ai-CAH type II, indicating that some cases of this form of chronic hepatitis might be HCV-mediated [60]. On the other hand, low titers of ANA and/or SMA can be detected in around 20% of patients with chronic hepatitis B or C.

Primary biliary cirrhosis (PBC) can present with histologic features of CAH. In fact a disease overlapping PBC and CAH has been described. In this condition liver biopsy shows lesions typical of CAH together with those of PBC, and both antimitochondrial antibodies (AMA) and ANA are detected in serum [61].

### 2.3 Chronic Hepatitis of Metabolic Origin

This group includes $\alpha_1$-antitrypsin deficiency [62], Wilson's disease [63], and porphyria cutanea tarda (Chaps. 23, 25, 26). Wilson's disease is usually seen before 25 years of age, but it must be taken into consideration until the age of 40 [64]. $\alpha_1$-Antitrypsin deficiency can make its clinical presentation at any age. Porphyria cutanea tarda is more common in adults.

In these diseases, specific biochemical changes and characteristic clinicopathologic findings are essential clues to the diagnosis.

### 2.4 Drug-Induced Chronic Hepatitis (see also Chap. 19)

Patients with drug-related chronic hepatitis have usually taken the drug for months or even years. The drugs that are known to cause this disorder include: oxyphenisatin, α-methyldopa, isoniazid, nitrofurantoin, methotrexate, perhexilene maleate, dantrolene sodium, and aspirin [65]. The occurrence of chronic liver disease (chronic hepatitis or cirrhosis) following such agents is rare. An increased idiosyncratic susceptibility to the drug must therefore be present. Identification of the offending agent by careful history taking (or, occasionally, by search of the patient's drug cupboard) is essential since clinical, biochemical, and pathologic recovery takes place when the drug is withdrawn.

## 3 Pathogenesis

It is currently thought that chronic hepatitis results from a cellular immune response against antigens expressed on the hepatocellular membrane. In hepatitis B the nucleocapsid protein HBcAg (expressed in the nucleus and cytoplasm of infected hepatocytes) acts as an efficient T-cell antigen [66]. It has been proposed that peptide fragments of HBcAg bind to major histocompatibility complex (MHC) class I molecules and are thus displayed on the liver cell membrane, serving as target for class I-restricted cytotoxic T lymphocytes. In fact, in chronic hepatitis B several studies have revealed the presence of HBcAg-specific CD4+ and CD8+ T cells in the liver [67, 68]. Immunocytochemistry techniques have shown that CD4+ cells predominate in the central part of portal tracts while CD8+ lymphocytes are found in the lobular and periportal parenchyma, in close contact with hepatocytes [69]. Interestingly, dendritic cells expressing DR antigens and serving as antigen-presenting cells are detected among T cells [70]. Adhesion molecules are displayed by hepatocytes in periportal areas, contributing to the retention of effector T cells in this zone [71]. Such cytotoxic lymphocytes would mediate hepatocellular injury and the elimination of infected cells. Thus, chronic hepatitis B may presumably reflect an ongoing HBV immune response that causes liver cell damage but is insufficient to eliminate the infection completely [66].

As regards hepatitis C virus, little is known about mechanisms of pathogenicity. One of the most outstanding features of this agent is the tendency to chronic infection. It is now thought that persistent HCV infection, either quiescent or active, might occur in the majority of subjects who have been exposed to the virus. This concept is supported by the observation that chronic hepatitis is found not only in anti-HCV positive patients with elevated aminotransferase levels, but also in some seropositive subjects with sustained normotransaminasemia [72]. On the other hand, studies in chimpanzees have shown that persistent viremia may prevail in the absence of increased aminotransferase values [73]. How HCV modulates its lytic potential and avoids elimination by the host's immune response is currently unknown [40]. An interesting fact, recently reported, is the finding of an increased expression of transforming growth factor beta (TGF β) in liver biopsies in patients with chronic hepatitis C [74]. This cytokine is a potent mediator of fibrogenesis and at the same time antagonizes many of the responses of lymphocytes, including the maturation of cytotoxic T cells. Thus it seems possible that this cytokine might be involved both in the chronification of the infection and in the frequent progression to cirrhosis of chronic hepatitis C.

In Ai-CAH it is believed that a basic defect in immunoregulatory mechanisms leads to abnormal activation of CD4+ lymphocytes and the appearance of autoreactive T cell clones. Normal components of hepatocellular membrane, such as the asialoglycoprotein receptor, seem to be the target for cytotoxic T cells [75]. Circulating liver cell membrane-specific activated T cells are found in this condition [76]. The role of environmental agents in the development of Ai-CAH remains unknown.

It has been reported that patients with porphyria cutanea tarda who show histologic features of chronic hepatitis exhibit serum antibodies reacting with porphyric but not with normal liver cells [77]. Although these antibodies might conceivably be secondary to liver damage, and hence of no pathogenetic importance, it has also been proposed that haptenization of liver cell membrane proteins by porphyrin metabolites might lead to autoantibody formation and cell lysis through an ADCC (antibody-dependent cell cytotoxicity) mechanism. Similar haptenization of liver cell proteins by reactive metabolites might take place in some forms or drug-induced chronic hepatitis.

## 4 Clinical Features

Chronic hepatitis may range from an asymptomatic state of relatively benign evolution to an incapacitating disease due to an aggressive course, rapidly evolving to liver failure. Usually the presence of symptoms and physical findings suggests an inflammatory process of moderate to severe intensity [78].

The symptoms of chronic hepatitis have little specificity. Fatigue is the major complaint, being observed in the majority of patients with severe CAH. However, this symptom does not correlate with the histologic activity or biochemical abnormalities, since patients with CAH and high aminotransferase values may be asymptomatic and subjects with CPH and mildly elevated aminotransferase values may present with incapacitating fatigability. Discomfort or a dull or sharp pain in the right hypochondrium occurs in half of the patients. It has been suggested that the distension of the liver capsule by hepatic inflammation may cause this symptom, but the increased awareness of the patient of this region might also be important. Other causes of abdominal pain should be excluded. Severe forms of hepatitis or reactivations may lead to jaundice and pruritus. Anorexia is not a usual symptom. Somnolence is frequent.

Patients with chronic hepatitis without cirrhosis may lack physical manifestations of the disease. Hepatomegaly is the most common finding. Liver volume usually is normal or increased in chronic hepatitis C, while in a significant proportion of patients with chronic hepatitis B it tends to diminish. Splenomegaly bears a strong association with cirrhosis, but as many as 30% of patients without cirrhosis may have mild splenomegaly. Jaundice may be seen in severe forms of Ai-CAH and during reactivations of the underlying disease. Ascites has been reported in some cases of severe Ai-CAH without cirrhosis. Spider nevi are seen in half the patients with severe inflammatory changes in the liver.

Some symptoms and physical findings such as sicca syndrome, thyromegaly, synovitis, pleuritis, amenorrhea, facial rounding, acne, and hirsutism are characteristic of Ai-CAH [58]. Exacerbations of chronic hepatitis B may be due to superinfection with other viral agents (hepatitis D, hepatitis C, hepatitis A), clearance of HBeAg, or spontaneous reactivation of hepatitis B [79]. Corticosteroid withdrawal, alcohol consumption, hepatotoxic drugs, and hepatocellular carcinoma may also lead to an exacerbation of the disease. Serologic markers of hepatitis B, D, C, and A and epidemiologic questioning usually establish the differential diagnosis.

Polyarteritis nodosa has been associated with hepatitis B [80]. As many as 30% of patients with polyarteritis nodosa are carriers of HBsAg (they are usually HBeAg positive). However, this vasculitis is uncommon among patients with chronic hepatitis B. Fever, arthritis, myalgia, rash, purpura, renal impairment, hypertension, abdominal pain, and peripheral neuropathy are common manifestations of polyarteritis nodosa. Circulatory immune complexes composed of HBsAg/anti-HBs have been isolated in these patients, as have HBsAg, IgM, and complement fractions in the blood vessel walls. Other conditions that have been associated with immune complexes in hepatitis B are membranous and membranoproliferative glomerulonephritis, mixed cryoglobulinemia, the papular acrodermatitis of childhood, and polymyalgia rheumatica.

Extrahepatic manifestations of chronic non-A, non-B hepatitis are exceptional, although circulating immune complexes have been observed. The serum sickness syndrome and mixed cryoglobulinemia have been described [81]. Cases of aplastic anemia have been reported during acute resolving non-A, non-B hepatitis.

Wilsonian CAH may be suspected by the presence of neurologic manifestations and of the Kayser-Fleischer ring. However, this latter finding may be observed in severe cholestatic forms of liver disease. Chronic hepatitis related to $\alpha_1$-antitrypsin deficiency may be associated with pulmonary emphysema.

Drug-induced chronic hepatitis usually is clinically comparable to other forms of CAH. Rash and arthritis may be seen, as well as other physical findings of Ai-CAH [65]. The diagnosis is based on the improvement of the liver disease upon withdrawal of the implicated agent.

The physical findings and symptoms of ulcerative colitis suggest that chronic hepatitis may coexist with sclerosing cholangitis [82].

## 5 Biochemical Findings

The level of serum aminotransferases is the major biochemical marker of inflammatory activity in the liver. It correlates with the degree of hepatic inflammation but cannot serve as a basis for histologic characterization (CPH–CAH) [78]. In most cases of chronic hepatitis aminotransferase values do not exceed 500 IU/liter. The ALT/AST ratio is usually higher than 1. Aminotransferase levels higher than 1000 IU/liter may be seen in severe forms of Ai-CAH, in exacerbations of chronic hepatitis B, and in drug-induced hepatitis. Frequently, chronic non-A, non-B hepatitis has a fluctuating pattern, with marked changes in the aminotransferase values [41]. They can range from normal to more than 20 times the normal limit. Patients are not usually subjectively aware of these changes. The demonstration of an extreme aminotransferase elevation requires the exclusion of acute hepatitis by appropriate clinical and serologic means. Patients with chronic hepatitis B or C generally have lower levels of aminotransferase activity than do patients with Ai-CAH. High aminotransferase levels in chronic hepatitis B may be due to superinfection with another viral agent, but also may precede viral clearance. In this context, high aminotransferase values are usually associated with low levels of viral replication. Cholestatic findings such as hyperbilirubinemia and elevation of serum alkaline phosphatase are common in severe forms of Ai-CAH, while they are unusual in chronic hepatitis B and C, unless severe hepatocellular inflammation is present. Serum gammaglobulin reflects the severity and duration of liver inflammation. Hypergammaglobulinemia is one of the characteristic findings of Ai-CAH, being present in the majority of patients. Serum levels higher than 3 g/dl are seen in half of the patients [78]. Hypergammaglobulinemia is not so frequent and is less marked in viral forms of chronic hepatitis. Hypoprothrombinemia, hypoalbuminemia, and thrombocytopenia are usually associated with liver cirrhosis. However, severe forms of CAH may show such disorders. Anemia usually reflects hypersplenism, but a Coombs-positive hemolytic anemia has been reported in Ai-CAH. α-Fetoprotein has been used as a screening marker of hepatocellular carcinoma in patients with chronic hepatitis B. However, some patients exhibit elevated levels of α-fetoprotein without underlying hepatocellular carcinoma. In such cases α-fetoprotein levels correlate with the presence of bridging necrosis [83]. Serum procollagen type III levels correlate with the inflammatory and fibrogenic activity of the liver disease [74, 84]. They are useful in distinguishing patients with active disease from those in remission, and in assessing the efficacy of treatment. The pattern of autoantibodies in Ai-CAH is described in Chap. 21. Drug-induced chronic hepatitis may present with high titers of ANA and SMA. Ticrynafen-induced liver injury has been associated with anti-LKM2 antibodies and anti-LKM3 antibodies have been found in patients with chronic delta hepatitis. Low titers of ANA and/or SMA have been observed in 10%–20% of chronic hepatitis B and C patients.

Other blood tests can establish the diagnosis of Wilson's disease, primary biliary cirrhosis, $\alpha_1$-antitrypsin deficiency, and hemochromatosis (Chaps. 22–26).

## 6 Diagnosis

Hypertransaminasemia lasting for at least 6 months together with characteristic histologic features in the liver biopsy form the basis for the diagnosis of chronic hepatitis. Specific serologic tests (Table 3), and sometimes typical pathologic findings, allow etiologic categorization to be made in the majority of cases. The viral serology useful in the diagnosis of chronic hepatitis includes the testing of HBsAg and of anti-HCV. If the patient is HBsAg positive, testing of HBeAg and HBV DNA is appropriate to determine whether or not there is active viral replication. Anti-HDV should be investigated to assess whether there is coexisting delta hepatitis. PCR for HCV RNA should be performed in cases of suspected viral origin which are negative for both HBsAg and anti-HCV. Serum autoantibodies, if present at high titer, indicate Ai-CAH. However, it must be kept in mind that anti-LKM1 at high titers may be present in patients with chronic hepatitis C. Determination of $\alpha_1$-antitrypsin, ceruloplasmin, and urinary copper should allow identification of $\alpha_1$-antitrypsin deficiency and wilsonian chronic hepatitis. The presence of characteristic skin lesions and quantitation of urinary uroporphyrin are major clues in the diagnosis of porphyria cutanea tarda.

Liver biopsy is essential to differentiate chronic hepatitis from other diseases that may cause chronic hypertransaminasemia, such as alcoholic liver disease, nonalcoholic steatohepatitis, hemochromatosis, primary biliary

**Table 3.** Laboratory tests in suspected chronic hepatitis

| | |
|---|---|
| *Basic biochemistry and assessment of liver dysfunction* | |
| Hemoglobin | Aminotransferases (AST, ALT) |
| White cell count | Alkaline phosphatase |
| Platelet count | Bilirubin |
| Albumin | Gamma globulins |
| Prothrombin time | |
| *Investigation of causes of chronic ALT elevation*[a] | |
| Iron, transferrin | Glucose, triglycerides |
| HBsAg | α1-Antitrypsin |
| Anti-HCV | Ceruloplasmin, urinary copper |
| ANA, AMA, SMA | Urinary uroporphyrin |
| *If HBsAg positive* | |
| HBeAg, anti-HBe, HBV DNA, anti-HDV | |
| *Other tests* | |
| HCV RNA by PCR. HDV RNA and Ag. Anti-HIV (in high risk groups) | |
| Anti-LKM1 | |
| α-Fetoprotein | |
| Procollagen-III-peptide | |

[a] With HBsAg, anti-HCV, and ANA, 97% of cases of chronic hepatitis are diagnosed

**Table 4.** Clinical, biochemical, and histologic features in chronic hepatitis

| | Ai-CAH | CHB | CHC | Wilson's disease | Drug-induced |
|---|---|---|---|---|---|
| Age | 20–40<br>50% children in anti-LKM1 (+) | >35<br>Younger in endemic areas | >35<br>Younger in high risk groups | <35 | Higher incidence in >40 |
| Sex (M/F ratio) | 1/9 | 8/2 | 1/1 | 1/1 | 2/8 |
| Mode of onset | Insidious<br>35% acute in anti-LKM1 (+) | 30% asymptomatic onset | 70% asymptomatic onset | Insidious | Usually acute |
| Systemic manifestations | Usually present<br>Thyroid disease, synovitis<br>Sjögren syndrome | Unusual or mild, unless advanced disease | Unusual | Neurologic and psychiatric manifestations | Sometimes similar to Ai-CAH |
| Histologic findings | Chronic active hepatitis with moderate to severe necrosis | Chronic persistent and chronic active hepatitis.<br>Ground-glass cells | Usually mild chronic active hepatitis.<br>Steatosis, sinusoidal cell activation, and eosinophilic bodies | Chronic active hepatitis.<br>Glycogen in the nucleus of hepatocytes; fatty infiltration and fibrosis | Features resembling Ai-CAH |
| Aminotransferase levels | Moderately elevated.<br>Markedly elevated in severe forms | Mildly to moderately elevated.<br>Usually higher with HDV infection | Mildly to moderately elevated. Fluctuating pattern in 20% | Mildly elevated.<br>AST > ALT | Mildly to moderately elevated |
| Gammaglobulins | Marked hypergammaglo-bulinemia | Normal or mildly elevated | Normal or mildly elevated | Usually normal | Hypergammaglo-bulinemia |
| Non-organ-specific autoantibodies | ANA, SMA, anti-LKM1, anti-SLA | Low titers of ANA, SMA in 20%.<br>Anti-LKM3 in some CHD cases | Low titers of ANA, SMA in 15%–20% | – | ANA, SMA, may be present |
| HLA associations | $A_1$, $B_8$, DRw3/DRw4 | BW15, BW17, BW35 | – | – | – |

*Abbreviations*: Ai-CAH, autoimmune chronic active hepatitis; CHB, chronic hepatitis B; CHC, chronic hepatitis C; CHD: chronic hepatitis D cirrhosis, and sclerosing cholangitis. Although alcoholic liver disease has distinctive histopathologic features, alcohol was in the past also thought to cause chronic hepatitis in some cases. Recent evidence, however, has shown that most of the alcoholic patients (HBsAg negative) with histologic signs of CAH are anti-HCV positive [46], indicating a significant role for HCV in the genesis of the hepatic lesion in alcoholics with advanced liver disease. Nonalcoholic steatohepatitis and liver steatosis may have different etiologies but they are frequently associated with overweight, diabetes, or hyperlipidemia. Hemochromatosis is evidenced by histopathologic and biochemical signs of iron overload. In idiopathic hemochromatosis there is chronic hepatic inflammation and fibrosis but features of CAH are normally absent. In stage II primary biliary cirrhosis liver biopsy may show changes similar to those of chronic hepatitis. Differentiation, however, can be made on the basis of positive AMA and of the increase in both alkaline phosphatase and IgM. In sclerosing cholangitis biochemical signs of cholestasis together with liver histology and endoscopic cholangiography usually establish the diagnosis. Occasionally, radiologic and/or endoscopic studies of the colon and small bowel are of importance in identifying cases of chronic hepatitis accompanying inflammatory bowel disease (ulcerative colitis, Crohn's disease, celiac disease). PAS-positive globules in the hepatic tissue, increased liver copper content, and autofluorescence of the liver biopsy are indicators of $\alpha_1$-antitrypsin deficiency, Wilson's disease, and porphyria cutanea tarda, respectively. Table 4 summarizes some of the clinical, biochemical, and histologic features that are of interest in the differential diagnosis of chronic hepatitis.

## 7 Natural History and Prognosis

### 7.1 Chronic Hepatitis B

#### *7.1.1 Natural History*

The natural history and prognosis of CAH are determined more by its etiology than by its histologic classification.

In HBV infection, liver damage is caused by immune lysis of the infected hepatocytes and a direct cytopathic effect does not seem to play a significant role. Age at the time of infection, sex, and immune status have been identified as important factors in the development of chronic HBV infection [14, 85]. Age has been shown to be the most important factor favoring HBV chronicity; 95% of neonates born to HBeAg positive mothers develop chronic HBV infection. In preschool children the rate of progress to chronic disease is around 25% and in the adult immunocompetent population it ranges from 5% to 10% in most series [14], although some have reported much lower rates [85–87]. A mild acute illness seems to predispose to the development of chronicity. Males appear to be more susceptible to

HBV infection that females. Patients immunosuppressed (chemotherapy, hemodialysis, Down's syndrome) have an increased risk of developing the chronic carrier state after acute HBV infection. Evidence suggests that immune alterations may facilitate the development of the chronic carrier state during adult life. Subnormal production of interferon-α by peripheral blood mononuclear cells has been reported [88]. Diminished interferon production would lead to an abnormal activation of hepatocytes by this cytokine. Accordingly, a substantial decrease in the expression of MHC class I proteins by infected hepatocytes has been documented in chronic hepatitis B [89]. This would make liver cells less susceptible to lysis by cytotoxic T cells.

The long-term natural history of chronic HBV infection has not been completely defined. Most chronic carriers suffer the infection for many years or decades, and some do so for their whole lifetime. However, HBV replication tends to diminish over a period of years, and in most patients seroconversion to the anti-HBe status eventually occurs [28]. Fluctuations of HBV replication can be seen, and even reactivations of the HBV replication after seroconversion. Factors that determine the span of time between the onset of infection and the loss of HBV replication markers are not well known. Age, sex, and immunologic status may influence the rate of spontaneous seroconversion. Some exogenous factors can also affect the natural course of chronic HBV infection. Corticosteroid administration is followed by a rise in HBV replication [90]. Suppression of the immune response and activation of the steroid-responsive element of the HBV genome might be implicated in the genesis of this effect. Intercurrent infections with HDV and HAV tend to suppress HBV replication [91, 92]. Finally, antiviral agents such as interferon-α and adenine arabinoside inhibit HBV replication and sometimes lead to seroconversion [93, 94].

In chronic HBV carriers seroconversion from HBeAg to anti-HBe status occurs after a fall in HBV replication. In this context the expression of MHC proteins increases and cytotoxic T cells eliminate the hepatocytes harboring replicating viruses. Seroconversion may represent the transition from chronic hepatitis to a healthy carrier state with the resolution of necroinflammatory activity. However, hepatocytes that contain HBV integrated forms do not express HBcAg and avoid immune lysis.

The annual rate of seroconversion to anti-HBe ranges from 2% to 25% [28, 95]. Some parameters have been found to be predictors of seroconversion: aminotransferase levels higher than 300 IU/liter, α-fetoprotein values higher than 100 ng/ml, and the presence of significant hepatic inflammation (CAH and CLH versus CPH) [28]. Reversion to the HBeAg status can be frequent during the "e window" period, just after clearance of HBeAg and before the appearance of anti-HBe [95]. Some of these reversions are transient. A further seroconversion to anti-HBs with the previous loss of HBsAg occurs annually in 1%–2% of the chronic anti-HBe carriers [96].

It has been shown that after successful interferon-α treatment most patients who cleared HBeAg and HBV DNA continued to have HBV DNA detectable by PCR. Years later, the further loss of HBsAg was preceded in most of them by HBV DNA being no longer detectable by PCR. However, in some cases the presence of HBV DNA persisted after seroconversion to anti-HBs [97]. This clearly shows that HBV replication persists to some degree even when HBsAg has fallen to undetectable levels. Reappearance of HBsAg and viral replication in anti-HBs patients during immunosuppression might be explained by these findings [98].

Several mechanisms may account for acute exacerbations of the liver disease in chronic HBsAg carriers. Reactivations of HBV infection with the reappearance of viral replication in patients who had seroconverted may mimic acute viral hepatitis. However, such episodes frequently go unnoticed. Lobular hepatitis is the histologic hallmark of these events. Sometimes the reactivation may be severe or even fatal in patients with cirrhosis [99, 100]. The rates of reactivation episodes have varied between studies, but they might account for 30% of the exacerbation bouts [31, 95]. Recurrent reactivations have been associated with significant progression of the liver damage. Increases in viral replication in HBeAg positive patients may also account for these flares of disease activity. The causes of spontaneous reactivations are not known, although they have been more frequently observed in male homosexuals [101]. Transient immunosuppression by intercurrent infections, surgery, and drugs has also been implicated in their pathogenesis [31]. Reactivations are accompanied by the appearance of anti-HBc IgM.

Superinfection with other hepatitis viruses accounts for a significant proportion of exacerbations. Infection with HDV may lead to fulminant hepatitis or to the establishment of severe CAH [54]. The serologic profile of HDV superinfection is characterized by the presence of HBsAg, anti-HBc IgG, and anti-HDV. Superimposition of hepatitis A may cause severe or even fulminant hepatitis [102]. Non-A, non-B hepatitis superinfection is frequently seen in high-risk groups such as drug abusers and male homosexuals [103]. The diagnosis during the acute phase needs to exclude HAV and HDV superinfection (anti-HAV IgM and anti-HDV), as well as reactivation (anti-HBc IgM and HBV DNA). Later, the usually delayed appearance of antibodies against HCV may confirm the diagnosis.

Corticosteroid or chemotherapy withdrawal, high alcohol consumption, drug-induced hepatic injury, and hepatocellular carcinoma are also causes of hepatic deterioration in chronic hepatitis B.

Clearance of HBeAg is usually preceded (in 60% of cases) by a peak of aminotransferase activity. Although seroconversion frequently remains unnoticed, severe and even fatal outcomes have been documented in cirrhotic patients [104]. It has been estimated that nearly 40% of the exacerbations in HBeAg positive patients are caused by seroconversion episodes [79].

Markers of viral replication (HBV DNA in serum and HBcAg in liver) have been detected in HBsAg(+), anti-HBe(+) patients with chronic liver disease [105]. This form of chronic hepatitis B is common in the Mediterranean basin (20%–30% of anti-HBe patients), and its natural history and prognosis differ from those of the classic chronic hepatitis B. A low rate of spontaneous remission, a tendency to evolve to cirrhosis, and a high relapse rate after interferon therapy are characteristic features of this variant of chronic hepatitis B [106]. A point mutation from guanine to adenine at nucleotide 1896 (precore region) that converts the codon for tryptophan (TGG) to a stop codon (TAG), thus preventing the expression of the precore sequence, has been found in the majority of these patients. As a consequence HBeAg is not produced. Severe forms of acute hepatitis have been associated with this mutant. Mixed types of infection involving the precore mutant and the wild-type HBV can occur, and during the course of the disease the precore mutant/wild type ratio increases in some patients [107]. The natural history of infection by this HBV mutant shows that the outcome of chronic hepatitis B is influenced not only by the host's immune response but also by the genetic heterogeneity of the virus.

### *7.1.2 Prognosis*

The 5-year survival rates for chronic hepatitis B have been estimated to be 97% for patients with CPH, 86% for those with CAH, and 55% for those with CAH with cirrhosis. In the study in question, the usual cause of death was liver failure [108]. Other studies have shown that HBeAg positive patients had the highest risk of dying from liver cancer or liver failure [29]. Factors that have been found to identify patients with a higher risk of death are an age of more than 40 years, bilirubin higher than 1.5 mg/dl, ascites, and spider nevi [108]. Among patients with CAH, HBV infection represents a predictor of a higher mortality [109]. The development of cirrhosis in chronic hepatitis B has been associated with repeated episodes of acute exacerbation, without the subsequent clearance of HBeAg, and with reactivations of viral replication. Mild to moderate forms of CAH are not particularly prone to evolve to liver cirrhosis [110].

In children, mild and stable disease has been observed despite high levels of HBV replication [17]. However, some of them develop cirrhosis at very early ages. Male sex and perinatal infection have been found to predict the overt development of chronic liver disease in children [111].

Hepatitis B carriers have 200 times more chance than noncarriers of developing hepatocellular carcinoma [33]. HBeAg positive patients are at greater risk than HBeAg negative patients. Usually the appearance of hepatocellular carcinoma occurs several decades after the onset of HBV infection. Integration of HBV DNA into the host genome is thought to promote cellular transformation, but the exact pathogenetic mechanism of hepatocellular carcinoma remains unknown [112].

## 7.2 Chronic Hepatitis Delta

Hepatitis delta infection can be acquired by two mechanisms: coinfection with HBV in the normal person and superinfection of HBsAg carriers. In coinfection, the HBV helper virus is received together with HDV in the original inoculum, while in superinfection with HDV the hepatocytes infected by HBV in the HBsAg carrier provide the environment required for the proliferation of hepatitis delta virus [54].

Coinfection may range from mild to fulminant illness. While acute hepatitis B leads to fulminant liver failure in 1% of the cases, it has been estimated that coinfection may evolve to fulminant hepatitis in 3% of the subjects. A bimodal course, with two peaks of aminotransferase activity, is frequently seen in coinfection. Since hepatitis delta replication depends upon the persistence of HBV infection, the termination of the latter leads to the clearance of the former. Prospective studies have shown that the risk of developing chronic HBV infection after acute HBV–HDV coinfection is not increased compared with that of ordinary hepatitis B [54].

Superinfection represents the usual setting for the development of delta-related chronic liver disease. It may present as a flare-up of the underlying chronic hepatitis B process or as an intercurrent non-B illness in the setting of a healthy carrier. Hepatitis delta virus usually adds further damage to the liver in patients with chronic hepatitis B. Fulminant liver failure may be seen following HDV superinfection. This is a severe condition but it can be self-limited and sometimes eliminates the HBV. Although it has been thought that HDV superinfection invariably accelerates underlying HBV-induced chronic hepatitis [113], recent data show that only a subgroup of patients superinfected with HDV develop a significantly more severe form of liver disease, compared with chronic hepatitis B [114]. In some series, no significant differences have been observed in survival rate or histologic activity among patients with and without HDV. However, other studies have revealed a significantly higher morbidity and mortality in patients with HDV chronic infection [115]. It has been suggested that the maximal pathogenic action of HDV takes place during the early stages of superinfection. The persistence of HBV replication has been associated with a more severe and progressive disease, compared with delta superinfections without HBV replication [116]. While in chronic hepatitis B the histologic activity normally ranges from mild to moderate, in HDV-infected patients moderate to severe degrees of liver disease activity are frequently found [117]. In Italy almost all cases of HBsAg rapidly progressive liver disease are due to HDV infection.

## 7.3 Chronic Hepatitis C

Chronicity is one of the most outstanding features of HCV infection [41]. Several prospective studies of posttransfusion acute non-A, non-B hepatitis have shown that about 50% of the patients do not show normalization of the aminotransferase levels and develop chronic hepatitis. In community-acquired non-A, non-B hepatitis, similar rates of progression to chronicity have been reported. From these studies it has been shown that the majority of patients with persistent HCV infection develop significant liver damage; CAH has been reported in 41% of cases and cirrhosis in another 20% [118]. However, the inflammatory activity usually ranges from mild to moderate. Progression from minimal hepatitis or CPH to CAH and cirrhosis has been reported, and it seems that this is not exceptional [119]. Remissions can be seen in 20% of cases, but later reactivations of cytolytic activity may occur. In chronic hepatitis C, liver damage usually progresses over several years or even decades before the development of advanced forms of liver disease, such as cirrhosis or hepatocellular carcinoma. In one study, the mean time span from transfusion to the detection of cirrhosis was 17.8 years [120]. Nevertheless, rapid progression from acute non-A, non-B hepatitis to liver cirrhosis has been documented, in some instances in HIV-infected patients [121]. Hepatitis C-related cirrhosis is usually asymptomatic for a number of years or may exist with only minor symptoms. Advanced forms, with complications derived from hepatocellular failure or portal hypertension, are only observed in a minority of patients with cirrhosis. It is estimated that most patients with chronic HCV infection acquired in adult life do not live long enough to die from liver disease. On the other hand, however, many patients with hepatitis C-related terminal liver disease are being included in liver transplant programs. In addition, epidemiologic studies based on the prevalence of anti-HCV antibodies show evidence for HCV involvement in the pathogenesis of hepatocellular carcinoma in HBsAg negative patients with chronic liver disease [122].

### 7.4 Autoimmune Chronic Active Hepatitis

The overall natural course and prognosis of Ai-CAH remain obscure [58]. Several reasons account for this. Firstly, since an effective therapy is available for this condition, most patients have been treated, and this has altered the natural course of the disease. Secondly, in early studies on Ai-CAH almost all patients showed severe forms of the disease. Furthermore in some of these trials, other forms of liver disease were not excluded (HBsAg carriers). On the other hand, patients with cryptogenic chronic hepatitis also participated in some of these series and it has recently been demonstrated that most of these patients may represent sporadic or community-acquired cases of chronic hepatitis C. The subdivisions of Ai-CAH that have emerged in the last decade (see Chap. 21) and the presence of antibodies against HCV in Ai-CAH type II (anti-LKM1 positive) add further difficulties to the evaluation of the natural course of Ai-CAH. In spite of these pitfalls it has been estimated that piecemeal necrosis is almost universal in the early stages of the disease [59]. Severe forms with bridging necrosis and multilobular necrosis may be seen and imply a poor prognosis, unless treated [58]. Progression to cirrhosis is the rule without appropriate therapy, although successful treatment assessed by biochemical tests does not prevent smouldering progression to cirrhosis [58]. Some patients may enter spontaneous remission when cirrhosis develops, leading to inactive cirrhosis [58]. Mild forms of Ai-CAH have been shown to be less aggressive, but progression to cirrhosis and death from ensuing complications are possible. In one study involving 71 untreated patients followed for an average of 7.5 years, progression to cirrhosis and death were seen in 83% and 46%, respectively, of patients with severe disease, while cirrhosis was observed in 64% of patients with less severe activity, of whom 23% died [123]. Studies concerning mild forms of the disease probably included chronic hepatitis C patients. Therefore, conclusions cannot be deduced. Spontaneous remissions have been documented in 20% of the patients.

Treatment leads to remission in the majority (85%) of patients with severe Ai-CAH. Some of them (17%) have sustained remission after withdrawal of immunosuppresive therapy, others (59%) relapse within 6 months after drug withdrawal, requiring retreatment, and finally 24% continue to have mild inflammatory activity [124, 125]. Systemic manifestations of the disease usually respond to therapy in the same way as the liver disease. Relapses may be severe, thus worsening the prognosis. Prognosis of unresponsive patients remains dismal, liver transplantation being the only chance of cure. Survival is mainly influenced by the presence or absence of cirrhosis prior to therapy. A study has shown that the 10-year probability of survival is 98% without cirrhosis and 65% with cirrhosis [126]. Therefore early diagnosis and prompt therapy enhance survival.

## 7.5 Wilsonian Chronic Hepatitis

Copper-chelating therapy of Wilson's disease in the stage of chronic hepatitis brings about complete remission [63]. A normal longevity can be achieved if treatment is continued for the entire life span. If treatment is not applied, a fatal outcome is certain.

## 7.6 Drug-Induced Chronic Hepatitis

The withdrawal of the offending drug is usually followed by a rapid reversal of the hepatic lesion [65]. The continued administration of the causative drug may finally lead to severe liver damage with the complications of liver failure and portal hypertension. However, this evolution has only occasionally been reported.

# 8 Management

Therapy of chronic hepatitis depends on its etiology. Therefore, a precise and accurate diagnosis is a prerequisite for correct treatment. As a general rule hepatotoxic drugs and alcohol should be avoided, as should exhausting exercise.

## 8.1 Chronic Hepatitis B

In the last two decades several antiviral agents and immunomodulators have been investigated in the treatment of chronic hepatitis B, but only interferon-α has demonstrated effectiveness in the majority of trials [127]. The antiviral agent adenine arabinoside and its monophosphate hydrosoluble derivative have been assessed on the basis of their capacity to inhibit HBV DNA polymerase. However, while some trials carried out in Europe have shown promising results, in others, mainly performed in the United States, the proportion of successful outcomes has been disappointing. Although the effectiveness of interferon-α seems unquestionable at the present time, the results obtained are far from satisfactory. This is the reason why several combination therapies have been tried in the last few years.

The aim of treatment is the termination of viral replication with seroconversion to anti-HBe status [128]. It must be borne in mind that spontaneous seroconversion occurs in 5%–15% of patients per year. Therefore clinical trials should be randomized and should include a control group. It is now considered that treatment should be applied early in the course of the disease, before significant integration of the HBV genome takes place. In these cases HBsAg can be lost with seroconversion to anti-HBs. Treatment should also improve symptoms, decrease the rate of progression of the disease and the incidence of hepatocellular carcinoma, and finally improve survival.

Monitoring of the patients before treatment is necessary to assess the stability of replication, since patients with high aminotransferase values may seroconvert spontaneously. During antiviral treatment and in the following months, markers of replication (HBeAg and HBV DNA) should be serially assessed.

### *8.1.1 Immunomodulators*

Several studies have shown that long-term corticosteroid treatment enhances viral replication and prevents spontaneous seroconversion to anti-HBe. A deleterious effect on the natural course of the disease has also been demonstrated in prospective controlled trials [129, 130]. Short-term corticosteroid treatment followed by a sudden withdrawal has been shown to trigger an immunologic rebound phenomenon, probably due to an increase in the expression of HBV antigens in hepatocytes (HBcAg) which are the target of cytotoxic specific T cells. This immunologic response is associated with a peak in aminotransferase levels, a worsening of liver histology, and a decrease or cessation of viral replication. However, sustained seroconversions are not frequent and serious decompensations of the liver disease (variceal bleeding, ascites, encephalopathy) have been recorded, especially in patients with established cirrhosis [131]. Therefore corticosteroids as single agents should be avoided in chronic hepatitis B.

Other immunomodulators, such as levamisole and interleukin-2, have been ineffective or associated with adverse effects.

### *8.1.2 Antiviral Agents*

#### *8.1.2.1 Adenine Arabinoside*

Adenine arabinoside (ARA-A) is a synthetic nucleoside, an adenosine analogue, which has the ability to inhibit several DNA polymerases, including that of HBV [94]. Its low solubility makes its intravenous administration with large volumes of fluid solvent mandatory. A monophosphate derivative of ARA-A, adenine arabinoside monophosphate (ARA-AMP), is hydrosoluble and shares the same antiviral spectrum. It can be administered by intramuscular injection, twice daily, in an outpatient regimen. Several studies have shown a decline of HBV replication with ARA-AMP treatment (5 mg/kg daily for 1 month); however long-term responses have varied between trials [127, 132]. Some trials have shown effectiveness, especially among the heterosexual population [133]. Neuromuscular side-effects have further dampened the enthusiasm for administering this drug.

#### *8.1.2.2 Acyclovir*

Acyclovir is a guanosine analogue with antiviral activity, mainly against herpesviruses. Its activity depends upon its activation by the viral thymidine kinase. HBV does not possess a thymidine kinase. However, intravenous acyclovir administration results in a mild to moderate reduction in HBV replication [134]. Long-term responses have not been attained with acyclovir, used as a single agent. Therefore its use is now being investigated in combination with interferon [135]. Deoxyacyclovir, an acyclovir derivative which can be administered by the oral route, has been tested with disappointing results [136].

#### *8.1.2.3 Foscarnet*

Foscarnet (trisodium phosphonoformate) is an antiviral agent that inhibits viral-specific DNA polymerases, mainly those of the herpesvirus and hepadnavirus families. It also inhibits reverse transcriptases. Currently it is used in the treatment of cytomegalovirus retinitis. In vitro and in vivo inhibitory effects against the DNA polymerases of hepadnaviruses have been documented [137]. Foscarnet has been successfully used in fulminant hepatitis B. A pilot study in which eight patients with HBeAg positive chronic hepatitis B were treated with intravenous foscarnet (160 mg/kg/day) for 15 days showed only a mild decrease in serum HBV DNA during therapy [138].

#### *8.1.2.4 Other Antiviral Agents*

Several drugs possess inhibitory activity against HBV DNA polymerase (primaquine, quinacrine, suramin). However, their partial and transitory effect and their adverse effects have led to their abandonment. Other antiviral agents have been investigated more recently (3′-azydo-3′-deoxythymidine, 2′,3′-dideoxycitidine, and gancyclovir) but clinical trials have not been reported.

### *8.1.3 Interferons*

Interferon activity was first identified in 1957 by ISAACS and LINDENMANN. The interferons are glycoproteins that combine antiviral, immunomodulatory, and antiproliferative activities [139, 140]. There are three types of interferon: interferon-α or leukocyte interferon, interferon-β or fibroblast interferon, and interferon-γ or immune interferon. Interferon-α and interferon-β share many properties and the same cellular receptor, and both have been categorized as type I interferons. Details about the characteristics of interferons are given in Table 5. Currently, large amounts of highly purified

**Table 5.** Classification and characteristics of interferons

| | Interferon type I | | Interferon type II Gamma (immune) |
|---|---|---|---|
| | Alpha (leukocyte) | Beta (fibroblast) | |
| Source | Monocytes and B cells | Fibroblasts | T Cells |
| Subtypes | 24 | 1 | 1 |
| Molecular weight | 16000–27000 | 20000 | 15000–25000 |
| Glycosylation | Variable | Yes | Yes |
| pH2 stability | Yes | Yes | No |
| Chromosome | 9 | 9 | 12 |
| Inducers | Viruses<br>Antigens | Viruses<br>ds-RNA<br>Polyribonucleotides | Antigens<br>Mitogens |
| Biologic activities | Antiviral<br>Antiproliferative<br>Immunomodulation | Antiviral<br>Antiproliferative<br>Immunomodulation | Mainly immunomodulation |

**Table 6.** Adverse effects of interferon-α

| | | |
|---|---|---|
| Transient[b] | | Fever (chills)[a] |
| | | Myalgias[a] |
| | | Arthralgias[a] |
| | | Headache |
| | | Nausea |
| | | Diarrhea |
| | | Anorexia[a] |
| | | Fatigue |
| Persistent: | Systemic | Fatigue[a] |
| | | Low grade fever |
| | | Myalgias (back and thighs)[a] |
| | | Arthralgias (erratic)[a] |
| | | Headache |
| | | Weight loss |
| | | Hair loss (usually mild)[a] |
| | | Decreased libido |
| | Gastrointestinal | Anorexia[a] |
| | | Nausea |
| | | Diarrhea |
| | Psychiatric | Irritability[a] |
| | | Anxiety |
| | | Depressión[a] |
| | | Psychosis[c] |
| | | Phobias |
| | Neurologic | Insomnia |
| | | Hypersomnia |
| | | Clouding of consciousness[c] |
| | | Convulsions[c] |
| | Autoimmune | Thyroiditis |
| | | Vasculitis |
| | | Non-organ-specific autoantibody formation |
| | Hematologic | Neutropenia[a] |
| | | Thrombocytopenia[a] |
| | Infections | Increased susceptibility to bacterial infections |

[a] The most common adverse effects
[b] Usually only seen during the 1st week of therapy
[c] Almost only observed with high doses

recombinant interferon-α, -β, and -γ and lymphoblastoid interferon-α are available for clinical use.

Although results have not been uniform, several reports have documented a suboptimal activation of the interferon system in chronic hepatitis B patients [88]. This has been considered to be an explanation for the progression to chronicity of HBV infection and represents a rationale for the use of interferon in this disease. Adverse effects of interferon-α therapy are listed in Table 6.

Interferons act through their interaction with specific receptors located in the surface of the cells. Interferon-α and interferon-β share the same

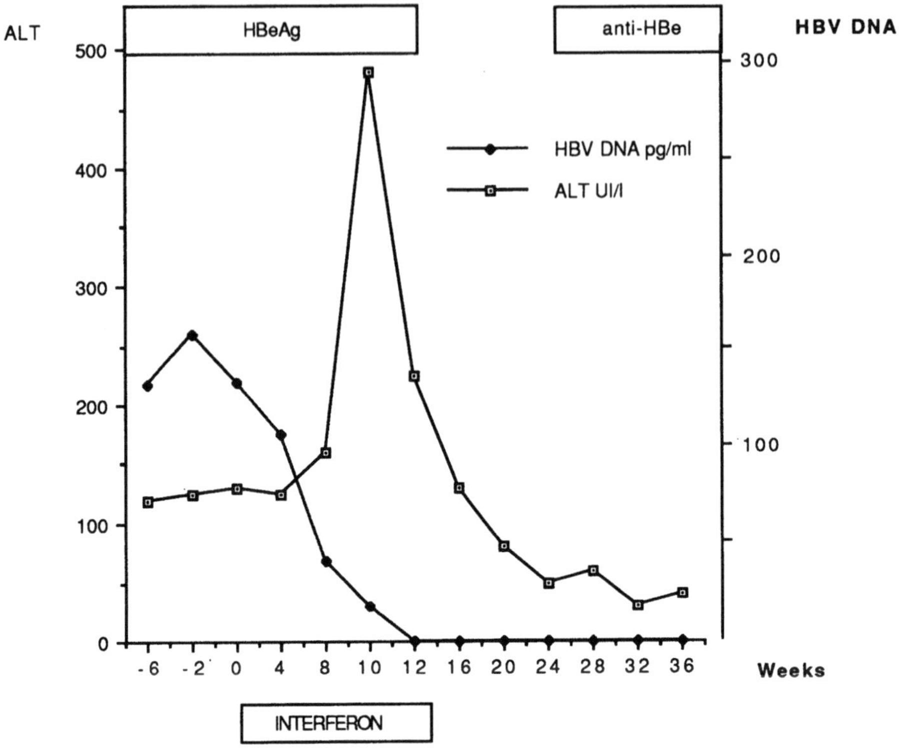


**Fig. 5.** Evolution of ALT and HBV serum markers in a typical favorable response to interferon therapy in a patient with chronic hepatitis B. Seroconversion to anti-HBe is heralded by an aminotransferase peak, reflecting lysis of hepatocytes harboring replicating viruses

receptor while interferon-γ acts through its own specific receptor. Its interaction with the receptor induces the synthesis of several proteins by means of second messengers [140]. These proteins, mainly 2′, 5′-oligoadenylate synthetase and several protein kinases, exert antiviral properties at several levels of the viral replicative process. The immunomodulatory activity of interferon may also have a significant role in stopping HBV replication in chronic hepatitis B. Interferon stimulates natural killer lymphocytes, as well as cytotoxic T cells, and induces the expression of proteins of the major histocompatibility complex (MHC) [141]. Viral antigens are expressed on the surface of hepatocytes in association with MHC type I proteins. This complex is the target of cytotoxic T cells. By all these mechanisms interferon can facilitate the lysis of hepatocytes harboring replicating viruses [142]. This is reflected in the aminotransferase peak that usually precedes interferon-induced seroconversion (Fig. 5).

Both recombinant and lymphoblastoid interferon-α have been extensively used in chronic hepatitis B. Between 30% and 50% of adult patients in Western countries seroconvert to anti-HBe with interferon-α treatment and enter a remission phase of the disease [128, 143, 144]. Some of these patients, usually those with a shorter evolution, may subsequently lose HBsAg and seroconvert to anti-HBs [97]. Intermediate doses of interferon-α (5–15 MU) are used, usually on a three times per week schedule. The optimum duration of the therapy has not been established, but 3- to 6-month courses have frequently been applied. A longer duration does not improve results but less than 2 months of therapy has been associated with poor results.

From several clinical trials, some pretreatment variables have been shown to predict response [26, 145]. Low levels of viral replication measured by HBV DNA and high aminotransferase levels (more than 3 times the normal value) have been considered to be the better predictors of response in most studies. Other variables that predict response are significant histologic inflammatory activity, the absence of anti-HIV antibodies or immunosuppression, female sex, and the acquisition of the infection during adult life. The poor response rates among Asiatic patients have been related to the acquisition of the disease perinatally or during early childhood; however, genetic factors cannot be excluded. Anti-interferon antibodies have been associated with a lack of response. Most patients with highly replicative chronic hepatitis B and with mild cytolytic activity are not responsive to interferon. Two ways of enhancing the effectiveness of interferon in such cases have been investigated: the immunostimulation which follows the withdrawal of a short course of corticosteroids and the use of antiviral agents to reduce viral replication. Prednisone withdrawal followed by interferon-α has not improved the overall results but seems to be more effective in the subgroup of patients with low aminotransferase values [146]. The concomitant use of antiviral agents such as adenine arabinoside and acyclovir has not increased the number of seroconversions [135, 147].

A synergistic action of interferon-α and -γ has been proposed. However, the combination of both has not been effective, and substantial side-effects of interferon-γ have been reported [148].

Chronic hepatitis B patients infected by the precore mutant that does not secrete HBeAg can respond to interferon with disappearance of HBV DNA and an associated fall in aminotransferase levels. Nevertheless, reactivation of the disease has been frequently reported in these patients [106]. Low doses of interferon could be effective in decreasing the progression of liver damage in patients with cirrhosis and low HBV replication. Adverse side-effects can be severe in this group of patients, and thus interferon treatment should be monitored carefully.

The majority of patients infected with HBV live in Asia, mostly in China and in the Southeast region, and in Africa. Interferon treatment has been of little benefit in these patients, probably because most of them share predictive factors of no response [145]. The most important factor is the poor immunologic response against HBV due to the early exposure to the virus (perinatally or in early childhood). This induces immunotolerance and therefore high replication of HBV together with low inflammatory activity in the liver and low aminotransferase levels. Asiatic patients with low replication of the HBV can be responsive to interferon.

Interferon treatment of children chronically infected by HBV has yielded poor results, probably for reasons similar to those mentioned for Asiatic patients [149].

## 8.2 Chronic Hepatitis D

Chronic hepatitis D has been associated with a rapid progression to cirrhosis in some patients. At the present time there is no effective therapy for this condition. Immunomodulators such as corticosteroids, azathioprine, and levamisole are not useful. Interferon-α treatment has shown promising results in some controlled trials [150, 151]. Its administration has been followed by a clearance of HDV RNA and antigenemia in a significant proportion of patients (50%), associated with a significant improvement in aminotransferase levels and liver histology. Disappearance of the delta antigen in liver tissue has also been reported.

The main problems of interferon treatment in chronic hepatitis D are the almost universal relapse of the disease once interferon administration is stopped or the dose diminished, and the poor tolerance of long-term treatment with intermediate doses of interferon (5–15 MU daily or three times per week). Long-term treatment with the minimum effective dose is recommended in those who respond to interferon in order to prevent the progression of the disease.

Anti-HIV antibodies and anti-LKM1 autoantibodies have been reported to be negative predictors of response to interferon.

## 8.3 Chronic Hepatitis C

In the past, the only means of evaluating the effectiveness of the therapeutic agents in chronic non-A, non-B hepatitis were serial aminotransferase determinations and examination of the liver biopsy. The latter is impractical for close control, while aminotransferase levels tend to fluctuate markedly in some patients with this form of chronic hepatitis. It has been the discovery of HCV which has settled the basis for a correct assessment of antiviral strategies.

Corticosteroids did not prove to be useful [152], and a trial of short-term intravenous acyclovir also showed a lack of effectiveness [153]. The first report of interferon-α came in 1986, when a pilot trial that included ten patients showed that low doses of interferon-α normalized or nearly normalized the aminotransferase values in eight. An improvement in the liver histology was also seen in the patients who responded to interferon [154].

Other pilot studies and randomized controlled trials have yielded similar results [155–157]. It has been shown that between 50% and 70% of patients with chronic hepatitis C respond to interferon (1.5–5 MU) given daily or on a three times per week basis. Lower doses seem to be associated with an inferior percentage of responses and with higher rates of relapse. However, still higher doses have not improved the results. At the present time, relapses after the discontinuation of interferon treatment are frequently seen (35%–80%) among those who have shown a sustained response during therapy. More prolonged treatment might reduce the number of relapses. Criteria for when interferon can be withdrawn have not yet been defined. Clearance of the viremia might predict a sustained remission [158]. Patients who relapse usually respond to another cycle of interferon.

Recently, it has been reported that interferon responders show a marked reduction of tumor growth factor beta mRNA levels in the liver [74]. This cytokine has been implicated in the pathogenesis of liver cirrhosis, as a promoter of fibrogenesis.

Some pretreatment variables could be predictive of response to interferon-α. The most important one seems to be the absence of cirrhosis. In one study that included 100 patients treated with the same schedule of lymphoblastoid interferon-α, the overall response rate was 70%, but only 37.5% of the patients with cirrhosis ($n = 24$) responded, while interferon was effective in 80% of those with CAH without cirrhosis ($n = 76$) [159].

Beta interferon seems to be as effective as interferon-α in chronic hepatitis C. The use of other antiviral agents need to be investigated, since a significant proportion of patients are unresponsive to interferon. In a recent pilot study, serum aminotransferase concentrations were significantly reduced during oral ribavirin therapy [160]. Caution is needed when interferon treatment is applied to chronic non-A, non-B hepatitis negative for anti-HCV antibodies. Ai-CAH can be severely exacerbated by interferon therapy. Therefore this condition should be carefully excluded [161].

## 8.4 Autoimmune Chronic Active Hepatitis

Autoimmunity against some antigens expressed on the surface of hepatocytes has been incriminated as the cause of the chronic inflammation of the liver in patients with Ai-CAH [162]. This condition has been associated with a quite uniform progression to cirrhosis and a poor prognosis in terms of survival, if treatment is not applied. One of the characteristic features of this disease, which is almost definitive, is the good response to immunosuppressive therapy. Corticosteroids induce a remission of the disease (defined as a fall in aminotransferase values to less than twice the normal value) in approximately 80% of the patients [58]. The addition of azathioprine allows a reduction in the dose of corticosteroids by virtue of its

**Table 7.** Immunosuppressive treatment of Ai-CAH

| | | | |
|---|---|---|---|
| *Classic* | | | |
| Induction phase: | Prednisone[a] | 60 mg/day 1st week | |
| | | 60 mg/day 2nd week | |
| | | 40 mg/day 3rd week | + azathioprine 50 mg/day |
| | | 30 mg/day 4th week | |
| | | 20 mg/day 5th week | |
| Maintenance phase: | Prednisone | 10 mg/day + azathioprine 50 mg/day (for 2–3 years)[b] | |
| *Prednisone alone* | | | |
| Induction phase: | Prednisone | 60 mg/day 1st week | |
| | | 50 mg/day 2nd week | |
| | | 40 mg/day 3rd week | |
| | | 30 mg/day 4th week | |
| Maintenance phase: | Prednisone | 15 mg/day | |

[a] Other corticosteroids may be used in an equivalent dose
[b] After prednisone withdrawal azathioprine alone (2 mg/kg/day) may be used to avert reactivation

corticosteroid-sparing effect [58]. Systemic manifestations of disease also enter remission with therapy, and survival improves significantly. However, slow progression to cirrhosis cannot be excluded, even when aminotransferase levels are normal or near normal.

The classic therapeutic protocol includes prednisone or methyl prednisolone and azathioprine. Some patients who do not tolerate azathioprine need a higher dose of corticosteroids to maintain the remission (Table 7). Corticosteroid boluses and cyclosporine could be effective in resistant cases [163].

Discontinuation of the immunosuppression is followed by reactivation in nearly 65% of the patients. Maintenance of remission has been achieved with azathioprine alone (2 mg/kg/day) [164].

### 8.5 Drug-Related Chronic Hepatitis

Chronic hepatitis secondary to drug toxicity is a reversible condition when the incriminated drug is withdrawn [65]. If cirrhosis is already present, this lesion persists in its inactive form. Thus, the management of drug-related chronic hepatitis consists in stopping the administration of the drug involved unless its administration is mandatory and no alternatives are available. In such exceptional cases, close monitoring of the hepatic function, including serial liver biopsies, is necessary.

### 8.6 Wilsonian Chronic Active Hepatitis

Wilson's disease should be considered in any patient with CAH of unknown etiology below the age of 40 years. This is underscored by the fact that untreated Wilson's disease is always fatal and that D-penicillamine or trientine treatment brings about a clinical remission. Long-term survival can be achieved, even when cirrhosis is already present [63] (see Chap. 23).

## 8.7 Other Causes of Chronic Hepatitis

Other causes of chronic hepatitis need to be properly diagnosed and managed. In its initial stages, primary biliary cirrhosis may present with the histologic picture of chronic hepatitis. In these cases ursodeoxycholic acid appears to be the most promising therapy (Chap. 22). Porphyria cutanea tarda sometimes shows features of chronic hepatitis. Phlebotomies are indicated in this condition (Chap. 26). Chronic hepatitis associated with ulcerative colitis can revert when appropriate therapy for the intestinal disease (corticosteroids, sulfasalazine) is instituted. Colectomy has ameliorated liver tests in some cases.

## References


1. De Groote J, Gedigk P, Popper H et al. (1968) A classification of chronic hepatitis. Lancet II:626–628
2. Leevy CM, Popper H, Sherlock S (1976) Diseases of the liver and biliary tract. Standardization of nomenclature, diagnostic criteria, and diagnostic methodology. US Government Printing Office, Washington DC
3. Bianchi L (1986) Necroinflammatory liver diseases. Semin Liver Dis 6:185–198
4. Eileen Hay J, Czaja AJ, Rakela J, Ludwig J (1989) The nature of unexplained chronic aminotransferase elevations of a mild to moderate degree in asymptomatic patients. Hepatology 9:193–197
5. Sherlock S (1989) Classifying chronic hepatitis. Lancet II:1168–1170
6. Liaw Y-F, Chu C-M, Chen T-J, Lin D-Y, Change-Chien C-S, Wu C-S (1982) Chronic lobular hepatitis: a clinicopathological and prognostic study. Hepatology 2:258–262
7. Popper H (1983) Changing concepts of the evolution of chronic hepatitis and the role of piecemeal necrosis. Hepatology 3:758–762
8. Scheuer PJ (1986) Changing views on chronic hepatitis. Histopathology 10:1–4
9. Boyer JL (1976) Chronic hepatitis. A perspective on classification and determinants of prognosis. Gastroenterology 70:1161–1171
10. Knodell RG, Ishak KG, Black WC et al. (1981) Formulation and application of a numerical scoring system for assessing histological activity in asymptomatic chronic active hepatitis. Hepatology 1:431–435
11. Hoofnagle JH, Alter HJ (1984) Chronic viral hepatitis. In: Vyas GN, Dienstag JL, Hoofnagle JH (eds) Viral hepatitis and liver disease. Grune & Stratton, New York, pp 97–113
12. Hoofnagle JH (1990) Chronic hepatitis B. N Engl J Med 323:337–339
13. Margolis HS, Alter MS, Hadler SC (1991) Hepatitis B: evolving epidemiology and implications for control. Semin Liver Dis 11:84–92
14. Schalm SW, Thomas HC, Hadziyannis SJ (1990) Chronic hepatitis B. In: Popper H, Schaffner F (eds) Progress in liver diseases. Grune & Stratton, New York, pp 443–462
15. Hoofnagle JH, Shafritz DA, Popper H (1987) Chronic type B hepatitis and the "healthy" HBsAg carrier state. Hepatology 7:758–763

16. Naoumov NV, Portmann BC, Tedder RS et al. (1990) Detection of hepatitis B virus antigens in liver tissue. A relation to viral replication and histology in chronic hepatitis B infection. Gastroenterology 99:1248–1253
17. Lok ASF, Lai C-L (1988) A longitudinal follow-up of asymptomatic hepatitis B surface antigen-positive Chinese children. Hepatology 8:1130–1133
18. Schalm SW (1990) Treatment of chronic viral hepatitis. Anno 1990. Scand J Gastroenterol 25 [Suppl 178]:111–118
19. Jauregui JI, Serrano M, Civeira MP, Prieto J (1987) Correlación entre los distintos marcadores de replicación del virus de la hepatitis B. Gastroenterología y hepatología 10:105–109
20. Brunetto MR, Stemler M, Bonino F et al. (1990) A new hepatitis B virus strain in patients with severe anti-HBe positive chronic hepatitis B. J Hepatol 10:258–261
21. Carman WF, Hadziyannis S, McGarvey ML et al. (1989) Mutation preventing formation of hepatitis B e antigen in patients with chronic hepatitis B infection. Lancet II:588–590
22. Lieberman HM, Labrecque DR, Kew MC, Hadziyannis SJ, Shafritz DA (1983) Detection of hepatitis B virus DNA directly in human serum by a simplified molecular hybridization test: comparison to HBeAg/anti-HBe status in HBsAg carriers. Hepatology 3:285–289
23. Kaneko S, Miler RH, Feinstone SM et al. (1989) Detection of serum hepatitis B virus DNA in patients with chronic hepatitis using the polymerase chain reaction assay. Proc Natl Acad Sci USA 86:312–316
24. Liang TJ, Isselbacher KJ, Wands JR (1989) Rapid identification of low level hepatitis B-related viral genome in serum. J Clin Invest 84:1367–1371
25. Hadziyannis SJ, Lieberman HM, Karvountzis GG et al. (1983) Analysis of liver disease, nuclear HBcAg, viral replication and hepatitis B virus DNA in liver and serum of HBeAg vs. antiHBe positive carriers of hepatitis B virus. Hepatology 3:656–662
26. Brook MG, Karayiannis P, Thomas HC (1989) Which patients with chronic hepatitis B virus infection will respond to alpha-interferon therapy? A statistical analysis of predictive factors. Hepatology 10:761–763
27. Levy P, Marcellin P, Martinot-Peignoux M et al. (1990) Clinical course of spontaneous reactivation of hepatitis B virus infection in patients with chronic hepatitis B. Hepatology 12:570–574
28. Liaw YF, Chu CM, Su IJ, Huang MJ, Lin DY, Chang-Chien CS (1983) Clinical and histological events preceding hepatitis B e antigen seroconversion in chronic type B hepatitis. Gastroenterology 84:216–219
29. Sakuma K, Saitoh N, Kasai M et al. (1988) Relative risks of death due to liver disease among Japanese male adults having various statuses for hepatitis B s and e antigen/antibody in serum: a prospective study. Hepatology 8:1642–1646
30. Sumazaki R, Motz M, Wolf H, Heinig J, Jilg W, Deinhardt F (1989) Detection of hepatitis B virus in serum using amplification of viral DNA by means of the polymerase chain reaction. J Med Virol 27:304–308
31. Davis GL, Hoofnagle JH (1987) Reactivation of chronic hepatitis B virus infection. Gastroenterology 92:2028–2031
32. Thiers V, Kremsdorf D, Schellekens H et al. (1988) Transmission of hepatitis B from hepatitis-B-seronegative subjects. Lancet II:1273–1276
33. Liang TJ, Blum HE, Wands JR (1990) Characterization and biological properties of a hepatitis B virus isolated from a patient without hepatitis B virus serologic markers. Hepatology 12:204–212
34. Lai MY, Chen PJ, Yang PM et al. (1990) Identification and characterization of intrahepatic hepatitis B virus DNA in HBsAg-seronegative patients with chronic liver disease and hepatocellular carcinoma in Taiwan. Hepatology 12:575–581

35. Beasley RP, Hwang L-Y, Lin C-C, Chien C-S (1981) Hepatocellular carcinoma and hepatitis B virus: a prospective study of 22707 men in Taiwan. Lancet II:1129–1133
36. Choo QL, Kuo G, Weiner AJ et al. (1989) Isolation of a cDNA clone derived from a blood-borne non-A, non-B viral hepatitis genome. Science 244:359–362
37. Kuo G, Choo QL, Alter HJ et al. (1989) An assay for circulating antibodies to a major etiologic virus of human non-A, non-B hepatitis. Science 244:362–364
38. Choo QL, Weiner AJ, Overby LR et al. (1990) Hepatitis C virus: the major causative agent of viral non-A, non-B hepatitis. Br Med Bull 46:423–441
39. Bradley DW, Krawczynski K, Beach MS, Purdy MA (1991) Non-A, non-B hepatitis: toward the discovery of hepatitis C and E viruses. Semin Liver Dis 11:128–146
40. Genesca J, Esteban JI, Alter HJ (1991) Blood-borne non-A, non-B hepatitis: hepatitis C. Semin Liver Dis 11:147–164
41. Dienstag JL (1983) Non-A, non-B hepatitis. I. Recognition, epidemiology, and clinical features. Gastroenterology 85:439–462
42. Alter MJ, Sampliner RE (1989) Hepatitis C and miles to go before we sleep. N Engl J Med 321:1538–1539
43. Hoofnagle JH, Di Bisceglie A (1991) Serologic diagnosis of acute and chronic viral hepatitis. Semin Liver Dis 11:73–83
44. Sanchez Tapias JM Barrera JM, Costa J et al. (1990) Hepatitis C virus infection in patients with nonalcoholic chronic liver disease. Ann Intern Med 112:921–924
45. Samsomo D, Dammaceo F (1989) Antibodies to hepatitis C virus in non-A, non-B post transfusion and cryptogenetic chronic liver disease. Lancet II:798–799
46. Parés A, Barrera JM, Caballería J et al. (1990) Hepatitis C virus antibodies in chronic alcoholic patients: association with severity of liver injury. Hepatology 12:1295–1299
47. Takase S, Takada N, Enomoto N et al. (1991) Different types of chronic hepatitis in alcoholic patients: Does chronic hepatitis induced by alcohol exist? Hepatology 13:876–881
48. Van Der Poel CL, Reesink HW, Schaasberg W et al. (1990) Infectivity of blood seropositive for hepatitis C virus antibodies. Lancet 335:558–560
49. Mac Farlane IG, Smith HH, Johnson PJ et al. (1990) Hepatitis C virus antibodies in chronic ative hepatitis: pathogenic factor or false-positive result? Lancet 335:754–757
50. Garson JA, Tuke PW, Makris M et al. (1990) Demonstration of viraemia patterns in haemophiliacs treated with hepatitis-C-virus-contaminated factor VIII concentrates. Lancet 336:1022–1025
51. Mattsson L, Weiland O, Glaumann H (1989) Chronic non A-non B hepatitis developed after transfusion, illicit self injections or sporadically outcome during long-term follow up. A comparison. Liver 9:120–127
52. Hopf U, Möller B, Küther D et al. (1990) Long term follow up of posttransfusion and sporadic chronic hepatitis non A non B and frequency of circulating antibodies to hepatitis C virus (HCV). J Hepatol 10:69–76
53. Alter HJ (1989) Chronic sequences of non A, non B hepatitis. In: Seef LB, Lewis JH (eds) Current perspectives in hepatology. Plenum, New York, pp 83–97
54. Bonino F, Negro F, Brunetto MR, Verme G (1990) Hepatitis delta virus infection. In: Popper H, Schaffner F (eds) Progress in liver diseases. WB Saunders, Philadelphia, pp 485–496
55. Hoofnagle JH (1989) Type D (delta) hepatitis. JAMA 261:1321–1325
56. Aldrete JS, Sterling WA, Hathaway BH et al. (1975) Gastrointestinal and hepatic complications affecting patients with renal allografts. Am J Surg 129:115–124

57. Phillips MS, Blendis LM, Poucell S et al. (1991) Syncytial giant-cell hepatitis. Sporadic hepatitis with distinctive pathological features, a severe clinical course and paramyxoviral features. N Engl J Med 324:455–460
58. Czaja AJ (1984) Natural history, clinical features and treatment of autoimmune hepatitis. Semin Liver Dis 4:1–12
59. Schalm SW, Korman MG, Summerskill WHJ et al. (1977) Severe chronic active liver disease. Prognostic significance of initial morphologic patterns. Am J Dig Dis 22:973–980
60. Lenzi M, Ballardini G, Fusconi M et al. (1990) Type 2 autoimmune hepatitis and hepatitis C virus infection. Lancet 335:258–259
61. Berg PA, Klein R (1987) Immunology of primary biliary cirrhosis. Bailliere's Clin Gastroenterol 1:675–706
62. Berg NO, Eriksson S (1972) Liver disease in adults with alpha-1-antitrypsin deficiency. N Engl J Med 287:1264–1267
63. Schilsky ML, Scheinberg IH, Sternlieb I (1991) Prognosis of wilsonian chronic active hepatitis. Gastroenterology 100:762–767
64. Sternlieb I, Scheinberg IH (1972) Chronic hepatitis as a first manifestation of Wilson's disease. Ann Intern Med 76:59–64
65. Seeff LB (1981) Drug-induced chronic liver disease, with emphasis on chronic active hepatitis. Semin Liver Dis 1:104–115
66. Milich DR (1991) Immune response to hepatitis B virus proteins: relevance of the murine model. Semin Liver Dis 11:93–112
67. Ferrari C, Penna A, Giuberti T et al. (1987) Intrahepatic, nucleocapsid antigen-specific T cells in chronic active hepatitis B. J Immunol 139:2050–2060
68. Ferrari C, Mondelli MU, Penna A et al. (1987) Functional characterization of cloned intrahepatic hepatitis B virus nucleoprotein-specific helper T cell lines. J Immunol 139:539–548
69. Chu CM, Liaw YF (1989) Studies on the composition of the mononuclear cell infiltrates in liver from patients with chronic active delta hepatitis. Hepatology 10:911–915
70. Van den Oord JJ, De Vos R, Facchetti F et al. (1990) Distribution of non-lymphoid, inflammatory cells in chronic HBV infection. J Pathol 160:223–230
71. Volpes R, Van den Oord JJ, Desmet VJ (1990) Hepatic expression of intercellular adhesion molecule-1 (ICAM-1) in viral hepatitis B. Hepatology 12:148–154
72. López-Talavera JC, Esteban JI, Hernandez JH et al. (1990) Evaluation of anti-HCV positive donors identified during routine screening. J Hepatol 11 [Suppl 2]:540
73. Bradley DW, Maynard JE, Krawczynski K et al. (1982) Non A, non B hepatitis in chimpanzees infected with a factor VIII agent: evidence of persistent hepatic disease. In: Symunness W, Alter HJ, Maynard JE (eds) Viral hepatitis 1981 International Symposium. Franklin Institute Press, Philadelphia, pp 319–329
74. Castilla A, Prieto J, Fausto N (1991) Expression of transforming growth factors beta 1 and alpha in chronic liver disease. Effects of alpha interferon therapy. N Engl J Med 324:933–940
75. Löhr H, Treichel U, Poralla T et al. (1990) The human hepatic asialoglycoprotein receptor is a target antigen for liver-infiltrating T cells in autoimmune chronic active hepatitis and primary biliary cirrhosis. Hepatology 12:1314–1320
76. Wen L, Peakman M, Yeo AL et al. (1990) T-cell-directed hepatocyte damage in autoimmune chronic active hepatitis. Lancet 336:1527–1530
77. Baravalle E, Prieto J (1983) Serum antibodies against porphyric hepatocytes in patients with porphyria cutanea tarda and liver disease. Gastroenterology 83:1483–1491
78. Czaja AJ, Wolf AM, Baggenstoss AH (1980) Clinical assessment of cirrhosis in severe chronic active liver disease. Specificity and sensitivity of physical and laboratory findings. Mayo Clin Proc 55:360–364

79. Chu CM, Liaw YF, Pao CP et al. (1989) The etiology of acute hepatitis superimposed upon previously unrecognized asymptomatic HBsAg carriers. Hepatology 9:452–456
80. McMahon BJ, Heyward WL, Templin DW, Clement D, Lanier AP (1989) Hepatitis B-associated polyarteritis nodosa in Alaskan Eskimos: clinical and epidemiologic features and long-term follow-up. Hepatology 9:97–101
81. Castilla A, Cuende JI, Camps J et al. (1989) Crioglobulinemia mixta y hepatitis crónica no A, no B. Rev Clin Esp 184:390–391
82. Chapman RWG, Marborgh BA, Rhodes JM et al. (1980) Primary sclerosing cholangitis: a review of its clinical features, cholangiography, and hepatic histology. Gut 21:870–877
83. Lok ASF, Lai C-L (1989) Alpha-fetoprotein monitoring in Chinese patients with chronic hepatitis B virus infection: role in the early detection of hepatocellular carcinoma. Hepatology 9:110–115
84. McCullough AJ, Stassen WN, Wiesner RH, Czaja AJ (1987) Serum type III procollagen peptide concentrations in severe chronic active hepatitis: relationship to cirrhosis and disease activity. Hepatology 7:49–54
85. Bortolotti F, Bertaggia A, Crivellaro C et al. (1986) Chronic evolution of acute type B hepatitis: prevalence and predictive markers. Infection 14:64–67
86. Tassopoulos NC, Papaevangelou GJ, Sjogren MH, Roumeliotou-Karayannis A, Gerin JL, Purcell RH (1987) Natural history of acute hepatitis B surface antigen-positive hepatitis in Greek adults. Gastroenterology 92:1844–1850
87. Seef LB, Beebe GW, Hoofnagle JH et al. (1987) A serologic follow-up of the 1942 epidemic of post-vaccination hepatitis in the United States Army. N Engl J Med 316:965–970
88. Ikeda T, Lever AML, Thomas HC (1986) Evidence for a deficiency of interferon production in patients with chronic hepatitis B virus infection acquired in adult life. Hepatology 6:962–965
89. Montano L, Miescher GC, Goodhall AH et al. (1982) Hepatitis B virus and HLA display in the liver during chronic hepatitis B virus infection. Hepatology 2:557–561
90. Rakela J, Redeker AG, Weliky B (1983) Effect of short term prednisone therapy on aminotransferase levels and HBV markers in chronic type B hepatitis. Gastroenterology 84:956–960
91. Zachoval R, Roggendorf M, Deinhardt F (1983) Hepatitis A infection in chronic carriers of hepatitis B virus. Hepatology 3:528–531
92. Krogsgaard K, Kryger P, Aldershvile J et al. (1987) Delta-infection and suppression of hepatitis B virus replication in chronic HBsAg carriers. Hepatology 7:42–45
93. Perrillo RP (1989) Treatment of chronic hepatitis B with interferon: experience in Western countries. Semin Liver Dis 9:240–248
94. Whitley R, Tucker B, Kinkel A et al. (1980) Pharmacology, tolerance and antiviral activity of vidarabine monophosphate in humans. Antimicrob Agents Chemother 18:709–715
95. Lok ASF, Lai C-L, Wu P-C, Leung EKY, Lam T-S (1987) Spontaneous hepatitis B e antigen to antibody seroconversion and reversion in Chinese patients with chronic hepatitis B virus infection. Gastroenterology 92:1839–1843
96. Sampliner RE, Hamilton FA, Iseri OA, Tabor E, Boitnott J (1979) The liver histology and frequency of clearance of the hepatitis B surface antigen in chronic carriers. Am J Med Sci 277:17–22
97. Korenman J, Baker B, Waggoner J, Everhart JE, Di Bisceglie AM, Hoofnagle JH (1991) Long-term remission of chronic hepatitis B after alpha-interferon therapy. Ann Intern Med 114:629–634
98. Degos F, Lugassy C, Degott C et al. (1988) Hepatitis B virus and hepatitis B-related viral infection in renal transplant recipients. A prospective study of 90 patients. Gastroenterology 94:151–156

99. Davis GL, Hoofnagle JH, Waggoner JG (1984) Spontaneous reactivation of chronic hepatitis B virus infection. Gastroenterology 86:230–235
100. Davis GL, Hoofnagle JH (1985) Reactivation of chronic type B hepatitis presenting as acute hepatitis. Ann Intern Med 102:762–765
101. Perrillo RP, Campbell CR, Sanders GE et al. (1984) Spontaneous clearance and reactivation of hepatitis B virus infection among male homosexuals with chronic hepatitis B virus infection. Ann Intern Med 100:43–46
102. Conteas C, Kao H, Rakela J et al. (1983) Acute type A hepatitis in three patients with chronic HBV infection. Dig Dis Sci 28:684–686
103. Tsiquaye KN, Portmann B, Tovey G et al. (1983) Non-A, non-B hepatitis in persistent carriers of hepatitis B virus. J Med Virol 11:179–189
104. Sheen IS, Liaw YF, Tai DI, Chu CM (1985) Hepatic decompensation associated with hepatitis B e antigen clearance in chronic type B hepatitis. Gastroenterology 89:732–735
105. Bonino F, Brunetto MR, Rizzetto M, Will H (1991) Hepatitis B virus unable to secrete e antigen. Gastroenterology 100:1138–1141
106. Brunetto MR, Oliveri F, Bonino F et al. (1989) Natural course and response to interferon of chronic hepatitis B accompanied by antibody to hepatitis B e antigen. Hepatology 10:198–202
107. Okamoto H, Yotsumoto S, Akahane Y et al. (1990) Hepatitis B viruses with precore region defects prevail in persistently infected hosts along with seroconversion to the antibody against e antigen. J Virol 64:1298–1303
108. Weissberg JI, Andres LL, Smith CI et al. (1984) Survival in chronic hepatitis B. An analysis of 379 patients. Ann Intern Med 101:613–616
109. Lashner BA, Jonas RB, Tang H-S, Evans AA, Ozeran SE, Baker AL (1988) Chronic hepatitis: disease factors at diagnosis predictive of mortality. Am J Med 85:609–614
110. Liaw Y-F, Tai D-I, Chu C-M, Chen T-J (1988) The development of cirrhosis in patients with chronic type B hepatitis: a prospective study. Hepatology 8:493–496
111. Hsu H-C, Lin Y-H, Chang M-H, Su I-J, Chen D-S (1988) Pathology of chronic hepatitis B virus infection in children: with special reference to the intrahepatic expression of hepatitis B virus antigens. Hepatology 8:378–382
112. Popper H, Shafritz DA, Hoofnagle JH (1987) Relation of the hepatitis B virus carrier state to hepatocellular carcinoma. Hepatology 7:764–772
113. Rizzetto M, Bonino F, Verme G (1988) Hepatitis delta virus infection of the liver: progress in virology, pathobiology, and diagnosis. Semin Liver Dis 8:350–356
114. Bonino F, Negro F, Baldi M et al. (1987) The natural history of chronic delta hepatitis. Prog Clin Biol Res 234:145–152
115. Fattovich G, Boscaro S, Noventa F et al. (1987) Influence of hepatitis delta virus infection on progression to cirrhosis in chronic hepatitis B. J Infect Dis 155:931–935
116. Smedile A, Rosina F, Saracco G et al. (1991) Hepatitis B virus replication modulates pathogenesis of hepatitis D virus in chronic hepatitis D. Hepatology 13:413–416
117. Sagnelli E, Felaco FM, Filippini P et al. (1989) Influence of HDV infection on clinical, biochemical and histological presentation of HBsAg positive chronic hepatitis. Liver 9:229–234
118. Shih W-K, Esteban Mur JI, Alter HJ (1986) Non-A, non-B hepatitis: advances and unfulfilled expectations of the first decade. In: Popper H, Schaffner F (eds) Progress in liver diseases. Grune & Stratton, New York, pp 433–452
119. Realdi G, Alberti A, Rugge M et al. (1982) Long-term follow-up of acute and chronic non-A, non-B post-transfusion hepatitis: evidence of progression to liver cirrhosis. Gut 23:270–275
120. Kiyosawa K, Akahane Y, Nogata A et al. (1982) Significance of blood transfusion in non-A, non-B chronic liver diseases in Japan. Vox Sang 43:45–52

121. Martin P, Di Bisceglie AM, Kassianides C, Lisker-Melman M, Hoofnagle JH (1989) Rapidly progressive non-A, non-B hepatitis in patients with human immunodeficiency virus infection. Gastroenterology 97:1559–1561
122. Bruix J, Barrera JM, Calvet X et al. (1989) Prevalecence of antibodies to hepatitis C virus in Spanish patients with hepatocellular carcinoma and hepatic cirrhosis. Lancet II:1004–1006
123. Thaler H (1974) The natural history of chronic hepatitis. In Schaffner F, Sherlock S, Leevy CM (eds) The liver and its diseases. Stratton Intercontinental Medical Books, New York, pp 207–215
124. Soloway RD, Summerskill WHJ, Baggenstoss AH et al. (1972) Clinical, biochemical, and histological remission of severe chronic active liver disease: a controlled study of treatments and early prognosis. Gastroenterology 63:820–833
125. Czaja AJ (1986) Treatment strategies in chronic active hepatitis. In: Czaja AJ, Dickson ER (eds) Chronic active hepatitis: the Mayo Clinic experience. Marcel Dekker, New York, pp 247–267
126. Baggenstoss AH, Soloway RD, Summerskill WHJ et al. (1972) Chronic active liver disease. The range of histologic lesions, their response to treatment, and evolution. Hum Pathol 3:183–198
127. Di Bisceglie AM, Hoofnagle JH (1990) Antiviral therapy of chronic viral hepatitis. Am J Gastroenterol 85:650–654
128. Hoofnagle JH (1990) Alpha-interferon therapy of chronic hepatitis B. Current status and recommendations. J Hepatol 11:S100–107
129. Lam KC, Lai CL, Ng RP, Trepo C, Wu PC (1981) Deleterious effect of prednisolone in HBsAg-positive chronic active hepatitis. N Engl J Med 304:380–386
130. A Trial Group of the European Association for the Study of the Liver (1986) Steroids in chronic B-hepatitis. A randomized, double-blind multinational trial on the effect of low-dose, long-term treatment on survival. Liver 6:227–232
131. Nair PV, Tong MJ, Stevenson D, Roskamp D, Boone C (1985) Effects of short-term high-dose prednisone treatment of patients with HBsAg-positive chronic active hepatitis. Liver 5:8–12
132. Hoofnagle JH, Hanson RG, Minuk GY et al. (1984) Randomized controlled trial of adenine arabinoside monophosphate for chronic type B hepatitis. Gastroenterology 86:150–157
133. Novick DM, Lok ASF, Thomas HC et al. (1984) Diminished responsiveness of homosexual men to antiviral therapy in HBsAg positive chronic liver disease. J Hepatol 1:29–35
134. Weller IVD, Carreño V, Fowler MJF et al. (1982) Acyclovir inhibits hepatitis B virus replication in man. Lancet I:273
135. Schalm SW, Heytink RA, Van Buuren HR, de Man RA (1985) Acyclovir enhances the antiviral effect of interferon in chronic hepatitis B. Lancet II:358–360
136. Weller IVD, Tedder RS, Karayannis P, Thomas HC, Fiddian AP (1986) A pilot study of BW A5I5U (6-deoxyacyclovir) in chronic hepatitis B virus infection. J Hepatol 3 [Suppl 2]:S119
137. Sherker AH, Hirota K, Omata M, Okuda K (1986) Foscarnet decreases serum and liver duck hepatitis B virus DNA in chronically infected ducks. Gastroenterology 91:818–824
138. Bain VG, Daniels HM, Chanas A, Alexander GJ, Williams R (1989) Foscarnet therapy in chronic hepatitis B virus e antigen carriers. J Med Virol 29:152–155
139. Zoon KC (1988) Human interferons: structure and function. Interferon 9:1–11
140. Peters M (1989) Mechanisms of action of interferons. Semin Liver Dis 9:235–239
141. De Maeyer-Guignard J, De Maeyer E (1985) Immunomodulation by interferons: recent developments. Interferon 6:69–91

142. Peters M, Davis GL, Dooley JS, Hoofnagle JH (1986) The interferon system in acute and chronic viral hepatitis. In: Popper H, Schaffner F (eds) Progress in liver diseases. Grune & Stratton, Orlando, pp 453–467
143. Castilla A, Civeira MP, Jáuregui JI et al. (1989) Tratamiento de la hepatitis crónica B con interferón alfa linfoblastoide. Med Clin (Barc) 93:601–603
144. Hoofnagle JH, Peters M, Mullen KD et al. (1988) Randomized, controlled trial of recombinant human alpha interferon in patients with chronic hepatitis B. Gastroenterology 95:1318–1325
145. Perrillo RP (1990) Factors influencing response to interferon in chronic hepatitis B: implications for Asian and Western populations. Hepatology 12:1433–1435
146. Perrillo RP, Schiff ER, Davis GL et al. (1990) A randomized, controlled trial of interferon alpha-2b, alone and following prednisone withdrawal, in the treatment of chronic hepatitis B. N Engl J Med 323:295–301
147. García G, Smith CI, Weissberg JI et al. (1987) Adenine arabinoside monophosphate (vidarabine phosphate) in combination with human leukocyte interferon in the treatment of chronic hepatitis B: a randomized, double-blinded, placebo-controlled trial. Ann Intern Med 107:278–285
148. Di Bisceglie AM, Rustgi VK, Kassianides C et al. (1990) Therapy of chronic hepatitis B with recombinant human alpha and gamma interferon. Hepatology 11:266–270
149. Lai CL, Lok ASF, Lin HJ, Wu PC, Yeoh EK, Yeung CY (1987) Placebo-controlled trial of recombinant alpha-interferon in Chinese HBsAg carrier children. Lancet II:877–880
150. Rosina F, Rizzetto M (1989) Treatment of chronic type D (delta) hepatitis with alpha interferon. Semin Liver Dis 9:264–266
151. Rosina F, Pintus C, Rizzetto M et al. (1990) Long-term interferon treatment of chronic hepatitis D: a multicentre Italian study. J Hepatol 11:S149–S150
152. Stokes P, Lopez WC, Balart L (1987) Effects of short-term corticosteroid therapy in patients with chronic non-A, non-B hepatitis. Gastroenterology 92:1783
153. Pappas SC, Hoofnagle JH, Young N et al. (1985) Treatment of chronic non-A, non-B hepatitis with acyclovir: a pilot study. J Med Virol 15:1–9
154. Hoofnagle JH, Mullen KD, Jones DB et al. (1986) Treatment of chronic non-A, non-B hepatitis with recombinant human alpha interferon: a preliminary report. N Engl J Med 315:1575–1578
155. Davis GL, Balart L, Schiff E et al. (1989) Treatment of chronic hepatitis C with recombinant interferon alpha: a multicenter randomized controlled trial. N Engl J Med 321:1501–1506
156. Di Bisceglie AM, Martin P, Kassianides C et al. (1989) Recombinant interferon alpha therapy for chronic hepatitis C: a randomized, double-blind, placebo-controlled trial. N Engl J Med 321:1506–1510
157. Camps J, Castilla A, Civeira MP, Serrano M, Prieto J (1989) Randomized trial of lymphoblastoid alpha interferon in chronic non-A, non-B hepatitis: effects on inflammation and fibrogenesis. J Hepatol 9:S17
158. Camps J, García-Granero M, Riezu-Boj JI et al. (1991) Predictive factors of disease relapse after therapy with lymphoblastoid interferon in chronic hepatitis C. J Hepatol 13:516
159. Camps J, Crisóstomo S, García-Granero M et al. (1991) Predictive factors of response to lymphoblastoid interferon in chronic hepatitis C: a statistical analysis. J Hepatol 13:5106
160. Reichard O, Andersson J, Schvarcz R, Weiland O (1991) Ribavirin treatment for chronic hepatitis C. Lancet 337:1058–1061
161. Vento S, Di Perri G, Garofano T et al. (1989) Hazards of interferon therapy for HBV-seronegative chronic hepatitis. Lancet II:926
162. Meyer zum Büschenfelde K-H, Lohse AW, Manns M, Poralla T (1990) Autoimmunity and liver disease. Hepatology 12:354–363

163. Hyams JS, Ballow M, Liechtern AM (1987) Cyclosporine treatment of autoimmune chronic active hepatitis. Gastroenterology 93:890–893
164. Stellon AJ, Keating JJ, Johnsons PJ (1988) Maintenance of remission in autoimmune chronic active hepatitis with azathioprine after corticosteroid withdrawal. Hepatology 8:781–784

# B. Cirrhosis

J. Quiroga, O. Beloqui, and A. Castilla

## 1 Definition

Cirrhosis is a chronic and diffuse process occurring in the liver which alters the structural and functional properties of the organ. It cannot be considered a single entity since it represents the irreversible end-stage of different chronic liver diseases of various etiology. The WHO has defined cirrhosis as "a diffuse process characterized by fibrosis and the conversion of normal liver architecture into structurally abnormal nodules" [1, 2]. Independently of morphologic or etiologic factors, the triad of parenchymal cell necrosis, nodular liver cell regeneration and liver fibrosis constitutes the hallmark of any cirrhotic process. The three components of the triad are frequently present simultaneously, their relative contribution varying according to the type of cirrhosis and the stage of the disease.

The diffuse character of the lesion and the existence of fibrosis and abnormal nodules are essential for diagnosis, but the presence of necrosis and nodular regeneration is no longer regarded as necessary [3]. Because the definition of cirrhosis is morphologically based, a liver biopsy is always needed for a definite diagnosis. In a needle biopsy specimen, the presence of at least two parenchymal nodules surrounded by fibrous septa is virtually diagnostic [4].

Clinical manifestations of liver cirrhosis are independent of its etiology and are principally related to the degree of liver dysfunction and the severity of the intrahepatic circulatory impairment which results from the loss of normal liver architecture. Although liver cirrhosis is frequently associated with characteristic clinical features and suggestive radiologic findings, it may be asymptomatic and consequently pass unnoticed.

## 2 Epidemiology

Cirrhosis of the liver shows a worldwide distribution and affects all races and ages and both sexes. Nevertheless, few epidemiologic studies have been performed and most available data are based on autopsy records or mortality rates. In a prospective study conducted in Birmingham [5], the annual incidence of cirrhosis (number of new cases diagnosed per million person-year) rose from 56 in 1959 to 153 in 1974, and that of cirrhosis of alcoholic origin from 23 to 95. In Baltimore the annual incidence of cirrhosis in 1973 was estimated as 192 (150 alcohol related) [6]. A recent report from Denmark [7] has shown that a total of 6160 cases of cirrhosis were registered in the period 1981–1985, representing a global annual incidence of 242 per million. In the same study the incidence of alcoholic cirrhosis was 190 in males and 85 in females (over-all incidence: 137), that of primary biliary cirrhosis 4 in males and 14 in females (overall incidence: 9), and that of nonalcoholic–nonbiliary cirrhosis 110 in males and 82 in females (overall incidence: 96).

Between 0.17% and 0.4% of hospital admissions are due to cirrhosis of the liver [5, 8]. The incidence of cirrhosis in the apparently healthy population is not known. In 512 cirrhotic patients, the diagnosis of cirrhosis was an incidental finding at autopsy in 58 cases (11.3%) [5].

Although several reports had shown the prevalence of cirrhosis in autopsy studies to be around 3.5% [8], a more recent report from Italy disclosed that over a 10-year period, 2563 cirrhotic livers were identified in a total of 26879 autopsies; this represented a prevalence of 9.5% among autopsied cases [9].

Cirrhosis of the liver ranked as the ninth most common cause of death in the United States in 1984, and was the fifth most common cause in the 45- to 64-year-old group [10]. In the present century, mortality due to cirrhosis progressively increased in the United States until 1973, when it reached a peak of 15.0 per 100000 population. A steady decline ensued, the figure falling to 10.1 per 100000 population in 1984 [10]. The increase in mortality due to cirrhosis was observed independently of age, race, and sex (Table 1) [11]. Similar patterns of cirrhosis-related mortality were observed in France and Spain [12, 13]. The worldwide increase in cirrhosis-related mortality clearly correlates, in both sexes, with a parallel increase in alcohol consumption [10]. Other nutritional factors (protein, fat, calcium, vitamin A, and vitamin $B_2$) have also been associated with the mortality due to liver cirrhosis in different countries [14].

All the above studies have shown that, at any age, the incidence of and mortality due to cirrhosis are consistently approximately twice as high for

**Table 1.** Age-specific death rates (per 100000 population) for liver cirrhosis by sex and age (whites): United States, 1961–1985[a]

| | Male | | | | | Female | | | | |
|---|---|---|---|---|---|---|---|---|---|---|
| | 25–34 years | 35–44 years | 45–54 years | 55–64 years | 65–74 years | 25–34 years | 35–44 years | 45–54 years | 55–64 years | 65–74 years |
| 1985 | 3.1 | 11.1 | 28.0 | 47.1 | 53.1 | 1.3 | 4.2 | 11.9 | 20.1 | 26.0 |
| 1975 | 3.2 | 18.2 | 44.7 | 66.3 | 67.2 | 1.3 | 8.0 | 21.5 | 29.7 | 24.7 |
| 1967 | 3.0 | 18.1 | 43.1 | 65.1 | 62.7 | 1.8 | 10.0 | 23.7 | 27.9 | 24.2 |
| 1961 | 2.5 | 13.3 | 35.8 | 50.3 | 56.9 | 1.6 | 8.6 | 18.7 | 20.1 | 19.5 |

[a] Modified with permission from Hasin et al. [11]

males as for females. In both sexes the peak frequency of cirrhosis is in the fifth and sixth decades.

## 3 Classification

Currently, the classification of liver cirrhosis remains a subject of debate, since the ideal system should provide information about the etiology, pathogenesis, and prognosis of the disease [3]. It is worth noting that cirrhosis of identical etiology may show different histologic appearances, while different etiologies may produce the same morphologic pattern. Moreover, occasionally a certain morphologic type varies with time, and in the terminal stage most cases of cirrhosis look alike. Since there is not a definite system for classification, the complete diagnosis of cirrhosis has to be based on a combination of clinical, biochemical, serologic, and morphologic data [15]. In fact in the classification of liver cirrhosis morphologic and etiologic criteria are not mutually exclusive and they are the most widely used.

In morphologic terms three types of liver cirrhosis can be distinguished: micronodular, macronodular, and mixed. Micronodular cirrhosis has also been known as portal, diffuse septal, Laënnec's, or nutritional cirrhosis. The liver may be enlarged or of normal size (in rare instances its size is reduced) and firm or even hard. The nodules are small (less than 3 mm in diameter) and regular in size, giving rise to a uniform granular appearance on the external and cut surface. Macroscopically fine and regular fibrous septa are diffusely present. Alcohol is the leading cause of micronodular cirrhosis, although hemochromatosis, drugs, chronic venous obstruction, chronic biliary disease, and Indian childhood cirrhosis may show the same morphology [3, 15]. Although it is of limited informational value, the color of the liver (tan or yellow in alcohol-related cirrhosis, dark reddish brown in hemochromatosis, olive green to brown in biliary cirrhosis) may help in the etiologic diagnosis [3].

Macronodular, or postnecrotic, cirrhosis is characterized by large nodules (greater than 3 mm in diameter), generally of variable size, that are separated by fibrous bands of different widths and lead to an irregular appearance of the liver (Fig. 1). In long-standing disease the organ is shrunken with broad, depressed, connective scars between nodules. Chronic viral hepatitis, autoimmune chronic active hepatitis, cryptogenic cirrhosis, and most cases of end-stage cirrhosis of whatever cause are macronodular. When micronodular cirrhosis changes to the macronodular type, a mixed form may be seen, where smaller and larger nodules coexist in the same liver [3, 15].

The etiologic classification of cirrhosis is shown in Table 2. The clinical and histologic features of the diverse entities are considered in other chapters.

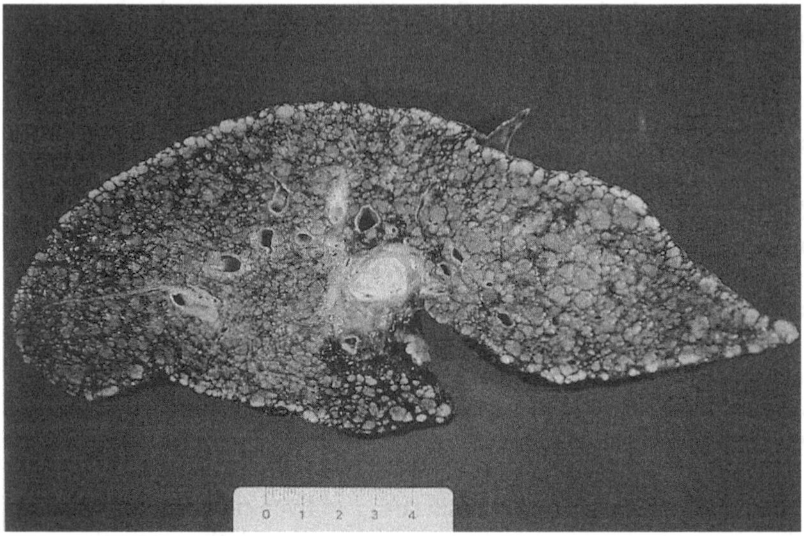


**Fig. 1.** Macronodular cirrhosis. Macroscopic appearance of the cut surface of the liver

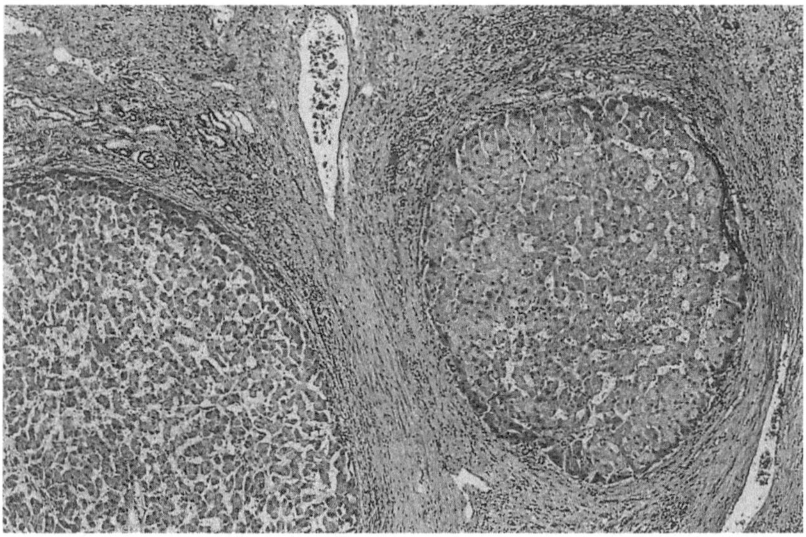

**Fig. 2.** Nodules of parenchymal cells surrounded by fibrous septa serve as a definitional criterion for cirrhosis

As mentioned above, the histologic diagnosis of liver cirrhosis is based on the presence of abnormal nodules surrounded by fibrous septa (Fig. 2) [4]. Although the size of the liver specimen analyzed is crucial, an adequate needle biopsy, in combination with macroscopic features (as revealed by

**Table 2.** Etiologic classification of liver cirrhosis

| | |
|---|---|
| Drugs and toxins | Alcohol |
| | Methotrexate |
| | Amiodarone |
| | Others |
| Viruses | Hepatitis B |
| | Hepatitis C |
| | Hepatitis D |
| Biliary obstruction | |
| Primary | PBC |
| | Sclerosing cholangitis |
| | Atresia |
| Secondary | Gallstones and carcinoma |
| | Stricture |
| | Cystic fibrosis |
| Metals | Hemochromatosis |
| | Wilson's disease |
| Vascular | |
| Primary | Budd-Chiari syndrome |
| | Veno-occlusive disease |
| Secondary | Right heart failure |
| | Inferior vena cava obstruction |
| Genetic | |
| Proteins | $\alpha_1$-Antitrypsin deficiency |
| Amino acids | Tyrosinemia |
| Urea cycle | Ornithine transcarbamylase |
| Carbohydrate | Glycogen storage |
| | Galactosemia |
| | Fructose intolerance |
| Lipid | Abetalipoproteinemia |
| Porphyria | Erythropoietic protoporphyria |
| Idiopathic | Autoimmune hepatitis |
| | Indian childhood cirrhosis |
| Miscellaneous | Cryptogenic |
| | Sarcoidosis |
| | Schistosomiasis |
| | Intestinal bypass |
| | Hereditary hemorrhagic telangiectasia |

peritoneoscopy), gives an accurate diagnosis in most cases [16]. Microscopically, micronodular cirrhosis is easier to identify since nodules and fibrous septa are usually present in the needle sample. However, in the macronodular form the whole needle biopsy may show only part of a single nodule with no fibrous component [15]. Fragmentation of the needle sample is frequent in cirrhosis and this event is of diagnostic value. In the diagnosis of liver cirrhosis a good reticulin preparation is essential since it discloses minimal alterations in the amount and distribution of fibrotic tissue and helps in the distinction from bridging necrosis, for which cirrhosis is easily mistaken [16].

In cirrhotic livers, hepatocytes may look normal. Active regeneration is recognized by a variable thickening of the liver cell plates, which exhibit little lipofuscin content. Regenerated areas may compress the neighboring parenchyma. In a needle sample, the existence of different populations of hepatocytes showing variable cellular and nuclear appearances together with reticulin fibers disposed in various directions strongly suggests cirrhosis [16]. Findings of hepatic veins in contact with septa, fibrous septa traversing the specimen, or an altered relationship between vessels and other architectural components point to the presence of cirrhosis [4].

Finally, the intensity of the inflammatory infiltrate and the degree of hepatocellular necrosis indicate the activity of the lesion, although a single liver sample might not be fully representative of the entire organ [16].

## 4 Pathogenesis

As mentioned above, liver cirrhosis is characterized by cell necrosis, regeneration, and fibrosis. Different etiologic agents may induce hepatocellular necrosis. This is the initial event that, when chronic, triggers nodular regeneration and fibrosis. Acute and massive liver necrosis, if not lethal, is followed by regeneration of the liver in a normal fashion, without fibrosis. Only chronic liver disease produces cirrhosis. The period required for cirrhosis to develop varies depending on its etiology, its activity, and individual factors.

### 4.1 Necrosis

Although necrosis of hepatocytes is considered a basic factor in the development of liver cirrhosis, the physiopathologic processes leading to cell death are, at present, still poorly understood.

Cell death has been defined as a state of equilibrium precluding any vital function. All normal structures or functions are ultimately irreversibly perturbed. Hepatocytes may disappear or persist as remnants or debris [17].

Morphologically three types of cell death are recognized. The first, *apoptosis*, represents the mechanism for physiologic cell turnover. The initial event in apoptosis is unknown. Scattered cells show nuclear and cytoplasmic degeneration by an energy-dependent mechanism and through the action of endogenous endonucleases. These cells may appear as round acidophilic bodies on light microscopy. Although apoptotic cells are digested by phagocytic cells, inflammation is absent.

*Cytolysis*, the second form of cell necrosis, is characterized by rupture of hepatocytes and replacement of the normal cell population by reactive inflammatory cells, including lymphocytes and macrophages. This type of cell death can be seen in cases of immunologic damage of the liver.

Finally, *coagulative necrosis* of cells is identified by the presence of eosinophilic cytoplasm and pyknotic nuclei. It is characteristic of hypoxia or toxic liver injury. Once cell death has occurred, macrophage, rather than lymphocyte, infiltration may take place [18].

Several mechanisms of liver cell death have been described and a huge body of experimental data is currently available. In situations involving hypoxia, the ATP/ADP ratio is reduced and all the energy-dependent cellular functions are disturbed. In other instances, free radicals are generated. These may attack a great variety of cellular macromolecules and produce lipid peroxidation in plasma membrane and in organelles. In still other cases, the exposure to xenobiotics, or their metabolic products, may inhibit critical enzymatic activities or induce cellular depletion of vital cofactors. In general, several of these necrogenic mechanisms are initially or sequentially involved in a single type of injury. For example, in alcohol-related liver damage there is a zonal hypoxia due to a hypermetabolic state, but alcohol itself or acetaldehyde also induces cytoskeletal alterations and may trigger fibrogenesis and the release of chemoattractant factors. Moreover, chronic alcohol consumption increases cytochrome P-450 activity and depletes reduced glutathione, both factors favoring oxidative stress and free radical damage [18].

Liver injury may be initiated by several mechanisms but, in later stages, the influx of calcium ions represents the final common pathway leading to cell death. The lethal effect of high calcium concentrations is not fully understood [19].

### 4.2 Fibrosis

Liver fibrosis may be defined as the pathologic situation characterized by the accumulation of newly synthesized extracellular matrix (ECM) within the organ. Morphologically, it is recognized by the presence of excessive connective tissue. Liver fibrosis is the end-result of a complex and dynamic process, called fibrogenesis, which includes the synthesis of a great variety of macromolecules, the participation of most of the normal cell subpopulations, and the secretion of soluble and insoluble factors. The degradation of the excessive connective tissue is known as fibrolysis [20, 21].

Although an excess of ECM is present in liver fibrosis, the structure of the organ is preserved and the process is still potentially reversible. In chronic liver disease, fibrosis may progress to cirrhosis. In this situation the normal parenchymal structure is lost and the lesion is regarded as irreversible. The clinical differentiation between extensive fibrosis and established cirrhosis is frequently difficult.

*Structure and Function of the Extracellular Matrix*

Extracellular matrix represents the insoluble portion of the extracellular milieu. In the liver, it is possible to distinguish between pericellular matrix, in relation with integral cell membranes, interstitial matrix, present in intercellular spaces, and, basement membrane matrix, which supports epithelial, endothelial, and certain mesenchymal cells [22] (Fig. 3).

Extracellular matrix is composed by three different classes of macromolecules: proteins (collagens and elastin), glycoconjugates (glycoproteins and proteoglycans), and a pure glycosaminoglycan (hyaluronidate) [23]. The proportions and characteristics of these components may differ in various tissues and in different regions within an individual tissue [24, 25], possibly in accordance with matrix-specific functions.

Collagens, the most abundant components of ECM, consist of one or more triple-helical structures formed by three polypeptide chains [20]. At least 13 distinct types of collagen have been described [26]. In normal liver, collagens type I, III, IV, V, and VI have been found, accounting for 2–8 mg/g wet weight or 20–80 mg/g protein [20].

Collagens type I and III each represent about 33% of the total collagen content of the normal liver. They represent the fibrillar, interstitial collagen, mainly present within portal areas. Fibrillar collagens provide tensile strength and help to maintain tissue architecture [24]. Type VI collagen codistributes with types I and III.

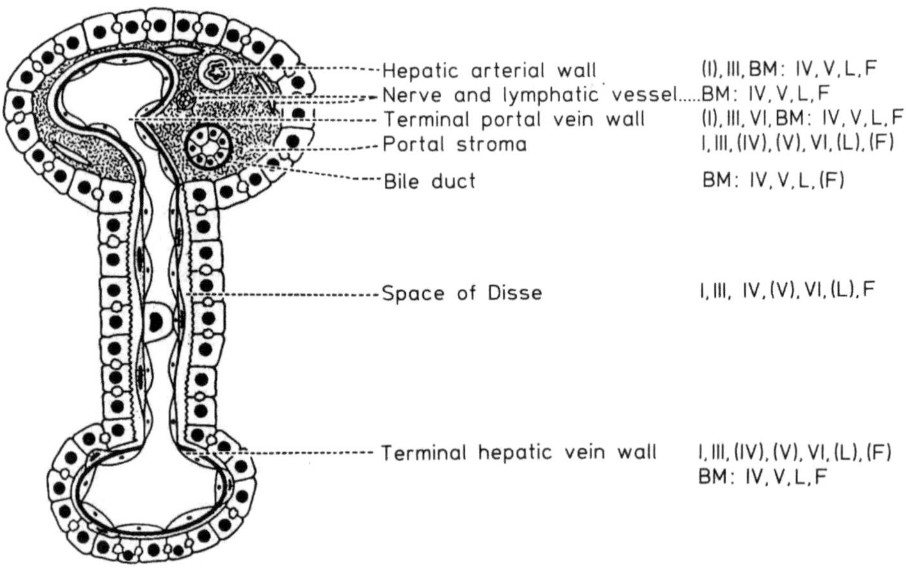


**Fig. 3.** Distribution of collagen and other ECM components in normal liver. *BM*, basement membrane; *L*, laminin; *F*, fibronectin. (Reproduced with permission from HAHN and SCHUPPAN [21])

Type IV collagen, predominantly located in the subendothelial space of Disse, forms a lattice-like structure also present in the basement membranes of lobular vessels and bile ductules [27]. It accounts for 7% of collagen content in normal liver. The interstitial collagen type V has a pericellular distribution and represents 5%–15% of total collagen.

Elastin is a minor component of ECM in the liver. In normal conditions it is found in portal tracts and vessel walls [21].

Proteoglycans, the second most abundant component of ECM, are large molecules consisting of a core of protein and a variable number of covalently linked side chains of glycosaminoglycans. Their classification is based on the predominant disaccharide of the side chains. Normal liver contains especially heparan sulfate, followed by chondroitin sulfate and dermatan sulfate. Proteoglycans are found in all ECM, interact with collagens and elastin, and play a role in tissue growth, differentiation, and organization. Moreover, liver cell-associated proteoglycans, such as heparan sulfate, may be involved in transmembrane signaling and cell adhesion. In normal rat liver heparan sulfate is detected in sinusoids and portal basement membranes [20, 28].

The noncollagenous glycoproteins may account for 40%–50% of the total protein content of ECM and in the liver are represented by fibronectin, vitronectin, laminin, undulin, and nidogen (entactin) [22]. Fibronectin is constituted by subunits of 220 kd linked by a disulfide bond. There are two forms: plasma (soluble) fibronectin, which is secreted by the liver, and cellular (insoluble) fibronectin [20]. In the normal liver, fibronectin is detectable in all extracellular compartments, including basement membranes [22]. Fibronectin not only mediates cellular adhesion to collagens, but is a potent chemoattractant and acts as a growth factor for mesenchymal cells [22]. Vitronectin, another adhesion glycoprotein, codistributes with fibronectin within the liver [22].

Laminin is a cross-shaped molecule of 900 kd consisting of three subunits linked by disulfide bonds [28]. It is the major glycoprotein in basement membranes. It specifically binds type IV collagen, heparan sulfate, nidogen, and at least two classes of membrane receptors on epithelial and endothelial cells [22], anchoring cells to basement membrane and modulating epithelial growth and differentiation.

Undulin, another glycoprotein of liver ECM, is present in the contact regions between thick collagenous fibers, playing a role in fibril bundle [22]. Nidogen specifically binds to laminin and probably modulates its interaction with cellular receptors [22].

The isolation of the various liver cell populations in a highly purified manner and their culture under controlled experimental conditions, coating the culture dishes with different types of matrix, have provided useful tools to study the cellular source of ECM components and their role in liver function. All liver cells (hepatocytes, lipocytes, and bile duct, endothelial, and Kupffer cells) produce one or more matrix components although their contribution in normal and pathologic situations has not been completely clarified [20]. Nevertheless, lipocytes seem to be the main source of ECM components (collagenous and noncollagenous proteins) in liver fibrosis [23, 29].

There is increasing evidence that ECM not only provides structural support to tissues but also has a biologic activity that may modify cell behavior. ECM induces polarization of cells and plays an essential role in gene expression and cell differentiation, modifying parenchymal and non-parenchymal cell functions [22, 30]. When culture dishes are coated with a basement membrane-like matrix, rat liver hepatocytes show a cuboidal morphology and the secretion of albumin is preserved at physiologic levels for several weeks. In contrast, cells layered on an interstitial-type matrix are flattened and albumin secretion is significantly depressed [31]. It has been shown that proteoglycans maintain liver-specific gene expression in cultured hepatocytes [32], and it has also been demonstrated that Ito cells in culture produce different amounts and types of collagen depending on the matrix to which they are attached [33].

At present the exact mechanism by which ECM exerts its biologic effects on adjacent cells is not well characterized, but it seems to be based on the direct contact between the two elements. Specific cell-binding domains have been described in laminin and fibronectin, and cell membrane receptors for matrix proteins have also been identified [28, 30].

It is currently believed that hepatic fibrosis might induce hepatocellular dysfunction through alterations in ECM. The functional impairment appears to be related not only to the amount of accumulated connective tissue but, even more critically, to its lobular localization. Local changes in matrix composition may result in modification of its normal biologic activity and consequently in disturbed behavior of the cells attached to it.

In liver fibrosis, the presence of fibroblast-like cells in areas neighboring fibrotic tissues suggests that these cells may be responsible for the characteristic accumulation of ECM. There is now compelling evidence that these fibroblast-like cells correspond to lipocytes. When exposed to certain stimuli, the cells undergo morphologic transformation and functional activation which ultimately leads to their proliferation and to increased synthesis and secretion of ECM components [23, 29].

The activation of lipocytes may represent the mechanism of initiation of liver fibrosis. Lipocyte activation can be induced in vitro by several cytokines. These cytokines are presumably produced in vivo by Kupffer and inflammatory cells, which are typically present in chronic liver disease.

One of these cytokines is transforming growth factor-β (TGF-β), which strongly stimulates the production of collagen and noncollagenous proteins by cultured lipocytes. It has been shown that the expression of TGF-β mRNA is significantly increased in liver samples from patients with chronic active liver disease and that it correlates directly with the fibrogenic activity as measured by several parameters (Fig. 4). Interestingly, in those patients

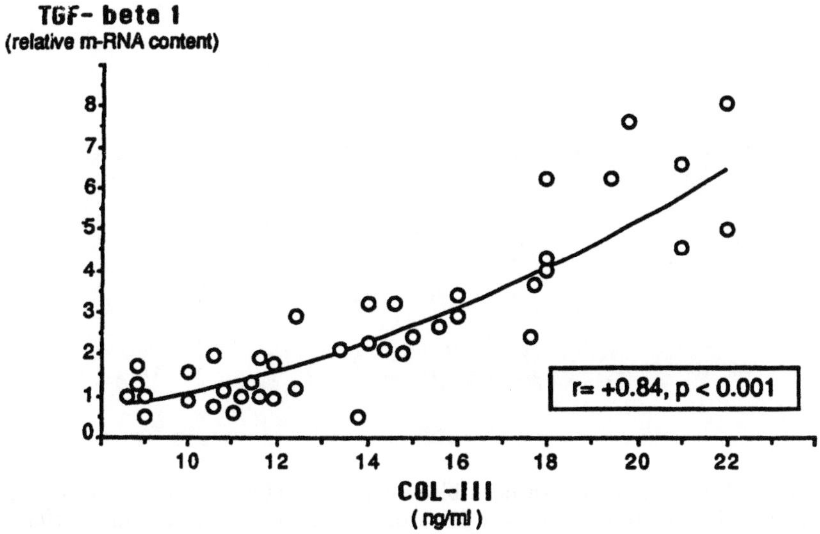


**Fig. 4.** Hepatic TGF-β1 mRNA expression in relation to the serum concentration of procollagen type III peptide in patients with chronic liver disease. (Reproduced with permission from CASTILLA et al. [34])

successfully treated with interferon-α, liver TGF-β mRNA levels are normal (Fig. 5) [34].

Collagen synthesis by cultured lipocytes is also activated by the addition of platelet-derived growth factor (PDGF), which has both proliferating and chemoattractant properties. The activation of lipocytes by PDGF seems to be mediated in vitro through a Kupffer cell-derived factor, not yet characterized, which stimulates the receptors for PDGF on the lipocyte membrane [29]. Several other cytokines (tumor necrosis factor-α, interleukin-1, epidermal growth factor, interferon-γ, hepatocyte-derived factors) may also modify the synthetic activity of lipocytes [29]. In addition other soluble factors (retinoids, glucocorticoids, acetaldehyde, iron, etc.) may modify collagen synthesis by lipocytes, although their role in fibrogenesis remains to be clarified [29].

Once initiated, the progression of liver fibrosis is also dependent on the interaction between the newly formed ECM and the resident lipocytes. The production of interstitial type collagen by activated lipocytes leads to collagenization and capillarization of the space of Disse, which, in turn, stimulate fibrogenesis. In vitro studies have shown that while basement membrane-like matrix keeps lipocytes in a quiescent state, their culture on the interstitial type results in activation [33].

In summary, liver fibrogenesis appears to be an active process in which the activation of quiescent lipocytes plays a determinant role. Lipocytes are maintained in an activated state by the action of a great variety of soluble and insoluble factors and the interrelation of different cell populations.

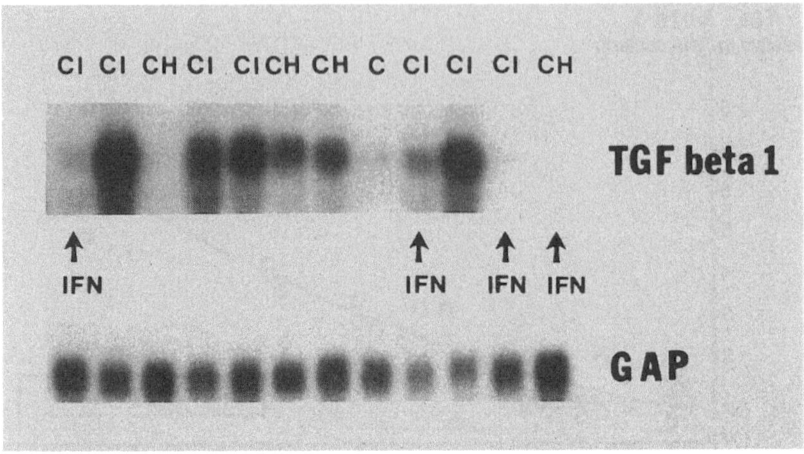


**Fig. 5.** Representative Northern blot analysis of TGF-β1 mRNA in liver specimens from patients with chronic liver disease, untreated or treated with interferon (IFN). The expression of glyceraldehyde 3-phosphate dehydrogenase (*GAP*) mRNA is shown for comparison. CI = cirrhosis; CH = chronic hepatitis (Reproduced with permission from CASTILLA et al. [34])

Ultimately liver fibrosis is a common feature of many chronic liver diseases. By itself, it may partially explain the clinically apparent hepatocellular dysfunction observed in these conditions.

### 4.3 Regeneration

Adult human hepatocytes have a long life span and under normal circumstances the mitotic activity of the organ is very low. Nevertheless, the liver has a tremendous regenerative capacity, as demonstrated by the rapid recovery of liver cell mass after subtotal hepatectomy. Liver cell regeneration after hepatocyte death probably follows the same pattern of gene activation described in the partial hepatectomy model (see Chap. 3), but with regeneration only occurring in the necrotic areas. The triggering mechanisms seem to be local, but at present they are unknown. The role of the ECM in hepatic regeneration remains to be established although matrix alterations secondary to cell necrosis and/or chronic liver disease may play a role [35].

## 5 Pathophysiology and Clinical Manifestations

When cirrhosis is established, parenchymal liver cell mass is reduced and, as a result of scarring, connective tissue forms fibrous septa which disrupt the plates of hepatocytes and disarrange the liver acini. Regenerated hepatocytes cannot be normally disposed in plates; rather they fill the irregular spaces delimited by connective tissue so that regeneration occurs in a nodular fashion. Intrahepatic branches of the portal vein and the hepatic artery lose their normal distribution. Terminal portal branches are constricted within the septa. Sinusoids may collapse or are compressed between nodules. Radicles of the hepatic artery are the only vessels supplying hepatocytes inside the nodular areas. The intrahepatic vascular resistance rises, thus increasing hydrostatic pressure backwards in the portal system. This anatomic and functional derangement of the intrahepatic circulation is an essential characteristic of liver cirrhosis.

Structural changes determine two essential features: reduction in hepatocellular function and development of portal hypertension. The intensity of each of these disorders ranges from very mild, with no clinical manifestations, to extremely severe, leading to death. Although they do not run parallel, hepatocellular failure and portal hypertension are closely linked in determining the course of the disease [1–4].

## 5.1 Hepatocellular Failure

### *Pathogenesis*

#### *Factors Responsible for Impaired Liver Cell Function*

*Reduced Parenchymal Liver Cell Mass.* According to the "intact hepatocyte theory," cirrhotic livers contain hepatocytes which are functionally normal but reduced in number as compared with weight-matched normal livers [36]. Hepatocytes isolated from cirrhotic and normal livers are functionally similar when evaluated in vitro [37]. However, the in vitro function of isolated hepatocytes cannot be extrapolated to "organ function." The function of otherwise normal hepatocytes is dependent on the preservation of the liver structure, and this structure is lost in the cirrhotic liver.

*Reduced "Effective Liver Blood Flow" and "Sinusoidal Blood–Hepatocyte Mismatching."* The structure of the normal liver is highly specialized to allow parenchymal cells to come into direct contact with the sinusoidal blood. This makes possible an intense bidirectional traffic between sinusoidal blood and the basolateral surface of hepatocytes. This feature, which is essential for liver function, is impaired to a variable extent in the cirrhotic liver because of the following abnormalities [1–4]:

1. There is a certain degree of intrahepatic shunting of blood from portal radicles to terminal branches of the hepatic veins, bypassing the sinusoids. This fraction of the intrahepatic portal blood flow is functionally ineffective.

2. The sinusoidal wall is thickened, with loss of fenestrae, formation of a basement membrane-like structure (sinusoidal capillarization), and deposition of collagen in the space of Disse. As a result, macromolecules in the sinusoidal blood cannot pass freely into and through the space of Disse. Furthermore, the intrahepatic resistance to blood flow increases.

3. Regenerative nodules receive blood flow from terminal branches of the hepatic artery but perfusion to hepatocytes in the center of the nodules may be reduced.

Overall these alterations might be defined as sinusoidal blood–hepatocyte mismatching.

*Other Factors Influencing Liver Function.* These include:

1. Mechanical compression of the intrahepatic biliary tree, with possible collapse of some small- and medium-sized ductules due to regenerating nodules.

2. Accumulation in hepatocytes of products that cannot be secreted to sinusoids (bile salts, proteins).

3. Parenchymal collapse, abnormal rearrangement of the plates of hepatocytes, and deficient hepatocyte–sinusoidal interaction. These factors cause alterations in the lobular gradient which influence uptake and secretion processes in the liver acini (see Chap. 8).

*Relationship Between Liver Size and the Severity of Hepatocellular Failure.* In general, liver enlargement is seen in early cirrhosis due to inflammation, edema, and liver cell regeneration. As cirrhosis advances liver volume tends to decrease progressively, so that small livers are characteristic of end-stage cirrhosis. A preliminary study from CASTILLA et al. showed that liver volume roughly parallels hepatic function and regenerative activity in cirrhosis of viral origin [38]. Small cirrhotic livers are associated with low regenerative activity and poor liver function.

*Progression of Liver Cirrhosis, Fibrogenesis, and Regenerative Activity: The Role of Transforming Growth Factors.* The rate at which hepatocytes regenerate, on the one hand, and the rate of collagen synthesis and deposition, on the other, are opposite forces governing the course of liver cirrhosis. It is well known that 70% partial hepatectomy in the rat is followed by complete restoration of liver mass within 10 days. This fascinating property of the liver is partly dependent on soluble mediators, called growth factors, which are able to modify the rate of cell proliferation. The isolation and characterization of these factors, such as TGF-α, TGF-β, and human hepatocyte growth factor, has added to our understanding of the pathobiology of liver cirrhosis [35, 39]. As already mentioned, TGF-β stimulates the synthesis of collagen by lipocytes, while TGF-α, as well as other hepatocyte growth factors, stimulates parenchymal cell proliferation. In a recent study TGF-α mRNA was detected exclusively in cirrhotic livers showing signs of regeneration [34]. In general terms, it seems possible that the course of liver cirrhosis may depend on factors that influence liver fibrogenesis and regenerative activity.

### *Consequences of Hepatocellular Failure* [40, 41]

In cirrhosis resulting from direct hepatocellular damage (viral, alcoholic, or metabolic) the impairment of the various liver functions parallels quite closely the progression of the cirrhosis. In contrast, in cirrhosis secondary to chronic cholestasis (primary and secondary biliary cirrhosis, sclerosing cholangitis), the failure of biliary excretion is already evident at early (precirrhotic) stages of the disease.

Hepatocellular failure in chronic liver disease is manifested by disturbances of the following functions:

1. Regulation of energy metabolism and of the intermediary metabolism of carbohydrate, fat, and protein
2. Synthesis of all the major serum proteins, including clotting factors, anticoagulant proteins, and proteins of the fibrinolytic system
3. Synthesis of urea
4. Synthesis of all major lipids and lipoproteins
5. Synthesis of bile salts, generation of bile flow, and maintenance of the enterohepatic circulation of bile salts
6. Clearance, biotransformation, and biliary excretion of a large number of endogenous and exogenous compounds, especially lipophilic molecules (including most of the drugs in common use)
7. Degradation and elimination of a variety of hormones and hormonal metabolites
8. Storage and biotransformation of some vitamins (i.e., A, D, $B_{12}$, folic acid)
9. Extracellular fluid volume homeostasis

## 5.2 Portal Hypertension

### *Pathogenesis*

Pressure in a vascular system depends on blood flow and vascular resistances. Accordingly, portal hypertension can be due to increases in portal blood flow, portal vascular resistance, or both. Normal portal pressure is below 10 mmHg. Portal pressure is measured by means of hepatic vein catheterization as the pressure gradient between free and wedged pressures in the hepatic vein. This gradient is thought to represent sinusoidal pressure which is transmitted backwards in the portal system. In patients with advanced cirrhosis, portal pressure may reach more than 30 mmHg and this is due to increases in both intrahepatic vascular resistance and portal blood inflow.

*Increased Intrahepatic Vascular Resistance*

In liver cirrhosis, mechanical and functional factors contribute to increase the intrahepatic resistance to portal flow. The increased resistance is located at the sinusoidal and often the postsinusoidal level [42–44]. Compression of portal endings by fibrous septa, compression and collapse of sinusoids by regenerative nodules, sinusoidal capillarization, and collagenization of the space of Disse (which renders sinusoids more rigid) are the principal factors generating a mechanical ("fixed") portal resistance. In alcoholic subjects, perivenous (pericentral) fibrosis in the acinar area 3 may increase the resistance to liver outflow by compressing hepatic vein terminals [45]. This resistance is transmitted backwards, increasing portal resistance within the liver. Perivenous central fibrosis may be the only lesion produced by alcohol in some individuals and is able to produce portal hypertension in the absence of cirrhosis. In alcoholic cirrhosis, abstention is followed weeks to months later by a fall in intrahepatic vascular resistance. The size and volume of hepatocytes are augmented by the effect of alcohol, so that total parenchymal cell volume increases during active drinking. Abstention allows reversal of this lesion. As a result sinusoidal compression decreases and sinusoidal resistance falls. The precise mechanism is nevertheless the subject of controversy since the various studies [42–46] have yielded equivocal results.

In cirrhosis, intrahepatic resistance rises when catecholamines are infused. This shows that structures sensitive to pressor agents may participate in the elevation of intrahepatic resistance.

It is widely accepted that the increased intrahepatic vascular resistance is the main factor determining portal hypertension in cirrhosis [42–44].

*Increased Portal Blood Flow*

Portal hypertension leads to the opening of portal-systemic collaterals which connect the portal system with veins of the systemic circulation (see Chap. 11). One would expect portal-systemic collaterals to attenuate portal hypertension by lowering portal blood flow to the liver. However, in cirrhotics with extensive portal-systemic collateral circulation, portal pressure is in fact even higher than in patients without portal collateralization [42–44]. This apparent paradox is explained by the concomitant increase in arterial splanchnic blood flow. Thus portal liver inflow is maintained or even increased in spite of the diversion of large amounts of portal blood through collateral veins. The increase in arterial blood flow to the splanchnic vascular bed is due to marked vasodilation in this area (see Sect. 7.1 for details).

***Pathophysiology*** (see Chaps. 10, 11, and 12)

As a consequence of portal hypertension, the following disturbances occur:

1. Development of vasodilation and opening of arteriovenous fistulae in the splanchnic vascular bed.

2. Increase in sinusoidal hydrostatic pressure with subsequent overproduction of hepatic lymph and formation of ascites (see Chap. 12). This complication occurs when a significant degree of hepatocellular dysfunction is also present.

3. Splenomegaly, which is partly due to the retrograde increase in pressure in the portal system but is also dependent on the high arterial flow entering the splenic artery. Hypersplenism with excessive destruction or abnormal splenic pooling of peripheral blood cells is a consequence of the increased activity of the splenic reticuloendothelial system rather than of the splenomegaly. The final clinical consequence is pancytopenia.

4. Opening of portal-systemic collateral circulation. Portal-systemic collaterals connect the portal system (hypertensive) with the venous plexus ending in the superior and inferior vena cava, and, to a much lesser extent, with the pulmonary venous system [42–44]. Thus, a fraction of the portal blood flow is diverted through these collaterals, bypassing the liver. In addition, shunting from portal branches to the central veins takes place within the liver. Portal-systemic collateral blood flow in the presence of a patent portal vein bearing hepatopetal blood flow may reach up to 5 liters/min and may account for 80% of total portal inflow [47]. Thus, although it varies widely, portasystemic shunting is relevant from a quantitative viewpoint.

The opening of portal-systemic collateral circulation has a series of implications, including: (a) reopening (or de novo formation) of formerly inactive veno-venous shunts in the splanchnic area, which increases the pooling capacity of the splanchnic venous vascular bed; (b) diversion of a variable (but often high) amount of portal blood to veins which under normal conditions receive a considerably lower flow [pathophysiologically, the most important are the venous plexus located in the walls of the esophagus and the stomach (esophageal and gastric varices)]; and (c) shunting of a fraction of the portal blood flow directly from the portal vein to the systemic circulation, bypassing the liver. Such shunting has four consequences. *First*, substances that normally undergo complete hepatic clearance gain access to the systemic circulation (e.g., antigens of intestinal origin, endotoxins). This is aggravated by the existence of intrahepatic shunting and by the abnormal functioning of the mononuclear phagocyte system. These alterations are the basis for frequent episodes of bacteremia and for the continuous antigenic stimulation which is thought to be involved in the characteristic hyperglobulinemia of cirrhosis. *Second*, substances (various hormonal and nonhormonal compounds) physiologically present in systemic blood and normally subjected to liver degradation may be found in abnormally high serum concentrations. This is especially important in the case of substances having either vasoactive properties or potentially toxic effects on the CNS. The same applies for ingested drugs normally metabolized by the liver. *Third*, portalsystemic shunting disrupts the complex equilibrium governing the intermediate metabolism of nutrients. *Fourth*, portopulmonary shunts contribute to the arterial hypoxemia often found in cirrhosis.

## 5.3 Clinical Presentation

Liver cirrhosis may have various clinical presentations [48–50].

### *Patients with Clinically Latent Cirrhosis*

In patients with clinically latent cirrhosis, the disease is first suspected during medical examination, laboratory screening, or surgery due to a condition unrelated to liver disease. The patient may report no symptoms or may have minor and nonspecific complaints. Some patients complain of fatigue, slight abdominal discomfort, mild deterioration of health, or some loss of physical strength. Not infrequently there is a decrease in libido and sexual potency; this is especially common in alcoholics. Women may have unexplained menstrual alterations or amenorrhea. Easy bruising, epistaxis, petechiae, or gingivorrhagia may have occurred. On physical examination an enlarged hard liver and mild splenomegaly may be found. Less frequently, vascular spiders or palmar erythema are seen.

Some patients are discovered to have liver disease when routine biochemical examination reveals elevated aminotransferase levels. There is a subgroup of patients, growing in number in recent years, in which cirrhosis is diagnosed after a variable follow-up period because of chronic active hepatitis; in such cases there may have been no change in the subjective health of the patient. The diagnosis depends on the liver biopsy.

### *Patients with Decompensated Cirrhosis*

Patients with decompensated cirrhosis seek medical attention because of some major complication of the disease. Their general state of health is poor. Jaundice, abdominal distention with progressive weight gain, peripheral edema, episodes of agitation, disorientation, changes in mood or sleep pattern, and upper gastrointestinal bleeding are major complications that may require hospital admission. In general these patients have a poor outcome, with a mean life expectancy of about 5 years.

Some patients present with a major infectious episode such as septicemia or pneumonia. A minority show an abrupt general deterioration due to the development of hepatocellular carcinoma over a preexistent silent cirrhosis.

### *Patients with Diagnosis of Cirrhosis at Autopsy*

In a substantial number of patients liver cirrhosis is only discovered at autopsy. Reported estimations suggest that 15%–25% of all cases of cirrhosis are not detected during the patient's lifetime [51].

## 5.4 Approach to the Patient

In patients suspected of having liver cirrhosis the clinical history should cover familial history of liver disease, epidemiologic data regarding contact with hepatitis viruses, previous consumption of hepatotoxic drugs (isoniazid, oxyphenisatin, methotrexate, nifedipine, halothane anesthesia, etc.), and detailed documentation of alcohol intake (in terms of grams of alcohol/day and length of drinking habit).

### *Physical Examination*

The general aspect of patients varies widely. Compensated cirrhotics may present some skin changes (see below), hepatomegaly, and splenomegaly. Patients with far-advanced cirrhosis usually show jaundice of variable degree, muscle wasting, and a distended abdomen. The frequency of the main physical findings is summarized in Table 3.

Some of the findings regarding the habitus are related to endocrine changes. Both hypogonadism and feminization may occur. Their effects are

**Table 3.** Main physical findings in cirrhosis (data are given as a percentage of the total number of patients)

| Signs | Powell and Klatskin ($n = 283$)[a] | Ratnoff and Patek [188] ($n = 388$) | Galambos [48][b] ($n = 3785$) |
|---|---|---|---|
| Jaundice | 75.0 | 65.3 | 49.0 |
| Vascular spiders | 48.8 | 15.0 | 38.0 |
| Palmar erythema | 37.1 | 4.2 | ND |
| Hepatomegaly | 95.8 | 75.4 | 72.0 |
| Splenomegaly | 45.6 | 44.0 | 40.0 |
| Ascites | 66.1 | 78.0 | 58.0 |
| Superficial abdominal collateral veins | 47.0 | 23.6 | ND |
| Gynecomastia | 15.0 | ND | ND |
| Testicular atrophy | 45.0 | ND | ND |
| Dupuytren's contracture | 4.6 | 4.6 | ND |
| Noninfectious fever | 21.6 | 24.5 | |

ND, No data in the original source
[a] Am J Med (1968) 44:406–420
[b] Patients from ten cumulated clinical series

especially evident in young and middle-aged patients. If severe, these changes include in men a reduction in the size and consistency of the testes, loss of secondary sexual hair, and feminine distribution of public hair. Facial hair is scarce and less strong. Mono- or bilateral gynecomastia due to glandular hyperplasia may develop, especially in patients with alcoholic cirrhosis or receiving spironolactone. Gynecomastia is often tender and variable in size; in some patients surgical correction is required to avoid psychological problems. Regression of gynecomastia (sometimes incomplete) occurs after liver transplantation.

In women, the breasts and uterus tend to be atrophic although signs of hypogonadism are less evident than in males since a majority of females with cirrhosis are in the perimenopausal period of life.

Circulatory hyperkinesia is manifested by bounding peripheral pulses, mild tachycardia, and ejection systolic murmur. In a few cases, cyanosis and clubbing of the fingers may be observed as manifestations of the hepatopulmonary syndrome. Bone pain in the distal portions of the extremities due to hypoxemic osteoarthropathy is infrequent. Both systolic and diastolic arterial pressures are slightly reduced. Signs of clinically overt cardiac failure are not seen unless cardiomyopathy due to alcohol or hemochromatosis coexists.

The abdominal examination may disclose hepatomegaly, splenomegaly, superficial portal-systemic collaterals, and ascites. Secondary findings are umbilical herniation, testicular edema, and edema of the abdominal wall.

Liver enlargement, often marked, is commonly observed. The increase in the size of the caudate lobe predominates over the enlargement of the remaining liver. Missing an enlarged left lobe occupying the epigastrium and extending to the left hypochondrium is a frequent mistake in the examination of the liver. Liver size is estimated as the distance between the upper and the lower margin of the hepatic dullness. Some patients with advanced disease have no palpable liver since its size is reduced. Consistency of the liver is firm and hard but not stony, the latter finding suggesting malignancy. The cirrhotic liver is not tender. Tenderness indicates acute distention of the Glisson's capsule and suggests the coexistence of acute inflammation, mechanical distention by stasis of blood (cardiac failure, constrictive pericarditis, or venous outflow block in the Budd-Chiari syndrome), or a rapidly expanding intrahepatic process (hematoma, abscess, ruptured adenoma). Auscultation over the liver surface may detect murmurs which suggest the existence of vascular malformations, vascular tumors, and especially liver cancer.

Mild to moderate splenomegaly is found in about half of the cases. The spleen is of intermediate consistency and is not tender. An enlarged area of splenic dullness reveals mild splenomegaly when the spleen is impalpable below the costal margin.

The presence of ascites may be easily detected by physical examination (see Chap. 12).

Collateral venous circulation is more often seen on both sides of the abdomen. Venous blood flow stops if pressure is exerted over these veins, a maneuver which reveals the direction of blood flow. This may be useful in differentiating caval-caval anastomoses, which show ascending flow, from portacaval shunts, which tend to be centrifugal from the umbilicus. Recanalization of the umbilical vein may be identified by the presence of several veins converging in a larger vein in the umbilical area. This sign is called caput medusae or Cruveilhier-Baumgarten's sign. Umbilical herniation and testicular edema may be present in patients with tense ascites. Peripheral or sacral edema may be found, sometimes in association with ascites.

The skin of cirrhotic patients is a rich source of physical signs. Although not specific to liver cirrhosis, these signs are so characteristic that their presence always raises suspicion of underlying cirrhosis.

Jaundice is observed, with serum bilirubin levels above 2.5 mg/dl. Pallor is seen in anemic patients, although it may be masked by jaundice or by hyperpigmentation. Hyperpigmentation in scratched areas is characteristic of patients with pruritus (cholestatic disorders). Hyperpigmentation of hemochromatosis makes the skin grayish due to hemosiderin deposition. White nails occur in 80% of cirrhotic patients due to opacity of the nailbed. Muerhrcke's lines, transverse pale bands in the nails, may be present; they are also often seen in patients with the nephrotic syndrome. Patients with porphyria cutanea tarda, a rare cause of liver cirrhosis, show facial hypertrichosis. In porphyric patients, vesicular lesions develop in the areas of the skin exposed to sunlight. Residual scars on the face and the dorsum of the hands are very useful for the diagnosis.

Vascular changes on the skin such as telangiectasia, vascular spiders (spider angiomas, spider nevi, nevi aranei), and palmar erythema (hepatic palms) are characteristic findings. Malar telangiectasia is frequent in alcoholic cirrhosis but is unspecific. Vascular spiders are lesions constituted by multiple dilated capillaries radiating from a dilated, pulsatile, and protuberant (palpable) central arteriole. Histologically, they resemble the short corkscrew endometrial arteries that develop and slough rapidly during the menstrual cycle [50]. These lesions are found on the face, the neck, the upper extremities, and the upper chest, an area roughly corresponding to the superior vena cava territory. Vascular spiders collapse and disappear when the central arteriole is compressed. They may appear in chronic active hepatitis, in acute hepatitis, in women taking estrogens, during the second and the third trimester of pregnancy (disappearing 2 months after delivery), and more rarely in healthy non pregnant people. Patients showing a rapid increase in the size and number of vascular spiders are likely to have liver cirrhosis with rapidly worsening liver function. In general, cirrhotic patients with vascular spiders have a more severe derangement of the systemic and pulmonary circulations than patients without these lesions [52]. If they are accidentally damaged, vascular spiders may bleed with noticeable intensity for such small lesions. Regression of vascular spiders is completed some weeks after successful liver transplantation. Although they are very easy to identify, vascular spiders must be differentiated from other vascular lesions such as those of hereditary hemorrhagic telangiectasia (Rendu-Osler-Weber disease), telangiectasia in the CRST syndrome, venous stars, and Campbell de Morgan's spots [49].

A lesion associated with vascular spiders has been called "paper money skin." This cutaneous change is distributed in the same areas as vascular spiders and consists of multiple small vessels scattered randomly through the skin which resemble the silk threads in US dollar bills [49].

Palmar erythema is characterized by a change in the color of parts of the palms (and soles), which become reddish and warm. The thenar and hypothenar eminences and the distal pads of the fingers are the areas especially involved. Pressure with a glass over the palms allows one to see skin flushes coupled with pulse beats. This lesion represents an extensive collection of arteriovenous anastomoses [50]. Palmar erythema predominates in cirrhosis of alcoholic etiology. Similar changes may appear in pregnancy and in patients with rheumatoid arthritis. Some families show palmar erythema unrelated to any known disease. Dupuytren's contracture is a contraction of the palmar fascia of the hands which leads to progressive flexion of the digits. It occurs predominantly in alcoholic cirrhosis. It affects a variable number of fingers and may be uni- or bilateral.

## 6 Metabolic Disturbances

### 6.1 Disorders of Energy Metabolism and Nutrition

The liver plays a central role in the regulation of fuel metabolism and in the integration of intermediary metabolism of carbohydrate, fat, and protein [40, 41]. These functions are impaired in advanced cirrhosis.

In hospitalized cirrhotics evaluated by objective nutritional parameters, the prevalence of protein-calorie malnutrition is 88%–100% [53]. Patients with this nutritional disorder have a poor short-term outcome and an increased risk of developing major complications and infections.

Muscular wasting is the most obvious manifestation of malnutrition. In general, it is associated with weakness and easy fatigability on mild exertion. Body composition shows an increase in total body water, a decrease in total protein, and a variable proportion of body fat [54, 55]. The clinical correlates of these changes are ascites and edema, decreased muscle mass, and reduced skinfold thickness [54–56].

Factors thought to cause protein-calorie malnutrition in cirrhosis include poor dietary intake, nutrient malabsorption or maldigestion, intestinal protein loss, impaired hepatic synthesis of protein, increased energy requirements, and changes in the intermediary metabolism.

Factors directly related to low intake are anorexia, nausea, vomiting, and sometimes diarrhea, especially in alcoholic patients. In addition, the handling of food nutrients is altered by anatomic and functional factors. Portal-collateral circulation permits the escape of nutrients to the systemic blood before reaching the liver. On the other hand, the chief hormones controlling intermediary metabolism such as insulin and glucagon but also growth hormone, insulin-like growth factors I and II, thyroid hormones, cortisol, and catecholamines may show alterations in secretion, rate of degradation, or both, resulting in alterations in their serum concentrations. Moreover, target organ responses to some of these hormones are often inadequate. The overall result of these alterations is a predominance of catabolic over anabolic functions.

Both a reduction in protein synthesis and an increase in its breakdown may be mechanisms underlying muscular wasting in cirrhosis. Thus, the urinary excretion of 3-methylhistidine, a marker of muscle myofibrillar breakdown, was found to be increased [57], suggesting that degradation of muscle protein is accelerated. However, additional sources of this amino acid exist which may contribute to its urinary excretion [58]. Other authors have found no modification in the rate of protein breakdown, but a reduction in muscle protein synthesis in association with an overall fall in whole body protein turnover [59, 60].

### *Oxygen Consumption and Resting Energy Expenditure*

Resting energy expenditure and oxygen consumption have been found to be normal, increased, or decreased in cirrhotic patients as compared with control subjects [61–63]. These differences may arise for two reasons: (a) the classic Harris-Benedict equation to predict energy expenditure yields large errors in advanced cirrhotics and (b) changes in body composition in cirrhosis lead to inaccuracies when values are referred to body weight, body surface area, lean body mass, or 24-hour creatinine excretion. Despite these limitations, recent studies in cirrhotic patients have shown that oxygen consumption and resting energy expenditure are inversely correlated with the Child score [61], suggesting that there is progressive impairment of energy production as cirrhosis advances.

Interestingly, Dolz et al. have demonstrated that removal of ascites (mean 16.6 liters, ten patients) is associated with a decrease of more than 10% in resting energy expenditure. Specifically, these authors observed a reduction of 9.6 kcal/day per liter of ascites removed [64]. These data indicate that ascites is not an inert volume and add support to the convenience of its removal.

### *Substrate Utilization*

It is possible that a shift of intermediary metabolism towards the catabolic side is a critical factor in the progressive deterioration of cirrhotics. These patients obtain only 15%–20% of calories from carbohydrate while the degradation of free fatty acids is markedly increased as compared with normal subjects. This change is extreme in short-term starvation (16 h), when glucose utilization in cirrhotics becomes virtually "zero" [65]. This has been interpreted as a mechanism to avoid hypoglycemia (see below); however, it may also reflect alterations in glucose metabolism. Glucose intake in normal subjects induces a manifest increase in the acetoacetate to β-hydroxybutyrate ratio in serum, indicating changes in the redox state as a result of mitochondrial activity and ATP synthesis. In advanced cirrhosis, glucose administration has virtually no effect on this ratio, suggesting that glucose cannot be used normally [66]. On the other hand, in cirrhosis a catabolic state may be determined by the marked predominance of catabolic over anabolic hormones.

## 6.2 Carbohydrate Metabolism

### *Carbohydrate Intolerance and Diabetes*

Hyperinsulinism, insulin resistance, and carbohydrate intolerance are frequent findings in cirrhotics. The association of cirrhosis and diabetes is well established. The extent of this association varies widely in diverse studies, probably reflecting differences in methodology and selection of population [67, 68]. About 80% of cirrhotics display glucose intolerance. The prevalence of diabetes in cirrhotic patients has been reported as 5%–40% in different series while the prevalence of cirrhosis in diabetic patients is about 3% [69]. Among cirrhotics, the higher the patient's age and the more developed the cirrhosis, the higher is the prevalence of diabetes [67].

Several mechanisms may contribute to the development of hyperinsulinemia and diabetes in cirrhosis. Hyperinsulinemia is due to not only reduced hepatic degradation of insulin but also insulin hypersecretion, as has recently been demonstrated [70]. Decreased insulin degradation is due both to hepatocellular failure and to portasystemic shunting of this hormone. Carbohydrate intolerance is manifested by normal fasting blood glucose in the presence of hyperinsulinemia and by abnormally high glucose levels after food intake or glucose loading. Fasting hyperglucemia is indicative of diabetes. In these cases there is peripheral resistance to insulin because of down-regulation of insulin receptors secondary to hyperinsulinemia, but also because of postreceptor events [71]. Hyperglucagonemia, which is common in cirrhosis, as well as elevations in growth hormone, cortisol, and catecholamines add to carbohydrate intolerance [72, 73].

### *Decreased Consumption of Glucose as a Fuel*

Despite liver failure, advanced cirrhotics show a certain protection against the development of hypoglycemia, in contrast with patients with acute liver failure.

During starvation serum glucose levels reflect the balance between endogenous glucose production and peripheral glucose utilization.

In healthy individuals, short-term starvation increases free fatty acid (FFA) concentration, FFA turnover rates, and net fat oxidation rates, with a concomitant increase in plasma ketone body concentrations. In the same period, serum glucose levels, glucose turnover, and glucose clearance rates decrease and net glucose oxidation is reduced. Similar but more intense changes maintain glucose levels during fasting in cirrhotics. In these patients FFA concentration and FFA oxidation rates increase more than in controls, whereas net glucose oxidation is much lower. Thus, the maintenance of normal glucose levels in cirrhotics during fasting is achieved by a shift of fuel source from glucose to fat, thus reducing glucose utilization while lipolysis and fat oxidation are clearly increased [65]. Renal gluconeogenesis may contribute to the defense of cirrhotics from hypoglycemia.

The occurrence of alcohol-induced hypoglycemia is similar in alcoholics with and without liver disease.

### 6.3 Metabolism of Fat and Lipoproteins

The liver synthesizes triglyceride, cholesterol, and phospholipid and degrades fatty acids into smaller molecules able to be used as a source of energy. Cholesterol, cholesterol ester, triglyceride, and phospholipids are the major plasma lipids. All of them are water insoluble. These lipids are transported in plasma by means of their inclusion in macromolecules called lipoproteins which allow these lipidic compounds to remain soluble in an aqueous medium [40, 41].

Cirrhosis leads to changes in the serum levels of lipids and lipoproteins and to alterations in the activity of enzymes involved in the homeostasis of these substances. In chronic parenchymal liver disease, serum levels of triglyceride and cholesterol are initially normal and decrease in the advanced stages of the disease, whereas the ratio of free to cholesterol ester is already increased in the early stages of cirrhosis. Concerning lipoproteins, VLDL and especially HDL are reduced while triglyceride-rich LDL accumulates to above normal levels in serum. The activities of lecithin-cholesterol acyl transferase (LCAT) and hepatic lipase are decreased [74].

In patients with primary biliary cirrhosis, free and total cholesterol levels are elevated in serum whereas cholesterol ester is decreased. Serum concentrations of HDL are reduced and accumulation of APO E-rich particles (intermediate between LDL and HDL) may be detected. LCAT activity tends to fall with the progression of the disease. Lipoprotein-X, absent in sera from control subjects, can be found in sera from these patients (see Chap. 8).

## 6.4 Protein Synthesis and Metabolism

### *Changes in Protein Metabolism*

The liver synthesizes about 50 g protein daily. Most of the proteins are export proteins which are released into the blood. The liver synthesizes many of the major circulating proteins such as albumin, $\alpha_1$- and $\alpha_2$-globulins, fibrinogen, lipoproteins, transport proteins, ceruloplasmin, transferrin, haptoglobin, proteins belonging to the clotting cascade and the fibrinolytic and antifibrinolytic systems, and proteins limiting the procoagulant activity (Sect. 7.8). The only quantitatively relevant serum proteins not synthesized by the liver are immunoglobulins [40, 41].

In liver cirrhosis the rate of synthesis of proteins is maintained until advanced stages of the disease. However, plasma levels of some of these proteins (e.g., albumin) may be low due to dilution because of increase plasma volume. The release of synthesized protein may be deficient in intermediate stages of cirrhosis, contributing to the fall in blood levels. In advanced stages of cirrhosis, when the parenchymal cell mass is clearly reduced, the production of protein by the liver falls markedly.

Synthesis of proteins belonging to the "acute phase response" is accelerated due to inflammatory activity in the liver. Thus, these proteins may be increased in plasma even in well-advanced disease [75].

### *Changes in Amino Acid Metabolism*

Methionine and the aromatic amino acids phenylalanine, tyrosine, and free tryptophan are increased, whereas the three branched chain amino acids valine, leucine, and isoleucine are decreased. The lowering of the ratio of branched chain to aromatic amino acids is thought to play a role in the development of hepatic encephalopathy [76].

### *Ammonia Metabolism and Synthesis of Urea*

Ammonia is generated from digested protein by the action of bacterial urease in the colon. In healthy subjects, ammonia enters the urea cycle in the liver as substrate for urea formation. In cirrhotic patients, portasystemic shunting and hepatocellular failure allow high amounts of ammonia to enter the systemic circulation. Physiologically, skeletal muscle, and to a lesser extent the brain and other tissues, takes up ammonia to form glutamine. Muscle wasting reduces the amount of ammonia taken up by muscle and blood ammonia levels increase to levels potentially toxic for the central nervous system [40, 41]. Neurotoxicity of ammonia through several mechanisms has been demonstrated, and alterations in ammonia metabolism in cirrhosis are important in the development of hepatic encephalopathy. Since ammonia is an end product of protein catabolism, conditions increasing protein degradation, urea formation, and passage of urea to the colon lead to a greater generation of ammonia by intestinal flora. This is the mechanism by which gastrointestinal bleeding or excessive protein intake can initiate hepatic encephalopathy [77].

### 6.5 Metabolism of Bile Acids and Bile Flow Pathophysiology

See Chap. 8.

### 6.6 Porphyrin Metabolism

See Chap. 26.

### 6.7 Drug Metabolism and Drug Action

A substantial proportion of the commonly used therapeutic agents are taken up and metabolized by the liver. In some cases the biochemical transformation inactivates the drug, while some agents are converted to more active compounds. Metabolites can be returned to the blood in a water-soluble form and eliminated in urine. Other drugs or their derivatives undergo biliary excretion which in most cases is followed by cycling in the enterohepatic circulation. Fecal elimination completes the biliary excretion [78].

#### *Pharmacodynamics and Pharmacokinetics*

In cirrhotic patients, absorption of orally administered drugs may be impaired. On the other hand, a decrease in protein binding with a concomitant increase in free drug levels may occur when serum albumin falls. The volume of distribution may increase owing to the expansion of plasma volume. Hepatic extraction of drugs is reduced because of portasystemic and intrahepatic shunting. Metabolism of drugs in the liver is compromised when the activity of the drug-metabolizing systems decreases. Biliary excretion is especially impaired if a cholestatic component coexists. Consequently, cycling in the enterohepatic circulation, a feature common to many drugs, will be disturbed in cirrhosis. The overall consequence of these alterations is prolongation of the half-lives of many drugs. Therefore, drug overdose may occur with administration of standard doses. Some representative drugs whose half-lives are prolonged in cirrhosis are heparin, propranolol, nifedipine, furosemide, valproic acid, some barbiturates, the benzodiazepines (excluding oxazepam), methadone, meperidine, pentazocine, and a large majority of antibiotics and other drugs of general use [79].

### *Supranormal Responsiveness to Particular Drugs*

Cirrhotic patients are hypersensitive to some drugs whose administration results in effects out of proportion to the dose administered or the serum level attained. Abnormality of the organ(s) targeted by the drug as a consequence of liver cirrhosis is responsible for these unexpected responses. This holds true especially for the effects of CNS depressants on the level of consciousness and for the alterations in renal function induced by nonsteroidal anti-inflammatory drugs. Administration of standard or even reduced doses of CNS depressants such as chlorpromazine, morphine, diazepam, or triazolam to cirrhotic patients may cause responses ranging from slowing of the EEG to precipitation of hepatic encephalopathy and deep coma. These alterations are attributable not to changes in the plasma levels or prolonged half-lives of these drugs but rather to alterations in the target organ secondary to liver cirrhosis. Although the mechanisms of this exaggerated response are unknown, it has been hypothesized that an up-regulation of the GABA–benzodiazepine–barbiturate receptor complex increases the susceptibility of the CNS to agonists [80].

Nonsteroidal anti-inflammatory drugs inhibit prostaglandin synthesis in both healthy and cirrhotic individuals. However, in cirrhotics with ascites, renal function is critically dependent on enhanced synthesis of these vasodilators by the kidney. Prostaglandin inhibition reduces renal blood flow and renal function in cirrhotic patients with ascites but not in normal subjects [81].

### *Drug-Induced Hepatotoxicity*

Because of their role in drug metabolism and/or excretion, the liver and the kidney are especially exposed to drug toxicity. The use of potentially hepatotoxic drugs in cirrhotics must be carefully balanced against the benefits of their administration. The possibility of using safer alternative compounds must always be considered. The development of acute drug toxicity in an already seriously damaged liver may convert a self-limited and moderate hepatotoxic episode into fatal liver failure. The same cautionary note has to be voiced in respect of nephrotoxic drugs, especially in patients with ascites, in whom the development of renal failure increases the risk of death.

### *Enzymatic Induction*

The ability of drugs to induce various forms of cytochrome P-450 is affected by liver disease. In general, normal induction is preserved in early, well-compensated cirrhosis, whereas no or very reduced induction is observed in far-advanced, decompensated disease. This difference is observed with various inducers such as phenobarbital, glutethimide, and phenytoin. It may influence the therapeutic effects of drugs, modify drug–drug interactions, and amplify or limit their toxic effects [82, 83].

# 7 Systemic Derangements

In advanced cirrhosis, the combined effects of portal hypertension and hepatocellular failure have deleterious effects on whole body homeostasis. Virtually no organ or system remains functionally normal. The intensity of the alterations varies widely. Patients with cirrhosis form a wide spectrum ranging from those with a subclinical course to those with progressive multi-systemic dysfunction who ultimately die as a result of major complications of the disease.

## 7.1 Circulatory System

In cirrhotics, derangements of systemic hemodynamics are closely associated with alterations in renal function (Fig. 6) and with changes in the activity of neurohumoral systems controlling extracellular fluid volume homeostasis.

It has been a matter of debate whether the retention of sodium and water in liver cirrhosis is primary or secondary to ascites formation. Both concepts were apparently supported by clinical and experimental data so that two opposite views, the so-called underfilling and overflow theories, were proposed (see Chap. 12). Recently a third explanation [84], the peripheral arterial vasodilation hypothesis, has reconciled elements of the two previous theories. This hypothesis considers that the key factor in the initiation and progression of sodium and water retention in cirrhosis is the alteration in systemic hemodynamics.

The essential circulatory changes are: (a) a hyperdynamic circulatory state characterized by decreased total systemic vascular resistance, increased cardiac output, and decreased blood pressure; (b) expansion of plasma volume; and (c) activation of the sympathetic nervous system (SNS), activation of the renin-angiotensin-aldosterone system (RAAS), and, in advanced stages, increased serum levels of arginine vasopressin (AVP), which is released by a nonosmotic mechanism [85–90]. The intensity of these changes varies from patient to patient but roughly parallels the severity of the liver disease. The hyperdynamic circulatory state is mild or even absent in patients with early cirrhosis without ascites, but severe in those with far-advanced disease, intense sodium retention, and massive ascites.

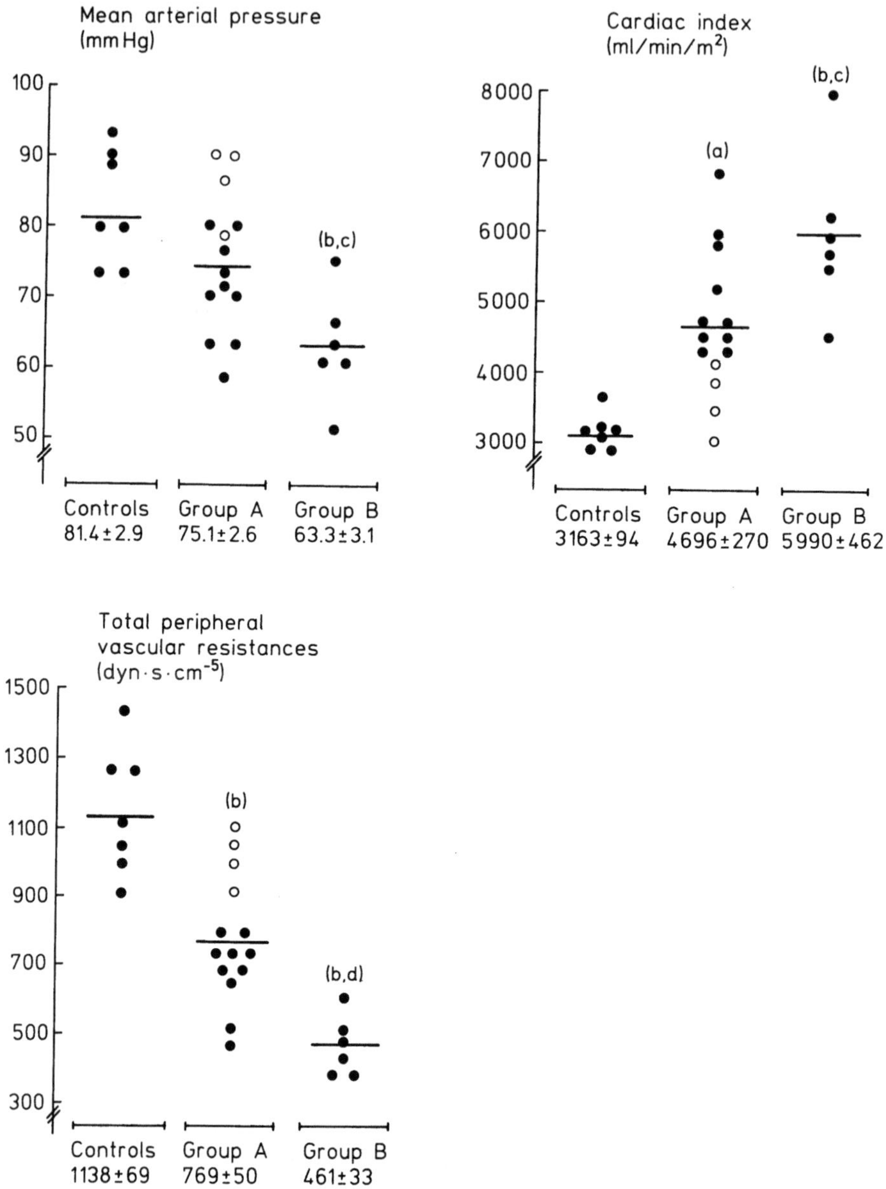


**Fig. 6.** Parameters of systemic hemodynamics in control subjects and in cirrhotic patients with ascites. Values are mean ±SEM. *Group A*: patients with preserved renal function. *Group B*: patients with functional renal failure. In group A, *open circles* denote patients who underwent spontaneous natriuresis and lost weight during the 5-day equilibration period preceding the study. Statistical significance: (*a*) $P < 0.05$ vs controls; (*b*) $P < 0.01$ vs controls; (*c*) $P < 0.05$ vs group A; (*d*) $P < 0.01$ vs group A. (Reproduced with permission from FERNANDEZ-SEARA et al. [90])

***Pathogenesis of the Hyperdynamic Circulation***

*Peripheral Vasodilation.* A decrease in systemic vascular resistance is the initial change that leads to the hyperdynamic circulation. When systemic vascular resistance falls, blood pressure drops and cardiac output increases in compensation. The fall in systemic vascular resistance is due to an abnormal peripheral arterial vasodilation and to the opening of arteriovenous fistulae [84] which takes place predominantly but not exclusively in the splanchnic vascular bed [84, 91]. Extrasplanchnic vasodilation has also been observed in human and experimental cirrhosis [89–92]. Pioneer hemodynamic studies in cirrhotics had already demonstrated increased blood flow to the cutaneous and muscular vascular beds together with hot skin and a bounding pulse [93].

The peripheral arterial vasodilation causes an imbalance between the holding capacity of the vasculature (which increases) and the intravascular content (which is initially normal). As a result, the fraction of the total blood volume filling the central areas of the arterial tree (the so-called effective blood volume) decreases. Direct estimation of central blood volume confirmed its low value in cirrhotic patients [94]. Clinically, the first effect of peripheral vasodilation is a small reduction in blood pressure which triggers the activation of compensatory mechanisms.

*Homeostatic Response and the Onset of Sodium Retention.* The "central arterial underfilling" stimulates carotid and aortic high-pressure receptors and probably baroceptors or volume receptors located in the kidneys and other areas of the vascular bed [95]. The homeostatic response is directed to the restoration of blood pressure to normal through the activation of the SNS and RAAS and consequent increases in plasma norepinephrine, plasma renin activity, and plasma aldosterone concentration [96, 97]. These systems increase vascular tone and induce renal retention of sodium and water, thus expanding plasma volume. In patients with early cirrhosis this response returns blood pressure to normal, thereby attenuating the activity of the RAAS and SNS. However, the hemodynamic equilibrium is established at a level of intravascular volume above physiologic values. This excess of fluid is necessary to normalize blood pressure. In nonascitic cirrhotics, if plasma volume is lowered by decreasing sodium intake, blood pressure falls and the SNS and RAAS are again activated, as has recently been demonstrated [98]. Therefore, the maintenance of normal blood pressure in cirrhotic patients requires expansion of the plasma volume and the extent of this expansion will depend on the intensity of peripheral vasodilation.

*Progression of the Hemodynamic Disturbances and Ascites Formation.* Plasma volume cannot be expanded indefinitely. Rather, the upper limit for volume expansion is determined by the equilibrium of the Starling forces at capillary level [95]. Edema develops when hydrostatic pressure exceeds plasma oncotic pressure. In liver cirrhosis, portal hypertension localizes the edema in the peritoneal cavity in the form of ascites. This takes place when the imbalance of the Starling forces occurs at sinusoidal level (see Chap. 12).

*Chronology of Changes in Circulation, Renal Function, and Neurohumoral Systems.* Arterial vasodilation is an early event in the evolution of cirrhosis which precedes the overactivation of the pressor and sodium-retaining systems, the onset of renal sodium retention, the expansion of the plasma volume, and the formation of ascites [84]. In cirrhotic rats the fall in blood pressure occurs before hyperaldosteronism is observed, and the latter, in turn, heralds the onset of renal sodium retention. Ascites formation starts after several days of positive sodium balance [99, 100].

*The Spectrum of the Hyperdynamic Circulation.* The intensity of hemodynamic disturbances is greater in patients with ascites than in non-ascitic patients. The most severe hyperdynamic state has been described in ascitic subjects with functional renal failure [90].

### *Mechanisms of Vasodilation*

Splanchnic vasodilation is likely to account for most of the reduction in systemic vascular resistance in cirrhosis. The cause of this vasodilation is unknown. However, it has been shown experimentally that the graded interruption of portal blood flow to the liver is followed immediately by proportional increases in hepatic artery blood flow [101]. This suggests that splanchnic vasodilation may be a compensatory phenomenon to maintain liver blood flow. According to experimental data and indirect calculations in patients, vascular resistance in the splanchnic vascular bed decreases progressively from the initial to the final stages of cirrhosis.

Splanchnic blood flow has been estimated in cirrhotic patients and directly measured in cirrhotic animals. In both cases, variable but large increases above normal values have been observed. Vasodilation of nonsplanchnic territories has also been demonstrated in animals with experimental cirrhosis. In cirrhotic patients the number of studies evaluating extrasplanchnic flows is very limited. However, high cutaneous and muscular blood flow has been reported [93], and recently vasodilation and increased blood flow to the femoral territory were observed in cirrhotic patients with ascites [90].

### *Mediators of Vasodilation*

*Increased Vasodilator Activity.* Vasodilators such as prostacyclin, glucagon, vasoactive intestinal polypeptide, substance P, histamine, GABA, and enkephalins, are elevated in systemic blood of patients and animals with liver cirrhosis [102]. These compounds, which are mainly generated in the splanchnic area, are elevated in blood due to portal-collateral shunting, deficient hepatic degradation, and, in some cases, overproduction [103]. It is thought that they contribute to the vasodilation of cirrhosis. Glucagon appears to be the most relevant quantitatively [104]. Preliminary studies in cirrhotic rats suggest that the endothelium-derived relaxing factor (nitric oxide), a powerful vasodilator, may be involved in the vasodilation of cirrhosis, since its inhibition reverses the hemodynamic disturbances in these animals [105].

*Altered Vasopressor Activity.* The main known vasoconstrictors, angiotensin II, catecholamines, and AVP, display high levels in cirrhosis [84]. Exogenous endothelin given to cirrhotic rats decreases the intensity of the hyperdynamic circulation [106]. The role of endothelin in the hemodynamic changes of cirrhosis remains to be established; however, endothelin has been found to be increased in the kidney in patients with functional renal failure [107], probably contributing to renal vasoconstriction.

*Impaired Vascular Response to Vasoconstrictors.* Angiotensin II and norepinephrine have a lesser hypertensive effect in cirrhotics than in normal subjects [106]. Whether this is due to a true resistance of the vascular wall or to the counteracting effect of high concentrations of vasodilators remains to be established.

*The Cause of Peripheral Arterial Vasodilation.* The primary cause of peripheral arterial vasodilation in cirrhosis remains unknown: it is not clear whether portal hypertension or hepatocellular failure is predominantly responsible. Since a hyperdynamic circulation also occurs in prehepatic portal hypertension, the increase in portal pressure appears to be critical in the induction of splanchnic vasodilation. However, it has been shown in cirrhotic rats that the onset of vasodilation occurs just after liver function falls below a critical threshold [108], and that the same is true of renal sodium retention [109]. These findings are in keeping with previous studies demonstrating that renal sodium retention in alcoholic cirrhotics is more closely correlated with liver function than with portal hypertension [110].

## 7.2 **Renal Function** (see Chap. 12)

Renal sodium retention, renal water retention, and the development of a particular form of renal failure, so-called functional renal failure or the hepatorenal syndrome, are the abnormalities of renal function characteristic of patients with liver cirrhosis.

Renal sodium retention in cirrhosis occurs in the presence of a normal glomerular filtration rate and is due to renal sodium hyperreabsorption in both the proximal and the distal tubules. The tendency to retain sodium may be without clinical consequences if the patient is receiving a low sodium diet but it may lead to edema formation if sodium intake is high. A positive sodium balance occurs in patients who are unable to excrete all the ingested sodium; such a balance is found in the preascitic phase and during active ascites formation. Renal sodium output is virtually absent in some patients. A negative sodium balance is observed during elimination of ascites either spontaneously or through the effect of diuretics [110].

Renal water retention always occurs in cirrhotics with ascites and reflects a noticeable degree of arterial underfilling which leads to nonosmotic activation of AVP release. Mechanisms of renal water retention include: (a) diminished delivery of fluid to the diluting segments of the nephron, (b) increased AVP levels, and (c) reduced renal synthesis of prostaglandin $E_2$. This prostaglandin is important in that it antagonizes the distal tubular effects of AVP. Patients who retain water frequently develop hyponatremia, which may be aggravated by vigorous diuretic therapy [111].

Functional renal insufficiency or HRS refers to a particular type of renal failure developing essentially in cirrhotics with ascites. HRS occurs in the absence of structural renal damage; it is associated with avid renal sodium retention, preserved tubular function, and a tendency toward oliguria. Patients with HRS show an extreme activation of the RAAS, the SNS, and AVP. The hallmark of HRS is severe renal vasoconstriction with reduced renal blood flow. The cause of renal vasoconstriction seems to be an imbalance between vasoconstrictor and vasodilator forces acting on the kidney, since pressor systems are highly activated while the compensatory increase in the renal synthesis of kinins and vasodilative prostaglandins is abolished, with values of these substances in the range of control subjects or even lower [112].

## 7.3 Respiratory System

### *Respiratory Diseases Associated with Specific Forms of Cirrhosis*

Panacinar pulmonary emphysema develops in patients homozygous for the ZZ or the SS variants of the $\alpha_1$-antitrypsin phenotype. The prevalence of fibrosing alveolitis is higher in patients with chronic active hepatitis or primary biliary cirrhosis than in the general population, an association thought to have an immunologic basis. In a large series of patients with primary biliary cirrhosis there was an impairment in $DL_{CO}$ (carbon monoxide diffusing capacity) and its intensity was directly correlated with the histopathologic stage and with the "Mayo Clinic risk score" [113]. No patient in this series had reduced lung volumes or radiologic signs of interstitial lung disease [113]. The mechanism of this disorder remains to be explained.

### *Idiopathic Pulmonary Hypertension*

On the basis of autopsy data, idiopathic pulmonary hypertension was reported to be more prevalent in cirrhotics (0.63%) than in the general population (0.13%). Recently, pulmonary hypertension was observed in 2% of 507 patients with portal hypertension. The risk of developing pulmonary hypertension seems to increase with the duration of portal hypertension without displaying any significant relationship with its severity, the degree of hepatic failure, or the extent of portasystemic shunting [114].

### *Respiratory Disorders Related to the Presence of Ascites*

*Ascitic Hydrothorax ("Pleural Ascites").* A particular form of pleural effusion due to accumulation of ascitic fluid in the pleural space can occur in cirrhotics with ascites in whom defects in the diaphragm allow direct thoracoabdominal communication. During inspiration, intrathoracic pressure becomes negative whereas intra-abdominal pressure increases, leading to aspiration of ascites into the pleural space. Rarely, large pleural effusions are present without clinically detectable ascites. The presence in the pleural space of labeled serum albumin shortly after its injection into the peritoneal cavity confirms the abdominal origin of the pleural fluid. If isotope scanning is used for detection, selective accumulation of the tracer in the pleural space is demonstrated [115].

*Pleural Effusion.* Pleural effusion unrelated to anatomic failure of the diaphragm is found in about 5% of cirrhotics; it is most common in those with advanced disease and ascites or with generalized edema. Pleural effusion may be unilateral or bilateral, with predominance of the right side. It must be differentiated from pleural effusions of infectious or neoplastic origin.

*Atelectasis.* Atelectasis of areas of the lung parenchyma near the diaphragm is frequent in patients with tense ascites, especially when pleural effusion is present. Poor ventilation and compression of these areas by the elevated diaphragm lead to mechanical atelectasis. In general, linear or segmental atelectasis is seen, although in severe cases lobar collapse may occur. Local accumulation of secretions may contribute to atelectasis and to superinfection.

Patients with atelectasis show tachypnea, shortness of breath, and a tendency to develop fatigue of the respiratory muscles, especially if the nutritional state is deficient or hypokalemia is present. Dyspnea at rest is very frequent. It worsens with decubitus and with very mild physical activity. Patients with tense ascites may show a similar clinical picture despite the absence of atelectasis.

### *The Hepatopulmonary Syndrome*

Arterial hypoxemia without evidence of respiratory or cardiac disease is detected in about one-third of patients with cirrhosis and constitutes the hallmark of the so-called hepatopulmonary syndrome (HPS) [116]. One of the characteristics of this syndrome is its reversibility after liver transplantation [52, 116–125].

On clinical grounds, exertional dyspnea occurs in about one-third of cirrhotics with moderate to advanced disease, but only a minority of patients are cyanosed (cyanosis may be easily missed in jaundiced patients). Finger clubbing and, rarely, hypoxic osteoarthropathy may be observed in cases with severe hypoxemia [48–50, 113].

The pathogenesis of HPS is incompletely understood. Although signs of respiratory dysfunction were described in cirrhotics more than a century ago, this issue has received little attention until recent years. The multiple inert gases elimination technique has been especially valuable in the elucidation of mechanisms implicated in HPS [117].

#### *Blood Gases*

In the majority of patients there is a mild to moderate resting arterial hypoxemia. In different series of patients evaluated for liver transplantation, $PaO_2$ below 70 mmHg was observed in 18%–28% of the cases. Arterial hypoxemia is worsened by physical exertion [119, 120]. Hyperventilation at rest associated with mild hypocapnia ($PaCO_2$: 30–35 mmHg) and respiratory alkalosis (pH up to 7.50) is a frequent finding, even in normoxemic cirrhotics. A widened alveolar–arterial difference in $PO_2$ [$P(A\text{-}a)O_2$] is present in more than 50% of cirrhotics regardless of the presence or absence of arterial hypoxemia [52, 121].

#### *Lung Volumes, Ventilatory Patterns, and Diffusion of Gases*

Obstructive airways disease plays no significant role in HPS. A mild to moderate decrease in FEF25–FEF75 indicating peripheral airways obstruction, and a closing volume in the range of the tidal volume have been reported in some cirrhotics [123–125]. Severe airways obstruction with $FEV_1/FVC$ less than 50% is extremely infrequent; even in subjects who have been or are smokers, it is found in only 5% and 8% respectively [118]. It is of clinical interest that although propranolol slightly decreases FEF25–75 in cirrhotics, it is well tolerated, improves $P(A\text{-}a)O_2$, and does not cause a deterioration in $PaO_2$ [122].

A restrictive ventilatory pattern (total lung capacity ≤80% of predicted value) was observed in 25% of 116 patients with advanced liver disease [118]. However, only a minority of those concerned had an associated impairment of $DL_{CO}$. All patients with decreased total lung capacity and normal $DL_{CO}$ values had ascites, often in association with pleural effusion. Thus, mechanical restriction of obvious origin occurs in most cirrhotic patients with decreased lung volumes.

Variable results have been reported concerning pulmonary diffusion in liver cirrhosis. A reduced $DL_{CO}$ was observed in 0%–52% of the patients evaluated in recently published series [58, 118–121, 123–125]. However, an isolated impairment of $DL_{CO}$ seems to lack clinical relevance.

### *Pulmonary Circulation*

Abnormalities in the pulmonary circulation are likely to be the major determining factor of HPS. At rest the pulmonary circulation is hyperkinetic due to pulmonary vasodilation and, in some patients, opening of arteriovenous shunts. Pulmonary vascular resistance is less than half of normal values. Cardiac output is proportionally increased [58, 117, 123, 125]. Pulmonary vasoconstriction occurs physiologically in response to alveolar hypoxia. This mechanism, which prevents $\mathring{V}/\mathring{Q}$ mismatching, is impaired in cirrhotic patients [117, 125]. During physical exertion normal subjects meet the increased oxygen demand by increasing cardiac output together with pulmonary vasodilation. This response is absent or reduced in patients with cirrhosis in whom pulmonary vasodilation at rest is so extreme that no further decrease in pulmonary vascular resistance can be achieved [117, 126].

Anatomic abnormalities of the pulmonary vascular bed, such as telangiectasia, vascular spiders, arteriovenous communications, and markedly dilated vessels have been demonstrated in liver cirrhosis, especially in the basal lobes of the lungs. Pleural vessels may show similar abnormalities [48–50].

## ***Mechanisms of Arterial Hypoxemia***

*Ventilation/Perfusion ($\mathring{V}/\mathring{Q}$) Mismatching* [117, 121–128]. The reduction in pulmonary vasoconstriction in response to alveolar hypoxia in an already abnormally vasodilated pulmonary vascular bed implies that nonventilated areas will be overperfused. The resulting $\mathring{V}/\mathring{Q}$ mismatching generates functional right-to-left shunting which leads to arterial hypoxemia. In liver cirrhosis, the existence of nonventilated respiratory units is mainly due to the presence of tense ascites, pleural effusion, and, occasionally, atelectasis in the lung bases. However, even in the absence of nonventilated units, disproportionately high perfusion to some lung areas may alter $\mathring{V}/\mathring{Q}$ matching. Cirrhotic patients show the most markedly dilated pulmonary vessels at the lung bases. This may explain why hypoxemia worsens in cirrhotics when they move from decubitus to the standing position. This phenomenon, which has been called orthodeoxia by ROBIN et al. [123], is due to blood redistribution to dependent areas of the lungs as a result of the postural change. Orthodeoxia is observed in 10%–20% of cirrhotics. Platypnea refers to the dyspnea occurring in less than 10% of the patients upon assumption of the standing position. $\mathring{V}/\mathring{Q}$ mismatching is thought to be the main mechanism responsible for arterial hypoxemia in subjects with moderately advanced cirrhosis.

*Right-to-Left Shunting (Anatomic).* Right-to-left shunting due to pulmonary arteriovenous communications contributes to arterial deoxygenation in some patients. Anatomic and functional evidence of the presence of anatomic right-to-left shunts of variable size has been obtained. As a rule, the extent of shunting is small, although figures higher than 20% of the cardiac output have been reported. Shunting is greater in advanced than in early stages of cirrhosis and may be the leading cause of hypoxemia in the former group of patients.

*Portal-Pulmonary Shunting.* Portal-pulmonary shunting is quantitatively not important in a vast majority of cirrhotics and plays a minor role in arterial hypoxemia.

*Abnormalities in Oxygen Diffusion.* An increased alveolar–arterial $PO_2$ difference is a characteristic finding in cirrhotics. The apparent disturbance in oxygen diffusion is not due to alterations of the alveolar–arterial membrane; rather it is secondary to marked pulmonary vasodilation and high blood flow. Studies using the multiple inert gases elimination technique have been of particular value in the characterization of this abnormality. The normal diameter of gas-exchanging capillaries is about 8–15 μm, while in cirrhotics it may reach up to 60 μm. It is thought that red blood cells in the midstream of these extremely dilated pulmonary capillaries cannot be oxygenated due to the increased diffusion distance and the shortened transit time of the blood in the pulmonary circulation. In fact, only a few cirrhotic patients show findings of interstitial lung disease on chest radiographs.

*Decreased Hemoglobin–Oxygen Affinity.* Hemoglobin from cirrhotic patients has a decreased affinity for oxygen, due to an increased erythrocyte content of 2,3-diphosphoglycerate [129]. As a result, the hemoglobin–oxygen dissociation curve is shifted to the right.

### *The Spectrum of HPS*

The pulmonary and systemic circulations show parallel degrees of hyperkinesis. In one study, patients were grouped according to the presence or absence of vascular spiders on the skin [58]. It was shown that patients with vascular spiders had more severe hepatocellular dysfunction, greater disturbance of systemic and pulmonary hemodynamics, a greater reduction in the hypoxia-induced pulmonary vasoconstriction, and more severe arterial hypoxemia.

#### *HPS and Liver Transplantation*

Clinically, problems arising from HPS are restricted to patients with severe arterial hypoxemia or with associated respiratory diseases. It is important to emphasize that the HPS is fully reversed after successful liver grafting [130], and that severe HPS may therefore now represent an indication for liver transplantation rather than a contraindication.

### 7.4 Central Nervous System

***Hepatic Encephalopathy/Portal-Systemic Encephalopathy*** (see also Chap. 10)

Hepatic encephalopathy is a general term usually employed with reference to the alterations in the level of consciousness or higher cerebral functions that occur in cirrhotic patients in the absence of signs of structural brain damage. Hepatic encephalopathy is caused by metabolic disturbances; it is "functional" and reversible, although anatomic correlates have been described [131, 132].

The prototype of hepatic encephalopathy is portal-systemic encephalopathy (PSE), which occurs almost exclusively in patients with advanced cirrhosis and portal hypertension. Although clinically indistinguishable from encephalopathies caused by different mechanisms and from the encephalopathy of fulminant hepatic failure, PSE has individual pathogenetic and pathophysiologic features. It is dependent on the extent of portasystemic shunting, which allows substances toxic to the CNS to gain access directly to the systemic blood, bypassing the liver. Indeed, patients undergoing surgical portasystemic shunts frequently develop PSE. This complication occurs not only in patients with portacaval anastomosis but also in those with splenorenal shunts. The severity of hepatocellular failure also influences the development of this complication.

Recently Conn has proposed that hepatic encephalopathy should be classified into different categories [131]. According to this author, true PSE is induced by nitrogenous compounds, as in cases of azotemia, gastrointestinal bleeding, dietary protein excess, constipation, or diuretic-induced hypokalemic alkalosis. In all of these conditions PSE is associated with abnormally high blood ammonia levels. PSE accounts for up to 60% of episodes of encephalopathy in cirrhotic patients. The remaining episodes are induced by factors which do not increase the blood ammonia concentration and are classified as pseudo-PSE. Principal among these latter factors is the administration of CNS depressants, especially benzodiazepines and barbiturates. Other causes are metabolic, such as acid-base disturbances, hypoglycemia, hypomagnesemia, hyponatremia, and hypokalemia [131, 132].

Clinically, PSE may be acute or chronic; the latter form is seen predominantly in cirrhotic patients with surgical portasystemic shunts. Patients with hepatofugal portal-collateral circulation and large gastric varices with spontaneous splenorenal shunts are more prone to develop PSE than patients with hepatopetal portal blood flow and high flow towards the esophageal plexus and the azygos vein [133].

The clinical spectrum of PSE varies from no detectable abnormality to irreversible coma. Compromised functions include the state of consciousness, intellectual performance, behavior and personality, and neuromuscular activities. The severity of PSE ranges from grade I (mild) to grade IV (deep coma). Initial PSE is difficult to recognize unless a detailed history is taken and a full neurologic examination performed. Data provided by relatives of the patient are very useful in evaluating changes in mood, behavior, and personality. Subtle disturbances in several areas of intellectual function (memory, visual-spatial ability, problem-solving capacity, calculation, etc.) and changes in sleep pattern should be sought. In more advanced stages, neurologic impairment is easily recognizable. However, the immediate diagnosis of PSE in any cirrhotic presenting with a diminished level of consciousness is a not uncommon, and sometimes fatal, clinical error. In addition to metabolic disturbances which may mimic PSE, subarachnoid hemorrhage, subdural hematoma, CNS infections, and cerebral masses should be ruled out.

Typically, patients present asterixis (flapping tremor) (see Chap. 10). Asterixis is not specific to PSE and may occur in other metabolic encephalopathies.

Other methods of assessing the presence and the severity of PSE include the use of neuropsychological tests which can detect subclinical alterations of mental function, the determination of blood ammonia levels, and EEG registration, which shows diffuse slowing with waves of increased amplitude and decreased frequency associated with the occurrence of triphasic waves. None of these signs is specific. The usefulness of visual evoked potentials for the diagnosis of PSE is under study [134]. In recent years attention has focused on auditory evoked potentials. The latency of the P-300 event-related potential was found to be significantly increased in encephalopathic patients as compared with nonecephalopathic cirrhotics and control subjects [135]. The search for rapid, specific, and sensitive methods to diagnose PSE continues. It should be recalled that several studies have demonstrated that making use of neuropsychological tests and EEG 30%–60% of cirrhotic patients regarded as neurogically normal show abnormalities related to subclinical PSE.

Recently, BERNTHAL et al. have reported cerebral CT scan abnormalities in cirrhotics which correlated with deficiencies in neuropsychological testing

[136]. Specifically, the bicaudate diameter and the bicaudate index were both significantly reduced as compared with normal values. Overall, these observations indicate the presence of cerebral atrophy confined to the anterior cortical region. It is currently considered that some degree of structural CNS damage results from long-term cirrhosis even in patients with no clinical evidence of PSE. Pathologic changes in the brain are mild in most of the patients. Alzheimer's type II astrocytes are present in most cases of long-standing cirrhosis.

#### *Hepatocerebral Degeneration and Portal-Systemic Myelopathy*

A few cirrhotic patients develop serious histopathologic lesions of the CNS affecting the gray matter, which may suffer severe neuron loss. Basal ganglia are predominantly affected although lesions may be diffuse, resembling spongiform encephalopathies. This picture constitutes the so-called hepatocerebral degeneration, which occurs in cases of chronic and severe PSE and, most frequently, in subjects with surgical portasystemic anastomoses. Frequent manifestations are dementia of variable degree, athetosis, dystonia, or other abnormalities of motion due to lesions in the basal ganglia, although other deficits may also occur [137].

A rare condition known as portal-systemic myelopathy, which develops in patients with protracted PSE, may lead to demyelination of the pyramidal tracts, causing spastic paraplegia due to transverse myelitis. Milder forms may show any combination of signs of pyramidal involvement [138].

In spite of the presence of structural lesions, patients with the hepatocerebral syndrome may improve considerably after liver transplantation. Thus hepatocerebral degeneration must not be regarded as an absolute contraindication to liver grafting [139].

#### *CNS Damage Associated with Particular Etiologies of Cirrhosis*

Damage to the CNS in Wilson's disease (Chap. 23) arises due to copper deposition in the brain. Alcoholic cirrhosis may be associated with several CNS syndromes due to alcohol toxicity or to secondary nutritional deficiencies. Wernicke's encephalopathy, Korsakoff's dementia, and alcoholic cerebellar degeneration are the commonest forms. In addition, alcoholic polyneuropathy may also occur.

### 7.5 Digestive System

#### *Lesions with a Potential for Bleeding*

Upper gastrointestinal hemorrhage is a life-threatening complication of liver cirrhosis. Esophageal and gastric varices, congestive gastropathy, peptic ulcers, and the mucosal tears of Mallory-Weiss syndrome account for the vast majority of bleeding episodes in cirrhotics. Bleeding from the hemorrhoidal venous plexus is rarely severe, and rupture of varices at other atypical anatomic sites (duodenum, jejunum, gallbladder, colon) is very infrequent. Regardless of the bleeding lesion, the final outcome in patients with upper gastrointestinal hemorrhage is influenced by the function of the hemostatic and clotting mechanisms.

*Esophageal and Gastric Varices.* Variceal rupture is the most important cause of acute hemorrhage and one of the leading causes of death in cirrhosis. This complication is extensively covered in Chap. 11.

*Peptic Ulcers.* Peptic ulcers are two to three times more frequent in cirrhotics than in the general population, so that 10%–15% of cirrhotics have this additional source of bleeding [140]. These ulcers were once tentatively attributed to gastric hypersecretion induced by the high serum levels of histamine and gastrin due to the impaired hepatic degradation of these secretagogues. However, hyposecretion rather than hypersecretion of gastric acid predominates in these patients. Recent studies have demonstrated decreased synthesis of prostaglandin $E_2$ in the gastric mucosa of cirrhotics with portal hypertension. The lowest values of prostaglandin $E_2$ were observed in patients with ulcers and especially in those with mucosal congestion [141]. Since prostaglandin $E_2$ has a well-known cytoprotective and antiulcerogenic effect, its deficient production may be important in the pathogenesis of ulcers.

*Mallory-Weiss Syndrome.* Acute arterial bleeding from lacerations in the mucosa of the gastroesophageal junction (Mallory-Weiss syndrome) is more prevalent in cirrhotics than in noncirrhotic subjects. From less than 1% to 16% of all episodes of upper gastrointestinal bleeding have been reported to be due to Mallory-Weiss syndrome by different authors [142]. Retching (39%), alcohol consumption (58%), and intake of nonsteroidal anti-inflammatory drugs (9%) have been identified as potential predisposing factors. In general, Mallory-Weiss syndrome is not life threatening, and it is the most easily controllable form of gastrointestinal bleeding in cirrhotics.

*Congestive Gastropathy.* Congestive gastropathy is characterized by the presence of vascular ectasias in the gastric mucosa with no or mild inflammation. This condition has recently been identified as a specific cause of bleeding in liver cirrhosis [143]. Mucosal changes have been related to the severity of portal hypertension and reflect the abnormal vascularization of the entire wall of the stomach, which has been previously demonstrated by anatomic studies [144]. In a recent report, congestive gastropathy was found at admission in 53 of 212 (27%) cirrhotics and developed in 73 additional patients (33%) during a mean follow-up of 46 months [145]. The prevalence of *Helicobacter pylori* is the same in cirrhotics with and without congestive gastropathy, suggesting that this agent plays no pathogenetic role [145]. Endoscopically, mild congestive gastropathy consists of multiple erythematous areas outlined by a white reticular network (mosaic-like pattern) or fine pink speckling (scarlatina-like pattern) [143, 145]. In severe forms, cherry red spots on a finely granular mucosa with or without associated spontaneous bleeding are seen. Mucosal involvement may be generalized (as in about 40%–50%) or restricted to the antrum (50%–55%) or, very rarely, to the fundus and fornix [145]. Histopathologically, superficial capillary vessels are congestive and increased in number. In severe forms this picture changes towards an architectural distortion of the mucosa with more congestion and ectasia in the small vessels, development of gland atrophy, hyperplasia of the muscularis mucosae, and presence of edema. Clinically, congestive gastropathy may cause chronic bleeding and recurrent iron-deficient anemia, although overt bleeding may also occur. Prior variceal sclerotherapy appears to be a significant risk factor for the development of congestive gastropathy [145].

*Other Causes of Gastrointestinal Bleeding.* Varices atypically located in the digestive tract, in the gallbladder, on the peritoneal surface, or in the hemorrhoidal venous plexus are possible but very infrequent sources of bleeding in cirrhosis. Acute erosive gastritis, especially in alcoholic patients, is common and may cause severe hemorrhage.

### *Cholelithiasis*

The prevalence of cholelithiasis is increased among cirrhotics. Stones are predominantly of calcium bilirubinate.

Mechanisms leading to the formation of this kind of gallstone in patients with liver cirrhosis remain to be defined. However, the most likely predisposing factor is chronic hemolysis secondary to hypersplenism [48–50].

### *Malabsorption and Diarrhea*

In cirrhotics the size of the bile salt pool is reduced and the excretion of bile salts by the liver is impaired. Deficiency of these compounds in the intestine may compromise fat digestion and absorption. Many cirrhotics have subclinical fat malabsorption, which may contribute to malnutrition. In primary biliary cirrhosis and other cholestatic disorders, malabsorption of fat and fat-soluble vitamins may be sufficiently severe to produce steatorrhea and deficiency of fat-soluble vitamins (see Chap. 8). In alcoholic cirrhosis the effect of alcohol on the intestinal mucosa may reduce the absorption of some nutrients. Folate malabsorption is common and this leads to folate deficiency, which may cause mucosal damage besides its hematologic effects. In advanced cirrhosis with severe portal hypertension and hypoalbuminemia, the intestinal mucosa may be edematous and this may be partly responsible for malabsorption and diarrhea. Serum electrolyte disturbances, especially hyponatremia, alter normal intestinal peristalsis and may predispose to bacterial overgrowth which in turn may provoke diarrhea and malabsorption [48–50].

*Pancreatic Function*

Bouts of acute pancreatitis and exocrine pancreatic insufficiency due to chronic pancreatitis may be seen in patients with alcoholic cirrhosis. Mucoviscidosis is able to produce both chronic pancreatitis and secondary biliary cirrhosis. Hemochromatosis affects both divisions of the pancreatic function. Alterations of the exocrine secretion pass unnoticed, whereas endocrine damage leads to diabetes.

*Other Disorders of the Digestive System*

*Parotid enlargement* due to gland hypertrophy is typical of alcoholic cirrhosis, but it may develop early in cirrhosis of other etiology. It has been attributed to nutritional deficiencies and is associated with salivary hypersecretion. The parotid is soft and nontender and is not adhered to underlying tissues [50]. *Vomiting and nonspecific abdominal discomfort* are frequent, especially in alcoholic cirrhotics. Alcohol directly damages gastric mucosa and is probably responsible for some episodes of acute erosive gastritis. Hydroelectrolytic disorders, abnormal transit time of meals in the intestine, and distention due to ascites or accumulation of gases may cause unspecific abdominal complaints. Umbilical, scrotal, or inguinal herniations may occur secondary to ascites.

## 7.6 Endocrine System

Cirrhotic patients show abnormalities at various levels in the endocrine system, reflecting either secondary adaptive changes or primary gland malfunction.

***Hypothalamus-Pituitary-Gonadal Axis***

*Gonadal Failure and Feminization*

Males with liver cirrhosis exhibit clinical evidence of hypogonadism and feminization. Hypogonadism is manifested in men by loss of libido and sexual potency. Oligo- and azoospermia are very common, and prostatic hyperplasia is less prevalent in cirrhotics than in healthy men of similar age. In women, hypogonadism causes loss of libido, amenorrhea or erratic and sparse menstruation, ovulatory failure with sterility, and early occurrence of menopause. The biochemical hallmark of hypogonadism is the underproduction of testosterone in men and of estradiol and progesterone in women [146, 147].

The presence of feminine habitus and hair distribution and the development of gynecomastia (seen in 20%–30% of patients) are the main manifestations of feminization in cirrhotic males. It should be noted, however, that spironolactone therapy accounts for a significant proportion of cases of gynecomastia. The presence of vascular spiders and palmar erythema are also thought to be consequences of feminization but their origin is less clear.

### *Mechanisms of Hypogonadism*

Disturbed function of the hypothalamus, pituitary, and testes is responsible for hypogonadism. These endocrine changes are secondary to cirrhosis but they are much more prominent in alcoholic cirrhotics and alcohol is considered to play a major role in their development [146–148].

Alcoholic cirrhotics show testicular atrophy with failure of both the endocrine and the reproductive functions. The seminiferous tubules are reduced in size and contain few or no germ cells. Serum testosterone levels are low in about half of the cases, and borderline values are seen in most of the remainder. Testosterone-binding globulin is increased, further reducing free testosterone values. Alcohol is metabolized in the testes, as in other tissues. The failure of Leydig cells to produce testosterone has been attributed to the toxicity of alcohol or its metabolites. Alcohol inhibits local retinol bioconversion within the testes, alters the testicular redox state (the NAD/NADH ratio is decreased), and inhibits 3β-hydroxysteroid dehydrogenase and isomerase activities. All these changes impair testosterone synthesis. In addition, alcohol depletes Leydig cells of LH receptors and disturbs the function of the hypothalamic-pituitary axis. Serum levels of follicle stimulating hormone (FSH) and luteinizing hormone (LH) are normal or minimally increased in the vast majority of cirrhotics, despite the fact that they exhibit low testosterone levels and oligo- or azoospermia. Thus, the feedback response of the high centers is deficient. The causes of gonadotropin failure are incompletely defined. Gonadotropin releasing hormone (GnRH) is modulated through negative feedback by peripheral hormones. The mediator acting on the hypothalamus is not testosterone but estradiol arising from the peripheral conversion of testosterone. It is possible that increased serum estradiol inhibits GnRH release in cirrhosis. However, in this condition, the response to clomiphene may also be impaired (clomiphene is a nonsteroidal compound with "weak" estrogenic activity which displaces estradiol from its hypothalamic receptors).

Androgen receptors in target tissues are reduced in alcoholic cirrhosis. Thus, tissue insensitivity to testosterone may complement testosterone deficiency in determining hypogonadism [146–149].

Van Thiel et al. [150] observed spontaneous reversal of gonadal failure in 25% of a series of alcoholic men who had abstained from alcohol for at least 6 months. Markers predicting hypogonadism reversal were the absence of testicular atrophy and normal gonadotropin responses to GnRH and clomiphene. Interestingly, administration of exogenous androgens to patients without reversal of hypogonadism resulted in weaker than expected responses, in agreement with the existence of reduced androgen sensitivity [150].

In addition to endocrine and reproductive failure, hypogonadism may contribute to osteopenia, muscular wasting, and progressive weakness.

### *Mechanisms of Feminization*

Feminization of male cirrhotics is more dependent on cirrhosis in itself than on its alcoholic etiology. The mechanisms of feminization are still unclear. Theoretically, estrogen excess, tissue hypersensitivity to estrogen, or both may be involved. Estrone degradation in the liver is decreased due to portasystemic shunting of a fraction of estrone which undergoes enterohepatic circulation. Additional estrone arises from androstenedione, which, leaving the enterohepatic circulation, is converted to estrone in nonendocrine tissues. Thus, serum levels of estrone tend to be increased. It has been proposed that nonsteroid compounds of dietary origin possessing estrogenic activity (isoflavones) might accumulate in cirrhotics, contributing to feminization. Decreased levels of an estrogen binding protein of hepatic origin [146, 147, 151] may also play a role in estrogen hypersensitivity.

### *Gonadal Function in Nonalcoholic Cirrhosis*

Few studies have evaluated hypogonadism and feminization in patients with cirrhosis due to causes other than alcohol, but some differences are known to exist. Fifty percent of patients with hemochromatosis have associated testicular atrophy and gonadal failure. Iron deposition affects the hypothalamus, the hypophysis, and the testes; thus hypogonadism in hemochromatosis has primary and secondary components. The rare occurrence of feminization in hemochromatosis has been tentatively attributed to the low tendency of these patients to develop large-volume collateral circulation [146, 147, 152].

Those forms of liver cirrhosis characterized by increased copper tissue levels, such as Wilson's disease and chronic cholestatic disorders, are associated with increased serum gonadotropin levels but with little or no evidence of gonadal failure. This may be due to the copper-stimulated release of anterior pituitary hormones, an unspecific and well-known effect of this metal [146, 147, 152].

The few studies evaluating gonadal function in postnecrotic cirrhosis suggest that in these patients gonadal failure is less frequent and less severe than in alcoholic cirrhotics [146, 147, 152].

*Gonadal Failure and Liver Transplantation*

Liver transplantation leads to a rapid improvement in gonadal function, with recovery of libido and sexual functioning in men and of normal menstrual cycles in women. Successful pregnancy has been reported in these patients. The stigmata of feminization in cirrhotic men disappear weeks to months after the operation [153, 154].

***Growth Hormone and Insulin-Like Growth Factors I and II***

Growth hormone (GH) is released by the anterior pituitary in an irregular and intermittent fashion, with peak levels occurring during stages 3 and 4 of sleep. It is under stimulatory (GRH) and inhibitory (somatostatin) hormonal control. GH stimulates the release of two polypeptides which mediate most of its peripheral actions. These substances, formerly called somatomedins C and A, and now known as insulin-like growth factor I (IGF-I) and II (IGF-II), share the anabolic properties of insulin and may bind to its receptor. Both IGF-I and IGF-II are synthesized in several peripheral tissues, including bone, brain, gastrointestinal tract, kidney, fibroblasts, and chondrocytes. However, the main source of IGF-I is the liver, where IGF-I is synthesized and released in response to the binding of GH to its hepatic receptors. Synthesis of IGF-II has also been demonstrated in fetal liver [155, 156].

Serum GH levels are increased severalfold in cirrhotic patients [157] and are not suppressed by glucose injection. GH receptors are reduced in the cirrhotic liver and serum IGF-I levels are markedly diminished. IGF-I deficiency parallels the severity of hepatocellular failure [158, 159]. Whether the increase in serum GH represents a feedback response to IGF-I deficiency is unknown. The increase in GH in cirrhosis has been attributed to hyperestrogenemia since estrogen is a well-known stimulator of GH release. The consequences of GH excess and IGF-I deficiency in liver cirrhosis have not been extensively evaluated.

Increased GH levels decrease carbohydrate utilization because of the induction of insulin resistance acting at a postreceptor level, and this causes hyperinsulinemia. However, the deficiency of IGF-I may be expected to blunt the actions of GH that depend on this mediator. Effects of IGF-I include enhancement of protein synthesis and reduction of protein breakdown with incorporation of amino acid into protein, incorporation of glucose into adipose tissue, and inhibition of lipolysis. In addition, IGF-I mediates the stimulatory action of GH on bone formation through its actions on the renal metabolism of vitamin D precursors and on renal phosphate reabsorption. Furthermore, IGF-I increases both renal blood flow and glomerular filtration rate by a mechanism dependent on the renal synthesis of endothelium-derived relaxing factor and prostaglandins [160]. In summary, IGF-I displays metabolic actions, shifting intermediary metabolism to its anabolic side, promotes renal vasodilation, has plastic actions on bone, and in general stimulates tissue growth and protein synthesis. Therefore, the deficiency of IGF-I may be of pathophysiologic importance in liver cirrhosis.

## *Thyroid Hormones*

### *Thyroid Function in Cirrhosis*

Synthesis and secretion of thyroxine ($T_4$) and triiodothyronine ($T_3$) are normal. Serum thyroid-stimulating hormone (TSH) levels are normal or minimally elevated (probably due to stimulation by increased serum estrogen), and the TSH response to the administration of thyrotropin-releasing hormone (TRH) is also normal. The response to TRH may be impaired in some alcoholic subjects. In most patients with advanced cirrhosis, serum levels of $T_4$ and $T_3$ are moderately abnormal. $T_4$ is most often mildly decreased due to the fall in thyroxine-binding globulin (TBG), which is synthesized in the liver. However, free $T_4$ levels are normal or slightly raised. The conversion of $T_4$ to $T_3$ is impaired because of hepatocellular failure; hence, serum $T_3$ levels are frequently decreased in cirrhotics. In fact, it has been proposed that measurement of serum $T_3$ may be an accurate test of liver function [161]. However, clinically overt thyroid dysfunction is not more prevalent in cirrhotics than in healthy people.

On the other hand, it has been postulated that hepatocellular necrosis in the acinar area 3, characteristically seen in alcoholic cirrhotics, could be due to hypoxia resulting from a hypercatabolic state mimicking the metabolic picture of hyperthyroidism. This theory provided the basis for the use of antithyroid drugs in the treatment of alcoholic hepatitis. However, the results obtained by different authors have been controversial [146, 147].

### *Thyroid Disease Associated with Specific Etiologies of Cirrhosis*

Patients with cirrhosis secondary to autoimmune chronic hepatitis or primary biliary cirrhosis have an increased rate of autoimmune thyroiditis (up to 20% in patients with primary biliary cirrhosis in some series), leading to hypo- or hyperthyroidism. This condition is associated with other manifestations of autoimmunity.

## *Other Hormones*

In cirrhosis, ACTH levels are normal and cortisol clearance is decreased. Degradation of this hormone is shifted to 20α reduction instead of A-ring reduction, so that tetrahydrocortisol formation is reduced and 20α cortolone synthesis increases. Free cortisol levels are normal due to a concomitant increase in cortisol-binding globulin. Urinary free cortisol is useful in establishing the existence of primary alterations in cortisol production [162].

Hepatic metabolism of exogenous steroids is also affected in cirrhosis. The degradation of prednisone is diminished so that administration of this drug to cirrhotics may result in serum levels several times above those expected. This may lead to immunodepression and hydromineral imbalance [163].

Insulin and glucagon have been considered previously, and the renin-angiotensin-aldosterone axis, catecholamines, arginine vasopressin, and atrial natriuretic peptide are dealt with in Chap. 12.

## 7.7 Hemopoietic System

Patients with liver cirrhosis may present with quantitative and/or qualitative alterations in the peripheral blood picture affecting red cells, leukocytes, and platelets. Deficient production of precursors in the bone marrow and increased destruction of mature cells in the peripheral blood may account for these disorders.

***Impaired Bone Marrow Function*** [48–50, 164, 165]

Factors which may impair bone marrow function include "inflammatory" iron sequestration in cells of the mononuclear phagocyte system, iron deficiency, folate deficiency, and, infrequently, vitamin $B_{12}$ deficiency. In cirrhosis, dysfunction of bone marrow affects mainly the erythroid series.

Bone marrow function becomes critically important in cirrhosis since the half-lives of peripheral blood cells are frequently shortened and activation of hemopoiesis is the only compensatory mechanism. In this setting, the deficiency of some nutrients makes the bone marrow unable to achieve compensation. Low hemoglobin values are found in 70% of cirrhotics, but in about one-third of these patients total red cell mass is normal and anemia is due to dilution.

Anemia of the inflammatory processes is characterized by low serum iron, low serum transferrin, normal to increased ferritin levels, and the presence of iron in the bone marrow. Iron administration is ineffective. This form of anemia may be observed in cirrhosis.

Iron deficiency is common in liver cirrhosis due to bleeding, which occurs almost exclusively in the gastrointestinal tract. Gastrointestinal bleeding may be acute or chronic. Acute bleeding leads to acute hemorrhagic anemia. Iron deficiency anemia may occur thereafter if adequate iron supplementation is not given. Occasionally, patients may present with acute severe anemia with no noticeable previous bleeding episode. If acute hemolysis is excluded, occult bleeding into the peritoneum must be ruled out, especially if invasive procedures such as needle liver biopsy have been performed. Chronic and progressive iron deficiency anemia in cirrhosis is due to chronic blood loss because of congestive gastropathy or peptic ulcer.

In females with impaired coagulation, exaggerated menstrual blood loss should be considered even though menstruation tends to be sparse in cirrhotic women.

Iron deficiency anemia is microcytic and is associated with very low serum iron and ferritin levels and with a high total iron-binding capacity. No iron is seen in the bone marrow smear. Characteristically, reticulocytosis develops some days after iron supplementation. In cirrhotics, however, microcytosis may be masked by folate deficiency or alcohol toxicity and the response to iron administration may be blunted by the associated inflammatory defect in iron utilization.

Folate deficiency is the commonest cause of macrocytic anemia in cirrhosis. It may occur in all types of cirrhosis but it is characteristically more frequent and severe in alcoholic cirrhotics, because of the direct toxicity of alcohol on the bone marrow. The folate stored in the liver averages 5–10 mg, which is sufficient to supply the bone marrow for 3 months. Poor nutrition, partial folate malabsorption, interruption of the folate enterohepatic cycle, and direct antagonism of the folic acid metabolism by alcohol account for folate deficiency in cirrhosis. In the bone marrow, folate deficiency leads to megaloblastic hemopoiesis affecting the three series. In peripheral blood its earliest manifestation is macrocytosis with no or only mild macrocytic anemia. Multilobed neutrophils in blood and macrocytic megakaryocytes in the bone marrow smear are also seen in these patients. Slight macrocytic anemia is frequent in cirrhosis regardless of folate levels, suggesting that additional nutritional deficiencies may be involved. Vitamin $B_{12}$ deficiency is rare in liver cirrhosis, since the amount of vitamin $B_{12}$ normally stored in the liver (about 10 mg) represents a 5-year reserve.

### *Decreased Survival of Peripheral Blood Cells* [48–50, 164, 165]

In liver cirrhosis, a decreased half-life of peripheral blood cells may lead to anemia, leukopenia, and/or thrombocytopenia when the rate of cell destruction exceeds the bone marrow's capacity for compensation. Hypersplenism is the main cause of hemocatheresis. It is related more to the activity of the splenic reticuloendothelial system than to the size of the spleen.

Modification of the cholesterol/phospholipid ratio in the erythrocyte membrane contributes to hemolysis and results in the formation of "target cells," "thin macrocytes," and "spur cells," also called "burr cells" and "acanthocytes." In addition, immune-mediated hemolysis with a positive Coombs' test may be seen in primary biliary cirrhosis and in cirrhosis secondary to autoimmune chronic active hepatitis. Hemolytic crises may occur in patients with Wilson's disease as the first manifestation of the disease or after discontinuation of D-penicillamine therapy. Acute hemolysis also occurs in patients with Zieve's syndrome, in which alcoholic hepatitis is associated with hypercholesterolemia.

Dyserythropoiesis may also be found in liver cirrhosis, especially in alcoholics. Polycythemia, due to the secretion of an erythropoietin-like substance, can occur as a paraneoplastic sign in 5%–10% of patients developing hepatocarcinoma.

Leukopenia and/or thrombocytopenia can result from hypersplenism in the absence of significant anemia. These alterations may have clinical relevance in patients with far-advanced cirrhosis in whom levels of leukocytes and platelets below $1500/mm^3$ and $20\,000/mm^3$, respectively, can be seen. In general thrombocytopenia is moderate but represents a risk at the time of surgery or when invasive procedures have to be performed. Since the splenic pooling of platelets is greatly increased, it is doubtful whether platelet transfusions will be effective.

The increased susceptibility to infections in cirrhotics is related to functional deficiencies of leukocytes rather than to their reduced number. However, leukopenia affects predominantly the polymorphonuclear cells, so that opportunistic infections may occur in a small proportion of patients in whom leukopenia is abnormally severe. Leukocytosis is usually associated with acute infection.

## 7.8 Hemostasis and Coagulation

Bleeding is a frequent complication of liver cirrhosis. The commonest forms of bleeding are easy bruising, petechiae, ecchymoses, gingivorrhagia, and epistaxis. Prolonged bleeding after tooth extraction or venipuncture is also common. Hemostatic function must be checked before liver biopsy or other invasive procedures.

Upper gastrointestinal bleeding due to a variety of lesions is the commonest major form of bleeding in liver cirrhosis. This complication has a high mortality, especially in patients with impaired hemostasis.

### *Mechanisms*

#### *Primary Hemostasis*

After vascular injury, blood comes into contact with subendothelial connective tissue; platelets then adhere to exposed subendothelial collagen and release a series of substances which initiate the reversible phase of platelet aggregation. Specifically, secreted ADP promotes the binding of fibrinogen to a receptor on the platelet surface membrane. Subsequent release of thrombospondin induces irreversible aggregation. More ADP is discharged with resulting amplification of the aggregation process, which is directed toward sealing the area of endothelial injury. Thromboxane $A_2$, a cyclooxygenase arachidonic acid derivative, is released from platelets at this time. This substance is a powerful inducer of platelet aggregation and also a vasoconstrictor which contributes to effective hemostasis. The von Willebrand factor binds to both platelets and subendothelial collagen, thus mediating the attachment of the hemostatic plug to the vessel wall.

### *Clotting Mechanisms and Definitive Hemostasis*

Essentially coagulation consists in the conversion of prothrombin to thrombin, which catalyzes fibrinogen cleavage to form fibrin. The first reaction is triggered by activated factor X (factor Xa), which, in turn, is activated by a cascade of proteolytic reactions through the intrinsic and extrinsic pathways of coagulation (Fig. 7). Fibrin monomers polymerize, forming a meshwork that embraces the hemostatic plug. Solid covalent bonds within subunits in the fibrin polymer are provided by factor XIII. By this means, definitive hemostasis is achieved.

In the presence of procoagulant activity, physiologic inhibitors of coagulation are activated to restrict the clotting process to the damaged area. The fibrinolytic system, which degrades the fibrin meshwork and reduces fibrin formation from fibrinogen, also controls the clotting process.

### ***Disorders*** [166–168]

In early cirrhosis the clotting system and platelet count are normal or mildly altered but in advanced cirrhosis marked defects in the clotting system may coexist with a low platelet count and altered platelet function. Changes in hemostasis and coagulation in liver cirrhosis are complex. The following points are worth bearing in mind:

1. The impairment of the hemostatic function tends to parallel the severity of the disease. Patients with compensated cirrhosis have mild to moderate hemostatic deficiencies which in general are of limited clinical relevance. In patients with advanced cirrhosis, deterioration of hemostatic mechanisms is severe but the clinical relevance of these disorders cannot be accurately predicted from biologic tests.

2. There is no single "coagulation disorder of liver cirrhosis" but rather a group of several disorders affecting all procoagulant pathways, the fibrinolytic system, and the clotting inhibitors. These different systems are not necessarily affected to the same extent, so that any combination is possible. This picture is compounded by the inability of the cirrhotic liver to adequately clear activated clotting proteins, which may promote a variety of secondary disorders in hemostatic function.

3. In liver cirrhosis, disorders of hemostasis and coagulation are not the primary cause of major bleeding but they are the major factor aggravating blood loss through any bleeding lesion and in fact may cause the death of the patient.

4. Finally, it should be kept in mind that in cirrhotic patients undergoing any invasive procedure, careful and simple prevention of bleeding is more effective than the most brilliant therapy for active bleeding.

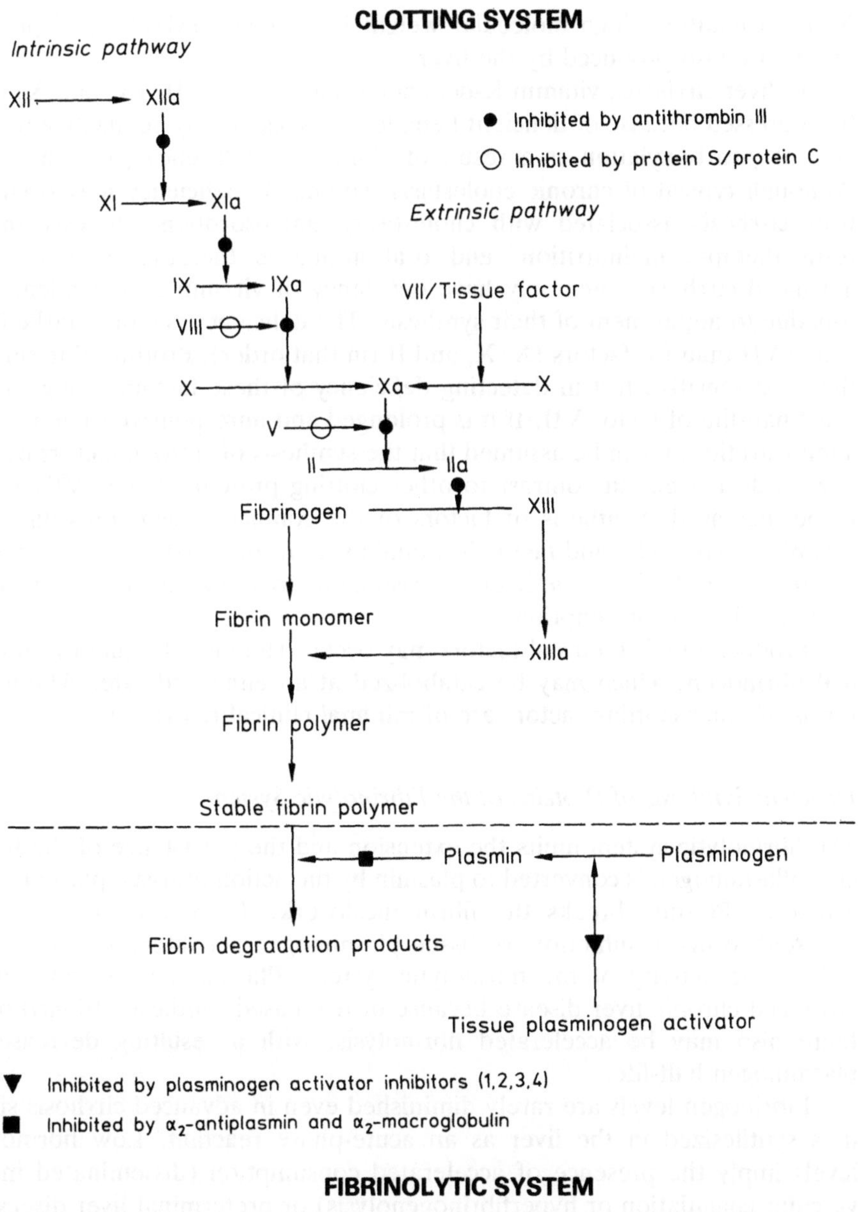


**Fig. 7.** Clotting cascade, fibrinolytic system, and physiologic inhibitory systems

Various disorders of hemostasis and coagulation will now be discussed in turn.

### *Deficient or Abnormal Synthesis of Clotting Factors*

The liver synthesizes vitamin K-dependent factors, contact system factors, fibrinogen, factor V, a subunit of factor VIII (factor VIIIC), and factor

XIII. In addition, high molecular weight kininogen (HMWK) and prekallikrein are also produced by the liver.

In liver cirrhosis, vitamin K-dependent factors (II, VII, IX, and X) may be depressed because of deficient hepatic synthesis or may be inactive due to lack of γ-carboxylation as a result of vitamin K deficiency (see Chap. 8). Although typical of chronic cholestasis, vitamin K deficiency may occur in liver cirrhosis associated with cholestasis, malabsorption, cholestyramine resin therapy, malnutrition, and oral antibiotic therapy. Patients with advanced cirrhosis commonly have deficiency of vitamin K-dependent factors due to impairment of their synthesis. The deficiency is more marked for factor VII than for factors IX, X, and II (in that order). Prothrombin time is the most sensitive test in detecting deficiency of these factors owing to the short half-life of factor VII. If it is prolonged and unresponsive to vitamin K administration, it can be assumed that the synthesis of clotting factors by the liver is decreased. In contrast to other clotting proteins, factor VIII tends to be increased. Synthesis of factors of the contact system, prekallikrein, HMWK, factor XII, and factor XI, diminishes in proportion to impairment of protein synthesis by the liver. Occasionally prekallikrein shows a further decrease due to consumption.

Production of abnormal factors may occur. The most frequent is abnormal fibrinogen, which may be catabolized at an enhanced rate. Abnormal forms of other clotting factors are of minimal clinical relevance.

### *Deficient Synthesis of Proteins of the Fibrinolytic System*

The fibrinolytic system limits the extension and the persistence of the fibrin clot. Plasminogen is converted to plasmin by the action of tissue plasminogen activator. Plasmin breaks the fibrin meshwork. There are at least four different forms of inhibitors of tissue plasminogen activator, which in turn reduce the activity of the fibrinolytic system. Plasminogen is reduced in advanced chronic liver disease because of decreased synthesis. In cirrhotics there also may be accelerated fibrinolysis, with a resulting decrease in plasminogen half-life.

Fibrinogen levels are rarely diminished even in advanced cirrhosis since it is synthesized in the liver as an acute-phase reactant. Low fibrinogen levels imply the presence of accelerated consumption (disseminated intravascular coagulation or hyperfibrinogenolysis) or preterminal liver disease.

### *Deficient Synthesis of Inhibitors of the Clotting Cascade*

A series of proteins synthesized in the liver counterbalance procoagulant activity, limiting the extent of fibrin formation when the clotting cascade is activated. These proteins include antithrombin III, protein C, and protein S.

Antithrombin III is the major blood inhibitor of thrombin, factor Xa, and factor IXa. Its deficiency is associated with thrombotic diathesis.

Deficiency of antithrombin III may be congenital or secondary to liver failure. Antithrombin III production is depressed in cirrhosis. The thrombotic tendency that would result is equilibrated by a roughly parallel deficient synthesis of clotting factors. $\alpha_2$-Macroglobulin, which also possesses antithrombin activity, is normal or increased in cirrhosis and may help to compensate antithrombin III deficiency. In general, antithrombin III levels in cirrhotics are lower than expected from the severity of liver failure, suggesting that increased consumption contributes to its deficiency.

Protein C limits thrombin formation by inhibiting activated factors VIII and V. Protein S is a cofactor for protein C. These anticoagulant proteins are vitamin K dependent. They are reduced in liver cirrhosis, and as in the case of antithrombin III, their deficiency is not associated with increased thrombotic events probably owing to the coexistence of alterations in the clotting system.

$\alpha_2$-Antiplasmin levels may be low in patients with cirrhosis because of deficient hepatic synthesis. Its deficiency parallels that of albumin, plasminogen, and antithrombin III. This protein is a powerful inhibitor of plasmin, thus preventing the degradation of the fibrin mesh. It has been suggested that the low-grade disseminated intravascular coagulation (DIC) observed in liver cirrhosis is partly responsible for $\alpha_2$-antiplasmin deficiency.

*Deficient Blood Clearance of Activated Clotting Factors, Fibrin, and Fibrinogen Degradation Products* [166, 170]

In advanced chronic liver disease, activated proteases of the clotting cascade are less efficiently removed by the liver than in normal subjects. The presence of these activated proteases in the circulation represents a continuous stimulus for coagulation and may lead to DIC. On the other hand, the deficient clearance of plasminogen activators and plasmin may contribute to the development of primary hyperfibrinogenolysis.

A common finding in advanced cirrhosis is elevated blood levels of fibrin and fibrinogen degradation products (FDPs). This is due to impaired removal by the liver of these substances and also to their enhanced generation. The excessive production of FDPs is probably secondary to several mechanisms, such as accelerated catabolism of abnormal fibrinogen, low-grade DIC, primary fibrinolysis, and the degradation of fibrinogen present in the ascitic fluid.

Abnormally high FDP levels further impair coagulation in cirrhosis, since FDPs inhibit fibrin polymerization, hinder platelet aggregation, and possess antithrombin activity. Thus, FDPs prolong thrombin time and bleeding time.

*Disseminated Intravascular Coagulation* [169, 170]

Patients with liver cirrhosis may exhibit biologic evidence of DIC as a result of several abnormalities in the clotting cascade. The only difference between classic DIC and the DIC state of cirrhosis is the elevation of serum factor VIII in the latter condition, in contrast with its low levels in other cases. Conversely, cirrhotic patients have decreased levels of factor VII, a factor which is not so reduced in classic DIC. However, the two main features of DIC, increased procoagulant and fibrinolytic activities, are present in most cirrhotic patients even though the synthesis of the proteins involved in both cascades is depressed. Results of clotting tests that allow the diagnosis of DIC include prolongation of the prothrombin time, thrombin time, and partial thromboplastin time, decreased survival of fibrinogen, and increased degradation of fibrin as demonstrated by the increased levels of FDPs.

*Accelerated Fibrinolysis* [169, 170]

Cirrhotic patients with advanced disease display an increased rate of fibrin degradation, manifested by increased serum levels of fibrin degradation products and shortening of the euglobulin clot lysis time, implying abnormal activation of the fibrinolytic system. Decreased clearance of the plasminogen activator from plasma by the diseased liver is mainly responsible for this disturbance. This leads to an increased rate of plasmin generation from plasminogen and thus to enhanced fibrin degradation. It has been suggested that a deficiency of inhibitors of the fibrinolytic cascade, such as plasminogen activator inhibitor types 1,2,3,4 and $\alpha_2$-antiplasmin, is also involved in this disorder.

Enhanced fibrinolytic activity in patients with cirrhosis is expected to increase the risk of bleeding or the intensity of bleeding episodes. In addition, fibrin degradation products are deficiently cleared from plasma by the cirrhotic liver and these substances further reduce the effectiveness of both the clotting cascade and platelet aggregation. These alterations may have their greatest importance at the time of surgery because they can increase blood loss.

*Thrombocytopenia and Abnormal Platelet Function* [166–168]

Thrombocytopenia of cirrhosis is essentially secondary to hypersplenism. In massively enlarged spleens, up to 90% of platelets may be sequestered, but rarely does this lead to a hemostatic problem. However, hypersplenism may be severe in advanced cirrhosis and the platelet count may fall below 50 000/$mm^3$. The clinical severity of thrombocytopenia is best evaluated by the degree of spontaneous cutaneous or mucosal bleeding.

Thrombocytopenia in cirrhosis also may be due to folic acid deficiency, toxic effects of alcohol on the bone marrow, sepsis, and peripheral consumption because of subclinical DIC. The contribution of alterations in platelet function to the hemostatic disorders of cirrhosis remains controversial. A recent study failed to demonstrate abnormal platelet function in a series of 60 cirrhotic patients. Nevertheless, there have been reports in cirrhotic patients of alterations able to impair platelet function, such as deficient platelet production of thromboxane $A_2$ (proaggregating agent) and increased systemic synthesis of prostacyclin (antiaggregating agent). In addition, in patients with DIC or hyperfibrinolysis, the accumulation in blood of fibrin or fibrinogen degradation products may reduce platelet aggregation. This function also may be altered by massive hypergammaglobulinemia, a situation comparable to that which occurs in patients with multiple myeloma. It has been postulated that other unidentified factors, dialyzable from cirrhotic plasma, may play a role in disturbing platelet function. Clinically, bleeding in excess of what is expected from deficiencies in platelet count and clotting tests should raise concern about platelet dysfunction.

***Evaluation of Hemostasis*** [48–50, 166–170]

In most cases the hemostatic performance of cirrhotics represents the combined effect of alterations at various levels. Notwithstanding this fact, routine hemostatic evaluation of cirrhotic patients is quite simple. Determination of individual clotting factors is rarely needed for clinical purposes. However, it can prove very difficult to identify the specific alterations which lead rare patients to manifest abnormally easy and prolonged bleeding which is not justified on the basis of the alterations revealed by routine tests.

Clinically, disturbances of hemostasis in liver cirrhosis are especially important in the setting of lesions leading to serious hemorrhage, at the time of invasive diagnostic or therapeutic procedures, and in patients undergoing liver transplantation.

Prothrombin time, activated partial thromboplastin time, thrombin time, bleeding time, and platelet count are the tests routinely used for hemostatic evaluation in cirrhosis. Determination of fibrinogen and FDPs or D-dimer is also useful. If bleeding time is more prolonged than expected on the basis of the intensity of thrombocytopenia, a study of platelet aggregation is indicated.

## 7.9 Locomotor System

***Osteopenia*** [171–173]

Osteopenia is a potential complication of any type of liver cirrhosis and not only of cholestatic chronic liver disease. Its prevalence in patients with cirrhosis is about 30% regardless of the etiology. (Osteopenia is usually defined by a bone mineral density value below the limit represented by the mean minus 2 SD in a sex- and age-matched control population).

Osteopenia in cirrhotic individuals may affect trabecular bone (i.e., lumbar spine) and mixed trabecular and cortical bone (i.e., femoral neck).

The skeletal site where the prevalence of osteopenia is highest (39%, in a recent study) is the triangle of Ward (the specific site of the femoral neck particularly prone to fracture) [171].

*Mechanisms*

The pathogenesis of osteopenia in cirrhosis is poorly understood although osteoporosis rather than osteomalacia is its essential feature. The role of vitamin D malabsorption has been overemphasized in the past. In fact, vitamin D deficiency and hypocalcemia occur in only a minority of patients. Vitamin D supplementation has had no, or merely a questionable, beneficial effect in most trials. Exceptions are severe chronic cholestatic disorders which lead to the development of rickets (children) or osteomalacia (adults), for which vitamin D and calcium are the only effective therapy (see Chap. 8). Ethanol toxicity may play a role in the osteopenia of alcoholic cirrhotics. In patients with protein-calorie malnutrition and muscle wasting it is likely that formation of the protein-bone matrix is disturbed. Indeed, bone density and urinary creatinine excretion (which reflects muscle mass) were found to be directly correlated in cirrhotic patients. Gonadal failure, a well-recognized cause of osteoporosis in the general population, has been found to be an independent and significant risk factor for the development of osteoporosis and bone fractures in cirrhotics. Physical inactivity, which is the rule in advanced cirrhotics, is also a cause of osteoporosis.

As noted earlier, serum levels of IGF-I are decreased in advanced cirrhotics. In addition to the cirtical role of GH and IGF-I in mediating growth in early life, adults are partially dependent on IGF-I for the preservation of bone mass. Thus the contribution of IGF-I deficiency to osteopenia should be evaluated.

A failure in osteocalcin carboxylation due to vitamin K deficiency might be an additional factor in osteopenia. Noncarboxylated osteocalcin is inactive and unable to retain calcium, and thus not useful for bone formation (see Chap. 8).

*Clinical Manifestations* [171–173]

Bone pain, predominantly in the spine, and bone fractures involving the hip, the vertebrae, and the forearms are the essential clinical manifestations of cirrhotic osteopenia.

The prevalence of bone fractures in cirrhosis has been reported to be as high as 31% for eugonadal patients and 71% for patients with hypogonadism [172]. Decreased spinal bone density, hypogonadism, and liver insufficiency (as evaluated by the antipyrine clearance rate) were the disorders significantly related to the occurrence of spinal fractures in a recent study, whereas peripheral fractures were associated only with the existence of hypogonadism [172]. The etiology of cirrhosis has no influence on the occurrence of spinal fractures [172].

Osteopenia cannot be accurately evaluated by conventional bone radiology or biochemical tests. The only reliable method for its assessment is the measurement of bone density by dual photon absorptiometry. The increased hydroxyprolinuria which has been observed in cirrhotics is thought to reflect increased collagen turnover in the liver rather than in bone. Indeed, low collagen turnover in bone has been observed in cirrhotic osteopenia.

#### *Arthropathy Associated with Specific Liver Diseases*

Arthralgia and arthritis may be seen in patients with hemochromatosis as a result of chondrocalcinosis. In cirrhosis due to autoimmune chronic active hepatitis, arthritis (synovitis) is very common. Primary biliary cirrhosis may be associated with autoimmune disorders involving joints (synovitis).

#### *Muscle Wasting*

Advanced cirrhosis is accompanied by marked muscle wasting. Most but not all studies suggest that reduced synthesis of muscle protein rather than increased degradation of myofibrils is the mechanism chiefly responsible. Factors probably involved in low protein synthesis include: protein-calorie malnutrition, altered composition of the plasma amino acid profile (increased aromatic and reduced branched chain amino acids), alcoholic myopathy, and partial denervation of muscle fibers because of alcoholic polyneuropathy and immobilization. Hormonal changes like hypogonadism and IGF-I deficiency may be implicated. Alterations in the intermediary metabolism, which is switched from equilibrium to catabolic conditions, resembling a state of starvation, may be the ultimate underlying mechanism of muscle wasting (see Sect. 6).

## 8 Infections and Noninfectious Fever

Cirrhotic patients are especially prone to develop bacterial infections, which account for 7% of the deaths of compensated cirrhotics and contribute to death in more than 20% of decompensated patients [174]. The most common infections in cirrhosis are bacteremia, urinary tract infections, pneumonia, and spontaneous bacterial peritonitis (SBP); endocarditis and meningitis are seen rather less frequently. Decompensated subjects are predominantly infected by Gram-negative bacteria, while Gram-positive organisms predominate in compensated patients [175]. Malnutrition, ascites, and upper gastrointestinal hemorrhage are conditions predisposing to infection, as are any invasive diagnostic or therapeutic procedures. With regard to the etiology, alcoholic cirrhosis and primary biliary cirrhosis are associated, respectively, with the highest and the lowest risk of infection.

## 8.1 Alterations of the Immune System [174–176]

Cirrhotic patients, especially alcoholics and those with far-advanced disease, exhibit disturbances in the defense mechanisms against bacterial infections. Components of the complement system are decreased in serum and in ascitic fluid owing to diminished hepatic synthesis. This contributes to the deficient chemoattractant and opsonic activities observed in these fluids. Neutrophil phagocytic activity and intracellular killing of bacteria are diminished. Low serum fibronectin levels add to the impairment of opsonic activity. The antibactericidal activity of IgM is also reduced in cirrhosis. The mononuclear phagocyte system is functionally defective. Clearance of bacteria and endotoxin from portal blood is inefficient due to intrahepatic shunting and abnormal Kupffer cell function. Thus, endotoxin and bacteria of intestinal origin may reach the systemic circulation, leaving the portal blood by portal collaterals or directly crossing the cirrhotic liver. RIMOLA et al. demonstrated that impairment of the phagocytic activity of the mononuclear phagocyte system is a determinant factor for the development of bacteremia and/or SBP [176]. Among patients in whom this function was altered, 24% developed bacteremia and/or SBP during hospital admission and 33% did so during an immediate follow-up period of 28 months whereas no patient with normal mononuclear phagocyte activity experienced infection [176].

## 8.2 Major Infections

The urinary tract is the commonest location of infectious episodes in cirrhotics. Asymptomatic bacteriuria may be detected in up to 20% of cirrhotic women. Gram-negative bacteria, especially *E. coli*, predominate as etiologic agents. Urinary tract infections are the source of microorganisms causing bacteremia and SBP in 50% and 20% of the episodes, respectively [174, 175].

Alcoholic cirrhotics are especially prone to develop pneumonia. Balloon tamponade of bleeding esophageal varices is an important risk factor. *Haemophilus influenzae* and *Klebsiella pneumoniae* are the predominant agents. Alcoholism predisposes to pneumococcal pneumonia and is also associated with an increased incidence of aspiration pneumonia, in which anaerobic bacteria are the commonest organisms [177].

Bacterial endocarditis occurs in less than 2% of cirrhotic patients. It entails an almost 40% mortality. *Streptococcus pneumoniae* and enteric Gram-negative bacteria are often isolated. Mitral and aortic valves are the sites most frequently involved [178].

Patients with hemochromatosis seem to have a special susceptibility to become infected with *Yersinia enterocolitica*, other *Yersinia* species, *Listeria monocytogenes*, and other agents which are atypical in the general cirrhotic population [179]. The reason for this suspected predisposition is unknown.

## 8.3 Spontaneous Bacterial Peritonitis

Spontaneous bacterial peritonitis is a life-threatening complication of cirrhosis. It is defined as infection of the ascitic fluid without any apparent intra-abdominal source of infection. The mean incidence of SBP is ascitic patients is about 15% and it is still associated with an overall mortality of 25%–50%. These data represent a marked improvement in the outcome of patients with SBP as compared with survival rates observed 10 years ago, when most series reported 70%–90% mortality [180, 181]. Gastrointestinal bleeding, a protein concentration in the ascitic fluid of less than 1 g/dl, impaired function of the mononuclear phagocyte system, and low opsonic activity of the ascitic fluid are determinant factors in the development of SBP [180, 181]. Patients who recover from their first SBP episode have a high risk of recurrence. Recurrence rates of 43%, 69%, and 74% at 6, 12, and 24 months after the first episode have been reported by TITÓ et al. [182]. Gram-negative enteric bacteria account for more than 70% of SBP episodes. *Staphylococci* species are the leading agents among Gram-positive microorganisms [180–184]. Simultaneous infection with two or more bacteria occurs in less than 10% of the cases of SBP. In patients undergoing prophylactic intestinal decontamination with daily oral norfloxacin, the incidence of SBP is markedly reduced [183], and staphylococci and streptococci become the most frequent infective agents. The intestine and the urinary tract are the sites of origin of bacteria, which may reach the peritoneal cavity by local spread or, much more commonly, through hematogenous spread during a bacteremic episode. Translocation of enteric bacteria across the intestinal mucosa is favored by bacterial overgrowth in the gut, hemorrhagic shock, and immunodeficiency induced by cancer chemotherapy. Deficient function of the mononuclear phagocytes allows spreading of germs into the systemic circulation. A low protein concentration in the ascitic fluid facilitates bacterial invasion and proliferation.

Early clinical suspicion of SBP permits rapid diagnosis and institution of therapy, thus improving survival of patients. Classic signs of peritoneal irritation are not reliable. RUNYON has compared the signs and symptoms in patients with SBP in series reported in 1985 and in 1990 [181]. Abdominal pain (60% in 1985 vs 49% in 1990), abdominal tenderness (50% vs 39%), rebound tenderness (42% vs 10%), and decreased bowel sounds (42% vs 12%) were present with higher frequency in the earlier series of patients [181]. Prompt diagnosis of SBP in the most recent series was probably responsible for these differences and had a determinant influence on the difference in survival rate (about 20%–25% vs 55%–60%). Abdominal pain and/or fever are the first clinical manifestations in most cases and their presence makes analysis of ascitic fluid mandatory. However, both pain and fever may be absent in a substantial proportion of cases [180, 181, 183]. Any abrupt deterioration of a cirrhotic patient with no clear explanation should also raise suspicion of SBP; this is especially the case when there is unexpected occurrence of renal failure, hepatic encephalopathy, or, to a lesser extent, gastrointestinal bleeding [183]. When SBP is suspected, diagnostic paracentesis must be performed. Ascitic fluid is inoculated directly into culture vials at bedside, a technique which increases the number of positive cultures to about 90%. A sample of ascitic fluid can be centrifuged and the pellet used for Gram staining. The polymorphonuclear leukocyte (PMN) content of the ascitic fluid is the most sensitive and specific method in early diagnosis [181, 183]. Sterile ascitic fluid contains no more than 250 PMNs/$mm^3$. True SBP requires PMNs >250/$mm^3$ and positive ascitic fluid culture. The variant called "nonneutrocytic bacterascites" is diagnosed in cases with positive culture and PMNs <250/$mm^3$, and "culture-negative neutrocytic ascites" is diagnosed when culture is negative and PMNs >250/$mm^3$ [180, 181, 183].

An additional consideration is whether the episode is true SBP or secondary bacterial peritonitis. Secondary peritonitis (mainly due to viscus perforation) is suspected and must be ruled out if ascitic fluid with PMNs >250/$mm^3$ meets at least two of the following three criteria: (a) total protein >10 g/liter, glucose <50 mg/dl, LDH > the upper limit of normal serum; (b) multiple organisms seen on Gram's stain; (c) bilirubin concentration in ascites >6 mg/dl or greater than serum bilirubin levels [181].

### 8.4 Noninfectious Fever

Approximately one-third of patients with advanced cirrhosis may show low-grade fever unrelated to infection. Fever ranges from 37° to 38°C and is rarely accompanied by systemic manifestations. Rigors or rapid peaking of fever, as in bacteremia, are absent. The fever may persist for weeks or months and in some cases is continuous. This type of fever is related to cirrhosis itself, but the mechanism has not yet been defined. Classically, it was attributed to alterations in the hepatic metabolism of sexual steroids (e.g., etiocholanolone).

Differential diagnosis of this "cirrhotic fever" includes any febrile illness, especially those of infectious or paraneoplastic (hepatocellular carcinoma) origin.

## 9 Diagnosis

Liver cirrhosis may be suspected in patients with clinical or biochemical manifestations of hepatocellular failure, portal hypertension, or both, but the definitive diagnosis requires morphologic confirmation. Macroscopically, it may be diagnosed by means of laparoscopy or in the course of a laparotomy. Microcopic diagnosis requires liver biopsy.

### 9.1 Diagnostic Workup

After the diagnosis of liver cirrhosis has been definitely confirmed, a full evaluation of the cirrhotic patient should yield information on the following issues: (a) etiology of cirrhosis; (b) histopathologic staging and activity of the primary disease; (c) degree of liver dysfunction; (d) degree of portal hypertension; (e) existence of major complications; (f) existence of associated disorders related to the primary disease; and (g) definition of patient status according to Child's classification (or another scoring system).

### 9.2 Laboratory Findings

***Liver Function Tests and Other Biochemical Parameters*** [48–50]

In cirrhotics, serum aminotransferase levels are usually mildly to moderately elevated (up to five times normal values), reflecting low-grade but sustained hepatocellular necrosis. Aminotransferase levels roughly reflect the activity of the primary disorder. Nevertheless, parallelism between aminotransferase levels and histopathologic activity is lacking in some cases, and serum aminotransferases may be markedly elevated in patients with chronic active hepatitis and initial cirrhosis but normal or only slightly elevated in patients with end-stage disease. Serum bilirubin is a good marker of liver function and has prognostic value in cirrhotic patients. Predominantly unconjugated hyperbilirubinemia is most often associated with hemolysis and is not an indication of liver failure. No or very mild hyperbilirubinemia is seen in early cirrhosis. Hyperbilirubinemia is characteristically of mixed type and values as low as 2–3 mg/dl signal a substantial reduction in liver function. An exception is cirrhosis secondary to chronic cholestatic disorders, which may show mild to moderate hyperbilirubinemia (largely conjugated) in association with increased serum levels of alkaline phosphatase, $\gamma$-glutamyltransferase (GGT), 5′-nucleotidase, and leucine aminopeptidase from the initial stages of the disease onward (see Chap. 8). This cholestatic pattern is unusual in other types of cirrhosis, in which levels of canalicular enzymes are normal in the vast majority of patients. An exception is the elevation in serum GGT with no proportional increase in alkaline phosphatase observed in some alcoholic cirrhotics. This elevation in GGT is due to enzymatic induction and is a typical, albeit unspecific, finding of active drinking with or without associated alcoholic hepatitis (see Chap. 8). The elevation of canalicular enzymes (especially if progressive) in other types of cirrhosis suggests the existence of associated complications and should be investigated. Specifically, hepatocellular carcinoma and biliary tract disease should be ruled out.

Fasting and postprandial serum bile acid levels are almost invariably increased in cirrhotic patients. The ratio of trihydroxy to dihydroxy bile acids in serum is reduced. Urinary bile acid excretion is increased. The ratio of bile acids to creatinine in urine has been claimed to be a sensitive index of the severity of the liver disease. However, bile acid determinations are not used routinely in the evaluation of cirrhotic patients because of their lack of specificity (see Chap. 8).

Hypoalbuminemia and hypergammaglobulinemia are characteristic of established liver cirrhosis. Serum albumin below 3 g/dl indicates advanced disease. Hypoalbuminemia reflects the combined effects of impaired hepatic synthesis and fluid retention. Hypergammaglobulinemia of cirrhosis is typically polyclonal; only occasionally is monoclonal hyperglobulinemia seen. $\gamma$-Globulin values twice normal are frequently observed. Hypergammaglobulinemia is thought to arise as a result of a continuous stimulation of the immune system by antigens of intestinal origin which escape hepatic clearance through portal collaterals. Defects in immunoregulation may play a role in hypergammaglobulinemia of autoimmune chronic hepatitis and primary biliary cirrhosis. Patients with autoimmune ("lupoid") chronic hepatitis show the highest levels of immunoglobulins (up to four times the upper limits of normal values). Marked increases in serum IgA and IgM are characteristic of alcoholic cirrhosis and primary biliary cirrhosis, respectively. In advanced chronic liver disease, proteins acting as acute phase reactants tend to be increased while proteins of the complement system are reduced. As the disease progresses, levels of serum cholesterol and serum triglycerides decline slowly.

### *Hydromineral Equilibrium and Renal Function* [48–50]

In patients without ascites, serum electrolytes, serum osmolarity, and parameters of renal function are essentially normal. Routine urinalysis is normal. In these patients the 24-hour urinary sodium output matches daily sodium intake and the sodium to potassium ratio in urine is above 1.

A sodium to potassium urinary ratio below 1 indicates sodium retention or dietary sodium restriction. This is a well-accepted indirect sign of hyperaldosteronism. Interpretation of 24-hour natriuresis is only possible with the patient under controlled sodium intake. In this manner, sodium balance can be calculated.

In patients with ascites who are not receiving diuretics, urinary sodium excretion is low; indeed, it can be virtually absent. In general, serum creatinine is normal. Most of these patients show hyperaldosteronism.

Patients with far-advanced disease and ascites tend to develop spontaneous hyponatremia and hypo-osmolarity as a result of active renal water retention. This may be aggravated by vigorous diuretic therapy. Creatinine clearance should be monitored periodically in ascitic patients since it is more accurate in assessing renal function than are creatinine and BUN serum levels. Paradoxically, patients with severe hyponatremia and thus with low serum osmolarity exhibit very high values of arginine vasopressin, which is released by a nonosmotic mechanism and is out of osmotic control. If these patients are given a water overload, they exhibit negative free water clearance.

Hyperkalemia may be induced by spironolactone therapy in patients with ascites and borderline and unstable renal function. Hypokalemia occurs secondary to the administration of loop diuretics, which may also induce hypochloremic alkalosis. Ammonia levels in arterial blood are increased in about 60% of patients with hepatic encephalopathy [48–50].

#### *Acid-Base status*

Mild arterial hypoxemia with moderate hypocapnia and respiratory alkalosis are characteristic findings in cirrhosis. In some patients $PaO_2$ may fall below 50 mmHg. Metabolic acidosis may be seen in patients with renal failure and azotemia or in the course of severe systemic infections.

#### *The Hemopoietic System and Coagulation*

Alterations in coagulation and the hemopoietic system have been previously considered in this chapter.

#### *Laboratory Testing for the Etiologic Diagnosis of Cirrhosis*

The etiology of cirrhosis may be ascertained by means of specific laboratory determinations in many cases. The most relevant of them are summarized in Table 4.

#### *Special Tests for the Evaluation of Liver Function*

There are a series of tests designed to evaluate the functional reserve of the liver. Although most of them were in the past thought to be useful in the detection of liver disease and in the appraisal of the degree of hepatic dysfunction, their true usefulness is limited. No functional test has been shown to be superior to classic liver function tests in assessing liver function.

The essential characteristics of these tests are discussed in Chap. 2.

**Table 4.** Laboratory testing for the etiologic diagnosis of cirrhosis

| Etiology | Laboratory marker |
|---|---|
| Alcoholic | None |
| HBV | HBV serology, HBV-DNA, in serum or in tissue |
| HCV | HCV serology, HCV-RNA, in serum or in tissue |
| PBC | AMA (+) |
| | High IgM levels |
| | Compatible histopathology |
| Autoimmune | ANA (+) |
| | $LKM_1$ antibodies |
| Hemochromatosis | Serum ferritin >1000 ng/ml |
| | Serum iron binding capacity saturation >80% |
| | HII >1.9 (homozygotes)[a] |
| Wilson's disease | Serum ceruloplasmin <20 mg/dl |
| | $Cu^{2+}$ in dry liver tissue >250 μg/g |
| $\alpha_1$-Antitrypsin deficiency | $\alpha_1$-AT <105 mg/dl |
| | $\alpha_1$-AT phenotype PiZZ |
| | Liver biopsy with diastase-resistant PAS (+) granules |
| Porphyria cutanea tarda | Increased uroporphyrin excretion in 24-hour urine[b] |
| | Liver biopsy with red fluorescence under UV light |
| Toxic/drugs | None |

[a] HII, hepatic iron index = μmol $Fe^{2+}$·g dry liver weight·age (years)$^{-1}$
[b] In general >1000 μg/24 h

## 9.3 Imaging Studies

### *Conventional Radiography*

Abdominal plain films with the patient in the upright position may show splenomegaly and enlargement of the liver, which displaces the colon downward. Ascites is manifested by diffuse attenuation of the contours of anatomic structures.

Chest radiography is essentially normal in most cirrhotic patients. However, some characteristic findings may be observed. A recent study has shown the following abnormalities on chest x-ray films of patients with end-stage cirrhosis: decreased lung volumes (66%), pleural effusions (19.3%) (right-sided: 6.9%; left-sided: 4.4%; bilateral: 7.8%), increased interstitial markings (13.8%), and increased pulmonary vascularity (3.7%) [118].

Studies of the esophagus with barium meal for the evaluation of esophageal varices are obsolete, having been superseded by endoscopy. However, they are still useful in nonbleeding patients in whom upper endoscopy is contraindicated. Conventional radiology of the small bowel and the colon has the same indications in cirrhotics as in the general population.

**Table 5.** Effectiveness of imaging studies in liver cirrhosis

| | Presumptive diagnosis of cirrhosis[a] | Evaluation of the portal system | | | Detection of complicating malignancy |
|---|---|---|---|---|---|
| | | Portal vein | Collateral circulation | Spleen | |
| Doppler ultrasound | ++ | ++ | ++ | +++ | ++ |
| CT scan | ++ | ++ | ++ | +++ | ++<br>+++[b] |
| Nuclear magnetic resonance | ++ | +++ | +++ | +++ | ++ |
| Angiography | + | +++ | +++ | +++ | +++ |
| Radionuclide scan[c] | +/− | − | − | ++ | +/− |

Effectiveness: +/−, poor; +++, very good
[a] Based on parenchymal changes
[b] With previous Lipiodol injection
[c] Evaluates activity of the mononuclear phagocyte system

***Ultrasonography, Computed Tomography, Nuclear Magnetic Resonance, Isotope Scanning, and Angiography***

These procedures provide information related to the following issues: diagnosis of cirrhosis, calculation of liver size and volume, liver morphology, detection of portal hypertension and examination of the portal system, evaluation of complications of cirrhosis such as splenomegaly, ascites, portal-collateral circulation, and hepatocellular carcinoma and other associated processes. Isotope scanning is of less value than the other techniques. It provides semiquantitative information about the degree of impairment of the reticuloendothelial system by estimating the amount of the tracer detected outside the liver, especially in the spleen and bones. Angiography provides a most accurate information, since it delineates both the arterial and the portal circulation. Angiography shows the intrahepatic circulatory pattern, the characteristics of the portal vein, and the portal-collateral circulation. In addition it is the most sensitive technique in detecting small hepatocellular carcinomas and permits immediate therapeutic intervention. Table 5 summarizes the usefulness and limitations of ultrasonography, computed tomography, nuclear magnetic resonance, isotope scanning, and angiography in the evaluation of cirrhotic patients (see Chap. 5).

## 9.4 Hemodynamic Measurements

See Chap. 11.

## 9.5 Histopathologic Diagnosis

Definitive diagnosis of liver cirrhosis should be obtained by biopsy, laparoscopy, or laparoscopy-guided biopsy. Liver biopsy is commonly performed with needles of the TruCut or the Menghini type. Ultrasound-guided needle biopsy of the liver prevents the accidental puncture of abnormal vascular formations or parasitic cysts within the liver and the lesion of the extrahepatic biliary tree, all of which are infrequent but potential complications of percutaneous needle liver biopsy. In addition, biopsy is taken from the desired site of the liver parenchyma. The risk of severe hemorrhage as a result of liver biopsy is very low (0.1%–0.3%), although cases of fatal bleeding do occur (0.04%–0.1%) [185, 186]. If coagulopathy is severe enough to contraindicate percutaneous liver biopsy, the transjugular route may be used. Requirements and advantages of laparoscopy-guided biopsy are described in Chap. 6.

False positive and false negative results from liver biopsy in the diagnosis of cirrhosis may occur. A study comparing the accuracy of percutaneous biopsy versus laparoscopy plus liver biopsy yielded false negative rates of 20% and 6%, respectively [187].

### *Information Obtained from Liver Biopsy*

Liver biopsy provides the definitive diagnosis of liver cirrhosis and, in addition, gives important, often definitive, information regarding the etiology, the activity, and the stage of the hepatic lesion. In addition, it may identify associated conditions, such as hepatocellular carcinoma.

Processing of liver tissue for histopathologic study is standardized and should include special stainings if required (see Chap. 6). Conventional light microscopic examination is used for standard diagnosis. Occasionally electron microscopic studies of liver tissue are required for clinical purposes. Liver specimens can be used for purposes other than morphologic examination. Measurements of iron and copper in liver tissue remain the gold standards for the diagnosis of hemochromatosis and Wilson's disease, respectively. The presence of viral antigens in the liver tissue may be assessed by immunofluorescence staining using monoclonal antibodies. In situ hybridization using liver slices allows rapid diagnosis of some viral infections. Although not yet standardized for general use, the detection of minimal amounts of viral genomic material is now possible after amplification of a fraction of the genomic sequence by means of the polymerase chain reaction.

Histopathologic requirements for the diagnosis of liver cirrhosis have been cited previously in this chapter (see also Chap. 6). The specific histopathologic pictures for each etiology of liver cirrhosis are given in the corresponding chapters.

***First Diagnostic Evaluation and Follow-up Studies***

In all patients with biopsy-proven liver cirrhosis the presence of major complications should be investigated. These include ascites, esophageal and/or gastric varices, hyperemic (congestive) gastropathy, PSE and abnormalities of renal function, fluid balance, and blood gases. In the presence of ascites, the ascitic fluid should be examined. However, each patient has to be evaluated on an individual basis.

Follow-up studies in cirrhotic patients should be planned to cover the following main goals: (a) prevention (if possible) of major complications or, alternatively, early diagnosis and treatment; (b) surveillance for the possible development of hepatocellular carcinoma, aiming at its early detection and the implementation of effective therapy; (c) assessment of the progression of cirrhosis; and (d) periodic reevaluation of prognosis, including the possibility of candidacy for liver transplantation.

## 10 Prognosis

In 1942 RATNOFF and PATEK reported an overall 5-year survival of 7% for alcoholic cirrhotics with ascites [188]. Although this figure has improved, reaching 50% in some series, the life expectancy of cirrhotic patients is clearly reduced after the first major complication has developed. To establish the prognosis for individual patients is a difficult task since the course of the disease is quite variable. Liver function cannot be defined on the basis of a single objective parameter (there is no "creatinine clearance" for the assessment of liver function) and because of this, the prognosis of liver cirrhosis is more often based on combinations of several parameters.

**Table 6.** Child-Turcotte classification (Pugh's modification) for cirrhotic patients

| Variables | Score (points) | | |
|---|---|---|---|
| | 1 | 2 | 3 |
| Ascites | Absent | Slight–moderate | Tense |
| Encephalopathy | None | Grades I–II | Grades II–IV |
| Serum albumin (g/dl) | >3.5 | 2.8–3.5 | <2.8 |
| Serum bilirubin (mg/dl)[a] | <2.0 | 2.0–3.0 | >3.0 |
| Prothrombin time (seconds above control value) | <4.0 | 4.0–6.0 | >6.0 |

Grading: A: 5–6 points
B: 7–9 points
C: 10–15 points

[a] For primary biliary cirrhosis, bilirubin values (mg/dl) are: <4, 4–10, and >10, respectively

The acceptance of liver transplantation as the treatment of choice for advanced cirrhosis has led to a renewal of interest in prognostic methods in recent years. The number of medical institutions performing transplantation has expanded worldwide, and thousands of patients have undergone liver grafting. The wide experience thereby obtained has clearly shown that patients who are critically ill at the time of surgery have a less favorable outcome, but also that well-compensated patients may die early after transplantation. This prompted studies searching for accurate predictors of the short-term outcome of cirrhotic patients in an attempt to optimize the timing of liver transplantation.

**Table 7.** Clinical and biochemical variables with prognostic value in compensated cirrhosis[a]

| Variables[b] | 10 years' survival (% of patients) | *P*< |
|---|---|---|
| Etiology | | |
| Nonalcoholic | 55 | 0.005 |
| Alcoholic | 39 | |
| Gender | | |
| Male | 50 | 0.025 |
| Female | 48 | |
| Age | | |
| <60 yr | 52 | 0.025 |
| >60 yr | 25 | |
| Hepatic stigmata[c] | | |
| Absent | 57 | 0.015 |
| Present | 34 | |
| Alkaline phosphatase | | |
| Normal | 62 | 0.05 |
| High | 37 | |
| Bilirubin | | |
| <1 mg/dl | 62 | 0.001 |
| >1 mg/dl | 31 | |
| Albumin | | |
| >35 g/dl | 52 | 0.025 |
| <35 g/dl | 32 | |
| γ-Globulin | | |
| <18 g/dl | 59 | 0.025 |
| >18 g/dl | 37 | |
| Prothrombin time | | |
| >80% | 56 | 0.025 |
| <80% | 31 | |

[a] Modified with permission from GINÉS et al. [193]
[b] The presence of hepatomegaly or splenomegaly and the serum levels of aspartate transferase, alanine aminotransferase, and γ-glutamyltransferase were without significant prognostic value
[c] Presence of vascular spiders and/or palmar erythema

The prognosis of patients with liver cirrhosis may be viewed from a variety of perspectives: etiology, stage of disease, presence of major complications, influence of treatments, and the impact of new treatments on the natural history of the disease.

## 10.1 Prognostic Classification of Cirrhotic Patients

Several systems are used to classify cirrhotic patients according to their probability of survival at a given time on the basis of clinical and biochemical parameters. Equations including several parameters have been developed to estimate the expected time of survival of a patient at a certain phase of the disease.

### *The Child-Pugh Classification*

The classic scoring system designed nearly 30 years ago by CHILD and TURCOTTE [189] and then modified by PUGH et al. [190] (the CTPC classification) remains the most widely used prognostic tool in cirrhosis. The CTPC was conceived to define the operative risk of patients undergoing surgery for portal hypertension but it was thereafter generalized for prognostic appraisal of cirrhotic subjects. As shown in Table 6, the variables included in CTPC are very simple. The CTPC may be used as an ordinal scale (gradings A, B, and C), as a continuous scale (a score from 5 to 15 points), or as a multivariate model with indicator and continuous variables [191]. A recent study has demonstrated that the third of these possibilities yields the highest prognostic power (specificity and sensitivity were both 80%) in predicting short-term survival (1 year) [191]. At present this system is widely accepted as a method for classification in prospective or retrospective studies and can be used to assess whether populations evaluated at different times or by different authors are or are not comparable.

## 10.2 Variables with Prognostic Value Identified by Univariate Analysis

Table 7 summarizes data from several authors on the influence of the most frequently investigated variables on the survival of cirrhotic patients.

## 10.3 Prognostic Models Based on Multivariate Analysis of Variables

### *Chronic Cholestatic Liver Diseases (Primary Biliary Cirrhosis)*

Prognostic factors with independent prognostic value have been identified in different investigations. Serum bilirubin is the most powerful discriminant

**Table 8.** Risk score for patients with cirrhosis and ascites[a]

| *r* equal to: | Key |
|---|---|
| −0.690 × hepatomegaly | Absent = 0; present = 1 |
| −0.131 × serum albumin | g/liter |
| +0.698 × nutritional status | Good = 0; poor = 1 |
| −0.036 × mean arterial pressure | 1/3 (systolic + 2 diastolic) mmHg |
| +0.024 × blood urea nitrogen | mg/dl |
| −0.043 × serum sodium | mEq/liter |
| −0.041 × urinary sodium excretion | mEq/day |
| *r* value interval | 1-year survival |
| <−11.7 | 83% |
| −11.7 to −10.8 | 69% |
| >−10.8 | 17% |

[a] Adapted with permission from LLACH et al. [194]

parameter in all studies. A serum bilirubin level above 7 mg/dl is consistently associated with a life expectancy of less than 2 years, while a level above 13 mg/dl accurately predicts survival for less than 1 year (Fig. 8).

Recently the "Mayo Clinic score" has been elaborated on the basis of a retrospective analysis of more than 300 patients with primary biliary cirrhosis. This score, which is easy to use, served to demonstrate statistically for the first time that liver transplantation significantly improves patient survival [192].

### *Chronic Parenchymal Liver Diseases*

In cirrhosis secondary to chronic parenchymal liver diseases such as those due to alcohol, viral infection, autoimmunity, and metabolic disorders as well as those of cryptogenic origin, the critical issue regarding prognosis is whether cirrhosis is "compensated" or "decompensated." The word "decompensation" makes reference primarily to patients with "hydropic" decompensation (ascites) but frequently it is generalized to include cirrhotic patients who have had at least one episode of one of the major complications of liver cirrhosis (overt jaundice, ascites, functional renal failure, encephalopathy, or upper gastrointestinal bleeding).

#### *Compensated Cirrhosis*

Survival of compensated cirrhotics is quite good and the disease usually remains stable for years. Unexpected fatalities are infrequent since rarely do these subjects die from the first episode of an acute complication. However, the death rate increases sharply after the first major complication has occurred.

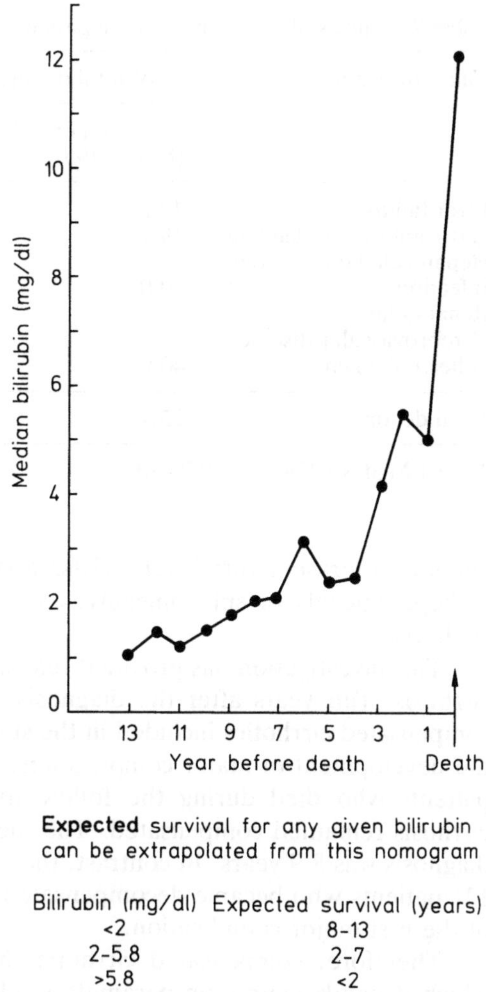


**Fig. 8.** The evolution of liver failure in primary biliary cirrhosis. This nomogram is derived from the medians of pooled serum bilirubin results in patients followed serially from diagnosis to death. (Serum bilirubin: 17 μmol/liter = 1 mg/dl). (Reproduced with permission from SHERLOCK [49])

Recently, GINÉS et al. [193] published an extensive study evaluating the natural history of compensated cirrhosis by analyzing a series of 293 consecutive patients with no history of major complications. The mean follow-up was 63 months and 21 variables were evaluated with regard to their influence on survival. From ten variables with a significant value in the univariate analysis, seven retained statistical significance in the multivariate analysis and were included in an equation which indicates the relative risk of death (Table 8). Variables lacking an independent influence on survival were: the degree of inflammatory activity (liver biopsy), the presence of either intranodular necrosis or piecemeal necrosis (liver biopsy), GGT and

**Table 9.** Causes of death in cirrhotic patients

| Cause of death | % of total deaths | | |
|---|---|---|---|
| | WALLACH et al.[a] (before 1957) | GALAMBOS [48] (1957–1980) | GINÉS et al. [193] (1987) |
| Liver failure | 19.2 | 28.3 | 27.2 |
| Gastrointestinal bleeding | 19.7 | 19.1 | 19.1 |
| Hepatocellular carcinoma | – | – | 14.5 |
| Infection | 20.0 | 6.2 | 7.3 |
| Renal failure | – | 2.6 | 5.5 |
| Cerebrovascular disease | | | |
| Other/unknown | 40.9 | 39.0 | 26.4 |
| Total deaths | 2314 | 2141 | 121 |

[a] Am J Med Sci (1957) 234:56–61

aminotransferase serum levels, HBsAg status, platelet count, the presence of hepatomegaly or splenomegaly, and abstinence in the case of alcoholic cirrhotics.

This investigation has provided relevant data on the natural evolution of cirrhosis. Ten years after the diagnosis, the probability of survival of the compensated cirrhotics included in the study was 47% and the probability of the development of major complications was 58%. Interestingly, of the 110 patients who died during the follow-up period, only six died while the cirrhosis remained compensated. The median survival for all patients after diagnosis was 8.9 years. In contrast, the median survival for the subgroup of 121 patients who became decompensated was only 1.6 years from the onset of the first major complication.

Therefore, compensated cirrhotics have a reasonably good prognosis which depends mainly on parameters related to liver function. In general, the occurrence of a major complication heralds a poor life expectancy.

### *Decompensated Cirrhosis*

*Ascites.* Ascites is the earliest of the major complications in a substantial proportion of patients. LLACH et al. [194] evaluated 38 parameters with potential prognostic influence in 139 cirrhotics admitted to the hospital because of ascites. A univariate analysis disclosed 18 variables with prognostic significance but only seven retained independent significance after a multivariate analysis. In the whole series, the probability of survival at 6, 12, and 24 months was 62%, 56%, and 49%, respectively. Interestingly, four of the seven parameters with predictive value were related to changes in systemic hemodynamics and renal function. The seven parameters were: mean arterial pressure, plasma norepinephrine, nutritional status, hepatomegaly, serum albumin, urinary sodium excretion, and glomerular filtration rate. Taken in isolation, the indicators with the greatest influence on 1-year survival were a mean arterial pressure of less than 82 mmHg (60% mortality), "poor" nutritional status as assessed by physical examination (75% mortality), and urinary sodium excretion of less than 1.5 mmol/day (55% mortality).

*Spontaneous Bacterial Peritonitis.* Cirrhotic patients with ascites have the additional risk of developing SBP. This complication has been reported to be present in 10%–22% of ascitic patients at admission [180–183]. The mortality in patients with SBP was 70% in some series, ranging from 50% in patients with relatively well-preserved hepatic and renal function to more than 90% in those with severely impaired liver function and renal insufficiency [180–183].

*Renal Failure.* Impairment of renal function is frequent in cirrhotics with ascites. In the series of LLACH et al., patients with a glomerular filtration rate (GFR) of more than 50 ml/min had survival rates of 81%, 61%, and 53% at 3, 12, and 24 months, respectively, whereas the corresponding values in patients with lower GFR values were 54%, 39%, and 33% respectively [194]. Renal failure due to the hepatorenal syndrome is considered to be irreversible and its mortality is close to 100% in days to months following its onset. The inability of the kidneys to excrete free water is a bad prognostic sign in cirrhotics with ascites. Patients who excrete less than 20% of a standard water load in the 5 h following its administration have a life expectancy of less than 6 months [195]. The relevance of renal failure in cirrhosis is highlighted by the fact that the preoperative parameter having the greatest predictive value for a fatal outcome following liver transplantation is a serum creatinine level above 1.7 mg/dl [196].

*Variceal Bleeding.* The mortality of the first episode of variceal bleeding is about 30%. The risk of rebleeding in survivors within the subsequent 6 months is as high as 50% and such rebleeding is associated with a similar or an even higher death rate (see Chap. 11). A recent analysis of four randomized clinical trials shows that either propranolol or nadolol is effective in preventing initial variceal bleeding as compared with placebo. Of 286 patients treated with β-blockers, 78% were free of bleeding and 90% free of fatal bleeding after 2 years, whereas the figures for 303 patients who were given placebo were 65% and 82%, respectively. However, survival rates after 2 years were 71% and 68% in the treated and placebo groups, respectively. The main factors identified as predictors of death in these patients were the presence of ascites and the severity of cirrhosis (Child's C patients) [197].

More dramatic were the results of a prophylactic sclerotherapy trial in 143 patients who were compared with 138 who received sham therapy.

Sclerotherapy effectively prevented initial bleeding but was associated with a significant increase in mortality (32.2%) as compared with the sham-treated group (17.4%). This result forced the termination of the study 22.5 months after it began [198]. Thus, after decompensation cirrhotics have a clinical course which, at least at present, cannot be modified substantially by available medical treatments.

*Hepatic Encephalopathy.* The occurrence of hepatic encephalopathy has a variable effect on survival in different series depending on the type of encephalopathy. If encephalopathy occurs acutely and a correctable triggering factor can be identified, its influence on prognosis is small. However, chronic encephalopathy or multiple recurrent episodes without a clear precipitating factor signal the existence of far-advanced disease and portend a poor prognosis.

*Jaundice.* Hyperbilirubinemia, even if moderate, denotes substantial liver dysfunction, especially if it is not associated with cholestasis. The prognostic significance of total bilirubin is improved by reference to the ratio of total bilirubin to GGT in serum (see below).

## 10.4 Prognosis Based on Selected Isolated Parameters

Some studies have tried to identify analytical parameters predictive of short-term survival in cirrhotics. Although none of them has an absolute discriminant value, they may be useful for an initial and rapid prognostic assessment.

*Ratio of Total Bilirubin to GGT in Serum (TSB/GGT).* This ratio, in which bilirubin is expressed in mmol/liter (value in mg/dl multiplied by 17), gave a mean value of 0.92 in a series of 127 consecutive cirrhotic patients (114 of whom were alcoholic). One-year survival was 66% for patients with a TSB/GGT ratio <1 and only 12% for those with higher values [199].

*Serum Bile Acids.* Normal serum bile acid concentrations in healthy people, after 12 hours' fasting, range from 5 to 10 mM. Higher values are found in patients with liver cirrhosis and are proportional to the degree of liver dysfunction. Fasting serum bile acid levels below 20 mM were found to be associated with a 1-year mortality of 7%, whereas the 1-year mortality was 67% in patients with values above 50 mM [200].

*Prothrombin Time plus Serum Bilirubin.* MADDREY et al. [201] obtained the so-called discriminant function in alcoholic liver disease: 4.6 × prothrombin time (s) + serum bilirubin (mg/dl). Patients yielding scores above 93 using this calculation have a very poor prognosis.

*Aminopyrine* N*-Demethylation.* Orally administered $^{14}$C-aminopyrine is demethylated by the hepatic microsomal oxidizing enzyme system and after intermediate transformations it finally yields $^{14}CO_2$, which is eliminated in breath. Thus, the metabolic capacity of the liver to metabolize this drug is reflected by the amount of expired $^{14}CO_2$. Several studies have demonstrated that measurement of the expired $^{14}CO_2$ in the 2 h following oral administration of a standard dose of $^{14}$C-aminopyrine (1–2 μCi) gives results which correlate closely with those obtained with methods using multiple and prolonged sampling. Normal people expire 6.6% ± 1.3% of the administered dose in 2 h, whereas cirrhotic patients expire 2.6% ± 1.2%. Patients with values below 1.0% have been reported to have a poor short-term outcome [202]. However, the accuracy of the $^{14}$C-aminopyrine breath test in predicting survival of cirrhotic patients was no greater than that of the Child-Turcotte classification or simply serum albumin. Other conceptually similar tests use caffeine, phenacetin, or lidocaine as substrate.

*Ketone Body Ratio.* The ratio of acetoacetate to β-hydroxybutyric acid in arterial blood indirectly reflects the redox potential of mitochondria and is a well-proven index of the ability of these organelles to synthesize ATP. In healthy people the acetoacetate/β-hydroxybutyric acid ratio shows a rapid increase after glucose intake and a decrease in the fasting state, so that marked fluctuations may be detected over a 24-hour period. In fasting cirrhotics the acetoacetate/β-hydroxybutyric acid ratio is lower than in controls and shows no or only a blunted increase in response to meals. Both the fall in the fasting value and the failure of the value to increase with glucose administration are more severe in Child C than in Child A and B patients [203]. Determination of the ketone body ratio may be important as a prognostic indicator in cirrhotic patients, but more validation studies remain to be done. This test has been applied to predict the function of the liver graft after liver transplantation with very promising results.

## 11 Treatment

At present the only treatment able to modify the prognosis of patients with advanced liver cirrhosis is liver transplantation. This therapeutic procedure is restricted to patients in whom a rapid fatal outcome may be anticipated but who are well enough to survive the ordeal. However, despite the enormous advance that liver transplantation represents, the very use of this procedure also shows how deficient are the prophylactic and therapeutic methods currently available for the control of liver cirrhosis.

Preventive measures and treatment of specific etiologies and of portal-systemic encephalopathy, portal hypertension, and ascites are covered elsewhere in this book. In this chapter, attention will be focused on general measures, general treatment of hepatocellular necrosis, inflammation, and fibrogenesis, and treatment of other complications not covered in other parts of the book.

## 11.1 General Measures [204, 205]

For patients with compensated cirrhosis, exercise should be encouraged to prevent osteopenia and loss of muscle mass and to improve general well-being. In cholestatic patients, sunlight exposure is beneficial because this facilitates vitamin D synthesis.

In uncomplicated cirrhotics a normal balanced diet providing a daily supply of 30–45 kcal/kg body wt. and 1–1.2 g protein/kg body wt. should be recommended. These patients do not require significant dietary constraints, although salt intake should be mildly restricted even in patients with no previous ascites. Loss of appetite, nausea, and unspecific dyspepsia are common. Not infrequently, patients with liver disease actually receive diets that contribute to the perpetuation of these complaints. These diets may worsen the nutritional status and the quality of life.

The nutritional guidelines for cirrhotic patients with associated cholestasis are outlined in Chap. 8.

Protein-calorie malnutrition is relatively common in patients with far-advanced cirrhosis and may occur in earlier stages in alcoholic cirrhosis. In these patients, assessment of nutritional status is necessary for adjustment of intake. Frequently, supplementation (or even substitution) of oral intake with enteral or parenteral alimentation is necessary. Total enteral alimentation has recently been tested in malnourished cirrhotics. Of the nutritional parameters measured, only serum albumin increased significantly in comparison with control patients (oral intake), but patient survival during hospitalization improved significantly in enterally fed patients [53].

Total parenteral alimentation is associated with a certain incidence of liver damage, metabolic or hydromineral disequilibrium, and catheter-related infections. In cirrhotics undergoing total parenteral alimentation, oligoelements must be supplied in amounts covering daily allowances. Special attention must be given to zinc supply since its deficiency has been reported to induce PSE in cirrhotics. Choline must also be supplemented since liver damage has followed choline-deficient total parenteral alimentation in recent series [206, 207].

Sodium intake must be restricted in ascitic patients. As a rule a total daily intake of 40 mmol sodium is sufficient and well tolerated. Greater restrictions complicate the elaboration of the diet, are not tolerable for the patient, and offer no clear advantages for the control of ascites. Sodium restriction should be maintained after the elimination of the ascites, to avoid relapse.

Water intake must be restricted to 500 ml daily in ascitic patients with severe hyponatremia, since hyponatremia is mainly due to renal water retention.

In patients with an acute episode of PSE total daily protein intake must be limited initially to 20 g. After recovery, additional protein is introduced progressively (10 g every third or fourth day) while tolerance is monitored. Some patients display an exquisite sensitivity to minor increases in protein ingestion, responding to them with the development of PSE. Protein of milk or vegetable origin is better tolerated than that of meat origin. Total daily protein intake should be distributed throughout the day. In addition, administration of branched chain amino acids has been claimed to be therapeutically useful in PSE, although definitive demonstration is still lacking [208].

## 11.2 Treatment of Hepatocellular Necrosis, Inflammation, and Fibrogenesis

### *Nonspecific Cytoprotection*

Various compounds, generically called "hepatoprotective agents," have been employed with no or little benefit. *3-Cyanydanol*, which gained some initial acceptance, was found to be ineffective and withdrawn. *Silymarin* caused some improvement in liver function tests in some series of patients but no long-term beneficial effect has been established [209]. Large doses of this drug are useful in diminishing liver damage after *Amanita phalloides* poisoning. *S-adenosylmethionine* has been reported to decrease aminotransferase levels in patients with chronic active hepatitis [210]. Although this drug may be of some benefit, long-term trials are needed to ascertain its influence on the progression and final outcome of the disease. *Prostaglandins* of the E series, which have been used with promising results in fulminant hepatitis, have never been employed in patients with chronic liver damage. In some countries "*vitamin cocktails*" are frequently given to cirrhotic patients. Except in very specific patients with proven vitamin deficiency this practice lacks any rational basis. Reduction of aminotransferase levels by *ursodeoxycholate* has recently been reported in a group of patients with chronic active hepatitis [211]. This effect may be related to alteration in the composition of bile acid pool since ursodeoxycholate may substitute toxic bile acids (see Chap. 8). Although it is a safe compound, its long-term effect on the evolution of noncholestatic diseases is at present unknown. Administration of *vitamin E*, a substance with antioxidant properties, has been observed to be of some benefit in isolated patients. *Choline* supplementation has proven to be beneficial in experimental models and in patients with total parenteral nutrition and choline deficiency [207].

### *Anti-inflammatory, Immunosuppressive, and Antifibrogenic Therapy*

Several drugs have been used in chronic liver diseases in an attempt to decrease the activity of the disease process by acting on pathogenic mechanisms. Some of these drugs are discussed below.

*Azathioprine.* This immunosuppressant has been used in combination with corticosteroids in the treatment of autoimmune chronic hepatitis at a dose of 2 mg/kg body wt. Azathioprine alone is ineffective in this condition [212].

*Colchicine.* The antimicrotubular agent colchicine inhibits the intracellular transport of several substances, and specifically that of collagen. In vitro studies showed colchicine to be effective in reducing liver fibrosis in $CCl_4$-treated rats [213]. These studies prompted its use as an antifibrogenic agent in alcoholic liver disease and primary biliary cirrhosis. The first colchicine trial in patients with cirrhosis was initiated by KERSHENOBICH et al. in 1978 [214]. The patients (50% alcoholics) were given colchicine (1 mg five times a week) or placebo. The treated group showed significantly higher cumulative 5-year survival (75%) and histologic improvement (18%) than those receiving placebo (34% and 0%, respectively). Results of this study are, however, controversial since the mortality of the control group was abnormally high. The value of colchicine in the treatment of alcoholic cirrhosis needs further assessment.

In primary biliary cirrhosis, colchicine ameliorated biochemical parameters but showed no influence on liver histology after 4 years of treatment [215].

*Chlorambucil.* This alkylating agent has been compared with placebo in a series of patients with primary biliary cirrhosis. After a follow-up of 4 years, there was an improvement in biochemical parameters in the treated group but not in the placebo group. Histologic progression of the disease and the degree of fibrosis were similar in the two groups [216]. In the group receiving the drug there were some instances of bone marrow depression and a non-significant increase in viral infections. The use of this drug requires reevaluation since in this study the number of patients in stages III and IV was greater in the placebo than in the chlorambucil group.

*Cyclosporine.* Cyclosporine is the most powerful immunosuppressant available. It was administered to patients with primary biliary cirrhosis at two different doses in different trials [217, 218]. Beneficial effects on biochemical parameters were seen but the frequency of hypertension and renal damage was significant at high doses.

*Corticosteroids.* Because of their powerful anti-inflammatory, antifibrogenic, and immunomodulatory activities, corticosteroids have been employed in several liver diseases. They are the drugs of choice for chronic autoimmune hepatitis, given alone or in combination with azathioprine [212]. If administered early in the disease, corticosteroids normalize aminotransferase and bilirubin levels, decrease the inflammatory activity in liver tissue, and control the extrahepatic manifestations in the majority of the patients. The risk of developing liver cirrhosis within 3 years after the initiation of therapy is about 40% but it does not increase substantially thereafter, so that the cumulative risk is below 50% after 10 years of therapy. Patients who are symptomatic at a premenopausal age, who display hyperglobulinemia, and who are at a precirrhotic stage with bridging necrosis at the commencement of treatment are more likely to show a good response. Prednisone (or methylprednisolone at equivalent doses) is given at an initial dose of 60 mg/day which is then tapered over 1 month to achieve a maintenance dose of 20 mg/day [212].

Although corticosteroids have been used in alcoholic hepatitis, the results are controversial and only the subgroup of patients with the most severe form of the disease show an improvement in survival. In a recent study, patients treated with prednisolone (40 mg/day) and placebo showed mortality rates of 12.5% and 55.8% respectively [219].

On the other hand, corticosteroid therapy has been proven to be deleterious in chronic hepatitis B, and at present there is no indication for the use of corticosteroids in chronic hepatitis C.

*D-Penicillamine.* This drug has immunomodulatory and antifibrogenic activities and is a copper chelating agent. It has been proposed as treatment for primary biliary cirrhosis because of its usefulness in Wilson's disease, since in both conditions there is increased copper deposition in the liver. Controlled trials have to date enrolled more than 800 patients. No beneficial effect of D-penicillamine has been demonstrated by reference to clinical, biochemical, or histopathologic data. Furthermore, 29%–46% of the patients treated with the drug have developed side-effects. Thus D-penicillamine therapy has to be avoided in patients with primary biliary cirrhosis [220]. In contrast, this drug is life-saving for patients with Wilson's disease, in which the ultimate mechanism of liver damage is related to copper toxicity.

*Interferon-α.* Interferon-α has been administered to patients with chronic hepatitis B and C. In addition to its antiviral effects it has been shown that interferon-α reduces fibrogenic activity as measured by various parameters [34] (see Sect. 4.2).

*Propylthiouracil.* This drug has been investigated in the treatment of alcoholic hepatitis since it was proposed that this condition showed features mimicking hyperthyroidism. In some studies it was found that propylthiouracil accelerated the rate of recovery of patients but did not influence short-term survival [221]. Orrego et al. reported a lower cumulative mortality (12%) in 157 patients taking propylthiouracil than in patients ($n$ = 157) given placebo (25%) [222]. However, other authors have not confirmed these results. Therefore, this drug requires further evaluation before it can be recommended in alcoholic hepatitis [223].

*Ursodeoxycholate.* This hypercholeretic bile salt has proven to be beneficial in primary biliary cirrhosis and in other chronic cholestatic disorders (see Chap. 8). A recent double-blind, placebo-controlled trial has demonstrated improvement in both biochemical and histologic parameters in patients with primary biliary cirrhosis [224].

## 11.3 Treatment and Prevention of Spontaneous Bacterial Peritonitis

Norfloxacin (400 mg/day) is effective in preventing the recurrence of SBP [183, 225]. In a multicenter double-blind, placebo-controlled trial the probability of SBP recurrence after 1-year of follow-up was 20% in the norfloxacin group and 68% in the placebo group. This difference was due to the virtual elimination in the treated group of SBP caused by enteric Gram-negative bacilli.

Treatment of SBP must be initiated immediately after the diagnosis is established, i.e., before bacteriologic data are available. Several antibiotic therapies have been demonstrated to be effective in achieving the resolution of SBP: tobramycin plus ampicillin (61%), ceftriaxone (83%), amoxicillin plus clavulanic acid (85%), cefotaxime (86%), and pefloxacin plus other antibiotics (87%). In one study, patient survival at the time of hospital discharge was highest with cefotaxime and no nephrotoxicity or superinfection was observed with its use [226]. Cefotaxime is administered at a dose of 2 g/4–6 h [183].

## 11.4 Treatment of the Hemostatic Disorder

The basic treatment is vitamin K. In patients who are to undergo invasive procedures or surgery, fresh-frozen plasma (12–20 ml/kg) and platelet concentrates are useful to prevent excessive bleeding. The administration of fresh-frozen plasma should provide clotting factors to obtain an additional 20% procoagulant activity. The main problems with this therapy are the induction of volume overload and its relatively transient effect because of the short half-life of factor VII. The effectiveness of platelet transfusions is limited by platelet sequestration in the enlarged spleen. The use of cryoprecipitate should be restricted to patients with fibrinogen deficiency not due to abnormal degradation but rather to reduced synthesis. This is an uncommon situation in liver cirrhosis. Administration of prothrombin complex is rarely indicated in patients with extreme deficiency of clotting factors. It is associated with a variety of complications, including the risk of parenterally transmitted diseases, anaphylactic reactions, and DIC. Some patients with accelerated fibrinolysis may benefit from the administration of ε-aminocaproic acid.

The use of 1-deamino-8-D-arginine-vasopressin (ddAVP) may shorten bleeding time and occasionally prothrombin time and activated partial thromboplastin time [166].

## References


1. Anthony PP, Ishak KG, Nayak NC, Poulsen HE, Scheuer PJ, Sobin LH (1977) The morphology of cirrhosis: definition, nomenclature and classification. Bull WHO 55:521–524
2. Anthony PP, Ishak KG, Nayak NC, Poulsen H, Scheuer PJ, Sobin LH (1978) The morphology of cirrhosis. J Clin Pathol 31:395–414
3. Millward-Sadler GH (1987) Cirrhosis. In: MacSween RNM, Anthony PP, Scheuer PJ (eds) Pathology of the liver. Churchill Livingston, Edinburgh, pp 342–363
4. Poulsen H (1987) Morphology: criteria for definition, diagnosis, typing, staining and morphogenesis. In: Tygstrup N, Orlandi F (eds) Cirrhosis of the liver: methods and fields of research. Elsevier, Amsterdam, pp 49–62
5. Saunders JB, Walters JRF, Davies P, Paton A (1981) A 20 year prospective study of cirrhosis. Br Med J 282:263–266
6. Garagliano CF, Lilienfeld AM, Mendeloff AI (1979) Incidence rates of liver cirrhosis and related diseases in Baltimore and selected areas of the United States. J Chronic Dis 32:543–554
7. Almdal TP, Sorensen TIA, The Danish Association for the Study of the Liver (1991) Incidence of parenchymal liver disease in Denmark, 1981 to 1985. Analysis of hospitalization registry data. Hepatology 13:650–655
8. Galambos JT (1979) Cirrhosis. Major problems in internal medicine, vol XVII. W.B. Saunders, Philadelphia, pp 91–127
9. Melato M, Mucli E (1989) Something new in liver cirrhosis epidemiology. Lancet 2:395–396
10. Grant BF, Dufour MC, Harford TC (1988) Epidemiology of alcoholic liver disease. Semin Liver Dis 8:12–25
11. Hasin DS, Grant B, Harford TC (1990) Male and female differences in liver cirrhosis mortality in the United States, 1961–1985. J Stud Alcohol 51:123–129
12. Coppere H, Audigier JC (1986) Evolution de la mortalité par cirrhose en France entre 1925 et 1982. Gastroenterol Clin Biol 10:468–474
13. Sanchez A, Gonzalez F, Pena Z, Castello B, Sarthou C (1989) Cirrosis hepatica: Estudio de la evolucion de la mortalidad en Espa ña (1951–1983). Rev Esp Ap Digest 76:367–374
14. Qiao ZQ, Halliday ML, Coates RA, Rankin JG (1988) Relationship between liver cirrhosis death rates and nutritional factors in 38 countries. Int J Epidemiol 17:414–418
15. Desmet VJ, Sciot R, Van Eyken P (1990) Differential diagnosis and prognosis of cirrhosis: role of liver biopsy. Acta Gastroenterol Belg LIII:198–208
16. Scheuer PJ (1988) Cirrhosis. In: Scheuer PJ (ed) Liver biopsy interpretation. Bailliere Tindall, London, pp 131–146
17. Popper H (1983) Introduction. In: Keppler D, Popper H, Bianchi L, Reutter W (eds) Mechanisms of hepatocyte injury and death. Falk Symposium 38. MTP Press, Lancaster, pp 1–10
18. Popper H (1988) Hepatocellular degeneration and death. In: Arias IM, Jakoby WB, Popper H, Schachter D, Shafritz DA (eds) The liver. Biology and pathobiology. Raven, New York, pp 1087–1103
19. Heilmann C, Spamer C, Gerok W (1990) Aspects of hepatic calcium metabolism. In: Popper H, Schaffner F (eds) Progress in liver disease, vol IX. W.B. Saunders, Philadelphia, pp 261–279

20. Biagini G, Ballardini G (1989) Liver fibrosis and extracellular matrix. J Hepatol 8:115–124
21. Hahn EG, Schuppan D (1987) Pathogenic mechanisms: fibrosis, fibrogenesis and fibrolysis. In: Tygstrup N, Orlandi F (eds) Cirrhosis of the liver: methods and fields of research. Elsevier, Amsterdam, pp 63–81
22. Shuppan D (1990) Structure of the extracellular matrix in normal and fibrotic liver: collagens and glycoproteins. Semin Liver Dis 10:1–10
23. Gressner AM, Bachem MG (1990) Cellular sources of noncollagenous matrix proteins: role of fat-storing cells in fibrogenesis. Semin Liver Dis 10:30–46
24. Martin GR, Kleinman HK (1985) The extracellular matrix components in development and in disease. Semin Liver Dis 5:147–156
25. Boot-Handford RP, Kurkinen M, Prockop DJ (1987) Steady-state levels of mRNAs coding for the type IV collagen and laminin polypeptide chains of basement membranes exhibit marked tissue-specific stoichiometric variations in the rat. J Biol Chem 262:12475–12478
26. Burgeson RE (1988) New collagens, new concepts. Annu Rev Cell Biol 4:551–557
27. Rojkind M, Ponce-Noyola P (1982) The extracellular matrix of the liver. Coll Relat Res 2:151–175
28. Bissell DM, Friedman SL, Maher JJ, Roll F (1990) Connective tissue biology and hepatic fibrosis: report of a conference. Hepatology 11:488–498
29. Friedman SL (1990) Cellular sources of collagen and regulation of collagen production in liver. Semin Liver Dis 10:20–29
30. Bissell DM (1990) Cell-matrix interaction and hepatic fibrosis. In: Popper H, Schaffner F (eds) Progress in liver disease, vol IX. W.B. Saunders, Philadelphia, pp 143–155
31. Bissell DM, Arenson DM, Maher JJ, Roll FJ (1987) Support of cultured hepatocytes by a laminin-rich gel: evidence for a functionally significant subendothelial matrix in normal rat liver. J Clin Invest 79:801–812
32. Fujita M, Spray DC, Choi H et al. (1987) Glycosaminoglycans and proteoglycans induce gap junction expression and restore transcription of tissue-specific mRNAs in primary liver cultures. Hepatology 7: 1S–9S
33. Friedman SL, Roll FJ, Boyles J, Arenson DM, Bissell DM (1989) Maintenance of differentiated phenotype of cultured rat hepatic lipocytes by basement membrane matrix. J Biol Chem 264:10756–10762
34. Castilla A, Prieto J, Fausto N (1991) Transforming growth factor β1 and α in chronic liver disease. Effects of interferon α therapy. N Engl J Med 324:933–940
35. Fausto N, Mead JE (1989) Regulation of liver growth: protooncogenes and transforming growth factors. Lab Invest 60:4–13
36. Wood AJJ, Villeneuve JP, Branch RA, Rogers LW, Shand DG (1979) Intact hepatocyte theory of impaired drug metabolism in experimental cirrhosis in the rat. Gastroenterology 76:1358–1362
37. Meyer B, Luo H, Bargetzi M, Renner EL, Stalder G (1991) Quantitation of intrinsic drug-metabolizing capacity in human liver biopsy specimens: support for the intact-hepatocyte theory. Hepatology 13:475–481
38. Castilla A, Vazquez J, Simón MA, Prieto J, Fausto N (1991) Liver cell proliferation in the natural history of chronic viral liver disease. J Hepatol 13 [Suppl 2]:S18
39. Roberts AB, Sporn MB (1989) The transforming growth factors. In: Sporn MB, Roberts AB (eds) Peptide growth factors and their receptors. I. Springer, Berlin Heidelberg New York (Handbook of experimental pharmacology, vol 95, pp 419–472)
40. Zakim D (1981) Pathophysiology of liver disease. In: Smith LH, Thier SO (eds) Pathophysiology: the biological principles of disease. W.B. Saunders, Philadelphia, pp 1960–1744

41. Jenkins W, Billing B (1985) Physiology of the liver. In: Berk JE, Haubrich WS, Kalser MH, Roth JLA, Schaffner F (eds) Bockus gastroenterology, 4th edn. W.B. Saunders, Philadelphia, pp 2666–2696
42. Boyer TD (1990) Portal hypertension and bleeding esophageal varices. In: Zakim D, Boyer TD (eds) Hepatology: a textbook of liver disease, 2nd edn. W.B. Saunders, Philadelphia, pp 572–615
43. Bosch J, Navasa M, García-Pagán J, DeLacy AM, Rodés J (1989) Portal hypertension. Med Clin North Am 73:931–953
44. Groszmann RJ, Atterbury CE (1982) The pathophysiology of portal hypertension. A basis for classification. Semin Liver Dis 2:117–186
45. Garcia-Tsao G, Groszmann RJ, Fisher RL et al. (1960) Spontaneous decrease in portal pressure with clinical improvement in cirrhosis. N Engl J Med 263:734–739
46. Blendis LM, Orrego, H, Crossley IR, et al. (1982) The role of hepatocyte enlargement and hepatic pressure in cirrhotic and non-cirrhotic alcoholic liver disease. Hepatology 2:539–544
47. Bosch J, Mastai R, Kravetz D et al. (1985) Measurement of azygos venous blood flow in the evaluation of portal hypertension in patients with cirrhosis. Clinical and haemodynamic correlation in 100 patients. J Hepatol 1:125–139
48. Galambos JT (1985) Alcoholic liver disease: fatty liver, hepatitis and cirrhosis. In: Berk JE, Haubrich WS, Kalser MH, Roth JLA, Schaffner F (eds) Bockus gastroenterology, 4th edn. W.B. Saunders, Philadelphia, pp 2985–3048
49. Sherlock S (1989) Diseases of the liver and biliary system, 8th edn. Blackwell Scientific, Oxford
50. Conn HO, Atterbury CE (1987) Cirrhosis. In: Schiff L, Schiff ER (eds) Diseases of the liver, 6th edn. J.B. Lippincott, Philadelphia, pp 725–864
51. Hallen J, Norden J (1964) Liver cirrhosis unsuspected during life: a series of 79 cases. J Chronic Dis 17:951–958
52. Rodriguez-Roisin R, Roca J, Agustí AGN, Mastai R, Wagner PD, Bosch J (1987) Gas exchange and pulmonary vascular reactivity in patients with liver cirrhosis. Am Rev Respir Dis 134:1085–1092
53. Cabre E, Gonzalez-Huix F, Abad-Lacruz A et al. (1990) Effect of total enteral nutrition on the short-term outcome of severely malnourished cirrhotics. A randomized controlled trial. Gastroenterology 98:715–720
54. Ekbom K, Hed R, Kirstein L, Astrom KE (1964) Muscular affections in chronic alcoholism. Arch Neurol 10:449–458
55. Waterlow JC, Garlick PJ, Millward DJ (1978) Protein turnover in mammalian tissues and in the whole body. Elsevier/North Holland Biochemical Press, Amsterdam
56. Marchesini G, Zoli M, Angiolini A, Dondi C, Bianchi FB, Pisi E (1981) Muscle protein breakdown in liver cirrhosis and the role of altered carbohydrate metabolism. 1:294–299
57. Zoli M, Marchesini G, Diondi C, Branchi GP, Pisi E (1982) Myofibrillar protein catabolic rates in cirrhotic patients with and without muscle wasting. Clin Sci 62:683–686
58. Emery PW, Cotellessa L, Holness M, Egan C, Rennie MJ (1986) Different patterns of protein turnover in skeletal and gastrointestinal smooth muscle and the production of *N*-methyl-histidine during fasting in the rat. Biosci Rep 6:143–153
59. Morrison WL, Bouchier IAD, Gipson JNA, Rennie MJ (1990) Skeletal muscle and whole body protein turnover in cirrhosis. Clin Sci 78:613–619
60. Moreau R, Lee SS, Soupison T, Roche-Sicot J, Sicot C (1988) Abnormal tissue oxygenation in patients with cirrhosis and liver failure. J Hepatol 7:98–105
61. Schneeweiss B, Graninger W, Ferenci P et al. (1990) Energy metabolism in patients with acute and chronic liver disease. Hepatology 11:387–393
62. Campillo B, Fouet P, Bonnet JC, Atlan G (1990) Submaximal oxygen consumption in liver cirrhosis. Evidence of severe functional aerobic impairment. J Hepatol 10:163–167

63. Shanbhogue RLK, Bistrian BR, Jenkins RL et al. (1987) Resting energy expenditure in patients with end-stage liver disease and in normal population. J Parenter Enteral Nutr 11:305–308
64. Dolz C, Raurich JM, Ibañez J, Obrador A, Marse P, Gaya J (1991) Ascites increases the resting energy expenditure in liver cirrhosis. Gastroenterology 100:738–744
65. Romijn JA, Endaert E, Sauerwein HP (1991) Glucose and fat metabolism during short-term acute starvation in cirrhosis. Gastroenterology 100:731–737
66. Iwata S, Ozawa K, Shimahara Y et al. (1991) Diurnal fluctuations of arterial ketone body ratio in normal subjects and patients with liver dysfunction. Castroenterology 100:1371–1378
67. Alberti KGMM, Johnston DG, Taylor R (1985) Carbohydrate metabolism in liver disease. In: Wright R, Millward-Sadler GH, Alberti KGM, Karran S (eds) Liver and biliary disease. W B Saunders Company, London 1985, pp 45–64
68. Creutzfeldt W, Frerichs H, Sickinger K (1970) Liver diseases and diabetes mellitus. In: Popper H, Schaffner F (eds) Progress in liver diseases, vol III. Grune and Stratton, New York, pp 371–407
69. Kingston ME, Ali MA, Atiyeh M, Donnelly RJ (1984) Diabetes mellitus in chronic active hepatitis and cirrhosis. Gastroenterology 87:688–694
70. Kruszynska Y, Home PD, McIntyre N (1991) Relationship between insulin sensitivity, insulin secretion and glucose tolerance in cirrhosis. Hepatology 14:103–111
71. Cavallo-Perin P, Cassader M, Bozzo C et al. (1985) Mechanism of insulin resistance in human liver cirrhosis: evidence of a combined receptor and postreceptor defect. J Clin Invest 75:1659–1665
72. Marco J, Diego J, Villanueva ML, Diaz-Fierros M, Valverde I, Segovia JM (1973) Elevated plasma glucagon levels in cirrhosis of the liver. N Engl J Med 289:1107–1111
73. Van Thiel DH (1988) The liver and the endocrine system. In: Arias IM, Jacoby WB, Popper H, Schachter D, Shafritz DA (eds) The liver: biology and pathobiology, 2nd edn. Raven, New York, pp 1007–1032
74. Calandra S, Martin MJ, McIntyre M (1971) Plasma lecitin: cholesterol acyltransferase activity in liver disease. Eur J Clin Invest 1:352–360
75. Schreiber G (1987) Synthesis, processing and secretion of plasma proteins by the liver (and other organs) and their regulation. In: Putnam FW (ed) The plasma proteins. Academic, New York
76. Fischer JE, Yoshimura N, Aguirre A et al. (1974) Plasma aminoacids in patients with hepatic encephalopathy. Effect of aminoacid infusions. Am J Surg 127:40–47
77. Shenker S, Brady CE (1989) Pathogenesis of hepatic encephalopathy. In: Conn HO, Bircher J (eds) Hepatic encephalopathy. Medi-Ed, Michigan, pp 15–30
78. Bass NM, Williams RL (1990) Hepatic function and pharmacokinetics. In: Zakim D, Boyer TD (eds) Hepatology: a textbook of liver disease, 2nd edn. W.B. Saunders, Philadelpia, pp 235–253
79. Reed D (1990) Chemical mechanism in drug-induced liver injury. In: Zakim D, Boyer TD (eds) Hepatology. WB Saunders, Philadelphia, pp 737–753
80. Ferenci P (1989) GABA in human hepatic encephalopathy. In: Conn HO, Bircher J (eds) Hepatic encephalopathy. Medi-Ed, Michigan, pp 53–60
81. Arroyo V, Ginés P, Rimola A, Gaya J (1986) Renal function abnormalities, prostaglandins and effects of nonsteroidal antiinflammatory drugs. Am J Med 81 [Suppl 2B]:104–122
82. Brodie MJ, Boobis AR, Bulpitt CJ et al. (1981) Influence of liver disease and environmental factors on hepatic monooxygenase activity in vitro. Eur J Clin Pharmacol 20:39–46
83. Farrell GC, Cooksley WGE, Powell LW (1979) Drug metabolism in liver disease: activity of hepatic microsomal metabolizing enzymes. Clin Pharmacol Ther 26:483–492

84. Schrier RW, Arroyo V, Bernardi M, Epstein M, Henriksen JH, Rodes J (1988) Peripheral arterial vasodilatation hypothesis: a proposal for the initiation of renal sodium and water retention in cirrhosis. Hepatology 8:1151–1157
85. Bosch J, Gines P, Arroyo V, Navasa M, Rodes J (1988) Hepatic and systemic hemodynamics and the neurohumoral systems in cirrhosis. In: Epstein M (ed) The kidney in liver diseases. Williams & Wilkins, Baltimore, pp 286–305
86. Kowalski HJ, Abelmann WH (1953) Cardiac output at rest in Laennec's cirrhosis. J Clin Invest 32:1025–1033
87. Benoit JN, Granger DN (1986) Splanchnic hemodynamics in chronic portal venous hypertension. Semin Liver Dis 6:287–298
88. Lieberman FL, Reynolds TB (1967) Plasma volume in cirrhosis of the liver. Its relation to portal hypertension, ascites and renal failure. J Clin Invest 46:1297–1308
89. Kontos HA, Shapiro W, Mauck HP et al. (1964) General and regional circulatory alterations in cirrhosis of the liver. Am J Med 37:526–535
90. Fernandez-Seara J, Prieto J, Quiroga J et al. (1989) Systemic and regional hemodynamics in patients with liver cirrhosis and ascites with and without functional renal failure. Gastroenterology 97:1304–1312
91. Vorobioff J, Bredfeldt JE, Groszmann RJ (1984) Increased blood flow through the portal system in cirrhotic rats. Gastroenterology 87:1120–1126
92. De Vusser P, Bounameaux H, Verhaeghe R et al. (1985) Liver cirrhosis, ascites and peripheral vascular resistance (letter). Lancet II:1078
93. Murray JF, Dawson AM, Sherlock S (1958) Circulatory changes in chronic liver disease. Am J Med 24:358–367
94. Henriksen JH, Bendtsen F, Sorensen TIA, Stadeager C, Ring-Larsen H (1990) Reduced central blood volume in cirrhosis. Gastroenterology 97:1506–1513
95. Moe GW, Legault L, Skorecki KL (1991) Control of extracellular fluid volume and pathophysiology of edema. In: Brenner BM, Rector FC (eds) The kidney, 4th edn. W.B. Saunders, Philadelphia, pp 623–676
96. Macgilchrist AJ, Howes LG, Hawks BYC, Reid JL (1991) Plasma noradrenaline in cirrhosis: a study of kinetics and temporal relationship to ascites formation. Eur J Clin Invest 21:238–243
97. Arroyo V, Bosch J, Mauri M et al. (1979) Renin, aldosterone and renal hemodynamics in cirrhotics with ascites. Eur J Clin Invest 9:69–73
98. Simon MA, Diez J, Prieto J (1991) Abnormal sympathetic and renal response to sodium restriction in compensated cirrhosis. Gastroenterology 101:1354–1360
99. Jiménez W, Martínez-Pardo A, Arroyo V et al. (1985) Temporal relationship between hyperaldosteronism, sodium retention and ascites formation in rats with experimental cirrhosis. Hepatology 5:245–250
100. López C, Jiménez W, Arroyo V et al. (1990) Temporal relationship between the decrease in arterial pressure and sodium retention in conscious spontaneously hypertensive rats with carbon tetrachloride-induced cirrhosis. Hepatology 13:585–589
101. Lautt W, Legare DJ, Ezzat WR (1990) Quantitation of the hepatic arterial buffer response to graded changes in portal blood flow. Gastroenterology 1024–1028
102. Pizcueta PM, Bosch J (1990) Role of vasoactive systems in the pathogenesis of circulatory abnormalities in cirrhosis. Liver disease and renal complications. In: Frati L, Aaronson SA (eds) Advances in experimental medicine. Raven, New York, pp 247–254
103. Guarner F, Guarner C, Prieto J et al. (1986) Increased synthesis of systemic prostacyclin in cirrhotic patients. Gastroenterology 90:687–694
104. Silva G, Navasa M, Bosch J et al. (1990) Hemodynamic effect of glucagon in portal hypertension. Hepatology 11:668–673
105. Pizcueta P, Piqué JM, Fernandez M, Bosch J, Rodés J, Whittle BJR, Moncada S (eds) Endogenous nitric oxide is involved in hemodynamic disturbances in portal hypertensive rats (abstract). J Hepatol 13 [Suppl 2]:S61

106. Claria J, Jimenez W, Arroyo V et al. (1990) Endothelin (ET) has natriuretic effect in conscious cirrhotic rats with ascites (abstract). J Hepatol 11 [Suppl 2]:S17
107. Moore KP, Wendon J, Fraser M et al. (1991) High plasma endothelin in hepatorenal syndrome (abstract). J Hepatol 13 [Suppl 2]:S54
108. Wensing G, Sabra R, Branch RA (1990) Renal and systemic hemodynamics in experimental cirrhosis in rats: relation to hepatic function. Hepatology 12; 13–19
109. Wensing G, Sabra R, Branch RA (1990) The onset of sodium retention in experimental cirrhosis in rats is related to a clinical threshold of liver function. Hepatology 11:779–786
110. Rector WG Jr, Lewis F, Robertson AD, Everson GT (1990) Renal sodium retention complicating alcoholic liver disease: relation to portosystemic shunting and liver function. Hepatology 12:445–449
111. Vaamonde CA (1988) Renal water handling in liver disease. In: Epstein M (ed) The kidney and liver disease, 3rd edn. Williams and Wilkins, Baltimore, pp 31–72
112. Epstein M (1988) Hepatorenal syndrome. In: Epstein M (ed) The kidney and liver disease, 3rd edn. Williams and Wilkins, Baltimore, pp 89–118
113. Dicksson ER, Grambsch PM, Fleming TR, Fisher LD, Langworthy A (1989) Prognosis in primary biliary cirrhosis: model for decision making. Hepatology 10:1–7
114. Hadengue A, Benhayoun HK, Lebrel D, Benhamou JP (1991) Pulmonary hypertension complicating portal hypertension: prevalence and relation to splanchnic hemodynamics. Gastroenterology 100:520–528
115. Singer JA, Kaplan MM, Katz RL (1977) Cirrhotic pleural effusion in the absence of ascites. Gastroenterology 73:575–581
116. Robin ED, Horn B, Goris ML et al. (1975) Detection, quantitation and pathophysiology of lung "spiders". Trans Assoc Am Phys 88:202–215
117. Agustí AGN, Roca J, Bosch J, Rodriguez-Roisin R (1990) The lung in patients with cirrhosis. J Hepatol 10:251–257
118. Hourani JM, Bellamy PE, Tashkin DP, Batra P, Simmons S (1991) Pulmonary dysfunction in advanced liver disease: frequent occurrence of an abnormal diffusing capacity. Am J Med 90:693–700
119. Naeije R, Melot C, Hallemans R et al. (1985) Pulmonary hemodynamics in liver cirrhosis. Semin Resp Med 7:164–169
120. Rakela J, Krowka MJ (1990) Cardiovascular and pulmonary complications of liver diseases. In: Zakim D, Boyer TD (eds) Hepatology. WB Saunders, Philadelphia, pp 530–537
121. Davis HH, Schwartz DJ, Lefrac SS, Susman N, Schainker A (1978) Alveolar-capillary oxygen disequilibrium in hepatic cirrhosis. Chest 73:507–511
122. Scemama-Clergue J, Piquet J, Clerici C, Harf A, Dhumeaux D (1989) Effect of propranolol on pulmonary gas exchange in patients with cirrhosis. J Hepatol 9:234–239
123. Robin ED, Laman D, Horn BR et al. (1976) Platypnea related to orthodeoxia caused by true vascular lung shunts. N Engl J Med 294:941–945
124. Naeijie R, Hallemans R, Mols P, Melot C. Hypoxic pulmonary vasoconstriction in liver cirrhosis. Chest 80:570–574
125. Castaing Y, Manier G (1989) Hemodynamic disturbances and $\mathring{V}a/\mathring{Q}$ matching in hypoxemic cirrhotic patients. Chest 96:1064–1069
126. Rodriguez-Roisin R, Roca J, Guitart R et al. (1986) Measurements of distributions of ventilation-perfusion ratios: multiple inert gases elimination technique. Rev Esp Fisiol 42:465–482
127. Agustí AGN, Roca J, Rodríguez-Roisin R et al. (1989) Pulmonary hemodynamics and gas exchange during exercise in liver cirrhosis. Am Rev Respir Dis 139:485–491

128. Dantzker DR (1987) Ventilation-perfusion inequality in lung disease. Chest 91:749–754
129. Astrup J, Rorth M (1973) Oxygen affinity of hemoglobin and red cell 2,3-diphosphoglycerate in hepatic cirrhosis. Scand J Clin Lab Invest 31:311–315
130. Eriksson LS, Söderman C, Ericzon BG, Eleborg L, Wahren J, Hedenstierna G (1990) Normalization of ventilation/perfusion relationships after liver transplantation in patients with decompensated cirrhosis: evidence for a hepatopulmonary syndrome. Hepatology 12:1350–1357
131. Conn HO (1989) The hepatic encephalopaties. In: Conn HO, Bircher J (eds) Hepatic encephalopathy. Medi-Ed, Michigan, pp 3–14
132. Jones EA, Schafer DF, Ferenci P et al. (1984) The neurobiology of hepatic encephalopathy. Hepatology 4:1235–1242
133. Gaiani S, Bolondi L, Bassi SL, Zironi G, Siringo S, Barbara L (1991) Prevalence of spontaneous hepatofugal portal flow in liver cirrhosis. Clinical and endoscopic correlation in 228 patients. Gastroenterology 100:160–167
134. Johansson U, Andersson T, Persson A, Eriksson LS (1989) Visual evoked potential – a tool in the diagnosis of hepatic encephalopathy?. J Hepatol 9:227–233
135. Davies MG, Rowan MJ, MacMathuna P, Keeling PWN, Weir DG, Feely J (1990) The auditory P300 event-related potential: an objective marker of the encephalopathy of chronic liver disease. Hepatology 12:688–694
136. Bernthanl P, Hays A, Tarter RE, Van Thiel D, Lecky J, Hegedus A (1987) Cerebral CT scan abnormalities in cholestatic and hepatocellular disease and their relationship to neuropsychologic test performance. Hepatology 7:107–114
137. Victor M, Adams R, Cole M (1965) The acquired (non-wilsonian) type of chronic hepatocerebral degeneration. Medicine 44:345–396
138. Pant S, Rebeiz J, Richardson E (1986) Spastic paraparesis following portacaval shunts. Neurology 18:134–141
139. Powell EE, Pender MP, Chalk JB et al. (1990) Improvement in chronic hepatocerebral degeneration following liver transplantation. Gastroenterology 98:1079–1082
140. Kirk AP, Dooley JS, Hunt RH (1980) Peptic ulceration in patients with chronic liver disease. Dig Dis 25:756–761
141. Weiler H, Weiler C, Gerok W (1990) Gastric mucosal prostaglandin $E_2$ levels in cirrhosis and portal hypertension. J Hepatol 11:58–64
142. Paquet KJ, Mercado-Diaz M, Kalk JF (1990) Frequency, significance and therapy of the Mallory-Weiss syndrome in patients with portal hypertension. Hepatology 11:879–883
143. Quintero E, Piqué JM, Bombi JA et al. (1987) Gastric mucosal vascular ectasias causing bleeding in cirrhosis. Gastroenterology 93:1054–1061
144. Hashizume M, Tanaka K, Inokuchi K (1983) Morphology of gastric microcirculation in cirrhosis. Hepatology 3:1008–1012
145. D'Amico G, Montalbano L, Traina M et al. (1990) Natural history of congestive gastropathy in cirrhosis. Gastroenterology 99:1558–1564
146. Van Thiel DH, Gavaler JS, Schade RR (1985) Liver disese and the hypothalamic pituitary gonadal axis. Semin Liver Dis 5:35–45
147. Becker U, Gluud C, Farholt S et al. (1991) Menopausal age and sex hormones in postmenopausal women with alcoholic and nonalcoholic liver disease. J Hepatol 13:25–32
148. Van Thiel DH, Stone BG, Schade RR (1987) The liver and its effect on endocrine function in health and diseases. In: Schiff L, Schiff ER (eds) Diseases of the liver. Lippincott, Philadelphia, pp 129–162
149. Van Thiel DH (1990) Disorders of the hypothalamic pituitary gonadal and thyroidal axes in patients with liver disease. In: Zakim D, Boyer TD (eds) Hepatology: a textbook of liver disease, 2nd edn. W.B. Saunders, Philadelphia, pp 513–529

150. Van Thiel DH, Gavaler JS, Sanghvi A (1982) Recovery of sexual function in abstinent alcoholic men. Gastroenterology 84:677–682
151. Lester R, Van Thiel DA, Eagon PK, et al. (1979) Hypothesis concerning the effects of dietary non-steroidal estrogen on the feminization of male alcoholics. Research Monograph 2. Alcohol and Nutrition, DHEW Publication
152. Van Thiel DH, Gavaler JS, Spero JA et al. (1981) Patterns of hypothalamic pituitary gonadal dysfunction in men with liver disease due to different etiologies. Hepatology 1:39–46
153. Newton ER, Turksoy N, Kaplan M et al. (1988) Pregnancy and liver transplantation. Obstet Gynecol 71:499–500
154. Shaw BW, Stratta RJ, Donovan JP et al. (1989) Postoperative care after liver transplantation. Semin Liver Dis 9:202–230
155. Findling JW, Tyrrell JB (1991) Anterior pituitary gland. In: Greenspan FS (ed) Basic and clinical endocrinology, 3rd edn. Prentice Hall, London, pp 79–132
156. Spencer EM (1991) Somatomedins. In: Greenspan FS (ed) Basic and clinical endocrinology, 3rd edn. Prentice Hall, London, pp 133–146
157. Zanoboni A, Zanoboni-Muciaccia W (1977) Elevated basal growth hormone levels and growth hormone responses to TRH in alcoholic patients with cirrhosis. J Clin Endocrinol Metab 45:576–582
158. Wu A, Grant DB, Hambley J, Levy AT (1974) Reduced somatomedin activity in patients with chronic liver disease. Clin Sci Mol Med 47:359–364
159. Wiedemann E, Schwartz E, Frantz AG (1976) Acute and chronic estrogen effects upon serum somatomedin activity, growth hormone and prolactin in man. J Clin Endocrinol Metab 42:942–949
160. Haylor J, Singh I, Nahas AME (1991) Nitric oxide synthesis inhibitor prevents vasodilation by insulin-like growth factor I. Kidney Int 39:333–335
161. Van Thiel DH, Udani N, Schade RR et al. (1985) Prognostic value of thyroid hormones in patients evaluated for liver transplantation. Hepatology 5:862–866
162. Zumoff B, Bradlow HL, Gallagher TF (1967) Cortisol metabolism in cirrhosis. J Clin Invest 46:1735–1743
163. Renner E, Horber FF, Jost G et al. (1986) Effect of liver function on the metabolism of prednisone and prednisolone in humans. Gastroenterology 90:819–828
164. Steinberg SE, Hillman RS (1990) The liver and hematopoiesis. In: Zakim D, Boyer TD (eds) Hepatology: a textbook of liver disease, 2nd edn. W.B. Saunders, Philadelphia, pp 537–545
165. Erslev AJ (1988) Hemopoietic functions of the liver. In: Arias IM, Jacoby WB, Popper H, Schachter D, Shafritz DA (eds) The liver: biology and pathobiology, 2nd edn. Raven, New York, pp 1073–1082
166. Fiore L, Levine J, Deykin D (1990) Alterations of hemostasis in patients with liver disease. In: Zakim D, Boyer TD (eds) Hepatology: a textbook of liver disease, 2nd edn. W.B. Saunders, Philadelphia, pp 546–571
167. Colman RW, Rubin RN (1988) Blood coagulation. In: Arias IM, Jacoby WB, Popper H, Schachter D, Shafritz DA (eds) The liver: biology and pathobiology, 2nd edn. Raven, New York, pp 1033–1042
168. Bowie EJW, Owen CA Jr (1980) The significance of abnormal preoperative hemostasis tests. Prog Hemost Thromb 5:179–209
169. Kelly DA, Tuddenham EGD (1986) Haemostatic problems in liver disease. Gut 27:339–349
170. Carr JM (1989) Disseminated intravascular coagulation in cirrhosis. Hepatology 10:103–110
171. Bonkovsky HL, Hawkins M, Steinberg K et al. (1990) Prevalence and prediction of osteopenia in chronic liver disease. Hepatology 12:273–280
172. Diamond T, Stiel D, Lunzer M, Wilkinson M, Roche J, Posen S (1990) Osteoporosis and skeletal fractures in chronic liver disease. Gut 31:82–87
173. Diamond TH, Stiel D, Lunzer M, McDowall D, Ekcstein RP, Posen S (1989) Hepatic osteodystrophy: static and dynamic bone histomorphometry and serum

bone gla-protein in 80 patients with chronic liver disease. Gastroenterology 96:213–221
174. Fierer J, Finley F (1979) Deficient serum bactericidal activity against *E. coli* in patients with cirrhosis of the liver. J Clin Invest 63:912–921
175. Rolando N, Wyke RJ (1991) Infections. Gut 32 [Suppl]:S25–S28
176. Rimola A, Soto R, Bory F et al. (1984) Reticuloendothelial system phagocytic activity in cirrhosis and its relation to bacterial infections and prognosis. Hepatology 4:53–58
177. Billie J, Glauser MP, Freeman LR (1980) Risk of death in adult pneumococcal bacteraemia. In: Lambert MP, Caldwell APS (eds) Pneumonia and pneumococcal infection. Academic, London. Royal Society of Medicine and Symposium series No. 27
178. Snyder N, Attebury CE, Correia JP, Conn HO (1977) Increased concurrence of cirrhosis and bacterial endocarditis, a clinical and post-mortem study. Gastroenterology 73:1107–1113
179. Tavill AS, Bacon BR (1990) Hemochromatosis: iron metabolism and the iron overload syndromes. In: Zakim D, Boyer TD (eds) Hepatology. W.B. Saunders, Philadelphia, pp 1273–1299
180. Wright TL, Boyer TD (1990) Diagnosis and management of cirrhotic ascites. In: Zakim D, Boyer TD (eds) Hepatology. W.B. Saunders, Philadelphia, pp 616–636
181. Runyon BA (1991) Pathogenesis and diagnosis of spontaneous bacterial peritonitis in cirrhosis. In: Rodés J, Arroyo V (eds) Therapy in liver diseases. Doyma, Barcelona, pp 388–396
182. Titó L, Rimola A, Ginés P, Llach J, Arroyo V, Rodés J (1988) Recurrence of spontaneous bacterial peritonitis in cirrhosis: frequency and predictive factors. Hepatology 8:27–31
183. Rimola A (1991) Treatment and prophylaxis of spontaneous bacterial peritonitis. In Rodés J, Arroyo V (eds) Therapy in liver diseases. Doyma, Barcelona, pp 397–406
184. Tavill AS, Bacon BR (1990) Hemochromatosis: iron metabolism and the iron overload syndromes. In: Zakim D, Boyer TD (eds) Hepatology: a textbook of liver disease, 2nd edn. W.B. Saunders, Philadelphia, pp 1273–1299
185. McGill DB, Rakela J, Zinsmeister AR, Ott BJ (1990) A 21-year experience with major hemorrhage after percutaneous liver biopsy. Gastroenterology 99:1396–1400
186. Piccinino F, Sagnelli E, Pasquale G, Giusti G (1986) Complications following percutaneous liver biopsy: a multicentre retrospective study on 68276 biopsies. J Hepatol 2:165–173
187. Pagliari L, Rinaldi F, Craxi A (1983) Percutaneous blind biopsy versus laparoscopy with guided biopsy in diagnosis of cirrhosis. A prospective randomized trial. Dig Dis Sci 28:39–46
188. Ratnoff OD, Patek AJ Jr (1942) The natural history of Laennec's cirrhosis of liver. Medicine 21:207–223
189. Child CG III, Turcotte J (1964) The liver and portal hypertension. In: Child CG III (ed) W.B. Saunders, Philadelphia, p 50
190. Pugh RNH, Murray-Lyon IM, Dawson SL, Pietroni ML, Williams R (1973) Transection of the oesophagus for bleeding oesophageal varices. Br J Surg 60:646–649
191. Infante-Rivard C, Esnaola S, Villeneuve JP (1987) Clinical and statistical validity of conventional prognostic factors in predicting short-term survival among cirrhotics. Hepatology 7:660–664
192. Markus BH, Dickson ER, Grambsch PM et al. (1989) Efficacy of liver transplantation in patients with primary biliary cirrhosis. N Engl J Med 320:1709–1713
193. Ginés P, Quintero E, Arroyo V et al. (1987) Compensated cirrhosis: natural history and prognostic factors. Hepatology 7:122–128

194. Llach J, Ginés P, Arroyo V et al. (1988) Prognostic value of arterial pressure, endogenous vasoactive systems, and renal function in cirrhotic patients admitted to the hospital for the treatment of ascites. Gastroenterology 94:482–487
195. Shear L, Hall PW, Gabuzda GJ et al. (1965) Renal failure in patients with cirrhosis of the liver. II. Factors influencing maximal urine flow rate. Am J Med 39:199–209
196. Cuervas-Mons V, Millan I, Gavalerl JS et al. (1986) Prognostic value of preoperatively obtained clinical and laboratory data in predicting survival following orthotopic liver transplantation. Hepatology 6:922–927
197. Poynard T, Cales P, Pasta L et al. (1991) Beta-adrenergic antagonist drugs in the prevention of gastrointestinal bleeding in patients with cirrhosis and esophageal varices. An analysis of data and prognostic factors in 589 patients from four randomized clinical trials. N Engl J Med 324:1532–1538
198. The Veterans Affairs Cooperative Variceal Sclerotherapy Group (1991) Prophylactic sclerotherapy for esophageal varices in men with alcoholic liver disease. A randomized single-blind, multicenter clinical trial. N Engl J Med 324:1779–1784
199. Poynard T, Zourabichvili O, Hilpert G et al. (1984) Prognostic value of total bilirubin/γ-glutamyl transpeptidase ratio in cirrhotic patients. Hepatology 4:324–327
200. Mannes GA, Thieme C, Stellaard F et al. (1986) Prognostic significance of serum bile acids in cirrhosis. Hepatology 6:50–53
201. Maddrey WC, Bointnott K, Bedline MS, Weber FL, Mezey E, White RI Jr (1978) Corticosteroid therapy of alcoholic hepatitis. Gastroenterology 75:193–199
202. Schneider JF, Baker AL, Haines NW et al. (1980) Aminopyrine *N*-demethylation: a prognostic test of liver function in patients with alcoholic liver disease. Gastroenterology 79:1145–1150
203. Taki Y, Ukikusa M, Morimoto T et al. (1987) Short-term changes in blood ketone body ratio in the phase immediately after liver transplantation. Transplantation 43:350–353
204. McIntyre N (1991) The management of patients with liver disease. In: Rodés J, Arroyo V (eds) Therapy in liver diseases. Doyma, Barcelona, pp 1–8
205. Silk DBA, O'Keefe JD, Wicks C (1991) Nutritional support in liver disease. Gut [Suppl]:S29–S33
206. Van Der Rijt CCD, Schalm SW, Schat H, Foeken K, De Jong G (1991) Overt hepatic encephalopathy precipitated by zinc deficiency. Gastroenterology 100:1114–1118
207. Chawla RK, Wolf DC, Kutner MH et al. (1989) Choline may be an essential in malnourished patients with cirrhosis. Gastroenterology 97:1514–1520
208. Eriksson LS, Conn HO (1989) Branched-chain amino acids in the management of hepatic encephalopathy: an analysis of variants. Hepatology 10:228–246
209. Ferenci P, Dragosics B, Dittrich H et al. (1989) Randomised controlled trial of silymarin treatment in patients with cirrhosis of the liver. J Hepatol 9:105–113
210. Rafique S, Guardascione M, Imai I, Burrhoughs K, Owen JS (1991) Plasma membrane lipid abnormalities and cellular dysfunction in liver disease and the protective role of *S*-adenosyl-L-methionine (SAMe). In: Rodés J, Arroyo V (eds) Therapy in liver diseases. Doyma, Barcelona, pp 374–384
211. Crosignani A, Battezzati PM, Setchell KDR et al. (1991) Effects of ursodeoxycholic acid on serum liver enzymes and bile acid metabolism in chronic active hepatitis: a dose response study. Hepatology 13:339–344
212. Ammon HV (1986) Assessment of treatment regimens. In: Czaja AJ, Dickson ER (eds) Chronic active hepatitis: the Mayo Clinic experience. Dekker, New York, pp 33–57
213. Mourelle M, Villalon C, Amezcoa JL (1988) Protective effect of colchicine on acute liver damage induced by carbon tetrachloride. J Hepatol 6:337–342

214. Kershenobich D, Vargas F, Garcia-Tsao G et al. (1988) Colchicine in the treatment of cirrhosis of the liver. N Engl J Med 318:1709–1713
215. Kaplan MM, Alling DW, Zimermann HJ et al. (1986) A prospective trial of colchicine for primary biliary cirrhosis. N Engl J Med 315:1448–1454
216. Hoofnagle J, David GL, Schnafer D et al. (1986). Randomized trial of chlorambucil for primary biliary cirrhosis. Gastroenterology 91:1327–1334
217. Weisner RH, Ludwig J, Klindon KD et al. (1990) A controlled clinical trial of cyclosporin in the treatment of primary biliary cirrhosis. N Engl J Med 322:1419–1429
218. Lombard M, Portmann R, Neuberger J et al. (1990) Cyclosporin A treatment in primary biliary cirrhosis (abstract). Hepatology 12:872
219. Ramond MJ, Poynard T, Rueff B et al. (1991) Prednisolone markedly improves short-term survival of patients with severe biopsy-proven alcoholic hepatitis. A double randomized bicenter trial (abstract). J Hepatol 13 [Suppl 2]:S63
220. Vierling JM (1990) Primary biliary cirrhosis. In: Zakim D, Boyer TD (eds) Hepatology: a textbook of liver disease, 2nd edn. W.B. Saunders, Philadelpia, pp 1158–1205
221. Orrego H, Kalant H, Israel Y et al. (1979) Effect of short-term therapy with propylthiouracil in patients with alcoholic liver disease. Gastroenterology 76:105–115
222. Orrego H, Blake JE, Blendis LM et al. (1987) Long-term treatment of alcoholic liver disease with propylthiouracil. N Engl J Med 317:1421–1426
223. Halle P, Paré P, Kaptein E, Kanel G, Redeher AG, Reynolds TB (1982) Double-blind, controlled trial of propylthiouracil in patients with severe acute alcoholic hepatitis. Gastroenterology 82:925–931
224. Poupon RE, Balkau B, Eschwege E, Poupon R, and the UDCA-PBC Study Group (1991) A multicenter, controlled trial of ursodiol for the treatment of primary biliary cirrhosis. N Engl J Med 324:1548–1554
225. Ginés P, Rimola A, Planas R et al. (1990) Norfloxacin prevents spontaneous bacterial peritonitis recurrence in cirrhotics: results of a double-blind, placebo-controlled trial. Hepatology 12:716–724
226. Felisart J, Rimola A, Arroyo V et al. (1985) Cefotaxime is more effective than is ampicillin-tobramycin in cirrhotics with severe infections. Hepatology 5:457–462

# 10 Portal-Systemic Encephalopathy

J. BIRCHER and W. SOMMER

## 1 Introduction

Portal-systemic encephalopathy (PSE) is usually a complication of late and advanced liver disease. It may present either as insidious and slow deterioration in mental function or with variable waxing and waning severity. Alternatively acute exacerbations including frank coma may follow complications of cirrhosis or ill-advised therapy. Since several moderately effective methods of treatment are now available, it is important to look for PSE in every patient with advanced chronic liver disease, particularly if precipitating causes may be present. It should be ensured that such patients are adequately cared for. PSE may be diagnosed if a patient has chronic liver disease and a mental disturbance. Hyperammonemia may be regarded as confirmatory. Other causes of cerebral dysfunction, particularly metabolic encephalopathies (Table 1) and neurologic diseases, must be excluded in every case.

## 2 Pathogenesis

Normal brain function is highly dependent on a normal composition of the blood supplying the brain. The liver is somehow essential for the maintenance of the postulated normal blood composition. Unfortunately it is not known which abnormal components of the blood are responsible for the PSE in patients with advanced liver disease. Consequently, several hypotheses regarding the pathogenesis for PSE coexist and are not mutually exclusive [1].

*Synergism Theory.* Although ammonia is known to be neurotoxic and levels are elevated to some degree in almost all cases of PSE, the correlation of ammonia levels and severity of PSE is not close. In liver failure mercaptans, medium chain fatty acids, and phenols accumulate in addition to ammonia. In experimental animals subcomatous doses of these compounds can induce coma, when given together. Thus, the synergism theory states that the combined effects of these compounds produce coma at concentrations at which a single agent is harmless. Since some of the above neurotoxins also

**Table 1.** Metabolic encephalopathies which must be distinguished from PSE

| |
|---|
| Diabetic coma |
| Hypoglycemia |
| Azotemia |
| Carbon dioxide narcosis |
| Urea cycle enzyme deficiencies |
| Reye's syndrome |

have excitatory effects and since in some experiments seizures have been observed preceding the coma, the relevance of the theory for PSE has been questioned.

It has been postulated that zinc deficiency, due to diuretic treatment and inadequate nutrition, may aggravate hyperammonemia and thereby contribute to the severity of PSE [2].

*False Neurotransmitter Theory.* In advanced liver disease concentrations of branched chain amino acids (BCAAs) in plasma may fall, whereas aromatic amino acids (AAAs) may accumulate. Under these circumstances more AAAs are thought to pass across the blood-brain barrier. This process is further favored by increased amounts of glutamine being transported from the brain to the blood. In the brain excess AAAs may serve as precursors for the false neurotransmitters octopamine and phenylethanolamine which reduce neural excitation and thereby increase neural inhibition. Although this theory has been the basis for treatments of PSE with BCAAs, the ratio of BCAAs to AAAs in blood correlates poorly with the severity of PSE. This observation and other physiologic studies in rats have cast doubt on the validity of the false neurotransmitter hypothesis.

*GABA-ergic Theory.* Several lines of evidence implicate an increased GABA-ergic tone as a component of PSE. This idea is related also to the pharmacology of benzodiazepines which bind to the GABA-benzodiazepine receptor complex, thereby increasing GABA-ergic tone. Although this theory has been extensively studied in many experimental models, the results have been somewhat inconsistent and most studies have used models of acute liver failure rather than chronic liver disease. Nevertheless, accumulation in brain of a ligand with high affinity for benzodiazepine receptors has been more pronounced in cirrhotics with recent PSE than in controls, when studied by positron emission tomography [3]. Furthermore, sensitivity of the brain to triazolam was higher in patients with advanced cirrhosis than in control subjects [4]. Finally, several studies have shown some improvement in PSE immediately after the intravenous administration of the benzodiazepine receptor antagonist flumazenil [5]. Recently, small amounts of many benzodiazepines have been identified in plants which serve as ordinary foods [6]. It is conceivable, but has not been established, that the quantities present in foods can accumulate in blood when the metabolic capacity of the liver is poor and may contribute to PSE in the presence of hypersensitivity of the brain. At least some accumulation of benzodiazepine receptor ligands is likely [7]. Nevertheless, it seems that increased GABA-ergic tone explains only a part of the cerebral dysfunction in PSE.

*Role of Portal-Systemic Circulation and the Gut.* Long-standing clinical experience has established that gut-derived factors are important, since blood in the gastrointestinal tract may acutely precipitate severe PSE. In addition, a high protein diet and constipation may aggravate it. Furthermore, large spontaneous splenorenal shunts are frequently associated with spontaneous episodes of PSE. Large quantities of ammonia originating from urease activity of the intestinal flora are cleared in a single passage through the normal liver but may reach the systemic circulation in patients with cirrhosis and portal-systemic shunting. GABA also arises in the bowel and is removed by the normal liver. Whether or not in cirrhotics GABA originating from the intestine reaches GABA-receptors in the brain has not been established. It is possible that other gut-derived compounds contributing to PSE are yet to be identified.

## 3 Clinical Presentation

The chronic form of PSE initially manifests itself as subclinical encephalopathy. Even in the absence of gross abnormalities in consciousness or alertness, up to 50% of cirrhotics with Child C severity have abnormalities on psychometric testing [8]. These may be interpreted as PSE, because they are related to the severity of the liver disease rather than to its etiology. Upon progression of the disease the patient may become lethargic or undergo changes in personality. At this stage other clinical signs are usually present, such as fetor hepaticus, asterixis, and some degree of ataxia. The clinical course of chronic PSE often varies in intensity depending on the patient's intake of proteins, on his bowel habits, and on other unknown factors. The different stages of PSE are listed in Table 2. A patient in frank coma generally exhibits hyperreflexia, good peripheral circulation, and some degree of hyperventilation.

Fetor hepaticus is a special aromatic and sweet odor of exhaled air. Its cause may be related to volatile mercaptans. This sign is useful for the detection of PSE by experienced clinicians, but due to its subjective nature confirmatory evidence for the diagnosis is required.

Asterixis results from short interruptions of a sustained and continuous muscular effort. It is usually tested by having the patient extend his arm

**Table 2.** Assessment of severity of PSE

| Stage | Mental state | Neurologic abnormalities |
|---|---|---|
| 0–1 | Subclinical PSE documented only by psychometric tests | None |
| 1 | Mild change in personality, euphoria or depression, decreased attention, forgetfulness, day–night reversal | Slight ataxia or tremor |
| 2 | Drowsiness, lethargy, obvious personality changes, inappropriate behavior, intermittent loss of orientation | Asterixis[a]<br>Hyperactive reflexes |
| 3 | Somnolent but rousable, loss of meaningful communication, speech incomprehensible, disorientation, marked confusion | Asterixis[a]<br>Hyperactive tendon reflexes |
| 4 | Coma | Babinski's sign ±<br>Preserved pupillary responses<br>Hyperventilation<br>Good peripheral circulation |

[a] "Flapping tremor"

and maintain dorsal flexion of the hand for as long as possible. Due to intermittent losses of muscular tone the hand repeatedly droops down and immediately thereafter is hyperextended again by a voluntary effort on the part of the patient. Upon repetition of this phenomenon, its severe form may appear as a flapping tremor. Most of the time only minor intermittent interruptions of muscular tone are seen.

Acute episodes of PSE are usually precipitated by complications of cirrhosis or by overly aggressive medical therapy (Table 3). Blood in the gastrointestinal tract resulting from an upper gastrointestinal hemorrhage may, in predisposed patients, lead to frank coma within 24 h. Similarly aggressive diuretic therapy often precipitates functional renal failure or hypokalemia, conditions which tend to aggravate PSE. Patients with advanced cirrhosis are likely to display a disproportionate response to all sedative drugs, including benzodiazepines [4], phenothiazines, and opiates. In addition, their elimination from the circulation may be markedly slowed. For this reason, episodes of coma induced by sedatives may be not only quite severe but also unusually prolonged. Infections such as spontaneous bacterial peritonitis, but also all other infections, may aggravate PSE. Finally in some sensitive patients, high protein intake or constipation may induce episodes of disorientation.

Rarely, patients with chronic PSE develop irreversible neurologic complications such as spastic paraplegia [9].

**Table 3.** Factors which may aggravate or precipitate PSE

| |
|---|
| Gastrointestinal hemorrhage |
| Diuretic therapy |
| Hypokalemia (± metabolic alkalosis) |
| Administration of sedative drugs |
| Infections (e.g., spontaneous bacterial peritonitis) |
| High protein intake |
| Constipation |

## 4 Clinical Investigation

When investigating a patient suspected of having PSE it is important to verify the liver disease, to assess the severity of the PSE, and to exclude other causes of abnormal mental function.

### 4.1 Verification of Liver Disease

In some patients the presence of advanced liver disease may not be obvious. Therefore, upon initial clinical examination spider angiomas, fetor hepaticus, hepatosplenomegaly, and ascites are important clues to be looked for. Abnormal laboratory tests often include hypoprothrombinemia, hypoalbuminemia, and hypergammaglobulinemia. Fasting venous ammonia determinations are useful if levels are frankly elevated. Normal ammonia concentrations, however, do not exclude PSE.

### 4.2 Assessment of Severity

The severity of PSE may be graded as shown in Table 2. Although the mental state has to be assessed clinically at each visit, psychometric testing is quite useful, particularly for a more objective documentation of the effects of therapy. The Reitan trail test has been used most extensively, but the digit symbol substitution test, reaction time, and other methods may also be useful. All of them are nonspecific and may become abnormal in any condition which affects mental function. The advantage of such tests compared to the drawing of a star or an analysis of the handwriting consists in the possibility of diagnosing subclinical PSE [8, 10] and in the quantitative expression of their results.

Once a patient is drowsy or unconscious, psychometric testing becomes impossible. For such patients the EEG provides objective evidence of the severity of the disease. It may be graded clinically (from 0 to 4) or subjected to Fourier transformation for the estimation of the mean dominant fre-

**Table 4.** Differential diagnosis of PSE

| |
|---|
| Intracranial lesions |
| Contusion of brain |
| Subdural hemorrhage |
| Subarachnoid hemorrhage |
| Brain tumors |
| Cerebrovascular disease |
| Intracranial infections |
| Toxic encephalopathies (alcohol, etc.) |
| Postseizure encephalopathy |
| Metabolic encephalopathies (Table 1) |
| Drug intoxications |

quency. It has not as yet been established that visual-evoked potentials or somatosensory-evoked potentials are superior to the ordinary EEG [10].

### 4.3 Exclusion of Other Causes of Abnormal Mental Function

In each patient it is important to exclude other causes of mental disturbances, as enumerated in Tables 1 and 4. For this purpose a careful history of precipitating factors (Table 3) should be obtained and a complete neurologic examination is to be performed. If, for example, a patient has decreased or absent tendon reflexes, poor peripheral circulation, or hypoventilation, other diseases must be looked for. Laboratory screening should exclude disturbances in carbohydrate metabolism and fluid and electrolyte balance and intoxications. Infections should be looked for, including spontaneous bacterial peritonitis and pneumonia. Finally, imaging of the skull to rule out intracranial lesions may be needed.

## 5 Management

Treatment of PSE is primarily concerned with the elimination of precipitating factors and of colonic breakdown of nitrogenous compounds. In practice, the approach differs depending on whether the patient presents with an acute episode of PSE or with chronic PSE (Table 5).

### 5.1 Acute Episodes of PSE

Severe PSE of rapid onset requires the urgent treatment of, for example, blood in the gastrointestinal tract, hypokalemia, and functional renal failure. To clear blood from the bowel, lactulose or lactitol may be used. If the patient tolerates oral administration (e.g., by nasogastric tube), laxative doses of 20–30 g may be given every 2 h until the patient experiences the

**Table 5.** Treatment of PSE

*Acute episodes of PSE*
1. Elimination of precipitating factors
   - Empty bowel of blood
   - Cessation of diuretics and restoration of fluid and electrolyte balance
   - Treatment of infections
   - Low protein intake (40 g/day)
   - Avoidance of sedative drugs
2. Drug treatment
   - Lactulose, lactitol, or neomycin
   - Flumazenil if history of benzodiazepine administration (otherwise its use is experimental)

*Chronic PSE*
1. Diet
   - Protein intake of 60 g/day or more
   - Lactovegetarian diet preferable
   - Only in severe protein intolerance replace part of oral proteins by branched chain amino acids
2. Drugs
   - Nonabsorbable disaccharide in doses sufficient to produce two soft bowel movements/day
   - Diuretics reduced to a minimum
   - Sedatives to be avoided
     (Exception: small doses of oxazepam if absolutely needed)

first diarrhea. Thereafter doses are adjusted to yield two soft bowel movements per day. Alternatively, 20–30 g lactulose may be added to water used for high enemas which are used to empty the colon. If excessive diuresis is at fault, fluid and electrolyte balance must be restored. Infections must be treated vigorously. Administration of branched chain amino acids has the advantage that these amino acids can serve as a nitrogen source without aggravating the encephalopathy. Evidence, however, that branched chain amino acids are beneficial for the PSE itself is still weak [11]. Therefore, the indication for BCAAs is nutritional [12]. Sedative drugs are to be withheld. If the patient has been receiving a benzodiazepine, he may benefit from the administration of the antagonist flumazenil. Upon intravenous injection of less than 1 mg the patient may wake up immediately. This drug, however, has a short half-life (Table 6) and therefore must be administered repeatedly or by intravenous infusion, until the agonist benzodiazepine is eliminated from the organism [13]. Since in these patients liver function is often markedly diminished, it may take weeks or months until long-acting benzodiazepines (such as nordiazepam) are completely cleared.

## 5.2 Chronic PSE

In patients with chronic PSE efforts should be made to achieve two goals: optimization of the metabolic situation for the patient and administration

**Table 6.** Pharmacology of the benzodiazepine antagonist Flumazenil

| | |
|---|---|
| Oral bioavailability | 15% |
| Protein binding | 40% |
| Volume of distribution | 0.8 liters/kg |
| Half-life | 1.0 h |
| Elimination | Hepatic metabolism |
| Normal i.v. dose | 0.3–0.6 mg |

Reproduced from KLOTZ U, KANTO J (1988) Clin Pharmacokinet 14:1–12

of individualized doses of nonabsorbable disaccharides. Although dietary proteins should be restricted, cirrhotics require a higher protein intake to stay in nitrogen balance than normal subjects. For this reason, optimal long-term diets should include at least 60 g protein per day. In general a lactovegetarian high residue diet has given better results than a diet which includes meat proteins. In the rare patient who does not tolerate a nutritionally adequate diet, a negative nitrogen balance may aggravate muscle wasting and hyperammonemia. Only for such cases may supplementation of a protein-restricted diet by oral branched chain amino acids be cost-effective. Since zinc deficiency may aggravate hyperammonemia, it has been postulated that zinc supplements may be beneficial for patients with PSE. These should be based on zinc serum levels. Experience, however, with zinc supplements is quite limited [2].

Since patients with chronic PSE generally tolerate the nonabsorbable disaccharides lactulose or lactitol quite well, it has become customary to prescribe these drugs on a long-term basis [14, 15]. The daily maintenance doses should be individually titrated in such a way that the patient has two soft bowel movements per day. Ideally, fecal pH, measured with a pH-sensitive paper, should be around 5.0 and at least below 6.0 [16]. In patients who have lactase deficiency, the same results may be achieved with lactose.

The mode of action of nonabsorbable disaccharides in PSE is not known. Nevertheless, many pharmacologic effects of these drugs have been studied, particularly with lactulose as model drug. Both lactulose and lactitol are not hydrolyzed by intestinal disaccharidases. Since intact disaccharides are not appreciably absorbed from the small bowel, they reach the cecum intact, where they are broken down rapidly by the bacterial flora to acetic, propionic, butyric, and lactic acid. In addition, molecular hydrogen ($H_2$) and in some subjects methane are formed and can be measured in exhaled air. The fatty acids result in acidification of cecal contents from normal values around pH 6.0 to around pH 4.8 with occasional falls as low as pH 3.5. In the left colon the pH falls only provided that doses are sufficient to result at least in mild diarrhea. This is due to the fact that most of the short chain fatty acids formed in the cecum are absorbed and do not reach the left colon, unless bowel passage is accelerated. The caloric value of lactitol is about 8.5 kJ/g or 2 kcal/g. The rapid laxative effects of nonabsorbable disaccharides are due to the osmotic load which occurs as a result of the breakdown of one molecule of lactulose or lactitol to four molecules of fatty acids. Consequently, upon overdosage watery diarrhea results with fluid and electrolyte losses, often leading to hypovolemia, azotemia, hypernatremia, and hypokalemia.

Upon chronic administration of lactulose it appears that the colonic flora becomes more efficient in its metabolism. While abdominal pains and meteorism decrease, acidification of cecal contents is more pronounced. It also appears that colonic bacteria exposed to an excess of carbohydrates are in need of nitrogen for growth and under these circumstances use up ammonia and amino acids [17]. Consequently fecal mass and fecal output of nitrogen increase, whereas urinary output of nitrogen decreases.

These observations suggest that nonabsorbable disaccharides have at least two potentially beneficial effects in PSE. Acidification of colonic contents prevents nonionic diffusion of ammonia from the colon to the blood and may even move ammonia from the blood to the colonic lumen. Furthermore, use of ammonia and amino acids by colonic bacteria as a nitrogen source renders ammonia less available for absorption. It may be assumed that ammonia is only a model compound for other unknown potential toxins which share their fate with ammonia. Thus, lactulose and its analogs may act on many other unidentified substances which are formed in the colon and aggravate PSE.

Minor adverse effects of lactulose include aversion to its sweet taste, which may lead to noncompliance and treatment failures. It is postulated that lactitol, being less sweet than lactulose, may be better tolerated [15]. Nausea and vomiting probably can be avoided if the hyperosmolar drug is not given on an empty stomach. The only severe side-effects, watery diarrhea and its consequences, can be avoided by careful dose titration. Since acidification of colonic contents is thought to be important for the action of nonabsorbable disaccharides, they should not be combined with antacids.

### 5.3 Neomycin

Neomycin is not absorbed appreciably and has been effective in PSE when given by mouth or nasogastric tube in doses of 1 g four to six times daily. Its mode of action is not understood, because it is not primarily effective against the anaerobic flora of the colon. However, it reproducibly lowers blood ammonia, produces malabsorption by damaging small intestinal mucosa, and has a tendency to induce loose bowel movements. It is adequate treatment for acute episodes of PSE, but upon long-term administration may lead to ototoxicity. It has not been established that the combination of neomycin with a nonabsorbable disaccharide is superior to either alone given in optimal doses.

### 5.4 Flumazenil

Although several studies have unequivocally shown that intravenous administration of the benzodiazepine antagonist flumazenil may be followed by an immediate improvement in PSE experimentally and clinically [5], in the absence of prior benzodiazepine administration its use in acute or chronic PSE must still be considered experimental.

## References


1. Jones EA, Gammal SH (1990) Hepatic encephalopathy. In: Cohen RD, Lewis B, Alberti KGMM, Denman AM (eds) The metabolic and molecular basis of acquired disease. Baillière Tindall, London, p 1246
2. Grüngreiff K, Pressner HJ, Franke D et al. (1989) Correlations between zinc, amino acids and ammonia in liver cirrhosis. Z Gastroenterol 27:731–735
3. Samson Y, Bernuau J, Pappata S et al. (1987) Cerebral uptake of benzodiazepine measured by positron emission tomography in hepatic encephalopathy. N Engl J Med 316:414–415
4. Bakti G, Fisch HU, Karlaganis G et al. (1987) Mechanism of the excessive sedative response of cirrhotics to benzodiazepines: model experiments with triazolam. Hepatology 7:629–638
5. Gammal SH, Basile AS, Geller D et al. (1990) Reversal of the behavioral and electrophysiological abnormalities of an animal model of hepatic encephalopathy by benzodiazepine receptor ligands. Hepatology 11:371–378
6. Wildmann J, Vetter W, Ranalder UB et al. (1988) Occurrence of pharmacologically active benzodiazepines in trace amounts in wheat and potato. Biochem Pharmacol 37:3549–3559
7. Butterworth RF, Layrargues GP (1990) Benzodiazepine receptors and hepatic encephalopathy. Hepatology 11:499–501
8. Koch H, Schauder P, Schäfer G et al. (1990) Diagnosis and prevalence of latent hepatic encephalopathy. Z Gastroenterol 28:610–615
9. Read AE, Sherlock S, Laidlow J et al. (1967) The neuropsychiatric syndromes associated with chronic liver disease and an extensive portal-systemic collateral circulation. QJ Med 36:135–150
10. Johansson U, Andersson T, Persson A et al. (1989) Visual evoked potential – a tool in the diagnosis of hepatic encephalopathy? J Hepatol 9:227–233
11. Naylor CD, O'Rourke K, Detsky AS et al. (1989) Parenteral nutrition with branched chain amino acids in hepatic encephalopathy. A meta-analysis. Gastroenterology 97:1033–1042
12. Horst D, Grace ND, Conn HO et al. (1984) Comparison of dietary protein with an oral, branched chain-enriched amino acid supplement in chronic portal-systemic encephalopathy: a randomized controlled trial. Hepatology 4:279–287
13. Klotz U, Kanto J (1988) Pharmacokinetics and clinical use of flumazenil (Ro 15-1788). Clin Pharmacokinet 14:1–12
14. Heredia D, Teres J, Orteu N et al. (1988) Lactilol vs. lactulose in the treatment of chronic recurrent portal-systemic encephalopathy. J Hepatol 7:106–110
15. Morgan MY, Alonso M, Stanger LC (1989) Lactilol and lactulose for the treatment of subclinical hepatic encephalopathy in cirrhotic patients. A randomized, cross-over study. J Hepatol 8:208–217
16. Bircher J, Haemmerli UP, Trabert E et al. (1971) The mechanism of action of lactulose in portal-systemic encephalopathy. Rev Eur Etudes Clin Biol 16:352–357

17. Mortensen PB, Holtug K, Bonnen H et al. (1990) The degradation of amino acids, proteins, and blood to short-chain fatty acids in colon is prevented by lactulose. Gastroenterology 98:353–360

# 11 Portal Hypertension

J. BOSCH, J.C. GARCIA-PAGÁN, F. FEU, and M.P. PIZCUETA

Portal hypertension is a common syndrome characterized by a chronic increase in the portal venous pressure [1]. This increases the pressure gradient between the portal vein and the inferior vena cava (the so-called *portal pressure gradient*, which represents the portal perfusion pressure of the liver) above the normal range of 1–5 mmHg [1]. Portal hypertension promotes the formation of collateral vessels that shunt portal blood to the systemic circulation, bypassing the liver. These portal–systemic collaterals form by the opening and dilatation of preexisting vascular channels connecting the portal venous system and the superior and inferior vena cava, which are closed under normal conditions and which dilate because of the high portal pressure. Other factors, such as active angiogenesis, may also be involved in the development of the collateral circulation. The main anastomotic systems are schematically represented in Fig. 1. The gastroesophageal collateral system draining in the azygos vein, which includes the esophageal varices, is responsible for the main complication of portal hypertension: massive bleeding from ruptured gastroesophageal varices. Other manifestations of the portal hypertension syndrome, such as ascites, hepatic encephalopathy, disturbances in the metabolism of drugs and endogenous compounds, and bacteremia, are discussed in other chapters of this book.

## 1 Etiology

Any disease interfering with portal blood flow can lead to portal hypertension. Causes of portal hypertension are usually classified according to their location as *prehepatic*, *intrahepatic*, or *posthepatic* [2] (Table 1). All can cause the formation of varices and bleeding. However, there are some differences in other clinical manifestations. Thus, ascites is a prominent finding in posthepatic portal hypertension but very rare in cases of prehepatic portal hypertension. This latter group is characterized by the formation of "bridging" collaterals carrying portal blood to the liver ("hepatopetal" collaterals), which often give rise to large gastric varices. The peculiarities of prehepatic portal hypertension are discussed at the end of this chapter. Intrahepatic portal hypertension can be caused by many liver diseases (Table 1). Cirrhosis accounts for more than 90% of the cases in developed

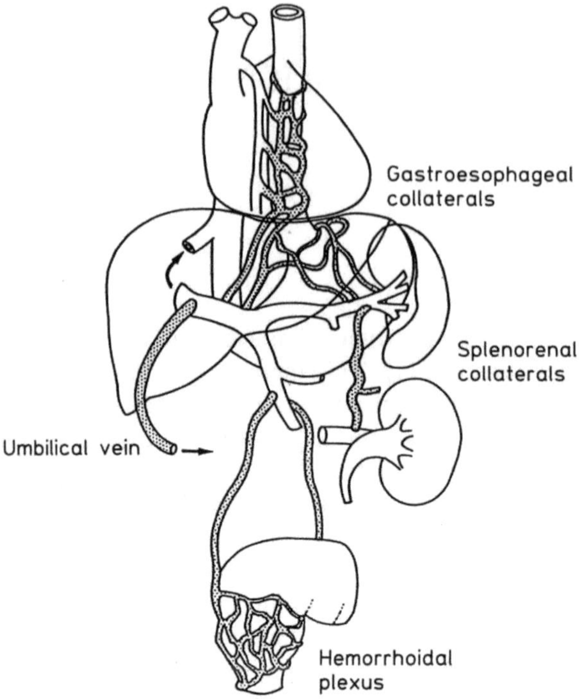


**Fig. 1.** Schematic representation of the main anastomotic portal–systemic systems in man [reproduced with permission from Bosch J et al. (1989) Med Clin North Am 73:931–953]

countries, to the point that all other intrahepatic causes have often been grouped as "noncirrhotic portal hypertension" [3]. This is clearly inadequate, since it includes schistosomiasis, which is probably the main cause of portal hypertension worldwide. Posthepatic portal hypertension is caused by diseases creating a hepatic outflow block; its prototype is the Budd-Chiari syndrome, in which ascites is the main clinical manifestation.

## 2 Pathophysiology

Portal pressure is determined by the interrelationship between portal blood flow and the vascular resistance that opposes that flow. These parameters are mathematically related by the equation:

$$\Delta P = Q \times R$$

In this equation, $\Delta P$ is the perfusion pressure gradient in the portal venous system (the difference between portal pressure and the inferior vena cava pressure), $Q$ is blood flow, and $R$ is the vascular resistance to portal blood flow. It follows that portal pressure can increase as a result of an

**Table 1.** Etiology of portal hypertension

| |
|---|
| *a) Prehepatic:* |
| Portal vein thrombosis |
| Splenic vein thrombosis |
| *b) Intrahepatic:* |
| Partial nodular transformation |
| Nodular regenerative hyperplasia |
| Congenital hepatic fibrosis |
| Peliosis hepatis |
| Polycystic disease |
| Idiopathic portal hypertension |
| Hypervitaminosis A |
| Arsenic, copper sulfate, and vinyl chloride monomer poisoning |
| Sarcoidosis |
| Tuberculosis |
| Primary biliary cirrhosis |
| Schistosomiasis |
| Amyloidosis |
| Mastocytosis |
| Rendu-Osler-Weber disease |
| Hematologic liver disease |
| Acute fatty liver of pregnancy |
| Severe viral hepatitis |
| Chronic active hepatitis |
| Hepatocellular carcinoma |
| Nonalcoholic cirrhosis |
| Alcoholic cirrhosis |
| Acute alcoholic hepatitis |
| Veno-occlusive disease |
| *c) Posthepatic:* |
| Budd-Chiari syndrome |
| Congenital malformations and thrombosis of the inferior vena cava |
| Constrictive pericarditis |
| Tricuspid valve diseases |
| *d) Miscellaneous:* |
| Arteriovenous fistulas (splenic, aortomesenteric, aortoportal, and hepatic artery–portal vein) |

increase in either blood flow or vascular resistance or both. Under normal conditions, the portohepatic circulation is highly compliant and can accommodate large variations in blood flow with only minor changes in portal pressure. This is the reason why portal hypertension is always initiated by an increased vascular resistance to portal blood flow. Increased resistance can be located at any point along the splenoportal axis (causing prehepatic portal hypertension), at the intrahepatic circulation (intrahepatic portal hypertension), or at the hepatic outflow (posthepatic portal hypertension) (Table 1). However, it is now well stablished that in chronic, advanced portal hypertension with marked portal–systemic collaterals, there is also a marked increase in portal blood inflow. Thus, the splanchnic circulation is not "congested" in portal hypertension, but hyperemic [4]. This increased blood flow contributes to the aggravation and maintenance of chronic portal hypertension, and explains in part why portal pressure remains elevated even after the formation of extensive collaterals that may shunt more than 90% of portal blood flow [5].

### 2.1 Increased Vascular Resistance

In recent years, new concepts have emerged in respect of the crucial role of increased vascular resistance in the pathogenesis of portal hypertension. Thus, it has been shown that, contrary to past assumptions, the vascular resistance of the cirrhotic liver is not a fixed, mechanical consequence of the vascular architectural distortion caused by nodule formation and collagenization of the sinusoids, but that there is also an active component, caused by the presence in the connective tissue of abundant myofibroblasts that undergo active constriction [6]. Other contractive elements may be located at the sinusoids. This "active" component of the hepatic vascular resistance of the cirrhotic liver may be modified by vasoactive compounds. Vasodilators decrease vascular resistance and portal pressure by this mechanism, which has provided the rationale for the use of vasodilators in the pharmacologic treatment of portal hypertension [6]. Theoretically, these agents may cause not only a decrease in portal pressure but also an improvement in hepatic perfusion. By contrast, vasoconstrictors have the potential to increase hepatic resistance and to further impair the liver perfusion [7]. This is especially evident with α-adrenergic stimulation.

In addition, recent research has shown that increased resistance at the portal vein and portal–systemic collaterals may further increase the overall resistance of the portohepatic circulation, thus aggravating the portal hypertension. It should be emphasized that in portal hypertension, the portal–collateral system is not only dilated but also hypertrophic, with a large muscle layer; this makes it likely that vasoactive compounds acting on vascular smooth muscle will also affect the portocollateral circulation, which may modify the net response to some pharmacologic agents, especially those aimed at reducing portal pressure by decreasing portal venous inflow [7]. Moreover, it has been shown that the mesenteric vascular bed is hypersensitive to serotonin (5-HT) in portal hypertension, and that the administration of 5-HT2 blockers significantly decreases portal pressure without causing any other hemodynamic effect.

### 2.2 Increased Splanchnic Blood Flow

Splanchnic hyperemia is mainly mediated by vasodilating transferable agents, as indicated by cross-circulation experiments showing splanchnic vasodilation in normal animals cross-circulated with portal hypertensive rats

[8]. Many candidate substances have been proposed. These are increased in portal hypertension either because of increased production or because they escape hepatic inactivation by being shunted to the systemic circulation through the portal–systemic collaterals. In addition to anatomic shunting through portal–systemic collaterals, functional intrahepatic shunts can be very important in diseases causing intrahepatic portal hypertension, such as cirrhosis. The only vasodilator for which there is experimental evidence supporting an important role in splanchnic hyperemia is glucagon, a powerful vasodilator which is markedly increased in portal hypertension and after portasystemic shunts [9, 10]. The splanchnic hyperemia is accompanied, and to some extent supported, by a hyperkinetic systemic circulation, with increased cardiac output and plasma volume, reduced systemic vascular resistance, and low arterial blood pressure. An abnormal vascular sensitivity to endogenous vasoactive compounds can also contribute to the arteriolar vasodilation. This may be favored by hyperglucagonemia [11]. More recently, abnormalities in the release of and/or response to endothelial-derived relaxing factor (nitric oxide) have been suggested to contribute to the splanchnic and systemic vasodilation. In summary, portal hypertension is determined by the interaction of an increased vascular resistance at the intrahepatic and portocollateral bed and an increased portal venous inflow. Knowledge regarding these events is very important for the understanding and development of new pharmacologic approaches that will achieve a dramatic change in the natural history of portal hypertension.

## 3 Evaluation of the Portal Hypertensive Patient

The evaluation of the portal hypertensive patient is based on the visualization of varices at endoscopy, on the definition of the portocollateral anatomy by ultrasonography and/or angiography, and on the measurement of portal pressure. Recently, techniques have been introduced that allow assessment of changes in pressure and blood flow in the collateral circulation. These have resulted in a better understanding of the hemodynamic changes associated with portal hypertension, of the mechanism of bleeding, and of the effects of new forms of pharmacologic therapy [1].

### 3.1 Measurement of Portal Pressure (Fig. 2)

The measurement of portal pressure is still the single more important hemodynamic measurement in portal hypertension. Other methods provide additional information but do not substitute for measurements of portal pressure. Portal pressure should be expressed in terms of the *pressure gradient* with the inferior vena cava (IVC), since this gradient is not modified by changes in intra-abdominal pressure [1]. Clinically significant portal hypertension,

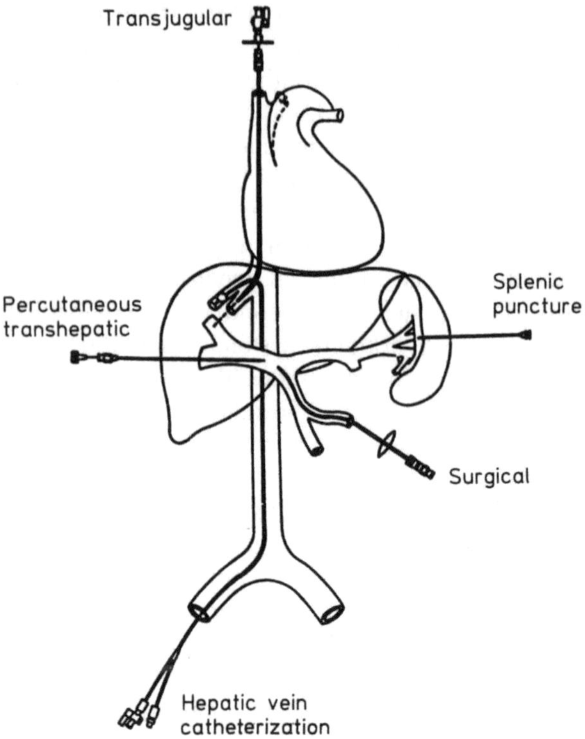


**Fig. 2.** Methods for the direct or indirect measurement of portal venous pressure [modified with permission from Bosch J et al. (1986) Semin Liver Dis 6:309–317]

with formation of esophageal varices, requires this gradient to increase above 10 mmHg. Variceal bleeding is rarely, if ever, observed if the gradient is less than 12 mmHg [12]. Moreover, patients with a high portal pressure gradient become completely protected against the risk of variceal bleeding when the portal pressure gradient is decreased to values equal to or lower than 12 mmHg [13].

Direct measurements of portal pressure involve invasive investigations based on the surgical, percutaneous transhepatic, or transvenous (transjugular) catheterization of the portal vein. Except when the transjugular approach is adopted, measurement of IVC pressure will require a separate simultaneous procedure [1].

Because of these disadvantages of direct measurements, the indirect approach of hepatic vein catheterization, with measurements of the wedged and free hepatic venous pressure (WHVP and FHVP), is the preferred technique for determination of portal pressure. WHVP is measured by occluding the hepatic vein, either by inflating a balloon at the tip of the catheter or by advancing the catheter until it becomes "wedged" into a small branch of a hepatic vein [1, 14]. When blood flow in a hepatic vein is stopped by a wedged catheter, the static column of blood transmits the pressure existing in the preceding communicated vascular territory (the hepatic sinusoids). Thus, WHVP is a measurement of the hepatic sinusoidal pressure and not of portal pressure itself [1]. When portal hypertension is due to increased sinusoidal resistance (*sinusoidal portal hypertension*) – as happens in alcoholic liver disease – WHVP is equal to portal pressure. However, when increased resistance is located at presinusoidal sites (*presinusoidal portal hypertension*), WHVP underestimates portal pressure. This happens in prehepatic diseases causing portal hypertension. In addition, some liver diseases affecting predominantly the portal tracts also cause presinusoidal portal hypertension [3]. The more frequent examples are schistosomiasis, initial stages of primary biliary cirrhosis, and idiopathic portal hypertension. Also, in nonalcoholic cirrhosis there may be such a presinusoidal component to the portal hypertension. In these cases, direct measurement of portal pressure may be preferable [15]. We recommended percutaneous transhepatic puncture with thin needles under ultrasonographic and radiologic guidance because this technique is easier to perform and more acceptable to the patient than other ways of obtaining a direct measurement. The form of hypertension found in diseases causing a hepatic outflow block, such as the Budd-Chiari syndrome, is classified as *postsinusoidal, posthepatic portal hypertension*.

Hepatic vein catheterization is a simple and safe technique. Complications of the procedure in a series of 2500 consecutive studies performed in our laboratory were limited to one femoral arteriovenous fistula, one leakage requiring blood transfusion, and the rupture of a venous introducer requiring phlebotomy and surgical reconstruction of the femoral vein under local anesthesia. There were no fatalities. An additional advantage of the technique is that it allows in the same procedure the measurement of portal pressure in absolute values, as WHVP, and as the pressure gradient WHVP–FHVP (the so-called hepatic vein pressure gradient, HVPG). When employing hepatic vein catheterization it is also possible to measure the hepatic blood flow using indocyanine green as the indicator [1], as well as the intrinsic clearance of indocyanine green, a valuable quantitative liver function test assessing overall liver metabolic activity. Finally, HVPG has been found to be closely related with prognosis in patients with cirrhosis, suggesting that its measurement can be used to monitor the course of the disease and to decide upon the correct time for liver transplantation.

### 3.2 Measurement of Azygos Blood Flow

Measurements of azygos blood flow represents an index of blood flow through the gastroesophageal collaterals and esophageal varices in portal hypertension [16, 17]. This technique is based on the well-known fact that most gastroesophageal collaterals drain into the azygos venous system; therefore, an increased azygos blood flow in patients with portal hypertension reflects the collateral blood flow emptying in the azygos vein. Obviously, the technique does not enable one to distinguish how much of the increase in azygos blood flow is contributed by esophageal varices and how much by periesophageal collaterals also draining into the azygos vein. It should be noted that in up to 25% of cases these cephalad collaterals drain into other thoracic veins (subclavian, innominate, and pulmonary) instead of the azygos vein. Therefore, the absence of an increase in azygos blood flow does not indicate the absence of esophageal varices [17].

Measurement of azygos flow requires the retrograde catheterization of the azygos vein using a continuous thermal dilution catheter. This is a very simple procedure in the course of routine hemodynamic investigations using the femoral vein approach, but much more difficult from the jugular vein. Measurement of blood flow is performed by indicator dilution during a constant infusion of isotonic glucose solution at room temperature, while simultaneously recording the temperature of the indicator and of azygos blood. The whole procedure, including repeated measurements of blood flow, does not take more than 15 min. The technique is accurate and reproducible: the variation in repeated measurements is less than 10%. Technical aspects of measurements of azygos blood flow have been reviewed recently [18].

Azygos blood flow is usually markedly increased in portal hypertension. Values in normal subjects range between 0.15 and 0.25 liters/min, whereas in patients with cirrhosis and portal hypertension they are increased on average to 0.65 liters/min [17]. Patients with noncirrhotic portal hypertension also have increased azygos flow (Table 2). These increased values are markedly reduced following surgical portacaval shunt or esophageal tamponade with a Sengstaken-Blakemore tube [17], and significantly correlate with portal pressure and with the size and extent of the esophageal varices. However, as already mentioned, these correlations are not helpful in assessing the risk of bleeding in individual patients.

The main application of measurements of azygos blood flow is in monitoring the effects of pharmacologic therapy for portal hypertension. The ability of the technique to detect changes in portal–collateral blood flow has allowed a better understanding of the beneficial effects of vasoactive drugs currently used in the medical treatment of portal hypertension. In addition, it has been demonstrated that some of these drugs, such as propranolol, cause greater decreases in azygos blood flow than in portal pressure, and that with equal falls in portal pressure there can be different effects on azygos blood flow [19, 20]. These findings have given rise to the important concept that vasoactive agents may have specific effects at the collaterals which cannot be assessed adequately by measurements of portal pressure.

**Table 2.** Azygos blood flow and hepatic venous pressure gradient (HVPG) in diseases causing portal hypertension

| Etiology | Azygos blood flow (ml/min) | HVPG (mmHg) |
|---|---|---|
| Alcoholic cirrhosis ($n = 54$) | 722 ± 41 | 19.3 ± 0.7 |
| Nonalcoholic cirrhosis ($n = 35$) | 646 ± 42 | 19.3 ± 0.8 |
| Primary biliary cirrhosis: | | |
| –with portal hypertension ($n = 7$) | 647 ± 321 | 14.1 ± 6.2[b] |
| –without portal hypertension ($n = 9$) | 319 ± 121[a] | 5.1 ± 2.3[c] |
| Idiopathic portal hypertension ($n = 4$) | 480 ± 256 | 6.1 ± 2.8[c] |
| Portal vein thrombosis ($n = 7$) | 519 ± 192 | 3.1 ± 1.7[c] |

[a] Significantly lower than in patients with portal hypertension of any origin ($P < 0.01$)
[b] Significantly lower than in alcoholic and nonalcoholic cirrhosis ($P < 0.05$)
[c] Significantly lower than in diseases causing intrahepatic portal hypertension ($P < 0.001$)
Reproduced from Bosch J, Feu F, Garciá-Pagán JC. In: Okuda K, Benhamou JP (eds) Portal hypertension–clinical and physiological aspects. Springer, Berlin Heidelberg New York Tokyo

### 3.3 Endoscopy

Esophagoscopy is the best method for evaluating the presence of varices and should be performed in every patient suspected of having portal hypertension. Endoscopy provides important prognostic information: variceal bleeding will not occur if there are no varices, which is not unusual even in the presence of other complications of portal hypertension such as ascites. Actually, it has been shown that varices are present in only 60% of cirrhotics at diagnosis, although this percentage increases to up to 90% on long-term follow-up. In addition to demonstrating the presence of varices, it is possible by means of endoscopy to grade variceal size on a I–IV scale. This is important because bleeding is directly related to the size of the varices [1]. Also, the endoscopic appearance of the wall of the varices is important: bleeding is more common in varices with "red signs" [telangiectasias, red wale marking (whip-like marks representing longitudinal dilated venules), and cherry red spots]. A recent multicenter prospective study has shown that the risk of variceal hemorrhage in patients with cirrhosis and esophageal varices is significantly related to the size of the varices, to the presence of red color signs, and to liver function, evaluated by the Child-Pugh classification [21]. On the basis of these three variables a prognostic index (the so-called NIEC index) was derived and validated prospectively [21]. This index allows identification of groups of patients with a high or low risk of variceal hemorrhage; however, its value in individual subjects has been questioned.

### 3.4 Measurement of Variceal Pressure

The pressure of the esophageal varices can be measured at endoscopy using two different approaches: direct variceal puncture [22], which has been used increasingly since the popularization of sclerotherapy, and by means of endoscopic pressure-sensitive gauges [23], which allow measurement of variceal pressure without puncturing the varices, and therefore without the risk of precipitating variceal hemorrhage. The endoscopic gauge technique is based on the assumption that, because of their thin walls and lack of external tissue support, the varices behave as an elastic structure; thus, the pressure needed to compress a varix equals the pressure inside the varix. We have demonstrated excellent agreement between measurements by both methods both in in vitro studies using artificial varices and in vivo, in patients with cirrhosis in whom measurements by both methods were performed during the course of the first session of sclerotherapy [24].

Measurements of variceal pressure are, for the moment, research procedures. The results may be difficult to interpret because of artifacts caused by esophageal peristalsis. In addition, there are limitations inherent to each of the proposed techniques. Thus, the real risk of measurements involving the puncture of the varices (bleeding, bacteremia, etc.) is still unknown. Probably, such techniques are only justified in patients undergoing therapeutic sclerotherapy. Endoscopic pressure-sensitive ("capsule") measurements can be influenced by the construction of the capsule and by the skill of the physician performing the measurements. Recent studies from our laboratory using an improved, miniaturized, pressure-sensitive capsule evaluated under double-blind conditions have shown that this technique is highly reproducible when strict criteria are adopted to define a satisfactory measurement [25].

The main findings of studies measuring variceal pressure in patients with cirrhosis are:

1. Variceal pressure is significantly lower than portal pressure; this is due to the resistance offered by the collaterals feeding the varices and indicates that measurements of variceal pressure cannot be used to estimate portal pressure [22–24].
2. Variceal pressure is greater in patients who have bled from the varices than in those who have not [23], suggesting that increased variceal pressure plays a key role in the mechanism of bleeding and that measurement of variceal pressure may be of value in assessing the risk of

bleeding, although this has still not been proved by prospective longitudinal studies.

3. The technique may be useful for assessing the effects of pharmacologic agents; however, due to the technical limitations outlined above, such investigations should be performed under strict double-blind conditions by critical investigators.

It should be emphasized that these measurements are carried out in conditions far from physiologic, and that they complement, rather than substitute for, the information obtained by conventional hemodynamic studies [25].

### 3.5 Ultrasonography and Pulsed-Doppler Measurements of Portal Blood Flow

Ultrasonography has found increasing application in the evaluation of the portal hypertensive patient. Ultrasonography is almost as accurate as angiography, CT scans, and magnetic resonance imaging in detecting the patency of the portal vein or the presence of portal vein thrombosis [1], which should be investigated in any patient with suspected portal hypertension. Accuracy in detecting portal vein thrombosis is increased by the concomitant use of pulsed-Doppler flowmeters (the so-called duplex technique). This permits determination of the presence, direction, and velocity of portal blood flow. The latter measurement can be used to estimate portal blood flow. This is done by multiplying portal flow velocity by the cross-sectional area of the portal vein, estimated by planimetry on the ultrasound imaging. This method is subject to many sources of error and should thus be used with caution. A recent study showed high variability in such estimations of portal blood flow, especially when comparing measurements by different observers [26]. Variation is reduced with skill and by careful selection of patients but is still considerable, which makes mandatory critical evaluation and a double-blind study design. The fact that ultrasonography is totally noninvasive makes it attractive, and despite its limitations it is being increasingly used. It is hoped that the rapid technologic improvement as well as the advent of instruments using the "compensated attenuation" method will increase its accuracy, thus making it suitable for physiologic and pharmacologic research. Ultrasonography and Doppler flow measurements are also useful in assessing the patency of surgical portacaval or splenorenal shunts, and in evaluating the patency of arterial and venous anastomoses after orthotopic liver transplantation [27].

## 4 Natural History of Esophageal Varices

Esophageal varices are responsible for the main complication of portal hypertension, namely massive upper gastrointestinal hemorrhage. This is one of the more dramatic medical emergencies and represents a leading cause of death in patients with cirrhosis. The mortality of the first bleeding episode ranges between 20% and 80%; the average in most recent series is ca. 30%. This poor prognosis is aggravated by the fact that about 50% of patients rebleed within 6 months and 75% within 1 year.

The prognosis of the bleeding episode is determined by two factors: the magnitude of blood loss and the degree of liver failure. Except in the case of patients with massive, exsanguinating bleeding, at risk of dying before reaching hospital, the degree of liver failure is by far the more important determinant of prognosis. This is well illustrated by the fact that while mortality exceeds 70% in patients with advanced liver failure, it is below 15% in previously compensated patients. The most usual and easiest way of assessing prognosis is the modified Child's classification (Table 3). Although this classification was initially devised to assess the operative risk of patients with cirrhosis, it has subsequently been shown to be an easy and very valuable prognostic marker in other situations, to the extent that none of the new and sophisticated quantitative liver function tests has been shown to be better than the Child-Pugh score in assessing prognosis. However, not all patients with portal hypertension will experience variceal hemorrhage, even though the vast majority will develop esophageal varices.

Many studies have shown that the risk of variceal hemorrhage is, on average, 10%–20% per year. As already stated, the risk of bleeding correlates with the degree of impairment of liver function, with the size of the varices, and with the presence on the varices of the "red color" signs, as shown by the NIEC study [21] (Table 4).

Recent studies incorporating measurements of variceal pressure have furthered our understanding of how these different factors interact, increasing the risk of variceal hemorrhage [23]. This is briefly discussed below.

### 4.1 Pathophysiology of Variceal Hemorrhage

Two theories have been proposed to explain variceal bleeding [22–24]. The *erosion theory* suggests that varices bleed because of external trauma to the thin, fragile walls of the varices caused by deglutition of solid food and/or by gastroesophageal reflux. This theory has been abandoned because of the lack of objective evidence supporting it. There is no proven relationship between eating and bleeding; neither the incidence of reflux nor that of esophagitis is greater in patients with bleeding varices than in those without. By contrast, the so-called *explosion* hypothesis suggests that the main event leading to bleeding is excessive hydrostatic pressure inside the varices due to

**Table 3.** Clinical assessment of the degree of liver failure (Child-Pugh's score)[a]

| Parameter | Range | Points |
|---|---|---|
| 1. Encephalopathy (grade) | Absent | 1 |
| | I and II | 2 |
| | III and IV | 3 |
| 2. Ascites | Absent | 1 |
| | Mild | 2 |
| | Moderate | 3 |
| 3. Bilirubin (mg/dl)[b] | <2 | 1 |
| | 2–3 | 2 |
| | >3 | 3 |
| 4. Albumin (g/dl) | >3.5 | 1 |
| | 2.8–3.5 | 2 |
| | <2.8 | 3 |
| 5. Prothrombin ratio (%) | >50 | 1 |
| | 30–50 | 2 |
| | <30 | 3 |

Group A: 5–6 points
Group B: 7–9 points
Group C: 10–15 points

[a] The original Child's classification included nutritional status evaluated as excellent, fair, and poor instead of prothrombin ratio
[b] Correction for bilirubin in primary biliary cirrhosis: <4 mg/dl (1 point), 4–10 mg/dl (2 points), >10 mg/dl (3 points)
Based on Pugh RNH, Murray-Lyon IM, Dawson JL, Pietroni MC, Williams R (1973) Br J Surg 60:646–664

portal hypertension. In support of this, a recent study showed that variceal pressure was substantially greater in portal hypertensive patients who had bled from the varices than in those who had not [23]. Moreover, it should be pointed out that more important than intravariceal pressure is the tension exerted on the walls of the varices: bleeding probably occurs when the varices break because of excessive wall tension. The factors regulating the tension on the walls of the varices are interrelated according to Laplace's law in the equation:

$$\text{Tension} = (P1 - P2) \times r/w$$

in which *P1* is the intravariceal pressure, *P2* the pressure in the esophageal lumen, *r* the radius of the varix, and *w* the thickness of its wall. This equation indicates that a large variceal size multiplies the deleterious effects of a high intravariceal pressure, increasing the tension exerted on the walls of the varices; a size IV varix with thin walls (indicated by red signs on endoscopy) can have a high risk of bleeding even at relatively low variceal pressure. The sequence of events leading to variceal hemoorhage is there-

**Table 4.** Estimated 1-year percentage probability of bleeding as a function of two endoscopic variables (size and red wale markings) for patients in Child class A, B, or C

| Red wale markings | Child class A | | | Child class B | | | Child class C | | |
|---|---|---|---|---|---|---|---|---|---|
| | Small | Medium | Large | Small | Medium | Large | Small | Medium | Large |
| Absent | 6 | 10 | 15 | 10 | 16 | 26 | 20 | 30 | 42 |
| Mild | 8 | 12 | 19 | 15 | 23 | 33 | 28 | 38 | 54 |
| Moderate | 12 | 16 | 24 | 20 | 30 | 42 | 36 | 48 | 64 |
| Severe | 16 | 23 | 34 | 28 | 40 | 52 | 44 | 60 | 76 |

Reproduced from The North Italian Endoscopic Club for the Study and Treatment of Esophageal Varices (1988) N Engl J Med 319:983–989

fore initiated by a high portal pressure, which promotes the opening of collaterals and the formation of varices. The maintenance of an increased pressure, together with a high blood flow, causes the dilatation of the varices, and as the varices dilate, their walls will become thinner. Any further increase in variceal pressure or size, or any defect in the variceal walls, will then cause leakage of the varices and clinical hemorrhage (Fig. 3).

It is likely that the factors determining bleeding are not the same as those influencing the severity of the subsequent hemorrhage. In addition to the transmural pressure at the varices, other important factors influencing the magnitude and duration of the hemorrhage include the area of the variceal tear, blood viscosity, and the degree of impairment of hemostasis.

## 5 Management of Variceal Hemorrhage

Acute variceal bleeding is a medical emergency that should be managed under intensive care facilities by a team of experienced medical staff, including an endoscopist, a clinical hepatologist, and a surgeon. It is essential to have well-trained nurses. Therapy should not be improvised for every new patient, but planned in a specifically designed protocol adapted to the human and technical resources available in the hospital; this is greatly facilitated by establishing gastrointestinal bleeding units.

The initial therapy is aimed at correcting hypovolemic shock, at preventing complications associated with gastrointestinal bleeding, and at achieving hemostasis at the bleeding site. The first two goals, which are independent of the cause of the hemorrhage, demand immediate management. Specific therapy to stop bleeding is usually given when the patient has had initial resuscitation and following emergency endoscopy.

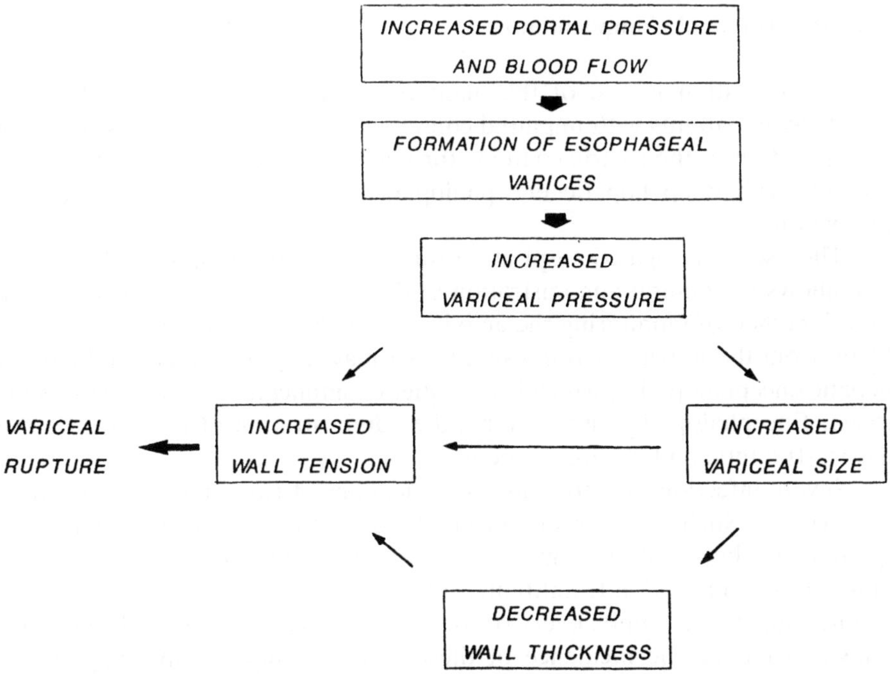


**Fig. 3.** Schematic representation of the pathophysiology of variceal hemorrhage. The figure illustrates the key role of increased variceal pressure interacting with the other factors that influence the tension of the variceal wall

## 5.1 Replacement of Blood Volume

Variceal bleeding is often massive; it is therefore essential to introduce a large-bore i.v. cannula to allow rapid blood transfusion if required. In addition, a central venous line should be placed. The blood bank should be contacted and 4–6 units of blood should be kept cross-matched ready for transfusion at any time. After restoring blood pressure to normal values by infusing plasma expanders or by blood transfusion, whole blood or packed red cells are transfused to keep the hematocrit at approximately 30%. Overtransfusion should be avoided, not only because of the risks inherent with blood transfusion but also because there may be a rebound increase in portal pressure with a consequent risk of continued bleeding or rebleeding. Experimental studies in rats with portal hypertension have shown an increase in portal pressure beyond basal values when restoring blood volume [28]. Furthermore, hypovolemia and low blood pressure are very powerful stimuli promoting a marked splanchnic vasoconstriction resulting in a reduction in portal pressure. Thus, variceal bleeding tends to stop spontaneously during hypovolemia but may continue or start up again with overtransfusion [28].

### 5.2 Prevention of Complications

Airway aspiration is one of the main complications of variceal bleeding, especially in patients with impaired consciousness. Its prevention is based on the aspiration of the gastric contents through an indwelling nasogastric tube. Patients with deep hepatic encephalopathy should also have orotracheal intubation.

The use of nasogastric aspiration through an indwelling large-bore tube also allows the enteral administration of drugs in comatose patients and is a useful method of monitoring the activity of bleeding. In addition, removal of blood from the upper gastrointestinal tract may help to prevent and correct hepatic encephalopathy, which is a frequent complication of variceal hemorrhage. Encephalopathy also requires the administration of lactulose via the nasogastric tube and cleansing enemas.

Severe infections are common complications of gastrointestinal bleeding in cirrhosis. Such patients are prone to develop systemic infections and spontaneous bacterial peritonitis due to enteric organisms. The administration of oral nonabsorbable antibiotics (colistin $1.5 \times 10^6$ units, neomycin 1 g, and nystatin $1 \times 10^6$ units every 6 h or of norfloxacin 400 mg b.i.d) has been shown to reduce the incidence of these serious complications. Support of renal function is also very important. This is based on maintaining adequate renal perfusion (i.e., avoiding hypotension) and maintaining hydroelectrolyte balance. It is crucial to avoid the administration of nephrotoxic drugs, especially aminoglycosides and nonsteroidal anti-inflammatory agents.

### 5.3 Diagnosis

As soon as the patient is stabilized, *emergency endoscopy* should be performed. This is the only way of ascertaining the bleeding site. This is very important, since these patients frequently bleed from lesions other than varices, in particular from gastric erosions, peptic ulcers, and portal hypertensive gastropathy. The diagnosis of bleeding varices is made (a) if there is a venous (nonpulsatile) spurt or a venous ooze, (b) if there is an adherent clot, or (c) if a platelet aggregate or fibrin clot (white in color) is seen on a varix. In the absence of these signs, variceal bleeding can only be diagnosed in the absence of other lesions in the stomach or duodenum. If more than one nonbleeding lesion is seen, immediate reendoscopy is mandatory if rebleeding occurs. Bleeding will have stopped spontaneously in approximately one-third of patients at the time of emergency endoscopy; however, about half of them will have recurrent bleeding within 48 h.

### 5.4 Specific Therapy

Several therapeutic procedures have been used. The main ones are discussed below.

#### *Balloon Tamponade*

Balloon tamponade controls bleeding by direct compression of the varices at the bleeding site. This is best achieved by the Sengstaken-Blakemore tube in esophageal varices, and by the single-balloon Linton-Nachlas tube in gastric varices [29]. Before passage of the tube, the stomach should be emptied to reduce the possibility of vomiting and aspiration, the channels of the tube checked for patency, and the balloons checked for leaks. The tube is lubricated and passed through the nose into the stomach. When using the Sengstaken-Blakemore tube, the gastric balloon is first inflated with 100 ml of air. The tube is then slowly withdrawn until firm resistance is encountered at the esophagogastric junction; thereafter the esophageal balloon is inflated at a pressure of 60 mmHg, and the tube is kept in place by fixing it to the nose, or preferably to a baseball mask or similar device. When using the Linton-Nachlas tube, the single, large gastric balloon is inflated with 600 ml of air and the tube is kept under external traction of 1 kg to compress gastric varices at the fornix. Tamponade is highly effective; the rate of control of bleeding ranges between 80% and 90% in experienced centers [29]. The two main drawbacks of this form of therapy are: (a) its effects are limited to the period for which the balloons are inflated and compress the varices (24–36 h); (b) there is a high rate of complications, which may be lethal. The most frequent severe complication is aspiration pneumonia, which occurs in more than 10% of patients even in experienced centers; this figure may be reduced if orotracheal intubation is performed prior to tamponade in patients with encephalopathy, if continuous aspiration of oropharyngeal secretions is performed, and if patients are kept under close supervision by an experienced nursing team. The most frequent side-effect is thoracic pain; this appears in one-fourth of the patients and may require sedation or even withdrawal of the tube. Tolerance is improved by using the Sengstaken-Blakemore tube without external traction.

#### *Pharmacologic Therapy*

If a safe and effective drug were available, pharmacologic therapy would offer the unique advantage of enabling specific therapy to be initiated as soon as the patient arrives at the emergency room, even before diagnostic endoscopy. Currently available pharmacologic therapy is summarized below.

*Vasopressin* has been widely used in the treatment of variceal hemorrhage but is still controversial. Vasopressin is a powerful vasoconstrictor that reduces blood flow in all splanchnic organs and thereby decreases portal blood flow and portal pressure. This results in a fall in azygos blood flow and in variceal pressure [17, 22]. Administered by continuous intravenous infusion, it arrests variceal bleeding in approximately 60% of cases [30]. The infusion is started at a rate of 0.4 U/min, which may be increased stepwise up to 1 U/min if necessary. These high rates of infusion should be decreased as soon as bleeding is controlled. Therapy is usually maintained until bleeding has been controlled for 12 h.

The main disadvantage of vasopressin is that it is associated with many side-effects due to systemic vasoconstriction and cardiotoxicity; these include heart failure, bradycardia and arrhythmias, hypertension, ischemic abdominal pain, chest pain, and dilutional hyponatremia [30]. Superior mesenteric artery infusions of smaller doses of vasopressin have been used in an attempt to decrease the systemic toxicity of the drug; however, comparative studies have shown almost identical effects as with intravenous vasopressin. Severe side-effects requiring discontinuation of the infusion are observed in 20% of cases.

It has recently been shown that *combination therapy with nitroglycerin and vasopressin* enhances the reduction in portal pressure while decreasing the adverse effects on the heart and systemic circulation [31]. This drug combination has proved better than vasopressin alone in three controlled trials (Table 5). In the aforementioned recent double-blind investigation [31], combination therapy was found to decrease significantly transfusion requirements, as well as the need for esophageal tamponade and emergency surgery. Nitroglycerin can be given sublingually, intravenously, or percuta-

**Table 5.** Results of studies comparing the administration of vasopressin (VP) alone versus the combination of nitroglycerin (NTG) and vasopressin infusion in the treatment of variceal bleeding

| | Route | No. of patients | Control of hemorrhage | | Major complications | | |
|---|---|---|---|---|---|---|---|
| | | | VP | VP + NTG | VP | VP + NTG | |
| Tsai et al. (1986) | Sublingual | 39 | 9/19 | 11/20 (at 6 h) | 6/19 | 2/20 | ($P < 0.05$) |
| Gimson et al. (1986) | Intravenous | 72 | 14/34 | 24/38 (at 12 h) | 7/34 | 1/38 | ($P < 0.02$)[a] |
| Bosch et al. (1990) | Percutaneous | 65 | 19/35 | 22/30 (at 24 h) | 3/35 | 2/30 | NS[b] |
| Total | | 176 | 42/88 | 57/88 | 16/88 | 5/88 | |

[a] Both in respect to control of bleeding and incidence of complications
[b] Significant differences in esophageal tamponade and emergency surgery requirements

neously. The last-mentioned is the simplest route of administration. The efficacy of vasopressin plus nitroglycerin in controlling variceal hemorrhage is approximately 75% [31]. Vasopressin plus nitroglycerin was almost as effective as tamponade in the initial control of bleeding in another recent study [32], and its effectiveness was equivalent to that of emergency sclerotherapy. The results of these studies suggest that if vasopressin is used, it should always be combined with nitroglycerin.

*Glypressin or terlipressin* is a synthetic vasopressin analog with long-acting activity. Its hemodynamic effects are similar to those of vasopressin but it is perhaps less toxic. Two placebo-controlled trials have shown that it is effective. Glypressin is given as an intravenous injection at a dose of 2 mg/6 h. Glypressin may also be combined with nitroglycerin.

*Somatostatin* was introduced for the treatment of variceal hemorrhage because of its capacity to decrease portal pressure without the adverse effects of vasopressin on the systemic circulation [33]. Somatostatin reduces portal and collateral blood flow by causing selective splanchnic vasoconstriction. This is due to inhibition of the release of vasodilating peptides and also to direct vasoactive effects. The latter are more evident following bolus injections than during continuous infusions.

The lack of significant side-effects from somatostatin represents its major advantage over other agents. Because of this feature, somatostatin is the drug which comes closest to meeting the ideal requirements for the pharmacologic treatment of variceal bleeding.

Somatostatin is administered clinically by means of continuous intravenous infusion at a rate of 250 μg/h, after a bolus of 250 μg which is repeated if the infusion has been inadvertently stopped. Additional boluses may be given if there is clinical evidence of rebleeding. Because of the much greater fall in portal pressure and azygos blood flow following bolus injections than continuous infusions [33], it has been suggested that repeated somatostatin bolus administration is appropriate during the initial hours of therapy (i.e., three boluses of 250 μg in the initial 4–6 h). When successful, therapy is maintained for 2–5 days. If bleeding is not controlled by somatostatin, alternative therapy should be given quickly. Several randomized controlled trials have shown that somatostatin is at least as effective as vasopressin but has fewer side-effects [30] (Table 6). Two placebo-controlled trials have come to opposite conclusions: one showed a clear beneficial effect of somatostatin while the other did not. However, in the study in which somatostatin was not effective there was an extremely high rate of response in the placebo group. This study may thus constitute a false-negative investigation. Furthermore, trials versus sclerotherapy and balloon tamponade show somatostatin to be just as effective as these much more invasive and cumbersome therapies for active bleeding. So far, somatostatin has not been adequately compared with either vasopressin plus nitroglycerin or glypressin. Several somatostatin derivatives, with a longer half-life, are being investigated.

**Table 6.** Results of studies comparing the efficacy and side-effects of vasopressin (VP) and somatostatin (SMT) infusions in the treatment of variceal hemorrhage

| | No. of patients | Final control of bleeding | | Complications | |
|---|---|---|---|---|---|
| | | VP | SMT | VP | SMT |
| Kravetz et al. (1984) | 61 | 18/31 | 16/30 | 8/31 | 0/30 |
| Jenkins et al. (1985) | 22 | 4/12 | 10/10 | 2/12 | 0/10 |
| Bagarani et al. (1987) | 66 | 9/32 | 23/34 | 4/32 | 2/34 |
| Cardona et al. (1989) | 38 | 12/18 | 10/20 | 6/18 | 0/20 |
| Total | 187 | 43/93 | 59/94 | 20/93 | 2/94 |

### *Emergency Sclerotherapy*

Emergency sclerotherapy is performed at the same time as diagnostic endoscopy, or after the bleeding has been controlled by the use of drugs or balloon tamponade. Its efficacy is thought to be similar to that of tamponade, but it provides the possibility of starting long-term treatment at the time of endoscopy. Intravariceal, paravariceal, and combined injections of sclerosants have been used, the most common sclerosants being 5% ethanolamine, 5% sodium morrhuate, and 1% polidocanol. The immediate effect is mostly due to obliteration of the bleeding vessel by local edema; thrombosis of varices is probably a secondary effect. Sclerotherapy has been shown to stop variceal bleeding and reduce the frequency of early rebleeding. This represents an important advance in the management of acute variceal bleeding.

After the first emergency injection, the usual approach is to continue to inject electively at 7-day intervals. However, early rebleeding, even within 24 h, can occur following injection. Several studies suggest that due to the fact that if more sclerosant is used, more complications are likely (including rebleeding from sclerosis ulcers), no more than two injection sessions should be used to arrest variceal bleeding following admission. Thus, if bleeding recurs despite these two sessions an alternative treatment is required.

Technical variations in the site and schedule of injection and in the sclerosant used appear to have little influence on the overall efficacy of sclerotherapy.

The more common and severe complications of sclerotherapy are esophageal ulceration (20%–40%), bleeding from esophageal ulcers (5%–20%), esophageal stenosis (5%–10%), and less frequently perforation of the esophagus and sepsis. Sclerotherapy is usually performed under antibiotic protection. Less severe but more frequent complications are transient dysphagia (60%–80%), chest pain (40%–60%), and pleural effusions (20%–30%). All complications are seen more frequently with emergency than with elective injection. An increasingly recognized complication of emergency sclerotherapy is the development of portal vein thrombosis, which may aggravate the bleeding and interfere with surgical therapy. Such thrombosis is frequently missed on ultrasonography and angiography. This emphasizes the importance of not "oversclerosing" patients during the active bleeding period.

Fundal varices are not usually accessible to sclerotherapy. Recently, they have been injected with bucrylate. The ensuing "variceal casts" physically eliminate the gastric varices in the following days. Neither the precise treatment schedule, nor the complications, nor the applicability of this technique are well established.

### *Surgical Therapy*

Surgical therapy is used in two circumstances; when everything else has failed to control bleeding, and when there is recurrent, massive bleeding. Emergency distal splenorenal shunts have a higher risk of thrombosis than elective shunts. The more effective operation is terminolateral portacaval shunt [34]. Shunting operations carry the risk of encephalopathy and have a high mortality in Child's C patients. Nonshunting procedures, such as esophageal transection, are also effective; their main advantage is the lack of potential for encephalopathy, but they are less effective in preventing further bleeding episodes than portacaval shunts [34]. All surgery should be carefully considered in those who are potential transplant candidates as it may make subsequent surgery more difficult. Most surgeons prefer decompression surgery to nonshunting operations. It is generally agreed that the operation should be done as far as possible from the hepatic hilum. This has led to many centers increasingly performing calibrated mesocaval or portocaval shunts, using an interposed 8-mm Goretex prosthesis. These will have some of the hemodynamic advantages of "selective" shunts and rarely may be removed at transplantation. It has been suggested that the administration of heparin for 1 month will decrease the risk of thrombosis of these shunts.

### *Other Procedures*

Percutaneous embolization of varices through the catheterization of the portal vein has been shown to be useful in arresting bleeding but carries a high rate of complications. It represents a complicated way of performing sclerotherapy. Intrahepatic shunts created by passing expandable stents through the hepatic veins and into the portal venous radicles will stop bleeding but again represent a highly specialized and technically difficult treatment; little information is available on its complications or long-term effectiveness.

## 6 Prevention of Variceal Hemorrhage

Cirrhotics who survive the first variceal hemorrhage have a 70% risk of rebleeding from varices while the risk of bleeding in patients with varices that have never bled is less than 30% at 1 year of follow-up. Preventive therapy is aimed at improving survival by preventing variceal hemorrhage, which is one of the leading causes of death in cirrhosis. Prophylactic medical therapy, which is feasible at present, may have a major impact on the natural history of cirrhosis.

Long-term therapy is based on the use of pharmacologic agents that lower portal pressure, of endoscopic sclerotherapy, and of surgery. Theoretically, the same treatment as is used for primary prophylaxis in patients who have never bled can be appropriate to prevent further episodes of hemorrhage, and vice versa. However, this is not always the case: because of the lower risk of bleeding in patients treated prophylactically, aggressive therapies (surgery and sclerotherapy) should be restricted to the prevention of recurrent bleeding.

### 6.1 Prophylaxis of the First Variceal Hemorrhage

#### *Pharmacologic Therapy*

Drug therapy is based on the use of agents that cause a sustained reduction in portal pressure and in portal–collateral blood flow. There is a large body of experience with the use of propranolol [19] and other nonselective β-blockers such as nadolol. These agents reduce portal pressure by reducing portal and collateral blood flow. This is the result of (a) a decrease in cardiac output and heart rate due to the blockade of $\beta_1$-adrenoceptors and (b) splanchnic vasoconstriction due to the blockade of vasodilating $\beta_2$-adrenoceptors [19]. This may be the reason why atenolol and other cardioselective β-blockers have less potential in the treatment of portal hypertension. The fall in portal pressure is moderate, averaging 12%–16% in most published studies [14, 19], but there is a marked reduction in azygos blood flow, reflecting a marked reduction in blood flow through gastroesophageal collaterals and esophageal varices [19]. It has recently been shown that propranolol significantly reduces the pressure of the esophageal varices in patients with cirrhosis [25]. A major drawback of propranolol therapy is that more than one-third of the patients do not exhibit any decrease in portal pressure despite adequate β-blockade [13, 19]. The mechanism of non-response is not related to inadequate dose, to the etiology or severity of portal hypertension, to circulating levels of epinephrine and norepinephrine, or to down-regulation of $\beta_2$-adrenoceptors. The most likely explanation for nonresponse is that an increase in portal–

collateral vascular resistance attenuates the reduction in portal pressure promoted by a fall in portal venous inflow [7]. Such an increase in portal–collateral resistance has been well documented in experimental models and may depend on the extent of the collateral circulation. There is no way of predicting the portal pressure response to propranolol in a given patient, except by invasive hemodynamic studies. This may be important clinically, since it has been shown that patients in whom the hepatic venous pressure gradient is reduced to below 12 mmHg are completely protected from variceal hemorrhage and have a longer survival than those in whom the gradient exceeds 12 mmHg [13]. Therefore, it is probably appropriate to measure the effects of propranolol on portal pressure when selecting patients for therapy. This problem may be overcome in the future if new, noninvasive procedures are shown to depict adequately the response to propranolol, or by introducing more powerful agents (alone or in combination with propranolol) that may decrease the number of nonresponders.

*Propranolol.* Many randomized controlled trials have evaluated the clinical efficacy of propranolol as compared with a placebo in patients with cirrhosis and esophageal varices that have not bled previously. Only one of these studies was done double-blind. The results of these studies are quite homogeneous and demonstrate a substantial reduction in the risk of bleeding in the patients treated with propranolol. This was so even in patients with severe liver disease (i.e., among those with ascites (Table 7)).

Although only one study showed a significant improvement of survival in the patients treated with propranolol, there was a homogeneous trend in favor of therapy in the other studies as well. It is thus no surprise that a significant improvement in survival was found when the results of all published studies were combined in a meta-analysis [35].

Since side-effects from propranolol are not severe, and not a single lethal complication has been reported in these randomized controlled trials, it has been advised that propranolol therapy be given to all patients with cirrhosis with varices that have not bled and who have no contraindications to β-blockers. This recommendation has been reinforced by the fact that similar beneficial effects of propranolol were observed in trials using different entry criteria in relation to variceal size and etiology of cirrhosis (Table 7).

However, it is still unknown whether nonresponders to propranolol in terms of reduction in portal pressure do benefit from this therapy. In addition, once started, propranolol therapy should be maintained almost for ever, since the beneficial effects of propranolol are limited to the period of drug therapy. Nevertheless, it is widely accepted that there is no need for further trials against placebo in the prophylaxis of the first variceal hemorrhage. Furthermore, it is accepted that any new forms of therapy should be tested against propranolol.

**Table 7.** Results of published randomized controlled trials of β-blockers (β-bloc) versus placebo (Plac) for the prevention of the first variceal hemorrhage

| | No. of patients | Mean follow-up (months) | Liver function | Bleeding (%) | | Mortality (%) | | Side effects of β-blockers (%) |
|---|---|---|---|---|---|---|---|---|
| | | | | Plac | β-bloc | Plac | β-bloc | |
| Pascal et al. (1987) (propranolol) | 199 | 18 | Pugh's score <14 | 27 | 17[a] | 34 | 22[a] | 17 |
| Ideo et al. (1988) (nadolol) | 79 | 24 | 75% Pugh A or B | 11 | 3[a] | 18 | 10 | 3 |
| Lebrec et al. (1988) (nadolol) | 106 | 12 | Pugh A or B | 19 | 13 | 17 | 19 | 9 |
| Pagliaro et al. (1989) (propranolol) | 174 | 28 | Exclusion of ascites or biliru bin >54 μmol/liter | 35 | 21 | 31 | 44 | 27 |
| Andreani et al. (1990) (propranolol) | 76 | 24 | 70% Pugh A or B | 39 | 6[a] | 54 | 66 | 12 |
| Conn et al. (1991) (propranolol) | 102 | 16 | 94% Pugh A or B | 22 | 4[a] | 22 | 16 | 16 |

[a] Statistically significant differences on an intention to treat basis

From a practical point of view, we recommend treating with propranolol all compensated cirrhotics with esophageal varices who are not actively drinking and who can understand the goal of therapy and comply with it.

Propranolol is used at maximally tolerated doses. Adjustment of the dose is done by stepwise increases, carefully looking at clinical tolerance, heart rate, and arterial blood pressure. In general, a decrease in heart rate of 25% (but not below 55 per min) is considered adequate.

As already mentioned, patients in whom the hepatic venous pressure gradient falls to values of 12 mmHg or less are totally protected from the risk of bleeding. This provides a rationale for repeat invasive studies in patients on long-term pharmacologic therapy [13].

*Combination Therapy.* It has been proposed that the addition of a vasodilator may enhance the reduction in portal pressure seen with propranolol. The rationale for such combination therapy derives from the finding that propranolol increases portal–collateral resistance, which suggests that the addition of a venous dilator may cause a further fall in portal pressure. In this regard, recent studies have shown that the combination of isosorbide-5-mononitrate and propranolol results in a greater reduction in portal pressure than is observed with either drug alone [36]. This beneficial effect was particularly evident in patients who had not responded to propranolol. On long-term administration, this drug combination has been shown to be superior to propranolol in the reduction of portal pressure, in decreasing the number of nonresponders, and in preserving liver blood flow and hepatic function; however, its clinical efficacy is still under investigation.

### *Endoscopic Sclerotherapy*

Injection sclerotherapy of esophageal varices has become very popular in the past decade. Sclerotherapy is aimed at obliterating and eliminating the varices. This is accomplished in a high proportion of patients (averaging 70%) by repeated sessions of sclerotherapy, using either intravariceal or perivariceal injections. Sclerotherapy is performed at 1- to 2-week intervals until disappearance (or obliteration) of the varices, which usually requires four sessions. After the initial obliteration of the varices it is mandatory to perform frequent follow-up endoscopies (every 3–6 months) because most patients will have recurrence of the varices and require repeated sclerotherapy [35].

The high incidence of complications and the lifelong need for endoscopic controls and repeated sclerotherapy represent the main limitations of this otherwise effective procedure.

Prophylactic sclerotherapy is highly controversial because of the finding in some studies of an increased rather than a reduced incidence of bleeding [37]. Sclerotherapy is too invasive to use in asymptomatic patients, considering that bleeding will occur before eradication in a small minority.

Nowadays, there is no clear place for sclerotherapy in the prevention of variceal bleeding, especially considering the efficacy of propranolol.

### *Surgery*

Surgical protacaval anastomoses are highly effective in reducing portal pressure and in preventing variceal hemorrhage. However, this technique is of limited applicability because of the relatively high incidence of hepatic encephalopathy [35]. Also, the deprivation of portal blood flow to the liver may aggravate liver failure. It is now well established that shunts should not be performed prophylactically because of reduced survival. However, non-shunting operations such as the Sugiura procedure are being used in Japan, apparently with good results.

## 6.2 Prevention of Recurrent Variceal Hemorrhage

Patients surviving an episode of variceal hemorrhage have a 70% 1-year likelihood of recurrent bleeding. Because of this, it is universally accepted that these patients should receive effective therapy to prevent further bleeding episodes. Once again, this can be based on surgery, sclerotherapy, or pharmacologic therapy.

### *Surgery*

Surgery is still a good therapeutic alternative to prevent recurrent variceal hemorrhage in selected patients surviving the first bleeding episode. The distal splenorenal shunt probably offers the best protection, with less potential for severe portasystemic encephalopathy [38]. However, the "selective" decompression of the varices as well as portal liver perfusion is progressively lost during the years that follow the operation, which may explain why randomized controlled trials reveal only marginal differences when comparing portacaval and distal splenorenal shunts. As mentioned before, "calibrated" 8-mm Goretex interposition mesocaval or portacaval shunts are being increasingly used, with good results, although there is much less experience with their use than with the distal splenorenal shunt. Nonshunting operations (esophageal transection with variable degrees of devascularization) offer less protection from rebleeding but do not cause encephalopathy [35]. However, these operations are not adequate in potential transplant candidates.

### *Long-term Variceal Sclerotherapy*

Many studies have demonstrated that repeat sclerotherapy is an effective treatment to prevent recurrent variceal hemorrhage and to improve survival.

The technical aspects are similar to those for prophylactic sclerotherapy. It should be pointed out that the beneficial effects of sclerotherapy may have been overestimated in the past. Careful analysis of the published controlled trials suggests that the benefit of such therapy is related more to its use during rebleeding episodes (in which it may reduce mortality) than to a reduction in the number of patients experiencing further episodes of variceal hemorrhage [35]. Only two of the six studies published documented a statistically significant reduction in the number of patients rebleeding. However, these studies do document a decrease in the total number of rebleeding episodes; this is achieved when the varices are eradicated, a goal that is achieved in about 70% of patients after 1–2 months. Unfortunately, "eradication" of varices does not mean that these will not reappear; on the contrary, in one-third of patients new varices form and are found to bleed on long-term follow-up. This makes it mandatory to implement an active program of frequent follow-up endoscopy and repeat sclerotherapy [35].

Controlled studies have shown that minor complications are frequent; major complications, although uncommon, may be fatal. Complications contributed to death in 2%–11% of patients in the six aforementioned studies.

Four trials have compared sclerotherapy and distal splenorenal shunts. In all of them, rebleeding was much more frequent in patients who underwent sclerotherapy than in shunted patients, while encephalopathy was more frequent following distal splenorenal shunt. When the results are taken together, there was no difference in survival between shunted patients and sclerotherapy patients, although one trial suggested that patients on the sclerotherapy arm who experienced rebleeding and were "salvaged" by performing a distal splenorenal shunt had better survival [35].

#### *Propranolol and Other β-Blockers*

Eleven controlled trials evaluating propranolol, nadolol, or atenolol versus no specific therapy have been reported in full papers or abstracts. These studies have shown that propranolol significantly reduces the risk of recurrent bleeding and slightly improves survival [35]. It is important to remark that in none of these studies has there been a single patient with a fatal complication due to treatment with β-blockers.

In addition, six studies compared β-blockers with long-term sclerotherapy. These studies have shown that sclerotherapy is significantly better than propranolol in preventing recurrent variceal bleeding. However, this is not associated with any difference in survival, so the benefit attributable to sclerotherapy is only marginal. Moreover, there is a definite trend toward an increased risk of bleeding from lesions other than esophageal varices in patients treated by sclerotherapy, such as portal hypertensive gastropathy, but not in those receiving β-blockers. This may account for the absence of any difference in survival [35].

β-blockers have also been used in combination with sclerotherapy. Five studies have been reported comparing this combination with sclerotherapy alone. Overall, these studies do not show any advantage to accrue from combining these forms of therapy, in terms of either a reduction in recurrent bleeding or improved survival.

So far, there has been no report of a controlled comparison of β-blockers and surgery. Similarly, there are still no studies comparing propranolol alone with the combination of propranolol and isosorbide-5-mononitrate or another vasodilator.

### *Transplantation*

Orthotopic liver transplantation offers the opportunity of curing both portal hypertension and the liver disease, and represents the only way of dramatically improving the survival of patients with advanced cirrhosis. The increasing success in transplant surgery, as well as in the number of donors and of experienced centers, means that transplantation should be considered as a true therapeutic alternative in patients who have bled from varices and have a poor liver function.

Our recommendation is to consider as transplant candidates all Child's C cirrhotics who survive an episode of bleeding and are below 50, who have neither portal vein thrombosis nor hepatocellular carcinoma, and who are either nonalcoholics or have abstained from alcohol for the preceding 6 months.

## 7 Ectopic Varices

While in most instances portal hypertension leads to the formation of esophageal and gastric varices, some patients develop varices at unusual locations. Such "ectopic varices" are rarely the sole manifestation of portal hypertension: usually they are associated with esophageal varices. Anorectal varices are frequently found as they are easily accessible.

Ectopic varices can develop, and rupture, in many different places. There are anecdotal reports of bronchial, vaginal, vesical, gallbladder, and common bile duct varices. However, the more frequent locations of ectopic varices are at the stoma of an enterostomy (27%), the duodenum (18%), the jejunum and ileum (18%), the colon (15%), the rectum (9%), and the peritoneum (10%). Bleeding from ectopic varices may thus result in unusual manifestations (e.g., hemobilia, hemoperitoneum, hematuria).

It has been suggested that the overall incidence of ectopic varices ranges between 1% and 3% in patients with cirrhosis, whereas it is higher in extrahepatic portal hypertension (20%–30%). It is likely that previous operations favor the development of ectopic varices, since these are much more common in patients with portal hypertension and previous abdominal surgery.

Ectopic varices have frequently been treated by surgery, using local resection, ligation of the varices, or portacaval shunts. However, the simplest methods should be used when possible as varices always re-form. Local resection for anorectal varices is contraindicated as major bleeding complications may ensue.

## 8 Portal Hypertensive Gastropathy

Patients with cirrhosis frequently bleed from nonvariceal sources. Hemorrhagic gastritis, acute erosions, and peptic ulcer occur frequently in patients with alcoholic cirrhosis. In addition, these patients may have a peculiar gastric lesion, so-called *portal hypertensive gastropathy*, which is characterized by a diffuse gastric mucosal vascular ectasia that at endoscopy appears as multiple small flat red spots [39]. These lesions may be located anywhere in the stomach. When the lesions are severe, the gastric mucosa has a "watermelon" appearance. In earlier stages, endoscopy reveals a mucosa with a "mosaic" pattern. There is no conclusive evidence to clarify the pathogenesis of this lesion. However, experimental studies have shown that gastric mucosal blood flow is markedly increased in portal hypertension, suggesting that the gastric mucosa is hyperemic. This increased blood flow, combined with the increased outflow pressure caused by portal hypertension, may promote the dilatation of the mucosal capillaries characteristic of this lesion. This increased gastric mucosal blood flow is partially reversed by propranolol [40]. Development of portal hypertensive gastropathy is often associated with hypergastrinemia, reduced serum levels of pepsinogen I, and decreased acid secretion but not with *Helicobacter pylori*. Clinically, the disease may cause episodes of overt gastrointestinal hemorrhage (often only manifested by melena and usually less severe than variceal bleeds) or manifest as chronic occult blood loss and microcytic anemia requiring repeated blood transfusions and oral iron therapy [39]. A recent multicenter randomized controlled trial showed that propranolol therapy significantly reduced the incidence of recurrent bleeding and the transfusion requirements in patients who had bled from portal hypertensive gastropathy. Interestingly, the rate of recurrent bleeding in the control group was 70%, quite similar to the risk of recurrent variceal hemorrhage in untreated patients.

# 9 Extrahepatic Portal Hypertension

## 9.1 Portal Vein Thrombosis

Portal vein thrombosis is the most frequent cause of prehepatic portal hypertension and is mainly observed in children and teenagers, in whom a history of onphalitis and/or umbilical catheterization can be frequently obtained. In adults, the causes of portal thrombosis is not so frequently identified. This more common cause of portal vein thrombosis in adults are intra-abdominal infections, oral contraceptives, abdominal trauma, pancreatitis, pregnancy, or underlying disorders favoring a hypercoagulative state, such as blood dyscrasias, antithrombin III deficiency, the presence of antiphospholipid antibodies, protein C deficiency, and autoimmune disorders. In this regard, recent investigations have shown that 48% of patients with portal thrombosis in whom no favoring factor can be identified suffer a silent primary myeloproliferative disorder [3].

Portal vein thrombosis may be a complication of cirrhosis. However, the prevalence is low (0.6%) whereas it becomes a frequent event after splenectomy or in patients with hepatocellular carcinoma. Furthermore, recently several authors have pointed out that endoscopic sclerotherapy of the varices may promote portal vein thrombosis, a risk that should be taken into account in patients who may thereafter benefit from liver transplantation or require shunt surgery. In patients with cirrhosis the development of portal thrombosis may induce a further increase in portal hypertension and perhaps precipitate variceal hemorrhage.

In the majority of the adult cases, portal vein thrombosis is diagnosed after a bleeding episode. The tolerance to bleeding is much better in these patients than in cirrhotics. This is due to the lack of liver disease. Ultrasonographic examination of the portal system is usually enough for the diagnosis of portal thrombosis, especially if combined with pulsed Doppler flowmetry [1, 27]. However, in selected cases angiography may be needed as a confirmatory tool. In the chronic phase of portal thrombosis, the obstruction is associated with the development of new vascular channels aimed to bypass the vascular stop and giving a cavernomatous appearance to the portal vein. This is best shown by angiography [1].

Patients with portal vein thrombosis have hemodynamic abnormalities similar to those found in patients with liver cirrhosis and portal hypertension. Thus, they exhibit a hyperdynamic circulatory state with increased cardiac output and reduced arterial pressure and peripheral vascular resistance and also an increase in the portal venous inflow.

The underlying condition potentially responsible for portal thrombosis should be properly treated if possible. Only those patients who have suffered bleeding related to portal hypertension must be considered for treatment aimed at preventing rebleeding. Endoscopic sclerotherapy may reduce the proportion of patients needing surgery. The most useful operation is splenorenal shunt, but often it is precluded by extended thrombosis to the splenic vein. The same problem applies with respect to the applicability of other kinds of shunt [3]. Esophageal transection, ligation of varices, and splenectomy are less useful because of the high frequency of gastric varices and the high index of rebleeding due to reappearance of the varices. There is one clinical trial suggesting that propranolol may be useful in the treatment of this condition. Although still not adequately explored, there is a large amount of evidence in experimental prehepatic portal hypertension indicating that propranolol therapy decreases portal pressure and portal–collateral blood flow, and reduces the formation of portal–systemic collaterals in this situation.

### 9.2 Splenic Vein Thrombosis

The main causes of isolated splenic vein thrombosis are chronic pancreatitis and carcinoma of the pancreas [3]. In rare cases, it has been described in relation to retroperitoneal infections, renal neoplasms, or retroperitoneal fibrosis. Usually, splenic vein obstruction is diagnosed after a bleeding episode related to gastric varices, since development of esophageal varices is uncommon because of the possible drainage through the left coronary vein. The diagnosis is established by ultrasonography and by radiologic visualization at the venous phase of splenic artery angiography [1]. However, nonvisualization of the splenic vein does not represent unequivocal evidence of splenic vein thrombosis owing to the fact that in some patients with cirrhosis and severe portal hypertension, the presence of an extensive network of collaterals arising from the spleen and a slow retrograde portal blood flow may impede the filling of the vein, thus creating false-positive results. Therefore, in some cases definite diagnosis may require splenoportography, transhepatic catheterization of the portal vein, or even peroperative measurement of the pressures along the portal bed with simultaneous peroperative ultrasonographic examination of the splenic vein.

Since splenectomy is a curative operation and is not associated with a high morbidity and mortality, surgical treatment is clearly justified, even in patients who have not yet bled from varices [3].

## 10 Diagnostic and Therapeutic Approach to the Portal Hypertensive Patient

Patients suspected of having portal hypertension should undergo ultrasonography and upper gastrointestinal endoscopy [1]. At endoscopy particular attention should be paid to the presence, extent, size, and appearance of the wall of the varices. Ultrasonography, preferably combined with Doppler flowmetry, will show whether the portal vein is patent or not, and may disclose additional useful information on liver, biliary, or pancreatic diseases that may be the cause of portal hypertension [27]. Portal hypertensive patients with a patent portal vein should undergo hepatic vein catheterization [1]. If the patient has varices and the hepatic venous pressure gradient is less than 12 mmHg, presinusoidal intrahepatic portal hypertension is likely; this should be investigated by liver biopsy and percutaneous transhepatic measurement of portal pressure [1]. If the hepatic vein pressure gradient is above 12 mmHg and the patient has large esophageal varices, the possibility of instituting prophylactic medical therapy should be considered [35]. Finally, if the gradient is above 12 mmHg but endoscopy shows no varices, it is wise to reevaluate the patient at 12-month intervals because of the risk of developing varices and bleeding if portal pressure remains elevated. It should be emphasized that portal pressure does not remain steady during the evolution of cirrhosis. Actually, it usually varies in parallel with the severity of the disease. Many abstinent patients exhibit a spontaneous reduction in portal pressure, while alcoholic hepatitis and the development of hepatocellular carcinoma are associated with marked aggravations of the portal hypertension.

## References


1. Bosch J, Mastai R, Kravetz D, Navasa M, Rodés J (1986) Hemodynamic evaluation of the patient with portal hypertension. Semin Liver Dis 6:309–317
2. Groszmann RJ, Atterbury CE (1982) The pathophysiology of portal hypertension: a basis for classification. Semin Liver Dis 2:117–186
3. Lebrec D, Benhamou JP (1986) Noncirrhotic intrahepatic portal hypertension. Semin Liver Dis 6:332–340
4. Benoit JN, Granger DN (1986) Splanchnic hemodynamics in chronic portal venous hypertension. Semin Liver Dis 6:287–298
5. Vorobioff J, Bredfeldt JE, Groszmann RJ (1984) Increased blood flow through the portal system in cirrhotic rats. Gastroenterology 87:1120–1126
6. Bathal PS, Grossman HJ (1985) Reduction of the increased portal vascular resistance of the isolated perfused cirrhotic rat liver by vasodilators. J Hepatol 1:325–337
7. Kroeger RJ, Groszmann RJ (1985) Increased portal venous resistance hinders portal pressure reduction during the administration of beta-adrenergic blocking agents in a portal hypertensive model. Hepatology 5:97–101
8. Benoit JN, Barrowman JA, Harper SL, Kvietys PR, Granger DN (1984) Role of humoral factors in the intestinal hyperemia associated with chronic portal hypertension. Am J Physiol 247:G486–G493
9. Kravetz D, Arderiu MT, Bosch J et al. (1987) Hyperglucagonemia and hyperkinetic circulation following portocaval shunt in the rat. Am J Physiol 252:G257–G261
10. Silva G, Navasa M, Bosch J et al. (1990) Hemodynamic effects of glucagon in portal hypertension. Hepatology 11:668–673
11. Pizcueta MP, Casamitjana R, Bosch J, Rodés J (1990) Decreased systemic vascular sensitivity to norepinephrine in portal hypertensive rats: role of hyperglucagonism. Am J Physiol 258:G191–G195

12. García-Tsao G, Groszmann RJ, Fisher RL et al. (1985) Portal pressure, presence of gastoesophageal varices and variceal bleeding. Hepatology 5:419–424
13. Groszmann RJ, Bosch J, Grace ND et al. (1990) Hemodynamic events in a prospective randomized trial of propranolol versus placebo in the prevention of a first variceal hemorrhage. Gastroenterology 99:1401–1407
14. Groszmann RJ (1984) Reassessing portal venous pressure measurements. Gastroenterology 80:1611–1617
15. Pomier-Layrargues G, Kusielewicz D, Willems B, Villeneuve JP, Marleau D, Coté J, Huet PM (1985) Presinusoidal portal hypertension in non-alcoholic cirrhosis. Hepatology 5:415–418
16. Bosch J, Groszmann RJ (1984) Measurement of the azygos venous blood flow by a continuous thermal dilution technique. An index of blood flow through gastroesophageal collaterals in cirrhosis. Hepatology 4:424–429
17. Bosch J, Mastai R, Kravetz D, Bruix J, Rigau J, Rodés J (1985) Measurement of azygos venous blood flow in the evaluation of portal hypertension in patients with cirrhosis. Clinical and haemodynamic correlations in 100 patients. J Hepatol 1:125–139
18. Bosch J, Feu F, García-Pagán JC (1991) Measurement of azygos blood flow. In: Okuda K, Benhamou JP (eds) Portal hypertension – clinical and physiological aspects. Springer, Berlin Heidelberg New York Tokyo, pp 139–150
19. Bosch J, Mastai R, Kravetz D, Bruix J, Gaya J, Rigau J, Rodes J (1984) Effects of propranolol on azygos blood flow and hepatic and systemic hemodynamics in cirrhosis. Hepatology 4:1200–1205
20. Mastai R, Bosch J, Navasa M et al. (1987) Effects of alpha-adrenergic stimulation and beta-adrenergic blockade on azygos blood flow and splanchnic haemodynamics in patients with cirrhosis. J Hepatol 4:71–79
21. The North Italian Endoscopic Club for the Study and Treatment of Esophageal Varices (1988) Prediction of the first variceal hemorrhage in patients with cirrhosis of the liver and esophageal varices. N Engl J Med 319:983–989
22. Bosch J, Bordas JM, Mastai R et al. (1988) Effects of vasopressin on the intravariceal pressure in patients with cirrhosis: comparison with the effects on portal pressure. Hepatology 8:861–865
23. Rigau J, Bosch J, Bordas JM et al. (1989) Endoscopic measurement of variceal pressure in cirrhosis: correlation with portal and variceal hemorrhage. Gastroenterology 96:873–880
24. Bosch J, Bordas JM, Rigau J et al. (1986) Non-invasive measurement of the pressure of esophageal varices using an endoscopic gauge. Comparison with measurements by variceal puncture in patients undergoing sclerotherapy. Hepatology 6:667–672
25. Feu F, Bordas JM, García-Pagán JC, Bosch J, Rodés J (1991) Double-blind investigation of the effects of propranolol and placebo on the pressure of the esophageal varices in patients with portal hypertension. Hepatology 13:917–922
26. Sabbá C, Weltin GG, Ciccheti DV et al. (1990) Observer variability in echo-doppler measurements of portal flow in cirrhotic patients and normal volunteers. Gastroenterology 98:1603–1611
27. Consensus conference committee (1990) The value of Doppler US in the study of hepatic hemodynamics. Consensus conference (Bologna, Italy, 12 September 1989). J Hepatol 10:353–355
28. Kravetz D, Bosch J, Arderiu MT, Pizcueta MP, Rodés J (1989) Hemodynamic effects of blood volume restitution following a hemorrhage in rats with portal hypertension due to cirrhosis of the liver: influence of the extent of portal systemic shunting. Hepatology 9:808–814
29. Panés J, Terés J, Bosch J, Rodés J (1988) Efficacy of balloon tamponade in treatment of bleeding gastric and esophageal varices. Results in 151 consecutive patients. Dig Dis Sci 33:454–459

30. Kravetz D, Bosch J, Terés J et al. (1984) A controlled comparison of continuous somatostatin and vasopressin infusions in the treatment of acute variceal hemorrhage. Hepatology 4:442–446
31. Bosch J, Groszmann RJ, García-Pagán JC et al. (1989) Association of transdermal nitroglycerin to vasopressin infusion in the treatment of variceal hemorrhage: a placebo controlled clinical trial. Hepatology 10:962–968
32. Terés J, Planas R, Panés J et al. (1990) Vasopressin/nitroglycerin infusion vs. esophageal tamponade in the treatment of acute variceal bleeding: a randomized controlled trial. Hepatology 11:964–968
33. Bosch J, Kravetz D, Rodes J (1981) Effects of somatostatin on hepatic and systemic hemodynamics in patients with cirrhosis of the liver. Comparison with vasopressin. Gastroenterology 80:518–525
34. Terés J, Baroni R, Bordas JM, Visa J, Pera C, Rodés J (1987) Randomized trial of portacaval shunt, stapling transection and endoscopic sclerotherapy in uncontrolled variceal bleeding. J Hepatol 4:159–167
35. Pagliaro L, Burroughs AK, Sorensen TIA, Lebrec D, Morabito A, D'Amico G, Tinè F (1989) Therapeutic controversies and randomised controlled trials (RCTs): prevention of bleeding and rebleeding in cirrhosis. Gastroenterol Int 2:71–84
36. García-Pagán JC, Navasa M, Bosch J, Bru C, Pizcueta MP, Rodés J (1990) Enhancement of portal pressure reduction by the association of isosorbide-5-mononitrate to propranolol administration in patients with cirrhosis. Hepatology 11:230–238
37. Santangelo WC, Dueno MI, Estes BL, Krejs GJ (1988) Prophylactic sclerotherapy of large esophageal varices. N Engl J Med 318:814–818
38. Langer B, Taylor BR, Mackenzie DR et al. (1985) Further report of a prospective randomised trial comparing distal splenorenal shunt and end to side portacaval shunt. An analysis of encephalopathy, survival and quality of life. Gastroenterology 88:424–429
39. Quintero E, Piqué JM, Bombí JA et al. (1987) Gastric mucosal vascular ectasias causing bleeding in cirrhosis. A distinct entity associated with hypergastrinemia and low serum levels of pepsinogen I. Gastroenterology 93:1054–1061
40. Piqué JM, Pizcueta P, Pérez-Ayuso RM, Bosch J (1990) Effects of propranolol on gastric microcirculation and acid secretion in portal hypertensive rats. Hepatology 12:476–480

## Suggested Reading

Bosch J, Terés J (1986) Management of acute variceal bleeding. In: Williams R (ed) Liver failure. Churchill Livingstone, London, pp 124–143

Bosch J, Rodés J (eds) (1989) Recent advances in the pathophysiology and therapy of portal hypertension. Serono Symposia Review No. 22. Ares-Serono Symposia, Rome

Bosch J, Navasa M, García-Pagán JC, DeLacy AM, Rodés J (1989) Portal hypertension. Med Clin North Am 73:931–953

Bruix J, Bosch J (to be published) Prehepatic portal hypertension. In: McIntyre N, Benhamou JP, Bircher J, Rizzetto M, Rodés J (eds) Oxford textbook of clinical hepatology. Oxford University Press, Oxford

Burroughs AK (ed) Methodology and reviews of clinical trials in portal hypertension. Excerpta Medica, Amsterdam

Burroughs AK, Bosch J (to be published) Clinical manifestations and management of bleeding episodes in cirrhotics. In: McIntyre N, Behnamou JP, Bircher J, Rizzetto M, Rodés J (eds) Oxford textbook of clinical hepatology. Oxford University Press, Oxford

Navasa M, Bosch J, Rodés J (1991) Pharmacological agents and portal hypertension. In: Okuda K, Benhamou JP (eds) Portal hypertension – clinical and physiological aspects. Springer, Berlin Heidelberg New York Tokyo, pp 35–50
Terblanche J, Burroughs AK, Hobbs KEF (1989) Controversies in the management of bleeding esophageal varices (first of two parts). N Engl J Med 320:1393–1398
Terblanche J, Burroughs AK, Hobbs KEF (1989) Controversies in the management of bleeding esophageal varices (second of two parts). N Engl J Med 320:1469–1475
Terés J, Bordas JM, Bosch J (eds) (1991) Hemorragia digestiva. Doyma, Barcelona

# 12 Ascites and Renal and Electrolyte Abnormalities in Cirrhosis

V. Arroyo and P. Ginès

## 1 Detection of Ascites

The diagnosis of ascites is simple when large amounts of fluid accumulate in the peritoneal cavity. On physical examination the abdomen is distended, the flanks bulge, and a fluid wave may be demonstrable. Other characteristic signs of ascites, such as flank and shifting dullness, are also obvious. The diagnosis of ascites, however, is much more difficult by physical examination when there is a small volume of ascitic fluid. It has been suggested that the exploration for the puddle sign, a maneuver designed to identify an ascitic "puddle" around the umbilicus by combining percussion and auscultation of the abdomen with the patient on his hands and knees, can detect minimal amounts of ascites (less than 500 ml) [1]. However, in a recent study in which five physical signs (bulging flanks, flank dullness, shifting dullness, fluid wave, and puddle sign) were compared with ultrasonographic demonstration of ascites (ultrasonography can detect as little as 100–200 ml of intraperitoneal fluid) in patients in whom the bedside diagnosis of ascites was in question, the puddle sign did not show greater specificity and sensitivity than the other signs of ascites [2]. Ultrasonography, computed tomography, and magnetic resonance imaging are very useful methods in the assessment of patients with ascites. In addition to their sensitivity in detecting minimal amounts of ascites they may suggest the etiology of ascites based on the characteristics of the intra-abdominal organs and vessels and the appearance of the intra-abdominal fluid. Ultrasonography is the best of these methods since it is not expensive, is as reliable as computed tomography, and is free of radiation hazards.

## 2 Characteristics of Cirrhotic Ascites

The ascitic fluid in cirrhotics is transparent and yellow/amber. The total ascitic protein concentration may range from 0.5 to more than 6 g/dl and is greater than 3 g/dl ("exudative ascites") in up to 20% of otherwise uncomplicated cases of cirrhosis. The percentages of albumin and globulins over total protein concentration are approximately 45% and 55%, respectively. There is a close direct correlation between ascitic albumin and globulin concentrations, indicating that ascitic fluid proteins in cirrhosis derive from capillaries with relatively large pores, probably the hepatic sinusoids. The relative contribution of the sinusoids and the splanchnic capillaries (which are hardly permeable to plasma proteins) to the formation of ascites, however, varies markedly from patient to patient since the ascitic fluid–plasma ratios for total proteins, albumin, and globulins have been shown to range between 0.04 and 1.03 in patients with cirrhosis and ascites [3, 4]. The total protein, albumin, and globulin concentrations in ascitic fluid correlate directly with the corresponding plasma concentrations and inversely with portal pressure [4]. The mobilization of ascites with diuretics increases the concentration of proteins in the ascitic fluid [5]. The ascitic fluid possesses opsonic and bactericidal activities which seem to be mediated by complement and fibronectin. Since the concentrations of these proteins having antibacterial activity in ascitic fluid correlate with the total protein concentration, it is not surprising that spontaneous bacterial peritonitis usually occurs in cirrhotic patients with a low protein concentration in ascitic fluid (<1 g/dl) [6].

The ascitic fluid in the cirrhotic patient without spontaneous bacterial peritonitis usually has fewer than 300–500 white blood cells per $mm^3$; nevertheless, 10%–15% may have more than 500 cells and 5% may have more than 1000 cells. More than 70% of these white cells are mononuclear leukocytes. In contrast, in cirrhotic patients with spontaneous bacterial peritonitis the ascitic fluid usually contains more than 500 white blood cells per $mm^3$ (frequently more than 2000), with more than 70% of them being polymorphonuclear leukocytes [7]. The pH and the concentration of lactate in ascitic fluid in otherwise uncomplicated cirrhotic patients are similar to those in plasma. In patients with spontaneous bacterial peritonitis, the ascitic fluid pH is lower and the concentration of lactate higher than in plasma. These measurements, however, do not improve the diagnostic efficacy of leukocyte concentration in ascitic fluid [8]. The concentration of red blood cells in cirrhotic ascites is usually lower than 1000 cells per $mm^3$, yet higher concentrations may occasionally be detected. In fact, bloody ascitic fluid, which indicates more than 50000 red cells per $mm^3$ (hematocrit of about 0.5%), occurs in approximately 2% of cirrhotics [9]. In one-third of these patients, bloody ascites is secondary to a superimposed hepatocellular carcinoma bleeding into the peritoneal cavity [10]. The hepatic and thoracic lymph of cirrhotic patients is also often bloody.

The concentration of fibrinogen and plasminogen in ascitic fluid is lower than would be expected considering their molecular weights, whereas the levels of fibrin/fibrinogen degradation products are elevated in comparison with their levels in plasma [11]. On the other hand, the concentration of fibrin monomers in ascitic fluid is almost ten times higher than in plasma [12]. These abnormalities are consistent with intraperitoneal coagulation and primary and secondary fibrinolysis. The infusion of ascitic fluid into the general circulation is associated with disseminated intravascular coagulation, thus confirming the procoagulant activity of ascitic fluid. Several substances present in the ascites, such as tissue thromboplastin, endotoxin, collagen, activated clotting factors, and fibrin degradation products, may be related to this feature.

Pleural effusions in the absence of primary pulmonary or pleural disease occur in approximately 5% of patients with hepatic cirrhosis. Clinical ascites is almost always evident and the pleural effusion is usually right-sided. Occasionally, however, effusion develops in the left pleura, on both sides, or in the absence of detectable ascites. Cirrhotic hydrothorax is generally due to direct passage of ascitic fluid from the abdomen through acquired defects in the diaphragm into the pleural space, with the driving force being the hydrostatic gradient between the positive intra-abdominal pressure and the negative intrathoracic pressure. In cases of cirrhotic hydrothorax without detectable ascites, the transport of fluid into the pleural space probably equals the rate of ascites production. The biochemical and cytologic characteristics of cirrhotic hydrothorax, therefore, are similar to those of the simultaneously obtained ascitic fluid.

Chylous ("milky") ascites is an infrequent feature in patients with cirrhosis. It is probably caused by the spontaneous rupture of lymph vessels leading to the leakage of lymph into the peritoneal cavity, since the proportion of lipids in the ascitic fluid (high concentration of chylomicrons very rich in triglycerides and normal concentration of cholesterol and phospholipids) is very similar to that in intestinal and thoracic duct lymph. Chylous ascites may occur as a complication of operations that may damage the retroperitoneal lymphatics (splenorenal shunt, renal transplantation, aortic aneurysmectomy, retroperitoneal lymphadenectomy, and pancreatoduodenectomy). However, the main cause of chylous ascites in the adult is obstruction of the lymphatic system due to malignancies, especially lymphomas.

Ascites secondary to postsinusoidal portal hypertension (congestive heart failure, constrictive pericarditis, obstruction of the inferior vena cava, Budd-Chiari syndrome) generally shows a total protein concentration of more than 3 g/dl. Patients with ascites due to constrictive pericarditis often lack symptoms of congestive heart failure and those with partial obstruction of the inferior vena cava usually do not present a clear cava–cava collateral circulation. Furthermore, patients with chronic Budd-Chiari syndrome may present hepatic stigmata, abnormal liver function tests, splenomegaly, and esophageal varices, suggesting hepatic cirrhosis. Ultrasonography to assess the patency of hepatic veins, echocardiography, hepatic and cardiac catheterization, inferior vena cavography, and, finally, liver biopsy, are frequently required to obtain a correct diagnosis in these patients.

## 3 Factors Involved in Ascites Formation in Cirrhosis

### 3.1 Portal Hypertension

The accumulation of ascites is a common complication in diseases causing sinusoidal portal hypertension (Budd-Chiari syndrome, acute alcoholic hepatitis, cirrhosis) but it is extraordinarily infrequent when portal hypertension is due to presinusoidal blockade of the portal venous flow (idiopathic portal hypertension, congenital hepatic fibrosis, portal venous thrombosis). Differences in anatomic and functional characteristics between the hepatic and splanchnic microvasculature are probably the reason for this feature.

#### *Effect of Sinusoidal Portal Hypertension on Transsinusoidal Fluid Exchange*

The hepatic sinusoids are structurally unique among microvessels since they do not have a basement membrane. They are lined mainly by endothelial cells which form a very porous wall with large apertures. This extremely porous membrane is almost completely permeable to macromolecules, including plasma proteins, so that the transsinusoidal oncotic gradient is virtually zero. Liver lymph formed in the space of Disse, with a protein concentration of approximately 95% of the simultaneously measured plasma, enters the lymphatics present in the portal tract and drains through vessels leaving at the porta hepatis into the thoracic duct. This is a 40 cm long lymphatic channel that ascends from the upper abdomen to the neck, where it joins the left subclavian or internal jugular vein. Lymph from pancreas, spleen, kidney, adrenals, stomach, large and small intestines, and mesentery also drains into the thoracic duct.

Constriction of the suprahepatic inferior vena cava or the hepatic veins in animals has been the most frequently used model to investigate the effect of sinusoidal portal hypertension on fluid exchange through the sinusoidal wall. The increased pressure in the hepatic veins is almost completely transmitted back to the hepatic sinusoids, indicating that capillary pressure is not autoregulated in the liver. Since no oncotic force opposes the elevation in sinusoidal pressure, there is a dramatic increase in the passage of fluid, with a protein concentration similar to plasma, from the sinusoidal lumen to the space of Disse [13, 14]. Because the compliance of the liver, that is the relationship between interstitial pressure and volume, is very low, the elevation of sinusoidal pressure gives rise to an increase in interstitial pressure, which explains the two major consequences of sinusoidal portal hypertension: a striking increase in lymph flow through the liver lymphatics and thoracic duct and the direct passage of hepatic lymph with very high protein concentration from the liver surface into the peritoneal cavity, forming ascites.

### *Effect of Portal Hypertension on the Splanchnic Transmicrovascular Fluid Exchange*

The structural and functional characteristics of the microvasculature of the stomach and intestines are very different from those in the liver. First, the splanchnic capillaries are much less porous than hepatic sinusoids (the estimated pore size is 50–100 times smaller than that in the sinusoids), have a well-defined basement membrane, and are hardly permeable to plasma proteins. This explains why the total protein concentration of the intestinal lymph is below 20% of the simultaneously measured plasma. Consequently, any increase in filtration is quickly counterbalanced by an increase in the oncotic pressure difference between capillary lumen and interstitial space. Second, there is evidence that the intestinal microvasculature autoregulates the capillary pressure and the capillary filtration coefficient (which depends on the size and number of pores and the filtration surface area) through a myogenic constriction of the arteriolar resistance and precapillary sphincters. Finally, the intestines have a very efficient lymphatic system to remove interstitial edema. In this respect, it is interesting to note that in normal conditions approximately 20% of the fluid absorbed by the small intestine is carried out to the general circulation by the lymphatics. These three features protect the intestine against edema formation following elevation in portal pressure and probably explain the infrequency of ascites in presinusoidal portal hypertension.

### *Source of Ascites in Cirrhotic Patients with Portal Hypertension*

From the above-mentioned data it appears clear that an imbalance between the hepatic lymph production and the ability of the lymphatic system of the liver and thoracic duct to return the hepatic lymph to the general circulation may be the predominant mechanism of ascites formation in patients with postsinusoidal portal hypertension (constrictive pericarditis, Budd-Chiari syndrome, and hepatic veno-occlusive disease) who show increased thoracic duct lymph flow and ascites with very high protein content. Hepatic cirrhosis, however, differs in many respects from experimental hepatic venous outflow block. Therefore, the mechanism of ascites formation in circumstances of hepatic venous outflow block cannot be extended to patients with chronic liver disease.

An important structural change in hepatic cirrhosis is the capillarization of the hepatic sinusoids. This abnormality consists in the transformation of the sinusoids into true capillaries with a continuous endothelial lining without fenestrae supported by a basement membrane and collagenous tissue [15]. (Fig. 1). This change occurs especially in the marginal areas of the regenerative nodules, but its distribution and extension vary markedly from patient to patient. The most important functional consequence of this abnormality is

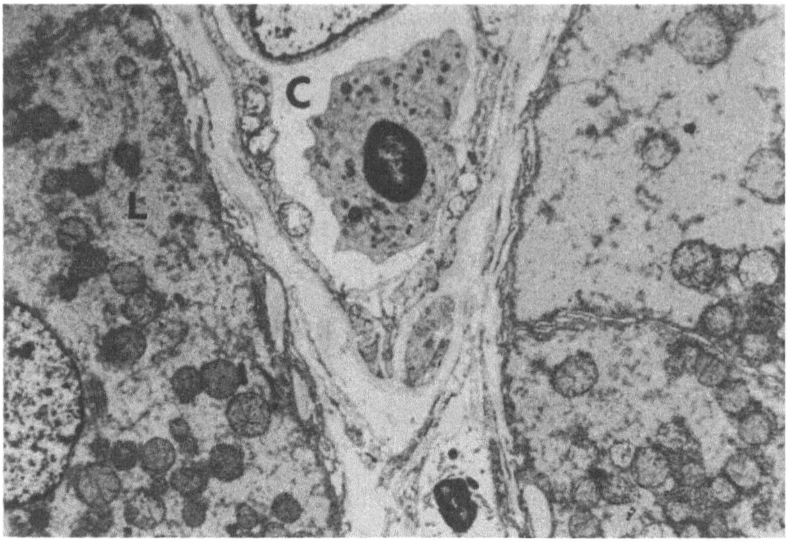


**Fig. 1.** Electron microscopic picture of changes in hepatic microcirculation in cirrhosis. The sinusoidal lumen (*C*) is separated from the liver cells (*L*) by a nonfenestrated endothelial cell membrane, a basement membrane, and a layer of fibrillary collagen. [Reproduced with permission from HUET PM et al. (1982) J Clin Invest 70:1234–1244]

a reduction in the sinusoidal permeability to plasma proteins. On the other hand, there is evidence that intestinal microvasculature does not autoregulate the capillary pressure or the capillary filtration coefficient in cirrhosis. Portal hypertension in cirrhotic patients and in animals with experimental portal hypertension is not associated with an increased splanchnic arteriolar resistance but rather with a generalized splanchnic arteriolar vasodilation [16]. Therefore, this important mechanism preventing edema formation in the intestine is not operative in cirrhosis. This may explain why interstitial edema in the mucosal, muscular, and serosal layers is prominent in human cirrhosis.

Increased flow of thoracic duct lymph (8–9 liters per day, normal < 1 liter/day), marked enlargement of thoracic duct, and high thoracic duct pressure are characteristic findings in cirrhotic patients with portal hypertension, whether or not ascites is present [17]. The total protein content in hepatic lymph in cirrhosis is remarkably lower than in experimental outflow block (between 20% and 80% of the plasma values), a feature probably related to the capillarization of the hepatic sinusoids. The total protein concentration of the intestinal lymph in cirrhotic patients with ascites is generally below 20% of that in plasma. Finally, the thoracic duct lymph and the ascitic fluid total protein concentrations are between that of the hepatic and that of the intestinal lymph. Therefore, it is very likely that ascites in cirrhosis derives from both the hepatic and the splanchnic vascular compartment. The lymphatic system is extremely efficient in returning most of the excessive hepatic and splanchnic lymph production to the general circulation in cirrhotic patients with ascites. The transvascular escape rate of radiolabeled albumin in these patients per hour, which permits estimation of the amount of fluid escaping from the intravascular compartment, represents 8.5% of the total intravascular mass of albumin. In contrast, the fraction of the transvascular escape of albumin passing into the peritoneal cavity is very low (0.2%) [18]. Ascites formation is therefore the consequence of a small spillover of the increased rate of hepatic and splanchnic lymph formation, most of which is returned directly to the circulation through the lymphatic system.

*Effect of Portal Hypertension on Splanchnic Arteriolar Circulation*

In addition to increasing hepatic and splanchnic lymph production, portal hypertension is also associated with a marked splanchnic arteriolar vasodilation which contributes to the increase in portal pressure. The high portal venous inflow probably explains why portal pressure remains elevated despite the development of marked collateral circulation. The mechanism of this splanchnic arteriolar vasodilation is not entirely understood. There is evidence indicating that some degree of portasystemic shunting is almost a sine qua non for its development [19]. The collateral circulation lowers the vascular resistance of the portal venous system, which may increase the inflow of blood through a myogenic reflex arteriolar vasodilation. In addition, portasystemic shunts allow the systemic delivery of vasodilating substances of splanchnic origin such as glucagon. Finally, a decreased vascular sensitivity of the splanchnic arterioles to the sympathetic nervous activity may also contribute to the splanchnic hyperemia associated with portal hypertension. The splanchnic arteriolar vasodilation is probably the cause of the hyperdynamic circulation that characterizes chronic liver diseases. Cirrhotic patients with portal hypertension with or without ascites present arterial hypotension, hypervolemia, high cardiac index, and low peripheral vascular resistance [20] (Fig. 2).

## 3.2 Renal Function Abnormalities

*Sodium Retention*

Sodium retention is constantly present in cirrhotic patients with ascites and plays a major role in the pathogenesis of this complication. The degree of sodium retention varies considerably from one patient to another and whereas sodium excretion is practically nonexistent in some cases it is relatively high in others [21]. Although azotemia may develop in patients with cirrhosis and ascites, the impairment of sodium excretion in most cases occurs in the setting of a normal glomerular filtration rate (GFR), indicating

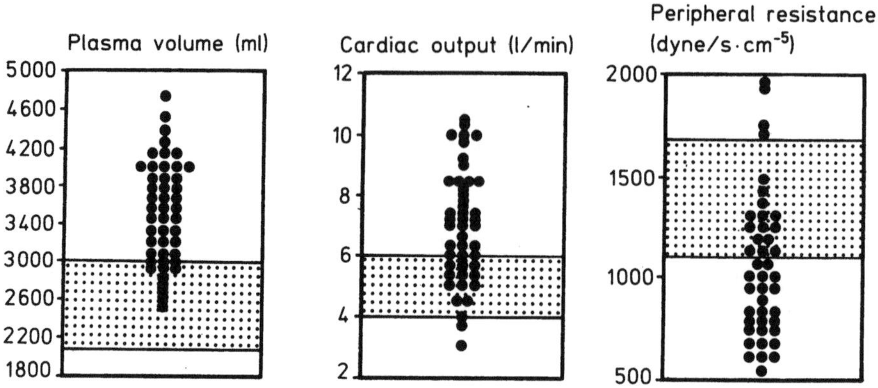


**Fig. 2.** Plasma volume, cardiac output, and peripheral vascular resistance in a series of patients with cirrhosis and ascites. The *shaded area* represents the normal range

that the predominant mechanism of sodium retention is an increased tubular sodium reabsorption. Longitudinal studies in animals with experimental cirrhosis have shown that sodium retention precedes ascites formation, supporting the view that this abnormality is a cause rather than a consequence of the accumulation of fluid within the abdominal cavity [22].

### *Water Retention*

An impairment in the renal ability to excrete free water is the second most frequent renal function abnormality in cirrhotic patients with ascites. In normal subjects, the oral administration of a water overload of 20 ml/kg body weight is followed by the excretion of a hypotonic urine (60–110 mOsm/kg) at a rate of 8–14 ml/min. Six to 12 ml/min of this volume is water free of solutes (free water clearance) and the remaining volume consists of water dissolving urinary solutes isosmotically with respect to plasma (osmolar clearance). Patients with compensated cirrhosis show a normal free water clearance after a water load. In contrast, free water clearance is reduced in most patients with cirrhosis and ascites [23]. As with sodium retention, the degree of impairment of water excretion varies markedly from patient to patient. Thus, whereas in some cirrhotics with ascites free water clearance after a water load is only slightly reduced, others present very low free water clearance or are even unable to dilute the urine after a water load (negative free water clearance). These latter patients retain most of the water taken in with the diet, causing a dilution of the interior milieu, hyponatremia, and hypo-osmolality. Hyponatremia in cirrhosis with ascites is, therefore, a consequence of an excess of water and not of sodium deficiency. This concept is important from a therapeutic point of view. Treatment of hyponatremia should be directed toward reducing total body water. The administration of sodium may produce a transient increase in serum sodium at the expense of increasing the rate of ascites formation.

***Functional Renal Failure***

Functional renal failure (FRF), a syndrome characterized by the spontaneous development of a marked reduction in renal blood flow and GFR, azotemia, and oliguria in the absence of significant histologic abnormalities of the kidney, is an outstanding feature in cirrhotics with ascites. It is present in approximately 17% of patients admitted to hospital with ascites and in more than 50% of the cirrhotics who die. The probability of developing FRF within 2 and 5 years after the onset of ascites in patients with cirrhosis is 32% and 41%, respectively. The mechanism of FRF in cirrhosis is an intense vasoconstriction of the renal arteries that impairs renal perfusion and GFR [24].

From a clinical point of view, there are two distinct types of FRF in cirrhosis [25]. The first is characterized by a rapid increase in blood urea nitrogen (BUN) and serum creatinine concentration, which reach very high levels within days after the onset of renal failure, progressive oliguria, dilutional hyponatremia, and hyperkalemia. This rapidly progressive FRF (also called hepatorenal syndrome) always occurs in patients with extremely poor hepatic function who, in addition to ascites, present other problems such as jaundice or hepatic encephalopathy. Progressive FRF is frequently observed in alcoholic cirrhotics with superimposed alcoholic hepatitis or in any etiologic type of cirrhosis with ascites in which hepatic function deteriorates rapidly as a consequence of a serious bacterial infection, gastrointestinal hemorrhage, or a major surgical procedure. Progressive FRF carries an ominous prognosis and most, if not all, patients die within days or weeks after the onset of the syndrome regardless of the therapy used (hemodialysis, plasma volume expansion, peritoneovenous shunt, vasoactive agents), with the mechanism of death being a combination of hepatic and renal failure and the precipitating event of the syndrome. The second type of FRF is characterized by a moderate increase in BUN and serum creatinine which remains steady over a period of months. This type of FRF usually occurs in cirrhotics with a relatively preserved hepatic function whose main clinical problem is an ascites refractory to diuretic treatment. The survival of these patients, however, is significantly shorter than that of nonazotemic cirrhotics with ascites.

## 4 Mechanism of Renal Function Abnormalities

### 4.1 The Renin-Angiotensin-Aldosterone System

Renin is produced in the kidney by specialized cells of the juxtaglomerular apparatus, which is in intimate contact with the vascular pole of the glomerulus and the convoluted distal tubule. Renin release is mediated by three mechanisms: (a) the renal baroreceptor mechanism sensitive to changes in renal perfusion; (b) the macula densa mechanism, which responds to changes in sodium delivery or transport within the distal tubule; and (c) the renal sympathetic nervous activity which directly stimulates renin release by operating upon $\beta_1$ receptors present in the juxtaglomerular apparatus. These three mechanisms usually operate in concert since they are influenced in the same direction by changes in effective circulating blood volume or arterial pressure. Renin transforms angiotensinogen into angiotensin I, which is subsequently converted to angiotensin II (A-II), the active component of the system, by specific converting enzymes present in many vascular territories, including the juxtaglomerular apparatus. Thus, significant amounts of A-II are generated locally immediately adjacent to the afferent and efferent glomerular arterioles and glomeruli. A-II is among the most active vasoconstrictors so far identified and stimulates aldosterone secretion, which increases sodium reabsorption in the distal and collecting tubules. The renal vasculature is especially sensitive to the vasoconstrictor effect of A-II since a striking reduction in renal blood flow occurs with doses of A-II well below those required to induce a pressor response. A-II reduces GFR as a consequence of the decrease in renal perfusion and also through a direct contracting effect on glomerular mesangial cells.

The renin-angiotensin-aldosterone system is activated in most cirrhotic patients with ascites and marked sodium retention and in all patients with FRF [26, 27] (Fig. 3). In cirrhotic patients with ascites and moderate sodium retention the plasma levels of renin and aldosterone may be normal or only slightly elevated. Three lines of evidence indicate that aldosterone plays a major role in the pathogenesis of sodium retention in cirrhotic patients with ascites: (a) urinary sodium excretion correlates closely with the degree of hyperaldosteronism [26]; (b) sodium retention can be reversed in many cases by blocking the effect of aldosterone with spironolactone [28]; (c) longitudinal studies in experimental cirrhosis have shown a close temporal

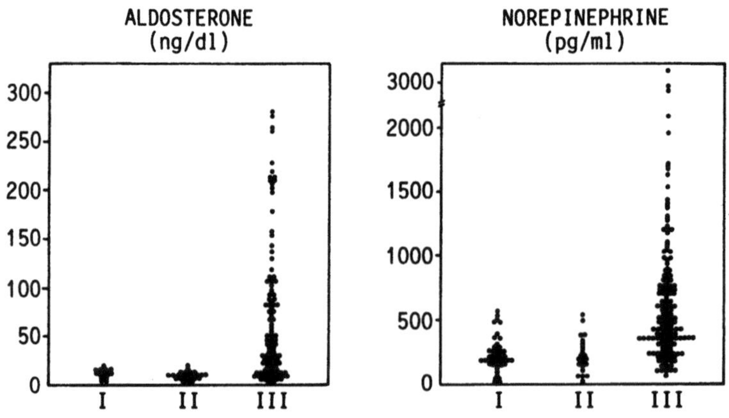


**Fig. 3.** Plasma aldosterone and norepinephrine concentrations in normal subjects (*I*), patients with cirrhosis without ascites (*II*), and patients with cirrhosis and ascites (*III*)

relationship between the development of hyperaldosteronism and the onset of sodium retention, both features preceding ascites formation [22]. The observation that some cirrhotics with ascites present sodium retention in the absence of hyperaldosteronism, however, indicates that other factors are also involved in the excessive tubular sodium reabsorption. Among cirrhotics with ascites, those with FRF present the highest values of plasma renin activity [26]. Therefore, it is reasonable to presume that endogenous A-II is involved in the pathogenesis of the active renal vasoconstriction causing FRF in cirrhosis.

Although renin and aldosterone are catabolized by the liver, it is clear that hyperreninism and hyperaldosteronism in cirrhosis are due to increased secretion and not to impaired hepatic metabolism. Plasma renin activity may be markedly increased in cirrhotic patients with ascites and normal renal blood flow and GFR, indicating that total renal perfusion is not a major determinant of renin secretion in these patients. Studies using saralasin, a specific antagonist of the vascular effect of A-II, indicate that the activation of renin-angiotensin-aldosterone system in cirrhosis with ascites is a homeostatic response to maintain arterial pressure within normal or near normal levels. The administration of saralasin to these patients produces arterial hypotension due to arteriolar vasodilation [29, 30]. The reduced arterial pressure and peripheral vascular resistance present in cirrhotic patients with ascites would, therefore, be even lower if endogenous A-II were not acting in the peripheral vasculature to maintain arterial pressure. It is important to note that saralasin does not affect arterial pressure in healthy subjects.

## 4.2 The Sympathetic Nervous System

The sympathetic nervous system is another important endogenous mechanism controlling systemic hemodynamics and renal function in man. This system is activated through high-pressure baroreceptors located in the carotid sinus and aortic arch, sensitive to changes in arterial pressure, and low-pressure baroreceptors (volume receptors) present in the cardiac atria, sensitive to alterations in intravascular volume. Afferent impulses arising from these structures travel to an integrative site in the medulla, which modifies the sympathetic nervous outflow according to the information received. Afferent impulses from high- and low-pressure baroreceptors are also sent to the supraoptic and paraventricular nuclei of the hypothalamus, thus modifying antidiuretic hormone secretion. Recent studies suggest that baroreceptors may also exist within the intrahepatic circulation. The hemodynamic effects of activation of the sympathetic nervous system result from a direct action of catecholamines (mainly norepinephrine) on the heart (increased cardiac rate and contractibility) and peripheral arterioles (vasoconstriction), and also from the stimulation of renin release and antidiuretic hormone secretion. In addition, the activation of the renal sympathetic nervous activity produces renal vasoconstriction and directly stimulates sodium reabsorption in the proximal tubule, loop of Henle, and distal nephron.

Plasma norepinephrine (NE) concentration is usually increased in cirrhotic patients with ascites [31, 32] (Fig. 3). Investigations using radiotracer techniques have conclusively demonstrated that the high circulating plasma levels of NE in cirrhosis with ascites are related to an increased release by the terminal ends of the postsynaptic sympathetic neurons due to a general activation of the sympathetic nervous system and not to impaired degradation [32, 33]. On the other hand, the renal venous – arterial difference for NE concentration, which is zero or slightly negative in normal subjects, is usually positive in cirrhotic patients with ascites, reflecting an increased renal sympathetic nervous activity [33, 34]. Several lines of evidence support the hypothesis that the sympathetic nervous activity is involved in the pathogenesis of sodium retention and FRF in cirrhosis: (a) plasma NE concentration is normal in compensated cirrhotics and increased in most patients with sodium retention and ascites [31, 32]; (b) in this latter group of patients, plasma NE correlates directly with urinary sodium retention and inversely with renal plasma flow and GFR [35]; and (c) bilateral renal surgical denervation in common bile duct-ligated miniature swine with cirrhosis and ascites is followed by a marked increase in urine volume and sodium excretion, a feature not observed in sham-operated animals [36]. If denervation is performed prior to the ligation of the common bile duct, animals do not develop sodium retention or ascites.

### 4.3 Antidiuretic Hormone

The kidney is constantly generating free water in the water-impermeable ascending limb of the loop of Henle by a process involving the reabsorption of sodium chloride without a concomitant reabsorption of water. The final excretion of free water depends on the plasma levels of antidiuretic hormone (ADH), which renders the collecting tubules highly permeable to water, thus allowing the passive reabsorption of water from the tubular lumen to the surrounding hypertonic medulla. In addition to osmotic stimuli, ADH secretion is influenced by changes in systemic hemodynamics. The reduction of effective blood volume or arterial pressure increase the release of ADH independently of changes in plasma osmolality. This effect is mediated by neurogenic stimuli that arise in high- and low-pressure baroreceptors. The physiologic effects of ADH depend on its interaction with V-1 receptors located in the vascular smooth muscle, resulting in arteriolar vasoconstriction, and on V-2 receptors present in the collecting tubules, resulting in antidiuresis.

Traditionally, the impairment of free water excretion in cirrhosis has been considered as secondary to a reduced delivery of sodium chloride to the ascending limb of the loop of Henle due to a decrease in filtered sodium and an increase in sodium reabsorption in the proximal tubule [37]. However, recent evidence indicates that ADH plays a major role in the pathogenesis of this abnormality. The plasma levels of ADH are increased in most patients with cirrhosis and ascites and correlate closely with the degree of impairment of free water excretion [38, 39]. Longitudinal studies in rats with experimental cirrhosis and ascites have shown that the impairment of water excretion appears in close chronological relationship with the onset of ADH hypersecretion [40]. Finally, the blockade of V-2 receptors with specific antagonists normalizes renal water metabolism in these animals [41]. ADH hypersecretion in cirrhotics with ascites is clearly mediated by a nonosmotic stimulus since most patients have hyponatremia and the plasma levels of ADH do not fall after further reducing plasma osmolality by a water load [39] (Fig. 4). The blockade of V-1 receptors with specific antagonists in rats with experimental cirrhosis, ascites, and ADH hypersecretion is followed by a significant decrease in arterial pressure, an effect not observed in control animals [42]. This indicates that ADH contributes to the maintenance of arterial pressure in cirrhosis with ascites and that the most likely mechanism of ADH hypersecretion in this condition is arterial hypotension.

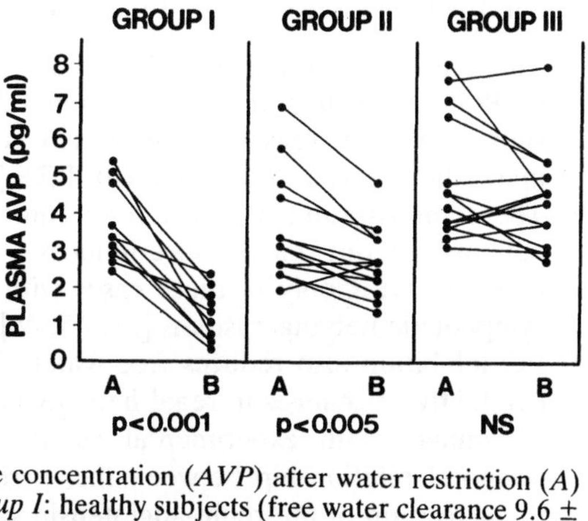


**Fig. 4.** Plasma antidiuretic hormone concentration (*AVP*) after water restriction (*A*) and after a water overload (*B*). *Group I*: healthy subjects (free water clearance 9.6 ± 0.8 ml/min). *Group II*: cirrhotics with ascites who were able to generate free water after the water load (3.6 ± 0.6 ml/min). *Group III*: cirrhotics with ascites who were unable to generate free water after the water load (0.37 ± 0.1 ml/min). [Reproduced with permission from PÉREZ-AYUSO et al. (1983) Kidney Int 26:72–80]

### 4.4 Arachidonic Acid Metabolites

The kidney contains several structures that are capable of synthesizing prostaglandins (PGs): epithelial cells of the collecting ducts, arterial vascular endothelial and smooth muscle cells, medullary interstitial cells, and mesangial cells. The initial step of PG synthesis is the interaction of a stimulus, commonly a hormone (A-II, NE, and ADH are powerful stimuli of PG synthesis), with a receptor on the cell surface, leading to activation of phospholipase $A_2$, which releases arachidonic acid from membrane phospholipids. Intracellular cyclooxygenase converts arachidonic acid on the endoperoxides $PGG_2$ and $PGH_2$. $PGH_2$ is subsequently converted into the active compounds $PGE_2$, $PGI_2$, $PGD_2$, and thromboxane $A_2$ by the action of specific enzymes. Once synthesized, PGs are rapidly metabolized so they exert their biologic actions only at the site of synthesis. $PGE_2$ and $PGI_2$ are powerful renal vasodilators and antagonize the renal vascular effect of A-II and NE. $PGE_2$ also antagonizes the hydroosmotic effect of ADH. Therefore PGs regulate renal function by modulating the renal effects of these endogenous hormonal systems. In fact, PG inhibition with nonsteroidal anti-inflammatory drugs, which decrease the cyclooxygenase activity, potentiates the renal vasoconstrictor effect of A-II and NE and the hydroosmotic effect of ADH and may induce renal failure and water retention in patients with high plasma levels of these substances.

The following data support the view that renal PGs play an important role in the homeostasis of renal function in cirrhotic patients with ascites:

1. The urinary excretion of $PGE_2$ and 6-keto-$PGF_{1\alpha}$ (a stable metabolite of $PGI_2$), which permits estimation of the renal production of these substances, is increased in nonazotemic cirrhotic patients with ascites and markedly reduced in patients with FRF [31, 43, 44].
2. The administration of nonsteroidal anti-inflammatory drugs to cirrhotic patients without renal failure induces a marked decrease in renal blood flow and GFR only in those cases with activated renin-angiotensin and sympathetic nervous systems [31, 45, 46] (Fig. 5).
3. PG inhibition also reduces free water clearance in these patients, independently of changes in renal hemodynamics [39].
4. In animals with experimental cirrhosis and ascites there is a close temporal relationship between the increased urinary PG excretion and the activation of the renin-angiotensin system [47].

Therefore, renal blood flow, GFR, and free water excretion are normal or only moderately decreased in nonazotemic patients with cirrhosis and ascites despite the stimulation of the renin-angiotensin and sympathetic nervous systems and ADH because an increased renal PG synthesis antagonizes the vascular and tubular effects of these systems.

In addition to the synthesis of the classical PGs, the kidney is able to produce leukotrienes (LTs) from arachidonic acid. These compounds are

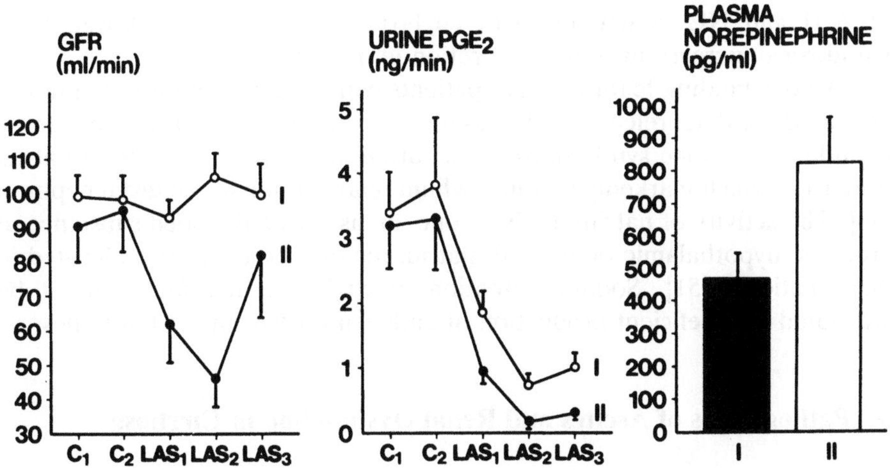


**Fig. 5.** Glomerular filtration rate and urinary excretion of $PGE_2$ (mean ± SEM) before and after the i.v. injection of 450 mg lysine acetylsalicylate in 19 patients with cirrhosis and ascites. Patients are divided into two groups according to whether they developed renal insufficiency (*II*: 11 patients) or not (*I*: 8 patients) after the administration of the drug. $C_1$ and $C_2$ represent two 30-min control periods before the administration of lysine acetylsalicylate. $LAS_1$, $LAS_2$, and $LAS_3$ represent three 30-min periods after the administration of lysine acetylsalicylate. Values of plasma norepinephrine correspond to samples obtained before lysine acetylsalicylate injection. [Reproduced with permission from Arroyo V et al. (1983) Eur J Clin Invest 13:271–278]

renal vasoconstrictors and may reduce the GFR by acting on the glomerular mesangial cells. Recent studies have shown that the urinary excretion of $LTE_4$ and *N*-acetyl-$LTE_4$ is markedly increased in cirrhotics with FRF [48, 49], suggesting that this syndrome may be related to an imbalance between the activity of endogenous vasoconstrictor substances (A-II, NE, and LTs) and the renal production of vasodilator PGs.

### 4.5 Alterations in Intrarenal Hemodynamics and Natriuretic Hormones

Under normal conditions, GFR and proximal tubule sodium reabsorption vary in parallel. This glomerular–tubular balance, which is related to alterations in physical factors in the peritubular capillaries (the elevation in GFR increases oncotic pressure and decreases hydrostatic pressure in these vessels), is disrupted when disturbances exist in the extracellular fluid volume or renal perfusion pressure. Therefore, changes in intrarenal physical factors secondary to arterial hypotension (the main determinant of renal perfusion pressure) or impaired renal perfusion may contribute to the pathogenesis of sodium retention in cirrhosis with ascites. In fact, the production of a moderate increase in mean arterial pressure by the intravenous infusion of A-II and NE in patients with cirrhosis and ascites is followed by a paradoxical increase in sodium excretion in most cases.

An outstanding feature is that patients with cirrhosis and ascites present increased cardiac release and plasma concentration of atrial natriuretic peptide, a hormone synthesized by the atrial myocytes in response to atrial distension which markedly inhibits sodium reabsorption in the distal nephron [50]. The activity of natriuretic hormone, an as yet unidentified substance of probable hypothalamic origin with natriuretic properties, is also elevated in these patients [51]. Sodium retention in cirrhosis, therefore, cannot be attributed to a deficient production of endogenous natriuretic hormones.

## 5 Pathogenesis of Ascites and Renal Dysfunction in Cirrhosis

In the analysis of the pathogenesis of ascites and renal dysfunction in cirrhosis, the following points should be taken into account:

1. Portal hypertension and renal sodium and water retention are sine qua non for ascites formation in cirrhosis.
2. Portal pressure correlates closely with the degree of stimulation of the renin-angiotensin system and sympathetic nervous system [20, 33].
3. Cirrhotic patients with portal hypertension without ascites present a high plasma volume and cardiac index. Despite this circulating hypervolemia, arterial pressure is not elevated, indicating a reduced peripheral vascular resistance. The plasma levels of renin, NE, and ADH are normal in these patients [20].
4. Patients with cirrhosis and ascites also show low arterial pressure, hypervolemia, high cardiac index, and low peripheral vascular resistance. In addition these patients also present marked overactivity of the renin-angiotensin system, sympathetic nervous system, and ADH, which are powerful arteriolar vasoconstrictors [20, 52]. The blockade of the vascular effect of A-II and ADH is associated with a further reduction in arterial pressure and peripheral vascular resistance, indicating that the reduced arterial pressure and peripheral vascular resistance would be even lower if endogenous vasoconstrictor systems were not acting in the peripheral arteriolar vascular resistance [29, 30]. Systemic hemodynamics are therefore more impaired in cirrhotic patients with ascites than in compensated cirrhotics.
5. Renal function abnormalities in cirrhosis correlate with the plasma levels of renin, aldosterone, NE, and ADH.

The traditional theory, which considers that ascites is solely a consequence of the rupture of Starling equilibrium within the hepatic and splanchnic capillaries and that renal sodium and water retention is the result of a contraction of the circulating blood volume secondary to ascites formation [17], and the "overflow" theory [53], which proposes that the accumulation of ascitic fluid is the consequence of a "primary" renal sodium and water retention leading to an expanded plasma volume that overflows in the peritoneal cavity due to portal hypertension, cannot satisfactorily explain all the above-described features. First, and contrary to what the traditional theory suggests, cirrhotic patients with ascites are not hypovolemic but rather present a circulating hypervolemia [54]. Second, whereas the overflow theory proposes that this circulating hypervolemia overfills the systemic circulation, the majority of evidence from clinical and experimental studies indicates that the systemic circulation is underfilled in cirrhotic patients with ascites, not because the circulating blood volume is reduced but rather because the arterial vascular compartment is enlarged.

Recently, a new theory on the pathogenesis of sodium and water retention and ascites formation in cirrhosis, the peripheral arterial vasodilation hypothesis, has been suggested [55] (Fig. 6). This hypothesis proposes that portal hypertension is the initial event in ascites formation, with splanchnic arterial vasodilation causing underfilling of the arterial vascular compartment and high-pressure baroreceptor-mediated stimulation of renin-angiotensin and sympathetic nervous systems and ADH being the intermediate step, and renal sodium and water retention the final consequence.

When sinusoidal portal hypertension is moderately increased, the systemic hemodynamic disturbance is corrected by transient periods of sodium and water retention. The fluid retained by the kidneys remains in the intravascular compartment, increases the intravascular volume and

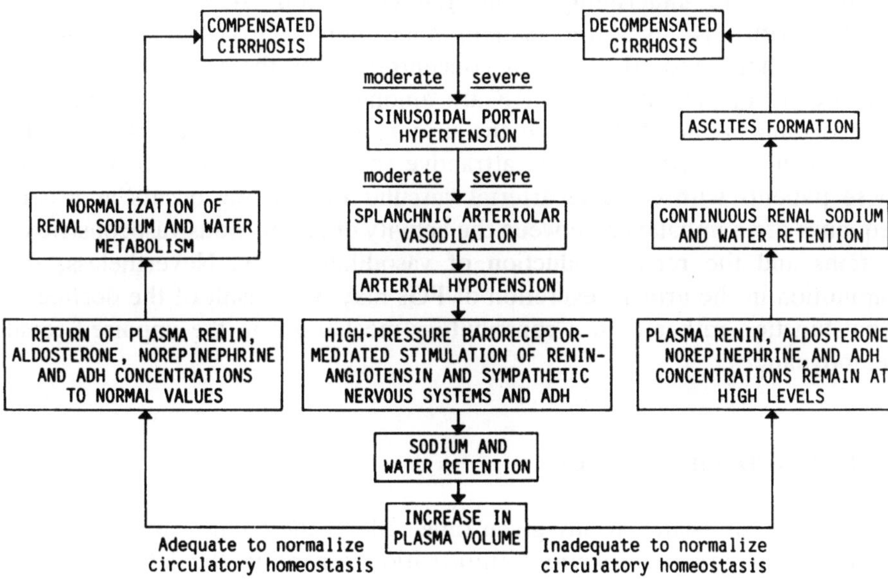


**Fig. 6.** Peripheral arteriolar vasodilation hypothesis of sodium and water retention and ascites formation in cirrhosis

cardiac output, refills the dilated arterial vascular bed, suppresses the signals stimulating the endogenous vasoactive systems, and normalizes sodium and water excretion. This sequence of events explains what occurs in patients with compensated cirrhosis, who show moderate portal hypertension, increased plasma volume and cardiac index, reduced peripheral vascular resistance, normal plasma levels of renin, aldosterone, NE, and ADH, preserved renal ability to excrete sodium and free water, and normal renal blood flow and GFR.

Nonazotemic cirrhotic patients with ascites represent a more advanced stage of the continuum in the process of portal hypertension-induced arterial vascular underfilling. At this stage of cirrhosis, the increase in cardiac output and blood volume secondary to renal sodium and water retention is no longer sufficient to maintain circulatory homeostasis. The progression of the liver disease causes a greater splanchnic arteriolar vasodilation and portal venous inflow, resulting in a more intense arterial vascular underfilling and, most importantly, in an increase in portal venous pressure. This latter event gives rise to the extravasation of fluid within the peritoneal cavity, so that the fluid retained by the kidneys is not effective in correcting the arterial underfilling. The activity of the renin-angiotensin and sympathetic nervous systems and the release of ADH remain increased to maintain arterial pressure, thus perpetuating sodium retention and ascites formation. Renal blood flow and GFR are normal or only moderately reduced in these patients despite the overactivity of these vasoconstrictor systems since they are antagonized by increased renal production of vasodilator PGs.

Functional renal failure of cirrhosis represents the most extreme manifestation in the underfilling of arterial circulation. Arterial pressure in patients with FRF is lower than in nonazotemic cirrhotics with ascites. On the other hand, the plasma concentration of the three major vasoconstrictors in patients with FRF are among the highest in patients with cirrhosis and ascites [52]. Since the urinary excretion of PGs is markedly reduced in these patients, it is attractive to consider that renal failure in these patients with extreme arterial vascular underfilling occurs as a consequence of an imbalance between the activity of endogenous vasoconstrictor systems and the renal production of vasodilator PGs. Nevertheless, the diminution in the urinary excretion of PGs may be a result of the decline in renal function rather than a contributory mechanism in the impaired renal hemodynamics.

## 6 Reabsorption of Ascites

The amount of ascites at any given time reflects the balance between rates of formation and reabsorption. Information regarding the latter process, however, is limited. It appears that the lymphatics on the undersurface of the diaphragm are especially important in removing ascitic fluid from the peritoneal cavity. The peritoneal surface of the diaphragm is covered by a single layer of mesothelial cells which rests on a connective tissue matrix containing a rich plexus of terminal lymphatic vessels (lymphatic lacunae). These lymphatic lacunae directly communicate with the peritoneal cavity through stomas, which are large enough to allow the passage of particles of India ink, colloidal carbon, and erythrocytes (Fig. 7). The submesothelial plexus of lymphatic vessels drains via parasternal trunks on the ventral thoracic wall into the right lymphatic duct and right subclavian or internal jugular veins. During inspiration, intercellular stomas close, intraperitoneal pressure is increased, and the lacunae are emptied through the combined effects of local compression and increased intra-abdominal and reduced intrathoracic pressures. During expiration, the stomas are opened and free communication is reestablished.

Reabsorption of ascites from the peritoneal cavity to the general circulation is a rate-limited phenomenon and varies markedly from patient to patient. The rate of ascitic fluid reabsorption, as estimated by the transport of radiolabeled proteins from the peritoneal cavity to circulating plasma, has been found to range from 0.5 to 5.3 liters/day [18, 56]. The time of appearance of radioactivity in plasma after the injection of radiolabeled albumin into the ascitic fluid is, on average, 0.5 h. This time lag suggest that the transport of ascitic fluid to the general circulation is slow and through tubes (lymphatic vessels) and not a transperitoneal absorption process. The low rate of ascites formation and ascites reabsorption in cirrhotic patients with ascites should not be taken as an indication that the intraperitoneal cavity is a segregated compartment isolated from the rest of the body. In fact, the transperitoneal exchange of water and water-soluble substances by diffusion is very rapid.

## 7 Treatment of Ascites

The appearance of ascites in patients with cirrhosis carries a poor prognosis. The probability of survival 1 and 5 years after the first episode of ascites has been estimated as 50% and 20%, respectively. Among cirrhotics with ascites, those with low arterial pressure (mean arterial pressure <82 mmHg), marked sodium retention (urinary sodium excretion <10 mEq/day), low GFR (<50 ml/min), and high plasma levels of renin and NE have the shortest survival [57]. Therefore, these patients should be considered as candidates for liver transplantation. At present, there is no effective therapy for FRF in cirrhotics with ascites. There is also no pharmacologic treatment for the impairment in free water excretion and dilutional hyponatremia in these patients. The treatment of cirrhotic patients with ascites, therefore, is directed toward eliminating the intra-abdominal fluid and increasing urinary sodium excretion.

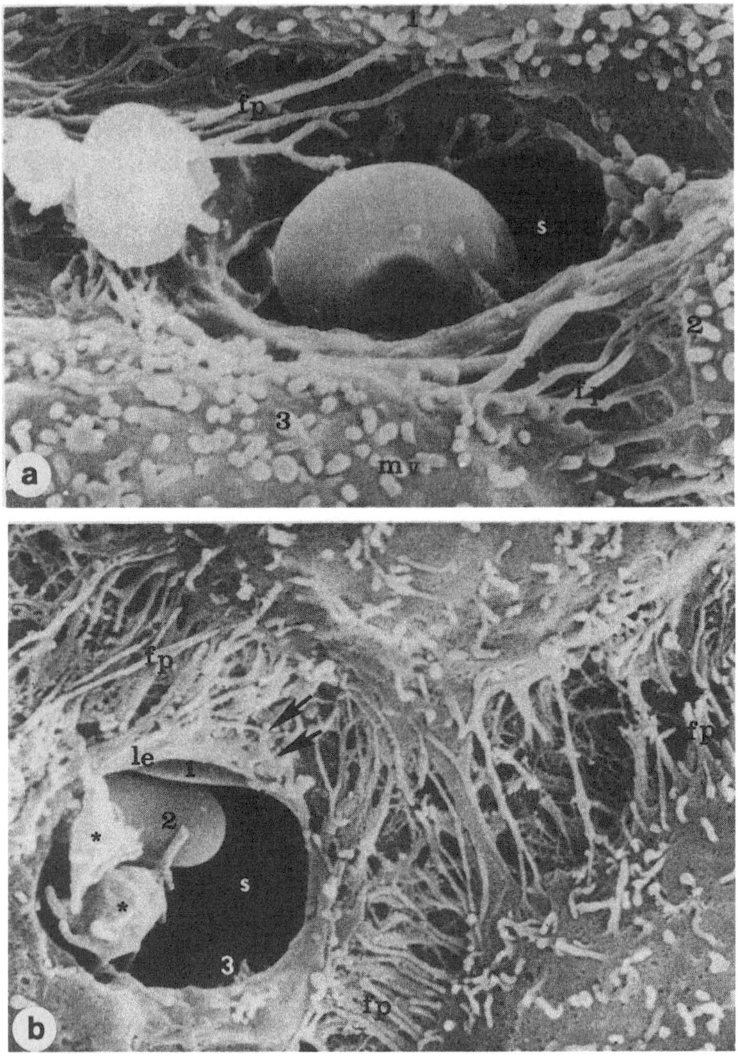


**Fig. 7a,b.** Scanning electron micrographs of the peritoneal surface of the diaphragm. The *upper figure* (**a**) shows a stoma (*s*) located at the junction of several cells (*numbered 1–3*). A red blood cell was caught in the process of entering the stoma. Numerous filamentous processes (*fp*) and intercellular gaps are also shown. In the *lower figure*, (**b**) three red blood cells (*numbered 1–3*) and two platelets are in the process of entering the stoma. Margins of the lymphatic endothelial cells (*le*) extend to the peritoneal surface and make contact with the margins and filamentous processes (*fp*) of cuboidal mesothelial cells (*arrows*). [Reproduced with permission from Leak LV and Rahill K (1978) Am J Anat 151:557–594]

### 7.1 Bed Rest and Low Sodium Diet

The assumption of an upright posture by patients with cirrhosis and ascites is associated with a striking activation of the renin-angiotensin-aldosterone and sympathetic nervous systems, a reduction in GFR and sodium excretion, and a decreased response to loop diuretics [58]. Therefore, from a theoretical point of view, bed rest could be useful for the treatment of ascites in cirrhosis.

The aim of the medical treatment of ascites is to mobilize the intra-abdominal fluid by creating a net negative balance of sodium. In the approximately 20% of cirrhotics with ascites who spontaneously excrete relatively high amounts of sodium in the urine, this can be achieved simply by reducing the sodium content in the diet to 40–60 mEq/day. In the remaining patients with marked sodium retention, a negative sodium balance cannot be achieved without the aid of diuretics to increase urinary sodium excretion over the sodium intake. However, even in these patients, dietary sodium restriction is essential. A frequent cause of diuretic-resistant ascites is an inadequate sodium restriction. This should be suspected when ascites volume does not decrease despite good natriuretic response to diuretics.

### 7.2 Diuretics

Loop diuretics, particularly furosemide, and distal diuretics, especially spironolactone, are the drugs most commonly used in the treatment of ascites in cirrhosis. Loop diuretics are the most potent diuretics available. They exert their primary action in the ascending limb of the loop of Henle and in high dosage can cause as much as 30% of filtered sodium to be excreted. The natriuretic action of loop diuretics is mainly related to their inhibitory effect on a specific cotransport system, the $Na^+2Cl^-K^+$ carrier, located in the luminal membrane of the ascending limb cells. Therefore, the pharmacologically active component of loop diuretics is that reaching the tubular lumen by active secretion in the proximal tubule. Spironolactone and other distal diuretics (triamterene, amiloride) have a much lower natriuretic potency than loop diuretics. Spironolactone can only cause up to 2% of the filtered sodium to be excreted. Spironolactone inhibits sodium reabsorption in the collecting tubules by antagonizing the effect of aldosterone and is therefore particularly effective in patients with hyperaldosteronism. The therapeutic dosage of spironolactone depends on the plasma aldosterone concentration. Patients with moderately increased plasma aldosterone levels require between 50 and 200 mg/day. However, as much as 500 mg/day may be required to antagonize the effect of aldosterone in patients with marked hyperaldosteronism. Furosemide and other loop diuretics are rapidly absorbed from the gut. Onset of action is extremely rapid (within 30 min after oral administration, with peak effect occurring within 1–2 h and most natriuretic activity having finished in 3–4 h). In contrast, there is a lag of 2–4 days between the initiation or discontinuation of spironolactone therapy and the onset or termination of the natriuretic effect.

Several studies in nonazotemic cirrhotic patients with ascites have shown that, unlike in normal subjects, spironolactone is more effective than loop diuretics. The administration of a loop diuretic alone gives rise to satisfactory diuretic response in only 50% cirrhotics without renal failure whereas spironolactone increases sodium excretion in most of these patients [28, 59–62]. Since loop diuretics do not inhibit sodium reabsorption in the distal and collecting tubules, it is possible that most sodium not reabsorbed in the loop of Henle by these drugs is subsequently reabsorbed along the distal nephron by the action of aldosterone. In fact, patients not responding to furosemide are those with higher plasma aldosterone levels. Therefore, the most rational treatment of cirrhotic patients with ascites is the administration of spironolactone alone or associated with furosemide. The simultaneous administration of furosemide and spironolactone increases the natriuretic effect of both drugs and reduces the incidence of hypokalemia or hyperkalemia frequently observed when these agents are given alone. A useful therapeutic schedule is to start with furosemide 40 mg/day and spironolactone 100 mg/day. If there is no response after 4 to 5 days, the dosage is increased stepwise up to furosemide 160 mg/day and spironolactone 400 mg/day. Patients not responding to this high dosage should be considered as having diuretic-resistant ascites. Once ascites has been mobilized, diuretic dosage should be adjusted to maintain patients without sodium retention.

The use of diuretics in cirrhotic patients with ascites is frequently associated with complications, which have been reported to occur in 11%–70% of the patients, depending on the type of diuretics used, the maximum dosage achieved, and the characteristics of the patients included in the study. Approximately 20% of these patients develop azotemia due to intravascular volume depletion. This diuretic-induced renal failure is usually moderate and always reversible after diuretic withdrawal; it occurs as a consequence of an imbalance between the intravascular fluid loss caused by the diuretics and the net passage of fluid (ascites reabsorption minus ascites formation) from the peritoneal cavity to the general circulation. Interstitial fluid accumulated as edema is more easily reabsorbed than ascites. This explains why diuretic-induced azotemia occurs less frequently in patients with both ascites and edema than in those having only ascites. Hyponatremia, occasionally severe, is another common complication of diuretic therapy. It is due to an impairment in the renal ability to excrete free water due to a direct effect of diuretic treatment on the renal diluting mechanism (loop diuretics) or to a nonosmotic hypersecretion of ADH secondary to intravascular volume depletion. The incidence of diuretic-induced azotemia or hyponatremia is low in patients loosing between 300–500 ml/day of ascitic fluid. Hyperkalemia and/or metabolic acidosis are common when high dosages of spironolactone are used, particularly in patients with FRF. Finally, diuretic therapy may cause hepatic encephalopathy by a mechanism still unknown.

Most cirrhotic patients with refractory ascites have FRF. The mechanism of refractory ascites in these patients is probably related to alterations in both the pharmacokinetics and the pharmacodynamics of diuretics. The access of loop diuretics to the organic acid secretory site and of spironolactone to the aldosterone receptors, which is mainly determined by the amount of blood flowing to the proximal tubule and distal nephron, respectively, is impaired in cirrhotic patients with FRF due to their low renal perfusion. On the other hand, the delivery of sodium chloride to the loop of Henle and distal nephron, which are the sites of action of furosemide and spironolactone, may be markedly reduced in cirrhotic patients with FRF secondary to low GFR and enhanced sodium reabsorption in the proximal tubule. Nonsteroidal anti-inflammatory drugs depress the diuretic response to furosemide and spironolactone in cirrhotic patients with ascites by a mechanism unrelated to the impairment in renal hemodynamics [63, 64]. The use of these agents should, therefore, be carefully investigated in any cirrhotic patient with refractory ascites.

### 7.3 Peritoneovenous Shunt

The LeVeen peritoneovenous shunt consists of a multiperforated intra-abdominal tube connected through a one-way valve to an outflow tube that traverses the subcutaneous tissue up to the neck (Fig. 8). The tip of the shunt is introduced through the internal jugular vein into the superior vena cava near the right atrium. Whenever intraperitoneal pressure exceeds right atrial pressure by 3–5 $cmH_2O$, the valve opens and ascitic fluid flows into the vascular compartment [65]. The aim of the shunt is therefore the continuous expansion of the plasma volume with ascitic fluid. Treatment with peritoneovenous shunting (PVS) increases plasma volume and cardiac output, suppresses renin, aldosterone, NE, and ADH, and increases urine volume, sodium excretion, and free water clearance. In patients with FRF, PVS may increase renal perfusion and GFR [66–69]. Finally, in patients with refractory ascites it increases the natriuretic effect of diuretics.

In the initial series of patients treated with PVS there was a high rate of early complications related to the procedure, particularly acute bacterial infections, usually caused by *Staphylococcus*, intravascular coagulation, pulmonary edema, and gastrointestinal hemorrhage [70]. The incidence of complications, however, has subsequently been considerably reduced by adequate perioperative management [71]. Bacterial infection is now an infrequent complication owing to the use of prophylactic antibiotics. The

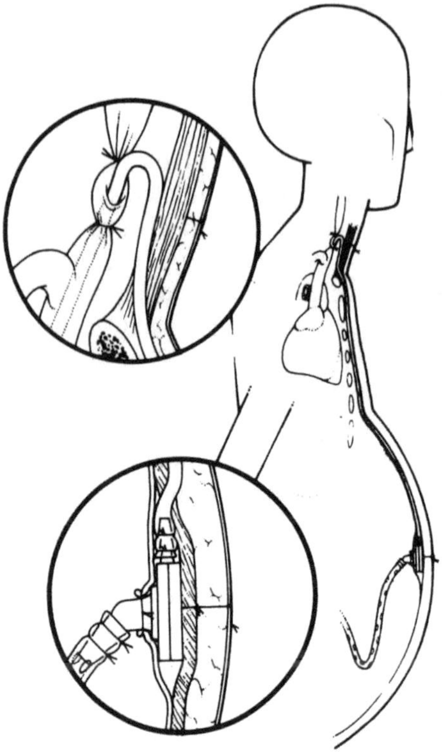

**Fig. 8.** Schematic drawing of the LeVeen shunt. The valve lies outside the peritoneum and deep to the abdominal muscles. The venous collecting tube traverses the subcutaneous tissue of the chest wall into the neck, where it enters the internal jugular vein. The tip of the tubing is pushed into the superior vena cava. The two detailed views illustrate the valve lying subcutaneously and the tip of the venous tube entering the internal jugular vein. [Reproduced with permission from LeVeen H et al. (1976) Ann Surg 184:574–581]

other complications, which are related to the massive passage of ascitic fluid to the general circulation, can be prevented by removing most ascitic fluid prior to the insertion of the shunt. At present, shunt obstruction is the most common complication, since it occurs in 30%–40% of patients within the 1st postoperative year [71]. It can be due to thrombosis of the superior vena cava, thrombosis of the venous limb of the prosthesis, or fibrin deposition within the valve. Shunt obstruction should be suspected in any patient developing reaccumulation of ascites. In these cases Doppler ultrasonography or scintigraphy after the intraperitoneal injection of technetium 99 m should be performed to confirm the absence of flow through the shunt. If shunt obstruction is confirmed, a shuntogram using fluoroscopically controlled injection of contrast media into the proximal venous limb should be carried out to determine the site of obstruction. In cases with obstruction of the venous limb of the shunt, intravenous digital subtraction angiography is required to rule out a thrombosis of the superior vena cava. Peritoneal fibrosis induced by the intra-abdominal tube, which may produce intestinal obstruction, is another unsolved problem of PVS.

Despite the extensive use of PVS during the last 15 years, the role of this prosthesis in the management of cirrhotics with ascites is still not well established. It does not increase the survival of these patients and in addition the improvement in the long-term control of ascites is counteracted by the high rate of complications, particularly shunt obstruction. Since morbidity and mortality in patients treated with PVS directly correlate with the degree of impairment of liver and renal function, the best results of PVS should be expected in those very few patients with refractory ascites and preserved hepatic function.

### 7.4 Paracentesis

Several studies have shown that repeated large volume paracentesis (4–6 liters per day until complete mobilization of ascites) or total paracentesis (complete mobilization of ascites in only one tap) in association with intravenous albumin infusion (8 g per liter of ascitic fluid removed) is a rapid, effective, and safe therapy for "tense" ascites in cirrhosis [72–75]. These therapeutic procedures were more effective than conventional diuretic therapy in eliminating the ascitic fluid, were associated with a lower incidence of complications, and considerably reduced the duration of hospital stay and the cost of treatment (Table 1). Therapeutic paracentesis is, therefore, the treatment of choice in cirrhotic patients admitted to hospital with tense ascites. It is important to note that this therapeutic procedure is a treatment of ascites but not of sodium retention. Consequently, patients treated with paracentesis require diuretic therapy to prevent reaccumulation of ascites. A recent multicenter controlled trial comparing paracentesis and PVS in patients with refractory ascites failed to find differences between the two therapeutic groups with respect to (a) the time spent in hospital after start of therapy and (b) survival [76]. Thus, therapeutic paracentesis represents an alternative to PVS in cirrhotic patients with refractory ascites.

Mobilization of ascites by paracentesis plus intravenous albumin does not produce significant changes in systemic and renal hemodynamics or in the plasma concentration of renin, aldosterone, NE, and ADH [72–74]. In contrast, therapeutic paracentesis without albumin infusion invariably produces a marked increase in plasma renin activity and aldosterone concentration, suggesting a deterioration in effective circulating blood volume, and is associated with hyponatremia and/or renal impairment in a significant proportion of patients [73]. The infusion of albumin is, therefore, essential to prevent the deterioration of systemic hemodynamics after paracentesis. Recent studies suggest that dextran 70 or Hemaccel is as effective as albumin in preventing electrolyte disturbances or renal impairment after paracentesis [77, 78].

**Table 1.** Complications during hospitalization in cirrhotics with ascites treated with four different treatment modalities: paracentesis plus iv albumin*, total paracentesis plus iv dextran-70, repeated paracentesis (4–6 L/day) without iv albumin, and diuretics

| | Paracentesis plus iv albumin* (n = 191) | | Total paracentesis plus iv dextran-70 (n = 45) | | Repeated paracentesis (4–6 L/day) without iv albumin (n = 53) | | Diuretics (n = 59) | |
|---|---|---|---|---|---|---|---|---|
| | No | (%) | No | (%) | No | (%) | No | (%) |
| Patients with complications | 32 | (17) | 10 | (22) | 16 | (30) | 36 | (61) |
| Hyponatremia | 8 | (4) | 4 | (9) | 9 | (17) | 18 | (30) |
| Renal impairment | 3 | (2) | 1 | (2) | 6 | (11) | 16 | (27) |
| Hyperkalemia | 2 | (1) | 0 | | 0 | | 7 | (12) |
| Encephalopathy | 19 | (10) | 3 | (7) | 3 | (6) | 17 | (29) |
| Gastrointestinal bleeding | 7 | (4) | 3 | (7) | 1 | (2) | 6 | (10) |
| Bacterial infection | 8 | (4) | 2 | (4) | 4 | (7) | 4 | (7) |

Data shown in this table are derived from four studies (Ginès et al., 1987, 1988; Planas et al., 1989; Titó et al., 1990). Criteria for including patients in these studies were identical. Hyponatremia was defined as a decrease in serum sodium concentration >5 mEq/L to a level <130 mEq/L; renal impairment ≥50% increase in serum cratinine or BUN, or both, to levels >1.5 mg/dl and 30 mg/dl, respectively; hyperkalemia, increase in serum potassium concentration >1.5 mEq/L to a level >5.5 mEq/L.

* Includes either total paracentesis or repeated paracentesis (4–6 L/day).

## References


1. Lawson MJ, Weissbein AS (1959) The puddle sign. An aid in the diagnosis of minimal ascites. N Engl J Med 260:652–654
2. Cattau EL, Benjamin SB, Knuff TE et al. (1982). The accuracy of the physical examination in the diagnosis of suspected ascites. JAMA 247:1164–1166
3. Wilson JAP, Suguitan EA, Cassidy WA et al. (1979) Characteristics of ascitic fluid in alcoholic cirrhosis. Dig Dis Sci 24:645–648
4. Hoefs JC (1983) Serum protein concentration and portal pressure determine the ascitic fluid protein concentration in patients with chronic liver disease. J Lab Clin Med 102, 260–273
5. Runyon BA, Van Eps DE (196) Diuresis of cirrhotic ascites increases its opsonic activity and may help to prevent spontaneous bacterial peritonitis. Hepatology 6:396–399
6. Runyon BA (1986) Low-protein-concentration ascitic fluid is predisposed to spontaneous bacterial peritonitis. Gastroenterology 91:1343–1346
7. Hoefs J, Runyon BA (1985) Spontaneous bacterial peritonitis. Disease-a-Month 31:1–48
8. Reynolds TB (1986) Rapid presumptive diagnosis of spontaneous bacterial peritonitis. Gastroenterology 90:1294–1297
9. Bar-Meir, Lerner E, Conn HO (1979) Analysis of ascitic fluid in cirrhosis. Dig Dis Sci 24:136–144

10. Desitter L, Rector WG Jr (1984) The significance of bloody ascites in patients with cirrhosis. Am J Gastroenterol 79:136–138
11. Baele G, Raskin K, Barbier F (1986) Coagulant, fibrinolytic, and aggregating activity in ascitic fluid. Am J Gastroenterol 81:440–443
12. Hoefs J, Barnes T, Halles P (1981) Intraperitoneal coagulation in chronic liver disease ascites. Dig Dis Sci 26:518–522
13. Laine GA, Hall JT, Laine SH et al. (1979) Transsinusoidal fluid dynamics in canine liver during venous hypertension. Circ Res 45:317–323
14. Greenway CV, Lautt WW (1970) Effects of hepatic venous pressure on transsinusoidal fluid transfer in the liver of the anaesthetized cat. Circ Res 26:697–703
15. Huet M, Goresky CA, Villeneuve JP et al. (1982) Assessment of liver microcirculation in human cirrhosis. J Clin Invest 70:1234–1244
16. Vorobioff J, Bredfeldt JE, Groszmann RJ (1984) Increased blood flow through the portal system in cirrhotic rats. Gastroenterology 87:1120–1126
17. Witte MH, Witte CL, Dumont AE (1971) Progress in liver disease: physiological factors involved in the causation of cirrhotic ascites. Gastroenterology 61:742–750
18. Henriksen JH, Lassen NA, Parving HH et al. (1980) Filtration as the main transport mechanism of protein exchange between plasma and the peritoneal cavity in hepatic cirrhosis. Scand J Clin Lab Invest 40:503–513
19. Sikuler E, Kravetz D, Groszman RJ (1985) Evolution of portal hypertension and mechanisms involved in its maintenance in a rat model. Am J Physiol 248:G618–G625
20. Bosch J, Arroyo V, Betriu A et al. (1980) Hepatic hemodynamics and the renin-angiotensin-aldosterone system in cirrhosis. Gastroenterology 78:92–99
21. Arroyo V, Rodés J (1975) A rational approach to the treatment of ascites. Postgrad Med J 51:558–562
22. Jimenez W, Martinez-Pardo A, Arroyo V et al. (1985) Temporal relationship between hyperaldosteronism, sodium retention and ascites formation in rats with experimental cirrhosis. Effect of spironolactone. Hepatology 5:245–250
23. Shear L, Hall PW, Gabuzda GJ (1966) Renal failure in patients with cirrhosis of the liver. II. Factors influencing maximal urinary flow rate. Am J Med 39:199–209
24. Epstein M, Berk DP, Hollengerg NK et al. (1970) Renal failure in the patient with cirrhosis. The role of active vasoconstriction. Am J Med 49:175–185
25. Rodés J, Bosch J, Arroyo V (1975) Clinical types and drug therapy of renal impairment in cirrhosis. Postgrad Med J 55:492–497
26. Arroyo V, Bosch J, Mauri M et al. (1979) Renin, aldosterone and renal hemodynamics in cirrhosis with ascites. Eur J Clin Invest 9:69–73
27. Rosoff L Jr, Zia P, Reynolds TB et al. (1975) Studies on renin and aldosterone in cirrhotic patients with ascites. Gastroenterology 69:698–705
28. Perez Ayuso RM, Arroyo V, Planas R et al. (1983) Randomized comparative study of efficacy of furosemide versus spironolactone in non-azotemic cirrhosis with ascites. Relationship between the diuretic response and the activity of the renin-angiotensin-aldosterone system. Gastroenterology 84:961–968
29. Schroeder ET, Anderson GH, Goldman SH et al. (1976) Effect of blockade of angiotensin II on blood pressure, renin and aldosterone in cirrhosis. Kidney Int 9:511–519
30. Arroyo V, Bosch J, Mauri M et al. (1981) Effect of angiotensin II blockade on systemic and hepatic hemodynamics and on the renin-angiotensin-aldosterone system in cirrhosis with ascites. Eur J Clin Invest 11:221–229
31. Arroyo V, Planas R, Gaya J et al. (1983) Sympathetic nervous activity, renin-angiotensin system and renal excretion of prostaglandin $E_2$ in cirrhosis. Relationship to functional renal failure and sodium and water excretion. Eur J Clin Invest 13:271–278

32. Henriksen J, Christensen N, Ring-Larsen H (1981) Noradrenaline and adrenaline concentrations in various vascular beds in patients with cirrhosis. Relation to haemodynamics. Clin Physiol 1:293–304
33. Henriksen J, Ring-Larsen H, Kanstrup IL et al. (1984) Splanchnic and renal elimination and release of catecholamines in cirrhosis. Evidence of enhanced sympathetic nervous activity in patients with decompensated cirrhosis. Gut 25:1034–1043
34. Ring-Larsen H, Hesse B, Henriksen JH et al. (1982) Sympathetic nervous activity and renal and systemic hemodynamics in cirrhosis: plasma norepinephrine concentration, hepatic extraction and renal release. Hepatology 2:304–310
35. Bichet DG, Van Putten VJ, Schrier RW (1982) Potential role of increased sympathetic activity in impaired sodium and water excretion in cirrhosis. N Engl J Med 307:1552–1557
36. Zambraski E (1985) Effects of acute renal denervation on sodium excretion in miniature swine with cirrhosis and ascites. Physiologist 28:268
37. Sheld HP, Bartter FC (1960) An explanation for and experimental correction of abnormal water diuresis in cirrhosis. J Clin Invest 39:2248–2258
38. Bichet D, Szatalowicz V, Chaimovitz C et al. (1982) Role of vasopressin in abnormal water excretion in cirrhotic patients. Ann Intern Med 96:413–417
39. Perez Ayuso RM, Arroyo V, Camps J et al. (1984) Evidence that renal prostaglandins are involved in renal water metabolism in cirrhosis. Kidney Int 26:72–80
40. Camps J, Solá J, Arroyo V et al. (1987) Temproal relationship between the impairment of free water excretion and antidiuretic hormone hypersecretion in rats with experimental cirrhosis. Gastroenterology 93:498–505
41. Clarià J, Jimenez W, Arroyo V et al. (1989) The blockade of the hydroosmotic effect of vasopressin normalizes water excretion in cirrhotic rats. Gastroenterology 97:1294–1299
42. Clarià J, Jimenez W, Arroyo V et al. (1991) Effect of V1-vasopressin receptor blockade on arterial pressure in conscious rats with cirrhosis and ascites. Gastroenterology 100:494–501
43. Rimola A, Ginès P, Arroyo V et al. (1986) Urinary excretion of 6-keto-prostaglandin-$F_{1\alpha}$, thromboxane $A_2$ and prostaglandin $E_2$ in cirrhosis with ascites. Relationship to functional renal failure (hepatorenal syndrome). J Hepatol 3:111–117
44. Guarner C, Colina J, Guarner F et al. (1986) Renal prostaglandins in cirrhosis of the liver. Clin Sci 70:477–484
45. Zipser RD, Hoefs JC, Speckart PF et al. (1979) Prostaglandins: modulators of renal function and pressor resistance in chronic liver disease. J Clin Endocrinol Metab 48:895–900
46. Boyer TD, Zia P, Reynolds TB (1979) Effects of indomethacin and prostaglandin $A_1$ in renal function and plasma renin activity in alcoholic liver disease. Gastroenterology 77:215–222
47. Sola J, Camps J, Arroyo V et al. (1988) Longitudinal study on renal prostaglandin excretion in cirrhotic rats. Relationship with the renin-aldosterone system. Clin Sci 75:263–269
48. Huber M, Kästner S, Schölmerich J et al. (1989) Analysis of cysteinyl leukotrienes in human urine: enhanced excretion in patients with liver cirrhosis and hepatorenal syndrome. Eur J Clin Invest 19:53–60
49. Moore KP, Taylor GW, Maltby N et al. (1990) Increased production of cysteinyl-leukotrienes in hepatorenal syndrome. J Hepatol 11:263–271
50. Ginès P, Jimenez W, Arroyo V et al. (1988) Atrial natriuretic factor in cirrhosis with ascites: plasma levels, cardiac release and splanchnic extraction. Hepatology 8:636–642
51. LaVilla G, Asbert M, Jiménez W et al. (1990) Natriuretic hormone activity in the urine of patients with cirrhosis of the liver. Hepatology 12:467–475

52. Arroyo V, Ginès P, Rimola A et al. (1986) Renal function abnormalities, prostaglandins and effects of non-steroidal antiinflammatory drugs in cirrhosis with ascites. An overview with emphasis on pathogenesis. Am J Med 81[Suppl 2B]:104–122
53. Lieberman FL, Denison EK, Reynolds TB (1970) The relationship of plasma volume, portal hypertension, ascites and renal sodium retention in cirrhosis: the overflow theory of ascites formation. Ann NY Acad Sci 170:202–212
54. Lieberman FL, Reynolds TB (1967) Plasma volume in cirrhosis of the liver: its relation to portal hypertension, ascites and renal failure. J Clin Invest 46: 1297–1310
55. Schrier RW, Arroyo V, Bernardi M et al. (1988) Peripheral arterial vasodilation hypothesis: a proposal for the initiation of renal sodium and water retention in cirrhosis. Hepatology 8:1151–1157
56. Buhac I, Flesh L, Kishore R (1984) Intraabdominal pressure and resorption of ascites in decompensated liver cirrhosis. J Lab Clin Med 104:264–270
57. Llach J, Ginès P, Arroyo V et al. (1988) Prognostic value of arterial pressure, endogenous vasoactive systems and renal function in cirrhosis with ascites. Gastroenterology 94:482–487
58. Bernardi M, Santini C, Trevisani F (1985) Renal function impairment induced by change in posture in patients with cirrhosis and ascites. Gut 26:629–635
59. Arroyo V, Bosch J, Casamitjana R et al (1980) Use of piretanide, a new loop diuretic, in cirrhosis with ascites. Gut 21:855–859
60. Moult PJA, Lunzer MR, Trash DB et al. (1974) Use of bumetanide in the treatment of ascites due to liver disease. Gut 15:988–992
61. Campra JL, Reynolds TB (1978) Effectiveness of high-dose spironolactone therapy in patients with chronic liver disease and relatively refractory ascites. Dig Dis Sci 23:1025–1030
62. Eggert RC (1970) Spironolactone diuresis in patients with cirrhosis and ascites. Br Med J 4:401–403
63. Planas R, Arroyo V, Rimola A et al. (1983) Acetylsalicylic acid suppresses the renal hemodynamic effect and reduces the diuretic action of furosemide in cirrhosis with ascites. Gastroenterology 84:247–252
64. Mirouze D, Zipser RD, Reynolds TB (1983) Effects of inhibitors of prostaglandin synthesis on induced diuresis in cirrhosis. Hepatology 3:50–55
65. LeVeen HH, Christoudias G, Moon JP et al. (1974) Peritoneovenous shunting for ascites. Ann Surg 180:580–591
66. Berkowitz DH, Mullen JL, Miller LD et al. (1978) Improved renal function and inhibition of renin and aldosterone secretion following peritoneovenous (LeVeen) shunt. Surgery 84:120–126
67. Blendis LM, Greig PD, Langer B et al. (1979) The renal and hemodynamic effects of the peritoneovenous shunt for intractable ascites. Gastroenterology 77:250–257
68. Blendis LM, Sole MJ, Campbell P et al. (1987) The effect of peritoneovenous shunting on catecholamine metabolism in patients with hepatic ascites. Hepatology 7:143–148
69. Klepetko W, Müller CH, Hartter E et al. (1988) Plasma atrial natriuretic factor in cirrhotic patients with ascites. Effect of peritoneovenous shunt implantation. Gastroenterology 95:764–770
70. Bernhoft RA, Pellegrini CA, Way LW (1982) Peritoneovenous shunt for refractory ascites. Operative complications and long-term results. Arch Surg 117:631–635
71. Smajda C, Franco D (1985) The LeVeen shunt in the elective treatment of intractable ascites in cirrhosis. A prospective study on 140 patients. Ann Surg 201:488–493
72. Ginès P, Arroyo V, Quintero E et al. (1987) Comparison of paracentesis and diuretics in the treatment of cirrhotics with tense ascrites. Results of a randomized study. Gastroenterology 93:234–241

73. Ginès P, Titó L1, Arroyo V et al. (1988) Randomized comparative study of therapeutic paracentesis with and without intravenous albumin in cirrhosis. Gastroenterology 94:1493–1502
74. Titó L1, Ginès P, Arroyo V et al. (1990) Total paracentesis associated with intravenous albumin in the management of patients with cirrhosis and ascites. Gastroenterology 98:146–152
75. Salerno F, Badalamenti S, Incerti P et al. (1987) Repeated paracentesis and i.v. albumin infusion to treat "tense" ascites in cirrhotic patients: a safe alternative therapy. J Hepatol 5:102–108
76. Ginès P, Arroyo V, Varges V et al. (1991) Paracentesis with intravenous infusion of albumin as compared with peritoneovenous shunting in cirrhosis with refractory ascites. N Engl J Med 325:829–835
77. Planas R, Ginès P, Arroyo V et al. (1990) Dextran-70 versus albumin as plasma expanders in cirrhotic patients with tense ascites treated with total paracentesis. Results of a randomized study. Gastroenterology 99:1736–1745
78. Salerno F, Badalamenti S, Lorenzano E et al. (1991) Randomized comparative study of hemaccel vs albumin infusion after total paracentesis in cirrhotic patients with refractory ascites. Hepatology 13:707–713

# 13 Viral Hepatitis A and E

## A. Type A Viral Hepatitis

S.M. LEMON

### 1 Introduction

Type A viral hepatitis results from an acute infection of the liver with a picornavirus, hepatitis A virus (HAV). The disease has a worldwide distribution but is more prevalent in developing and transitional regions where public health sanitation may be inadequate. HAV is usually transmitted by the fecal–oral route and is well known for its ability to cause impressive common source outbreaks of hepatitis. Infection with HAV leads to acute liver disease that is wide-ranging in terms of severity but never progresses to chronic hepatitis. Passive immunization with immune serum globulin provides high level protection against hepatitis A, but effective inactivated vaccines will soon be available for clinical use.

### 2 Etiologic Agent

Being a picornavirus, HAV is similar in many respects to viruses responsible for the common cold (rhinoviruses), poliomyelitis, and aseptic meningitis (enteroviruses). Although initially classified among the enteroviruses as enterovirus 72, HAV is now widely considered to represent a distinct genus (hepatoviruses) among the family Picornaviridae [1].

The RNA genome of HAV is approximately 7500 bases in length, polyadenylated at its 3′ end, and covalently linked to a small protein (VPg) at its 5′ end (Fig. 1) [2]. The 5′ end of the viral RNA contains a 735-base nontranslated region, which plays important roles in the control of virus translation and probably also replication of viral RNA. This is followed by a 3-kb region (P1) encoding three, or more likely four, capsid proteins. Downstream of this P1 domain are the P2 and P3 domains, which encode a variety of nonstructural proteins, including a virus-specific protease and an RNA replicase, followed by a short 3′ nontranslated region. This virion RNA is packaged within particles that are approximating 27 nm in diameter and which contain 60 copies of each of three capsid proteins ranging from 225 to 300 amino acids in length (VP1, VP2, VP3). One of these capsid proteins, VP3, has been shown to contribute to an immunodominant antigenic site on the surface of the virus capsid [3]. A smaller protein, VP4, is

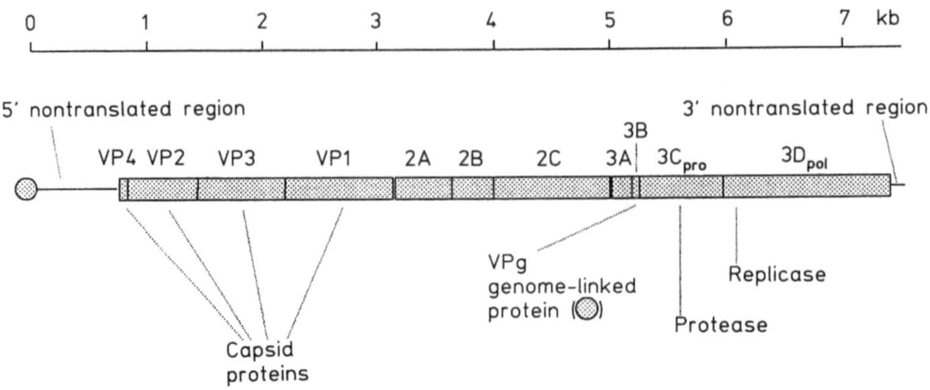


**Fig. 1.** The genomic organization of hepatitis A virus. Nontranslated regions of the genome appear as a *narrow line*, while *boxes* depict the proteins encoded by the large open reading frame. The P1 region encodes VP4, VP2, VP3, and VP1 (the capsid proteins), while the P2 and P3 domains represent the remainder of the large open reading frame

probably present within the interior of the capsid but has never been demonstrated directly. The capsid is of course not enveloped.

Compared with many other viruses, including poliovirus and other enteroviruses, HAV has remarkable thermostability [4]. Less than a one log drop in infectivity is noted when virus is held at 60°C for 10 min. Substantially greater resistance to thermal inactivation is noted in the presence of one molar magnesium chloride. At 37°C, virus present in fecal material may remain viable for many days. This capacity of the HAV virion to withstand environmental stresses contributes directly to its propensity for epidemic spread.

Unlike other human hepatitis viruses, HAV can be propagated in conventional cell cultures [5]. Primary isolation of the agent is usually made in African green monkey kidney cells, but this is a tedious, difficult, and uncertain process. As the infection is usually noncytopathic, demonstration of the presence of virus in infected cell cultures requires immunologic techniques such as radioimmunoassay or fluorescent antibody staining of cell cultures for detection of HAV antigen (Fig. 2). Generally speaking, only primate cells are permissive in cell culture, although limited replication of HAV has been noted in mouse hepatocyte cultures. While useful to research virologists, cell culture isolation has no role in clinical diagnosis.

## 3 Natural History

Hepatitis A virus infection is usually acquired by the oral route. Occasional cases have been associated with blood transfusion but this is rare. The virus presumably replicates at a primary site somewhere within the intestinal

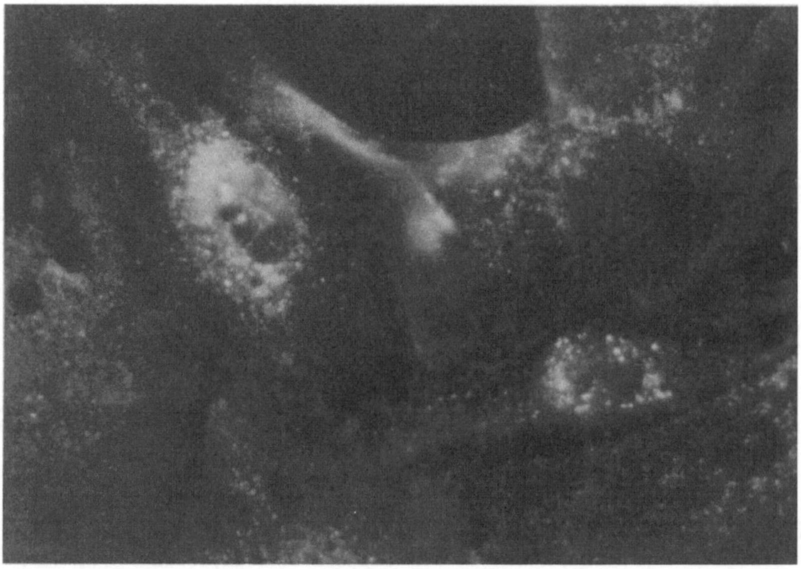

**Fig. 2.** Typical granular, cytoplasmic virus-specific HAV antigen present in infected monkey kidney cells in culture, demonstrated by direct immunofluorescence staining of acetone-fixed cells with fluorescein-conjugated human anti-HAV

tract, although this has never been clearly demonstrated. Most if not all virus shed in the feces appears to be replicated within the liver, from which it reaches the intestinal contents via the biliary system [6, 7].

The incubation period for hepatitis A, extending from exposure to the onset of disease, is approximately 4 weeks, with a range of 2–6 weeks (Fig. 3) [8]. The virus is not quiescent during the incubation period. In New World owl monkeys infected by the intravenous route, fecal shedding of virus has been noted within 4 days of challenge and persists until the onset of liver disease. Generally speaking, intravenous inoculation of virus does not lead to a shortened incubation period compared with challenge by the oral route in susceptible primates. This suggests that virus rapidly gains access to the liver when individuals are exposed orally. Both experiments in animals and clinical studies in humans indicate that fecal virus shedding reaches a maximum just prior to the onset of liver disease [6, 9, 10]. Thus individuals may shed virus in their feces and be potentially contagious for 3 or more weeks, through the end of the incubation period and extending into the acute illness. Viremia is also present during the incubation period, although the titer of viremia is usually 100- to 1000-fold lower than the titer of virus shed in feces [11]. It is likely that both the viremia and the fecally shed virus originate within infected hepatocytes, and that the sustained increases in levels of viremia and fecal virus shedding that are noted during the mid to late incubation period reflect the infection of increasing numbers

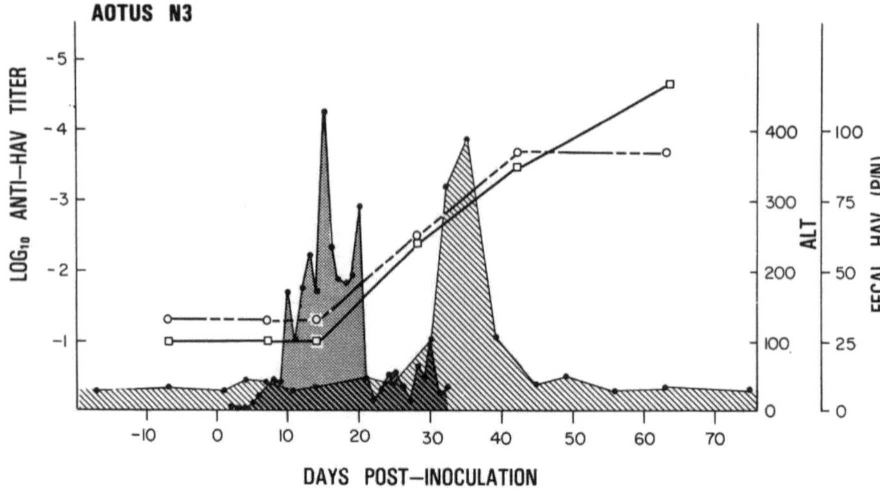


**Fig. 3.** Infection of a New World owl monkey with HAV. Virus was administered by intravenous injection on day 0. The *stippled area* represents fecal HAV antigen detected by a relatively insensitive radioimmunoassay, while the *striped area* represents serum ALT levels. *Open squares* represent the titers of neutralizing anti-HAV antibody detected by a radioimmunofocus inhibition assay, while the *open circles* are the corresponding antibody titers detected by a commercial competitive inhibition radioimmunoassay. [Reproduced with permission from Lemon SM and Binn LN (1983) J Infect Dis 148:1033–1039]

of hepatocytes, and a generally increasing intrahepatic virus load. Copious amounts of virus are found in the bile during this period [7].

Late in the incubation period, serum aminotransferases remain normal and the patient asymptomatic despite the fecal shedding of virus and the presence of viremia. Virus may also be present in saliva. The onset of symptoms and the earliest evidence of liver injury usually coincide with initial reductions in the amount of virus shed in feces and in the level of viremia [11]. At the same time, there is usually evidence of an emerging immune response, marked by the appearance of specific antibodies to the virus [12]. This sequence of events indicates that replication of the virus in the liver is not linked temporally to liver injury, and constitutes relatively strong evidence that hepatocellular injury is immunopathologically mediated [13]. In the early phase of the illness, both infectious virus and neutralizing anti-HAV antibodies may be present in serum. Immune complexes have been detected in serum from patients with hepatitis A, but their role in pathogenesis remains undefined [14].

Additional evidence for an immunopathologic basis for acute hepatitis A is the fact that HAV is almost always noncytopathic when grown in cell culture. Furthermore, the heavy infiltration of the liver with lymphocytes during hepatitis A [10] suggests that cellular immune mechanisms play an important role in this process. It has been shown that patients with hepatitis A develop at least two types of cytotoxic lymphocytes which are capable of killing virus-infected cells. The presence of natural killer cells (NK cells) which express cytotoxic activity against HAV-infected monkey kidney cell cultures probably represents an early, relatively nonspecific response to the infection [15]. CD8+, cytotoxic T lymphocytes which are capable of killing HAV-infected cells in a human leukocyte antigen (HLA)-restricted fashion represent a later and probably more specific immune response [16]. This cytotoxic T cell response may account for many of the lymphocytes found in the liver in hepatitis A and may in fact be largely responsible for the disease itself. These T cells have been shown capable of releasing interferon-$\gamma$ in an HLA-dependent but not HLA-restricted fashion upon exposure to HAV-infected cells [17]. While the antiviral activity of interferon-$\gamma$ is uncertain, this immune modulator may result in enhanced expression of HLA determinants by infected hepatocytes. As the display of HLA antigens by the normal hepatocyte is low or absent, this upregulating activity of interferon-$\gamma$ may promote the cytotoxic activity of the CD8+ cells and directly contribute to the killing of infected hepatocytes. Interferon-$\beta$, on the other hand, has been clearly shown to have an antiviral effect against HAV in infected cells in culture, although its role in vivo remains less certain.

The contemporary view of hepatitis A is that this cellular immune attack against the HAV-infected hepatocyte is of primary importance in the resolution of the infection. While antibody plays a major role in protection against reinfection, it is not clear that antibody is important in resolving infection once established. Antibody-dependent cellular cytotoxicity has not been demonstrated. As virus replication takes places exclusively in the cytoplasm, and because there is no state of latent HAV infection comparable to that seen with DNA viruses, the elimination of infected cells by T lymphocytes and/or the antiviral effects of interferon terminate the infection. With the exception of reports describing relatively lengthy infections in premature infants, this sequence of events seems to occur even in immunocompromised individuals. Perhaps the best evidence supporting this statement is the fact that HAV has not emerged as a threat to persons who are infected with the human immunodeficiency virus (HIV), nor has the HIV epidemic led to apparent increases in the prevalence of hepatitis A.

Much of the process underlying the resolution of HAV infections is poorly understood, however. HAV typically causes persistent infections in cell cultures and yet has not been shown to do so in people. It is not clear why the immune system should be so effective at eliminating HAV infection and apparently so ineffective at eliminating hepatitis C virus infection. Moreover, if a substantial majority of hepatocytes are infected with virus in some patients with hepatitis A, as studies with immunofluorescent probes have suggested, it is not clear why life-threatening liver disease does not accompany the immune elimination of virus-infected cells more often.

## 4 Clinical Findings

Although the typical case of hepatitis A is usually recognized as a form of acute viral hepatitis, it is not possible in the individual case to distinguish between acute hepatitis due to HAV and that due to other hepatitis viruses [13]. While clinical findings and epidemiologic associations may suggest HAV as the etiologic agent, serodiagnostic studies are necessary for specific diagnosis of the infection. Nonetheless, there are several clinical findings which are typical of hepatitis A.

The onset of hepatitis A is characteristically abrupt. Early symptoms include malaise, fatigue, nausea, vomiting, and right upper quadrant discomfort [13]. While fever occurs in about half of all patients and may be impressive in early stages of the disease, it is usually absent by the time the patient seeks medical attention. The first specific evidence that the illness relates to an intrahepatic process may be the onset of dark urine, light clay-colored stool, and/or scleral icterus. The urine typically acquires the color of Coca Cola and is characteristically frothy. Scleral icterus may be noted when the serum bilirubin exceeds 2.5–3.0 mg/dl. These signs typically appear during the first few days of illness but are usually absent at the onset. Diarrhea occurs in about one-half of all infected children but it is uncommon in adults.

The most stiking laboratory findings include elevations of serum aminotransferase activities, serum bilirubin (both total and direct), and serum alkaline phosphatase activity. The serum alanine aminotransferase (ALT) is usually elevated in excess of the aspartate aminotransferase. These enzyme activites may be minimally elevated, or in severe cases may be elevated over 100-fold the upper limit of normal. Characteristically, the ALT level exceeds 1000 IU/dl in individuals with typical symptoms of hepatitis A. Elevations of serum aminotransferase activity usually precede rises in the serum bilirubin level [8]. The same may be said for alkaline phosphatase activity, which rises relatively late in the course of the infection and tends to parallel serum bilirubin elevations. Other laboratory findings include nonspecific elevations of acute phase reactants, immunoglobulins, and the erythrocyte sedimentation rate. Total hemolytic complement levels may be depressed in acute hepatitis A, possibly reflecting the presence of circulating immune complexes described by some workers [18]. Rheumatoid factor (IgM anti-IgG) is often present.

The entire acute illness may last from 1 to several weeks. Resolution is marked by a return in the patient's general sense of well-being and appropriate declines in abnormal serum chemistries. Typically the aminotransferase activities may begin to resolve before the serum bilirubin. However, aminotransferase activities may remain abnormal for several months following acute HAV infection, although usually at relatively low levels. Abnormal ALT levels may persist after the serum bilirubin has returned to normal. However, it is probably safe to say that abnormalities in serum chemistries are seldom present beyond 6 months after the acute infection and virtually never after 1 year.

Extrahepatic manifestations of hepatitis A are uncommon. Urticarial rash and acute arthritis, such as may occur with acute hepatitis B, are not found in acute hepatitis A. Concomitant meningoencephalitis has been reported in several cases, possibly reflecting the fact that HAV is a picornavirus and thus relatively closely related to the enteroviruses, common causes of viral meningitis and meningoencephalitis in humans.

The severity of the liver injury associated with acute HAV infection ranges widely from asymptomatic infection, to full-blown, frank hepatitis, to fulminant hepatitis and death. The most important host determinant influencing the severity of disease and the ultimate outcome of the infection appears to be the age of the patient. There are very solid data collected in several epidemiologic settings which indicate that asymptomatic (or at least anicteric) infection is common in very young children infected with hepatitis A [19]. This may reflect relative immaturity of the immune system and the fact that hepatitis A is generally considered to be an immunopathologically mediated disease process. A recent report suggests that HAV infections may be very lengthy in premature infants and that some premature infants infected with HAV shed the virus in feces for a number of months. Further studies are required to confirm this finding, however. In general, children under the age of 2 years usually do not experience symptoms suggestive of acute hepatitis, even though they are readily infected and often transmit the infection to others. Less that 1 in 20 such children are recognized to have had HAV infection clinically, even in retrospect [19]. The situation is quite different in older individuals, including young adults. Studies carried out in closed military populations experiencing outbreaks of hepatitis A suggest that up to 90% of young adults who are infected with HAV have associated symptoms, and perhaps as many as two-thirds become frankly icteric [20]. Hepatitis A is particularly risky for the elderly individual. Several studies suggest a direct relationship between increasing age and the risk of developing fulminant hepatitis following acquisition of HAV infection.

Several unusual clinical manifestations of HAV infection are worth noting. The first of these is what has been termed "cholestatic hepatitis A" [21]. Patients with this syndrome have persistent jaundice and chemical evidence of intrahepatic cholestasis in the absence of substantial hepatocellular disease. Despite their jaundice, such patients typically feel quite well. Although few patients have been studied intensively, patients with cholestatic hepatitis A do not appear to be particularly infectious or to replicate large quantities of virus. The mechanisms underlying this response to HAV infection are not clear, although it is probable that this syndrome has an immunologic basis.

A second and very unusual manifestation of HAV infection is the occurrence of fulminant hepatitis [22]. Typically, HAV causes only a small proportion of all cases of fulminant viral hepatitis presenting to physicians in the United States and Western Europe. Such cases account for less than 0.2% of all hospitalized patients with hepatitis A, and an even smaller fraction of all hepatitis A infections. The occurrence of fulminant hepatitis A may be suggested by the onset of confusion or an otherwise altered sensorium, or a bleeding diathesis associated with an elevated prothrombin tine. Most patients with fulminant hepatitis A die as a result of the infection, despite the best supportive care. These patients are often but not always over the age of 50. Other than age, no factors predisposing to this kind of severe disease have been clearly delineated. The risk of fulminant hepatitis does not appear to be dependent upon the paticular strain of hepatitis A.

Yet a third unusual clinical outcome is the occurrence of relapsing hepatitis A. Patients with this entity experience a second discreet rise in serum aminotransferase activities, typically a symptomatic relapse, usually 2–3 months after the initial presentation. Some reports of "relapsing hepatitis A" undoubtedly reflect dual infections with two different hepatitis viruses. However, reports have occurred with sufficient frequency in recent years to suggest that relapsing hepatitis does occur in a small proportion of patients with hepatitis A. At least one report suggests that patients with relapsing hepatitis A may be replicating virus and have detectable fecal shedding of HAV [23]. The prognosis for such cases is uniformly excellent, however. As with typical acute hepatitis A, the symptoms of liver disease subside over 1–2 months, leading eventually to complete resolution of all clinical and chemical evidence of hepatitis.

## 5 Pathology

Histopathologic examination of the liver is usually not warranted in acute hepatitis A. A specific virus diagnosis with its attendant excellent prognosis is readily made by widely available serologic tests. Nonetheless, a considerable body of data exists concerning the pathology of the liver in acute hepatitis A, both in man and in experimentally infected chimpanzees, New World owl monkeys, or marmosets [10, 24, 25].

The predominant lesion in acute hepatitis A is hepatocellular degeneration and necrosis, associated with considerable mononuclear cell infiltration. Vacuolation of hepatocytes may be a prominent feature. These findings are usually most striking in the periportal regions (Fig. 4) and at times may be associated with piecemeal necrosis providing a histologic picture which resembles chronic active hepatitis. Clumps of Kupffer cells containing stainable iron were also noted in a large proportion of human liver biopsies in one series [10]. The extent of necrosis and inflammation correlate generally with the severity of serum aminotransferase abnormalities. Hepatocyte degeneration and necrosis as well as inflammation may also be present in centrilobular regions, particularly in older humans, and may be a marker of

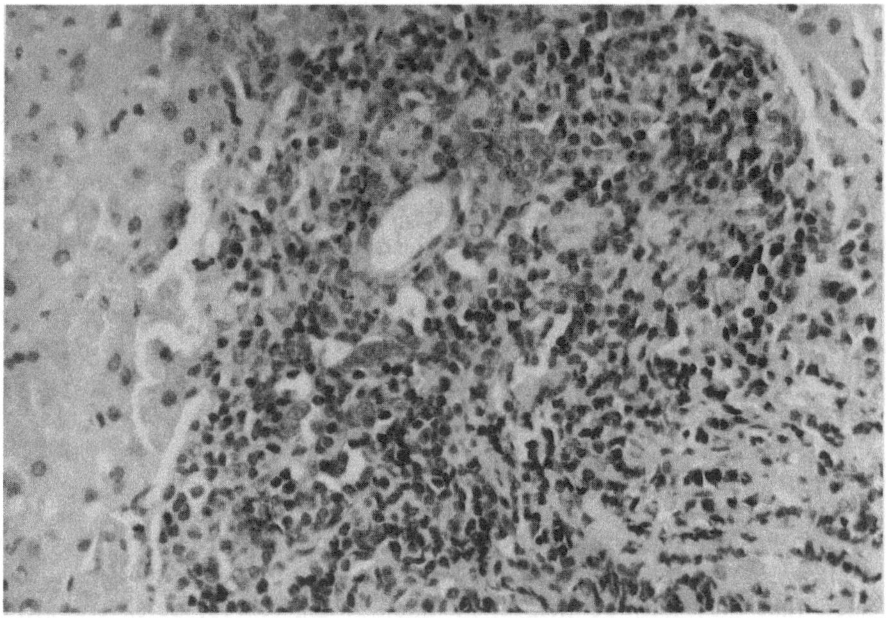

**Fig. 4.** Section of liver taken at open biopsy from an experimentally infected chimpanzee, showing an extensive periportal inflammatory infiltrate

more extensive liver damage. Centrilobular cholestasis is usually present and at times may be very prominent. None of these histologic changes become chronic, and resolution of the liver injury has typically been noted in follow-up examinations. During the acute period of hepatitis, viral antigen is present within the cytoplasm of the majority of hepatocytes, and virus particles may be seen by electron microscopy within cytoplasmic vesicles of hepatocytes [26].

## 6 Diagnosis

The diagnosis of hepatitis A is based on the serologic demonstration of IgM antibodies to the virus. Such antibodies are present in over 99% of individuals at the time of their initial presentation [27]. IgM anti-HAV usually peaks within the first month of illness and declines to nondetectable levels within 12 (usually 6) months. Virus-specific IgM antibody is usually detected by very sensitive and specific solid-phase antibody-capture immunoassays and is often found against a background of nonspecific increases in IgM. Total antibody to HAV, on the other hand, is measured in a separate competitive inhibition (blocking) radioimmunoassay or enzyme-linked immunosorbent assay (ELISA). Total antibody to HAV consists predominantly of IgG antibody except immediately after acute HAV infection, when IgM and IgA antibodies represent a greater proportion of the virus-specific antibody response. Like tests for IgM anti-HAV, tests for total anti-HAV are also positive at the onset of acute hepatitis A. A negative test for total antibodies to hepatitis A thus effectively excludes a diagnosis of acute HAV infection. However, a positive competitive inhibition test is unable to distinguish between acute (recent) and long past infection. Competitive inhibition immunoassays for total anti-HAV antibodies usually remain positive for life following acute infection and are a good marker of immunity. Neither tests for IgM anti-HAV nor tests for total anti-HAV are influenced by passive administration of immune globulin given in normal doses. Thus the administration of immune globulin does not complicate subsequent efforts at serologic diagnosis.

## 7 Treatment

There is no effective antiviral treatment for hepatitis A. Steroids are not beneficial even in severe forms of hepatitis A, although it has been suggested that they may be helpful in ameliorating severe, persistent intrahepatic cholestasis [21]. Even in this setting, steroids should be used with caution, as cholestatic hepatitis A is always a benign, self-limited condition. Enforced bedrest is of no benefit in promoting resolution of the infection and patients should be allowed to pursue activities as tolerated. Hospitalization is usually not required, except for the older patient whose fluid and/or nutritional status may be in question. Patients with fulminant forms of hepatitis A require hospitalization in an intensive care unit, however, and therapy with vitamin K and fresh frozen plasma to correct coagulation defects. Restriction of protein intake and oral administration of lactulose is indicated if encephalopathy or coma develops.

## 8 Epidemiology

As already mentioned, HAV is predominantly transmitted by the fecal–oral route. Large amounts of virus are shed in the feces of infected individuals, and thus it is not surprising that the most commonly reported risk factor responsible for acquisition of hepatitis A within well-developed countries is to have resided within the same household as another infected person. Specific activities which promote fecal–oral spread of virus may also contribute to transmission of the agent [28]. Thus, homosexual males who engage in oral–anal sexual activity are at increased risk for acquiring hepatitis A. Similarly, children attending preschool day-care centers caring for children under the age of 2 years are also at risk. Outbreaks of hepatitis A associated with transmission of virus within such day-care centers are common [19, 29]. The children most at risk for transmitting the infection are usually those who are not yet toilet trained, although frank hepatitis is not commonly associated with HAV infection in children of this age. The usual victims of day-care center-associated outbreaks of hepatitis A are parents, siblings, and other older contacts of these children attending the center, as well as center staff, who because of their age are more likely to develop symptoms of hepatitis when infected. Filter-feeding shellfish represent additional potential sources of infection, as they are capable of concentrating virus present in polluted waters. Contaminated shellfish must be thoroughly cooked in order to inactivate the virus.

Although a rare event, transfusion-associated hepatitis A has been reported on a number of occasions. These rare cases occur as a result of the fortuitous collection of blood from an asymptomatic individual during the late incubation period of hepatitis A when viremia is present. Blood-borne transmission may also account for recent increases in the number of hepatitis A cases related to drug use in the United States and elsewhere [30]. The viremia associated with hepatitis A may be up to several weeks in duration [11], providing an opportunity for transmission of virus among individuals who frequently use intravenous drugs and who share needles. It is not entirely clear, however, whether the association of hepatitis A with intravenous drug use reflects needle-borne transmission of virus or otherwise poor hygiene on the part of intravenous drug users.

One of the unique aspects of HAV is its propensity for epidemic spread. The most dramatic HAV outbreaks are common source epidemics associated with contaminated food or drink, often related to infection in an index case who happens to be a food handler. Such outbreaks account for only a small proportion of all hepatitis A infections but may be impressive events and involve several dozens if not hundreds of individuals. The hallmark of such outbreaks is the occurrence of a large number of cases within a period of only a very few weeks. Outbreaks lasting several months or longer are usually not associated with food handlers or contaminated food sources, but have been reported in association with sustained transmission within a day-care center [31] or transmission within the homosexual male population of a particular city [32].

The polymerase chain reaction (PCR) now affords the ability to detect and characterize viral nucleic acid present in clinical specimens collected from patients with hepatitis A. This approach is currently providing a new view of the epidemiology of HAV [33]. Sequencing of genomic cDNA transcripts that have been reverse transcribed and amplified by PCR provides a measure of the degree of genetic relatedness among different HAV strains. To date, these studies have linked different outbreaks that were previously thought to be unrelated to each other, and have demonstrated that genetically unique but antigenically indistinguishable strains of virus are circulating within different endemic regions.

Overall, the incidence of hepatitis A seems to be declining worldwide. This is most likely due to general improvements in public health sanitation and is leading to a generally lower seroprevalence of antibodies to the agent, particularly in developing countries that are in transition to higher socio-economic standards. In turn, this will result in enhanced susceptibility of most populations to hepatitis A, which in transitional countries may be associated with paradoxically increased disease activity. The reason for this surprising increase in disease activity relates to the age at which infection occurs. This age increases as HAV becomes less prevalent. In some transitional countries where virtually the entire population became infected during early childhood previously, many individuals are now becoming infected at older ages when they are more likely to develop jaundice and frank hepatitis. In addition, decreasing overall prevalence may be expected to lead to cyclic increases in disease activity, as greater population susceptibility may promote transmission of the agent. The most impressive example of HAV disease in a transitional country occurred recently in Shanghai. Over a period of 30 years, the mean age at HAV infection had risen from 7 to 20 years in the Shanghai region, as HAV infection became generally less common. This led to a large population of susceptible young adults in Shanghai by 1988, at which time HAV-contaminated clams were introduced on the food markets. Over a 3-month period, more than 300 000 cases of acute hepatitis A occurred within the Shanghai population. Most cases were in young adults. Thousands were hospitalized although only 32 cases were fatal. This outbreak demonstrates the special risk that developing nations may experience during their transition to conditions of improved sanitation and also bears testimony to the fact that filter-feeding shellfish may be important vectors for transmission of this agent. It is likely that vaccination against HAV, once available at reasonable cost, will prove most useful in transitional countries like China.

## 9 Prevention

For many years it has been possible to prevent hepatitis A by administration of immune serum globulin (ISG). The exact mechanism by which ISG confers protection is not known, but it is recognized that ISG may often prevent the disease without preventing the infection. ISG is most effective if given within 2 weeks of exposure. The dose recommended for persons who are household contacts of hepatitis A is 0.02 ml/kg administered intramuscularly as a single dose [34]. Other persons for whom postexposure prophylaxis may be indicated include sexual contacts of persons with acute hepatitis A, and persons with exposure to children attending a day-care center within which transmission of HAV has been documented (generally by the occurrence of more than one case of hepatitis A in staff, children, or their immediate families). Occasional outbreaks of hepatitis A in persons in other residential institutions (prisons, institutions for the mentally retarded) may warrant use of ISG. The use of ISG in individuals exposed to HAV in the setting of a common source outbreak of hepatitis A is somewhat controversial, as an incubation period has often elapsed by the time the exposure is recognized. However, most public health authorities use ISG liberally in such epidemic settings. For preexposure prophylaxis, such as for persons travelling overseas to regions where hepatitis A may be endemic, the recommended dose is 0.06 ml/kg. This higher dose may provide up to 80% protection against symptomatic infection with hepatitis A, for a period of 4–6 months. The administration of ISG is usually not associated with significant side-effects, although anaphylactic reactions may occur rarely. These are more common in individuals who are deficient in IgA. The absence of identifiable risk factors in up to 40% of all cases of hepatitis precludes their prevention by passive immunization and has prompted development of HAV vaccines.

Considerable progress has been made in recent years in the development of vaccines for hepatitis A [35]. This work began with recognition in the late 1970s that HAV could be propagated in conventional cell cultures and that it might be possible to develop both inactivated and attenuated types of vaccines resembling those used for poliovirus. It was shown that the passage of HAV in cell culture results in attenuation of the ability of the virus to cause liver injury in otherwise susceptible primates [36]. While this observation has been exploited in efforts to develop an attenuated HAV vaccine, vaccine candidates evaluated thus far have been poorly immunogenic and the future development of these vaccines remains problematic in the early 1990s. Greater progress has been made in development of formalin-inactivated HAV vaccines. Such vaccines are derived from virus grown in cell culture, inactivated in formalin over a period of many hours, and mixed with alum as an adjuvant [37]. The better of these vaccines are highly purified and contain less than 10% nonviral proteins. These products appear very safe and are highly immunogenic. Specific neutralizing antibody to HAV develops in the majority of individuals receiving a single 400 ng dose, raising the possibility that these vaccines may be utilized for preexposure prophylaxis on relatively short notice, for example, in travelers going overseas to regions of greater HAV endemicity. A more conventional schedule, however, would be a series of three immunizations given over a 6- to 12-month period.

While the level of antibody elicited by these formalin-inactivated vaccines is perhaps 10- to 100-fold less than that occurring after infection with wild-type virus, the levels of antibody achieved are far greater than those reached with passive administration of ISG [38]. Thus it is quite likely that these vaccines will be proven to be efficacious. Large-scale clinical trials are now in progress with at least two commercial products, and it is probable that both will be available for clinical practice within the relatively near future. While inactivated HAV vaccines, like inactivated poliovirus vaccines, will probably not elicit significant secretory immunity, currently available evidence suggests that secretory IgA plays little if any role in natural protection against hepatitis A [39].

There has been substantial interest in developing a vaccine containing HAV antigen expressed from recombinant cDNA. This has not been possible thus far, because the critical neutralizing epitopes of HAV are conformationally defined and not present in individually expressed capsid proteins. However, recent work involving the expression of the entire capsid-protein encoding region of the HAV genome in recombinant vaccinia virus suggests that such approaches may be possible in the future.

## References

1. Ticehurst JR, Cohen JI, Feinstone SM, Purcell RH, Jansen RW, Lemon SM (1989) Replication of hepatitis A virus: new ideas from studies with cloned cDNA. In: Ehrenfeld E, Semler BL (eds) Molecular aspects of picornavirus infection and detection. ASM, Washington DC, pp 27–50
2. Cohen JI, Ticehurst JR, Purcell RH, Buckler-White A, Baroudy BM (1987) Complete nucleotide sequence of wild-type hepatitis A virus: comparison with different strains of hepatitis A virus and other picornaviruses. J Virol 61:50–59
3. Ping L-H, Jansen RW, Stapleton JT, Cohen JI, Lemon SM (1988) Identification of an immunodominant antigenic site involving the capsid protein VP3 of hepatitis A virus. Proc Natl Acad Sci USA 85:8281–8285
4. Siegl G, Frosner GG, Gauss-Muller V, Tratschin J-D, Deinhardt F (1981) The physicochemical properties of infectious hepatitis A virions. J Gen Virol 57:331–341
5. Provost PJ, Hilleman MR (1979) Propagation of human hepatitis A virus in cell culture in vitro. Proc Soc Exp Biol Med 160:213–221
6. Dienstag JL, Feinstone SM, Purcell RH et al. (1975) Experimental infection of chimpanzees with hepatitis A virus. J Infect Dis 132:532–545
7. Schulman AN, Dienstag JL, Jackson DR et al. (1976) Hepatitis A antigen particles in liver, bile, and stool of chimpanzees. J Infect Dis 134:80–84
8. Boggs JD, Melnick JL, Conrad ME, Felsher BF (1970) Viral hepatitis: clinical and tissue culture studies. JAMA 214:1041–1046
9. Skinhoj P, Mathiesen LR, Kryger P, Muller AM (1981) Copenhagen Hepatitis Acuta Programme. Faecal excretion of hepatitis A virus in patients with symptomatic hepatitis A infection. Scand J Gastroenterol 16:1057–1059
10. Teixera MR Jr, Weller IVD, Murray A et al. (1982) The pathology of hepatitis A in man. Liver 2:53–60
11. Lemon SM, Binn LN, Marchwicki R et al. (1990) In vivo replication and reversion to wild-type of a neutralization-resistant variant of hepatitis A virus. J Infect Dis 161:7–13
12. Lemon SM, Binn LN (1983) Serum neutralizing antibody response to hepatitis A virus. J Infect Dis 148:1033–1039
13. Lemon SM (1985) Type A viral hepatitis: new developments in an old disease. N Engl J Med 313:1059–1067
14. Margolis HS, Nainan OV, Krawczynski K et al. (1988) Appearance of immune complexes during experimental hepatitis A infection in chimpanzees. J Med Virol 26:315–326
15. Kurane I, Binn LN, Bancroft WH, Ennis FA (1985) Human lymphocyte responses to hepatitis A virus-infected cells: interferon production and lysis of infected cells. J Immunol 135:2140–2144

16. Vallbracht A, Gabriel P, Maier K et al. (1986) Cell-mediated cytotoxicity in hepatitis A virus infection. Hepatology 6:1308–1314
17. Maier K, Gabriel P, Koscielniak E et al. (1988) Human gamma interferon production by cytotoxic T lymphocytes sensitized during hepatitis A virus infection. J Virol 62:3756–3763
18. Baer GM, Walker JA, Yager PA (1977) Studies of an outbreak of acute hepatitis A: I. Complement level fluctuation. J Med Virol 1:1–7
19. Hadler SC, Webster HM, Erben JJ, Swanson JE, Maynard JE (1980) Hepatitis A in day-care centers: a community-wide assessment. N Engl J Med 302:1222–1227
20. Lednar WM, Lemon SM, Kirkpatrick JW, Redfield RR, Fields ML, Kelley PW (1985) Frequency of illness associated with epidemic hepatitis A virus infections in adults. Am J Epidemiol 122:226–233
21. Gordon SC, Reddy KR, Schiff L, Schiff ER (1984) Prolonged intrahepatic cholestasis secondary to acute hepatitis A. Ann Intern Med 101:635–637
22. Rakela J, Redeker AG, Edwards VM, Decker RH, Overby LR, Mosley JW (1978) Hepatitis A virus infection in fulminant hepatitis and chronic active hepatitis. Gastroenterology 74:879–882
23. Sjogren MH, Tanno H, Fay O et al. (1987) Hepatitis A virus in stool during clinical relapse. Ann Intern Med 106:221–226
24. Dienstag JL, Popper H, Purcell RH (1976) The pathology of viral hepatitis types A and B in chimpanzees. Am J Pathol 85:131–144
25. Keenan CM, Lemon SM, LeDuc JW, McNamee GA, Binn LN (1984) Pathology of hepatitis A infection in the owl monkey (*Aotus trivirgatus*). Am J Pathol 115:1–8
26. Shimizu YK, Shikata T, Beninger PR et al. (1982) Detection of hepatitis A antigen in human liver. Infect Immun 36:320–324
27. Lemon SM, Brown CD, Brooks DS et al. (1980) Specific immunoglobulin M response to hepatitis A virus determined by solid-phase radioimmunoassay. Infect Immun 28:927–936
28. Francis DP, Hadler SC, Prendergast TJ et al. (1984) Occurrence of hepatitis A, B, and non-A/non-B in the United States: CDC Sentinel County Hepatitis Study I. Am J Med 76:69–74
29. Hadler SC, Erben JJ, Matthews R, Starko K, Francis DP, Maynard JE (1983) Effect of immunoglobulin on hepatitis A in day-care centers. JAMA 249:48–53
30. Center for Disease Control (1988) Hepatitis A among drug abusers. MMWR 37:297–305
31. Benenson MW, Takafuji ET, Bancroft WH, Lemon SM, Callahan MC, Leach DA (1980) A military community outbreak of hepatitis type A related to transmission in a child care facility. Am J Epidemiol 112:471–481
32. Christenson B, Brostrom C, Bottiger M et al. (1982) An epidemic outbreak of hepatitis A among homosexual men in Stockholm: hepatitis A, a special hazard for the male homosexual subpopulation in Sweden. Am J Epidemiol 116: 599–607
33. Jansen RW, Siegl G, Lemon SM (1990) Molecular epidemiology of human hepatitis A virus defined by an antigen-capture polymerase chain reaction method. Proc Matl Acad Sci USA 87:2867–2871
34. Advisory Committee on Immunization Practices CDC (1985) Recommendations for protection against viral hepatitis. MMWR 34:313–335
35. Siegl G, Lemon SM (1990) Recent advances in hepatitis A vaccine development. Virus Res 17:75–92
36. Provost PJ, Banker FS, Giesa PA, McAleer WJ, Buynak EB, Hilleman MR (1982) Progress toward a live, attenuated human hepatitis A vaccine. Proc Soc Exp Biol Med 170:8–14
37. Provost PJ, Emini EA, Lewis JA, Gerety RJ (1988) Progress toward the development of a hepatitis A vaccine. In; Zuckerman AJ (ed) Viral hepatitis and liver disease. Alan R. Liss, New York, pp 83–86

38. Stapleton JT, Jansen RW, Lemon SM (1985) Neutralizing antibody to hepatitis A virus in immune serum globulin and in the sera of human recipients of immune serum globulin. Gastroenterology 89:637–642
39. Stapleton JT, Lange DK, LeDuc JW, Binn LN, Jansen RW, Lemon SM (1991) The role of secretory immunity in hepatitis A virus infection. J Infect Dis 163:7–11

# B. Type E Viral Hepatitis

D.W. BRADLEY and K. KRAWCZYNSKI

## 1 Introduction

The enterically and parenterally transmitted forms of non-A, non-B hepatitis (ET-NANBH and PT-NANBH, respectively) have long been recognized as important causes of morbidity and mortality in man. Until recently, however, little was known about the etiology of either ET-NANBH or PT-NANBH except that viral agents were strongly suspected on the basis of the epidemiologic, clinical, and histologic features of each disease. The development of sensitive and specific serologic assays for markers of actue infection by hepatitis A virus (HAV) [1, 2] and hepatitis B virus (HBV) [3, 4] led to the realization that many epidemics of hepatitis associated with fecally contaminated water were not caused by HAV or HBV [5]. Earlier reviews of NANBH cover many historical aspects of this rapidly expanding area of medical research [6–8].

### 1.1 Natural History and Geographic Distribution

A substantial proportion of cases of acute viral hepatitis occurring in young to middle-aged adults in Asia and the Indian subcontinent appears to be caused by an agent that is serologically unrelated to either HAV or HBV [5]. This disease has been shown to occur in both epidemic and sporadic, endemic forms and is primarily associated with the ingestion of fecally contaminated drinking water. The term "enterically transmitted non-A, non-B hepatitis" has evolved from the waterborne mode of virus transmission and presumed enteric route of natural infection in humans [8]. This type of hepatitis was first documented in New Delhi, India in 1955, when 29 000 cases of icteric hepatitis were identified following widespread fecal contamination of the city's drinking water [9]. A similar epidemic of viral hepatitis occurred between December 1975 and January 1976 in Ahmedabad City, India, again due to contaminated water supplies [10]. Both outbreaks were thought originally to be caused by HAV; however, retrospective serologic analysis of paired serum specimens from documented cases revealed that neither HAV nor HBV could be implicated as the etiologic agent [5]. Large epidemics of enterically transmitted viral hepatitis have also been observed in the Kirgiz Republic, USSR [11]. Between 1955 and 1956 more than 10800 cases of acute viral hepatitis were documented there in young to middle-aged adults; approximately 18% of infected pregnant women died as a result of acute disease. The epidemiologic and clinical features of these outbreaks are remarkably similar to those associated with the 1955–56 New Delhi outbreak. Subsequent outbreaks of epidemic and sporadic NANBH were documented in North India [12] and in Kashmir, India [13]. Outbreaks of epidemiologically similar cases of ET-NANBH have also been reported in Southeast Asia, including Burma [14] and Nepal [15], and were associated with a high mortality in infected pregnant women. Between June 1976 and August 1977, more than 20000 icteric cases occurred in Mandalay, Burma, with a case fatality ratio of 18% in pregnant women (Schreeder, unpublished data). An epidemic of viral hepatitis involving 10000 cases in the Kathmandu Valley, Nepal, in 1973 was also reported to be associated with a high mortality in infected pregnant women [15, 16]. The occurrence of ET-NANBH in Pakistan has recently been inferred from the observation of cases of disease imported into the United States [17]. Outbreaks of ET-NANBH have also been reported in Africa, including Algeria [18], Ivory Coast [19], Eastern Sudan [20], and Somalia [20]. A high mortality among infected pregnant women was noted in most of these outbreaks.

Enterically transmitted NANBH does not appear to be confined to Asia, the Soviet Union, and North Africa, however. In fact, outbreaks of NANBH associated with fecally contaminated drinking water have been documented recently in Borneo (Lubis and Wuryadi, personal communication) and in two rural villages located south of Mexico City, Mexico [21]. Virologic and serologic studies of stool and serum specimens, respectively, obtained from affected persons suggested that the etiologic agent responsible for disease in North America might be similar or identical to that associated with ET-NANBH in other regions of the world (see below).

### 1.2 Clinical and Epidemiologic Features

Cases of ET-NANBH occur primarily in developing countries of the world. The disease is transmitted fecally/orally, and the highest attack rate is seen in young to middle-aged adults. The highest mortality is seen in pregnant women, but in most cases the disease is self-limiting; like hepatitis A, ET-NANBH is not associated with chronic liver disease or persistent viremia. The average incubation period for the disease is about 6 weeks after primary exposure. In the United States, the only cases seen have been imported by travelers who have contracted the disease in endemic areas [17], and no cases of secondary exposure have been reported in the United States.

Currently, a diagnosis of acute ET-NANBH is made by serologic exclusion complemented by supportive epidemiologic circumstances. The only laboratory tests available for the diagnosis of ET-NANBH are (a) immune electron microscopic (IEM) examination of patient stools for virus-like particles and (b) a fluorescent antibody blocking assay for the detection of virus-specific antibodies in patient sera. Neither is suitable for use in routine screening of patients.

## 2 The Agent of Enterically Transmitted non-A, non-B Hepatitis

### 2.1 Experimental Studies in Primates

Transmission of ET-NANBH to nonhuman primates was reported first by BALAYAN and co-workers in 1983 [22]. Two cynomolgus macaques ("cynos") were inoculated intravenously with a 10% w/v suspension of a human volunteer stool that was positive by IEM for 27–30 nm diameter virus-like particles (VLPs). In these animals, elevations in alanine aminotransferase (ALT) activity developed between 24 and 36 days after inoculation; they excreted 27–30 nm VLPs in their preacute-phase stools and seroconverted, as demonstrated by IEM, acquiring antibody to morphologically similar VLPs in the inoculum. ANDJAPARIDZE and co-workers later reported the successful transmission of ET-NANBH to African green monkeys, as well as cynos, using ET-NANBH case-derived stool specimens positive by IEM for 27–30 nm VLPs [23].

More recently, animal transmission studies have been conducted in cynos, tamarins, and chimpanzees using highly characterized inocula [24, 25]. These studies have provided preinoculation, acute-phase, and convalescent sera for use in coded serum panels, in immunofluorescence antibody assays (see below), and in immunoscreening studies of lambda gtll cDNA libraries. Intravenous inoculation of four tamarins with a 1982–1983 Burma outbreak stool pool (positive by IEM for 32–34 nm VLPs) caused elevated serum isocitrate dehydrogenase (SICD) activity in three animals, with peak values occurring between 70 and 80 days after inoculation [25]. Three of four cynos inoculated intravenously with the same material developed elevated ALT activity after an average incubation period of 38 days [25]. This ET-NANBH isolate was passaged in cynos using preacute-phase stool suspensions from animals exhibiting the highest elevations of ALT activity. The incubation period at each passage level appeared to be shorter, and all animals became infected. For example, third passage of ET-NANBH in five cynos resulted in elevated ALT activity in all animals, with an average incubation period of 20 days (Fig. 1). Intravenous inoculation of four cynos with a partially purified virus preparation (Mexico case stool; see below for details) containing a relatively large number of 32–34 nm VLPs

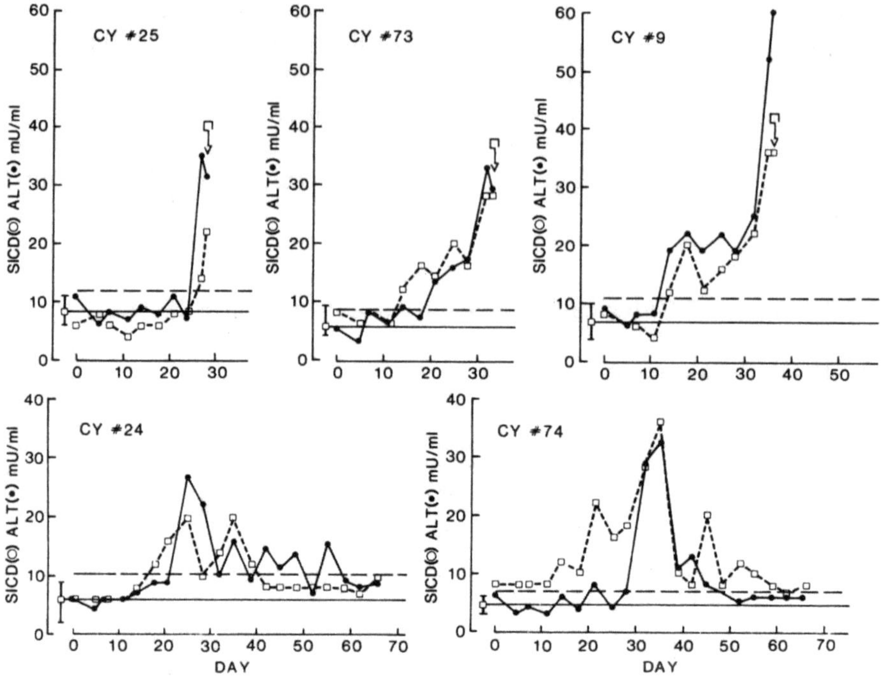


**Fig. 1.** Third passage of a Burmese HEV isolate in cynos. Each animal was intravenously inoculated with 1.0 ml of a 10% w/v stool suspension prepared from a collection of preacute-phase stools obtained from a second-passage cyno

resulted in elevated ALT activity after incubation periods of 5, 5, 8, and 12 days, respectively (Fig. 2). Inoculation of chimpanzees with ET-NANBH case-derived stools obtained from outbreaks in geographic areas other than Mexico or containing fewer numbers of 32–34 nm VLPs demonstrated less severe disease or no disease at all. The difficulties in recovering VLPs with a similar or identical morphology from proven infectious stool pools was consistent with the fact of the observed instability of virus particles in a high percentage of well-documented cases of severe disease. However, the results of one IEM study showed a consistent and specific relationship between ET-NANBH in primates (and humans) and 32–34 nm VLPs recovered from case stools in Mexico and the Soviet Union [26].

Studies using stools containing large numbers of 32–34 nm VLPs revealed that acute-phase sera from both human cases and experimentally infected primates were much more likely to aggregate virus than convalescent sera from the same individuals. This finding was considered to be significant in that it allowed us to demonstrate consistently a clear serologic relationship between 32–34 nm VLPs and experimentally induced disease in nonhuman primates.

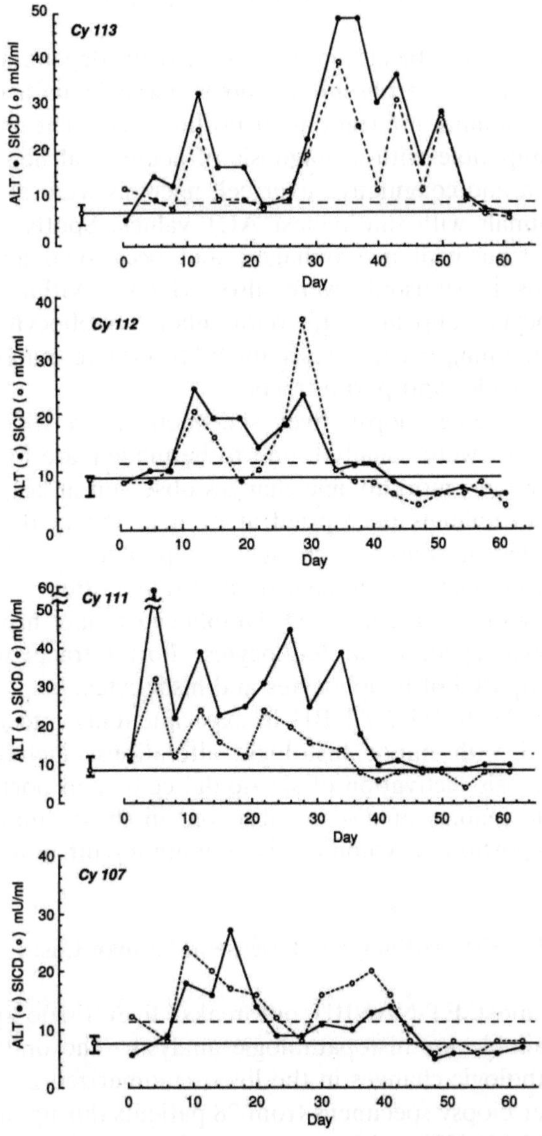


**Fig. 2.** First passage of ET-NANBH virus (HEV) in cynos after intravenous inoculation of partially purified virus from a Mexican case-derived stool specimen (see text for details). A very short incubation period was observed and a biphasic pattern of ALT was seen during the course of disease

### 2.2 Histopathology of Disease in Experimentally Infected Primates

In cynos with elevated ALT activity, degeneration and necroinflammatory changes were observed in liver parenchyma accompanied by inconspicuous or minimal infiltrations in portal tracts. The more advanced changes were compatible with a diagnosis of acute viral hepatitis. Acidophilic degeneration and coagulative liver cell necrosis were also prominent, particularly in animals with the highest ALT values. Spotty liver cell necrosis, activation of sinusoidal macrophages, and occasional accumulation of mononuclear cells in sinusoids were also evident. Within intralobular infiltrates, histiocytes appeared to outnumber lymphocytes. Sinusoidal macrophages containing diastase-resistant PAS-positive material were occasionally found in lobules and portal tracts.

Needle biopsy liver specimens from ET-NANBH infected *Saguinus mystax* were usually found to be inadequate for histopathologic evaluation; however, morphologic changes observed in larger tissue specimens obtained from animals necropsied at or near the peak of liver enzyme activity revealed morphologic changes compatible with those of acute viral hepatitis. Intralobular mononuclear infiltrates often delineated foci of liver cell necrosis and contained lymphocytes and histiocytes mixed with a few polymorphonuclear leukocytes. Portal tracts were enlarged by infiltrates composed of lymphocytes and histiocytes.

Acute ET-NANBH in experimentally infected chimpanzees was associated with minor histologic alterations, including limited areas of focal necrosis, activation of sinusoidal cells, and portal inflammation. A remarkable feature of disease observed in these animals was the relatively small proportion of lymphocytes seen among inflammatory cells.

### 2.3 Histopathology of Disease in Human Cases

In most ET-NANBH outbreaks, liver tissue specimens have rarely been available for histopathologic analysis. The only extensive studies of histopathologic changes in the liver, summarized in Table 1, were carried out in liver biopsy specimens from 78 patients during the large outbreak in Delhi in 1955–56 [27] and from endemically occurring ET-NANBH in 128 patients in Ghana (West Africa) in 1962–63 [28]. Two types of histopathologic changes were observed in the Indian outbreak, an "obstructive" or cholestatic type found in 58% of examined cases, and a "standard" type identified in 42% of cases [27]. The cholestatic type was characterized by bile stasis in canaliculi and parenchymal cells which were arranged in a gland-like fashion. Cholestasis and glandular transformation of liver cell plates were much more significant in the cases from West Africa (63% and 93%, respectively). Degenerative changes of liver cells (including acidophilic bodies) and focal necrosis were less frequently seen in the cholestatic type of ET-NANBH in

**Table 1.** Histopathologic features of ET-NANBH

| |
|---|
| A. *Intralobular changes*: |
| – Cholestasis (canalicular and cytoplasmic), ballooning of hepatocytes, pseudoglandular alterations of hepatocyte plates, focal necrosis |
| *or* |
| – Acidophilic degeneration, acidophilic bodies, ballooning of hepatocytes, focal necrosis |
| – Inflammatory infitrations: mononuclear macrophages, Kupffer cells, less frequent lymphocytes |
| B. *Portal inflammation*: monocytic (lymphocytes and monocytes) with polymorphonuclear leukocytes (in larger numbers sometimes) |

the Indian patients. Polymorphonuclear leukocytes were observed both in intralobular infiltrations and in portal tracts in larger amounts than seen in the classic acute viral hepatitis, although in portal tracts monocytes (lymphocytes) remained the predominant cell type. In the "standard" type of viral hepatitis, ballooned hepatocytes, acidophilic degeneration of hepatocytes, and acidophilic body formation were the most frequently encountered. Similarly, in experimental ET-NANBH in primates, the acidophilic type of hepatocytic degeneration was a characteristic morphologic feature, especially in cynomolgus macaques (see above). Focal necrosis was observed in both patients and infected primates with prominent accumulations of mononuclear macrophages and activated Kupffer cells and a much less striking presence of lymphocytes. In both human and experimental liver specimens, lymphocytes prevailed in portal infiltrations; in serial biopsies from infected macaques portal infiltrations seemed to occur later than intralobular changes. In summary, certain features of degenerative and necrotic changes in both humans and primates are reminiscent of a toxic type of parenchymal lesion.

### 2.4 Virus-like Particles

Although several reports of 27–30 nm VLPs associated with ET-NANBH have appeared in the literature, independent confirmation of the specificity of these candidate viruses for disease has been complicated by the limited availability of case-derived stool specimens and the relative instability of reagent virus. Our IEM studies of stool specimens for VLPs were initiated in 1982 when stools from cases of ET-NANBH occurring in Kathmandu Valley, Nepal were examined using convalescent serum as a source of antibody. One of nine stools was found to be positive for 27–32 nm VLPs; convalescent (but not preinoculation) serum from a tamarin in which NANBH had developed after inoculation with this stool specimen was shown to have antibody against these virus particles [15]. This finding suggested that the animal had seroconverted specifically by acquiring antibodies to VLPs contained in the inoculum and indicated further that these particles (or a related particle) might be causally related to disease. Subsequent serologic studies with these virus particles were compromised by the diminished number of particles found in stored and freeze-thawed stool suspensions. Stools from another outbreak of ET-NANBH occurring in 1982–1983 in Rangoon, Burma were made available to the CDC through collaboration with the Ministry of Health (H. Myint) [14, 25]. Four of 31 case-derived stools were found to be positive by IEM for 27–30 and 32–34 nm VLPs. Both sets of particles appeared to possess surface features that were morphologically similar to those found on the Nepal case-derived stool particles described above. One perplexing aspect of these studies was the notable discrepancy in the antibody coating of 27–30 and 32–34 nm VLPs; the smaller particles appeared to be minimally reactive with antibody contained in case sera, whereas the larger virus particles were found to be heavily coated.

Although our studies suggest that the larger, 32–34 nm VLP is responsible for all or nearly all cases of ET-NANBH, an inconsistency in reported particle diameters is evident. Proteolytic digestion or denaturation of the 32–34 nm virus during its passage through the gut may be responsible for some of the discrepancies in reported particle diameters [29].

More extensive IEM studies have recently been performed using stools obtained from outbreaks in the Soviet Union and Mexico. One stool recovered from a case of ET-NANBH occurring in Tashkent, USSR (1982–1983 epidemic) was found to contain large numbers of 32–34 nm diameter virus particles. These particles reacted specifically with acute-phase and convalescent sera from well-documented cases occurring in other regions of the world, including Burma, Pakistan, Nepal, Somalia, Sudan, Borneo, and Mexico [26]. In addition, sera from cases in the Soviet Union, Pakistan, Nepal, Burma, Borneo, Somalia, and Mexico were also capable of aggregating 32–34 nm VLPs in the Telixtac (Mexico) #14 stool; antibody coating on these particles was very heavy and was rated 4+ (scale: 0–4+) (Fig. 3). Seroconversion of experimentally infected primates was also clearly documented using both of the above virus preparations.

In short, it is clear that one virus or class of serologically related viruses is responsible for disease worldwide, including Soviet Asia, Asia, Southeast Asia, North Africa, and North America. Limited cross-challenge studies conducted in cynos suggest further that animals convalescent from a bout of ET-NANBH induced by an Asian isolate are protected from reinfection by a second (North American) isolate (D. BRADLEY, unpublished data). The latter finding is in agreement with the serologic (IEM) data showing that geographically distinct virus isolates react with antisera from a variety of ET-NANBH outbreaks. Figure 3 shows antibody-aggregated 32–34 nm VLPs typical of those found in stools of ET-NANBH cases in Borneo, Burma, Mexico, Pakistan, Somalia, and the Soviet Union. By consensus,

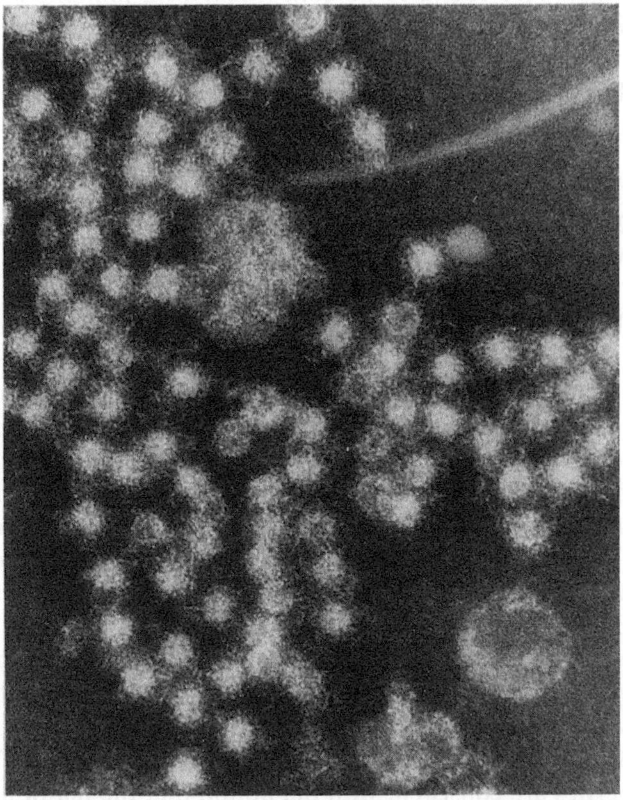

**Fig. 3.** Electron micrograph of typical 32–34 nm virus particles recovered from stool of a case of ET-NANBH occurring in Telixtac, Mexico during a 1986 outbreak. Particles are morphologically indistinguishable from those recovered from cases in Borneo, Burma, India, Somalia, and Tashkent. (*Bar* = 100 nm)

these virus particles have recently been designated hepatitis E virus, or HEV.

## 2.5 Identification of HEVAg in Hepatocytes

An antigen associated with ET-NANBH (HEVAg) has been identified in the cytoplasm of hepatocytes of experimentally infected cynos [30]. HEVAg was found in hepatocytes of infected cynos, chimpanzees, and aotus monkeys. The specificity of this antigen for hepatitis E was determined by blocking experiments with the use of acute- and convalescent-phase serum samples and by absorption experiments (normal liver and immunoglobulins). Positive results in the fluorescent antibody (FA) blocking assay were found to be concordant with immune aggregation of 32–34 nm HEV particles and suggested the existence of common antigenic determinants on HEVAg observed in hepatocytes. We conclude also that HEVAg dectected in liver cells by FA reflects the presence of HEV particles or their subcomponents.

### 2.6 Physiochemical Properties of ET-NANBH-Associated 32–34 nm Virus-like Particles

Table 2 summarizes what is known to date about the major etiologic agent of ET-NANBH. The virus appears to be extremely labile and will not tolerate exposure to high concentrations of salt, including CsCl. Pelleting of the virus from stool suspensions or gradient fractions frequently results in loss of detectable virus. Rate-zonal banding of 32–34 nm VLPs in linear, preformed sucrose gradients was found to yield partially purifed virus suitable for further IEM studies [26]. The computed sedimentation coefficient for the ET-NANBH-associated virus was approximately 183S, in contrast to 157S for that of HAV, a member of the Picornaviridae (Fig. 4). Sometimes ET-NANBH-associated virus particles sedimenting at 165S were found; these particles are presumed to be defective and probably lack a complete viral genome. Isopyknic banding of an aliquot of the Telixtac #14 stool suspension in a potassium tartrate/glycerol (KTar/Gly) gradient revealed 32–34 nm VLPs at a buoyant density of 1.29 g/cm$^3$. These biophysical properties are consistent with the notion that the major agent of ET-NANBH is calicivirus-like, for many caliciviruses sediment at approximately 183S and band at 1.29 g/cm$^3$ in KTar/Gly gradients.

Hepatitis A virus was found to have a mean diameter of 27.8 nm and HEV was found to have a mean diameter of 32.2 nm; 78% of HEVs had diameters between 31 and 35 nm, and there were no statistically significant differences in mean particle diameters in any of the four geographically different isolates (Fig. 5).

**Table 2.** Properties of HEV

1. *Size*: 32–34 nm in diameter [80% of virus particles visualized by IEM; 32.2 nm mean diameter (range: 27–38 nm)]
2. *Morphology*: spherical, nonenveloped particle; spikes and indentations visible on surface of virus
3. *Biophysical properties*: sedimentation coefficient = 183S (defectives, 165S); buoyant density = 1.29 g/cm$^3$ in KTar/Gly; sensitive to CsCl, freeze-thawing, pelleting
4. *Genome*: single-stranded, polyadenylated RNA of approx. 7.6 kb
5. *In vitro propagation*: unsuccessful (FRhK-4, AGMK, HEK, BSC-1, etc.)
6. *In vivo*: no effect on suckling mice inoculated intracerebrally with numerous case stool suspensions (10% w/v)

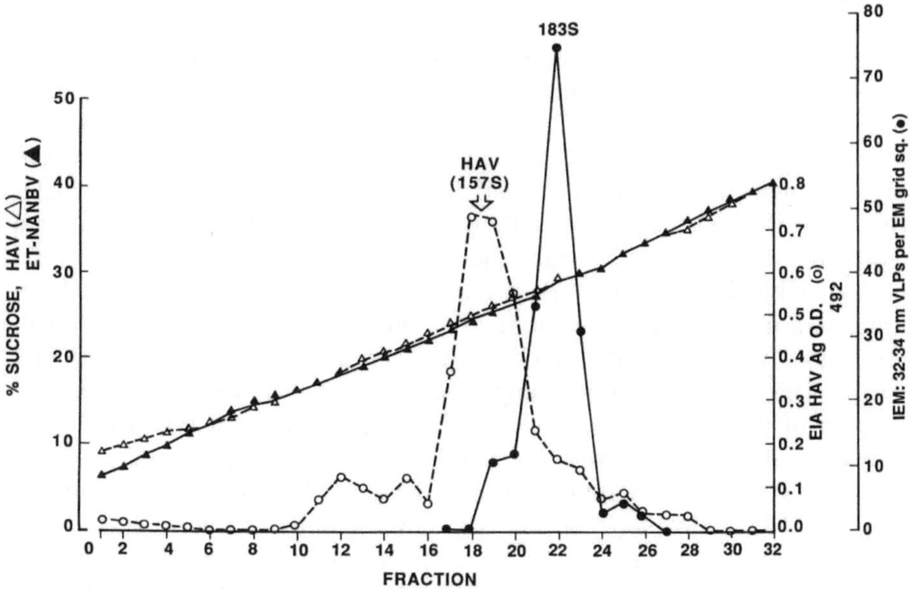


**Fig. 4.** Comparison of the sedimentation profiles (coefficients) of HEV and HAV in sucrose gradients

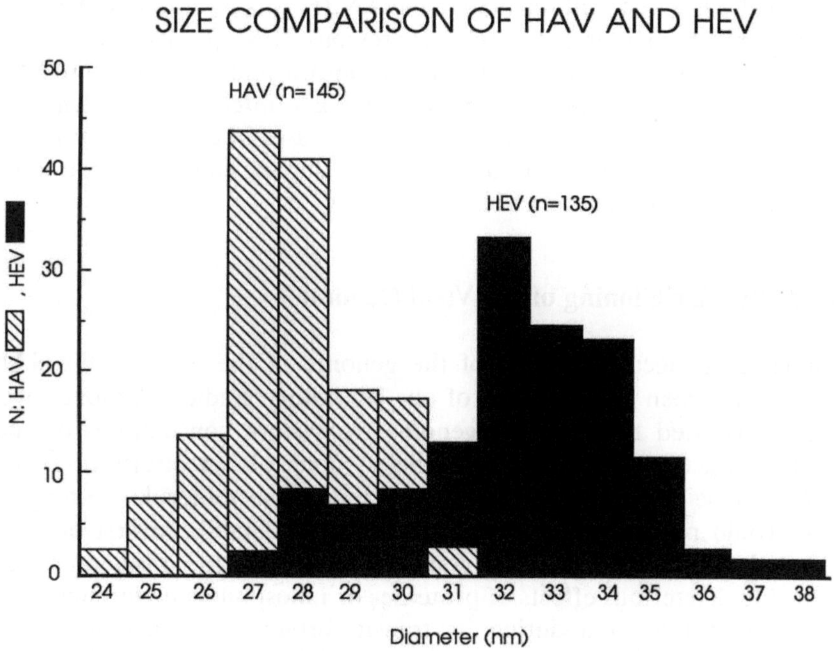


**Fig. 5.** Histogram comparing the ranges of HAV and HEV particle diameters observed by IEM

## 3 Serologic Assays and Immune Response

Attempts to develop a conventional radioimmunoassay (RIA) or enzyme-linked immunoassay (EIA) for ET-NANBH-associated antigen using acute-phase or convalescent-phase IgM or IgG, respectively, have met with failure in our laboratory. In fact, RIA analysis of separate gradient fractions containing equal numbers of HAV and ET-NANBH-associated virus particles (by IEM) showed that HAV could be easily detected using a conventional antibody "sandwich" assay, while no ET-NANBH-associated antigen could be found by this method. These results indicated that while antibody in some sera may be adequate for IEM or immunofluorescent antibody analysis, these same antibodies lack the avidity to function in RIA or EIA assays. This presumption was supported further by the finding that an IgG fraction of a convalescent serum obtained from a case of ET-NANBH in Mexico could be labeled with fluorescein isothiocyanate and used to detect ET-NANBH-associated antigen in liver tissue of infected cynos (see above) [30]. In 1989, an FA blocking assay was developed by KRAWCZYNSKI et al. as a prototype test for the identification and titration of anti-HEV in serum samples. The prevalence of anti-HEV in groups of patients from well-defined and geographically isolated outbreaks of ET-NANBH in Asia, Africa, and North America varied from 77% to 100% [31]. Although a relatively small number of serum samples were evaluated by FA for anti-HEV, an immunologic relationship between sera obtained from geographically isolated outbreaks of ET-NANBH was established. This finding is in complete agreement with our previous IEM results. Approximately 71% of sporadic cases of non-transfusion-transmitted, acute NANBH in Nepal, i.e., a geographic region where HEV infection is endemic, were positive for anti-HEV. In contrast, sporadic cases of acute, non-transfusion-transmitted NANBH in the United States, Japan, and Italy were found to be serologically unrelated to HEV infection.

## 4 Molecular Cloning of the Viral Genome

Successful molecular cloning of the genome of the virus of ET-NANBH (HEV) has been a major goal of our laboratory studies. Although we had previously tried to clone the genome from stool concentrates or sucrose gradient fractions rich in virus particles, none of our efforts resulted in a virus-specific clone. Therefore, we concluded that molecular cloning of the virus could not be achieved unless it could be stabilized first or another, more plentiful source of virus could be identified. In consideration of the probable deleterious effects of proteases or inhospitable environment on the integrity of the virus during its transit through the small intestine, we reasoned that large amounts of virus could be present in gallbladder bile prior to its discharge into the duodenum. Virus particles contained in gallbladder bile were found to have a diameter of 32–34 nm and were morphologically indistinguishable from those recovered from stool (D. BRADLEY, manuscript in preparation).

Molecular cloning of the viral genome of the 32–34 nm VLPs described above was carried out in collaboration with Genelabs, Inc., Redwood City, California [32]. A "plus-minus" (genomic) screening approach was used in this instance due to the availability of large amounts of virus in infected cyno bile. Briefly, cDNA libraries were made from RNA extracted from bile collected from cynos infected with a third-passage Burma HEV isolate. Libraries (in lambda gt10) were screened by differential hybridization with cDNA probes prepared from RNA extracted from uninfected and infected bile preparations. Several candidate clones were identified that hybridized only to the infected bile cDNA probe. One molecular clone, termed ET 1.1, was further characterized and shown to be approximately 1.3 kb in size. This clone did not hybridize to normal human placental DNA, DNA extracted from normal stools, or normal or infected cyno livers, nor did it hybridize to RNA extracted from normal cyno liver tissue or three normal human stool suspensions. This clone did hybridize, however, to cDNA prepared from RNA that had been extracted from HEV-positive stools from cases of ET-NANBH in Somalia, Borneo, Pakistan, and the Soviet Union. Also, ET 1.1 hybridized to an approximately 7.6-kb, single-stranded, polyadenylated RNA species in infected cyno livers. The latter finding is in keeping with our presumption that the major agent of ET-NANBH is calicivirus-like; caliciviruses possess an RNA genome with similar properties.

The HEV genome also appears to contain three separate open reading frames (G. REYES, personal communication), as does feline calicivirus (FCV) (J.D. NEILL, personal communication). The nonstructural genes appear to be located in the 5′ direction relative to the structural genes in HEV, as in FCV, which is the opposite orientation to that seen in picornaviruses (Fig. 6). We conclude that HEV is not a picornavirus and is more likely a distantly related member of the Caliciviridae family.

## 5 Unanswered Questions

In developing countries, more than 50% of acute viral hepatitis appears to be caused by agents other than HAV or HBV. It is assumed that a high proportion of NANBH in these countries is associated with an enterically transmitted agent, because environmental conditions in most endemic areas favor the fecal–oral route of transmission. In this regard, however, the preponderance of clinically apparent ET-NANBH cases in individuals between the ages of 15 and 40 years suggests that infection either occurs subclinically in younger individuals or does not occur at all. The latter presumption is difficult to justify in view of the fact that seroprevalence studies conducted in these countries clearly indicate that nearly all individ-

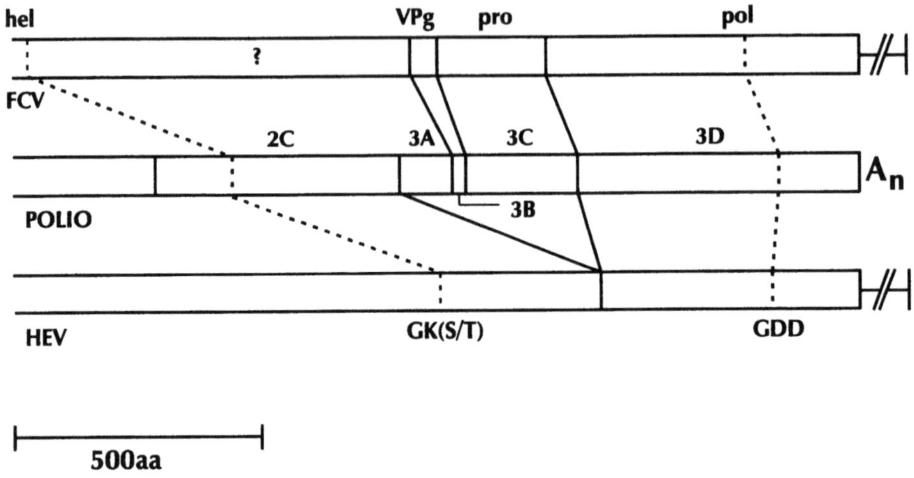


**Fig. 6.** Comparison of the carboxy termini of the nonstructural regions of feline calicivirus (FCV), the Sabin 1 vaccine strain of poliovirus, and a Burmese isolate of HEV. The *open-ended rectangles* represent the carboxyl regions of the nonstructural polyproteins from these viruses. The following domains have been identified by sequence comparison of FCV and HEV to a number of viral sequences, including that of poliovirus: *hel*, NTP binding protein (possibly a helicase); *?*, unknown function; *VPg*, genome linked protein; *pro*, proteinase; *pol*, RNA-directed RNA polymerase. The *vertical lines* represent the assumed boundaries of the nonstructural proteins. The amino terminus of the NTP binding protein for FCV and HEV could not be determined. The picornaviral genes 2C, 3A, 3B, 3C, and 3D are marked on the figure. The *even dashed lines* show the alignment of the consensus NTP binding protein —GK(S/T)— and RNA polymerase —GDD— peptide sequences in the three viruses. The *uneven dashed lines* represent a portion of the FCV sequence that has not yet been reported. At the *right of the figure*, $A_n$ indicates that the picornaviral nonstructural polyprotein sits at the 3′ end of the coding sequence, and the *broken line* indicates that the nonstructural polyprotein for FCV and HEV is followed by at least one more separate open reading frame, possibly encoding structural proteins. The *scale bar at the bottom of the figure* represents 500 amino acids

uals acquire anti-HAV before the age of 10. If, on the other hand, younger individuals exposed to HEV develop subclinical infection, and presumably protective antibody, outbreaks of ET-NANBH would not be expected to affect young to middle-aged adults disproportionately unless waning antibody levels permit reinfection. Clearly, further studies are needed to identify specific factors involved in the epidemiology and pathogenesis of hepatitis E.

Another important but unexplained observation is the unusually high mortality observed in infected pregnant women. Approximately 20% of women with ET-NANBH in their third trimester of pregnancy succumb, in contrast to 0.5%–3% of the local or general population suffering from ET-NANBH. The effect of pregnancy on viral hepatitis does not explain this observation for only negligible mortality is seen in infected pregnant women with other types of viral hepatitis. In this regard, the unexpectedly high mortality observed in HEV-infected pregnant women may reflect a unique feature of viral replication or disease pathogenesis in these individuals.

Another notable feature of hepatitis E is the relatively low frequency of clinical disease observed in case contacts, an unusual phenomenon for enterically transmitted agents. For example, among household contacts of hepatitis E cases during the 1981–82 epidemic in Kathmandu Valley, Nepal, clinical illness developed in only 2.4%. This is in sharp contrast to the much higher secondary attack rate of 10%–20% observed in household contacts of patients with hepatitis A occurring in the same region. The relative instability of the 32–34 nm VLPs described above may account for the decreased secondary transmission of hepatitis E; however, definitive studies of virus stability and infectivity will be required to support or refute this notion.

## References


1. Bradley DW, Maynard JE, Hindman SH et al. (1977) Serodiagnosis of viral hepatitis A: detection of acute phase IgM anti-HAV by radioimmunoassay. J Clin Microbiol 5:521–530
2. Bradley DW, Fields HA, McCaustland KA et al. (1979) Serodiagnosis of viral hepatitis A by a modified competitive binding radioimmunoassay for immunoglobulin M anti-hepatitis A virus. J Clin Microbiol 9:120–127
3. Walsh JH, Yalow R, Beeson SA (1970) Detection of Australia antigen and antibody by means of radioimmunoassay techniques. J Infect Dis 121:550–554
4. Bulletin WHO (1970) Viral hepatitis and tests for the Australia (hepatitis-associated) antigen and antibody. Bull WHO 42:957–962
5. Wong DC, Purcell RH, Sreenivasan MA et al. (1980) Epidemic and endemic hepatitis in India: evidence for non-A/non-B hepatitis virus etiology. Lancet II:876–878
6. Bradley DW, Maynard JE (1986) Etiology and natural history of posttransfusion and enterically-transmitted non-A, non-B hepatitis. Semin Liver Dis 6:56–66
7. Bradley DW, Krawczynski K, Kane MA (1991) Enterically-transmitted non-A, non-B hepatitis. In: Belshe RB (ed) Textbook of human virology, 2nd edn. Mosby Year Book, St. Louis, MO, pp 781–790
8. Bradley DW, Krawczynski K, Cook EH et al. (1988) Enterically transmitted non-A, non-B hepatitis: etiology of disease and laboratory studies in nonhuman primates. In: Zuckerman AJ (ed) Viral hepatitis and liver disease. Alan R. Liss, New York, pp 138–147
9. Viswanathan R (1957) Infectious hepatitis in Delhi (1955–56): a critical study: epidemiology. Indian J Med Res 45:1–30
10. Sreenivasan MA, Banerjee K, Pandya PG et al. (1978) Epidemiological investigations of an outbreak of infectious hepatitis in Ahmedabad city during 1975–76. Indian J Med Res 67:197–206
11. Sergeev NW, Paktoris EA, Ananev WA et al. (1957) General characteristics of Botkin's disease occurring in Kirgiz Republic of USSR in 1955–1956. Soviet Healthcare Kirgizii 5:16–23
12. Tandon BN, Joshi YK, Jain SK et al. (1982) An epidemic of non-A, non-B hepatitis in North India. Indian J Med Res 75:739–744
13. Khuroo SM, Duermeyer W, Zargar SA et al. (1983) Acute sporadic non-A/non-B hepatitis in India. Am J Epidemiol 118:360–364

14. Myint H, Soe MM, Khin T et al. (1985) A clinical and epidemiological study of an epidemic of non-A, non-B hepatitis in Rangoon. Am J Trop Med Hyg 34:1183–1189
15. Kane MA, Bradley DW, Shrestha SM et al. (1984) Epidemic non-A, non-B hepatitis in Nepal: recovery of a possible etiologic agent and transmission studies in marmosets. JAMA 252:3140–3145
16. Hillis A, Shrestha SM, Saha NK (1973) An epidemic of infectious hepatitis in the Kathmandu Valley. J Nepal Med Assoc 11:145–151
17. De Cock KM, Bradley DW, Sandford NL et al. (1987) Epidemic non-A, non-B hepatitis in patients from Pakistan. Ann Intern Med 106:227–230
18. Bellabes H, Benatallah A, Bourguermouh A (1984) Non-A/non-B epidemic viral hepatitis in Algeria: strong evidence for its water spread. In: Vyas GN, Dienstag JL, Hoofnagle JH (eds) Viral hepatitis and liver disease. Grune & Stratton, New York, p 637
19. Sarthou JL, Budkowska A, Sharma MD et al. (1976) Characterization of an antigen-antibody system associated with epidemic non-A, non-B hepatitis in West Africa and experimental transmission of an infectious agent to primates. Ann Inst Pasteur Virol 137E:225–232
20. Centers For Disease Control (1987) Enterically transmitted non-A, non-B hepatitis – East Africa. Morbidity and Mortality Weekly Report 36:241–244
21. Centers For Disease Control (1987) Enterically transmitted non-A, non-B hepatitis – Mexico. Morbidity and Mortality Weekly Report 36:597–602
22. Balayan MS, Andjaparidze AG, Savinskaya SS et al. (1983) Evidence for a virus in non-A, non-B hepatitis transmitted via the fecal-oral route. Intervirology 20:23–31
23. Andjaparidze AG, Balayan MS, Savinov AP et al. (1986) Fecal-orally tramsmitted non-A, non-B hepatitis induced in monkeys. Voprosy Virusologii 1:73–80
24. Arankalle VA, Ticehurst J, Sreenivasan MA et al. (1988) Etiological association of a virus-like particle with enterically-transmitted non-A, non-B hepatitis. Lancet II:550–554
25. Bradley DW, Krawczynski K, Cook EH et al. (1987) Enterically transmitted non-A, non-B hepatitis: serial passage of disease in cynomolgus macaques and tamarins and recovery of disease-associated 27–34 nm viruslike particles. Proc Natl Acad Sci USA 84:6277–6281
26. Bradley DW, Andjaparidze A, Cook EH et al. (1988) Aetiological agent of enterically transmitted non-A, non-B hepatitis. J Gen Virol 69:731–738
27. Gupta DN, Smetana HF (1957) The histopathology of viral hepatitis as seen in the Delhi epidemics. Indian J Med Res 45[Suppl]:101–113
28. Morrow RH, Smetana HF, Sai FT et al. (1968) Unusual features of viral hepatitis in Accra, Ghana. Ann Intern Med 68:1250–1264
29. Hillman B, Morris TJ, Kellen WR et al. (1982) An invertebrate calici-like virus: evidence for partial virion disintegration in host excreta. J Gen Virol 60:115–123
30. Krawczynski K, Bradley DW (1989) Enterically transmitted non-A, non-B hepatitis: identification of virus-associated antigen in experimentally infected cynomolgus macaques. J Infect Dis 159:1042–1049
31. Krawczynski K, Bradley DW, Ajdukiewicz A et al. (1991) Virus associated antigen and antibody of epidemic non-A, non-B hepatitis: serology of outbreaks and sporadic cases. In: Shikata T (ed) Proceedings of international symposium on non-A, non-B hepatitis and blood-borne infectious diseases, Tokyo 1989. Elsevier Scientific, Amsterdam, pp 229–236
32. Reyes GR, Purdy MA, Kim JP et al. (1990) Isolation of a cDNA from the virus responsible for enterically transmitted non-A, non-B hepatitis. Science 247:1335–1339

# 14 Viral Hepatitis B and D

S. Gupta and D.A. Shafritz

Although mankind has suffered the ravages of hepatitis from biblical times, it is only in the past three decades that we have begun to understand the nature of the viruses which infect the liver. We can now confidently talk of at least five viruses designated as hepatitis viruses (A, B, C or post-transfusion non-A non-B, D or delta, and E or water-borne epidemic non-A non-B). All cause acute hepatitis. Clinical manifestations alone are insufficient to allow distinction of one virus from another. However, an understanding of the biology and epidemiology of hepatitis viruses has greatly facilitated diagnosis. Hepatitis D virus (HDV) is unique because it is defective and requires hepatitis B virus (HBV) to survive. Both HBV and HDV (as well as HCV) can persist long-term and cause chronic hepatitis, cirrhosis, and/or death. Therefore, recognition of the onset and resolution of HBV or HDV infection are equally important. Moreover, highly effective vaccines against HBV have been developed and means are at hand to prevent HBV altogether and consequently, HDV.

## 1 Hepatitis B Virus and Viral Hepatitis B

In 1965, Blumberg and colleagues identified the surface antigen of HBV in the serum of an Australian Aborigine (originally called Australia antigen, now termed HBsAg) [1]. Following this seminal discovery, HBV was rapidly demonstrated by electron microscopy and recognized as the agent responsible for "serum hepatitis." Human HBV belongs to the hepadna (*hep*atitis-*a*ssociated *dna*) virus family [2]. Unique features of hepadnaviruses include silent infection (often early in life), indefinite viral persistence, curious genomic organization, and a complex replication strategy. Other members exist in the woodchuck, the ground squirrel, the tree squirrel, the heron, and the Pekin duck. Although hepadnaviruses exhibit predilection for hepatocytes, viral replication occurs in a variety of cell types, including hematopoietic cells, bile ductules, pancreas, and kidney.

Hepatitis B virus occurs primarily in liver and serum [3]. Purified preparations from serum demonstrate three types of HBV particle (Fig. 1). The infectious virion is the "Dane particle," which has a diameter of 42 nM. The outer envelope of protein and membrane lipids of this virus surrounds an

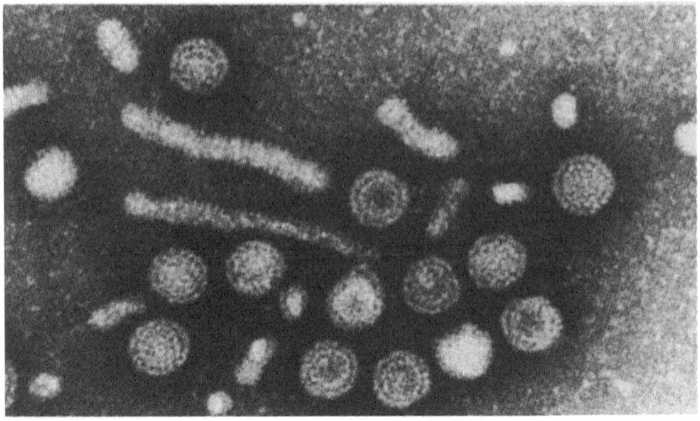

a

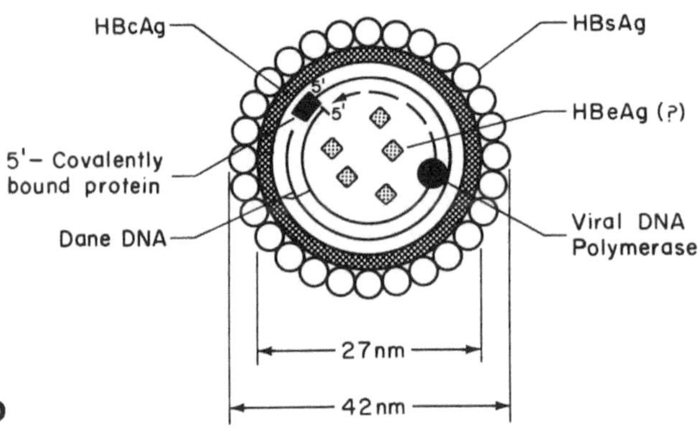


b

**Fig. 1a,b.** Hepatitis B virus particles as found in human serum. **a** Electron micrograph of virion particles (42 nM) and spherical and filamentous forms of HBsAg (22 mM in diameter). **b** A Dane particle (virion) shown schematically.

inner nucleocapsid (27 nM) containing the viral nucleic acid. Spherical particles (16–25 nM) and filaments (22 nM), which exist in $10^3$- to $10^6$-fold excess as compared to complete virions, contain viral proteins and lipids but no viral nucleic acids and are thus noninfectious. All three types of particle display the externally located 24-kd HBsAg glycoprotein. Detergent treatment of Dane particles releases an internal nucleocapsid core composed of a 21-kd basic phosphoprotein termed hepatitis B core antigen (HBcAg). Another protein called hepatitis B e antigen (HBeAg), initially distinguished from HBcAg serologically, may also circulate in patients with HBV. The HBeAg and HBcAg arise independently from a common gene by a unique expression mechanism utilizing an optional initiation site and containing a membrane signal sequence. Nucleocapsid cores are found within the nuclei of infected hepatocytes and are associated with HBV replication.

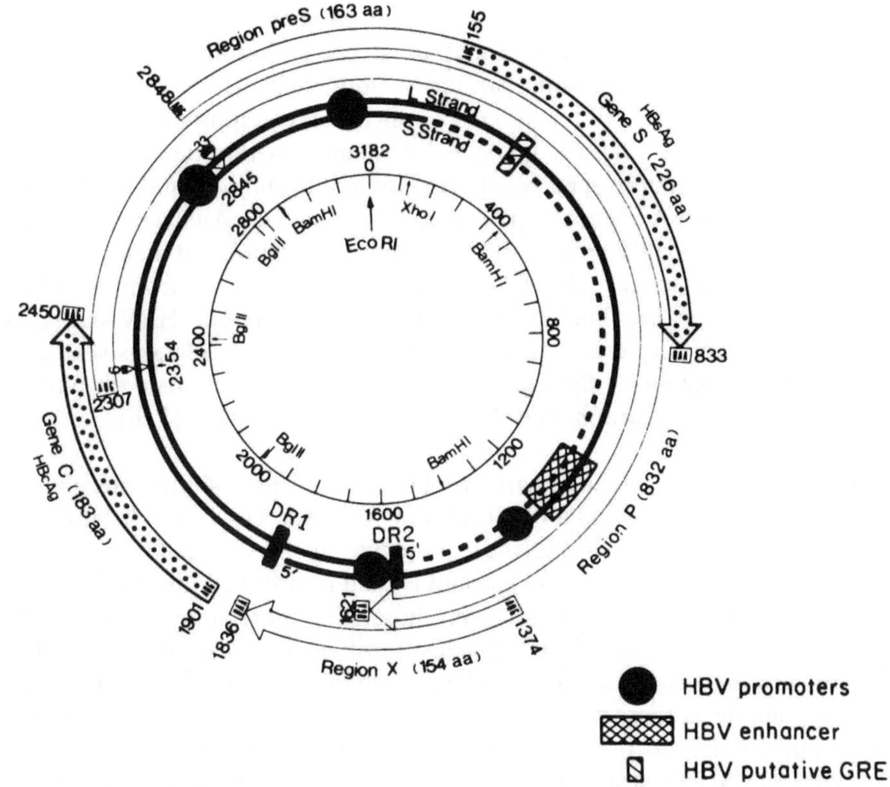


**Fig. 2.** A representative organization of the hepatitis B virus genome. The four transcriptional open reading frames S, C, P, and X are shown. The map positions are arbitrarily assigned, starting with the first nucleotide downstream of the *Eco*R1 cleavage site. The positions of HBV promoters, enhancer, and glucocorticoid responsive element are also indicated

*Genome Organization.* The DNA genome of HBV is circular and 3200–3300 base pairs long (Fig. 2) [4]. It is arranged in two strands, one of which is unit length while the other is shorter. The full-length DNA strand (L) is complementary to viral mRNAs and is designated as minus (−) strand. The short DNA strand (S), which is designated as plus (+) strand, lacks from 15%–50% of its potential sequence complement. Other asymmetries also exist in the HBV DNA molecule. The 5′ end of the (+) strand is located at nucleotide 1560 but its length and consequently the position of its 3′ end varies. The circular structure of the genome is maintained by base pairing of the 5′ termini of both DNA strands, which overlap by about 250–300 nucleotides to form the "cohesive end" region. Endogenous DNA polymerase associated with the nucleocapsid, which is distinct from other known DNA polymerases, repairs this single-stranded region of the (+) strand

DNA. Although in vitro the DNA polymerase does not yield a covalently closed HBV DNA circle, covalently closed circular (ccc) double-stranded DNAs (so-called superhelical forms) have been identified in chronically infected liver. Within the cohesive end region, there are two 11 base pair direct repeats, called DR1 and DR2, which serve important functions in HBV replication. A conserved TATAAA element within the 5′ end of the HBcAg coding sequence specifies the common 3′ termini of viral mRNAs by serving as an RNA cleavage/polyadenylation signal. Analysis of cloned HBV DNAs from different individuals indicates significant heterogeneity in nucleotide sequence. The DNA sequence of particles from an HBV isolate or subtype are homogeneous. However, different HBV subtypes exhibit significant sequence variation with additions and deletions scattered throughout the genome. Spontaneously arising HBV mutants with altered pathogenicity and natural history have also been recognized [5, 6].

*Genome Replication.* Hepadnavirus replication utilizes a unique mechanism (see ref. 2) and was originally elucidated for duck HBV [7]. Briefly, the asymmetric virion DNA inside the hepatocyte nucleus is first converted to ccc DNA. The circular DNA (−) strand is then transcribed into a full-length viral RNA transcript (+) strand, using host RNA polymerase. This RNA, termed the "pregenome," is 3.5 kb because of read-through past the initiation site, producing a terminal redundancy, and the addition of a 3′ poly A tail. The pregenome is then reverse transcribed in the cytoplasm, using a viral coded polymerase, to produce viral (−) strand DNA within core particles. The viral DNA (+) strand is then synthesized within these core particles, but remains incomplete, and the core particles are enveloped by HBs proteins to form virions. A number of complicated steps are involved in hepadnaviral replication, some of which have been partly elucidated. Analogies have been drawn between hepadnaviruses and other viruses, e.g., retroviruses and cauliflower mosaic viruses, because of a shared replication strategy involving reverse transcription. However, hepadnaviruses differ fundamentally from these other viruses, including an absence of long terminal repeats which are characteristic of retroviruses.

*Structural Genes.* Four translational open reading frames (ORFs) located on the (−) HBV DNA strand code for viral proteins [4]. The coding region for HBsAg (ORF S) extends over map positions (mp) 2848–833. An upstream reading frame (ORF pre-S) encodes HBsAg-related virion envelope proteins termed pre-S1 and pre-S2. The coding region for HBcAg (ORF C), mp 1836–2450, is further preceded by an upstream in-phase pre-C region capable of encoding a larger HBcAg-related polypeptide, the HBeAg. The presumptive viral polymerase is encoded by ORF P, mp 2357–1621. Another coding region overlapping ORFs P and C constitutes ORF X, mp 1374–1818. The (+) strand contains short ORFs, but these are not known to produce specific viral proteins.

Two classes of RNAs, 3.5 kb (genomic) and 2.4 or 2.1 kb (subgenomic), serve the replicative and transcription functions of hepadnaviruses [2, 4]. All reported HBV mRNAs are polyadenylated and are derived from the (−) strand. The 5′ end of the 3.5-kb genomic RNA has been mapped to the pre-C region and the 3′ end to the beginning of the C gene, where a specific polyadenylation signal is located. The 2.4-kb mRNAs encode the pre-S1 protein and possibly the pre-S2, S, and X proteins. The 2.1-kb mRNAs code for the pre-S2 and S proteins. Although minor RNA species of larger and smaller sizes have been recognized, specific mRNAs for ORF X or P are yet to be identified. Transcripts of HBV in livers from chronic HBV carriers demonstrate the two major classes of mRNA when both HBc and HBs proteins are expressed [8]. Presence of other candidate mRNAs is also suspected. Novel HBV transcripts, representing fusion mRNAs of viral DNA and flanking cellular sequences, may be found in liver or liver-derived cells containing integrated HBV DNA.

*HBV Gene Products* [2, 4, 9]. The *ORF S* encodes three coterminal proteins. Initially, only a *small* HBs protein (226 amino acids) was recognized in virions. Subsequently, two further proteins were detected, pre-S2 plus S or *middle* (281 amino acids) and pre-S1 plus pre-S2 plus S or *large* (389–400 amino acids, dependent upon viral subtype). Each of these polypeptides can be glycosylated and the native proteins found in virions are homodimers linked through disulfide bridges. The 3′ or S portion of these proteins is constant but the 5′ portion varies, because of the use of different S gene promoter–initiation sites (pre-S1 or pre-S2) or polypeptide processing. The HBs polypeptides are found mainly in 22-nM particles which contain about 25% lipid derived from host cytoplasmic phospholipids, free and esterified cholesterol, and small amounts of triglycerides [9]. Approximately 90% of the S gene product on the virion surface is small HBs. The filamentous forms of HBs in serum have a similar composition, but the 20-nM spherical particles contain very little large HBs. In the absence of viral replication, spherical particles contain less than 1% middle HBs and no large HBs. In highly viremic HBV carriers, the proportion of middle HBs may approach 5%–10% [9].

The HBs protein contains a major group-specific antigenic determinant called *a* and subtype determinants *d*, *y*, *w*, and *r*, producing four main serotypes *adw*, *ayw*, *adr*, and *ayr*. Each viral subtypes has a separate worldwide distribution and provides markers for epidemiologic studies. An exposed hydrophilic region of small HBs between amino acids 120 and 148 is responsible for the group and subtype specificity. Major B cell epitopes of this region are conformational and dependent upon disulfide bonds. However, development of HBV vaccines has required consideration of complexities related to antigen presentation, including molecular assembly, size, and denaturation state.

Various HBs proteins are secreted by different mechanisms. Small HBs protein is extruded into the endoplasmic reticulum with an amino-terminal signal peptide. Middle HBs protein utilizes the first signal sequence within the S domain for this translocation. Although small HBs is rapidly secreted from cells, as compared to pre-S1 protein, secretion of the viral particles may require up to 24 h [9]. In cells producing excess large HBs, the pre-S1 moiety may prevent secretion. Cells retaining large HBs comprise the "ground-glass" hepatocytes observed in long-term HBV carriers [10] and contain filamentous forms of HBsAg. A small proportion (<3%) of large HBs has no influence upon the morphology of spherical particles but a moderate proportion (10%–20%) generates filamentous structures. Particles containing >20% pre-S1 protein are probably not secreted [9]. However, regulation of large HBs expression is not fully understood.

The pre-S2 region encodes a species-specific receptor for polymerized serum albumin [9]. The role of the immune response elicited by the pre-S2 domain is unclear. Early or biphasic appearance of pre-S2 antibodies in acute hepatitis B, including persistence in chronic hepatitis, has been reported. The large pre-S1 polypeptide binds to hepatocyte membranes and is thought to be involved in attachment of virion particles to a specific hepatocyte receptor [9].

The *ORF C* contains two functional initiation codons which encode the HBc (22-kd) and HBe (15- to 16-kd) proteins [4]. Due to posttranslational modification and processing, a series of intermediate proteins are initially produced ranging from 15 to 25 kd. Nucleocapsids enclosing HBV DNA are composed primarily of HBc protein and are called core particles. The C-terminus of core antigen is rich in arginine, serine, and proline residues and contains a tandem repeat of an octapeptide which resembles protein sequences of DNA binding proteins. During viral replication, HBc protein packages the pregenomic RNA and viral polymerase. In addition, an endogenous protein kinase activity is present in hepadnavirus core particles. This leads to phosphorylation of the HBc protein at multiple residues, although its significance is unknown [4].

The 5′ end of ORF C (pre-C region) contains a short, in-phase sequence with an ATG codon ~80 nucleotides upstream of the core ATG that serves as the initiation site for HBeAg [9]. Initially, a 25-kd HBe protein is produced and enters the secretory pathway. The N-terminal residues are cleaved, resulting in a 23-kd protein (p23). The processed p23 is located transmembranously and is additionally modified to be secreted as p16–p20, dependent upon HBV subtype. Unlike HBc protein, the HBeAg does not contain glycosylation sites [9]. Although HBeAg was detected 20 years ago in sera from chronic hepatitis B carriers [11], its function remains unknown.

Much less is known about the expression of the *ORFs X and P* and their products [2, 4]. The ORF X could encode a polypeptide of 154 residues (~15 kd). Both genomic and subgenomic mRNAs contain X sequences. Evidence for X gene expression in natural HBV infection was recently obtained [12]. Antibodies against synthetic X-peptides recognize a 17-kd protein in infected livers. The ORF X is now known to encode two other proteins (8 and 6 kd). However, attempts to demonstrate either a nuclear or a cytoplasmic subcellular location for the putative X gene product have produced conflicting results. The ORF P protein product was recently identified as a putative 70-kd protein with reverse transcriptase activity [2]. Presence of antibodies in human sera against ORF P domains indicate that this ORF is expressed. Other viral proteins include a protein covalently bound to the (−) DNA strand which serves as a primer for viral replication and a protein kinase which can phosphorylate HBc protein. At least three additional viral proteins containing sequences from ORFs C and P are known.

*Cis- and Trans-Acting Elements Regulating HBV Gene Expression.* Several putative HBV promoters have been identified [2, 4]: pre-S1 (mp 2786–2791) with a TATAA element, pre-S2 (mp 3122–3130) with an SV40 promoter-like sequence, core (mp 1653–1660), which does not contain a TATAA element, and a promoter for X (mp 1374–1418). An enhancer element has been located at mp 1080–1234 [2]. The HBV enhancer regulates homologous (HBV) or heterologous (SV40) promoters and may confer tissue-specific expression. A second enhancer has recently been identified just proximal to the core gene. A glucocorticoid responsive element (GRE) is also present in HBV [13]. This GRE, located at mp 355–366, contains all but the first nucleotide of the core consensus sequence ACAA—GT$^{T}_{C}$CT found in the 5′-regulatory region of other glucocorticoid responsive genes. Termination of viral transcription may be regulated by a conserved TATAAA element within the ORF C [4] which is known to be critical for RNA cleavage and polyadenylation.

The ORF X of HBV occupies a position similar to the transactivating *tat* gene of HIV which is necessary for replication. The X protein may transactivate a variety of viral enhancer and promoter elements [14]. It has been suggested that the X protein interacts with other transcription factors, such as AP-1 or cEBP, which are DNA binding proteins that activate RNA polymerase II. A synergistic effect of X-transactivator or the HIV-1 *tat* gene may be governed by specific cellular factors. As the HBV enhancer influences surface and core promoters, stimulation of the HBV enhancer by X protein may have broad effects upon viral gene expression. Transactivating factors could play a major role in determining the hepatotropism and/or persistence of HBV by modulating viral gene expression. Similar mechanisms could interfere with HBV expression during intercurrent infection, such as with HDV. In view of the importance of these regulatory elements and factors, much current research is focused on the organization and function of regulatory sequences in the HBV genome.

### 1.1 Epidemiology

The high burden of HBV in certain parts of the world has assigned to hepatitis B a major public health importance. In addition, epidemiologic studies were pivotal in suggesting a relationship between HBV and hepatocellular carcinoma [15, 16].

The prevalence of HBV varies [16]. The HBsAg carrier rates in low endemic areas (e.g., 0.1%–0.2% in the United States, United Kingdom, and parts of Western Europe) contrast with areas of moderate endemicity (2%–5% in Spain, Italy, Japan, and Greece) or high endemicity (11%–15% in South Africa, Taiwan, and Hong Kong). In certain isolated communities, prevalence of HBV infection, indicated by any positive serologic marker, is astonishingly high (45%–76% by 19 years of age in Alaskan Eskimos [17] and Australian Aborigines [18]). The prevalence of antibody to HBsAg (anti-HBs), indicating past exposure to HBV, increases with age in the general population in a pattern consistent with the overall regional endemicity of HBV. Other apparent risk factors include situations where close interpersonal contact is inevitable, such as institutionalized individuals (mentally retarded, prisoners, etc.) or household contacts, intravenous drug abusers who share needles, hemodialysis patients in high-use units, intimate homo- or heterosexual contacts, frequent blood contact in a health-care setting, and poor socioeconomic circumstances. Despite screening of donor blood, 5%–10% of posttransfusion hepatitis is still HBV related.

The magnitude of the problem is indicated by the estimated annual incidence of about 200000 primary HBV infections in the United States alone. Over 10000 of these individuals require hospital care and 250 die of fulminant hepatitis. In the United States (a low-risk area), the lifetime risk of HBV infection for the general population is estimated at 5%, but this may approach 100% for high-risk populations. Some 6%–10% of cases develop chronic hepatitis B. As a result, there may be up to 800000 chronic HBV carriers in the United States and more than 250 million worldwide. Although about 1% chronic carriers may lose HBV annually, in most cases it is a lifelong affliction.

Very young age is a most important factor predisposing to persistent HBV infection. Before the introduction of HBsAg vaccine, persistent infection was virtually invariable in newborn or young infants born to HBV carrier mothers; such cases accounted for 40%–50% of HBV carriers in Taiwan [19]. The HBsAg carrier state is also frequent in immunosuppressed populations or patients with certain disorders, such as Down's syndrome, lepromatous leprosy, and chronic lymphocytic leukemia. The dose of infecting virus correlates with the probability of developing viral persistence. In experimental studies, lower doses of virus resulted in long incubation periods, anicteric or mild initial disease, and certain unexpected consequences, including chronic infection. There is no evidence that various HBV subtypes have different propensities for viral persistence. However, mutant forms of HBV were recently recognized in long-term carriers and can cause severe or fulminant hepatitis [5].

### *Routes of Transmission*

Humans constitute the source of infection. Infection is either blood-borne or through contaminated body fluids (saliva or semen) containing infectious virus. However, mere presence of the virus in a body fluid is insufficient for infection. Failure to detect HBsAg in blood does not exclude the presence of infectious HBV. There is no environmental reservoir of HBV and transmission is neither enteric nor respiratory. Contaminated razors, toothbrushes, needles, or sharp implements as for tattooing, acupuncture, ear piercing, or dental treatment have been incriminated.

Transmission is mainly either through percutaneous transfer or intimate, sexual contact. In homosexuals, who are particularly at risk for HBV, infection is related to the duration of homosexual activity, number of sexual partners, and frequency of anal contact. In households with infected members, transmission is commonest among sexual partners, although it also occurs between siblings. In populations with high HBV carrier rates, sexual transfer is probably a common source of infection. Health care personnel who are regularly exposed to infected material, e.g., workers in renal dialysis units, surgeons or dentists, etc., are at high risk for HBV infection. Conversely, chronic HBV-carrier health care workers have been implicated in transmission of HBV to patients, although such risk should be small. Contaminated endoscopes have also been incriminated.

Experimentally, HBV infection after oral intake of infectious material has been demonstrated, although this is not considered a significant route of transmission. Infection occurs due to transfer through breaks in mucosa. Insect vectors, such as mosquitoes, have not been shown to transmit HBV although mosquitoes and bedbugs containing HBsAg have been found.

In highly endemic areas, transmission from HBV carrier mothers to their progeny is important [19]. Only 5%–10% of these cases result from infection in utero. Exposure to maternal blood at the time of delivery or during the perinatal period is believed to be the commonest route of infection. Further intimate contact between mothers and infected siblings may account for transmission of infection during early childhood. High concentrations of circulating Dane particles during the last trimester of pregnancy or neonatal period and the late incubation period of acute hepatitis B correlate with infectivity [19].

## 1.2 Virus–Host Interactions

The host range of HBV is limited to humans and captive chimpanzees exposed to humans. Chimpanzees are highly susceptible to HBV and exhibit disease patterns similar to humans. Natural infection of animals with other hepadnaviruses, e.g., duck, groundsquirrel, or woodchuck, have provided much useful information regarding the replication and oncogenic potential of these viruses. Recently, systems have become available which provide powerful means for addressing questions including those related to virus–host interactions, i.e., transgenic mice containing integrated copies of cloned HBV genomes, HBV replication in successfully infected cultured primary hepatocytes, and chronic HBV carrier states in immunodeficient mice.

### *Patterns of HBV Infection and Serologic Responses*

The vast majority of HBV infections are anicteric and probably inapparent. Acute HBV infection involves the bulk of hepatocytes. Most primary acute infections are self-limited and resolve spontaneously. However, the spectrum of ensuing hepatitis ranges from mild with little morbidity to fatal fulminant hepatitis. In other instances, HBV is not cleared and leads to the asymptomatic carrier state, chronic hepatitis, or progression to cirrhosis and liver failure. Serologic testing has facilitated recognition of various outcomes. Chronic persistence may be associated with continued virus replication, inactivation of viral replication (latency) or reactivation – either spontaneously or due to immunosuppression. Hepatocellular carcinoma may develop; long-term male HBV carriers are at the greatest risk for hepatocellular carcinoma.

*Serologic Response to HBV.* In *acute HBV infection*, HBsAg is the first viral marker to appear in blood and may be detected within 1–2 weeks of exposure (Fig. 3). When HBV infection is self-limited, HBsAg generally persists for 1–6 weeks, although it may last longer. Clinical hepatitis usually manifests 1–7 weeks after appearance of HBsAg. Interestingly, if HBsAg remains positive for less than 7 weeks, symptomatic hepatitis is uncommon. The duration of HBsAg positivity tends to correlate with the severity of hepatitis. In symptomatic patients with hepatitis, HBsAg is usually cleared when symptoms and jaundice have resolved. At this time, antibody to HBsAg (anti-HBs) appears, although it may not peak for several months. Anti-HBs is of particular significance because it protects against subsequent HBV infection and lasts for years. In about 50% of patients with self-limited acute hepatitis, anti-HBs may not be detected for up to many months. In another 10%, in whom HBsAg is cleared rapidly, anti-HBs may never appear. The significance of this is unclear. In a number of cases, anti-HBs appears during the prodromal phase before the onset of clinical hepatitis. When this occurs, immune complexes form with HBsAg and patients may develop arthritis or skin rash as discussed below.

The second viral protein to appear in the circulation, HBeAg, appears either simultaneously or within a few days of HBsAg (Fig. 3). Subsequently, its concentration rises and declines concurrently with HBsAg. However,

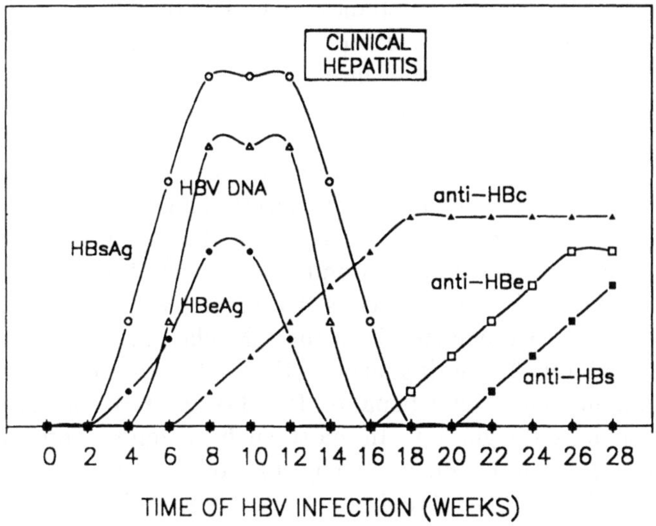


**Fig. 3.** A schematic depiction of the serologic response following initial exposure to HBV. See text for details

HBeAg disappears earlier than HBsAg, generally within the first 10 weeks from the onset of symptoms. In other instances, HBeAg/anti-HBe seroconversion may be delayed by several months. Longer persistence of HBeAg is associated with the onset of persistent infection. Anti-HBe appears either when HBeAg is cleared or within a few days. Presence of HBeAg and absence of anti-HBe indicates viral replication and infectivity. However, conclusions regarding the amount of virus production or HBV replication state on the basis of HBeAg/anti-HBe status are not entirely valid [20]. This was recently shown to be due to spontaneous mutations in the precore region of the HBV genome which prevented expression of the HBeAg but still permitted virus replication [5, 6].

Virion particles containing HBV DNA, as well as DNA polymerase, appear next. Detection of these markers requires assays for polymerase activity or molecular hybridization for HBV DNA. Unfortunately, these tests are technically complex and not available in most hospital laboratories. In self-limited HBV infection, HBV DNA and polymerase activity peak during the late incubation phase and disappear when hepatitis ensues (Fig. 3). Presence of HBV DNA correlates with replicating and infectious HBV; this marker is superior to the HBeAg/anti-HBe system [20]. Presence of HBV DNA beyond 4 weeks of acute hepatitis represents delayed clearance of virus and often leads to chronic persistence (defined as presence of HBsAg in serum for a period of 6 months or greater). In immunosuppressed patients, when viremia is marked, serum HBV DNA levels may be high, even though a relationship between liver necrosis or inflammation, cellular immune function, and circulating HBV DNA may be lacking. Antibodies against the middle or large HBs proteins, designated anti-pre-S, are also detected [10]. Initial studies suggested that these antibodies appear at the time HBV DNA is cleared in acute hepatitis. However, this response is of little prognostic significance because anti-pre-S may be present transiently or continuously in patients with high levels of serum HBV DNA and progression to cirrhosis.

Anti-HBc, which is directed against HBcAg located in hepatocyte nuclei, appears in all patients during the late incubation phase (Fig. 3). This antibody appears 3–5 weeks after HBsAg and peaks rapidly. Anti-HBc appears before anti-HBs and also persists for several years. Much of the anti-HBc is of the IgG class. However, early in the course of its evolution, the anti-HBc detected is of the IgM class [21]. The latter antibody is most useful for diagnosing acute HBV infection. For example, a number of patients with acute hepatitis B, who are HBsAg negative, may otherwise remain undiagnosed. In most such patients, anti-HBc IgM is positive. The IgM anti-HBc is also useful for recognizing acute exacerbations or recurrence of HBV replication in chronic HBV carriers, who remain HBsAg positive. However, as the half-life of IgM anti-HBc is prolonged, HBV DNA is superior for recognizing closely spaced, distinct episodes of hepatitis B reactivation [22].

Of various HBV markers, HBV DNA may be detected in patients who are either anti-HBs positive or without any serologic evidence of previous HBV infection. Amplification of HBV DNA by the polymerase chain reaction (PCR) may further increase test sensitivity (e.g., $\sim 10^4$ fold more sensitive than slot-blot hybridization). Therefore, immunologic tests of HBV have certain limitations, particularly when viral antigens and their specific antibodies coexist. The formation of immune complexes may interfere with competitive binding enzyme-linked immunosorbent assays or radioimmunoassays, although immune complexes may be detected with monoclonal antibodies to HBsAg.

*Persistent HBV infection* develops when HBsAg remains positive 24 weeks after acute hepatitis. Such individuals are designated chronic HBsAg carriers. The serologic evolution of the carrier state is depicted in Fig. 4. The patients carry HBsAg and anti-HBs does not appear, although the latter may be present at low levels in rare instances. Anti-HBc of the IgG class is found, often at high concentrations. In about 50% of these cases, HBV DNA or viral polymerase is found in the blood, at surprisingly high levels in about 10%. HBcAg is invariably detected in hepatocytes. With HBV replication, IgM anti-HBc is detected at high concentrations. In the absence of viral mutations described above, HBeAg is positive, whereas anti-HBe is absent. Patients who are positive for HBV DNA, IgM anti-HBc, or HBeAg may retain infectious potential, depending on the concentration of virion particles.

The natural history of persistent HBV infection encompasses a variety of outcomes, some of which are incompletely defined. The HBsAg titers and markers of viral replication may persist at a steady level for years, even

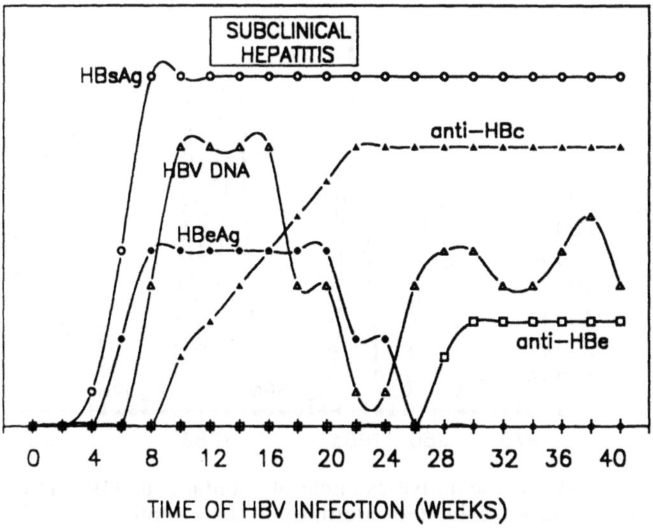


**Fig. 4.** Serologic pattern during development of persistent HBV infection. The replicative state of HBV determines the presence and concentration of HBV DNA, viral polymerase activity, HBeAg/anti-HBe, and IgM anti-HBc. These viral markers may persist unchanged, subside for variable periods, or reappear as a result of viral reactivation

lifelong, or somewhat more commonly, decline slowly. About 10% of the chronic HBV carriers spontaneously lose HBV DNA polymerase or HBeAg each year. Spontaneous clearance of all HBV markers, including HBsAg, occurs in about 1% each year. Spontaneous clearance of HBV may be quicker in females than in males, but the factors regulating this are unknown.

Replication of HBV may continue long-term in chronic HBV carriers or may resume following a period of interruption. Recently, spontaneous reactivation of HBV replication was recognized in chronic HBV carriers. Following initial loss of viral replication (with disappearance of HBV DNA, viral polymerase, HBeAg, or IgM anti-HBc), these markers reappear (Fig. 5) [22]. Spontaneous reactivation has epidemiologic and pathophysiologic significance. Various estimates suggest that reactivation in chronic HBsAg carriers may approach a 10%–35% annual incidence. In endemic areas, spontaneous reactivation may mimic primary acute HBV infection. Reactivation may lead to fatal fulminant hepatitis, a rapid downhill course, or worsening of chronic liver disease and could be recurrent. It is suggested that histologic progression of liver disease is particularly florid during, or as a consequence of, reactivation. Immunosuppression, cancer chemotherapy, or corticosteroids may also enhance viral replication, leading to secondary reactivation of HBV. Antiviral drugs, e.g., α-interferon or adenine arabinoside, have been demonstrated to inhibit HBV replication in chronic HBV carriers. Nevertheless, therapeutic trials of these and other agents in chronic

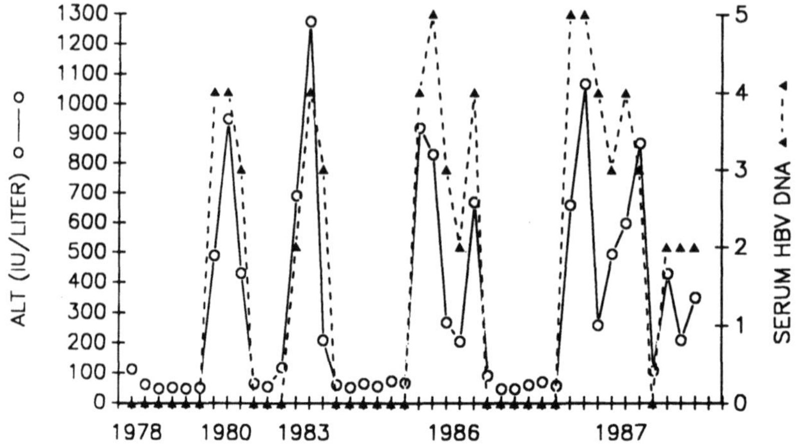


**Fig. 5.** A representative example of spontaneous HBV reactivation. This long-term HBsAg carrier exhibited intermittent HBV replication as indicated by serum HBV DNA (*dashed line*). Viral reactivation was accompanied by marked elevation of serum alanine aminotransferase (*solid line*). There were no significant symptoms during these episodes. Liver biopsies demonstrated chronic active hepatitis with progression of fibrosis over time. The last episode of reactivation caused unremitting subacute liver failure and proved fatal

hepatitis B may be confounded due to reactivation which may begin or terminate unpredictably.

Intercurrent infection may influence the natural history of the chronic HBV carrier state. In particular, HIV coinfection leads to increase in HBV replication, presumably due to depletion of immune effector cells. However, in homosexual men chronically infected with HIV and HBV, a relationship between cellular immune function and circulating HBV DNA is lacking. Simultaneous infection of chronic HBV carriers with HDV or hepatitis A virus, on the other hand, may suppress HBV replication. Understanding of mechanisms regulating these events requires further study.

Chronic HBV carriers may not have detectable HBsAg in blood and yet have persistent HBV infection. Recipients of blood from HBsAg negative and anti-HBc positive donor blood have been known to acquire HBV infection [23]. It is believed in such instances that HBV may be present intermittently and this can now be detected by sensitive PCR techniques. Other chronic HBV carriers have been reported who, during the course of several years, have lost all serologic markers of HBV. If encountered at this stage, liver disease in such patients would be considered as cryptogenic cirrhosis.

Once HBV is cleared with development of anti-HBs, lifelong immunity may be acquired against reinfection. Subsequent exposure to HBV results in a prompt and marked rise in anti-HBs titer. The *protective immune response* is the basis for the success of vaccination against HBV. Anti-HBs is primarily of anti-a specificity and provides protection against all HBV subtypes. Rarely, however, second infections with HBV have occurred either with the same or a different subtype. It is believed in these cases that a large viral load during reinfection could overcome the protective immune response. Following vaccination with an HBsAg vaccine, only anti-HBs is produced. Experimental studies indicate that anti-HBc or anti-HBe may also confer protection. However, the significance of this latter phenomenon in natural infection is not known.

### *Cellular Immune Response to HBV*

Absence of liver injury in some chronic HBV carriers suggested that HBV is not directly cytopathic. However, when liver cells were made to produce HBcAg in vitro, cell growth and function were impaired. Recently, transgenic mouse hepatocytes retaining filamentous forms of the large HBsAg were found to develop necrosis, degeneration, focal nodular hyperplasia, and liver cancer [24]. The precise mechanism for these events, however, remains unclear.

Specific cellular immune responses against HBV antigens have been described. Occurrence of severe hepatitis in agammaglobulinemic patients indicates that liver necrosis due to HBV is independent of the humoral immune response. Peripheral blood cells from chronic HBV carriers were shown to be cytotoxic to autologous hepatocytes in vitro, an event which was blocked by anti-HBs. Available evidence indicates that HBsAg proteins do not constitute a stimulus for cytotoxic T lymphocytes, although this has not been rigorously excluded. It is currently believed that HBcAg mediates cell lysis via cytotoxic T lymphocytes. During the latter part of the incubation period and early phase of acute hepatitis, immunofluorescence studies have shown that all infected hepatocytes express both HBsAg and HBcAg. Also, in chronic HBV carriers with no viral replication or HBcAg production, livers may be histologically normal. Sensitized cytotoxic T lymphocytes lyse hepatocytes displaying HBcAg in association with class I HLA molecules. One mechanism for viral persistence is believed to involve overproduction of HBeAg, which shares lymphocyte receptor sites with HBcAg [25]. Blockage of the receptor sites on cytotoxic T lymphocytes with HBeAg could lead to the infected cells escaping, even though HBcAg is displayed. However, virus–host interactions regulating persistence of HBV are poorly defined.

## 1.3 Replicating and Nonreplicating States of Persistent HBV Infection

Two states of HBV infection may occur during chronic persistence: permissive and nonpermissive [26]. During the replicating or permissive phase, serum HBsAg and HBV DNA are positive. Hepatocytes display HBsAg and HBcAg. Periportal lymphocytes are either helper T cells or cytotoxic/

suppressor T cells. Rapid progression of hepatic inflammation occurs and patients are infectious. During the nonpermissive phase, serum HBsAg is positive but HBV DNA is negative and HBcAg is not produced. Periportal infiltrates include helper T or B lymphocytes. Active liver inflammation is absent (histologic evidence of HBV may be limited to ground-glass hepatocytes or inactive cirrhosis) and HBcAg is usually negative with presence of anti-HBe.

In the replicative phase, HBV DNA in hepatocytes is mainly in free virion or replicating forms and integration into host genome is not evident. In the nonreplicating phase, random integrations occur, replicative forms of free virion DNA are not found, and HBV is not secreted. In some cases, unit length HBV molecules have been found in the liver. In other nonpermissive infections, clusters of HBsAg-producing cells, having the appearance of a focal clonal growth, have been noted. In these cases, HBV has been identified in liver DNA integrated into the host genome. A mixed type of persistent infection may also occur with features of both replicating and nonreplicating infection in the same liver. In cases with impaired or blocked secretion of HBV, replicative intermediates and extrachromosomal forms may accumulate, facilitating HBV DNA integration [27]. As discussed below, viral DNA integration has been associated with HCC in chronic HBV carriers.

### 1.4 HBV and Hepatocellular Carcinoma

Worldwide, increased HBsAg carrier rates are associated with a greater incidence of hepatocellular carcinoma (HCC). The most convincing epidemiologic evidence was obtained in 22707 Taiwanese government employees in whom HBV carriers had a 217-fold greater relative risk for HCC (113 cases) compared to HBsAg negative controls (3 cases) [16]. Similar conclusions were reached from a study of Japanese railroad workers. Conversely, patients with HCC demonstrated a high prevalence of HBV. Association between persistent hepadnavirus infection and HCC also exists in animal model systems, particularly in woodchucks. On average, HCC is detected 20 or more years after HBV infection. However, HCC has developed within 4 years from birth in a Japanese HBV carrier [28]. Integration of HBV DNA has been reported in HCC tissue and adjacent liver regions in most HBV carriers who develop tumors. Despite enormous efforts, however, the basis for this association remains obscure.

#### *HBV DNA Integration in Hepatocellular Carcinoma*

Most tumors from HBsAg positive patients show HBV DNA integrated in unique patterns varying with individual tumors [29]. Free viral DNA may be noted and indicates either continued viral replication or mingling of

HBV containing hepatocytes into the tumor tissue. Initial reports that HCC related to alcoholic cirrhosis with no HBV markers also contains integrated HBV DNA have not been confirmed [30].

Detailed analysis of integrated HBV DNA from tumor-derived cell lines, hepatic tumors, and chronically infected woodchuck livers has provided essentially similar information. The structure of integrated HBV DNA sequences varies from relatively simple unit length molecules to multiple rearrangements, including deletions of viral and/or adjacent cellular sequences, inversions, and direct or inverted duplications [2, 4]. In general, HBV DNA integrations are oriented such that the viral coding domains are often interrupted. Some HBV DNA integrations in HCC contain a greater than unit length HBV DNA sequence with an apparently intact copy of the genome. Extrachromosomal high molecular weight "novel" forms of viral DNA have also been reported. It has been suggested that these novel forms may represent by-products of defective genome replication during viral persistence and could represent precursors of integrations involved in HCC. Suggestions that a specific sequence within the DR1 and DR2 regions are frequently involved in a recombination event have not been substantiated. Whether specific cellular sites exist where HBV DNA preferentially integrates, such as in repetitive DNA sequences or specific histone-rich regions of cellular DNA, is unclear. Whether the X protein or transactivating fusion proteins arising from X and flanking cellular sequences play a role in oncogenesis is also unresolved.

### *HBV-Directed Mutagenesis*

Several tumor viruses function either by directly transferring oncogenes or activating proto-oncogenes in recipient cells. Recently, HBV integrations were found adjacent to or in the coding regions of *erbA* proto-oncogene [31], which is structurally related to the steroid receptor, or a cyclin gene, which regulates the cell cycle [32]. Nevertheless, augmented expression of these genes as a result of HBV DNA integration has not been demonstrated. Other HBV integrations in HCC have been found on a number of chromosomes, including 2, 3, 7, 9, 11, 12, 15, and 18, with also a translocation between chromosomes 17 q and 18 q [33]. However, hepadnaviruses do not contain an oncogene and HBV DNA has failed to transform cells in vitro, indicating that HBV is probably not directly oncogenic.

An alternative hypothesis has emerged with the recognition of recessive anti-oncogenes, loss of both alleles of which may lead to tumorigenesis [33]. This hypothesis gained substantiation in studies of retinoblastoma and Wilms' tumor when a recessive antioncogene was lost, leading to tumor development. An HBV integration has been found on chromosome 11p13, a region close to the Wilms' tumor locus. Loss of this region leads to Beckwith-Wiedemann syndrome (multisystem organomegaly, hepatoblastoma, and HCC). Loss of heterozygosity at chromosome 17p13, near the p53 locus which is a tumor suppressor gene, has also been found in HCC. Recent studies have shown enhanced expression of insulin-like growth factor II, which is normally expressed in fetal liver, in some HCCs in woodchuck hepatitis virus carriers [33]. Whether this increased expression is a cause or a result of hepatocellular transformation remains to be determined.

### *HBV, Proto-oncogenes, and Hepatocellular Carcinoma*

Among commonly expressed proto-oncogenes in HCC, genes of the *ras* and *myc* families are prevalent; several other genes have also been identified. C-Ha-*ras*, N-*ras*, and c-*myc* are expressed in HCC. Rearrangements or amplification of *ras* genes may be found. Another transforming gene, *hst*, which produces a putative growth factor, has been isolated from HCC. Besides known oncogenes which might be involved in HCC, a presumptive liver-derived oncogene, termed *lca*, was isolated from HCC. The transforming activity of *lca* is considerably less than that of other oncogenes. Whether this unique gene is involved in the pathogenesis of HCC also remains to be demonstrated.

To date, HBV DNA sequences have not been found to enhance proto-oncogene expression. In fact, expression of c-Ha-*ras* and c-*myc* genes in HCC is similar irrespective of the presence of integrated HBV DNA. This indicates that the probable mechanism by which HBV leads to HCC does not involve an effect of the virus upon these proto-oncogenes. The prolonged latency between HBV infection and HCC also argues that HBV does not carry an oncogene.

The demonstration that HBV DNA integrates into the host genome by itself does not prove that HBV is a complete carcinogen. Were neoplasia to occur frequently in HBV-infected livers and were HBV DNA integration to be equally frequent, then HCCs would often contain integrated HBV DNA by chance alone. This does not absolve HBV from a role in HCC but merely implies that neoplasia may result from epigenetic mechanisms.

## 1.5 Pathology

The essential pathologic features of viral hepatitis are independent of etiology. A combination of cell necrosis, inflammatory reaction, and hepatocellular regeneration is characteristic [35]. The overall histologic pattern is affected by the severity of viral hepatitis, age of the patient, integrity of immune function, and previous liver disease. Various criteria adopted have been generally adequate for diagnosis of viral hepatitis, but prognostic interpretation of changes has been difficult. Liver biopsy is only rarely necessary for diagnosing acute viral hepatitis.

In *acute viral hepatitis* (Fig. 6a), generalized hepatocyte necrosis occurs virtually simultaneously with the appearance of an inflammatory cell infiltrate. Cell necrosis tends to be accentuated in the centrilobular region. Surviving cells retain their glycogen. Fatty change is unusual. Cholestasis may be found. Necrotic hepatocytes may be densely eosinophilic, appear shrunken, may be surrounded by macrophages, and eventually drop out of the hepatic cords (apoptosis). The inflammatory infiltrate is composed predominantly of lymphocytes, monocytes, neutrophils, and eosinophils. Proliferation of existing lymphoid or Kupffer cells also occurs. The inflammatory cell exudate is marked in portal areas and often extends across the limiting plate into regions of cell necrosis within the lobule and sinusoidal spaces. The amount of inflammatory reaction varies from minimal to massive. Overzealous interpretation of marked necrosis and excessive inflammatory reaction may lead to a mistaken label of chronic active hepatitis. This difficulty may be compounded by the existence of substantial collagen due to preexisting liver disease.

Regenerative activity is noted by the time hepatitis becomes symptomatic. Ballooned, hydropic cells may disrupt the hepatic cord pattern [35]. Later in the course of acute hepatitis, hepatocytolysis may be circumscribed with further accentuation of the regenerative changes. The cholestatic variant of acute hepatitis is evidenced by bile plugs within dilated bile canaliculi, cholangiolar proliferation, and accumulation of lipofuscin pigment in Kupffer cells.

In *fulminant hepatitis*, extensive collapse of the hepatic stroma occurs, followed by exuberant regenerative activity at the time of recovery [35]. There is little or no continuing focal hepatocytolysis. The inflammatory response is not excessive, usually being attenuated. Several months later, the lobular architecture but not the cord pattern may be regained. However, despite this deviation from the normal architectural organization in fulminant hepatitis, recovery is complete and postnecrotic cirrhosis does not develop. Less severe hepatitis, which is not associated with hepatic coma, may demonstrate similar though relatively less marked changes. However, in the older patient the histologic pattern may differ. As a result of less active hepatocellular regeneration, recovery from severe hepatitis is slow and may be lacking. There is less distortion of hepatic architecture as the hepatic cord pattern is not altered by hepatocellular proliferation. Massive and submassive hepatic necrosis may cause a clinically fulminant course in patients over 40 years of age.

In severe hepatitis, the collapse of stroma may extend from portal to central areas of from portal to portal areas, a feature termed *bridging necrosis* (Fig. 6b). In a series including a large number of patients over 40 years of age, bridging hepatic necrosis was associated with a prolonged course and high mortality [36]. However, it is believed that bridging necrosis may not carry the same prognostic significance in younger patients, who have a greater regenerative potential [35]. Patients with submassive hepatic necrosis, especially when older, may exhibit less severe initial disease but have a slowly progressive course resulting in death. In these instances, little

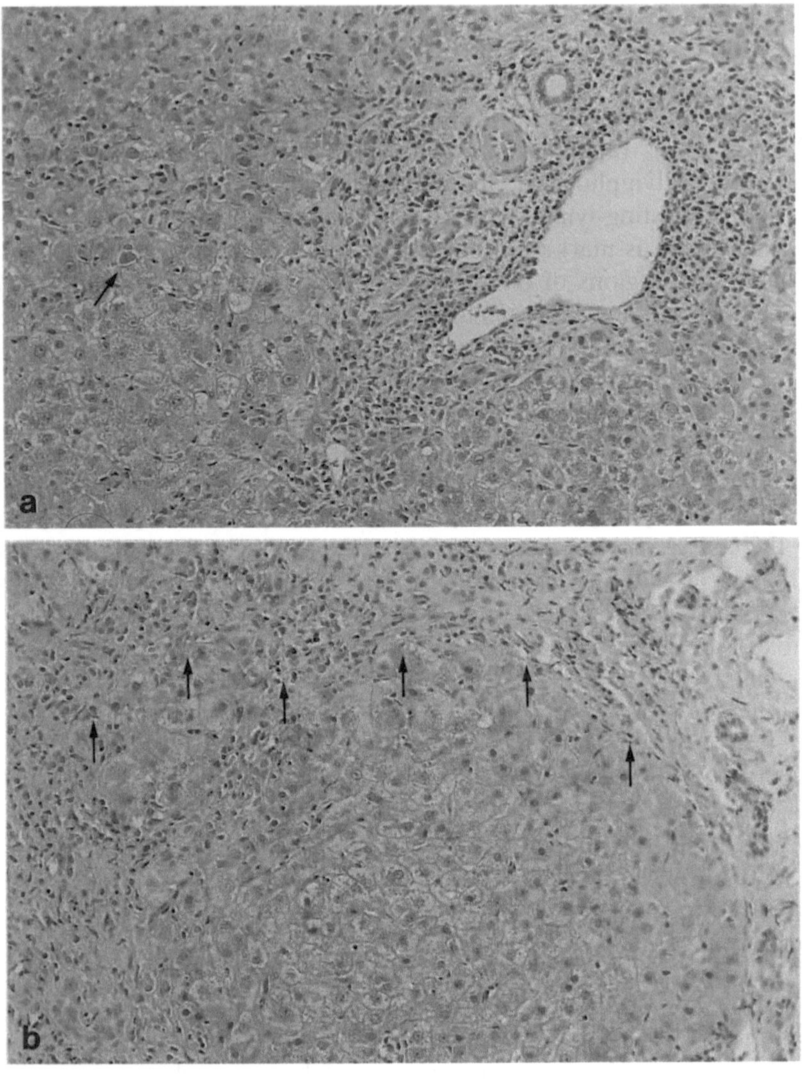

**Fig. 6. a** Acute hepatitis. The lobular parenchyma and portal tracts are diffusely infiltrated by lymphocytes. The hepatocytes demonstrate degenerative changes, including ballooning and acidophilic body formation (*arrow*). H&E, ×125. **b** Bridging hepatic necrosis. A curving bridge of inflammation and hepatocyte necrosis (*arrows*) extends from the portal tract at the upper right of this field into the centrilobular region, seen slightly *left of center*. H&E, ×125

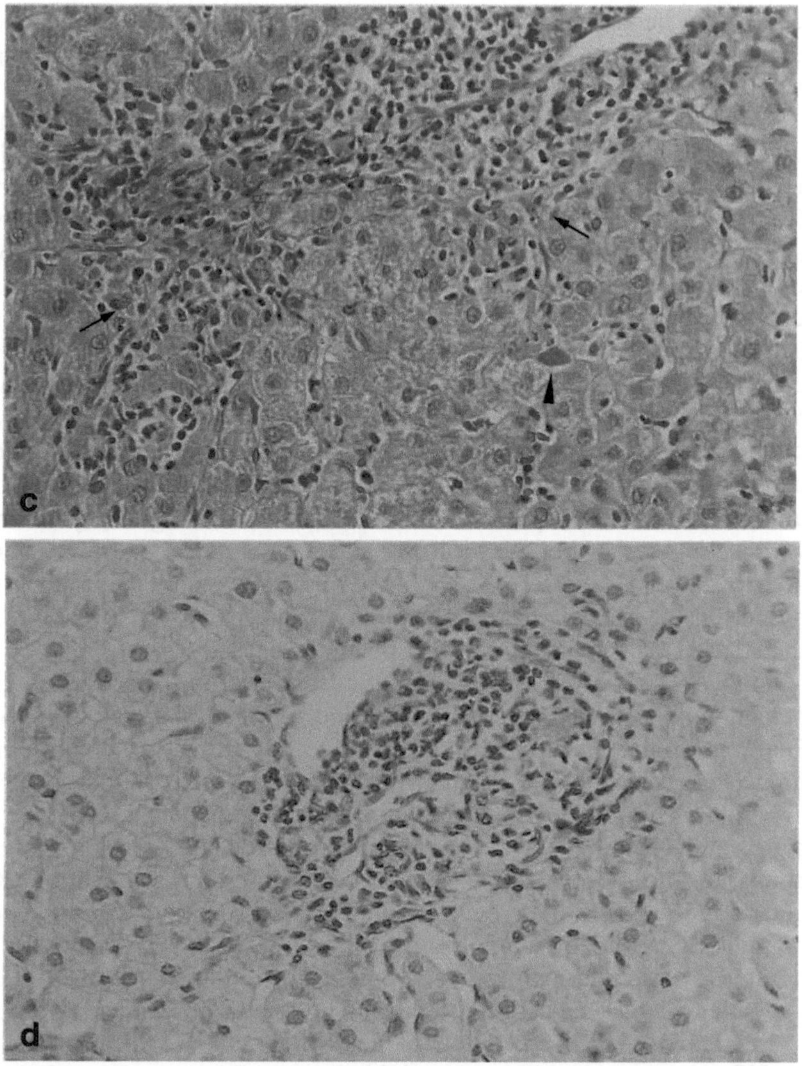

**Fig. 6. c** Chronic active hepatitis. The portal tract is enlarged and inflamed by lymphocytes and plasma cells which erode through the limiting plate into the periportal region (piecemeal necrosis) (*arrows*). Note the irregular edge of the portal tract produced by the piecemeal necrosis. The lobular parenchyma is also inflamed and an acidophilic body has formed (*arrowhead*). H&E, ×250. **d** Chronic persistent hepatitis. The portal area contains lymphocytes which are confined to the connective tissue and do not extend into the periportal region. H&E, ×250. (Reproduced by courtesy of Dr. J. Lefkowitch, Columbia Presbyterian Medical Center, New York)

continuing hepatocellular necrosis is found. However, liver regeneration is conspicuous by its impairment or absence. This pattern has been called *submassive necrosis, impaired regeneration* [35].

Progression of severe acute hepatitis B to chronicity is distinctly uncommon in well-studied cases, particularly those who are young [35, 37]. Disagreement with this finding may be ascribed to misdiagnosis resulting from a prominent degree of inflammation, residual focal hepatic necrosis, and preexisting disease, such as non-A, non-B hepatitis or alcoholic liver disease. When the inflammatory exudate extends beyond the portal areas due to irregular destruction of the limiting plates, the term *piecemeal necrosis* is applied. This feature, in association with hepatic necrosis and variable evidence of chronicity, is believed to be consistent with *chronic active hepatitis* (Fig. 6c). However, piecemeal necrosis is by no means pathognomonic of chronic active hepatitis. The inflammatory change and hepatic necrosis in chronic active hepatitis vary from one lobule to another and are no longer uniform as in acute hepatitis. In different lobules changes may be limited to various degrees of hepatic necrosis and inflammation or only regenerative activity. Over a long term, the course of chronic active hepatitis is marked by periods of greater or lesser inflammatory activity, most likely related to the state of viral replication, fibrosis, and eventually cirrhosis.

In 7%–12% of patients requiring hospitalization for acute hepatitis B, a benign condition develops called *chronic persistent hepatitis* (Fig. 6d) [37]. Features of this include focal hepatocytolysis, usually no more than one or two areas per lobule, slight hydropic change of hepatocytes, lymphoid hyperplasia limited to the portal areas without destruction of the limiting plate, and ground-glass hepatocytes containing HBsAg [35]. This corresponds to the nonreplicative phase of chronic HBV infection. Chronic persistent hepatitis may be asymptomatic with either normal liver tests or mild elevations of aminotransferases. Progression to cirrhosis does not occur. However, during periods of quiescence in the course of chronic active hepatitis, changes suggestive of chronic persistent hepatitis may occur.

In patients with resolution of acute hepatitis B, intracellular HBsAg or HBcAg are not demonstrated by immunofluorescence techniques. Of various HBs proteins, large and middle HBs are preferentially coexpressed with HBcAg, indicating their expression during viral replication. During progression of nonpermissive infection, hepatocytes containing intracytoplasmic HBsAg may be abundant within regenerative cirrhotic nodules. On the other hand, HBcAg positive nuclei are absent or uncommon and are not associated with HBsAg positive cells. In chronic active hepatitis, intranuclear HBcAg and intracytoplasmic HBsAg containing cells are frequently found and indicate active viral replication. In immunocompromised individuals, cells containing only intranuclear HBcAg, indicating viral replication, may be found.

## 1.6 Clinical Features

There are no distinguishing features to separate various causes of viral hepatitis. Epidemiological features were utilized before availability of serologic tests. This approach may be erroneous in about 25%, because epidemiologic features are not unique. Incubation periods overlap, rendering any possible distinction between, for example, hepatitis A and HBV, of little value. However, on some occasions, epidemiologic patterns provide important information.

In evaluating patients with acute hepatitis, it is useful to note the ethnic origin, recent travel, exposure to infected individuals, dental treatment in the preceding 6 months, injections, tattooing or acupuncture, homosexuality, heterosexual promiscuity, intravenous drug use, blood transfusions or receipt of blood products, including coagulation factor concentrates, ingestion of shellfish or clams, and drugs taken in the preceding 3 months.

The illness might by totally asymptomatic and unrecognized. Hepatitis may not be suspected unless a clear history of exposure exists, e.g., the patient is being followed after blood transfusion or blood is tested incidentally. Occasionally, during the *early prodromal phase*, in 10%–20% of patients, hepatitis may be heralded by a serum sickness-like syndrome caused by immune complexes of HBsAg and anti-HBs [34]. There may be moderate-grade fever, evanescent skin rash, transient symmetric polyarthritis involving small joints, angioneurotic edema, and lymphadenopathy. These symptoms appear 2–3 weeks before jaundice and usually disappear with the onset of overt hepatitis.

During the *prodromal phase*, usually lasting 3–4 days, nonspecific symptoms are frequent. Malaise, fatigue ranging from mild to profound, anorexia, nausea, and vomiting are most commonly described. Aversion to food, cigarettes, or alcohol may be marked. Mild to moderate diffuse, epigastric or right upper quadrant abdominal pain may develop. Weight loss is common. Occasionally, headache or respiratory symptoms, such as cough, may be prominent. Most patients feel markedly run down. The prodromal period is followed by the *icteric* phase, when urine becomes darker due to bilirubinuria. When cholestasis is a significant feature, stools lighten in color and pruritus may appear. With the onset of jaundice, symptoms decrease. Fever subsides. Appetite returns to normal and vomiting stops. Physical examination shows icterus in 70%; liver is palpable with a smooth, mildly tender edge in 40%; and spleen is occasionally palpable. Heavy percussion on the ribs overlying the liver may elicit a sickening sensation. Some spider nevi may appear transiently. The icteric phase lasts 1–4 weeks. During the *convalescent phase*, appetite improves further, fatigue lessens, and general well-being is restored. Recovery is quicker in younger patients. Hepatomegaly subsides and weight is gained. Lassitude and fatigue persist for a few weeks. Within 6 months from the onset of disease, full recovery is achieved.

Hepatitis B is frequently asymptomatic in the neonate, children, and immunosuppressed individuals, all of whom are at risk for chronic infection. The presentation may also be altered somewhat by coinfection with HDV, as discussed below. The clinical features of different hepatitis viruses are compared in Table 1.

### *Anicteric Hepatitis*

Prospective data regarding the incidence of icteric and anicteric hepatitis B are not available. Serologic surveys indicate high rates of anicteric hepatitis. Also, a large number of individuals positive for markers of HBV fail to recall hepatitis-like symptoms or jaundice. Anicteric hepatitis is milder than icteric hepatitis. The host factors determining whether hepatitis is anicteric or icteric are not clearly defined. Subclinical hepatitis B is more likely to cause chronic liver disease [38]. This is particularly so in immunocompromised individuals, e.g., in renal dialysis patients, organ transplant recipients or patients on chemotherapy, such as for hematologic disorders, or Down's syndrome [34]. Involvement of host factors regulating viral persistence is indicated by a self-limited and frequently icteric hepatitis occurring in health care workers in close contact with these patients.

### *Symptomatic Hepatitis*

Acute hepatitis B resolves with loss of symptoms and laboratory test abnormalities within 4 months in more than 90% of the patients [34, 37]. In about 10%, aminotransferases may remain abnormal after 3 months and chronic hepatitis develops. Fulminant or severe hepatitis occurs in about 1%. In severely ill patients, hemorrhagic acute gastritis may occur. Rapid onset of portal hypertension, leading to esophageal varices, has been reported. In some instances, hepatitis may take a protracted course, lasting 15–20 weeks. *Relapses*, which are frequent with hepatitis A or C, are uncommon in HBV infection. In the predisposed, e.g., intravenous drug abusers, exacerbations may be due to intercurrent A, non-A, non-B, or HDV infection. Such intercurrent infections may take multiple forms, including fatal hepatitis. Consequences of HDV infection are discussed below.

In addition to various factors discussed above, chronic hepatitis may result from corticosteroid therapy during acute HBV infection [38]. Chronic hepatitis is likely when HBsAg persists for longer than 13 weeks from the onset of hepatitis, HBeAg for longer than 10 weeks, and circulating immune complexes containing HBsAg for more than 5 weeks [34]. However, the age when infection is acquired is the single most important factor predicting chronicity. The HBV infection becomes chronic in 90%–95% of neonates born to carrier mothers, about 20% in children beyond the age of 1 year, and only 1%–10% adults [16, 19, 39]. In large series, about two-thirds of

**Table 1.** Comparison of the features of viral hepatitis

| Features | A | B | C | D | E |
|---|---|---|---|---|---|
| Type of virus | RNA | DNA | RNA | RNA | Unknown |
| Incubation (days) | 15–50 | 28–160 | 14–160 | ~20 | ~40 |
| Fecal excretion | + | − | − | − | + |
| Viremia | Transient | Prolonged | Prolonged | Prolonged | Probably transient |
| *Routes of transmission* | | | | | |
| Oral | + | − | − | − | + |
| Percutaneous | Rare | + | + | + | − |
| Sexual | + | + | − | − | Unknown |
| Perinatal | − | + | ± | − | Unknown |
| *Clinical features* | | | | | |
| Age at onset | Mostly young | All | All | All | Mostly adult |
| Rash or arthralgia | Uncommon | Frequent | Uncommon | Uncommon | Frequent |
| Fever | Frequent | Uncommon | Uncommon | Uncommon | Frequent |
| Waxing and waning hepatitis | − | − | + | − | − |
| Biphasic hepatitis | Rare | − | − | + | − |
| Cholestatic hepatits | + | − | − | − | + |
| *Outcome* | | | | | |
| Frequency of severe disease | Low | Moderate | Low | Moderate to high | High |
| Chronic carrier state | − | + | + | + | − |
| Hepatocellular carcinoma | − | + | + | ± | − |
| Mortality | Low | Low | Low | High | Moderate |

chronic carriers demonstrate changes of chronic persistent hepatitis and one-third chronic active hepatitis [37]. Chronic persistent hepatitis may have no or minimal symptoms. Liver tests are frequently mildly abnormal.

Chronic active hepatitis runs a protracted course, resulting in continuing liver injury, regeneration, and ultimately cirrhosis. Complications related to cirrhosis or chronic liver disease, such as portal hypertension, malnutrition, or hepatic failure, may supervene. Symptoms during chronic active hepatitis, therefore, may be protean and are related either to the severity of hepatitis or to other complications. During chronic active hepatitis, viral replication occurs for prolonged periods, even indefinitely. However, in other instances, HBV replication may cease, only to reappear either spontaneously or following immunomodulation, e.g., with drugs. The resultant reactivation of hepatitis may present with fever, fatigue, anorexia, or malaise [22]. Severe or fatal hepatitis may occur. During reactivation, patients with underlying chronic liver disease may have aggravation of portal hypertension with formation or worsening of ascites, variceal bleeding, and hepatic encephalopathy. Reactivation hepatitis may be asymptomatic and unrecognized in the absence of serial testing for viral markers of replication, e.g., HBeAg, IgM anti-HBc, or HBV DNA [22]. As discussed below, superinfection with HDV leads to a rapid, downhill course in patients with chronic HBV infection.

### *Cholestatic Hepatitis*

Cholestatic hepatitis is marked by development of fever, pruritus, marked hyperbilirubinemia, and prolonged cholestasis [34]. The latter implies impaired bile flow with elevated serum alkaline phosphatase and retention of bile salts. Hepatitis A is frequently the cause of cholestasis, although water-borne hepatitis E virus has been incriminated. Hepatitis B virus is not usually believed to be an etiologic factor for this disorder.

### *Pregnancy and Hepatitis B*

In well-nourished pregnant women, hepatitis B is no worse than in comparable nonpregnant women. However, poor nourishment, inadequate prenatal care, and low socioeconomic status adversely affect the outcome of hepatitis in pregnancy. The general effects of hepatitis on the fetus include excessive fetal wastage or intrauterine death, stillbirth, prematurity, and possibly congenital malformations. The most important consequence of maternal HBV infection is transmission of the virus to the offspring. This was suggested initially by the greater familial incidences of chronic HBV disease and HCC [19]. Subsequently, it was demonstrated that babies born to mothers with HBeAg positive acute hepatitis B or chronic HBV carriers became infected. The risk for transmitting the infection is greater if acute hepatitis occurs in the third trimester or the first 2 postpartum months

(66%–100%), as compared to the first or the second trimester. In endemic areas, maternal transmission to babies is significantly greater (HBsAg positive babies in Japan or Taiwan: 60%–74%, USA: 5%, Denmark: 0%, etc.) [34]. Available evidence indicates that the majority of neonatal HBV infection is acquired during delivery because of contact with contaminated maternal blood or following intimate contact during the nursing period. An ability to prevent 95% of the infections by passive–active immunoprophylaxis soon after birth is strong evidence for a perinatal route of transmission [40]. However, cesarian sections have not prevented transmission of HBV to the baby. The replicative state of HBV is most important in transmitting HBV. Neonatal transmission is greatest in areas of the world where HBeAg positivity is highest and may approach 100%. Serum HBV DNA is frequently detected in HBV carrier mothers and their offspring at birth. Measurement of maternal serum HBV DNA has been found to be predictive of the efficacy of HBV immunoprophylaxis for the newborn [41]. The outcome of neonatal HBV infection is a chronic carrier state, chronic active hepatitis, cirrhosis and HCC.

***HBV and Extrahepatic Associations***

Direct involvement of extrahepatic organs with HBV is uncommon (see ref. 34 for further details). A variety of disorders have been associated with circulating immune complexes of HBsAg and anti-HBs. A *serum sickness-like illness* may develop about a week before jaundice in acute hepatitis. Fever, urticaria, rarely papular acrodermatitis in children, and a symmetric nonmigratory arthritis may occur. The arthritis is seronegative, involving the small joints, and is usually transient. Low levels of complement are found in serum or synovial fluid from afflicted joints.

*Polyarteritis nodosa*, a multisystem disorder with vasculitis, is associated with chronic HBV infection in 10%–30% of patients. Serum complement levels are low and immune complexes containing HBsAg, IgG, and complement are found in vascular lesions. Circulating immune complexes correlate with disease activity. However, the frequency of polyarteritis in chronic HBV carriers is low.

*Membranous or membranoproliferative glomerulonephritis* has been associated rarely with chronic HBV infection. Deposits of immune complexes, HBsAg, or C3 complement may be found along the subepithelial surfaces of the glomerular basement membrane. The course of renal disease is gradually progressive. On the other hand, liver disease is not usually a clinical feature.

*Hematologic abnormalities* may be related to direct suppression of bone marrow, most commonly causing irreversible aplastic anemia, or rarely agranulocytosis. *Aplastic anemia* has been recorded in more than 200 cases. All formed elements of the blood may not be affected. The average time from the onset of hepatitis to pancytopenia is about 9 weeks. Hepatitis is usually mild and may have already resolved. The prognosis for aplastic anemia is poor. Hemolysis may cause extreme hyperbilirubinemia (up to 100 mg/dl) in sickle cell disease or in individuals with glucose-6-phosphate dehydrogenase deficiency.

*Cardiac abnormalities* may occur in fulminant hepatitis but are rare in uncomplicated hepatitis. Myocarditis, hypotension, acute pulmonary edema, conduction abnormalities, electrocardiographic changes, or cardiomegaly may occur. Pericarditis may occur and in the presence of diffuse intravascular coagulation, pericardial fluid may be hemorrhagic. *Pulmonary involvement* has been limited to rare pleural effusions. Serosal exudates may contain Dane particles or HBsAg and are potentially infectious. Involvement of the *gastrointestinal tract* is uncommon. Acute pancreatitis, ranging from edema to hemorrhagic necrosis, may occur in 12%–40% of fatal fulminant hepatitis. Serum amylase may be abnormal in up to 30% of the patients with acute hepatitis. A variety of *neurologic abnormalities* have been rarely reported, including aseptic meningitis, encephalitis, myelitis, seizures, Guillain-Barré syndrome, mono- or polyneuritis, and mononeuritis multiplex. Other poorly defined associations of HBV have been described with *essential mixed cryoglobulinemia* and *polymyalgia rheumatica*.

## 2 Hepatitis D Virus and Viral Hepatitis D

The HDV is a unique defective RNA virus related to viroids. It is hepatotropic and requires HBsAg for its assembly and virulence. This virus was found by Italian workers who in 1977 recognized a novel antigen in chronic hepatitis B carrier livers [42]. The antigen was purified, antibodies raised, and the virus itself cloned and sequenced [43–45]. HDV is capable of infecting primates, rodents, and ducks in the presence of appropriate hepadnaviruses. Recent studies indicate that HDV has peculiar biologic characteristics. Its natural history has been partly defined and clinical entities recognized.

*Biology*. Knowledge concerning the basic biology of HDV, its protein products, and its mechanism of replication is far less than for HBV. The virion particle is 36 nM in size (Fig. 7). An HBsAg envelope surrounds the nucleocapsid containing the hepatitis D antigen (HDAg) and an RNA genome of 1.7 kb. The HDV RNA is a single-stranded circular molecule with a high degree of self-complementarity. The HDV RNA contains the viroid and virusoid consensus sequences GAAAC and AGUUUU, which are believed to be important for their replication [45]. Viroids are non-encapsidated RNAs that never produce virions but produce infectious nucleic acids. In contrast to viroids, plant satellite viruses require a helper virus for replication and encapsidation. The GAAAC sequence is essential for the self-cleavage of virusoid RNA with somewhat similar implications for

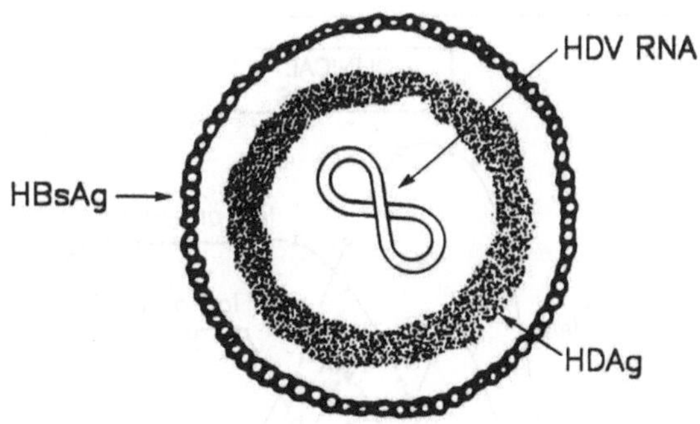


**Fig. 7.** Diagrammatic representation of the structural organization of hepatitis D virus. The genomic RNA is associated with HDAg and enclosed by an HBsAg envelope

HDV. However, HDV differs from these agents in important ways and to date represents the only identified member of a novel class of viruses.

In HDV, there are five ORFs capable of encoding polypeptides of more than 100 amino acids each [45]. The ORFs are organized in both orientations, potentially capable of bidirectional translation. So far, only HDAg has been identified. The HDAg contains two major polypeptides of 24 and 29 kd [46]. It has a specific HDV RNA binding activity conferred by the middle one-third of the HDAg molecule. Replication of HDV occurs in the nucleus of infected hepatocytes. The existence of a 0.8-kb antigenomic RNA, which is cytoplasmic and polyadenylated, was recently demonstrated [47]. This polyadenylated RNA is 500 times less abundant than the genomic RNA. It is believed to be responsible for the expression of the HDAg.

In vitro studies have demonstrated that HDV replicates in the absence of HBV in both liver- and non-liver-derived cells. Initiation of genome replication requires HDAg, probably to recruit other critically important factors by virtue of its transactivating function [48]. Of the two forms of HDAg, only the small form supports HDV genome replication. The large HDAg polypeptide acts as a dominant repressor of HDV replication. This has been taken to imply that synthesis of the large HDAg may suppress HDV replication, resulting in a clinically self-limited infection. In tissues supporting HDV replication, HDV RNA is present as monomers, dimers, and trimers of both strand polarities, consistent with a rolling circle model of replication [49].

The HDV adopts whichever HBsAg type is conveniently available for encapsidation. Transcapsidation studies have shown that when HDV from chimpanzees was passaged into woodchucks, it shed the HBsAg coat and acquired the WHBsAg coat [50]. It is not clear whether HDV is directly cytopathic. In vitro replication of HDV is not associated with cell lysis.

In susceptible hosts, HDV is highly infectious. It localizes to the nucleus of infected hepatocytes and can be easily demonstrated by immunohisto-

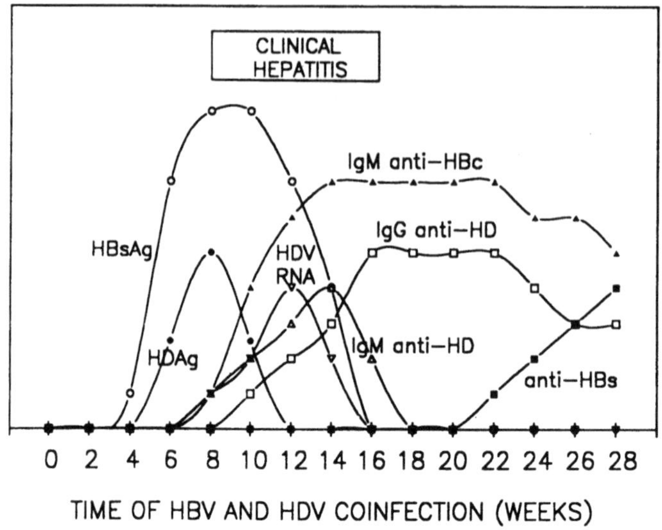


**Fig. 8.** Serologic evolution of acute hepatitis following coinfection with HBV and HDV. Diagnosis of HDV infection is often hampered by the transient nature of HDAg, HDV RNA, or IgM anti-HD response

chemical staining for HDAg. In comparison to HBV, its infectivity may be greater by four orders of magnitude [51]. Therefore, inocula which are insufficient to result in simultaneous HBV and HDV infection (coinfection) may be infectious in chronic HBV carriers (superinfection). Such carriers, e.g., hemophiliacs, are particularly prone to acquire HDV infection when blood products screened as negative for HBsAg contain infectious HDV. For coinfection to succeed, infection of hepatocytes with HBV is essential. When HBV is cleared, HDV cannot survive. Enhanced virulence of HDV during serial passages or due to unknown factors may cause severe or fulminant hepatitis.

Infection with HDV leads to suppression of HBV replication [52, 53]. The mechanism for this is not known. In patients with HDV superinfection, replicative intermediates of HBV and HBcAg are reduced or absent in hepatocytes [52, 54]. As a consequence, peripheral markers of HBV, including HBsAg, may disappear without actual virus clearance. In the presence of coexisting HIV infection or immunosuppression, HBV replication is augmented, but HDV replication is unchanged, suggesting that immune status has little effect on HDV [55]. However, as HBV infection in the immunosuppressed individual often persists, HDV coinfection is more likely to result in chronic hepatitis.

*Serologic Response to HDV.* In acute *coinfection*, HDAg is the first marker to appear peripherally, being detected 1–21 days after onset of dark urine, with mean duration of 6 days (Fig. 8). The titers decline rapidly and HDAg

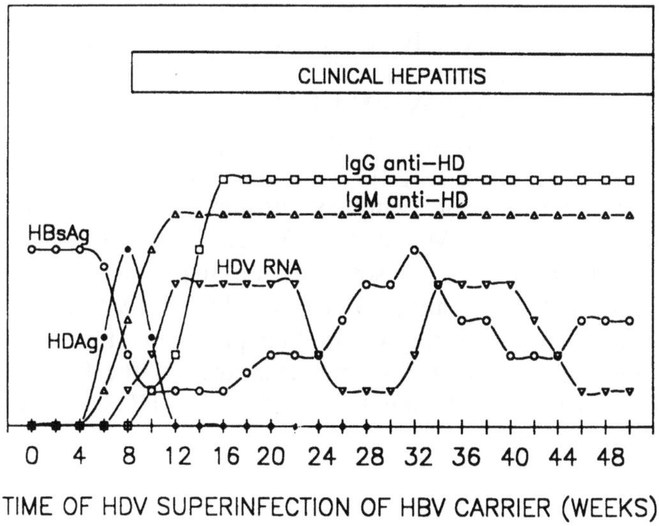


**Fig. 9.** Serologic development of chronic delta hepatitis following HDV infection in an HBV carrier. The acute-phase markers of HBV (e.g., IgM anti-HBc) are absent and HBV replication tends to be suppressed. Similar to some cases of chronic hepatitis B, there may be periods of HDV reactivation when HDAg or HDV RNA reappear. Persistence of HDV infection is characterized by rapid deterioration of liver disease in HBV carriers

is rarely detectable for more than 1–2 weeks. The HDAg was detected in 26%–100% of acute coinfection. The former number is more representative. Newer assay systems, e.g., immunoblot analysis, may improve detection of HDAg. Molecular hybridization with purified serum HDV RNA indicates its presence in about 60% of patients within the first week of illness. Antibodies to HDAg (anti-HD) are detected with radioimmunoassays and may be of either IgM or class. The IgM anti-HD appears within 2–3 weeks of the onset of illness. However, it is short-lived. Although the mean duration of persistence is 22 days, IgM anti-HD is rarely detected beyond 2–3 months from the onset of illness. The IgG anti-HD may be detected in only 50% of the patients with IgM anti-HD but remains positive for several months. In consecutive patients with coinfection, only 28% had HDAg followed by a primary IgM and a secondary IgG anti-HD response. In 60%, HDAg was absent and a primary IgM response within 1–4 weeks occurred with a secondary IgG response during convalescence. In the remainder, either a transient IgM or a delayed IgG response was noted. Unlike HBV, development of anti-HD does not confer immunity against reinfection [56].

In *superinfection*, the anti-HD response may be more consistent. High titers of IgM and IgG anti-HD are detected and may persist for years (Fig. 9) [57]. Serum HDV RNA is found in about 50%–60% of chronically infected patients. It correlates with intrahepatic HDAg and indicates active viral replication. The HDV replication may persist for prolonged periods or subside spontaneously only to be reactivated. This may be indicated by the presence of intrahepatic HDAg, which is the gold standard of HDV replication or serum HDV RNA [57].

Separation of monomeric 7s and pentameric 19s IgM anti-HD may be of prognostic value [58]. In patients with acute hepatitis D, only 19s IgM anti-HD was found whereas chronic HDV infection was associated with both forms of IgM anti-HD. When 7s and 19s IgM anti-HD were both present during the onset of acute hepatitis, patients developed chronic hepatitis D. Persistence of serum HDV RNA beyond 3 weeks of the onset of acute hepatitis may be another predictor of chronicity. Reinoculation of chimpanzees with HDV after clearance of the first experimental challenge is associated with low levels of serum HDV RNA and transient, mild hepatitis [59].

### 2.1 Epidemiology

Seroepidemiologic data indicate a wide distribution of HDV. In Southern Italy, the Mediterranean, North Africa, and the Middle East, HDV is highly endemic [60], while HBV is moderately so. In North America, HDV is sporadic and appears to be confined to high-risk groups, such as intravenous drug users, hemophiliacs, homosexuals, hemodialysis patients, or prison inmates [61, 62]. In developing countries with high HBV prevalence, HDV has been found in parts of West Africa, the South Pacific, and South America [60]. On the other hand, HDV is far less common in parts of Asia such as China, Taiwan, and Japan, where HBV is also highly endemic. Recent analysis of an epidemic in Yucpa Indians in Venezuela indicated the causative agent to be HDV [63]. So-called Labrea fever in the Brazilian Amazon valley and hepatitis of Sierra Nevada de Santa Marta in rural northern Colombia were due to HDV infection over the past several decades. Introduction of HDV in previously unexposed groups accounts for miniepidemics and development of new reservoirs. This is amply illustrated by a large increase (0% to 75%) in HDV infection among Swedish intravenous drug abusers during the last decade [64]. The endemicity of HDV infection is usually maintained by superinfected chronic HDV patients.

A less apparent source of transmission involves blood and blood products for transfusion. Screening of donor blood for HBsAg alone is still associated with some posttransfusion hepatitis B. This is believed to be due to insufficient sensitivity of the HBsAg assay, failure to detect HBsAg within immune complexes, or circulating infectious HBV particles even though HBsAg is undetected. Blood nonreactive to HBsAg is estimated to transmit HDV with a frequency of about 1 in 3000 transfusions. Presence of even low levels of HDV in such blood or blood products is particularly threatening to chronic HBV carriers in whom HDV superinfection occurs. Similarly infected pooled plasma products may transmit HDV to hemophiliacs or other groups. No satisfactory means are currently available to prevent such transmission. The major mechanism of HDV transmission is believed to be percutaneous, similar to that of HBV. In addition, homosexual as well as heterosexual transmission of HDV has been documented.

## 2.2 Clinical Manifestations

Symptomatic evolution of hepatitis is similar to that described above for HBV. As a result of the unique interactions between HBV and HDV, clinical illness may follow one of several possible courses.

*Coinfection*. When HDV replication is mild, usually minimal liver disease occurs. The HDAg is detected transiently in the liver but not the serum and HBsAg is rapidly cleared from the blood. Acute HBV infection is usually indicated by high titers of IgM anti-HBc. As almost 90% of the acute HBV infection resolves in the immunocompetent patient, HDV coinfection is limited, with little anti-HD response. In this situation, measurement of serum HDV RNA may be more useful. However, when more extensive HBV-HDV replication occurs, hepatitis may be severe or fulminant [65]. The HDV coinfection cannot be distinguished from primary HBV infection alone on clinical grounds.

Coinfection may result in a peculiar sequence of viral replication associated with a biphasic disease [66]. The initial peak of aminotransferases (AST/ALT) may be followed within 4 weeks by a relapse associated with a second peak. The first peak of ALT coincides with HDAg lasting 2–7 days followed by the appearance of anti-HD during the second ALT peak. The anti-HD appears 11–18 days after disappearance of HDAg. In biphasic hepatitis, the relapse is associated with greater prolongation of the prothrombin time and may result in severe or fulminant hepatitis. It is believed that HDV causes the initial hepatitis during which HBV replication is suppressed. When HDV is cleared, HBV replication ensues, resulting in the second phase of hepatitis.

*Superinfection*. Rescue of small amounts of HDV, rapid invasion of a large number of hepatocytes producing HBsAg, and development of chronic hepatitis D are devastating to the HBV carrier. The HDV infection in this setting is recognized by either intrahepatic HDAg or serologically (HDV RNA, high titer IgM or IgG anti-HD) [57]. Serum HBsAg is positive but high titer IgM anti-HBc is lacking. Superinfection with HDV, in general, causes a severe hepatitis with an aggressively downhill course. There may be periodic exacerbations or reactivations of hepatitis in association with the appearance of serum HDV RNA. Asymptomatic carriers of HBV with

HDV markers exhibit abnormal liver tests more frequently [67]. Histopathologic evidence of chronic active hepatitis or cirrhosis is also more frequent in asymptomatic carriers with abnormal liver tests and positive HDV markers (61%) compared to negative HDV markers (19%) [67]. Rapidly advancing liver disease terminating in advanced cirrhosis or liver failure within months is suggestive of chronic HDV. The IgM and IgG anti-HD persist at high titers indefinitely [57]. The histologic pattern is of continuing hepatitis, variable fibrosis, and widespread expression of HDAg in hepatocytes.

*Fulminant Hepatitis*. This is the least common but most dreaded form of acute viral hepatitis, leading to mortality in 80%. The term refers to abrupt onset of hepatic failure during acute hepatitis of less than 4 weeks' duration. Rapid hepatic encephalopathy associated with deteriorating liver function is characteristic. Throughout the world, hepatitis B is a common cause of fulminant hepatitis. Of hepatitis B-related fulminant hepatitis, 30%–40% cases are due to HDV [65].

The patient may exhibit repeated vomiting, altered sleep pattern, irritability, confusion, and coma. Liver size may decrease rapidly. Absence of glycogen stores predispose to hypoglycemia. Prothrombin time is progressively prolonged. Disseminated intravascular coagulation may result in hemorrhagic complications. Leukocytosis rather than the more usual leukopenia may be found. Hyperthermia and cerebral edema occur. Respiratory alkalosis due to hyperventilation and hypoxia due to intrapulmonary shunting are frequent. Sepsis, electrolyte disorders, hepatorenal syndrome, or adult respiratory distress syndrome may prove fatal. Most patients are deeply jaundiced. Recovery from fulminant hepatitis may be dramatic and is often heralded by steady improvement in prothrombin time. Recovery is slow and may take several months. Once recovered, sequelae are uncommon and recovery is complete. Fulminant hepatitis is uncommon in children and appears to be restricted at all ages to icteric hepatitis.

Prognostic factors indicating survival are only partially defined. The maximal degree of encephalopathy can be correlated with survival. As discussed earlier, hepatic regenerative potential is limited in patients older than 40 years. Mortality is thus highly correlated with age. Mortality is also high in preexisting malignancy or cirrhosis. Attempts to find reproducible, simple, and effective biochemical or serologic markers correlating with prognosis have not fully succeeded.

In fulminant hepatitis, viral replication is uncommon and HBV DNA or HDV RNA is found at low frequencies [68]. Therefore, liver transplantation for fulminant hepatitis is not associated with a high risk of HBV or HDV recurrence. The differential diagnosis of fulminant hepatitis should include toxins such as poisonous mushrooms, drugs such as acetaminophen, acute fatty liver and toxemia of pregnancy, Wilson's disease, and acute hepatic venous outflow obstruction.

**Table 2.** Serologic diagnosis of hepatitis B and D

| Serologic markers | Diagnostic significance |
|---|---|
| *Hepatitis B* | |
| HBsAg | Infection with HBV |
| HBV DNA | Active viral replication. Infectious. Acute, chronic, or reactivation hepatitis |
| HBeAg | Active viral replication. Infectious. Acute, chronic, or reactivation hepatitis |
| Anti-HBe | Convalescent phase or continued infectious state with viral replication |
| IgM anti-HBc (high titer) | Acute hepatitis B |
| IgG anti-HBc } IgM anti-HBc (low titer) | Past exposure (when HBsAg −ve) Chronic hepatitis (when HBsAg +ve) |
| Anti-HBs | Past exposure with immunity |
| *Hepatitis D* | |
| HD Ag | Acute infection. Active viral replication |
| HDV RNA | Active viral replication. Acute or chronic disease |
| IgM anti-delta | Acute or chronic disease |
| IgG anti-delta | Acute or chronic disease |

## 3 Laboratory Tests

Impairment of hepatic function results in a number of biochemical abnormalities [34]. However, tests which are useful for diagnosis of hepatitis are few. Diagnostic interpretation of HBV and HDV serologic markers is shown in Table 2.

*Serum Enzymes*. The most relevant abnormality occurs in alanine and aspartate aminotransferases (ALT and AST, respectively). Hepatocellular necrosis accompanies increased blood levels of these enzymes and is usually the first indicator of acute hepatitis. Blood levels of ALT and AST rise rapidly, preceding jaundice, and may be up to 100-fold high at the peak of hepatitis. However, the magnitude of this rise correlates poorly with the degree of cell necrosis. Most commonly, ALT and AST are elevated to about 300–400 IU/liter. In fulminant hepatitis, aminotransferase levels may be "low." The duration of the abnormality tends to last longer than hyperbilirubinemia. The AST levels decline earlier than ALT. Early in the disease, ALT values may decline to about 70% of the peak value after 1 week, although subsequent decline may be less swift. The ratio of ALT to AST is usually greater than 1 in acute viral hepatitis. However, this feature is not diagnostic as other conditions, such as alcoholic hepatitis, may occasionally present with this pattern. A mixed pattern may be found with an ALT to AST ratio of 0.5 or lower when viral hepatitis is superimposed on alcoholic liver disease. ALT or AST values higher than about 4000 IU/liter are uncommon but may occur occasionally. In this situation, toxic or vascular etiologies of hepatic necrosis should be considered. In chronic persistent hepatitis, ALT and AST are usually less than 100 IU/liter. In chronic active hepatitis, aminotransferases may be elevated during periods of exacerbation or viral reactivation, equivalent to those seen in acute hepatitis.

A number of other enzymes may be abnormally elevated. Of these, lactate dehydrogenase (LDH) is often a part of current automated blood testing procedures. The LDH levels are only mildly increased, usually no more than two- to threefold. Serum alkaline phosphatase levels are usually abnormal but no more than about twice above normal. Abnormal levels of these enzymes may rapidly decline to normal. In cholestatic hepatitis, alkaline phosphatase may rise to more than tenfold above normal. Abnormalities of isocitrate, sorbitol, malate, or glutamate dehydrogenase, ornithine carbamyltransferase, and a variety of other enzymes are of no value in the clinical management of hepatitis.

*Serum Bilirubin.* Jaundice is preceded by bilirubinuria. At the peak of jaundice, little bilirubin may reach the intestines and urobilinogen may disappear, to reappear in the late icteric phase. Serum bilirubin greater than 2.0 mg/dl manifests as detectable jaundice. In hepatitis, both conjugated and unconjugated forms of bilirubin are found. In the absence of hemolysis, cholestasis, or disorders of glucuronidation, serum bilirubin indicates severity of hepatitis. Total bilirubin is usually 3–6 mg/dl and levels rarely exceed 20 mg/dl. During recovery, serum bilirubin declines by about 50% of the peak value per week. Peak bilirubin levels greater than 30 mg/dl signify overproduction from hemolysis or impaired clearance due to renal failure.

*Hematologic Changes.* Leukopenia, lymphopenia, and neutropenia characterize the preicteric stage with rapid normalization. Leukocytosis ($>12\,000/mm^3$) may indicate associated sepsis or fulminant hepatitis. Mild anemia is due to shortened red blood cell life span. Macrocytosis or megaloblastosis and thrombocytopenia may be seen. Aplastic anemia may be a delayed feature. Erythrocyte sedimentation rate is of little significance.

Prothrombin time is prolonged early in the disease and indicates abnormal hepatic synthetic function. Progressive prothrombin prolongation may herald severe or fulminant hepatitis. Fibrinolysis and disseminated intravascular coagulation may occur in fulminant hepatitis.

*Miscellaneous Abnormalities.* Vitamin $B_{12}$ and other liver-stored substances may be released into the circulation. Serum iron levels may be high. Hypoglycemia or glucose intolerance and insulin resistance may occur.

Serum triglycerides may be increased and cholesterol synthesis or esterification impaired. Bile salts accumulate, particularly when cholestasis is prominent. Changes in serum immunoglobulin levels or complement may occur. Serum α-fetoprotein, an oncofetal protein, increases modestly with liver regeneration and indicates a good prognosis in acute hepatitis [69]. Serum albumin is unchanged in acute hepatitis with no preexisting disease. Acute phase reactant proteins such as c-reactive protein are not elevated in acute hepatitis.

*Other Tests*. Radiologic or other imaging modalities have no role in the diagnosis of acute hepatitis. Liver biopsy is not usually indicated in acute viral hepatitis, although evaluation of cholestasis or chronic hepatitis is often facilitated.

## 4 Treatment

No specific therapeutic measures are available. Fortunately, most cases of acute viral hepatitis resolve spontaneously. Treatment in these cases is mainly symptomatic. Patients recover at home or in domiciliary circumstances. In addition to evaluation of symptoms, liver tests should be performed (AST, ALT, bilirubin, alkaline phosphatase, and prothrombin time) twice weekly until the peak is passed. The frequency of testing should then be reduced. Patients should be followed until HBsAg is lost. If HBV infection persists, longer follow-up is required. Indicators of the onset of severe or fulminant hepatitis are shown in Table 3. In this situation, hospitalization and close observation are prudent. Avoidance of dehydration, hypoglycemia, and electrolyte imbalance may be important. Large firm liver, prominent splenomegaly, multiple spider nevi, collateral veins on the abdomen, and large ascites indicate preexisting liver disease. The mortality of fulminant hepatitis has changed in recent years owing to intensive care by staff especially knowledgeable in hepatic pathophysiology. Prompt treatment of sepsis, correction of acid-base disorders, circulatory and ventilatory support, monitoring of cerebral edema, and liver transplantation have contributed to this improvement. However, early indicators of mortality in fulminant

**Table 3.** Clinical indicators of severe or fulminant hepatitis

| |
|---|
| Persistent vomiting or anorexia |
| Rapid prolongation of prothrombin time >3 s above control |
| Persistent rise in bilirubin |
| Symptoms suggestive of hepatic precoma (e.g., irritability, confusion, or altered sleep pattern) |
| Rapid shrinkage of liver size |

hepatitis are still poorly defined. A full discussion of the management of fulminant hepatitis is beyond the scope of this chapter.

*Bed Rest.* In contrast to the past wisdom of strict bed rest, current evidence indicates that most patients can indulge in normal activity. However, physically exhaustive exercise during the preicteric phase may lead to severe or fulminant hepatitis [37]. Serum bilirubin of <4 mg/dl is associated with no significant effect of moderately severe exercise on recovery. Less strenuous physical exertion with higher bilirubin levels has caused relapses and slower resolution of hepatitis. In patients with severe symptoms and prolonged prothrombin time, excess physical strain may be deleterious. These patients should be allowed to rest with free movement within the room until hepatitis has peaked. Subsequently, activity should be increased as tolerated. Less severely ill patients need not restrict physical activity, but strenuous exercise should be avoided for 2–3 months or longer.

*Nutrition.* Anorexia, nausea, and vomiting may be problematic. Specific food aversions may occur. There is little evidence that limitation of fat benefits recovery. If hepatic precoma develops, protein intake should be restricted. Judicious timing of meals when nausea is least may help. Adequate intake of carbohydrates and calories may be important in patients with severe hepatitis. Vitamin supplements are of little value. In general, overly restrictive or compulsive dietary prescriptions tend to foster needless preoccupation with food. Alcohol should be avoided for at least 6 months although small amounts of alcohol may not hamper recovery.

*Medicines.* As liver is involved in metabolizing drugs, pharmacokinetics of drugs is frequently altered in liver disease. When there is a question of impending hepatic coma, narcotics, benzodiazepines, and other tranquilizers are particularly hazardous. Analgesics such as acetaminophen may cause superimposed drug hepatitis. For symptomatic control of nausea or vomiting, phenothiazines and metoclopramide may be used. Corticosteroid treatment has been shown to prolong HBV replication and foster development of a carrier state. Therefore, corticosteroids are contraindicated.

Unwitting or elective surgery during hepatitis is associated with exacerbation and severe or fulminant hepatitis [37].

*Specific Drugs.* No effective drugs are available to treat acute hepatitis B. Levamisole, an immunomodulatory drug with antiparasitic effects, was found to be of little value. Infusion of anti-HBs has also been ineffective. Recently, several agents have been utilized to treat chronic hepatitis. Among these, α-interferon has shown some antiviral activity and this may be a therapeutic option in patients with chronic hepatitis B and active viral replication. In these cases the outcome of the treatment is to accelerate transit from the replicating to the nonreplicating state of persistent HBV infection. Doses of 10 MU three times per week for 3 months are currently used. Prolonged α-interferon treatment may also be of benefit in chronic HDV patients. Further details on the use of interferon in chronic viral hepatitis are given in Chap. 9.

## 5 Prophylaxis

Development of highly effective vaccines against HBV is one of the successes of modern medicine. Prevention of HBV infection confers immunity against HDV also. The potential to control this major public health problem is limited only by the expense of available vaccines. Until economic means to accomplish universal immunization are found, other methods of prophylaxis will continue to be important.

Screening of donor blood for HBsAg has substantially reduced transfusion-related hepatitis B but has not eliminated it. On the other hand, public health measures have not been universally successful. This applies particularly to health care workers who in some instances may not be properly trained, refuse vaccination, or decline sensible precautions while dealing with needles, infectious blood, or body fluids. Here, a significant consideration is that infectious HBV particles occur virtually everywhere except for stool. Also, HBV is resistant to extremes of temperature and may survive for weeks on the surface of fomites. In health care settings dealing with large numbers of asymptomatic HBV carriers, casual practices may be particularly hazardous. These factors apply particularly to transmission of HBV in the institutionalized. In contrast, health care workers who are HBV carriers could pose a risk to predisposed patients. Adherence to standard practices for disposal of contaminated needles, use of protective gloves, and appropriate disinfection of reusable instruments is critical.

Spread of HBV from infected patients is commonest among either sexual partners or neonates. Abstinence during the acute illness should be practiced by the former. Immune serum globulin (ISG) and more specifically hepatitis B immune globulin (HBIG) may be useful in preventing symptomatic infection or seroconversion [34]. Neonatal HBV infection can be prevented by passive–active immunoprophylaxis, as discussed below.

*Passive immunization* with ISG prepared from pooled human plasma was unpredictable. It was later realized that the problem was due to inconsistent anti-HBs content. Use of pooled HBIG, containing high titer anti-HBs, has been more effective. Early preparations of ISG prepared by Conn fractionation were occasionally contaminated with infectious HBV particles. However, this is no longer a problem because several steps to denature HBV, HIV, and all known animal viruses have been introduced, and all lots of ISG and HBIG are prescreened. The prophylactic or postexposure efficacy of HBIG in decreasing transmission of HBV was demonstrated by several studies of patients undergoing hemodialysis, high-risk medical staff, accidental needle-stick, sexual contacts, and neonates [34]. HBIG was

**Table 4.** Immunoprophylaxis of hepatitis B

| Type of prophylaxis | Agent | Dose |
|---|---|---|
| I. Postexposure | | |
| A) HBsAg +ve blood Sexual partner | HBIG plus Recombinant hepatitis B vaccine | 0.06 ml/kg i.m. immediately; 10 μg i.m. within 7–10 days of exposure |
| Further action if recipient: | | |
| HBsAg +ve, anti-HBc + ve: | | None. Infected with HBV |
| HBsAg −ve, anti-HBc +ve: | | None. Immune |
| HBsAg −ve, anti-HBc +ve: | | Repeat hepatitis B vaccine at 1 and 6 months |
| B) Neonates born to HBsAg +ve mothers | HBIG plus Recombinant hepatitis B vaccine | 0.5 ml i.m. at birth; 10 μg i.m. (lateral thigh) within 7 days of birth, 1, and 6 months |
| II. Active | Recombinant hepatitis B vaccine | 10 μg i.m. (deltoid) initially and again at 1 and 6 months. May repeat one dose at 5 years |

shown to attenuate but not always prevent hepatitis B. This most possibly caused initial passive immunity followed by active immunization. Use of HBIG is now accepted for a variety of circumstances (Table 4).

*For active immunoprophylaxis*, it was recognized early that protective immunity resulted from injection of heated infectious serum [70]. Initially, vaccines were prepared with inactivated virus purified from pooled plasma of HBV carriers [71]. Subsequently, HBsAg was purified from plasma by physical methods and included several steps to inactivate residual virus [72]. Recombinant vaccines are now produced commercially from cloned HBV cDNA capable of expressing HBsAg in yeast [73]. The recombinant vaccine contains smaller HBsAg particles (17–25 nM) and is nonglycosylated in comparison to the natural vaccine. The final vaccine contains aluminum hydroxide as an adjuvant and thimerosal as a preservative [34].

The initial field trial in homosexual men proved that the vaccine (40 μg at 0, 1, and 6 months) was highly immunogenic, effective, and safe [72]. The immune response is expressed as ratio units (RU) of the anti-HBs assay (sample cpm – background cpm/negative control cpm; cpm: counts per minute of $^{125}$I). The response rate at 1 month was 76%, at 2 months, 78%, and at the end of 6 months, 95%. The degree of response at the end of 6 months was >20 RU (good) in 90%, 10–20 RU (fair) in 3%, and <10 RU (poor) in 2%. Several subsequent studies have confirmed these results with the plasma-derived or recombinant vaccines. It was learnt that the best results were obtained when the vaccine was stored at 2°–6°C and injected into the deltoid muscle (adults) or lateral thigh (neonates) rather than the gluteal region. In neonates, passive–active immunization with HBIG and vaccination has proven most effective [34, 40]. With this regimen, the HBV carrier rates in the offspring of infected mothers were reduced from 90% to 5%–10%. The immune response is greatest in immunocompetent patients and poor in immunodeficient individuals. Efficacy of the vaccines was 95%–100% in responders with anti-HBs of >10 RU. On the other hand, only 50% of patients on hemodialysis had a satisfactory response to vaccination, with no decrease in the incidence of hepatitis over the subsequent 25 months. The antibody following HBV vaccination persists for up to 5 years in 85% with a >10 RU response. Revaccination of the nonresponders results in a good response in 41% but after 18 months this response is maintained in only 8%. Poor responders fare better following revaccination. A second booster dose may be appropriate after 5 years to maintain the efficacy of vaccination, particularly in endemic areas. Occasional development of mutant HBV strains may be problematic [74].

HBV vaccines have proven to be safe. Except for pain at the local injection site, adverse reactions have been similar in recipients of the vaccines or placebo. Efforts to develop less expensive vaccines have included evaluation of synthetic peptides, but these have not yet produced satisfactory antibody titers.

## References

1. Blumberg BS, Alter HJ, Visnich S (1965) A "new" antigen in leukemia sera. JAMA 191:541–546
2. Ganem D, Varmus HE (1978) The molecular biology of the hepatitis B viruses. Annu Rev Biochem 56:651–693
3. Robinson WS, Lutwick LI (1987) The virus of hepatitis, type B. N Engl J Med 295:1168–1175, 1232–1236
4. Tiollais P, Purcell C, Dejean A (1985) The hepatitis B virus. Nature 317:489–495
5. Carman WF, Hadziyannis S, McGarvey MJ, Jacyna MR, Karayiannis P, Makris A, Thomas HC (1989) Mutation preventing formation of hepatitis B e antigen in patients with chronic hepatitis B infection. Lancet II:588–591
6. Okamoto H, Yotsumoto S, Akahane Y et al. (1990) Hepatitis B viruses with precore region defects prevail in persistently infected hosts along with seroconversion to the antibody against e antigen. J Virol 64:1298–1303
7. Summers J, Mason WS (1982) Replication of the genome of a hepatitis B-like virus by reverse transcription of an RNA intermediate. Cell 29:403–415
8. Yokosuka O, Omata M, Imazeki F, Ito Y, Okuda K (1986) Hepatitis B virus RNA transcripts and DNA in chronic liver disease. N Engl J Med 315:1187–1192
9. Gerlich WH, Harman KH, Bruss V et al. (1989) Structure, expression, and potential oncogenicity of hepatitis B virus proteins. In: Bannasch P, Keppler D, Weber G (eds) Liver cell carcinoma, Kluwer Academic, Dordrecht, pp 139–163
10. Hadziyannis SJ, Gerber MA, Vissoulis C et al. (1973) Cytoplasmic hepatitis B antigen in "ground-glass" hepatocytes of carriers. Arch Pathol 96:327–330

11. Magnius LO, Epsmark JA (1972) New specificities in Australia antigen positive sera distinct from the Le Bouviert determinants. J Immunol 109:1017–1021
12. Moriarty AM, Alexander H, Lerner RA (1985) Antibodies to peptides detect new hepatitis B antigen: serological correlation with hepatocellular carcinoma. Science 227:429–433
13. Tur-Kaspa R, Burk RD, Shaul Y, Shafritz DA (1986) Hepatitis B virus DNA contains a glucocorticoid responsive element. Proc Natl Acad Sci USA 83:1627–1631
14. Twu, JR-S, Schloemer RH (1987) Transcriptional *trans*-activating function of hepatitis B virus. J Virol 61:3448–3453
15. Szmuness W (1978) Hepatocellular carcinoma and the hepatitis B virus: evidence for a causal association. Prog Med Virol 24:40–69
16. Beasley RP, Hwang LY (1984) Epidemiology of hepatocellular carcinoma. In: Vyas GN, Dienstag JL, Hoofnagle JH (eds) Viral hepatitis and liver disease. Grune and Stratton, New York, pp 209–225
17. McMahon BJ, Rhoades ER, Heyward WL et al. (1987) A comprehensive program to reduce the incidence of hepatitis B virus infection and its sequelae in Alaskan natives. Lancet II:1134–1136
18. Gust ID (1984) The epidemiology of viral hepatitis. In: Vyas GN, Dienstag JL, Hoofnagle JH (eds) Viral hepatitis and liver disease. Grune and Stratton, New York, pp 415–421
19. Beasley RP, Trepo C, Stevens CE et al. (1977) The e antigen and vertical transmission of hepatitis B surface antigen. Am J Epidemiol 105:94–98
20. Lieberman HM, LaBrecque DR, Kew MC, Hadziyannis SJ, Shafritz DA (1983) Detection of hepatitis B virus DNA directly in human serum by a simplified molecular hybridization test: comparison to HBeAg/anti-HBe status in HBsAg carriers. Hepatology 3:285–291
21. Chau KH, Hargie MP, Decker RH et al. (1983) Serodiagnosis of recent hepatitis B infection by IgM class anti-HBc. Hepatology 3:142–149
22. Gupta S, Govindarajan S, Fong TL, Redeker AG (1990) Spontaneous reactivation in chronic type B hepatitis: patterns and natural history. J Clin Gastroenterol 12:562–568
23. Alter HJ, Holland PV, Purcell RH (1975) The emerging patterns of post-transfusion hepatitis. Am J Med Sci 270:329–334
24. Dunsford HA, Sell S, Chisari FV (1990) Hepatocarcinogenesis due to chronic liver cell injury in hepatitis B virus transgenic mice. Cancer Res 50:3400–3407
25. Milich DR, McLachlan A, Moriarty A, Thornton GB (1987) Immune response to hepatitis B virus core antigen (HBcAg): localization of T cell recognition sites within HBcAg/HBeAg. J Immunol 139:1223–1231
26. Shafritz DA, Hadziyannis SJ (1984) Hepatitis B virus DNA in liver and serum, viral antigens and antibodies, virus replication, and liver disease activity in patients with persistent hepatitis B virus infection. In: Chisari FV (ed) Advances in hepatitis research. Masson, New York, pp 80–90
27. Raimondo G, Burk RD, Lieberman HM et al. (1988) Interrupted replication of hepatitis D virus in liver tissue of HBsAg carriers with hepatocellular carcinoma. Virology 166:103–111
28. Tanaka T, Miyamoto H, Hino O et al. (1988) Primary hepatocellular carcinoma with hepatitis B virus – DNA integration in a 4 year old boy. Hum Pathol 17:202–204
29. Shafritz DA, Kew MC (1981) Identification of integrated hepatitis B virus DNA sequences in human hepatocellular carcinomas. Hepatology 1:1–8
30. Fong TL, Govindarajan S, Valinluck B, Redeker AG (1988) Status of hepatitis B virus DNA in alcoholic liver disease: a study of a large urban population in the United States. Hepatology 8:1602–1604
31. Dejean A, Bouguelert L, Grzeschik KH, Tiollais P (1986) Hepatitis B virus DNA integration in a sequence homologous to v-*erb-A* and steroid receptor genes in a hepatocellular carcinoma. Nature 322:70–72

32. Wang J, Chenivesse X, Henglein B, Brechot C (1990) Hepatitis B virus integration in a cyclin A gene in a hepatocellular carcinoma. Nature 343:555–557
33. Rogler CE, Hino O, Yang D, Shafritz DA (1989) Viral DNA integration, chromosome aberrations and growth factor activation in hepatocellular carcinomas of hepadnavirus carriers. In: Bannasch P, Keppler D, Weber G (eds) Liver cell carcinoma. Kluwer Academic, Dordrecht, pp 93–106
34. Seeff LB (1990) Diagnosis, therapy and prognosis of viral hepatitis. In: Zakim D, Boyer TD (eds) Hepatology. A textbook of liver disease. W.B. Saunders, Philadelphia, pp 958–1025
35. Peters RL (1975) Viral hepatitis: a pathologic spectrum. Am J Med Sci 270:17–31
36. Boyer JL, Klatskin G (1970) Pattern of necrosis in acute viral hepatitis. Prognostic value of bridging (subacute hepatic necrosis). N Engl J Med 283:1063–1071
37. Redeker AG (1975) Viral hepatitis: clinical aspects. Am J Med Sci 270:7–16
38. Sherlock S (1976) Predicting progression of acute type-B hepatitis to chronicity. Lancet 2:354–356
39. McMahon BJ, Alward WLM, Hall DB et al. (1985) Acute hepatitis B virus infection: relation of age to the clinical expression of disease and subsequent development of the carrier state. J Infect Dis 151:599–603
40. Beasley RP, Hwang LY, Lee GC et al. (1983) Prevention of perinatally transmitted hepatitis B virus infection with hepatitis B immune globulin and hepatitis B vaccine. Lancet II:1099–1102
41. Ip HM, Lelie PN, Wong VC, Kuhns MC, Reesink HW (1989) Prevention of hepatitis B virus carrier state in infants according to maternal serum levels of HBV DNA. Lancet I:406–410
42. Rizzetto M, Canese MG, Arico S et al. (1977) Immunofluorescence detection of a new antigen/antibody system (delta/anti-delta) associated with hepatitis B virus in liver and serum of HBsAg carriers. Gut 18:997–1003
43. Wang KS, Choo W-L, Weiner AJ et al. (1986) Structure, sequence and expression of the hapatitis delta (δ) viral genome. Nature 323:508–514
44. Chen P-J, Kalpana G, Goldberg J et al. (1986) Structure and replication of the genome of the hepatitis delta virus. Proc Natl Acad Sci USA 83:8774–8778
45. Makino S, Chang MF, Shieh CK et al. (1987) Molecular cloning, sequencing and replication of a human hepatitis delta virus RNA. Nature 329:343–346
46. Xia YP, Chang MF, Wei D, Govindarajan S, Lai MM (1990) Heterogeneity of hepatitis delta antigen. Virology 178:331–336
47. Hsieh SY, Chao M, Coates L, Taylor J (1990) Hepatitis delta virus genome replication: a polyadenylated mRNA for delta antigen. J Virol 64:3192–3198
48. Kuo MY, Chao M, Taylor J (1989) Initiation of replication of the human hepatitis delta virus genome from cloned DNA: role of delta antigen. J Virol 63:1945–1950
49. Negro F, Korba BE, Forzani B et al. (1989) Hepatitis delta virus (HDV) and woodchuck hepatitis virus (WHV) nucleic acids in tissues of HDV-infected chronic WHV carrier woodchucks. J Virol 63:1612–1618
50. Bergmann KF, Gerin JL (1986) Antigens of hepatitis delta virus in the liver and serum of humans and animals. J Infect Dis 154:702–706
51. Purcell RH, Gerin JL, Rizzetto M et al. (1983) Experimental transmission of delta agent to chimpanzees. Prog Clin Biol Res 143:79–89
52. Hadziyannis SJ, Sherman M, Lieberman HM, Shafritz DA (1985) Liver disease activity and hepatitis B virus replication in chronic delta antigen-positive hepatitis B virus carriers. Hepatology 5:544–547
53. Morante AL, De La Cruz F, DeLope CR, Echevarria S, Rodriguez GM, Pons-Romero F (1989) Hepatitis B virus replication in hepatitis B and D coninfection. Liver 9:65–70

54. Villari D, Raimondo G, Smedile V et al. (1989) Hepatitis B-DNA replication and histological patterns in liver biopsy specimens of chronic HBsAg positive patients with and without hepatitis delta virus superinfection. J Clin Pathol 42:689–693
55. Cassidy WM, Govindarajan S, Gupta S, Valinluck B, Redeker AG (1989) Influence of HIV on chronic hepatitis B and D infection. Hepatology 10:690
56. Karayiannis P, Saldanha J, Monjardino J et al. (1990) Immunization of woodchucks with recombinant hepatitis delta antigen does not protect against hepatitis delta virus infection. Hepatology 12:1125–1128
57. Govindarajan S, Gupta S, Valinluck B, Redeker AG (1989) Correlation of IgM anti-hepatitis D virus (HDV) to HBV RNA in sera of chronic HDV. Hepatology 10:34–35
58. Macagno S, Smedile A, Caredda F, Ottobrelli A, Rizzetto M (1990) Monomeric (7S) immunoglobulin M antibodies to hepatitis delta virus in hepatitis type D. Gastroenterology 98:1582–1586
59. Negro F, Shapiro M, Satterfield WC, Gerin GL, Purcell RH (1989) Reappearance of hepatitis D virus (HDV) replication in chronic hepatitis B carrier chimpanzees rechallenged with HDV. J Infect Dis 160:507–511
60. Rizzetto M, Verma G, Gerin JL, Purcell RH (1986) Hepatitis delta virus disease. Prog Liver Dis 8:417–431
61. Jacobson IM, Dienstag JL, Werner BG et al. (1985) Epidemiology and clinical impact of hepatitis D virus (delta) infection. Hepatology 5:188–191
62. DeCock KM, Jones B, Govindarajan S, Redeker AG (1988) Prevalence of hepatitis (delta) virus infection. A seroepidemiologic study. West Med J 148:307–309
63. Hadler SC, DeMonzon M, Ponzetto A et al. (1984) Delta virus infection and severe hepatitis. An epidemic in the Yucpa Indians of Venezuela. Ann Intern Med 100:339–344
64. Hansson BG, Moestrup T, Widell A, Nordenfelt E (1982) Infection with delta agent in Sweden: introduction of a new hepatitis agent. J Infect Dis 146:472–478
65. Govindarajan S, Chin KP, Redeker AG, Peters RL (1984) Fulminant B viral hepatitis: role of delta agent. Gastroenterology 86:1417–1420
66. Govindarajan S, Valinluck B, Peters RL (1986) Relapse of acute B viral hepatitis – role of delta agent. Gut 27:19–22
67. Arico S, Aragona M, Rizzeto M et al. (1985) Clinical significance of antibody to the hepatitis delta virus in symptomless HBsAg carriers. Lancet II:356–357
68. Mas A, Buti M, Esteban R et al. (1990) Hepatitis B virus and hepatitis D virus replication in HBsAg-positive fulminant hepatitis. Hepatology 11:1062–1065
69. Karvountsis GG, Redeker AG (1974) Relation of alpha-fetoprotein in acute hepatitis to severity and prognosis. Ann Intern Med 80:156–160
70. Krugman S, Giles JP, Hammond JP (1970) Hepatitis virus: effect of heat on the infectivity and antigenicity of the MS-1 and MS-2 strain. J Infect Dis 122:432–436
71. Buynak EB, Roehm RR, Tytell AA et al. (1976) Vaccine against human hepatitis B. JAMA 235:2832–2834
72. Szmuness W, Stevens CE, Harley EJ et al. (1980) Hepatitis B vaccine: demonstration of efficacy in a controlled trial in a high-risk population in the United States. N Engl J Med 303:833–841
73. Emini EA, Ellis RW, Miller WJ et al. (1986) Production and immunological analysis of recombinant hepatitis B vaccine. J Infect [Suppl A] 13:3
74. Carman WF, Zanetti AR, Karayiannis P et al. (1990) Vaccine-induced escape mutant of hepatitis B virus. Lancet 336:325–329

**Suggested Reading**

Ganem D, Varmus HE (1987) The molecular biology of the hepatitis B viruses. Annu Rev Biochem 56:651–693

Robinson WS (1990) Biology of human hepatitis viruses. In: Zakim D, Boyer TD (eds) Hepatology. A textbook of liver disease. W.B. Saunders, Philadelphia, pp 890–945

Seeff LB (1990) Diagnosis, therapy and prognosis of viral hepatitis. In: Zakim D, Boyer TD (eds) Hepatology. A textbook of liver disease. W.B. Saunders, Philadelphia, pp 958–1025

Tiollais P, Purcell C, Dejean A. (1985) The hepatitis B virus. Nature 317:489–495

# 15 Viral Hepatitis C

J.M. SÁNCHEZ-TAPIAS

By the middle of the 1970s, the application of serologic and virologic markers for hepatitis A virus and hepatitis B virus had made it clear that many cases of acute and chronic hepatitis are not caused by either of these two agents. The existence of other hepatotropic viruses, which were termed non-A, non-B hepatitis viruses, was first suspected and subsequently demonstrated in experiments on transmission to chimpanzees [1].

The importance of this virus or viruses as a cause of hepatitis in man came to light from seroepidemiologic surveys demonstrating that infection by non-A, non-B hepatitis virus or viruses accounts for 90% of posttransfusional and about one-third of sporadic hepatitis cases worldwide. In addition, follow-up studies of patients with acute non-A, non-B hepatitis, mainly of the posttransfusional type, revealed the alarming tendency of this infection to become chronic [2]. Furthermore, a possible role of these viruses in cryptogenic chronic hepatitis and cirrhosis was suspected because many of these patients had evidence of acute hepatitis in the past or had been exposed to parenterally transmitted viral diseases.

Awareness of the medical and social importance of non-A, non-B hepatitis prompted vigorous research to identify the responsible virus or viruses and to develop serologic assays for clinical diagnosis. However, none of the proposed agents or laboratory tests overcame the criticism of the scientific community, and particularly that of the United States' National Institutes of Heath [3]. Nevertheless, these efforts yielded abundant information on the nature of the causative agent and on the features of this disease. In addition, well-pedigreed serum samples from humans and experimentally infected chimpanzees, carefully collected over years of patient research, were invaluable in making possible the definite identification of the main agent of non-A, non-B hepatitis, which is now acknowledged worldwide as the hepatitis C virus (HCV) [4].

## 1 Identification of Hepatitis C Virus

The successful identification, cloning, and expression of proteins from the elusive non-A, non-B blood-borne hepatitis virus was announced by investigators from Chiron Corporation, a private company, at a press conference held in May 1988. This important discovery, however, did not reach the scientific literature until 1 year later, to the great disappointment of the medical and scientific community [5].

Chiron's investigators, in close cooperation with scientists from the United States' Centers for Disease Control, developed an entirely new strategy, based upon the combination of immunologic and genetic molecular technologies [6]. As starting material, these investigators chose the plasma of a highly infectious chimpanzee with well-documented non-A, non-B hepatitis. The presumption was that this plasma would contain a high number of infectious virions. After extensive ultracentrifugation, to recover any viral particle present in plasma, all the nucleic acids present in the pellet were extracted and the RNA was reverse transcribed into cDNA with random primers. Hypothetically, viral and chimpanzee genetic DNA should have been present in this material. To unmask the specific non-A, non-B genetic material, a cDNA library was constructed by inserting restriction cDNA fragments into the bacteriophage (lambd) GT-11, an efficient expression vector, followed by cloning and amplification in *E. coli*. The rationale was that some of these clones would contain genomic sequences of non-A, non-B hepatitis and, hopefully, would produce specific protein.

The next step was to identify which clones, among many thousands, contained specific non-A, non-B sequences. To this purpose, bacterial colonies were immunoscreened with sera from a patient with non-A, non-B hepatitis, which it was assumed would contain antibodies that might unveil specific antigens. Clone 5-1-1, which contained a 155-base pair (bp) cDNA, reacted with this antiserum but not with serum obtained from the same patient prior to development of hepatitis. The original cDNA library was then screened using the 155-bp sequence as a probe, and specific hybridization with a 353-bp larger clone, clone 81, was obtained. Further experiments demonstrated that clone 81 failed to hybridize with a large number of appropriate controls, including human placental DNA, DNA from a non-A, non-B hepatitis-infected chimpanzee liver, RNA from uninfected chimpanzee liver, and RNAse-digested liver RNA from a chimpanzee with hepatitis. In contrast, this clone did hybridize with undigested RNA from an infected liver and was homologous with a single-stranded RNA present in the pellet ultracentrifuged from the original infectious plasma. These data indicated that clones 5-1-1 and 81 were derived from the genome of a blood-borne non-A, non-B hepatitis virus which was termed hepatitis C virus. Studies aimed at characterizing further the complete genome indicated that it is a positive, single-stranded RNA which contains at least 10000 nucleotides [6].

By means of the cDNA HCV clone 5-1-1 three overlapping clones were isolated. These clones had one common open reading frame that encodes a viral antigen associated with non-A, non-B hepatitis. This open reading frame was reconstructed and expressed in yeast as a fusion protein with human superoxide dismutase, which facilitates expression of foreign proteins in cell cultures, to obtain large amounts of C-100, a 363 amino acid viral polypeptide. A radioimmunoassay was then developed by coating the wells of microtiter plates with C-100, to allow for capture of specific anti-HCV antibodies present in sera. The specificity of this test system was validated (a) by examining sera from patients and chimpanzees with well-documented non-A, non-B hepatitis and from blood donors implicated in hepatitis cases, and (b), very importantly, by blind examination of a panel of sera kept at the National Institutes of Health, a trial that several other non-A, non-B hepatitis candidate assays had previously failed. Finally, detection of anti-HCV antibodies in a large proportion of patients with posttransfusion and sporadic chronic non-A, non-B hepatitis from distant areas of the world underlined the pathogenic importance of this virus [7].

## 2 The Virus

Nowadays, because of the unusual route of discovery of this agent, which involved cloning without previous characterization, knowledge of the genomic organization of HCV is rapidly expanding, in contrast with the rather limited information concerning its physicochemical structure and functions. Almost 10 years ago, the loss of infectivity observed after treatment of infectious inocula with organic solvents indicated that a lipid-containing capsid is probably a biologically important component of the virus [8, 9]. More recently, extensive filtration studies through membranes of decreasing pore diameter showed that non-A, non-B virus was able to pass through 100-, 80-, and 50-nm filters but was retained by 30-nm filter, suggesting that the candidate non-A non-B virus is less than 60 nm in diameter [10]. These data, which were obtained a long time before the discovery of HCV, suggested to investigators that this small, lipid-encapsidated non-A, non-B virus candidate was probably a member of the flavivirus–togavirus family.

Data on the genomic structure indicate that the genome of HCV consists of a single 10000-nucleotide, positively stranded RNA molecule, which also suggests that this virus is related to the togavirus family [6]. Sequence analysis of the HCV genome and encoded proteins has shown that HCV has sequence similarities with a member of this family, the dengue 2 virus, and also that the degree of similarity is even greater with the bovine diarrhea virus and the hog cholera virus, which are members of the pestivirus group and distantly related to the flavivirus. HCV also shares sequence similarity with proteins encoded by members of the picornavirus-like and alphavirus-like plant virus supergroups, suggesting that HCV may be the result of evolution from animal and plant viruses [11].

Similarities with the above-mentioned viruses and sequence analysis suggest that the HCV genome, in addition to a noncoding region, contains several coding regions, termed C, M, E, NS1, NS2a, NS2b, NS3, NS4a,

NS4b, and NS5, which code for the nucleocapside, matrix, envelope, and several nonstructural proteins respectively [12].

Sequencing of clones isolated from different parts of the world has also shown a remarkable degree of heterogeneity in relation to the HCV genome prototype described by Chiron's investigators [13–15]. Heterogeneity, however, seems greater at the nucleotide level than at the amino acid level, suggesting that most of these mutations are silent. Mutations seem to be of epidemiologic interest [16]. Whether these different mutants have different pathogenic capacity and may influence the outcome of the infection and the response to antiviral therapy is currently unknown.

Sequence heterogeneity may also importantly affect the efficacy of molecular biologic polymerase chain reaction (PCR) techniques because mutants present in sera or other biologic specimens may not be detected if primers are not adequately selected. The sensitivity of PCR methods may be enhanced considerably if oligonucleotide sequences from highly conserved regions of HCV genome are chosen as primers [17].

## 3 Serologic Markers of Hepatitis C Virus

In clinical practice and in epidemiologic studies, the diagnosis of HCV infection is based mainly on immunologic assays aimed at unveiling the presence in serum of antibodies against HCV antigens. All the currently available assays use HCV antigens obtained by recombinant technology. Short-term development of laboratory procedures to detect circulating HCV antigens seems unlikely owing to the low amount of viral particles in serum, a feature of HCV infection which probably accounts for the failure of many immunoserologic and electron microscopic attempts carried out in the past. Nevertheless, antigen detection will probably be advantageously replaced by PCR detection of HCV RNA sequences. The presence of HCV RNA correlates well with infectivity and can thus be considered as a marker of viral replication and viremia. This sophisticated technique, however, cannot yet be used as a routine diagnostic procedure.

The immunologic and molecular biologic procedures have enormously contributed to our knowledge of many aspects of hepatitis C. The abovementioned procedures, however, are far from perfect. The ideal test to identify acute, chronic, and past HCV infection has not yet been developed and caution in interpreting the currently available assays must be recommended.

### 3.1 Tests for Anti-HCV Antibodies

#### *The Anti-C100-3 ELISA Test*

A radioimmunoassay to detect antibodies against the nonstructural C100-3 HCV antigen was the first laboratory technique used in the diagnosis of HCV infection. This antigen was soon incorporated into an ELISA assay which was rapidly validated and is now commercially available worldwide. In their initial report, Kuo and co-workers [7] highlighted the close association of the presence of anti-C100-3 antibodies with non-A, non-B hepatitis. Although many authors have consistently confirmed the observations of Kuo and co-workers, there is increasing evidence that, despite its intrinsic interest, the determination of anti-C100-3 antibodies may not be entirely adequate for a number of clinical, epidemiologic, and prophylactic purposes.

Posttransfusional hepatitis surveys have shown that most patients with posttransfusion hepatitis seroconvert to anti-C100-3 positive [18–20]. These studies have also made clear that most instances of posttransfusion hepatitis occur in recipients of anti-C100-3 positive blood, suggesting that anti-C100-3 is a marker of infectivity. Retrospective analysis of sera collected from donors and recipients included in prospective studies has shown that screening blood donors for anti-C100-3 and rejection positive donors would have prevented about 80% of cases of posttransfusional hepatitis with a minimal loss of blood donors, which represents a considerable improvement in comparison with screening for surrogate non-A, non-B hepatitis markers such as elevated alanine aminotransferase (ALT) and anti-HBc [20].

However, about 15% of cases of anti-C100-3 positive posttransfusion hepatitis occur in recipients of exclusively anti-C100-3 negative blood. Alter et al. [21] suggested that, as seroconversion to anti-C100-3 is often delayed in the course of hepatitis C, a blood donor may be infective if donation took place during the window period preceding seroconversion. However, Esteban et al. [19] have recently reported that several anti-C100-3 negative blood donors who were implicated in cases of posttransfusion hepatitis did not seroconvert after prolonged follow-up, a finding that indicates that HCV infection and the HCV carrier state may occur despite the absence of anti-C100-3 antibodies.

On the other hand, positivity for anti-C100-3 is not indefectibly associated with infectivity because about 30% of anti-C100-3 positive donors are not implicated in cases of posttransfusion hepatitis [20]. Usually, these donors do not present clinical or biochemical evidence of liver disease and it is difficult to ascertain whether positivity for anti-C100-3 reflects infection by HCV in the past or is a false-positive result of the ELISA technique. Whatever the reason, the finding of positivity for anti-C100-3 in an otherwise healthy person often leads to an amazing situation where to provide medical advice may be a difficult task. Thus, although screening blood donors for anti-C100-3 is certainly advantageous, there is no doubt that a more accurate marker of infectivity is still needed in blood transfusion centers.

Follow-up studies of experimentally infected chimpanzees [22] and persons with posttransfusional hepatitis C [21, 23] have yielded important information on the dynamics of the anti-C100-3 response in HCV infection, which seems similar in humans and animals. A small percentage of patients with posttransfusion hepatitis become anti-C100-3 positive shortly after transfusion, a phenomenon likely due to passive transfer of antibodies. More than 90%, however, develop a true seroconversion but the time lapse from the onset of hepatitis to detection of antibodies varies widely, from 2 weeks in some cases to 1 year or more in others. The mean time interval until seroconversion is about 15 weeks and about 80% of the patients have seroconverted at 6 months. The rate of anti-C100-3 positivity during the acute phase of the illness is slightly lower in patients who recover than in those progressing to chronicity. In general, the reactivity for anti-C100-3 is stronger in the latter than in the former, although anti-C100-3 may persist for years after the apparent resolution of the disease. Again, these data indicate that, although testing for anti-C100-3 may be useful, this test does not provide sufficient diagnostic or prognostic information in many patients with posttransfusional hepatitis.

In patients with sporadic acute non-A, non-B hepatitis, the fate of anti-C100-3 seems somewhat different [24]. The 26% rate of positivity observed in resolving cases was considerably lower than the 71% found in those progressing to chronicity. In addition, anti-C100-3 disappeared rapidly in the former but persisted in the latter. Thus, in acute, sporadic non-A, non-B hepatitis, testing for anti-C100-3 may provide useful prognostic information in some cases but it does not clarify whether anti-C100-3 negative cases are due to HCV infection with poor serologic response or are caused by another non-A, non-B unidentified agent.

Several groups have shown a high prevalence of anti-C100-3 antibodies in patients with chronic liver disease of unknown etiology [7, 25–28]. Among patients with a history of parenteral exposure, such as those who have received blood transfusions, hemophiliacs, and intravenous drug abusers, the proportion of anti-C100-3 positive cases is extremely high, 90% or more. In patients with no obvious parenteral exposure the prevalence of anti-C100-3 is also very high, ranging from 58% to 74%. These figures are much higher than those found in apparently healthy volunteer blood donors, which range from 0.5% to 1.5% [26, 27, 29–32]. This difference strongly suggests that HCV plays a very important role in cryptogenic chronic liver disease, where testing for anti-C100-3 may provide important diagnostic clues.

False-positive results, however, may restrict the diagnostic efficacy of the ELISA anti-C100-3 test in chronic liver disease. False-positive results have been described in a variety of conditions, including rheumatoid arthritis

[33], paraproteinemia [34], tropical populations [35], and, very importantly, autoimmune chronic liver diseases [36]. Since confirmatory tests are not yet readily available, interpretation of a positive test in some patients with chronic liver disease may be difficult. For this reason, urea treatment of microtiter wells, which washes out low-affinity antibodies and nonspecific reactants, has been recommended to enhance the specificity of the ELISA test [37, 38].

### *Other Anti-HCV Antibodies: The RIBA Tests*

The insufficient sensitivity and specificity of the anti-C100-3 ELISA test prompted investigators to develop more efficient immunoassays. Among these, the most commonly used is the recombinant immunoblot assay (RIBA). In this test diluted samples are layered over nitrocellulose strips where two recombinant HCV antigens, C100-3 and 5.1.1, which is a subsequence of C100-3, are immobilized as distinct antigenic bands. A third band consisting of human superoxide dismutase, a protein which is also present in HCV antigens, serves to control false-positive anti-HCV reactions and, finally, two additional bands containing high and low human IgG concentrations, respectively, serve as internal controls. The RIBA is considered positive when the reaction in the two HCV antigen bands is at least as intense as in the low concentration IgG band and there is no reaction in the superoxide dismutase band. RIBA is negative when there is no reaction in any of the HCV antigen bands or when the superoxide dismutase band reacts. If only one of the HCV antigen bands shows a reaction, RIBA is considered as indeterminate. The test is read by direct visualization of the strips and may therefore be subject to misinterpretation due to subjective observer errors. RIBA may serve as a supplementary test of the specificity of the ELISA anti-C100-3 but it cannot be considered as a true confirmatory test because both assays use the same antigen.

A fairly good correspondence usually exists between the results obtained with RIBA and the intensity of the anti-C100-3 reaction observed in the ELISA assay, which may be estimated from the ratio between the optical density of the sample and the cut-off, named the ELISA ratio. Most sera with an ELISA ratio higher than 4 are positive by RIBA while most weakly reactive sera, with an ELISA ratio lower than 1.5, are RIBA negative. However, there is not a perfect correlation between RIBA and ELISA because samples strongly reactive by ELISA may be negative by RIBA and, vice versa, RIBA positive samples may be weakly reactive by ELISA [39].

There is also a reasonably good correspondence between the results of RIBA and the presence of viremia since HCV RNA may be demonstrated by PCR in 70% of RIBA positive sera but is usually undetectable in RIBA indeterminate or negative sera [40]. Posttransfusional hepatitis studies have also shown a relatively good correspondence between infectivity and the results of RIBA because hepatitis is very common in recipients of RIBA positive blood [20, 41, 42]. However, hepatitis does not occur in all the patients transfused with RIBA positive blood while it may develop in recipients of RIBA negative or indeterminate blood. In other words, although RIBA may possibly improve the efficacy of blood donor screening for HCV infection, it does not obviate satisfactorily enough the deficiencies of the ELISA test. In addition, the high cost and the limited availability of RIBA reagents do not favor the use of this test for mass screening at blood banks.

Other assay systems using different recombinant HCV antigens are currently being developed. Promising results with a new recombinant immunoblot assay, named 4-RIBA, have very recently been reported [43]. This test uses four recombinant HCV antigens, the two C-100-3 and 5.1.1 antigens of the original RIBA plus two new antigens, an HCV core antigen, C22, and another nonstructural antigen, C33c. This new assay may be considered as a truly confirmatory test. The results obtained with 4-RIBA correlated well with the presence of viremia, as assessed by PCR, and also with infectivity, as shown by development of hepatitis in recipients of 4-RIBA positive blood. Furthermore, addition of C22 and C33c enabled earlier detection of HCV infection in patients with posttransfusion hepatitis. Ongoing studies with this and other second-generation immunoserologic tests will hopefully provide tools for more accurate diagnosis of HCV infection.

### 3.2 HCV RNA Sequences

Cloning and sequencing of the HCV genome have made possible the development of molecular biology techniques and probes that can be used to detect sequences of HCV RNA in plasma, serum, or liver tissue from infected or presumably infected persons and animals. Underlying viral replication and viremia may be inferred from the presence of HCV RNA sequences in blood, a finding with obvious diagnostic importance.

The minute amount of circulating virions present in the blood of HCV carriers does not permit detection of HCV RNA by conventional direct hybridization of RNA serum extracts with radiolabeled probes. This serious difficulty has been successfully circumvented by application of PCR, a sophisticated gene amplification technique which can produce thousands of copies of a single DNA molecule and, hence, facilitates detection by more ordinary procedures. In HCV RNA studies, extraction of RNA and reverse transcription into cDNA are mandatory steps prior to amplification by PCR.

The presence of HCV RNA sequences in plasma and liver tissue from patients and chimpanzees with non-A, non-B hepatitis was first reported by Weiner and co-workers [44]. These authors made several important observations using as primers a pair of oligonucleotides from two noncontiguous clones from the HCV genome flanking a region of 586 bp. PCR products were detected with a probe made by radiolabeling of an oligonucleotide sequence lying between the cDNA/PCR primers. HCV RNA was detected in the liver in seven of nine patients with anti-C100-3 positive chronic hepatitis and also in two of six with anti-C100-3 negative chronic hepatitis. It was also shown that the presence of HCV RNA in serum precedes seroconversion to anti-C100-3 in the acute phase of posttransfusional hepatitis. Existence of viremia in the absence of anti-C100-3 response may explain why some anti-C100-3 negative inocula are capable of transmitting HCV infection.

Shortly thereafter, GARSON and co-workers [14, 45] reported the results of their HCV RNA follow-up studies in hemophiliacs with non-A, non-B hepatitis related to treatment with factor VIII concentrates. These authors used a modification of the PCR technique in which the amplified DNA product is reamplified by a second PCR round with internal primers. After staining with ethidium bromide, the final product is detected by direct visualization under ultraviolet light [46]. The main advantage of this technique is the avoidance of potentially dangerous radiolabeled probes. The procedure is simpler and safer than the typical one-round PCR but the control of specificity is less strict. In "nested" PCR specificity is controlled by assessment of the size of the final product, which must have the expected length of the specifically amplified DNA region. Using this technique, GARSON and co-workers observed that several patterns of viremia may occur in HCV infection. Patients with acute resolving hepatitis present a transient period of viremia, preceding or at the time of ALT elevation and many weeks before seroconversion to anti-C100-3. Patients with chronic infection may have long-lasting, intermittent, or recurrent viremia and, interestingly, HCV RNA fluctuations do not parallel fluctuations in ALT activity (Fig. 1).

A few observations in posttransfusional hepatitis have shown a good association between presence of HCV RNA in transfused blood, either anti-C100-3 positive or negative, and development of hepatitis in the recipient [43, 45, 47]. Therefore, if it were technically feasible, PCR detection of HCV RNA might be a good method for screening individual blood donations but not for selecting blood donors because potentially infectious persons may escape detection owing to fluctuation of viremia in chronically infected persons.

Detection of HCV RNA is still a difficult procedure. In addition to the intrinsic complexity of PCR technology, important problems arise from the genetic heterogeneity of HCV, which may cause false-negative results if primers are not adequately chosen, a frustration that can be prevented if primers are selected from highly conserved regions of the HCV genome [17]. Nevertheless, HCV RNA studies are still beyond the capabilities of most clinical laboratories.

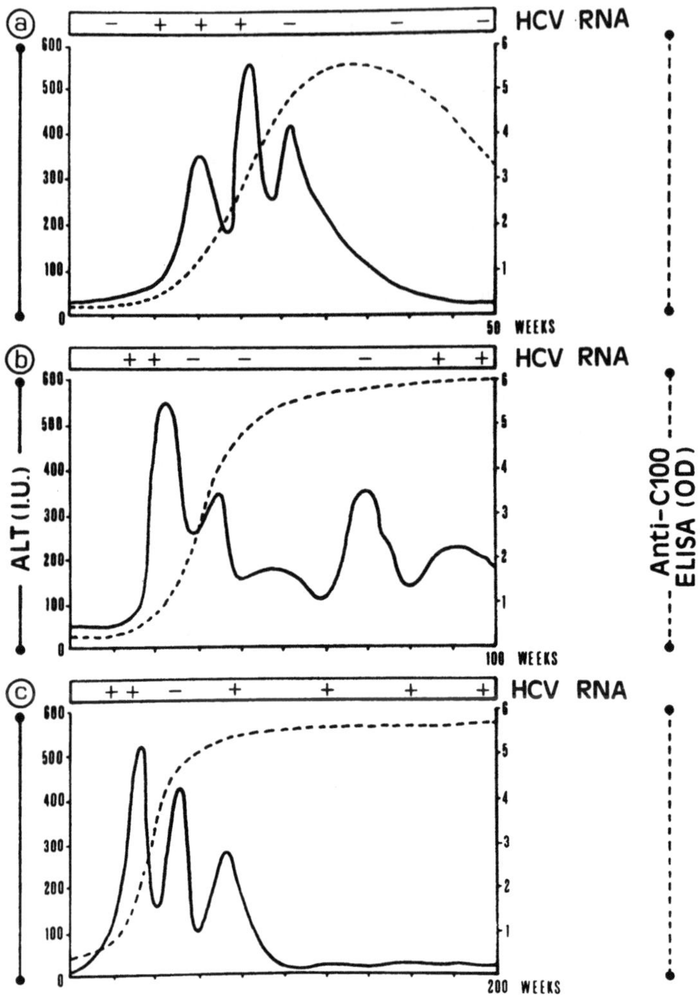


**Fig. 1a–c.** Biochemical and serologic patterns of HCV infection. **a** Resolving acute infection with decline in anti-HCV antibodies. **b** Acute hepatitis progressing to chronic hepatitis. **c** Acute infection progressing to chronicity with no biochemical evidence of hepatitis

## 4 Epidemiologic Aspects

### 4.1 Hepatitis C and Blood Transfusion

Viral hepatitis is a common complication of blood transfusion that occurs in 5%–15% of transfused patients. After implementation of HBsAg blood donor screening, more than 90% of cases of posttransfusion hepatitis are caused by non-A, non-B hepatitis virus or viruses [48–55]. The recent availability of serologic tests for HCV infection has made it possible to reexamine transfusion-related hepatitis, and important questions concerning the role of HCV infection and the prophylactic efficacy of screening for HCV markers are currently under active investigation.

At present, there is no doubt that HCV is responsible for most cases of non-A, non-B posttransfusion hepatitis. Whether other viruses may also be involved is as yet uncertain, but this possibility seems unlikely. Between 67% and 89% of patients with posttransfusion hepatitis develop anti-HCV antibodies [18–20] and, in some studies, this proportion approaches 100% in patients with hepatitis progressing to chronicity [21, 23]. In addition, 1%–2% of blood recipients seroconvert to anti-HCV positive in the absence of clinical or biochemical evidence of hepatitis. In some of the latter patients, transmission of HCV is demonstrated by emergence of HCV RNA in their sera [56].

As assessed by the anti-C100-3 ELISA test, about 10%–30% of patients with posttransfusion hepatitis do not develop anti-HCV antibodies, even if transfused with anti-HCV positive blood. Although infection by another unidentified virus cannot be excluded, there are also other possible explanations. First, ALT elevation may be of nonviral origin. Second, absence of anti-HCV does not necessarily rule out the responsibility of HCV because a weak serologic immune response may not be detected by the current ELISA assay or, alternatively, delayed seroconversion may pass unnoticed if sufficiently prolonged blood sampling is not performed on follow-up [21, 23]. Ongoing studies with recently developed serologic tests able to detect earlier serologic response to HCV antigens other than C100-3, as well as more extensive investigation of HCV RNA in recipients sera, will answer this question in the near future.

Transfusion with anti-HCV positive blood does not cause hepatitis in about one-third of recipients [19, 20]. Although some of these may be immune against HCV prior to transfusion, lack of infectivity of many anti-HCV positive blood units seems a more reasonable explanation. Analysis of anti-HCV positive donors implicated in hepatitis cases has shown that donors with persistent positivity for anti-HCV, a high ELISA ratio, a positive RIBA test, and elevated ALT levels are more likely infectious [18, 20], but absence of these conditions does not guarantee noninfectivity and hepatitis may develop following transfusion with low ELISA ratio, RIBA negative blood or with normal ALT, anti-HCV positive blood.

On the other hand, the observation that 15%–44% of patients with posttransfusion hepatitis C were transfused with exclusively ELISA anti-HCV negative blood [19, 20] clearly indicates that some infectious donors cannot be recognized by this test. As indicated previously, such donors may be identified by detection of HCV RNA in serum [45, 47], but this method is unsuitable for mass screening of blood donors.

From the above-mentioned studies it becomes apparent that most cases of posttransfusional hepatitis C might be prevented if blood donors were screened for anti-HCV antibodies and positive donors were excluded from

**Table 1.** Comparison of the efficacy of exclusion of blood donors after screening for anti-HCV, anti-HBc, elevated ALT (>40 IU/liter), and combinations to prevent post-transfusion hepatitis

| | Reason for exclusion | | | | | |
|---|---|---|---|---|---|---|
| | Anti-VHC + | Anti-HBc + | ALT >40 | Anti-VHC + Anti-HBc + | Anti-VHC + ALT >40 | Anti-HBc + ALT >40 |
| Absolute efficacy | 85% | 82.5% | 65% | 90% | 85% | 87.5% |
| Corrected efficacy | 80.5% | 52.5% | 45.4% | 70.4% | 72.8% | 61.1% |
| Donors to be excluded | 2.2% | 14% | 5.6% | 15.7% | 7.5% | 18.6% |

donation. This procedure, however, would probably not cause the complete disappearance of posttransfusion hepatitis and many noninfectious anti-HCV positive blood donations would unnecessarily be discarded.

Despite these limitations, screening of blood donors for anti-HCV antibodies by ELISA appears at present to be the most valuable method for preventing transfusion-associated hepatitis. Studies comparing the value of anti-HCV and non-A, non-B surrogate markers, i.e., anti-HBc and elevated ALT levels, for screening blood donors have shown that anti-HCV performs better than surrogate markers since it is more effective in preventing post-transfusion hepatitis and the proportion of donors who are rejected is lower (Table 1) [18, 20].

### 4.2 Hepatitis C in Hemophilia

Twenty years ago, replacement therapy with clotting factor concentrates prepared from large plasma pools became a great advance in the treatment of hemophiliac patients. This procedure, however, has been hampered by the occurrence in recipients of parenterally transmitted viral diseases, including hepatitis B, non-A, non-B hepatitis, and, more recently, the acquired immunodeficiency syndrome. Non-A, non-B hepatitis in hemophiliacs received little attention until recently, when the progressive character of the disease, leading to development of chronic active hepatitis and cirrhosis in a considerable proportion of patients, became apparent [57].

Infection with HCV appears to be by far the most important cause of hepatitis in hemophiliacs. The overall prevalence of anti-HCV antibodies, as assessed by the C100-3 ELISA test, is extremely high in these patients, ranging from 64% to 82% [25, 27, 58, 59]. The rate of positivity is higher in hemophiliacs with persistently elevated ALT serum levels than in those with intermittent ALT elevation. Furthermore, as many as 63% of hemophiliacs with normal ALT are anti-HCV positive [59] and in most of them the RIBA test is also positive [60], suggesting that positivity for anti-HCV is probably not due to the lack of specificity of the ELISA test.

As in other circumstances, the meaning of anti-HCV antibodies in hemophiliacs is uncertain. However, most anti-HCV positive hemophiliacs present abnormal liver function tests and their liver biopsies show lesions of chronic hepatitis with non-A, non-B hepatitis features [61]. These data suggest that positivity for anti-HCV truly reflects HCV infection in these patients.

The presence of anti-HCV antibodies in hemophiliacs is independent of the patient's age and type of hemophilia but correlates well with the amount of factor concentrates given in the past and also with the type of replacement therapy administered. The highest prevalence of anti-HCV occurs in the more heavily perfused patients while in untreated patients anti-HCV antibodies may be absent [61] or, when present, the prevalence is low [25]. Makris and co-workers [61] found that the prevalence of anti-HCV in patients treated with heated concentrates was only 22% and Noel and co-workers [59] did not detect anti-HCV antibodies in any of 16 children who had received exclusively solvent- and detergent-treated concentrates. In a prospective study, Mannucci and co-workers [62] did not observe hepatitis or seroconversion to anti-HCV in any of 26 patients treated with highly purified, pasteurized factor VIII. Thus, there is much less evidence of HCV infection in patients treated with products submitted to virucidal procedures than in those who have received conventional factor VIII concentrates. The decreased infectivity achieved by these procedures is due to destruction of viral particles which, as shown by HCV RNA studies, are invariably present in untreated concentrates.

At present, it is a matter of debate whether virucidal treatment of concentrates is more effective in preventing HCV infection in susceptible hemophiliacs than selection of donors by anti-HCV screening. This controversy, however, will be resolved in the near future when recombinant factor VIII, whose efficacy and safety have recently been demonstrated, becomes widely available [63].

### 4.3 Hepatitis C in Intravenous Drug Addicts

Infection with HCV is widespread among intravenous drug users. Several surveys have demonstrated that the prevalence of ELISA anti-HCV antibodies in these subjects is very high, ranging from 48% to more than 90% [25–27, 64, 65]. Differences are related to the composition of the population under study since the prevalence of anti-HCV is higher in addicts infected by HIV or with evidence of chronic liver disease. Among the latter, evidence of coexistent infection by two or more hepatitis viruses is frequently observed. For instance, in a recent study, Tító and co-workers found that more than two-thirds of drug addicts with chronic hepatitis attributed to hepatitis B virus and hepatitis D virus infection were also seropositive for anti-HCV antibodies [66]. These data, however, deserve further evaluation through the use of confirmatory assays because elevated serum globulin levels, which are very common among these patients, may cause falsely positive results in the ELISA test.

### 4.4 Hepatitis C and Hemodialysis

Patients on long-term hemodialysis are subjected to repeated venesections with reinfusion of blood and, additionally, many of them require blood transfusions. Because of these invasive therapeutic maneuvers these patients are heavily exposed to parenterally transmitted viral diseases. The fact that hemodialysis patients are at high risk of acquiring percutaneous viral infections was clearly demonstrated many years ago by their high rate of hepatitis B virus infection, which made it necessary to treat infected patients in physically separated units.

Many patients on chronic hemodialysis present biochemical evidence of chronic liver disease and their liver biopsies often show lesions typical of chronic hepatitis, which, in the absence of any other explanation, have been attributed to chronic non-A, non-B hepatitis virus infection [67, 68]. Recently, anti-HCV antibodies have been demonstrated by the ELISA assay in about 20% of patients on chronic hemodialysis [69–71]. Although there is a wide variation in the prevalence of anti-HCV antibodies among different units, which may be partially related to geographic differences in the prevalence of HCV infection, it seems reasonably clear that the rate of positivity of anti-HCV is mainly related to the duration of dialysis since patients on this therapy for 1 year or less only rarely present anti-HCV antibodies whereas they can be detected in almost 50% of patients on dialysis for 10 years or more [69]. Patients with a history of blood transfusion have a greater chance of being anti-HCV positive but a strict correlation has not been found between these two conditions [70]. In contrast, a good correlation has been observed between the presence of anti-HCV and the time on dialysis in nontransfused patients [71]. These data suggest that, in addition to blood transfusion, the intrinsic invasiveness of hemodialysis may, by itself or perhaps in association with the immune deficiency of chronic renal failure, facilitate the spread of HCV infection among these patients.

Again, the meaning of the ELISA positive anti-HCV test is not well understood. Although a good correspondence exists between a positive test and elevated ALT levels, some anti-HCV positive hemodialysis patients have normal liver function tests. As the presence of anti-HCV antibodies does not necessarily mean infectivity, creation of separate hemodialysis units to treat anti-HCV positive patients does not seem justified at present. Instead, prevention of HCV infection in hemodialysis patients should be attempted by means of very strict observance of physical safety measures, including barrier methods, and most judicious use of blood transfusion.

Improved selection of blood donors and the application of recombinant erythropoietin to treat renal failure-associated anemia will soon help to limit the incidence of HCV infection in hemodialysis units.

### 4.5 Sexual Transmission

Studies designed to investigate the role of sexual transmission of non-A, non-B hepatitis were hampered by the lack of appropriate serologic markers. Nevertheless, possible transmission by the sexual route was suggested by a recent epidemiologic survey in which multiple heterosexual contacts were significantly associated with acute non-A, non-B hepatitis in patients with no history of parenteral exposure [72]. In this study, increased risk for non-A, non-B hepatitis among male homosexuals was not observed.

Testing for anti-HCV antibodies has shed more light on this old problem but some doubt still persists. ESTEBAN and co-workers [25] observed a low prevalence of anti-HCV antibodies in male homosexuals and in sexual partners of drug addicts with HCV infection. On this basis, these authors suggested that the sexual route does not seem to play an important role in HCV transmission. A similar conclusion was reached by EVERHARDT and co-workers [73], who found neither clinical nor serologic evidence of hepatitis C among stable sexual partners of patients with anti-HCV positive chronic hepatitis. On the other hand, increased prevalence of anti-HCV antibodies *was* observed in HIV-infected male homosexuals [64], suggesting that sexual transmission of hepatitis C may occur under circumstances involving sexual promiscuity and immune depression. In any case, there is no doubt that hepatitis C is much less effectively transmitted by the sexual route than is hepatitis B.

### 4.6 Intrafamilial Transmission

Some serologic surveys of household contacts of patients with anti-HCV positive chronic liver disease have shown that the prevalence of anti-HCV antibodies in this population is about twice that in blood donors of the same geographic area [74, 75]. These findings suggest that HCV infection may spread through prolonged intimate contact with HCV carriers. However, this may not be so, given that comparison with blood donors is probably inappropriate because blood donors are a selected population that does not adequately represent HCV endemicity in the general population; moreover, other authors failed to observe clinical or serologic evidence of increased HCV infection among family members of patients with chronic hepatitis C [73]. On the other hand, some of the anti-HCV positive family contacts had a history of possible parenteral exposure. Thus, the presently available information indicates that, although intrafamilial HCV transmission cannot be excluded, it does not appear to be an important mechanism of HCV spreading.

### 4.7 Vertical Transmission

The role of vertical transmission of HCV infection is being examined by longitudinal serologic surveys of children born to anti-HCV positive mothers at the time of delivery. Most of these babies are anti-HCV positive at birth, suggesting that passive transmission of antibodies is very common. However, antibodies are progressively lost and, at 6 months, most babies are anti-HCV negative. These children do not present clinical or biochemical evidence of liver disease [76]. These data indicate that mother-to-child transmission of HCV infection does not usually occur. However, occasional cases of mother-to-child HCV transmission have been documented [77], particularly in children born to HIV-infected mothers [78]. Whether immunodeficiency enables HCV to replicate more actively and causes increased infectivity of anti-HIV positive mothers is now under investigation.

## 5 Hepatitis C Virus Infection in Chronic Liver Disease and Hepatocellular Carcinoma

Recent serologic surveys have shown the presence of HCV antibodies in the majority of patients with cryptogenic chronic active hepatitis and cirrhosis, in some patients with HBsAg positive chronic liver disease, and in a proportion of alcoholics with chronic liver disease. Furthermore, the finding of anti-HCV antibodies in many patients with primary hepatocellular carcinoma has elicited great interest in the possible role of hepatotropic viruses other than the hepatitis B virus in hepatic carcinogenesis.

### 5.1 Cryptogenic Chronic Liver Disease

Anti-HCV antibodies are detected in 42%–90% of patients with cryptogenic chronic hepatitis or cirrhosis [7, 25, 26, 79–82]. The prevalence of anti-HCV in patients with histories of blood transfusion, even in the very distant past, and in drug addicts was slightly higher than in those with no obvious source of exposure. These studies have also shown that a great difference exists in the anti-HCV positivity rate between patients with cryptogenic chronic liver disease and blood donors, and, hence, a possible role of HCV infection as a very important cause of chronic liver disease has vigorously emerged. This hypothesis is further supported by the different reactivity observed in the ELISA test in anti-HCV positive sera from chronic liver disease patients and blood donors. ELISA ratio values greater than 4 were observed in more

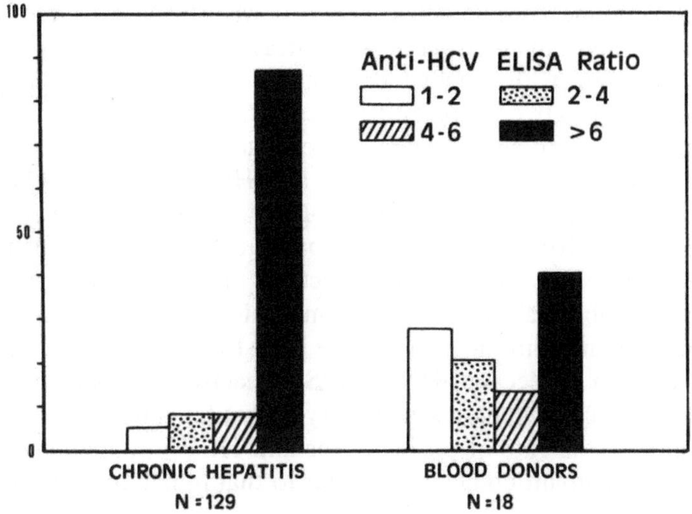


**Fig. 2.** Distribution of anti-HCV positive blood donors and patients with chronic hepatitis according to ELISA ratio values in the anti-HCV assay

than 90% of the former but in only one-half of the latter [26] (Fig. 2). Since a high ELISA ratio correlates reasonably well with the presence of HCV RNA sequences in sera [40], it may be speculated that continued antigenic stimulation resulting from persistent viral replication can explain the strong anti-C100-3 reactivity observed in most patients with cryptogenic non-A, non-B chronic liver disease. Nevertheless, the role of HCV infection in cryptogenic liver diseases deserves further evaluation with more direct diagnostic approaches.

### 5.2 Autoimmune Chronic Active Hepatitis

Recently, Lenzi and co-workers [83] described the presence of anti-HCV antibodies in 80% of patients with type 1 anti-LKM positive chronic hepatitis, a disease that was previously recognized as type 2 autoimmune chronic hepatitis [84]. In their series, sera from patients with very high titer anti-LKM autoantibodies did not react for anti-HCV in the ELISA test. Accordingly, these authors suggested that some cases of "autoimmune" chronic active hepatitis might indeed be due to chronic infection by HCV, which, as has been well documented in other chronic viral diseases of the liver, such as chronic delta hepatitis [85], would induce the emergence of anti-LKM autoantibodies.

However, this interpretation of the meaning of anti-HCV reactivity in the ELISA test in autoimmune chronic liver disease has been contested. McFarlane and co-workers [36] observed a positive reaction in the anti-

HCV ELISA assay in 20 of 31 patients with antinuclear autoantibody positive autoimmune chronic active hepatitis when tests were performed during an active phase of the disease. In contrast, anti-HCV was positive in only 1 of 22 patients with inactive disease and all the anti-HCV positive patients became negative on retesting once complete remission was achieved under immunosuppressive therapy. These authors also observed a strong correlation between positivity for anti-HCV and high globulin levels and suggested that positivity for anti-HCV in patients with severe autoimmune chronic active hepatitis was probably a false-positive result of the ELISA test caused by unidentified reactants present in hyperglobulinemic sera. Similar observations have been made in children with serologic markers of autoimmune chronic liver disease [86]. In our own series, however, we were unable to detect anti-HCV ELISA reactivity in patients with cryptogenic chronic active hepatitis with very high titer antinuclear autoantibodies. In contrast, the rate of positivity for anti-HCV in patients with low titer antinuclear autoantibodies was similar to that in patients with no autoantibodies [26].

Because it has important therapeutic implications, the differentiation of autoimmune from virus-induced chronic hepatitis cannot be considered as merely an academic exercise. Corticosteroids, which are highly effective in autoimmune hepatitis, should probably not be given to patients with viral disease, while interferon, which can be beneficial in some patients with chronic hepatitis C, may be detrimental if inadvertently administered to patients with autoimmune chronic active hepatitis [87]. Until more direct tests to identify HCV infection become widely available, distinction between autoimmune and HCV-induced chronic hepatitis may be difficult. In some cases, however, clinical and histopathologic data may guide the differential diagnosis and therapeutic management of these patients [88] (Table 2).

**Table 2.** Guidelines for etiologic diagnosis of chronic hepatitis in patients with a positive anti-HCV (ELISA) test and positive non-organ-specific autoantibodies

| Features | HCV induced | Autoimmune |
|---|---|---|
| History of parenteral exposure | Often present | Absent |
| Preferential age and sex | Any | Young females |
| Symptoms | Absent or mild | Usually present |
| Elevation of ALT and AST | Mild to moderate | Severe |
| Serum globulin levels | Normal or mildly elevated | Very elevated |
| Titer of autoantibodies (ANA, LKM) | Low | Usually high |
| Portal inflammation | Mild to moderate | Severe |
| Periportal changes | Mild to moderate | Severe |
| Lobular changes | Often present | Unconspicuous |

### 5.3 HBsAg Positive Chronic Liver Disease

Infection with HCV may also play a role in HBsAg positive chronic liver disease. Several studies have shown that 10%–15% patients with HBsAg chronic hepatitis and cirrhosis present anti-HCV ELISA antibodies [26, 82, 88]. The prevalence of anti-HCV, interestingly, is noticeably high, 30%–40%, among anti-HBe positive, HBV DNA negative carriers with chronic active hepatitis [26, 88]. Thus, HCV superinfection may account for persistence of disease activity in some HBsAg positive patients who do not present active replication of hepatitis B virus, but, again, this speculation awaits confirmation by more accurate assessment of HCV infection.

### 5.4 Alcoholic Liver Disease

Two studies including a large number of patients have recently shown that about 25% of chronic alcoholics with liver disease present antibodies against HCV [89, 90]. In one of these studies [89] positivity for anti-HCV was further supported by RIBA testing. In both studies, the observed prevalence of anti-HCV increased stepwise with the severity of liver damage, from 13% in patients with steatosis or fibrosis to 20% in patients with alcoholic hepatitis and about 40% in cirrhotics. In contrast, the prevalence of anti-HCV in alcoholics without evidence of liver damage was only 2%, similar to that in blood donors. Within the same histologic category, patients positive for anti-HCV showed a greater degree of impairment of liver function and, on histologic analysis, presented increased cellularity within the sinusoids more often than anti-HCV negative patients, a histologic trait which suggests non-A, non-B viral infection. These observations may indicate that superinfection by HCV is able to contribute to the development of liver lesions in a substantial proportion of chronic alcoholics with liver disease.

The reasons for the high prevalence of anti-HCV in alcoholics with cirrhosis are intriguing. One possible explanation is that these patients are at increased risk of becoming infected by HCV as a consequence of repeated hospitalizations, medical procedures, and blood transfusion. If so, HCV infection would be an indirect consequence of alcoholism and advanced liver disease. However, this may not be the correct explanation because many alcoholic patients with anti-HCV positive cirrhosis have never been hospitalized or had blood transfusions prior to the development of cirrhosis [89]. It is therefore possible that HCV infection has accelerated progression to cirrhosis in some cases. If this is so, these patients might have developed cirrhosis because, in addition to alcoholism, they are infected by HCV. Distinction between these possibilities may have important therapeutic implications in the future.

### 5.5 Hepatocellular Carcinoma

A few years ago, involvement of non-A, non-B hepatitis virus in the development of hepatocellular carcinoma became suspected on the basis of individual case reports [91–93] and occasional retrospective observations [94, 95]. However, further insight into this problem was prevented by the absence of serologic markers.

Identification of HCV was a crucial breakthrough that encouraged very active research in this field and, shortly thereafter, authors from Spain [89] and Italy [90] reported finding anti-HCV antibodies in 65%–75% of patients with hepatocellular carcinoma (Table 3). The prevalence of anti-HCV antibodies was particularly high among cancer patients with underlying non-A, non-B or cryptogenic chronic liver disease although, interestingly, it was also remarkably high in patients with underlying HBsAg positive or with alcoholic cirrhosis. Their data strongly suggested the involvement of HCV in the pathogenesis of hepatocellular carcinoma.

Further work from the United States [82], France [90], Italy [96], and Japan [82, 97] has shown rather similar figures in respect of the prevalence of anti-HCV antibodies in patients with hepatocellular carcinoma and cirrhosis of different etiology (Table 3). The rate of positivity for anti-HCV in cancer patients is approximately two to three times greater than in noncancer patients with HBsAg positive or alcoholic cirrhosis. Among patients with cryptogenic or posttransfusional chronic liver disease, most of whom have anti-HCV antibodies, the prevalence of anti-HCV is still higher in cancer patients, particularly those with a history of blood transfusion [82]. Thus, the accumulated evidence from these studies reinforces the idea that HCV is a very important factor in the development of hepatocellular carcinoma worldwide. Quantitatively, the role of HCV in hepatic carcinogenesis is relatively less important in countries with very high endemicity of hepatitis B virus infection, as has been shown in a recent study from South Africa, where the prevalence of anti-HCV in black patients with hepatocellular carcinoma is not as high as in countries with low or intermediate endemicity for hepatitis B [98].

The pathogenic mechanisms leading to development of hepatocellular carcinoma in patients infected by HCV are largely unknown. In most cases, the tumor develops on preexisting cirrhosis, and slow, often clinically silent, progression from chronic hepatitis to cirrhosis and then to cancer has already been well documented in patients with posttransfusional hepatitis C [82, 99]. It may thus be suspected that continued inflammation, liver cell necrosis, and regeneration may induce, after many years, malignant transformation of hepatocytes. Whether, in addition or alternatively, HCV itself acts as a direct initiator of mutagenesis is unknown. Since some HCV-infected patients with hepatocellular carcinoma do not have cirrhosis, a direct oncogenic capacity of HCV cannot be disregarded.

**Table 3.** Prevalence of anti-HCV antibodies in chronic liver disease patients, with or without hepatocellular carcinoma, according to the presumed etiology of the underlying liver disease[a]

| | Cryptogenic and non-A, non-B | | HBsAg positive | | Alcoholic | | |
|---|---|---|---|---|---|---|---|
| Authors, year [ref] | CH or cirrhosis | HCC | CH or cirrhosis | HCC | Cirrhosis | HCC | All HCC |
| Bruix et al. 1989 [79] | 38/49 (77) | 35/43 (81) | 2/8 (25) | 5/9 (55) | 19/49 (39) | 23/30 (77) | 60/82 (73) |
| Colombo et al. 1989 [80] | 103/139 (74) | 64/91 (70) | | 22/41 (54) | | 18/27 (67) | 104/159 (65) |
| Hasan et al. 1990 [81] | 32/76 (42) | 31/59 (53) | | 4/28 (14) | | | 35/87 (40) |
| Kiyosawa et al. 1990 [82] | 156/177 (88) | 51/54 (94) | 11/96 (12) | 10/29 (35) | | | 61/83 (73) |
| Kew et al. 1990 [97] | | 27/74 (36) | | 47/184 (25) | | | 110/380 (29) |
| Ohkoshi et al. 1990 [98] | | 50/58 (86) | | 8/42 (19) | | | 58/100 (58) |
| Nalpas et al. 1991 [90] | | 14/23 (60) | | | 28/78 (36) | 18/32 (56) | 32/55 (58) |
| Levrero et al. 1991 [96] | | 82/114 (72) | | 15/53 (28) | | 10/33 (30) | 97/167 (58) |

CH, chronic hepatitis; HCC, hepatocellular carcinoma
[a] Prevalence figures are given in parentheses

## 6 Pathogenesis of Hepatitis C

So far, studies on the pathogenic mechanisms that operate in hepatitis C have not been reported. However, since HCV infection accounts for most cases of non-A, non-B hepatitis, it seems reasonable to consider that available data on the pathogenesis of non-A, non-B hepatitis are also valid for hepatitis C. Unfortunately, only partial aspects have been studied and the limited and sometimes inconsistent information provided does not allow formulation of a complete pathogenic model of this disease.

A few years ago, data from histopathologic studies suggested that HCV may be directly cytopathic to liver cells [100]. However, recent surveys on posttransfusion non-A, non-B hepatitis have shown that hepatitis C may occur in recipients of anti-HCV positive blood from donors with normal ALT levels, suggesting that some persons infected by HCV do not have necroinflammatory liver damage. If this is so, mechanisms other than direct HCV cytotoxicity should operate in patients with hepatitis C.

Characterization with monoclonal antibodies of the phenotype of lymphocytes present in liver biopsies from patients with chronic non-A, non-B hepatitis has shown that the inflammatory infiltrates are mainly composed of CD8 positive T lymphocytes [101, 102]. Many of these cells bear activation epitopes, suggesting that they are functionally active [101, 102]. Under the electron microscope, some of these lymphocytes are in intimate contact with hepatocytes, suggesting that T cell-mediated cytotoxicity is involved in liver cell damage [101]. These in situ observations are in agreement with data from in vitro experiments demonstrating increased T lymphocyte toxicity against autologous hepatocytes in patients with chronic non-A, non-B hepatitis [103].

In addition to these hypothetical mechanisms of liver cell damage, there is clinical and experimental evidence indicating that the participation of the immune system in the pathogenesis of HCV infection is more complex. The dramatic response to interferon-α therapy observed in many patients with chronic hepatitis C leaves no doubt as to the crucial role of interferon in the pathogenesis of this disease. Interferon administration often induces a rapid normalization of serum aminotransferase levels with the disappearance of HCV RNA from serum [104], suggesting that adequate interferon production and function are important to control HCV replication and that deficiencies in the interferon system may be responsible, at least in part, for the "chronification" of HCV infection.

However, studies on interferon production by peripheral blood lymphocytes from patients with chronic non-A, non-B hepatitis have not yielded uniform results. Fuji and co-workers [105] observed that interferon-γ production was decreased in some patients with chronic active hepatitis while Zachoval and co-workers [106] found that interferon-α production was similar in patients and controls. In a provocative study, Serrano and co-workers [107] also observed a wide variation in interferon-γ production in patients with chronic non-A, non-B hepatitis but, interestingly, they found that interferon production was increased in patients with less active disease while in patients with more prominent hepatocellular necrosis and inflammation the interferon production was similar to that in controls. Furthermore, authors from the same group found that the degree of activity of monocytes and interleukin-1 production correlated directly with interferon-γ production and inversely with disease activity, suggesting that monocytes play an important role in the pathogenesis of this disease [108].

Availability of laboratory techniques has enabled investigators to examine other aspects of the immune response in chronic non-A, non-B hepatitis. Increased levels of soluble interleukin-2 receptor were observed in patients with chronic non-A, non-B hepatitis, which correlated with both serum aminotransferase activity and hepatocellular necrosis [109]. However, the pathogenic meaning of this finding is uncertain since the immunoregulatory role of soluble inteleukin-2 receptor is not yet well understood [110].

Attention has also been paid to tumor necrosis factor, a cytokine with a number of important immunoregulatory properties [111], but the role of this mediator in chronic non-A, non-B hepatitis has not been elucidated. YOSHIOKA and co-workers [112] observed increased production of tumor necrosis factor in interferon-γ-stimulated peripheral blood lymphocyte cultures, which was greater in patients with chronic active hepatitis than in those with chronic persistent hepatitis and correlated directly with the degree of activity of the disease. Recently, however, MULLER and ZIELINSKI [113] found decreased production of tumor necrosis factor in endotoxin-stimulated cultures of monocytes from patients with chronic viral hepatitis, which, like other studies [107, 108], suggested that monocyte functions are impaired in these patients.

## 7 Clinical and Histopathologic Aspects

### 7.1 Acute Infection

As in non-A, non-B hepatitis, the mean incubation period of posttransfusional hepatitis C is 7 weeks, ranging from 4 to 11 weeks [19, 21]. Characteristically, acute infection by HCV is a mild disease, and it very often runs a completely silent course. When present, symptoms are often nonspecific and only about one-third of the patients become jaundiced. Jaundice is usually mild and short-lived. Extrahepatic manifestations such as arthritis, which are fairly uncommon in non-A, non-B hepatitis, have not yet been described in patients with acute hepatitis C, although urticaria was reported in one case of posttransfusion hepatitis C [114].

There is little information concerning the role of HCV infection in fulminant hepatitis. Muto and co-workers [115] reported a high prevalence of anti-HCV antibodies in this condition but many of their patients also had evidence of hepatitis A virus or hepatitis B virus infection or drug-induced hepatotoxicity, suggesting that falsely positive anti-HCV reactions might have occurred. Since development of anti-C100-3 anti-HCV antibodies is a relatively late event in acute infection, examination of early markers of HCV infection is necessary in patients with fulminant hepatitis in order to evaluate the role of HCV.

Hepatitis-related aplastic anemia is mainly associated with non-A, non-B hepatitis. However, the prevalence of anti-HCV antibodies observed in a series of patients with aplastic anemia related to non-A, non-B hepatitis was similar to that in patients with aplastic anemia not associated with hepatitis [116]. This finding argues against a role of HCV in this condition, which might be caused by another unidentified hepatitis virus. However, the possible role of HCV cannot be excluded because immunologic defects that occur in patients with hepatitis-related aplastic anemia may cause a weak anti-HCV antibody response, undetectable by ELISA. This situation demonstrates again that the ELISA technique does not constitute an optimal diagnostic procedure, particularly in acute HCV infection.

## 7.2 Chronic Infection

### *Clinical Aspects*

A very long, clinically indolent course is characteristic of chronic HCV infection. About one-half of the patients are entirely asymptomatic and their liver disease comes to light by chance, as a result of an incidental medical examination for a variety of reasons. An increasing number of patients are recognized by routine anti-HCV screening of apparently healthy blood donors. Approximately another half of patients are diagnosed when they come to medical attention for a variety of nonspecific complaints, of which increased fatigability and vague pain over the right hypochondrium are the most common. Finally, in a minority of patients the diagnosis is not made until severe manifestations of cirrhosis or hepatocellular carcinoma develop.

Physical examination is often unrewarding, although an enlarged liver may be felt in about one-half of cases. Splenomegaly is also present in some cases. Stigmata of chronic liver disease can be found in advanced cases.

Abnormally increased serum aminotransferase levels are the most common biochemical alteration. ALT is usually higher than aspartate aminotransferase (AST). Values are extremely variable from patient to patient and fluctuations are characteristic. ALT and AST values may be transiently normal in some cases. Serum bilirubin, alkaline phosphatase, and $\gamma$-glutamyltranspeptidase are usually normal, but they may be elevated, mainly in patients with more advanced disease. Total serum proteins, albumin, and globulins are usually normal, although the last-mentioned may be increased in patients with very active disease or with cirrhosis. Prothrombin activity is usually normal but it may be low in patients with cirrhosis or, occasionally, in noncirrhotic patients with prominent hepatocellular necrosis. White and red blood cell counts are usually normal but in patients with advanced disease leukopenia and thrombocytopenia are very common. Less than 10% of the patients present non-organ-specific autoantibodies, such as antinuclear, or anti-liver and kidney microsomal autoantibodies. Autoantibodies may be detected only transiently and, when present, their titer is usually low. Sometimes, however, they may be present at high titer and differentiation from autoimmune hepatitis may be difficult, as discussed previously.

### *Histopathologic Aspects*

The histopathologic picture of hepatitis C has not yet been precisely described because some diagnostic difficulties still remain. However, histologic observations carried out in many patients with anti-HCV positive chronic hepatitis clearly indicate that the lesions present in the liver of these patients are closely similar to those found in non-A, non-B chronic hepatitis [61, 117]. The histopathologic spectrum of chronic HCV infection includes nonspecific and minimal changes, all the types of chronic hepatitis, liver cirrhosis, and hepatocellular carcinoma.

As in non-A, non-B hepatitis, liver biopsies of patients with hepatitis C often display some features which, although not exclusive to this disease, are less frequently found in other types of viral hepatitis [100, 118–121]. Hepatocytes of patients with hepatitis C often present fat droplets, microvesicular steatosis, or an eosinophilic cytoplasm. Councilman bodies may be conspicuous. In portal tracts, lymphocytes may aggregate to form lymphoid follicles or may surround bile ducts with abnormal epithelium. A frequent, but not constant, finding is the presence of increased mononuclear cellularity within the sinusoids. The presence of these lesions in patients with chronic liver disease must arouse suspicion of chronic HCV infection although none of these features is pathognomonic.

In a recent analysis (unpublished observations) we were unable to identify any histologic difference between patients with high ELISA ratio anti-HCV positive chronic hepatitis and patients with anti-HCV negative cryptogenic chronic hepatitis. Whether HCV is also responsible for these histologically C-like cases of chronic hepatitis or whether another hepatotropic virus may cause liver lesions similar to those of hepatitis C deserves further investigation.

### *Natural History*

Ten years ago, longitudinal surveys on patients with protracted elevation of serum aminotransferase levels as a result of non-A, non-B posttransfusional hepatitis revealed that this biochemical abnormality had a remarkable tendency to persist for months and years. Beside a variety of less important changes, liver biopsies showed chronic active hepatitis in about one-half of the cases and, after a relatively short follow-up, 10%–20% of the cases had already developed hepatic cirrhosis [122–127].

Recently, more information on the natural history of chronic hepatitis C has been obtained after prolonged observation of large series of patients with posttransfusional or community-acquired non-A, non-B chronic hepatitis [117, 128]. Initially, none of these patients had evidence of cirrhosis and about 80% of them had anti-HCV antibodies when retrospectively tested. These studies have confirmed that spontaneous, complete remission of chronic hepatitis C is fairly uncommon, in marked contrast with chronic hepatitis B. Transition to cirrhosis was documented in one-third of the cases after a mean follow-up of 9 years from diagnosis. Progression to cirrhosis was related to age, being higher in older patients, and also to the presence of bridging necrosis in the liver biopsy taken at the time of diagnosis. No clear-cut difference in outcome was observed between sporadic and post-transfusional patients. These findings suggest that chronic hepatitis C is a very long-lasting, slowly progressing disease, and that many years are necessary for cirrhosis to develop.

Despite its progressive character, patients with chronic hepatitis C remain asymptomatic or with minor symptoms for many years, even if cirrhosis has already developed. Some patients, however, are unable to perform normally because of increased tiredness, which is occasionally incapacitating. Major complications of cirrhosis, such as ascites, hepatic encephalopathy, variceal hemorrhage, and liver failure, do not occur until very late in the course of the disease. Among 300 patients with chronic hepatitis who were followed up for 2–20 years, only 10% developed complications and only 5% died as a consequence of their liver disease [128].

Development of hepatocellular carcinoma is another serious complication that threatens the insidious course of chronic HCV infection, particularly in patients with advanced, although otherwise asymptomatic, disease. In addition to the high frequency of anti-HCV antibodies in patients with hepatocellular carcinoma [79–81], there is increasing evidence from long-term longitudinal studies of patients with anti-HCV positive chronic hepatitis that unequivocally demonstrates the close association between these two conditions [82, 128].

## 8 Treatment of Hepatitis C Virus Infection

### 8.1 Chronic Hepatitis C

In the last few years, considerable progress has been achieved in the treatment of chronic liver diseases of viral origin, including hepatitis C. Nevertheless, many problems concerning the treatment of these diseases are still unsolved.

Prior to recognition of the precise nature of their disease, patients with non-A, non-B or cryptogenic chronic hepatitis were treated with immunosuppressive drugs, with little success, and often remained untreated. In 1985, Pappas and co-workers [129] reported the disappointing results obtained in a pilot study in which, for the first time, an antiviral agent, acyclovir, was given to patients with chronic non-A, non-B hepatitis.

Shortly thereafter, another pilot study conducted by Hoofnagle and co-workers [130] demonstrated that recombinant interferon-α, given at low doses, was able to induce substantial changes in patients with chronic non-A, non-B posttransfusion hepatitis. After a few weeks of therapy, most of the treated patients experienced a dramatic decrease in serum aminotransferase levels to normal or near normal values. However, there was a rapid return of serum enzymes to previous levels on withdrawal of the drug, which subsided again when interferon was reintroduced. After 1 year of therapy, liver biopsies showed a substantial improvement in lobular inflammation, liver cell necrosis, and portal tract infiltration.

Such encouraging results prompted numerous controlled therapeutic trials to evaluate the use of recombinant and lymphoblastoid interferon-α in chronic non-A, non-B hepatitis, which have recently been summarized [131, 132]. Retrospectively, the presence of anti-HCV antibodies was demonstrated in the majority of patients included in these studies, the main results of which are given in Table 4 [133–143].

In approximately one-half of treated patients serum aminotransferase levels became normal following administration of interferon (Fig. 3). In about one-third there was a consistent decrease in serum enzyme levels but complete normalization did not occur, and, finally, no response was observed in the remaining cases. The type of response during interferon administration seems related to dosage, since the rate of favorable responses was greater in patients treated with 3 MU than in those treated with 1 MU.

Predictive factors of response to interferon therapy have not been clearly identified. In some studies, advanced age, presence of cirrhosis [136, 144], long-lasting disease, and excessive body weight [133] were associated with a poor response rate, but these observations were not confirmed by others. Analysis of other factors such as presence of anti-HCV antibodies [145], sex, history of blood transfusion, degree of biochemical and histopathologic activity of the disease, presence of autoantibodies at low titer or emergence of these antibodies during therapy, and development of anti-

**Table 4.** Results of interferon therapy observed in controlled studies in patients with non-A, non-B chronic hepatitis

| Authors, year [ref] | Patients treated | Dose (MU, 3 × wk) | Duration (weeks) | Complete response (%) | Relapse upon withdrawal (%) |
|---|---|---|---|---|---|
| SCHVARCZ et al. 1989 [133] | 19 | 3 | 36 | 58 | 64 |
| DAVIS et al. 1989 [134] | 58 | 3 | 24 | 38 | 51 |
| | 57 | 1 | 24 | 16 | 44 |
| DI BISCEGLIE et al. 1989 [135] | 21 | 2 | 24 | 48 | 90 |
| SARACCO et al. 1990 [136] | 29 | 1 | 24 | 66 | 77 |
| | 26 | 3 | 24 | 68 | 60 |
| FERENCI et al. 1990 [137] | 24 | (a) | 52 | 58 | 57 |
| REALDI et al. 1990 [138] | 28 | (b) | 52 | 68 | Not given |
| MARCELLIN et al. 1990 [139] | 26 | 1 | 24 | 48 | 46 |
| | 24 | 3 | 24 | | |
| CERINI et al. 1990 [140] | 25 | (c) | 52 | 44 | 48 |
| CAMPS et al. 1990 [141] | 18 | (d) | 52 | 44 | 25 |
| IDEO et al. 1990 [142] | 30 | (e) | 52 | 45 | 60 |
| MULLER et al. 1990 [143] | 46 | 1 | 52 | 20 | 0 |

[a] 5 MU/day × 2 wk, 2 MU/day × 2 wk, and adjusted according to response thereafter
[b] 6 MU/3 × wk × 1 mo, 3 MU/3 × wk × 3 mo, 1 MU/3 × wk × 8 mo
[c] 5 MU/3 × wk × 6 mo, 3 MU/3 × wk × 3 mo, 1.5 MU/3 × wk × 3 mo
[d] 3 MU/d × 2 mo, 3 MU/3 × wk × 3 mo, 1.5 MU/3 × wk × 7 mo
[e] 3 MU/d × 2 wk, 3 MU/2 d × 6 wk, 3 MU/3 × wk × 10 mo

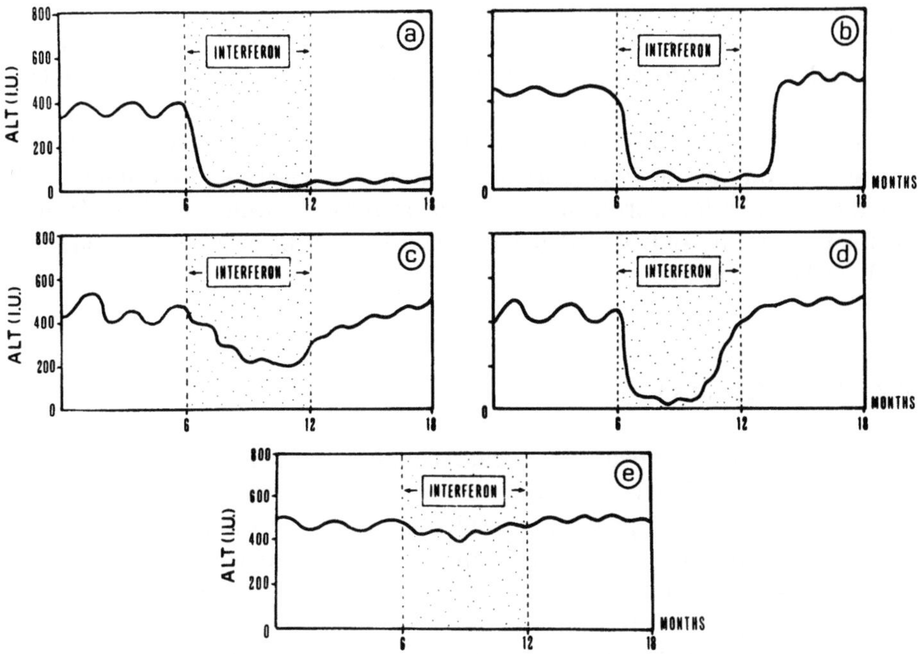


**Fig. 3a–e.** Schemes of the different types of response to interferon therapy in patients with chronic hepatitis C. A complete initial response is observed in about one-half of the cases (**a**) but many of them relapse on withdrawal (**b**). The remaining patients present either an incomplete response (**c** and **d**) or do not respond at all (**e**).

interferon antibodies suggests that none of these factors can be used as an independent prognostic marker of response to interferon therapy in this disease.

Despite the high rate of initially favorable responses, the rate of relapse following interferon withdrawal is also very high (Table 4). Relapse upon withdrawal is almost constant in patients exhibiting a partial response during therapy. Tapering of the drug is often followed by elevation of transaminases [138]. Although controlled studies have not yet been performed, the rate of relapse seems greater after 6 months than after 1 year of interferon therapy and in patients treated with a low dose than in those treated with a higher dose. Nevertheless, very low doses of interferon are able to induce sustained responses [143]. In some cases, discontinuation of interferon is followed by a transient rebound of transaminase activity which precedes prolonged inactivation of the disease [146].

The rapid effect of interferon administration in most patients with chronic hepatitis C is probably mediated by its direct antiviral activity, in contrast with its effects in hepatitis B, where the immunomodulatory activity of interferon seems more critical. The direct antiviral effect of interferon can be suggested by the rapid clearance of serum HCV RNA observed in patients on interferon therapy [104]. Unfortunately, however, preliminary information does not favor the use of HCV RNA to monitor accurately the effectiveness of interferon therapy, since relapse, with reappearance of HCV RNA in serum, may occur in patients who had apparently responded to therapy [147].

Beside a number of well-known undesirable side-effects, interferon administration, at the doses used in chronic hepatitis C, is usually well tolerated. Since interferon may cause a decrease in white blood cells and platelets, careful control and dose reduction may be required in patients with cirrhosis and hypersplenism.

## 8.2 Acute Hepatitis C

Despite its benign appearance, acute hepatitis caused by HCV infection has a marked tendency to become chronic, particularly when acquired by blood transfusion. The promising results obtained with the use of interferon in patients with chronic disease stimulated studies to assess the value of interferon administration to prevent development of chronic liver disease in patients with recent infection. So far, preliminary results of three studies have shown that, although interferon may favorably modify the course of the disease, none of the therapeutic regimes examined was clearly able to prevent progression to chronicity [148–150].

## References

1. Dienstag JL (1983) Non-A, non-B hepatitis. I. Recognition, epidemiology, and clinical features. Gastroenterology 84:439–462
2. Dienstag JL, Alter HJ (1986) Non-A, non-B hepatitis: evolving epidemiologic and clinical perspective. Semin Liver Dis 6:67–81
3. Alter HJ, Purcell RH, Feinstone SM, Tegtmeier GE (1982) Non-A, non-B hepatitis: its relationship to cytomegalovirus, to chronic hepatitis, and to direct and indirect test methods. In: Szmuness W, Alter HJ, Maynard JE (eds) Viral hepatitis: 1981 International Symposium. Franklin Institute, Philadelphia, pp 279–294
4. Anonymous (1990) Hepatitis C virus upstanding. Lancet 335:1431–1432
5. Zuckerman AJ (1990) Hepatitis C virus: a giant leap forward. Hepatology 11:320–322
6. Choo Q-L, Kuo G, Weiner AJ, Overby LR, Bradley DW, Houghton M (1989) Isolation of a cDNA clone derived form a blood-borne non-A, non-B viral hepatitis genome. Science 244:359–362
7. Kuo G, Choo Q-L, Alter HJ et al. (1989) An assay for circulating antibodies to a major etiologic virus of human non-A, non-B hepatitis. Science 244:362–364
8. Bradley DW, Maynard JE, Popper H et al. (1983) Post-transfusion non-A, non-B hepatitis: physicochemical properties of two distinct agents. J Infect Dis 148:254–265
9. Feinstone SM, Mihalik K, Kamimura T, Alter HJ, London WT, Purcell RH (1983) Inactivation of hepatitis B virus and non-A, non-B hepatitis by chloroform. Infect Immun 41:816–821

10. He L-F, Alling D, Popkin T, Shapiro M, Alter M, Purcell RH (1987) Determining the size of non-A, non-B hepatitis virus by filtration. J Infect Dis 156:636–640
11. Miller R, Purcell RH (1990) Hepatitis C virus shares amino acid sequence similarity with pestiviruses and flavoviruses as well as two plant virus supergroups. Proc Natl Acad Sci USA 87:2057–2061
12. Choo Q-L, Weiner AJ, Overby LR, Kuo G, Houghton M, Bradley DW (1990) Hepatitis C virus: the major causative agent of viral non-A, non-B hepatitis. Br Med Bull 46:423–441
13. Kubo Y, Takeuchi K, Boonmar S et al. (1989) A cDNA fragment of hepatitis C virus isolated from an implicated donor of post-transfusion non-A, non-B hepatitis in Japan. Nucleic Acid Res 17:10367–10372
14. Garson JA, Tuke PW, Makris M et al. (1990) Demonstration of viremia patterns in haemophiliacs treated with hepatitis-C-virus-contaminated factor VIII concentrates. Lancet II:1022–1025
15. Enomoto N, Takada A, Nakao T, Date T (1990) There are two major types of hepatitis C virus in Japan. Biochem Biophys Res Comm 170:1021–1025
16. Simmonds P, Zhang LQ, Watson HG et al. (1990) Hepatitis C quantification and sequencing in blood products, haemophiliacs, and drug users. Lancet II:1469–1472
17. Garson JA, Ring C, Tuke P, Tedder R (1990) Enhanced detection by PCR of hepatitis C virus RNA (letter). Lancet II:878–879
18. Van der Poel CL, Reesink HW, Schaasberg W et al. (1990) Infectivity of blood seropositive for hepatitis C virus antibodies. Lancet I:558–560
19. Esteban JI, Gonzalez A, Hernandez JM et al. (1990) Evaluation of antibodies to hepatitis C virus in a study of transfusion-associated hepatitis. N Engl J Med 323:1107–1112
20. Barrera JM, Bruguera M, Ercilla MG et al. (1991) Prevention of post-transfusion hepatitis by screening blood donors for antibodies to hepatitis C virus or surrogate markers: a comparative study. Ann Intern Med 115:596–600
21. Alter HJ, Purcell RH, Shih JW et al. (1989) Detection of antibody to hepatitis C virus in prospectively followed transfusion recipients with acute or chronic non-A, non-B hepatitis. N Engl J Med 321:1494–1500
22. Bradley DW, Krawczynski K, Ebert JW et al. (1990) Parenterally transmitted non-A, non-B hepatitis: virus specific antibody response patterns in hepatitis C virus infected chimpanzees. Gastroenterology 99:1054–1060
23. Tremolada F, Casarin C, Tagger A et al. (1991) Antibody to hepatitis C virus in post-transfusion hepatitis. Ann Intern Med 114:277–281
24. Bortolotti F, Tagger A, Cadrobbi P et al. (1991) Antibodies to hepatitis C in community acquired non-A, non-B hepatitis. J Hepatol 12:176–180
25. Esteban JI, Esteban R, Viladomiu L et al. (1989) Hepatitis C virus antibodies among risk groups in Spain. Lancet II:294–296
26. Sánchez-Tapias JM, Barrera JM, Costa J et al. (1990) Hepatitis C virus infection in non-alcoholic chronic liver disease. Ann Intern Med 112:921–924
27. Roggendorf M, Deinhardt F, Rasshofer R et al. (1989) Antibodies to hepatitis C virus. Lancet II:324–325
28. Sansonno D, Dammacco F (1989) Antibodies to hepatitis C virus in non-A, non-B post-transfusion and cryptogenic chronic liver disease. Lancet II:798–799
29. Kuhnl P, Seidl S, Stangel W, Beyer J, Sibrowsky W, Flik J (1989) Antibody to hepatitis C in German blood donors. Lancet II:324
30. Contreras M, Barbara JAJ (1989) Screening for hepatitis C virus antibody (letter). Lancet II:505
31. Janot C, Courouce AM, Maniez M (1989) Antibodies to hepatitis C virus in French blood donors. Lancet II:796–797
32. Sirchia G, Bellobuono A, Giovanetti A, Marconi M (1989) Antibodies to hepatitis C in Italian blood donors. Lancet II:797

33. Theilman L, Blazek M, Goeser T, Gmelin K, Kommerell B, Fiehn W (1990) False-positive anti-HCV tests in rheumatoid arthritis. Lancet I:1346
34. Boudart D, Lucas JC, Muller JY, Le Carrer D, Planchon B, Harousseau JL (1990) False-positive hepatitis C virus antibody tests in paraproteinaemia. Lancet II:63
35. Wong DC, Diwan AR, Rosen L et al. (1990) Non-specificity of anti-HCV test for seroepidemiological analysis. Lancet II:750–751
36. McFarlane IG, Smith HM, Johnson PJ, Bray GP, Vergani D, Williams R (1990) Hepatitis C virus antibodies in chronic active hepatitis: pathogenic factor or false-positive result? Lancet I:754–757
37. Gray JJ, Wreghitt TG, Friend PJ, Wight DGD, Sundaresan V, Calne RY (1990) Differentiation between specific and non-specific hepatitis C antibodies in chronic liver disease. Lancet I:609–610
38. Goeser T, Blazek M, Gmelin K, Kommerell B, Theilman L (1990) Washing with 8 mol/l urea to correct false-positive anti-HCV results. Lancet II:878
39. Menitove JE, Richards WA, Destree M (1990) Early US experience with anti-HCV kit in blood donors. Lancet II:244–245
40. Weiner AJ, Truett MA, Rosenblat J et al. (1990) HCV testing in low risk population. Lancet II:695
41. Ebeling F, Naukkarinen R, Leikola J (1990) Recombinant immunoblot assay for hepatitis C virus antibody as predictor of infectivity. Lancet I:982–983
42. Bellobuono A, Mozzi F, Petrini G, Zanella A, Sirchia S (1990) Infectivity of blood that is immunoblot intermediate reactive on hepatitis C virus antibody testing. Lancet II:309
43. Van der Poel CL, Cuypers HTM, Reesink HW et al. (1991) Confirmation of hepatitis C virus infection by new four-antigen recombinant immunoblot assay. Lancet I:317–319
44. Weiner A, Kuo G, Bradley DW et al. (1990) Detection of hepatitis C viral sequences in non-A, non-B hepatitis. Lancet I:1–3
45. Garson JA, Tedder RS, Briggs M et al. (1990) Detection of hepatitis C viral sequences in blood donations by "nested" polymerase chain reaction and prediction of infectivity. Lancet I:1419–1422
46. Kaneko S, Unoura M, Kobayashi K, Kuno K, Murakami S, Hattori N (1990) Detection of serum hepatitis C virus RNA. Lancet I:976
47. Zanetti AR, Tanzi E, Zehender G et al. (1990) Hepatitis C virus RNA in symptomless donors implicated in post-transfusion non-A, non-B hepatitis. Lancet II:448
48. Feinstone SM, Kapikian AZ, Purcell RH, Alter HJ, Holland PV (1975) Transfusion-associated hepatitis not due to viral hepatitis type A or B. N Engl J Med 292:767–770
49. Alter HJ, Holland PV, Morrow AG, Purcell RH, Feinstone SM, Moritsugu Y (1975) Clinical and serological analysis of transfusion-associated hepatitis. Lancet II:838–841
50. Aach RD, Lander JJ, Sherman LA (1978) Transfusion-transmitted viruses: interim analysis of hepatitis among transfused and not transfused patients. In: Vyas GN, Cohen SN, Schmid RD (eds) Viral hepatitis: a contemporary assessment of etiology, epidemiologty, pathogenesis and prevention. Franklin Institute, Philadelphia, pp 383–396
51. Hernandez JM, Piqueras J, Carrera A, Triginer J (1983) Post-transfusion hepatitis in Spain: a prospective study. Vox Sang 44:231–237
52. Bárcena R, Suárez-García E, Gil LA et al. (1985) Posttransfusion non-A, non-B hepatitis: a prospective study. Liver 5:71–76
53. Feinman SV, Berris B, Bojarski S (1988) Posttransfusion hepatitis in Toronto, Canada. Gastroenterology 95:464–469
54. Colombo M, Oldani S, Donato MF et al. (1987) A multicenter, prospective study of posttransfusion hepatitis in Milan. Hepatology 7:709–712

55. Barrera JM, Bruguera M, Ercilla MG et al. (1989) Hepatitis posttransfusional despues de cirugía cardíaca. Incidencia, clínica y pronóstico. Med Clin (Barc) 89:759–762
56. Van der Poel CL, Reesink HW, Cuypers HTM, Lelie PN, Schaasberg W (1990) Is anti-HCV screening useful? Lancet II:1193
57. Hay CRM, Preston FE, Triger DR, Underwood JCE (1985) Progressive liver disease in haemophilia: an understated problem. Lancet I:1495–1498
58. Rumi MG, Colombo M, Gringeri A, Mannucci PM (1990) High prevalence of antibody to hepatitis C virus in multitransfused hemophiliacs with normal transaminase levels. Ann Intern Med 112:379–380
59. Noel L, Guerois C, Maisonneuve P, Verroust F, Laurian Y (1989) Antibodies to hepatitis C virus in haemophilia. Lancet II:560
60. Colombo M, Rumi MG, Mannucci PM (1990) Specificity of hepatitis C antibody ELISA in patients with hemophilia. Lancet I:1345
61. Makris M, Preston FE, Triger DR et al. (1990) Hepatitis C antibody and chronic liver disease in haemophilia. Lancet I:1117–1119
62. Mannucci PM, Schimpf K, Brettler DB et al. (1990) Low risk for hepatitis C in hemophiliacs given a high-purity, pasteurized factor VIII concentrate. Ann Intern Med 113:27–32
63. Schwartz RS, Abildgaard CF, Aledort LM et al. (1990) Human recombinant DNA-derived antihemophilic factor (factor VIII) in the treatment of hemophilia A. N Engl J Med 323:1800–1805
64. Mortimer PP, Cohen BJ, Litton PA et al. (1989) Hepatitis C virus antibody. Lancet II:798
65. Huemer HP, Prodinger WM, Larcher C, Most J, Dierich MP (1990) Correlation of hepatitis C virus antibodies with HIV-1 seropositivity in intravenous drug addicts. Infection 18:122
66. Titó L, Sánchez-Tapias JM, Barrera JM et al. (1990) Infección por el virus de la hepatitis C en las enfermedades crónicas del hígado. Gastroenterol Hepatol 13:414–418
67. Galbraight R, Dienstag JL, Purcell RH, Gower PH, Zuckerman AJ, Williams R (1979) Non-A, non-B hepatitis associated with chronic liver disease in a hemodialysis unit. Lancet I:951–953
68. Bruguera M, Vidal L, Sánchez-Tapias JM, Costa J, Revert L, Rodes J (1990) Incidence and features of liver disease in patients on chronic hemodialysis. J Clin Gastroenterol 12:298–302
69. Schlipkoter U, Roggendorf M, Ernst G et al. (1990) Hepatitis C virus antibodies in haemodialysis patients. Lancet I:1409
70. Tamura I, Kobayashi Y, Koda T et al. (1990) Hepatitis C virus antibodies in haemodialysis patients. Lancet I:1409
71. Yamaguchi K, Nishimura N, Fukuoka N et al. (1990) Hepatitis C antibodies in haemodialysis patients. Lancet I:1409–1410
72. Alter M, Coleman PJ, Alexander J et al. (1989) Importance of heterosexual activity in the transmission of hepatitis B and non-A, non-B hepatitis. JAMA 262:1201–1205
73. Everhart JE, Di Bisceglie AM, Murray LM et al. (1990) Risk for non-A, non-B (type C) hepatitis through sexual or household contact with chronic carriers. Ann Intern Med 112:544–545
74. Kamitsukasa H, Harada H, Yakura M et al. (1989) Intrafamilial transmission of hepatitis C virus. Lancet II:978
75. Ideo G, Bellati G, Pedraglio E, Bottelli R, Donzelli T, Putignano G (1990) Intrafamilial transmission of hepatitis C virus. Lancet I:353
76. Fortuny C, Ercilla MG, Barrera JM et al. (1990) HCV vertical transmission. Prospective study in infants born to HCV positive mothers. The 1990 International Symposium on Viral Hepatitis and Liver Disease, Houston, p 158

77. Wejstal R, Hermodsson S, Iwarson S, Norkrans G (1990) Mother to infant transmission of hepatitis C virus infection. J Med Virol 30:178–180
78. Giovannini M, Tagger A, Ribero ML et al. (1990) Maternal-infant transmission of hepatitis C virus and HIV-infections: a possible interaction. Lancet I:1166
79. Bruix J, Barrera JM, Calvet X et al. (1989) Prevalence of antibodies to hepatitis C virus in Spanish patients with hepatocellular carcinoma and hepatic cirrhosis. Lancet II:1004–1006
80. Colombo M, Kuo G, Choo Q-L et al. (1989) Prevalence of antibodies to hepatitis C virus in Italian patients with hepatocellular carcinoma. Lancet II:1006–1008
81. Hasan F, Jeffers LJ, De Medina M et al. (1990) Hepatitis C-associated hepatocellular carcinoma. Hepatology 12:589–591
82. Kiyosawa K, Sodeyama T, Tanaka E et al. (1990) Interrelationship of blood transfusion and hepatocellular carcinoma: analysis by detection of antibody to hepatitis C virus. Hepatology 12:671–675
83. Lenzi M, Ballardini G, Fusconi M et al. (1990) Type 2 autoimmune hepatitis and hepatitis C virus infection. Lancet I:258–259
84. Homberg JC, Abuaf N, Bernard O et al. (1987) Chronic active hepatitis associated with antiliver/kidney microsome antibody type I: a second type of "autoimmune" hepatitis. Hepatology 6:1333–1339
85. Crivelli O, Lavarini C, Chiaberge E et al. (1983) Microsomal autoantibodies in chronic infections with the HBsAg associated delta antigen. Clin Exp Immunol 54:232–238
86. Dussaix E, Maggiore G, De Giacomo C, Mondelli M, Martres P, Alvarez F (1990) Autoimmune hepatitis in children and hepatitis C virus testing. Lancet I:1160–1161
87. Vento S, Di Perri G, Garofano T et al. (1989) Hazards of interferon therapy for HBV-seronegative chronic hepatitis. Lancet II:926
88. Fattovich G, Tagger A, Brollo L et al. (1989) Liver disease in anti-HBe positive chronic HBsAg carriers and hepatitis C virus. Lancet II:797–798
89. Pares A, Barrera JM, Caballeria J et al. (1990) Hepatitis C virus antibodies in chronic alcoholic patients: association with severity of liver injury. Hepatology 12:1295–1299
90. Nalpas B, Driss F, Pol S et al. (1991) Association between HCV and HBV infection in hepatocellular carcinoma and alcoholic liver disease. J Hepatol 12:70–74
91. Resnick RH, Stone K, Antonioli D (1983) Primary hepatocellular carcinoma following non-A, non-B post-transfusion hepatitis. Dig Dis Sci 28:908–911
92. Gillam JH, Geisinger KR, Richter JE (1984) Primary hepatocellular carcinoma after chronic non-A, non-B post-transfusion hepatitis. Ann Intern Med 101:794–795
93. Cohen EB, Gang DL, Zeldis JB (1987) Primary hepatocellular carcinoma following nonspecific non-B hepatitis with tumor DNA negative for HBV DNA. Dig Dis Sci 32:1428–1430
94. Okuda K, Fujimoto I, Hanai A, Urano Y (1987) Changing incidence of hepatocellular carcinoma in Japan. Cancer Res 47:4967–4972
95. Kiyosawa K, Akahane Y, Nagata A, Koike Y, Furuta S (1982) The significance of blood transfusion in non-A, non-B chronic liver disease in Japan. Vox Sang 43:45–52
96. Levrero M, Tagger A, Balsano C et al. (1991) Antibodies to hepatitis C virus in patients with hepatocellular carcinoma. J Hepatol 12:60–63
97. Kew MC, Houghton M, Choo Q-L, Kuo G (1990) Hepatitis C virus antibodies in southern African blacks with hepatocellular carcinoma. Lancet I:873–874
98. Ohkoshi S, Kojima H, Tawaraya H et al. (1990) Prevalence of antibody against non-A, non-B hepatitis virus in Japanese patients with hepatocellular carcinoma. Jpn J Cancer Res 81:550–553

99. Tremolada F, Benvegnu L, Casarin C et al. (1990) Antibodies to hepatitis C virus in hepatocellular carcinoma. Lancet I:300–301
100. Dienes HP, Popper H, Arnold W, Lobeck H (1982) Histologic observations in human hepatitis non-A, non-B. Hepatology 2:562–571
101. Dienes HP, Hutteroth T, Hess G, Meuer SC (1987) Immunoelectron microscopic observations on the inflammatory infiltrates and HLA antigens in hepatitis B and non-A, non-B. Hepatology 7:1317–1325
102. Garcia-Monzón C, Moreno-Otero R, Pajares JM et al. (1990) Expression of a novel activation antigen on intrahepatic CD8+ T lymphocytes in viral chronic active hepatitis. Gastroenterology 98:1029–1035
103. Mondelli M, Alberti A, Tremolada F, Williams R, Eddleston ALWF, Realdi G (1986) In vitro cell-mediated cytotoxicity for autologous liver cells in chronic non-A, non-B hepatitis. Clin Exp Immunol 63:147–155
104. Kanai K, Iwata K, Nakao K, Kako M, Okamoto H (1990) Suppression of hepatitis C virus by interferon-alpha. Lancet II:245
105. Fuji A, Kakumu S, Ohtani Y, Murase K, Hirofuji H, Tahara H (1987) Interferon gamma production by peripheral blood mononuclear cells of patients with chronic liver disease. Hepatology 7:577–581
106. Zachoval R, Abb J, Zachoval V et al. (1988) Interferon alpha in hepatitis type B and non-A, non-B. J Hepatol 6:364–368
107. Serrano M, Morte S, Castilla A, Civeira MP, Prieto J (1988) Gamma interferon production by peripheral mononuclear cells in patients with chronic non-A, non-B hepatitis. In: Zuckerman AJ (ed) Viral hepatitis and liver disease. Alan R Liss, New York, pp 572–575
108. Castilla A, Serrano M, Morte S, Subira ML, Civeira MP, Prieto J (1988) Monocyte function in chronic non-A, non-B hepatitis: relationship with the activity of liver disease. In: Zuckerman AJ (ed) Viral hepatitis and liver disease. Alan R Liss, New York, pp 568–571
109. Yamaguchi S, Onji M, Ohta Y (1988) Increased serum soluble interleukin 2 receptor levels in patients with viral liver diseases. Hepato-gastroenterology 35:245–248
110. Rubin LA, Nelson DL (1990) The soluble interleukin-2 receptor: biology, function, and clinical application. Ann Intern Med 113:619–627
111. Scheurich P, Thoma B, Ucer U, Pfizemaier K (1987) Immunoregulatory activity of recombinant human tumor necrosis factor (TNF)-alpha: induction of TNF receptors on human T-cell and TNF-alpha-mediated enhancement of T-cell responses. J Immunol 138:1786–1790
112. Yoshioka K, Kakumu S, Arao M, Tsutsumi Y, Inoue M (1989) Tumor necrosis factor alpha production by peripheral blood mononuclear cells of patients with chronic liver disease. Hepatology 10:769–773
113. Muller C, Zielinski CC (1990) Impaired lipopolysaccharide-inducible tumor necrosis factor production in vitro by peripheral blood monocytes of patients with viral hepatitis. Hepatology 12:1118–1124
114. Reichel M, Mauro TM (1990) Urticaria and hepatitis C. Lancet II:822–823
115. Muto Y, Sugihara J, Ohnishi H, Moriwaki H, Nishioka K (1990) Antihepatitis C antibody prevails in fulminant hepatic failure. Gastroenterol Jpn 25:32–35
116. Pol S, Driss F, Devergie A, Brechot C, Berthelot P, Gluckman E (1990) Is hepatitis C virus involved in hepatitis associated aplastic anemia? Ann Intern Med 113:435–437
117. Hopf U, Moller B, Kuther D et al. (1990) Long-term follow-up posttransfusion and sporadic chronic hepatitis non-A, non-B and frequency of circulating antibodies to hepatitis C virus (HCV). J Hepatol 10:69–76
118. Bamber M, Murray A, Arborgh BAM et al. (1981) Short-incubation non-A, non-B hepatitis transmitted by factor VIII concentrates in patients with congenital coagulation disorders. Gut 22:854–859

119. Schmid M, Pirovino M, Altorfer J, Gudat F, Bianchi L (1982) Acute non-A, non-B hepatitis: are there any specific light microscopic features? Liver 2:61–67
120. Lefkowitch JH, Apfelbaum TF (1989) Non-A, non-B hepatitis: characterization of liver biopsy pathology. J Clin Gastroenterol 11:225–232
121. Galbraith RM, Portman B, Eddleston ALWF, Williams R (1975) Chronic liver disease developing after outbreak of HBsAg-negative hepatitis in haemodialysis unit. Lancet II:886–889
122. Knodell RG, Conrad ME, Ishak KG (1977) Development of chronic liver disease after acute non-A, non-B posttransfusion hepatitis: role of γ-globulin prophylaxis in its prevention. Gastroenterology 72:902–909
123. Rakela J, Redeker AG (1979) Chronic liver disease after acute non-A, non-B viral hepatitis. Gastroenterology 77:1200–1202
124. Berman M, Alter HJ, Ishak KJ, Purcell RH, Jones EA (1979) The chronic sequelae of non-A, non-B hepatitis. Ann Intern Med 91:1–6
125. Koretz RL, Stone O, Gitnick G (1980) The long term course of non-A, non-B posttransfusion hepatitis. Gastroenterology 79:893–898
126. Realdi G, Tremolada F, Bortolotti F et al. (1983) The natural history of posttransfusion and sporadic non-A, non-B hepatitis in Italy. In: Verme G, Bonino F, Rizzetto M (eds) Viral hepatitis and delta infection. Alan R. Liss, New York, pp 55–66
127. Alter HJ, Hoofnagle JH (1984) Non-A, non-B hepatitis: observations on the first decade. In: Vyas GN, Dienstag JL, Hoofnagle JH (eds) Viral hepatitis and liver disease. Grune and Stratton, Orlando, FL, pp 345–354
128. Titó L, Sánchez-Tapias JM, Costa J et al. (1990) Long-term follow-up of chronic NANB (C) hepatitis. J Hepatol 11 [Suppl] 2:S61
129. Pappas SC, Hoofnagle JH, Young N, Straus SE, Jones EA (1985) Treatment of chronic non-A, non-B hepatitis with acyclovir: pilot study. J Med Virol 15:1–9
130. Hoofnagle HJ, Mullen KM, Jones DB et al. (1986) Treatment of chronic non-A, non-B hepatitis with recombinant human alpha interferon. A preliminary report. N Engl J Med 315:1575–1578
131. Hoofnagle HJ, Di Bisceglie AM (1989) Treatment of chronic type C hepatitis with alpha interferon. Semin Liver Dis 9:259–263
132. Davis GL (1990) Recombinant alpha-interferon treatment of non-A, non-B (type C) chronic active hepatitis: review of studies and recommendations for treatment. J Hepatol 11 [Suppl] 1:S72–S77
133. Schvarcz R, Weiland O, Wejstal R, Norkrans G, Fryden A, Foberg U (1989) A randomized controlled open study of interferon alpha-2b in chronic fon-A, non-B posttransfusion hepatitis: no correlation of outcome to the presence of hepatitis C virus antibodies. Scand J Infect Dis 21:617–625
134. Davis GL, Balart LA, Schiff ER et al. (1989) Treatment of chronic hepatitis C with recombinant interferon alpha. A multicenter randomized controlled trial. N Engl J Med 321:1501–1505
135. Di Bisceglie AM, Martin P, Kassianides C et al. (1989) Recombinant interferon alpha therapy for chronic hepatitis C. A randomized, double-blind, placebo-controlled trial. N Engl J Med 321:1506–1510
136. Saracco G, Rosina F, Torrani Cerenzia MR et al. (1990) A randomized controlled trial of interferon alpha 2b as therapy for chronic non-A, non-B hepatitis. J Hepatol 11[Suppl]1:S43–S49
137. Ferenci P, Vogel W, Pristautz H et al. (1990) One-year treatment of chronic non-A, non-B hepatitis with interferon alpha-2b. J Hepatol 11 [Suppl] 2:S50–S53
138. Realdi G, Diodati G, Bonetti P, Scaccabarozzi S, Alberti A, Ruol A (1990) Recombinant human interferon alpha-2a in community-acquired non-A, non-B chronic active hepatitis. Preliminary results of a randomized, controlled trial. J Hepatol 11 [Suppl] 2:S68–S71

139. Marcellin P, Boyer N, Giostra E et al. (1990) Long-term follow-up of patients with chronic non-A, non-B hepatitis with complete response to recombinant interferon alpha. Hepatology 12:847
140. Cerini R, Marcellin P, Antoniello S et al. (1990) Twelve months recombinant interferon alpha treatment in chronic non-A, non-B hepatitis. J Hepatol 12:961
141. Camps J, Castilla JI, Riezu-Boj JI, Civeira P, Prieto J (1990) Effectiveness of long-term lymphoblastoid interferon (L-Ifn) treatment in chronic hepatitis C. J Hepatol 11 [Suppl] 2:S15
142. Ideo G, Bellati G, Pedraglio E, Leandro G (1990) One year therapy of non-A, non-B/C chronic hepatitis with recombinant alpha-2a interferon or lymphoblastoid alpha interferon. J Hepatol 11 [Suppl] 2:S31
143. Muller R, Baumgarten R, Markus R et al. (1990) Long term treatment with low doses of alpha-2b interferon (rIFNα2b) in patients with chronic non-A, non-B hepatitis: data of a multicenter randomized prospectively controlled trial. J Hepatol 11 [Suppl] 2:S46
144. Metreau JM, Poupon R, Calmus Y et al. (1990) Factors predictive of a response to interferon therapy in chronic NANB hepatitis. J Hepatol 11 [Suppl] 2:S45
145. Marcellin P, Giostra E, Boyer N, Loriot MA, Martinot-Peignoux M, Benhamou JP (1990) Is the response to recombinant alpha interferon related to the presence of antibodies to hepatitis C virus in patients with chronic non-A, non-B hepatitis? J Hepatol 11:77–79
146. Hautekeete ML, Marcellin P, Giostra E et al. (1990) Rebound phenomenon after cessation of alpha-interferon therapy in chronic non-A, non-B (NANB) hepatitis. J Hepatol 11 [Suppl] 2:S29
147. Shindo M, Di Bisceglie AM, Cheung L et al. (1990) Changes in hepatitis C virus RNA in serum associated with alpha interferon therapy. Hepatology 12:884
148. Viladomiu L, Gonzalez A, Lopez-Talavera JC et al. (1990) A randomized controlled trial of alpha interferon in acute posttransfusion C hepatitis. J Hepatol 11 [Suppl] 2:S64
149. Omata M, Yokosuka O, Hosoda K, Kato N, Ohto M (1990) A control study of treatment for acute non-A, non-B hepatitis: effects on hepatitis C virus (abstr). Hepatology 12:883
150. Chemello L, Benvegnu L, Belussi F, Tagger A, Ruol A, Alberti A (1990) Pilot study of interferon alpha-2a therapy in preventing chronic evolution of acute hepatitis C. J Hepatol 11 [Suppl] 2:S81

# 16 Liver Involvement in Systemic Infection

J. GUARDIA, V. VARGAS, and R. ESTEBAN

The liver has a significant representation of the mononuclear phagocyte system and can, therefore, efficiently remove bacteria from the blood. However it can become involved during systemic infections when local or general conditions favor bacterial colonization. On the other hand it must be borne in mind that increased susceptibility to infection is common in patients with chronic liver disease due to impairment of the immune system and to malnutrition. In this chapter we discuss the involvement of the liver in systemic infections that have not been considered in other sections of the book.

## 1 Pyogenic Hepatic Abscess

Pyogenic hepatic abscess is a serious and not very common illness which accounts for around 15 per 100000 hospital admissions. The incidence in a series of postmortem examinations has been estimated to be between 0.29% and 1.47% [1]. It occurs most frequently between 40 and 60 years of age, predominantly in males.

### 1.1 Etiology and Pathogenesis

The pus-forming bacteria can reach the liver in various ways, but very often they do so as a direct extension of the infection from neighboring organs. However, in about 30%–50% of cases, and particularly in the elderly, the origin of the infection is not clear. In some of these cases, the development of abscesses is favored by diabetes or neoplastic disorders. In our series [2], 12% of the patients were diabetic.

The most common origin of infection is the biliary system; this is especially so when cholangitis occurs, be it secondary to choledocholithiasis or to other causes (tumors of the biliary system, surgical stenosis, chronic pancreatitis, cholestasis, post-sphincterotomy cholangitis). Hepatic abscesses may also occur after episodes of cholecystitis.

Abdominal infections are a major cause of hepatic abscesses; indeed, before the age of antibiotics they were the most common cause, usually following episodes of appendicitis. As a result of pylephlebitis or septic embolisms the organism(s) can colonize the liver; this occurs after acute appendicitis, diverticulitis, proctitis, pancreatitis, hemorrhoids, and outbreaks of inflammatory bowel disease.

Direct hepatic infection is also a cause of abscesses. They can result from abdominal trauma or liver-penetrating wounds, as well as from infection of hydatid cysts, neoplasia, hematomas after liver biopsy, and postoperative cavities in hepatic resections.

Infection via the hepatic artery can occur from any cause leading to bacteremia (e.g., endocarditis). Finally, as already mentioned, in a considerable number of cases no cause is discovered; such cases are considered cryptogenic.

The pathogenic mechanisms leading to the formation of hepatic abscesses are not clear. It is essentially unknown how obstruction of the biliary flow produces hepatic abscesses. One possibility is that the bacteria may ascend the common hepatic duct from the duodenum to the liver, where, in the presence of biliary obstruction, they would remain localized. Against this hypothesis is the fact that organisms of duodenal origin are not those which typically produce hepatic abscesses. Other theories suggest that the bacteria reach the liver after episodes of portal bacteremia; it must be borne in mind that low levels of bacteria are normally present in the portal vein being cleared by the normal liver [3]. Other factors that have been suggested to favor abscess formation include small areas of hepatic infarction caused by intrahepatic thromboembolism or tumoral necrosis.

Hepatic abscesses are more often single than multiple and more often affect the right lobe than the left. This can be explained by the greater size of the right lobe and the larger amount of portal blood which it receives. It has also been demonstrated that there is a characteristic flow in the portal circulation so that the blood from the superior mesenteric vein, which drains the majority of those areas whose infection leads to hepatic abscesses, mostly enters the right lobe, whereas blood from the splenic and inferior mesenteric vessels tends to enter the left lobe.

## 1.2 Bacteriology

In earlier series, up to 50% of pyogenic abscesses were considered sterile [5]. Currently, as a result of improved techniques, blood cultures are positive in almost 50% of cases and the pus culture in 67%–90% [1, 2, 6]. A large number of organisms have been isolated from hepatic abscesses; most frequent are the Gram-negative enteric bacilli, and in particular *Escherichia coli*. Less common are *Klebsiella*, *Proteus*, *Morganella*, *Citrobacter*, and *Pseudomonas*. *Streptococcus milleri*. Gram-negative anaerobic bacilli, and microaerophilic streptococci have also been isolated. *Streptococcus milleri*, an organism with a special tendency to form abscesses in various organs, is the most frequently isolated *Streptococcus* species in hepatic abscesses [8] and is only exceeded in frequency by *E. coli*. Other organisms more rarely isolated include *Staphylococcus*, *Salmonella*, *Yersinia*, *Mycobacterium tuberculosis*, and *Brucella* [9]. Abscesses due to *Actinomyces* and fungi, especially *Candida*, are rare and are usually observed in immunosuppressed patients. Cultures are frequently polymicrobial.

Table 1 shows the bacteriologic findings in our series of 33 cases of hepatic abscess.

### 1.3 Clinical Features

The clinical presentation of patients has changed over the last few decades. In the 1930s [5], the condition was mostly observed in young people, usually after postappendicitis pylephlebitis, with very symptomatic clinical features. Currently the condition is observed in elderly patients (average age between 40 and 60 years) and the clinical features are less dramatic [1, 2, 4, 7].

In the current series, the most common symptom was fever, followed by the presence of chills and abdominal pain. Constitutional symptoms (fatigue, anorexia, weight loss) were found in approximately half of the

**Table 1.** Microorganisms recovered from patients ($n$ = 33) with pyogenic hepatic abscesses

| | Blood | Pus |
|---|---|---|
| Enterobacteriaceae | 8 | 11 |
| *E. coli* | 3 | 6 |
| *Klebsiella* | 3 | 3 |
| *Proteus* | 0 | 1 |
| *Morganella* | 1 | 0 |
| *Citrobacter* | 1 | 1 |
| Streptococci | 5 | 8 |
| *S. milleri* | 4 | 5 |
| *S. sanguis* | 0 | 3 |
| Microaerophilic | 1 | 0 |
| Anaerobes | 6 | 4 |
| *Bacteroides* | 5 | 2 |
| *Fusobacterium* | 0 | 2 |
| *Clostridium* | 1 | 0 |
| Other Gram-negative RODS | 3 | 2 |
| *Acinetobacter* | 1 | 0 |
| *Haemophilus* | 1 | 1 |
| *Eikenella* | 1 | 0 |
| *Pseudomonas* | 0 | 1 |
| Other Gram-positive RODS | 0 | 2 |
| *Staph. epidermidis* | 0 | 2 |

Based on Comas P et al. (1989) Rev Clin Esp 185:225–230

patients. The most constant physical signs were hepatomegaly and tenderness in the right upper quadrant. Jaundice and thoracic signs such as hypophonesis or basal rales in the right hemithorax were less common. Patients with multiple abscesses more frequently presented constitutional signs, hepatomegaly, pain in the right upper quadrant, and jaundice (Table 2).

In the majority of cases the symptoms are of less than 3 weeks' duration. It should be noted that a minority of patients display symptoms which are not very expressive, such as malaise, weight loss, and slowly evolving low-grade fever, and only a few signs which are attributable to the hepatic lesion. These patients are normally elderly, and the lesion is often cryptogenic. On the other hand, cases in which the abscess is secondary to cholangitis normally have a very acute course with high fever and jaundice. The analytic data include an increase in ESR, leukocytosis with deviation to the left, and anemia. Liver function tests show an increase in alkaline phosphatase and/or γ-glutamyl transpeptidase in around 80%–90% of cases. Increases in serum bilirubin, aminotransferases, and/or γ-globulin are observed in 30%–50% of cases [1, 2, 6]; the increase in aminotransferases is not very significant, ranging between two and four times the normal values.

From a clinical point of view it is worth distinguishing between single and multiple hepatic abscesses. The latter have a more acute and serious course, and patients more frequently display jaundice and anemia and have higher levels of alkaline phosphatase and γ-glutamyl transpeptidase; the mortality associated with multiple abscesses is also higher. Multiple abscesses are often observed as a complication of another source of infection, while single abscesses have a cryptogenic origin in 25% of cases.

**Table 2.** Pyogenic hepatic abscess: signs and symptoms in 33 patients

| | |
|---|---|
| Symptoms | |
| Fever | 28 (85%) |
| Chills | 18 (55%) |
| Abdominal pain | 17 (52%) |
| Weight loss | 17 (52%) |
| Signs | |
| Febrile on admission | 25 (76%) |
| Fever (>37.5°C) | 28 (85%) |
| Hepatomegaly | 19 (58%) |
| Local abdominal tenderness | 21 (64%) |
| Jaundice | 5 (15%) |
| Chest signs | 6 (18%) |

Based on COMAS P et al. (1989) Rev Clin Esp 185:225–230

### 1.4 Diagnosis

The diagnosis of pyogenic hepatic abscess is often delayed and more than a third of patients are symptomatic more than 2 weeks before receiving medical therapy, probably due to their age and the existence of other illnesses which may mask the symptoms.

Between 35% and 75% of cases show abnormalities on chest x-ray films, which suggest an infradiaphragmatic process. Right pleural effusion, basal atelectases, or elevation of the right hemidiaphragm can be observed.

The new imaging techniques have revolutionized the diagnosis and management of pyogenic hepatic abscesses (Table 3). Radionuclide scanning within $^{99m}$Tc-sulfur colloid has a high sensitivity (80%–90%), displaying a "cold" area or an area where there is decreased uptake of $^{99m}$Tc. False-negatives most frequently occur when there are multiple abscesses and/or when the abscess diameter is less than 2 cm. Lack of specificity is the biggest drawback of this method, since there are numerous lesions which can produce a similar image. Gallium scintigraphy can increase specificity by showing "hot" areas that are only observed in tumors and abscesses; its main drawback is its slowness. Real-time ultrasonography and scanning by computed tomography (CT) (Fig. 1) have replaced radionuclide scanning as diagnostic procedures. Real-time gray-scale ultrasonography is a simple and rapid technique which visualizes the abscesses as rounded hypoechoic areas. Its sensitivity reaches about 80%, with false-negatives almost always being due either to abscesses in the hepatic cupula or to very small ones. CT is probably the most sensitive technique (up to 97%); abscesses are seen as rounded images which are less attenuated than the surrounding parenchyma [10]. While these last two techniques do lack specificity, the diagnosis of a suspected abscess can be completed with guided fine-needle aspiration. If pus is obtained, this will confirm the diagnosis and be very useful for culture to achieve an etiologic diagnosis. Arteriography is very rarely used in the diagnosis of hepatic abscesses. Probably, ultrasonography is the best initial diagnostic test, with CT serving as a means of confirmation or to clarify the diagnosis when multiple hepatic abscesses are suspected [3].

**Table 3.** Frequency of abnormal findings of chest roentgenography and modern diagnostic imaging procedures in patients ($n$ = 33) with pyogenic hepatic abscesses

| | Abnormal findings |
|---|---|
| Chest roentgenography | 12/33 (36%) |
| Ultrasonography | 27/30 (90%) |
| Radionuclide scanning | 19/21 (90%) |
| Computed tomography | 12/13 (92%) |

Based on Comas P et al. (1989) Rev Clin Esp 185:225–230

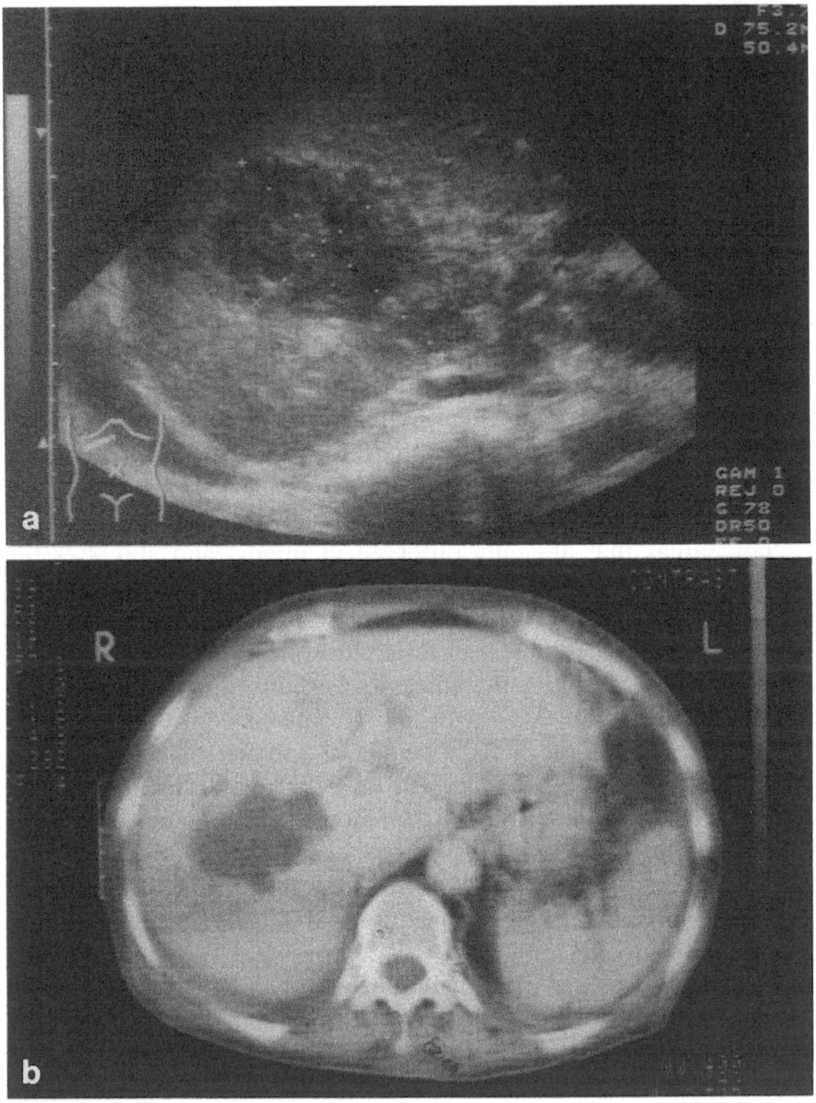

**Fig. 1.** **a** Ultrasonogram and **b** CT scan showing a pyogenic abscess in the right lobe of the liver

The pus culture obtained by needle aspiration and blood culture hold the clues to the correct etiologic diagnosis of the abscess. Aerobic, anaerobic, and *S. milleri* enriched medium cultures should be obtained. The pus culture from the abscess is positive in between 67% and 90% of cases and the blood culture in between 40% and 48% [1, 2, 6]. With one of the two methods the etiologic agent can be identified in 80% of cases. It is also essential to try to verify the cause of the abscess by studying the biliary tree;

if this proves fruitless, other possible origins, especially the gastrointestinal tract, should be investigated [11].

### 1.5 Treatment

Until recently, surgical drainage combined with broad-spectrum antibiotics was the usual treatment for abscesses. In recent years it has been suggested that medical treatment could avoid the need for surgery, which can entail significant morbidity. Although studies exist which suggest that treatment with broad-spectrum antibiotics (gentamicin and clindamycin) alone could be effective in uncomplicated hepatic abscesses [12], this has not been confirmed and the majority of authors consider that percutaneous drainage together with the administration of antibiotics is a good alternative treatment which could reduce the need for surgery [13–15].

The antibiotics used should be active against Gram-negative aerobic bacilli, microaerophilic streptococci, and anaerobes. This criterion is fulfilled by a combination of aminoglycosides, ampicillin and metronidazole or clindamycin; third-generation cephalosporins can substitute for aminoglycosides. Also, the combination of amoxicillin and clavulanic acid can be an effective alternative. When positive cultures are obtained, appropriate antibiotic treatment according to the susceptibility of the isolated organism should be instituted. Antibiotics should be administered parenterally for 15 days and then orally for a further 6 weeks. Percutaneous drainage is carried out using a pigtail catheter which is inserted employing ultrasonographic or CT guidance. The catheter can remain in place for between 3 and 20 days. With this procedure therapeutic success is achieved in 72%–90% of cases [16]. Complications of the procedure are few (occurring in less than 5% of cases) and can include perforation of other abdominal organs, pneumothorax, hemorrhage, and rupture of the abscess into neighboring areas, including the peritoneum. If there are multiple abscesses and one of these is large, an attempt to drain the largest one should be made. If all the abscesses are small and are located in one lobe or segment, then resection should be performed. If they are diffuse then only antibiotic treatment can be used.

In spite of all these forms of treatment, surgery continues to be appropriate in those cases where the primary abdominal disorder has a surgical solution and the laparotomy itself can solve both problems. Surgery may also be indicated in cases of suspected multiloculation or multiple abscesses when the anatomic location does not permit percutaneous drainage. In addition, surgery must be performed on patients who do not respond to 2 weeks of antibiotic treatment and percutaneous drainage. Surgical drainage provides certain advantages such as the capacity to explore the abdomen for the source of the abscess, good exposure of the whole liver, and the possibility of choosing the best place for drainage and access to the biliary tree [17].

### 1.6 Prognosis and Complications

Complications of pyogenic abscesses are observed in 10%–20% of patients and are related to the rupture of the abscess or its extension to adjacent structures. The most common complications are pleuropulmonary, with pleural effusion and empyema. Other complications are subphrenic abscess, hemobilia, peritonitis, and septic metastases. Septic endophthalmitis is a complication of pyogenic abscesses caused by *Klebsiella*, being observed in about 8% of such cases [18].

In the preantibiotic era, mortality in patients with hepatic abscesses reached nearly 60%. Currently, mortality in the case of a single abscess is 10%–15%. However, multiple abscesses continue to be associated with a mortality of 40% or more [3]. Other factors associated with high mortality are age, jaundice, polymicrobial infection, seriousness of the underlying illness, and the existence of associated neoplasia.

## 2 Systemic Bacterial Infections

In the course of bacterial infections, various clinical and biochemical disturbances indicative of liver involvement are frequently detected. In serious infections accompanied by hypotension and shock, liver ischemia may lead to an increase in serum bilirubin and aminotransferase levels [19]; other factors such as direct invasion of the liver by blood- or lymph-borne agents, endotoxin-induced liver cell injury, and nonspecific lesions related to malnutrition, hypoxia, and fever may also play a role in these biochemical alterations. Abnormal liver tests and jaundice are seen in newborns and infants, and less commonly in adults, with severe bacterial infections due to *E. coli*, *Klebsiella pneumoniae*, *Pseudomonas aeruginosa*, *Haemophilus influenzae*, *Proteus* spp, *Bacteroides* spp, *Staphylococcus aureus*, and aerobic and anaerobic *Streptococcus* spp. We will consider different types of hepatic lesions according to the causal organism.

### 2.1 Gram-Positive Cocci

In infections caused by *Streptococcus pneumoniae*, the serum levels of aminotransferases and alkaline phosphatase are frequently elevated and, in 20% of cases, hyperbilirubinemia also occurs. Jaundice may be seen as a consequence of hemolysis in cases of glucose-6-phosphate dehydrogenase deficiency, but in most instances it is of hepatic origin [20]. Hepatomegaly is often detected and the histologic picture is that of infiltrative focal hepatitis. In alcoholics, liver involvement is much more serious. The differential diagnosis includes the existence of a previous and undiagnosed liver disease;

any doubt is eliminated by the normalization of laboratory data when the infection resolves.

Infections caused by other streptococci often cause abnormalities in liver function tests without significant liver damage. Much less common is streptococcal septic hepatitis, with prolonged fever, perivascular infiltrative lesions, and hepatocellular necrosis at biopsy [21]. Biochemical changes and microabscess formation are more common in infections caused by staphlycocci.

## 2.2 Gram-Negative Cocci

Gram-negative cocci can cause septic shock and reduced liver perfusion resulting in changes in liver function tests [19]. Other causes of hepatic lesions are endotoxins and direct invasion by microorganisms. Cholangitis due to *E. coli* in the absence of biliary abnormalities has been described. In urinary infections and particularly in xanthogranulomatous pyelonephritis due to *E. coli*, a reactive hepatitis accompanied by biochemical abnormalities can be observed.

Women who suffer pelvic peritonitis due to *Neisseria gonorrhoeae* (sometimes subclinically) may develop a clinical condition characterized by the appearance of pain in the right hypochondrium (which can be similar to that produced by cholelithiasis), accompanied by fever, hepatomegaly, and the presence of a friction rub on the hepatic surface. This syndrome (Fitz-Hugh and Curtis syndrome) is diagnosed by identification of the gonococcus in vaginal exudate or by the observation of adhesions, pus, and fibrin on the liver capsule upon laparotomy (if surgery is erroneously performed) or laparoscopy. Similar cases have been observed in males and also as a result of *Chlamydia* infection [22]. In gonococcal septicemia and endocarditis, increases in hepatic enzymes and bilirubin have been observed, due to the existence of inflammatory infiltrates and areas of focal necrosis.

## 2.3 Salmonellae and Shigellae

There are healthy carriers of *Salmonella typhi* that harbour the microorganism in the gallbladder and who spread the illness in endemic zones. Both in typhoid and paratyphoid fever, enzimatic changes are normally found (increased levels of aminotransferases). Approximately a quarter of the patients exhibit hepatomegaly and a very small proportion, jaundice; exceptionally, hepatic involvement acquires clinical relevance. Histologically there is a reactive hepatitis with aggregates of Kupffer cells that do not, however, constitute granulomas. In shigellosis, similar lesions are found and some cases of clinical liver involvement with marked cholestasis have been described [23].

### 2.4 Brucella

Many patients suffering from brucellosis show irregularities in hepatic tests and some display jaundice; hepatomegaly is common. In infections due to *Brucella abortus*, liver biopsy shows marked granulomatous hepatitis with central necrosis. This is equally present, although without necrosis, in cases of infection by *Brucella melitensis* [24, 25]. Abscesses have rarely been described [9].

### 2.5 Legionella

Half of the patients with infections due to *Legionella* present biochemical changes secondary to focal hepatitis.

### 2.6 Clostridium Perfringens

In patients suffering from gas gangrene, hemolytic jaundice is common but in addition the liver can be affected by necrotic areas and abscesses which produce gas images on plain X-ray of the abdomen.

### 2.7 Actinomycosis and Nocardiosis

Infections due to *Actinomyces israelii*, which originate in the appendix or in the cecal region, can reach the liver via the portal system, by contiguity or, more rarely, via the arterial system. Clinically, they produce hepatomegaly, fever and abnormalities in hepatic tests (which, however, can be normal), most often without jaundice. The hepatomegaly can be irregular, and ultrasonography, CT, or laparoscopy reveals single or, rarely, multiple masses which can be erroneously interpreted as metastases. Diagnosis is obtained by culture of material derived from the hepatic aspirate, from the possible fistulas or pleural effusion, or from the material obtained at laparotomy [26]. In nocardiosis the liver is only affected in the disseminated forms which are observed in immunosuppressed patients.

### 2.8 Mycobacteria

Of the mycobacteria, it is *Mycobacterium tuberculosis* that most frequently infects man. Hepatotoxicity due to tuberculostatic drugs must be differentiated from the hepatic lesions due to the microorganism. Granulomatous hepatitis accompanies miliary tuberculosis in 90% of these cases; sometimes (in 20%–60% of cases) granulomatous hepatitis occurs in other forms of tuberculosis [27, 28]. Typical tuberculous granulomas show central caseous

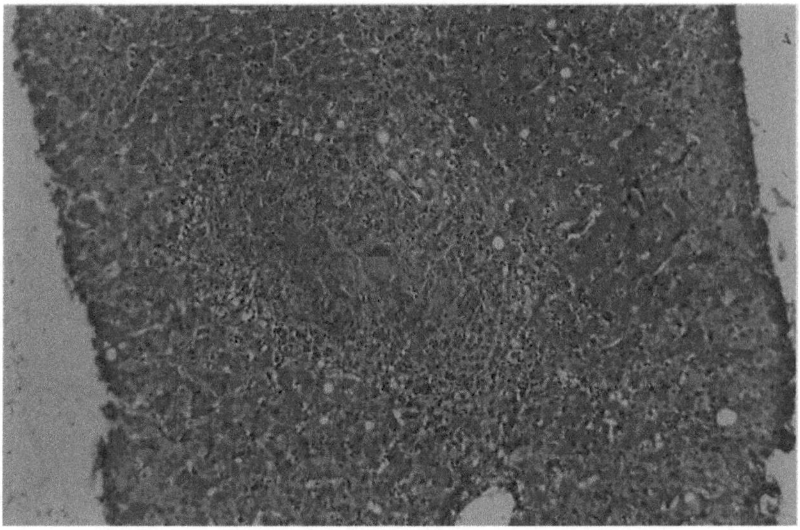

**Fig. 2.** Tuberculous granuloma of the liver. Central caseous necrosis, a multinucleated giant cell, and a lymphocytic rim can be seen. H&E, ×150

necrosis, epithelioid and multinucleated cells, and a rim of lymphocytes (Fig. 2). Tuberculoma, a hepatic mass formed by a conglomerate of granulomas, is rare and can be wrongly interpreted as a single or multiple hepatic tumor (Fig. 3); calcifications revealed by radiologic examination support the diagnosis but can also be observed in hepatocarcinoma, and for this reason histologic confirmation is essential [29]. Tuberculous cholangitis due to rupture of a tuberculoma in the biliary tree is an unusual clinical condition which causes fever, abdominal pain localized in the right hypochondrium, and jaundice, and is easily misinterpreted as choledocholithiasis [30]. Laparotomy can have fatal consequences and the diagnosis, which is generally difficult, must be based on clinical history (coexisting pulmonary tuberculosis) and biopsy (caseous granulomas). Cases of tuberculous cholecystitis and hemobilia have also been described.

Other mycobacteria (atypical, *M. leprae*) can be the cause of hepatic granuloma. The frequency of cases due to atypical mycobacteria, especially *Mycobacterium avium–intracellulare*, is increased in patients with AIDS [31].

## 2.9 Spirochetes

The liver is affected by all forms of syphilis; given the increase in the incidence of this infection and the variety of its clinical expression, syphilis must be taken into account in the differential diagnosis of hepatic disorders of no clear origin. Also to be considered is the association between syphilis,

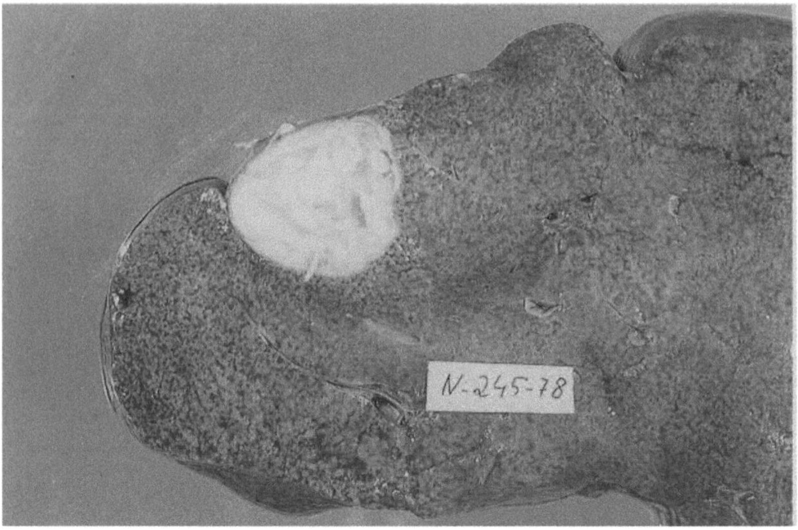


**Fig. 3.** Liver section showing a white round mass corresponding to a tuberculoma of the liver

hepatitis B, and AIDS among the homosexual community and drug addicts. In secondary syphilis, the presence of fever and rashes, can be associated with increases in the levels of aminotransferases and especially of alkaline phosphatase. Hepatic biopsy shows focal necrosis and sometimes cholestasis with a proliferation of intrahepatic bile ducts and granulomas [32].

In tertiary syphilis, gummas are found, especially in the right lobe; they are in general subclinical, although Budd-Chiari syndrome has been described due to suprahepatic compression. Jaundice, ascites, fever and constitutional symptoms with abdominal pain have also been found in association with syphilitic gummas.

*L. icterohaemorrhagiae* and *L. canicola* are, among more than 100 serogroups of Leptospira interrogans, the ones which possess clinical relevance. The most usual mode of spread is via rat urine (in paddy fields, sewers, etc.). Patients manifest high fever, myalgia and headache, accompanied by jaundice in a third of cases (Weil's disease), and occasionally by abdominal pain. The jaundice can be very marked (up to 40 mg/dl of bilirubin) but its course usually involves hardly any increase in alkaline phosphatase and aminotransferase levels. Hepatic biopsy shows cholestasis, signs of regeneration (mitosis), and, sometimes, steatosis. The diagnosis is established by isolating the microorganism in blood (1st week), cerebrospinal fluid (2nd week), or urine (3rd week) or by complement fixation using specific antigens [33].

In infections due to *Borrelia recurrentis* (recurrent fever) there is often hepatomegaly and an increase in aminotransferase levels; in some cases there is marked hyperbilirubinemia with almost normal hepatic enzymes. Enzyme increases and, more rarely, jaundice have also been described in Lyme disease due to *Borrelia burgdorferi* [34].

### 2.10 Rickettsiae and Mycoplasmas

During the course of Q fever there is an increase in hepatic enzymes and in less than 5% of cases jaundice may be found. Exceptional cases of cholangitis and fatal hepatitis have been described. The hepatic lesion is a granuloma characterized by the existence of a ring of fibrin (doughnut form) which, although very characteristic, can be observed exceptionally in tuberculosis and some lymphomas. The diagnosis is by epidemiologic data (contact with livestock) and by complement fixation [35, 36]. In boutonneuse fever [37] and in Rocky mountain spotted fever, there is a moderate increase in hepatic enzymes and nonspecific granulomas can be detected by hepatic biopsy.

During pneumonia due to *Mycoplasma pneumoniae*, changes in aminotransferase and alkaline phosphatase levels are found, without further implications.

### 2.11 Miscellaneous

In neonatal listeriosis, multiple granulomas can be found in the liver and cases of hepatic abscess have been described. In serious forms of tularemia aminotransferase levels are increased and foci of hepatic necrosis and/or granulomas are seen. In the rare disseminated forms of melioidosis (*Pseudomonas pseudomallei*) areas of hepatic necrosis exist.

## 3 Fungal Infections

Mycoses are especially observed in immunosuppressed patients and have a characteristic geographic distribution. The liver can be affected in a subclinical manner with unspecific lesions and occasionally abscesses, which are of greater clinical significance. Table 4 shows the hepatic lesions most common in each of the mycoses.

## 4 Viruses Other than Hepatitis Virus

In addition to hepatitis viruses, other viral agents can produce hepatic lesions, in general of nonspecific character (focal necrosis with lymphocytic infiltration) and with minimal biologic significance. Exceptions to this rule

**Table 4.** Frequency of liver involvement, type of lesion, and clinical picture in mycotic infections

| Fungi | Frequency of liver involvement | Type of lesion | Clinical picture |
|---|---|---|---|
| *Histoplasma capsulatum* | High in chronic forms | Granulomas | Subclinical<br>Rarely jaundice |
| *Cryptococcus* | High in disseminated forms | Caseous granulomas | Subclinical<br>Jaundice and liver failure rare |
| *Mucor* | Rare and in disseminated forms | Steatosis<br>Perivenular necrosis | Liver failure |
| *Aspergillus* | Rare and in systemic forms | Periportal abscesses | Jaundice, Budd-Chiari syndrome |
| *Coccidioides immitis* | 30% of patients | Granulomas | Subclinical |
| *Blastomyces dermatitidis* | In systemic forms | Granulomas | Subclinical |
| *Paracoccidioides brasiliensis* | 20% of systemic forms | Portal granulomas | Subclinical |
| *Candida albicans* | 50% of systemic forms | Granulomas and microabscesses | Hepatomegaly |
| *Sporothrix schenckii* | In systemic forms | Abscesses | Fever |
| *Trichosporon* | In the immunosuppressed | Granulomas | Jaundice and high aminotransferase values |

are the Epstein-Barr virus and yellow fever virus. These agents do induce hepatic lesions of clinical relevance.

In infectious mononucleosis, caused by the Epstein-Barr human herpetic virus IV (EBV), sinusoidal infiltration by atypical lymphocytes, proliferation of Kupffer cells, and polynuclear and lymphocytic infiltration with centers of isolated focal necrosis are observed. This lesion always regresses; clinically it typically develops with an increase in aminotransferases (to 10–20 times the normal value) and, in 30%–40% of cases, with jaundice. The presence of high fever, adenopathies, pharyngoamygdalitis and atypical lymphocytosis permits differential diagnosis from other types of viral hepatitis. The Paul-Bunnell-Davidson test, the "monospot" test, and the presence of IgM type antibodies against EBV capsid antigens are of diagnostic value.

Infection due to *Cytomegalovirus* in healthy adults produces a condition similar to infectious mononucleosis, without pharyngoamygdalitis or adenopathies and with a negative monospot test. Also, cases of granulomatous hepatitis, with prolonged fever and nonspecific histologic findings, have been described. In immunosuppressed patients (hepatic, renal, or bone marrow transplant patients and in those with leukemia) a disseminated picture can occur due to the reactivation of a previous infection or as a consequence of an infection from blood transfusion. The diagnosis may be established by serology (presence of IgM type antibodies), but a preferable means of diagnosis is either blood or culture of biopsy material or demonstration of the presence of the virus in hepatic tissue by means of immunohistochemistry or molecular hybridization (Fig. 4) [38].

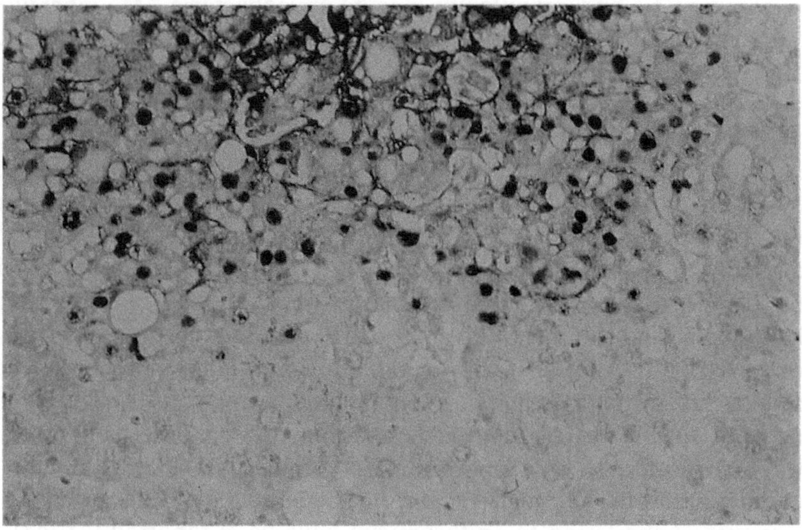

**Fig. 4.** Positive molecular hybridization in the nuclei of liver cells with a cytomegalovirus DNA probe

In immunosuppressed adults, herpes simplex virus 1 and 2 produces scattered infections with hepatic involvement. Histologically, centers of necrosis and hepatocytes with viral inclusions can be observed and verified by electron microscopy, immunohistochemistry, or molecular hybridization [39]. Cases similar to viral hepatitis have been described, sometimes with a fulminant course in previously healthy adults with or without previous genital herpes; in these cases leukopenia is common. The early administration of acyclovir can resolve the condition.

The yellow fever virus (arbovirus type B), which is transmitted by the *Aedes aegypti* mosquito and is endemic in South America and equatorial Africa, produces centrizonal acidophilic hepatic necrosis with the appearance of Councilman bodies and abundant ceroid deposits; if the patient survives, there is a complete regression of the lesion. Clinically, the condition is abrupt,with high fever, muscular pain, headache, vomiting which is often hematic, hypotension, jaundice, purpuric changes and hemorrhagic events. The illness evolves over 10 days; it either causes death by coma or gives way to a swift and complete recovery. Raised serum levels of alkaline phosphatase, aminotransferases, and bilirubin, and a reduction in prothrombin are found. The diagnosis is confirmed by intracerebral inoculation of mice with serum from the patient.

Other viruses capable of producing hepatic lesions are: Coxsackie B, adenovirus, varicella and varicella-zoster, measles and rubella, Lassa virus, Marburg virus, and Ebola virus. The last three viruses cause severe and frequent hepatic lesions in the course of hemorrhagic febrile diseases.

In patients infected by the human immunodeficiency virus (HIV) a great number of infections which affect the liver are observed [31]. Thus, it is common to find granulomas due to mycobacteria (*M. tuberculosis* and atypical) and infections due to fungi (*Cryptococcus*, *Histoplasma*, *Candida*, etc.), viruses (herpes, Epstein-Barr, cytomegalovirus), and bacteria. Due to the immunosuppression associated with the disease, granuloma formation may be absent even in the presence of these infective agents as demonstrated by specific techniques. Often, these patients are chronically infected by hepatitis viruses B, D, and C. They receive hepatotoxic drugs and require blood transfusions. All these factors sometimes make it difficult to attribute to a single agent the clinical and histologic hepatic lesion displayed by these patients. In addition, cases of Hodgkin's and non-Hodgkin's lymphoma and, more rarely, Kaposi's sarcoma in the liver have been observed [40]. Another form of hepatic lesion is the acalculous cholangitis similar to primary sclerosing cholangitis, which is attributed to cytomegalovirus. Cases of peliosis hepatis have been described; initially they were attributed to a cytopathic effect of the AIDS virus on the hepatic endothelial cells although recently a bacillary etiology and a favourable response of the lesion to erythromycin have been reported [41, 42].

## 5 Granulomas of the Liver

A large number of infectious illnesses can produce hepatic granulomas [43, 44]. In the majority of cases the lesion has no specific character although occasionally the causal germ can be located by staining techniques (Ziehl-Nielsen in tuberculosis, leprosy, and other mycobacterial diseases, Giemsa in kala-azar, and hematoxylin and eosin in schistosomiasis). In other cases the characteristics of the lesion (caseous necrosis in tuberculosis, fibrin ring in Q fever) are suggestive of a specific etiology. Histochemistry or molecular hybridization techniques may identify the cause of a granulomatous lesion if it is of infectious origin. Table 5 shows the causes of hepatic granuloma.

A picture of fever of unknown origin and abnormal liver test, associated with nonspecific granulomas in the hepatic biopsy, can be classified as idiopathic granulomatous hepatitis [45]. In some cases further investigation leads to an etiologic diagnosis (cytomegalovirus infection, lymphoma, tuberculosis); some other patients fully recover without therapy in weeks or months and still others respond to corticosteroids. An isolated form of sarcoidosis of the liver has been suggested as a cause of the disease in some patients.

**Table 5.** Etiology of hepatic granulomas

| | |
|---|---|
| I. Bacteria | VI. Fungi |
| Gram-negative cocci | Histoplasmosis |
| Tularemia | Cryptococcosis |
| Brucellosis | Coccidioidomycosis |
| Salmonellosis | Blastomycosis |
| Listeriosis | Candidiasis |
| Melioidosis | Trichosporosis |
| Granuloma inguinale | VII. Parasites |
| Actinomycosis | Schistosomiasis |
| II. Mycobacteria | Toxoplasmosis |
| Tuberculosis | Amebiasis |
| Atypical mycobacteria | Leishmaniasis |
| BCG | Oxyuriasis |
| Leprosy | Toxocariasis |
| III. Spirochetes | Ascaridiasis |
| Syphilis | Capillariasis |
| Lyme disease | VII. Other causes of hepatic granuloma |
| IV. Rickettsiae | Tumors |
| Q fever | Liver disease (primary biliary cirrhosis) |
| Boutonneuse fever | Drugs |
| | Systemic diseases (sarcoidosis, immune deficiencies, collagen diseases) |
| | Inflammatory bowel disease |
| | Foreign bodies (talc, silica, beryllium, silicone, copper) |
| | Chemical poisons |
| | Unknown causes |

Liver biopsy may be of assistance in patients with fever of unknown origin if a granuloma or a tumor (lymphoma) is found [46].

## References


1. McDonald MI, Corey CR, Gallis HA, Durack DT (1984) Single and multiple pyogenic liver abscesses. Natural history, diagnosis and treatment, with emphasis on percutaneous drainage. Medicine (Baltimore) 63:291–302
2. Comas P, Vargas V, Almirante B, González A, García-Sureda D, Esteban R, Guardia J (1989) Absceso piógeno hepático. Revisión de 33 casos. Rev Clin Esp 185:225–230
3. Rustgi AK, Richter JM (1989) Pyogenic and amebic liver abscess. Med Clin North Am 73:847–858
4. Lee JF, Block GE (1971) The changing clinical pattern of hepatic abscesses. Arch Surg 104:465–470
5. Oschner A, DeBakey M, Murray S (1938) Pyogenic abscess of the liver. II. An analysis of 47 cases with review of the literature. Am J Surg 40:292–329
6. Barnes PF, DeCock KM, Reynolds TN, Ralls PW (1987) A comparison of amebic and pyogenic abscess of the liver. Medicine (Baltimore) 66:472–483
7. Rubin RH, Swartz MN, Malt R (1974) Hepatic abscess: changes in clinical, bacteriologic and therapeutic aspects. Am J Med 57:601–610
8. Chua D, Reinhart HH, Sobel JD (1989) Liver abscess caused by *Streptococcus milleri*. Rev Infect Dis 11:197–202
9. Vargas V, Comas P, Gasser I, Lucea D, Esteban R, Guardia J (1991) Brucellar hepatic abscess. J Clin Gastroenterol 13:477–478
10. Halvorsen RA, Foster WL, Wilkinson RH, Silverman PM, Thompson WM (1988) Hepatic abscess: sensitivity of imaging tests and clinical findings. Gastrointest Radiol 13:135–141
11. Cohen JL, Martin FM, Rossi RL, Schoetz DJ (1989) Liver abscess. The need for complete gastrointestinal evaluation. Arch Surg 124:561–564
12. Herbert A, Fogel DA, Rothman J, Wilson S, Simmons F, Ruskin J (1982) Pyogenic liver abscesses: successful non-surgical therapy. Lancet I:134–136
13. Berger LA, Osborne DR (1982) Treatment of pyogenic liver abscesses by percutaneous needle aspiration. Lancet I:132–134
14. Gerzof SG, Johnson WC, Robbins AH, Nabseth DC (1985) Intrahepatic pyogenic abscesses: treatment by percutaneous drainage. Am J Surg 149:487–494
15. Bertel CK, Van Heerden JA, Sheedy PF (1986) Treatment of pyogenic hepatic abscesses. Arch Surg 121:554–558
16. Franquet T, Bescós JM, Barberena FJ, Mendioroz FJ (1989) Abscesos hepáticos piógenos: Valor de la ultrasonografia en su diagnóstico y tratamiento. Rev Esp Enf Ap Dig 76:461–464
17. Pitt HA (1990) Surgical management of hepatic abscesses. World J Surg 14:498–504
18. Chiu CT, Lin DY, Liaw YF (1988) Metastatic septic endophthalmitis in pyogenic liver abscess. J Clin Gastroenterol 10:524–527
19. Bank JG, Foulis AK, Ledingham IMcA et al. (1982) Liver function in septic shock. J Clin Pathol 35:1349–1352
20. Tugwell P, Williams AO (1977) Jaundice associated with lobar pneumonia. Q J Med 46:97–118
21. Weinstein L (1978) Bacterial hepatitis: a case report on an unrecognised cause of fever of unknown origin. N Engl J Med 299:1052–1054
22. Vickers FN, Maloney PJ (1964) Gonococcal perihepatitis. Arch Intern Med 114:120–123

23. Khosla SN, Singh R, Singh GPP et al. (1988) The spectrum of hepatic injury in enteric fever. Am J Gastroenterol 83:413–416
24. Williams RK, Crossley K (1982) Acute and chronic hepatic involvement of brucellosis. Gastroenterology 83:455–458
25. Cervantes F, Bruguera M, Force L, Webb S (1982) Liver disease in brucellosis. A clinical and pathological study of 40 cases. Postgrad Med J 58:346–350
26. Meade III RH (1980) Primary hepatic actinomycosis. Gastroenterology 78:355–359
27. Kim JH, Langston AA, Gallis HA (1990) Miliary tuberculosis: epidemiology, clinical manifestations, diagnosis and outcome. Rev Infect Dis 12:583–590
28. Masana L, Clotet B, Vilaseca J, Guardia J, Bacardí R, Martínez-Vázquez JM (1980) L'hépatite granulomateuse dans la tuberculose. Ann Gastroenterol Hepatol (Paris) 16:139–142
29. Oliva A, Duarte B, Jonasson O, Nadimpalli V (1990) The nodular form of local hepatic tuberculosis. A review. J Clin Gastroenterol 12:166–173
30. Maharaj B, Leary WP, Pudifin DJ (1987) A prospective study of hepatic tuberculosis in 41 black patients. Q J Med 63:517–522
31. Schaffner F (1990) The liver in HIV infection. Prog Liver Dis 9:505–522
32. Baker AL, Kaplan MM, Wolfe HJ, McGowan JA (1971) Liver disease associated with early syphilis. N Engl J Med 284:1422–1423
33. Heath CW Jr, Alexander AD, Galton MM (1965) Leptospirosis in the United States. Analysis of 483 cases in man, 1949–1961. N Engl J Med 273:857–864
34. Goellner MH, Agger WA, Burgess JH et al. (1988) Hepatitis due to recurrent Lyme disease. Ann Intern Med 108:707–709
35. Urso FP (1975) The pathologic findings in rickettsial pneumonia. Am J Clin Pathol 64:335–342
36. Turck WPG, Howitt G, Turnberg LA et al. (1976) Chronic Q fever. Q J Med 45:193–217
37. Guardia J, Vilaseca J, Moragas A, Martinez-Vazquez JM, Bombi JA, Calders J, Bacardí R (1981) Hepatitis in exanthematous Mediterranean fever. Hepatogastroenterology 21:81–83
38. Deny P, Debure A, Agut H et al. (1989) Detection of human cytomegalovirus DNA in liver biopsies from patients with cytomegalovirus-related liver disease. Res Virol 140:361–372
39. Lopez-Talavera JC, Allende H, Esteban R, Villegas G, Esteban JI, Guardia J (1990) Diagnóstico de hepatitis aguda por virus del *Herpes simplex* mediante hibridación in situ. Med Clin (Barc) 94:342–343
40. Capell MS, Schwartz MS, Biempica L (1990) Clinical utility of liver biopsy in patients with serum antibodies to the human immunodeficiency virus. Am J Med 88:123–130
41. Scoazec JY, Marche C, Girad PM et al. (1988) Peliosis hepatis and sinusoidal dilation during infection by the human immunodeficiency virus (HIV). An ultrastructural study. Am J Pathol 131:38–47
42. Perrocha LA, Geaghan SM, Yen TSB et al. (1991) Clinical and pathological features of bacillary peliosis hepatis in association with human immunodeficiency virus infection. N Engl J Med 323:1581–1586
43. Vilaseca J, Guardia J, Cuxart A et al. (1978) Hépatite granulomateuse: étude etiologique de 107 cas. Nouv Presse Med 7:323–325
44. Harrington PT, Gutiérrez JJ, Ramirez-Ronda CH, Quiñones-Soto R, Bermúdez RH, Chaffey J (1982) Granulomatous hepatitis. Rev Infect Dis 4:638-655
45. Telenti A, Hermans PE (1989) Idiopathic granulomatosis of the liver manifesting as fever of unknown origin. Mayo Clin Proc 64:44–50
46. Masana L, Guardia J, Clotet B, Cuxart A, Vilaseca J, Bacardí R (1980) Liver biopsy in fever of unknown origin. Gastroenterol Clin Biol 4:215–218

# 17 Protozoal and Helminthic Diseases of the Liver and Biliary Tract

L.C. DA SILVA, P.P. CHIEFFI, and F.J. CARRILHO

While there are a great number of parasitoses which can affect the liver throughout the world, certain protozoal and helminthic diseases deserve particular attention, especially in underdeveloped countries. Among the protozoal diseases, some involve primarily the liver parenchyma (e.g., amebiasis) whereas others are responsible for diffuse reticuloendothelial involvement (malaria and kala-azar). As to the helminthic diseases, some produce obstructive biliary lesions (ascariasis and liver fluke diseases, including fascioliasis, clonorchiasis and opisthorchiasis), whereas others cause obstructive vascular lesions (schistosomiasis). Parenchymal lesions may appear as cystic (hydatidosis) or granulomatous (toxocariasis, capillariasis, and strongyloidiasis). Finally, some helminths produce combined cystic and granulomatous lesions [1].

## 1 Amebiasis

The pathogenesis of tissue invasion by *Entamoeba histolytica* and the factors responsible for the different behavior of many strains isolated from infected persons are not well established. Recently published data have shed some light on this subject. SARGEAUNT [2] claims that it is possible to differentiate pathogenic from nonpathogenic *E. histolytica* strains through their zymodemes, which are characterized by the mobility of four isoenzymes on starch gel electrophoresis. However, in 1987 MIRELMAN [3] reported that isoenzymes of cloned cultures of "nonpathogenic" strains of *E. histolytica* can change their electrophoretic migration patterns if they are cocultured "in vitro" with some bacterial species. Moreover, these *E. histolytica* strains can also change their behavior in cell culture and present pathogenic features in inoculated hamsters.

Epidemiologic studies show that the majority of *E. histolytica* infected persons are asymptomatic, eliminating cysts for long periods of time. In South Africa, where amebiasis is an important cause of human disease, GATHIRAN and JACKSON [4] showed that 1% of *E. histolytica* infected persons develop invasive amebiasis. According to RAVDIN [5], there are certain factors that predispose to the occurrence of severe amebic disease; these include the use of corticosteroids, malnutrition, consumptive diseases, pregnancy, and puerperium, as well as infection in very young hosts.

### 1.1 Clinical and Pathologic Features

Amebic liver abscesses represent around 70% of all extraintestinal localizations of invasive amebiasis. There is evidence that extraintestinal localizations depend on circumstances that decrease the immune response and host defense mechanisms, such as malnutrition [6, 7].

Liver abscesses can present an acute or subacute onset. In the acute form, fever and abdominal pain are the most prominent symptoms; in the subacute form, weight loss is the main symptom and less than 50% of the patients report fever or abdominal pain. Abdominal pain is usually located in the right upper quadrant, with frequent irradiation to the shoulder; jaundice occurs in fewer than 10% of cases. Fever is usually not a prominent feature unless the abscess becomes secondarily infected [1].

In 23 patients with amebic liver abscesses Radin et al. [8] reported only one abscess in 74%; 22% had two to five abscesses, and 4% presented more than five. Seventy-eight percent of the patients had other extraintestinal amebic localizations, particularly right pleural and perihepatic.

Rupture is the main complication of liver abscess, with spontaneous drainage into thoracic, abdominal and pericardiac cavities, depending on the abscess localization in the liver parenchyma.

The pathology of liver amebiasis includes necrosis and, occasionally, periportal fibrosis. Abscess is characterized by the presence of acellular debris, leukocytes and a great number of *E. histolytica* trophozoites surrounding the lesion (Figs. 1 and 2).

### 1.2 Diagnosis

Laboratory findings of amebic liver disease are characterized by leukocytosis without eosinophilia, slight anemia, and high levels of serum alkaline phosphatase in 80% of the cases. Many patients show a high erythrocyte sedimentation rate and slightly increased serum aminotransferase levels. Serum electrophoretic patterns show significant changes, particularly hypoalbuminemia and an increase of alpha and gamma-globulins. Anti-*E. histolytica* antibodies are almost always present, often reaching high titers.

Modern imaging techniques, such as computed tomography (CT), magnetic resonance imaging (MRI), and ultrasound, are useful in the diagnosis of liver involvement by *E. histolytica* (Fig. 3), but, as a rule, they do not distinguish a pyogenic from an amebic abscess or, even, a tumoral lesion. The use of ultrasonography coupled to percutaneous puncture has been recommended for diagnosis, as well as for treatment.

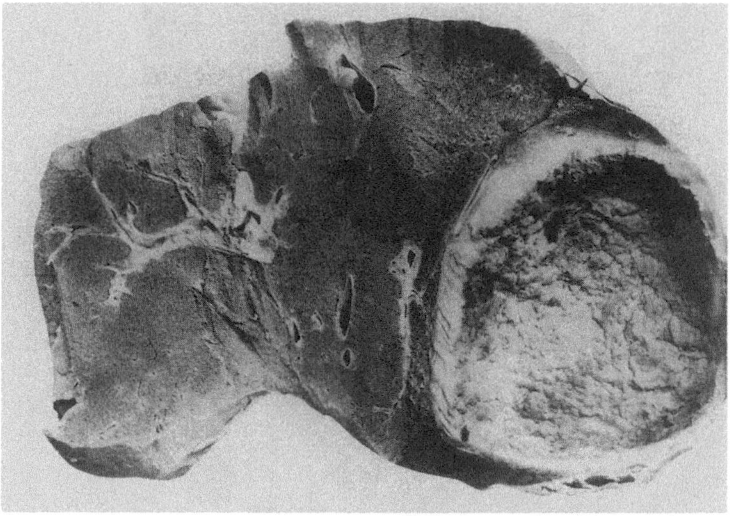

**Fig. 1.** Appearance at autopsy of an amebic abscess of the liver showing a partial destruction of the right lobe and a well-defined capsule around the abscess (by courtesy of the Department of Pathology, Santa Casa Medical Sciences School of Sao Paulo)

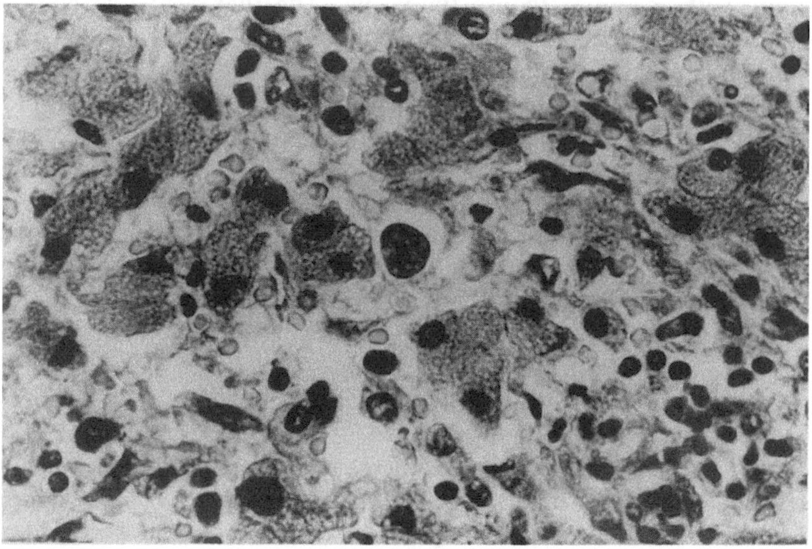

**Fig. 2.** Histologic appearance of the wall of an amebic abscess, showing an *E. histolytica* trophozoite (HE ×400) (by courtesy of the Department of Pathology, Santa Casa Medical Sciences School of São Paulo)

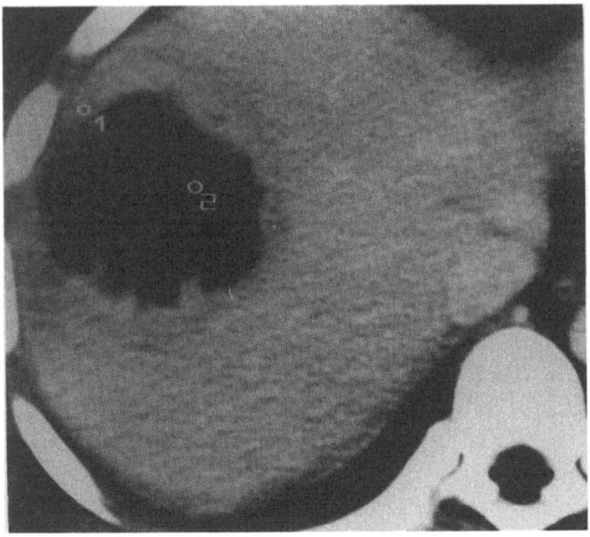

**Fig. 3.** CT scan of an amebic abscess of the liver (by courtesy of Dr. M. ROCHA)

### 1.3 Treatment

According to RALLS et al. [9] many amebic liver abscesses may be treated with drug therapy. In these cases, the drug of choice is metronidazole, but some authors prefer to use tinidazole. The therapeutic schedule is often similar to that used in intestinal cases, but it is more extended, and sometimes it is necessary to increase the dosage.

Patients with complications such as peritonitis or abscess rupture must be submitted to parenteral administration of emetine for some days (65 mg, two or three times a day).

In approximately 10–15% of the patients, complete resolution of amebic liver abscess is achieved by the combination of percutaneous drainage and drug therapy. This approach is particularly useful in cases of pyogenic secondary infection or juxtacardiac localization of the abscess.

## 2 Malaria

Malaria is caused by protozoa of the genus *Plasmodium*, which includes four species infective for man: *P. falciparum*, *P. vivax*, *P. malariae* and *P. ovale*. Malaria is the most important parasitic endemic disease worldwide; in fact, nearly two billion people are exposed to the infection [10].

The life cycle of the parasite consists of two phases: the asexual cycle, or schizogony, which takes place in humans, and the sexual cycle, or sporogony, which occurs in the female mosquito of the genus *Anopheles*. Malaria can also be transmitted by blood transfusion and by sharing of needles among drug addicts [11].

## 2.1 Clinical and Pathologic Features

The classic clinical tetrad in malaria comprises fever, usually with temperatures higher than 40°C, chills, headache, and variable gastrointestinal symptoms.

In a study of 121 patients carried out by DAHER et al. [12] hepatomegaly was observed in 84% and splenomegaly in 80%; neither was related to the degree of parasitemia. Jaundice was detected in 32% and its appearance correlated with the parasitic density. However, RAMACHANDRAN and PEREIRA observed jaundice in only 15.4% of 65 patients with primary uncomplicated malaria [13].

Histopathology of the liver in human malaria is characterized by Kupffer cell hyperplasia, mononuclear cell infiltration, and granuloma formation. Granulomatous lesions of small to moderate size with mononuclear cell infiltration and usually with hepatocyte necrosis ("malarial nodules") were described in 50% of biopsy specimens by RAMACHANDRAN and PEREIRA [13]. The "non-specific reactive hepatitis" observed in this study resembled closely the hepatic histology in typhoid fever, infectious mononucleosis, and Q fever, rather than that of viral hepatitis.

According to BOULOS [14] several degrees of liver involvement may be found in human malaria. The most severe is represented by an acute hepatitis.

In patients with low parasitemia, slight increases in serum aminotransferase activity and in nonconjugated bilirubin levels (hemolysis) are observed. With higher levels of parasitemia, serum enzyme changes are more pronounced; the elevation of conjugated bilirubinemia points to intrahepatic cholestasis.

In patients infected with *P. falciparum*, a clear relationship between malarial attacks and severe liver involvement is not observed. Thus PHILLIPS and WARRELL [15] did not detect clinical evidence of hepatic failure in more than 190 cases of cerebral malaria from Thailand.

Other features of liver damage have been reported in a small number of cases after the administration of antimalarial drugs. NEFTEL et al. [16] observed seven cases of agranulocytosis and two of hepatic lesions that had probably been induced by amodiaquine therapy, and ZITELLI et al. [17] reported a fatal case of hepatic necrosis after pyrimethamine-sulfadoxine treatment.

### 2.2 Diagnosis

The diagnosis of malaria depends on the demonstration of malarial parasites on a Giemsa-stained thick or thin blood smear; usually, the largest numbers are found during the highest fever spikes. The differentiation of the various species is beyond the scope of this presentation.

### 2.3 Treatment

The drug of choice for the treatment of all uncomplicated cases of malaria, except for chloroquine-resistant *P. falciparum*, is chloroquine phosphate [1].

## 3 Visceral leishmaniasis (Kala-azar)

Visceral leishmaniasis, or kala-azar, is caused by parasites of the genus *Leishmania* (*L. donovani*). Liver involvement is usually characterized by pronounced hyperplasia of the Kupffer cells; Kala-azar is essentially a disease of the reticuloendothelial system (RES).

The parasite is transmitted to humans by the bite of a sandfly of the genus *Phlebotomus* in the Old World and *Lutzomyia* in the New World. The parasites gain access to the bloodstream or lymphatics and are transported to the viscera, where they parasitize macrophages of the RES.

### 3.1 Clinical and Pathologic Features

Leishmanial parasitism of Kupffer cell and hypertrophy and hyperplasia of the RES cells are fundamental findings used to characterize visceral leishmaniasis.

According to Duarte and Corbett [18], this disease produces liver changes ranging from RES reactivity to a fibrogenic response which can progress to an intralobular diffuse fibrosis.

In 180 patients with visceral leishmaniasis, Khaldi et al. [19] found 16 cases with liver involvement, seven of which presented severe hepatitis, with cytolysis, cholestasis, and liver failure. Furthermore, an electron microscopic study by Duarte et al. [20] showed a direct involvement of the hepatocytes and the presence of *Leishmania* amastigote forms within these cells.

The disease may begin as an acute illness but usually has an insidious onset. The most common symptoms are fever, anorexia, abdominal pain, cough, weakness, marked weight loss, and diarrhea. Splenomegaly and hepatomegaly are variable but usually prominent (Fig. 4).

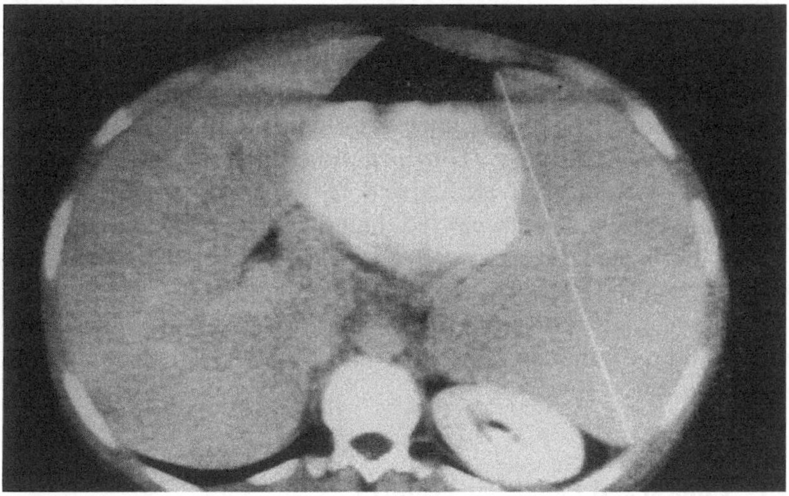

**Fig. 4.** CT appearance of visceral leishmaniasis showing very pronounced splenomegaly (by courtesy of Dr. M. ROCHA)

### 3.2 Diagnosis

The definite diagnosis of kala-azar is made by identifying the parasite in tissue sections or smears. Bone marrow aspiration yields the diagnosis in 90% of the cases, while liver biopsy is positive in 70% [1]. Splenic punctures are performed by some authors [21]. Sensitive immunoserologic tests such as the direct agglutination test and the immunofluorescence antibody test may also be used.

The routine clinical laboratory tests show pancytopenia, hypoalbuminemia, hypoprothrombinemia, and elevations in serum aspartate aminotransferase (AST), alanine aminotransferase (ALT), and alkaline phosphatase. A striking polyclonal hypergammaglobulinemia is usually observed.

### 3.3 Treatment

The drug of choice for visceral leishmaniasis is sodium stibogluconate, a pentavalent organic antimonial.

## 4 Ascariasis

Ascariasis is a helminthic infection of the small bowel caused by the nematode *Ascaris lumbricoides*. Its distribution is worldwide, with the highest prevalence in tropical countries. It can be acquired by the ingestion of vegetables, usually as salad, but in China, pickles are also implicated [22].

The adult worm measures from 15 to 35 cm. The female lays an average of more than 200 000 ova daily. After ingestion of fertilized eggs their shells are dissolved by the gastric juice and the larvae are released into the upper part of the small intestine. They penetrate the bowel wall, enter the veins of the portal system, and are carried to the liver. Some larvae may enter lymphatic vessels and are carried directly to the lungs.

In the liver, larvae move freely in the sinusoids and may subsequently pass through the hepatic veins to the heart and lungs.

Larvae are carried from the alveoli to the pharynx, where they molt and are swallowed. In the gastrointestinal tract they molt again and become mature worms.

### 4.1 Clinical and Pathologic Features

The commonest complications of ascariasis are due to the large number of parasites in the intestinal lumen, and their propensity to enter small orifices.

Hepatobiliary involvement may be due to the migration of larvae toward the lungs or, especially, to the obstruction of the biliary tree by adult worms (Fig. 17.5). Hepatobiliary symptoms are caused by the migration of the adult worm through the papilla to the biliary tree. The incidence is

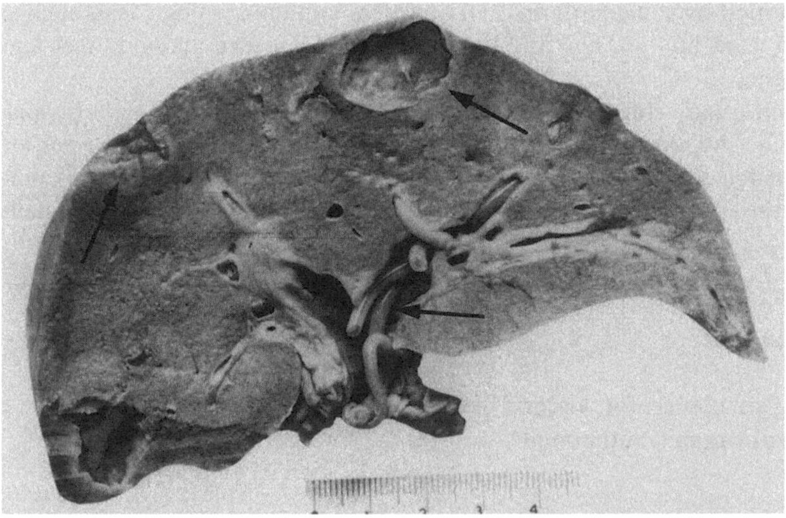

**Fig. 5.** Autopsy specimen from a patient with ascariasis of the biliary tract. Worms are seen in the bile duct and can also be seen in sections of liver abscesses (by courtesy of Deparment. of Pathology, Santa Casa Medical Sciences School of Sao Paulo)

greater in children and young adults. *Ascaris* may lodge in the intrahepatic ducts but is most frequently found in the common bile duct (Fig. 17.6). The living worm may lay eggs in the intrahepatic ducts and then migrate back to the duodenum through the ampulla of Vater. Some of them die in the bile duct, become fragmented and act as a nidus for stone formation. The main consequences of the obstruction of the biliary tree are cholangitis, liver abscesses (Fig. 5), and formation of calculi, but acute cholecystitis and pancreatitis may be observed as well; abscesses may rupture into the peritoneal cavity or into the subdiaphragmatic space. Through the diaphragm the worms may reach the pleural space and cause empyema [1]. Surgical exploration of the biliary tract frequently shows a single and alive worm, but cases with numerous worms have been described.

One of the most dreaded complications of ascaridian cholangitis is extension of the inflammatory process to the hepatic or portal veins, leading to a process of pylephlebitis [1].

### 4.2 Diagnosis

The clinical manifestations vary in severity, depending upon the number of parasites in the biliary system and whether they remain in the duct or return to the intestine. The migration of the worms into the biliary tract may

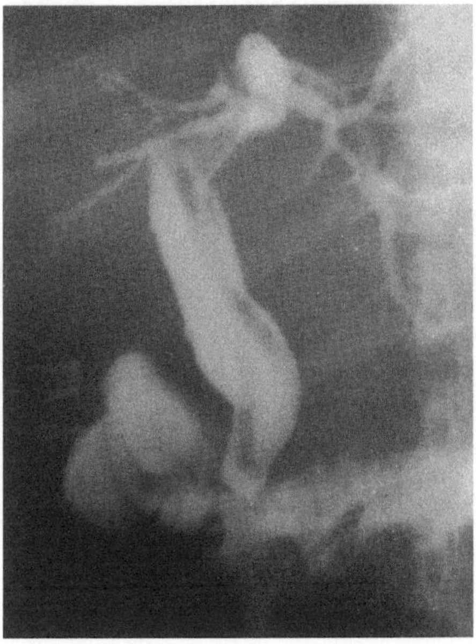

**Fig. 6.** Adult worms of *A. lumbricoides* in a dilated common bile duct as shown by endoscopic retrograde cholangiopancreatography (by courtesy of Dr. P. Sakai)

produce acute agonizing epigastric or right upper quadrant pain that radiates to the shoulder, back, or hypogastrium. This is accompanied by nausea and vomiting. Vomiting of roundworms occurs in a large number of cases [1]. The temperature may be subnormal, but pyrexia follows a bacterial infection [22].

Despite the obstruction of large bile ducts (Fig. 7), jaundice is observed in only 20% of cases. The low frequency of jaundice could be due to the intermittent nature of obstruction, as the parasites enter and leave the common duct [23].

The diagnosis of *Ascaris* migration to the biliary tract is difficult, but a history of vomiting of worms is helpful. In 85.7% of patients with a clinical diagnosis of biliary ascariasis, ultrasonography can detect worms in the biliary tree (Figs. 8 and 9) [24]. Real-time ultrasonography permits the demonstration of the characteristic morphology and motility of the worms [25].

### 4.3 Treatment

Supportive therapy includes intravenous fluids, antibiotics to treat cholangitis and antispasmodics to relieve pain. Surgery should be withheld initially unless there is associated cholangitis with jaundice and high fever. Some

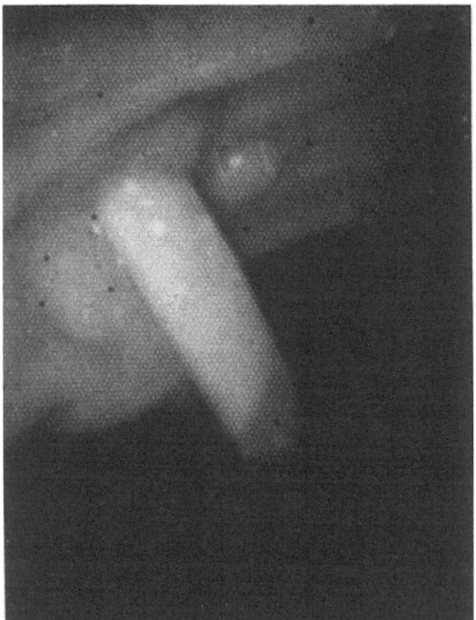

**Fig. 7.** Duodenoscopic view of the Vater's papilla containing an adult *Ascaris* worm (by courtesy of Dr. P. SAKAI)

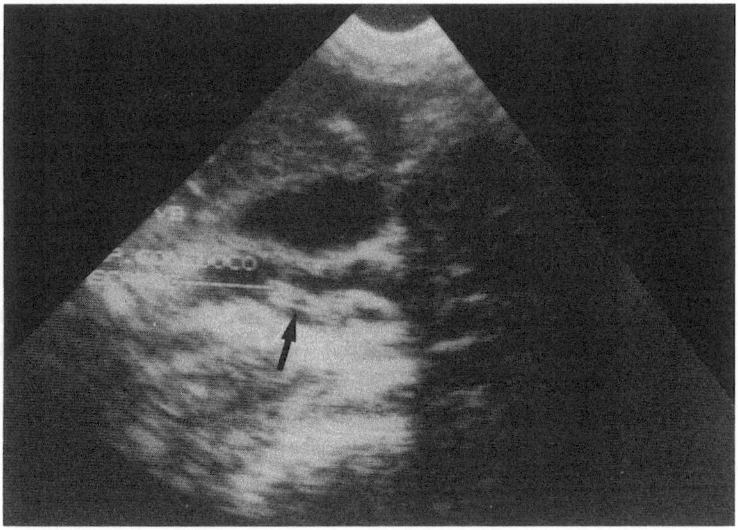

**Fig. 8.** Ultrasonography in a patient with ascariasis. The common bile duct is dilated owing to the presence of an adult *Ascaris*' worm (arrow) (By courtesy of Dr. G. CERRI)

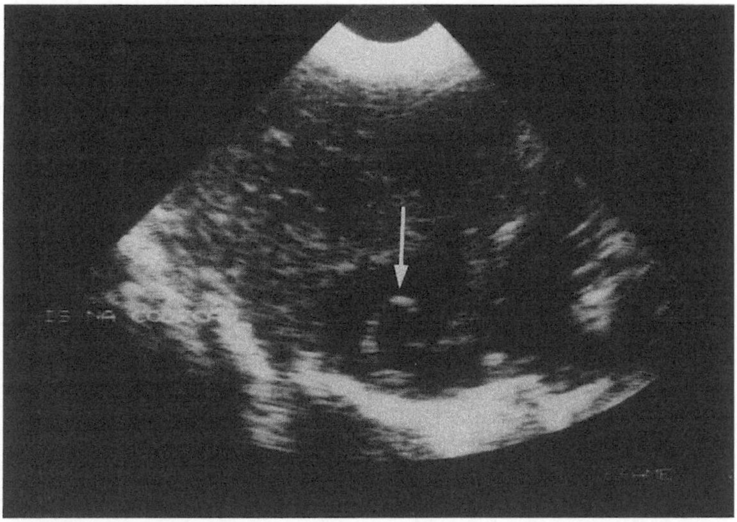

**Fig. 9.** Ultrasonogram revealing a liver abscess (arrow) in a patient with ascariasis (by courtesy of Dr. G. CERRI)

surgeons, however, recommend a more aggressive approach. Whenever surgical intervention is undertaken it is important to explore the whole abdomen before concentrating on the biliary tract [22]. If worms are found in the common bile duct they are removed through a choledochotomy and a T-tube is inserted. Instillation of ascaricides such as piperazine into the biliary tract has been recommended but, as mentioned above, a trapped dead worm can become fragmented and act as a nidus for stone formation. Furthermore, live worms may spontaneously move out of the biliary tract into the duodenum and become susceptible to antihelminthic therapy administered orally [23]. Obstructive cholangitis may be treated by endoscopic retrograde cholangiopancreatography with sphincterotomy and removal of worms with an endoscopic basket [26]. Treatment of intestinal ascariasis consists in the administration of levamisole or tetramisole, in a single dose of 150 mg for adults and 80 mg for children; the cure rate is above 90%. In cases of mixed nematode infections, mebendazole is especially useful.

## 5 Fascioliasis

The genus *Fasciola* comprises digenetic trematode parasites of herbivorous mammals, mainly domestic ruminants like sheep and cattle. *Fasciola hepatica* is the species most frequently found in human beings. *F. gigantica*, although a common parasite of herbivorous mammals from Africa and Asia, has rarely been found to parasitize human beings, in whom it gives rise to chronic cholecystitis [27].

The occurrence of fascioliasis depends on the ecological contact among infected sheep or cattle, snails of the genus *Lymnaea*, and human beings. Human transmission occurs by ingestion of raw vegetables where the metacercarie of *F. hepatica* usually encyst, after shedding by *Lymnaea* snails.

*Fasciola hepatica* has a cosmopolitan distribution; it is found in North, Central and South America, Europe, Australia and New Zealand. *F. gigantica*, on the other hand, has a more restricted distribution: Africa, India and the Far East [28].

### 5.1 Clinical and Pathologic Features

Human parasitism by *F. hepatica* is often asymptomatic or oligosymptomatic. Occasionally, however, it causes severe illness as a result of parasitic localization in the human biliary system and hypersensitivity to metabolic products produced by the worms.

Clinical manifestations of human fascioliasis include fever and digestive symptoms, mainly upper abdominal pain. Anemia, urticaria, loss of weight, and headache are other manifestations.

The liver is frequently enlarged, with a soft consistency. Months after infection, jaundice and, more rarely, cholecystitis and gallstones may appear. Acuna-Soto and Braun-Roth [29] described a rare and severe complication of human fascioliasis, represented by ulceration and bleeding of the common bile duct.

*Fasciola hepatica* can be found in extra hepatic areas: lungs, central nervous system, and skin are the main localizations. In human skin, *F. hepatica* produces painful subcutaneous nodules. In the Far East, as a consequence of consumption of raw liver of goats or other infected herbivorous mammals, a particular form of human fascioliasis that causes pharyngeal infection has been described.

### 5.2 Diagnosis

As regards laboratory data, a high degree of eosinophilia is the most frequent and early manifestation. However, specific diagnosis is based on fecal examinations and immunologic tests.

*Fasciola hepatica* eggs, discharged in the bile, reach the intestinal lumen and are discharged in the feces. Their size and morphologic features are characteristic, allowing easy identification. However, some individuals discharging *F. hepatica* eggs in the stool may be suffering from spurious parasitism due to consumption of raw liver of infected animals and to the escape of eggs via the intestinal tract. Therefore, the finding of *F. hepatica* eggs in the feces has diagnostic value only if confirmed by the examination of other fecal samples or by clinical and or epidemiologic data.

Several widely differing immunologic techniques have been recommended for the diagnosis of human fascioliasis. It is noteworthy that false positive immunologic reactions for fascioliasis are a frequent occurrence when the tests are performed in areas in which schistosomiasis is endemic.

### 5.3 Treatment

Nowadays, the drug of choice in the treatment of human fascioliasis is praziquantel, in single doses of 50–70 mg/kg body weight.

## 6 Clonorchiasis and Opisthorchiasis

Alongside *F. hepatica*, *Clonorchis sinensis, Opisthorchis viverrini* and *felineus*, are the most frequent trematode parasites of the human biliary tract.

Clonorchiasis is common in oriental countries like North and South Korea, Japan, Taiwan, Vietnam and the southern part of China. Human infection by *O. viverrini* has been found in Thailand and Laos, while human parasitism by *O. felineus* has a wider distribution reaching part of eastern Europe (Poland and USSR) besides Vietnam, India, Japan, and North Korea in Asia.

A trematode rarely found as a real parasite in the human biliary tract is *Dicrocoelium dendriticum*, a common parasite of the liver and biliary tract of herbivorous mammals. When human beings are shedding eggs of *D. dendriticum* in the stool, it should generally be considered as a case of spurious parasitism; such cases usually follow ingestion of infected animal livers.

Man seems to be the real definitive host of *C. sinensis*, although other mammals, such as dogs and cats, have been found to be naturally infected. On the other hand, dogs and cats are the most frequent definitive hosts of *O. viverrini* and *O. felineus*, and man is only an accidental host.

The life cycles of *Clonorchis* and *Opisthorchis* are similar, differing in only a few respects. In both cycles, embryonate eggs are deposited in the biliary tract of the definitive host, reaching the intestinal lumen with the bile to appear in the stool. The continuation of the cycle is observed when the eggs are ingested by susceptible snails (belonging to the genera *Parafossalurus* and *Bulinus* for *Clonorchis* and to the genus *Bulinus* for *Opisthorchis*), with the hatching of miracidia within the snail's body. In the tissues the miracidia give rise to sporocysts and rediae, and after some weeks of maturation, cercariae are shed by the infected snails, reach freshwater, and penetrate the second intermediate host. These hosts are represented by several freshwater fish species, mainly from the Cyprinidae family, where the metacercaria are formed and encysted. Man or other definitive hosts are infected by eating raw or uncooked fish. The metacercarie are then excysted in the duodenum; the freed larvae migrate to the common bile duct, through the ampulla of Vater, and reach the distal biliary ducts, where they become mature worms. This change is observed in 2 weeks for *Clonorchis* and in 3–4 weeks for *Opisthorchis*.

## 6.1 Clinical and Pathologic Features

Mild infections are frequently asymptomatic. However, the persistent habit of eating raw or uncooked fish may lead to a heavy worm load during the patient's life. Even asymptomatic patients can shed *Clonorchis* or *Opisthorchis* eggs in the stool over a long period, as a consequence of the great life span of the worms. Of 15 Korean patients examined in Sao Paulo state (Brazil), most were still shedding great numbers of *C. sinensis* eggs in the stool [30], more than 10 years after leaving the endemic area.

In symptomatic patients clonorchiasis usually causes anorexia, diarrhea and abdominal discomfort in the right upper quadrant. The liver is frequently enlarged, and jaundice is occasionally observed. Chronic infections due to heavy worm loads can produce severe complications, such as obstruction of bile ducts, suppurative cholangitis, pancreatitis, and cholangiocarcinoma.

In heavy infections the liver can be greatly enlarged and the bile ducts frequently show hyperplasia. Edema of the biliary epithelium and an increase in mucus production are usually observed. Sometimes patients with clonorchiasis display adenomatous proliferation of the biliary epithelium [31].

The extra hepatic bile ducts and the gallbladder show a normal aspect in clonorchiasis [32], but in opisthorchiasis the presence of worms in the gallbladder is a frequent finding and the gallbladder may be enlarged [33]. In chronic *Opisthorchis* infections complications such as chronic cholecystitis and purulent cholangitis are frequently observed.

### 6.2 Diagnosis

The laboratory diagnosis of human infections with *Clonorchis* or *Opisthorchis* is based on the demonstration of characteristic eggs in the stool or in the bile. It is important to distinguish these eggs from those of other trematodes, mainly from the family Heterophyidae. Besides the morphology of the egg, it is necessary to determine its length and width.

Quantitative coprologic techniques are important for evaluation of the worm load and provide useful information for clinical purposes and therapeutic control.

### 6.3 Treatment

Several drugs (trichloromethylbenzol, hexachloroparaxylol, dehydroemetine) have until recently been used for the treatment of clonorchiasis and opisthorchiasis [31]. Nowadays, the use of these drugs has been curtailed because of therapeutic failures and the appearance of severe side-effects. Praziquantel is now considered the drug of choice. Leite et al. [30] used praziquantel (60 mg/kg) in 15 patients infected with *C. sinensis* and obtained a 60% parasitologic cure rate. Even in patients who continued to pass *C. sinensis* eggs in the stool, an important decrease in the number of eggs was observed.

## 7 Schistosomiasis

Among the human diseases which are endemically found in different parts of the world, schistosomiasis is one of the most extensively studied and represents an important priority of the World Health Organization (WHO) [34]. Among the five species of *Schistosoma* that infect humans, *S. mansoni* and *S. japonicum* are associated with the most severe forms of liver disease and so far have been the main targets of clinical and experimental research.

## 7.1 Schistosomiasis mansoni

Despite the widespread distribution of schistosomiasis mansoni the last 10 years have witnessed a striking reduction in the severe forms of the disease in some parts of the world, particularly in Brazilian hyperendemic areas [35]. Many factors may be responsible for this decrease: large-scale treatment, a better awareness of the disease through public education, improved sanitation, and the migration of the population to urban areas [34].

The life cycle of the parasite in the host, which begins with penetration of cercariae into the skin and finishes with the adult worms living in the terminal branches of the portal vein, explains why *S. mansoni* can produce damage in several organs besides the intestines and liver.

### *Clinical Features*

Schistosomiasis mansoni shows a wide range of clinical manifestations, varying from asymptomatic to highly symptomatic forms. Sometimes the disease is accidentally discovered, either by a routine stool examination or by enlargement of the liver or spleen on physical examination [36].

The clinical forms of *S. mansoni* may be classified as follows: (1) acute, initial or toxemic form; (2) chronic forms, which include: (a) intestinal; (b) hepatointestinal; (c) hepatosplenic; (d) pulmonary ("cor pulmonale"); (e) other forms.

Intestinal manifestations, such as diarrhea and colicky pain, are occasionally observed, but asymptomatic forms are more frequent. The subdivision into an intestinal form (2a) and a hepatointestinal from (2b) is not uniformly accepted [36] but has practical implications.

Enlargement of the liver, mainly of the left lobe, is frequently seen in infected individuals living in highly endemic areas and characterizes the hepatointestinal form.

Symmers' fibrosis of the liver (Figs. 10 and 11), which may result in portal hypertension and congestive splenomegaly, occurs in the 6- to 20-year age group or 5–15 years after the onset of infection [37]. It is the most severe form and the most common cause of morbidity or death (Fig. 17.10).

It is worth mentioning that in heavily infected young patients there is a "noncongestive" phase of the disease with splenomegaly but with no evident signs of portal hypertension. Many data from Brazil show that in such cases the spleen may become impalpable after adequate chemotherapy.

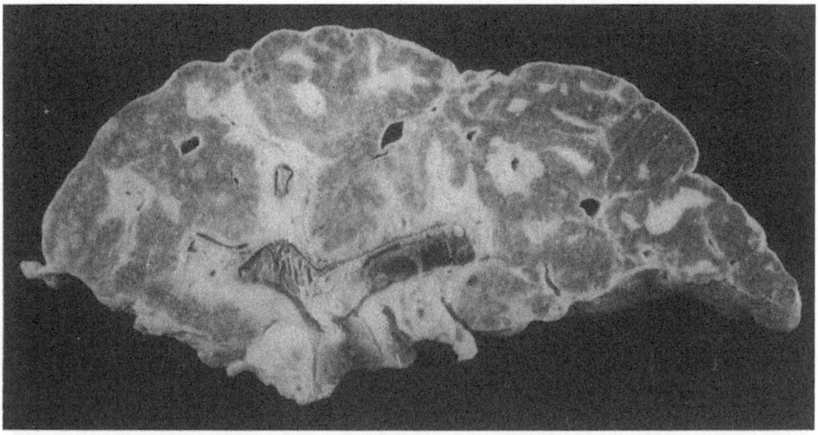

**Fig. 10.** Autopsy specimen from a patient with Symmers' (pipestem) fibrosis showing coarse fibrous bands irradiating from the porta hepatis (by courtesy of Department of the Pathology, Santa Casa Medical Sciences School of São Paulo)

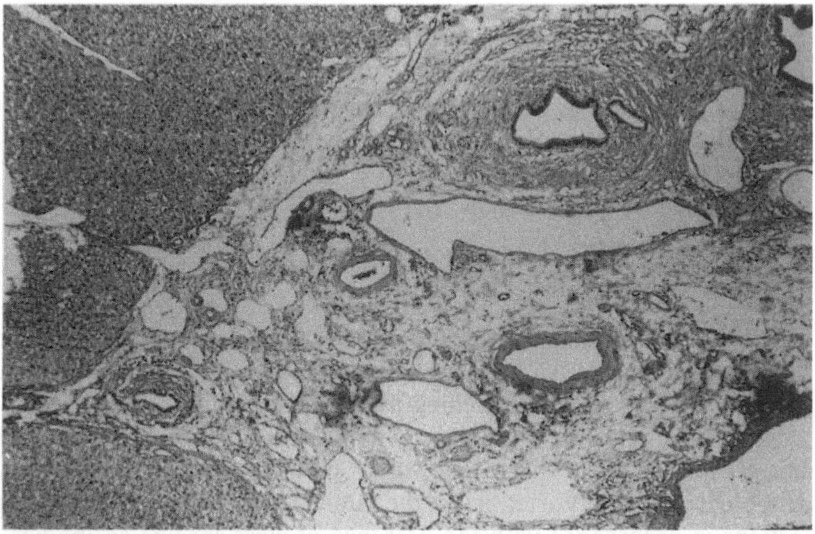

**Fig. 11.** Hepatosplenic form of schistosomiasis mansoni. Portal fibrosis is seen, and there is hypertrophy of the branches of the hepatic artery, with increased neovascularization (angiomatoid hyperplasia) (HE ×75)

### *Pathophysiology*

Egg granuloma (Fig. 12) is the main process responsible for the tissue damage in organs such as the liver, intestines, lungs, pancreas, and nervous system. However, immune-complexes derived from the parasite antigens are responsible for special forms of lesion, particularly glomerulopathy [38].

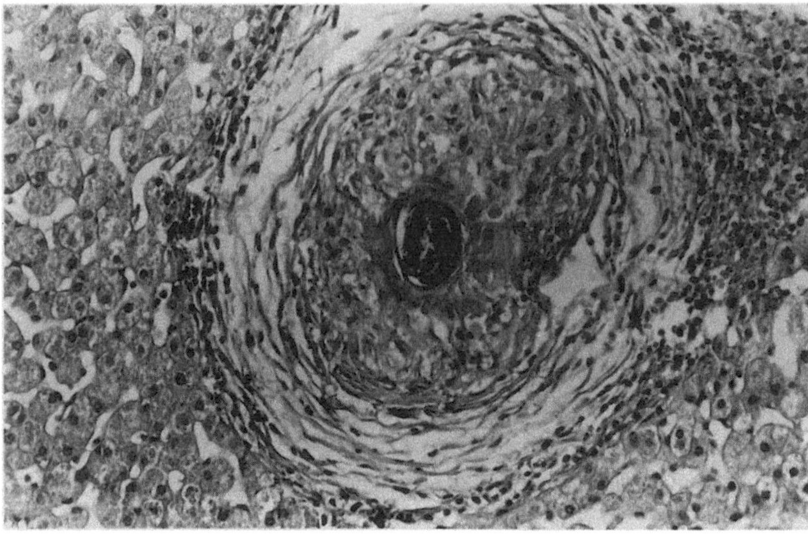

**Fig. 12.** Liver granuloma around *S. mansoni* egg with epithelioid cells circumscribed by a halo of elongated cells. The mononuclear cell infiltrate is located chiefly at the edge of the granulomatous reaction (HE ×120)

The pathogenesis of Symmers' fibrosis is not well established, but the worm load due to massive initial infection is considered a major pathogenetic factor. There are various opinions as to the associated factors, such as viral hepatitis (B and C), and their role is not well established.

### *Diagnosis*

The direct methods, based on the demonstration of eggs and miracidia, are the most important. We have used a combination of the Kato-Katz quantitative method [39] and the hatching test.

Serologic reactions, particularly immunofluorescence, hemagglutination, and ELISA tests, are used in some clinicaly obscure cases and in epidemiologic studies. Variations in the fluorescence patterns of worm and liver sections in accordance with the presence of class-specific antibodies, permit the differential diagnosis between acute and chronic forms [40].

As to the diagnosis of Symmers' fibrosis, Abdel-Wahab et al. [41] reported the ultrasonographic images in periportal fibrosis for the first time in 1979. Since then ultrasonography has become a reliable and sensitive method for demonstrating these lesions (Fig. 13) [42].

### *Treatment of the Helminthiasis*

Treatment of the helminthiasis is indicated in all stages and clinical forms of schistosomiasis mansoni, except in some special conditions such as severe

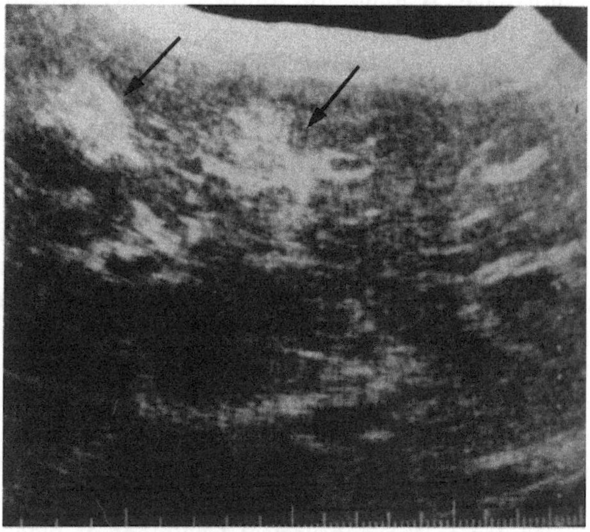

**Fig. 13.** Ultrasonographic appearance of Symmers' fibrosis, showing coarse fibrous bands (by courtesy of Dr. G. CERRI)

hepatic failure, renal and cardiac insufficiency, pregnancy, and in cases of other diseases more severe than schistosomiasis.

There are two highly effective drugs when given in a single oral dose: oxamniquine, with different dosages in Latin America (15–20 mg/kg) and Africa (30 mg/kg), and praziquantel, in a single dose of 40–50 mg/kg for adults and 60 mg/kg for children. A double-blind trial published by us in 1986 [43] showed that the two drugs have the same efficacy and produce similar side-effects, but that dizziness is more severe after oxamniquine. Furthermore, praziquantel is also effective against other species of *Schistosoma*. Chemotherapy is useful not only on an individual basis but also for the control of morbidity in hyperendemic areas.

The criteria of cure after chemotherapy include: (a) the absence of *S. mansoni* eggs in fecal examinations up to 6 months after chemotherapy and (b) the absence of viable eggs in material obtained from rectal biopsies (not routinely used).

### *Treatment of Portal Hypertension*

Up to 1977, the main operations used for the surgical treatment of portal hypertension in schistosomiasis mansoni were esophagogastric devascularization with splenectomy, classical (proximal) splenorenal shunt with splenectomy, and distal splenorenal shunt (or selective shunt).

From 1977 to 1983 our group [44, 45] performed a prospective trial comparing these three operations in 94 patients with previous gastrointestinal hemorrhage. A long-term follow-up study showed that classical splenorenal shunt with splenectomy produces portal-systemic encephalopathy at a prohibitive frequency (39%) and that this complication appeared in 15% of cases after distal splenorenal shunt. Recurrence of upper gastrointestinal hemorrhage occurred in about 24% of the patients, without significant statistical differences among the three types of surgery, although the reduction in the number and size of the varices was less marked after esophagogastric devascularization with splenectomy. The mortality was also significantly higher after classical splenorenal shunt with splenectomy. This prospective study showed that: (a) the best operation for the treatment of variceal bleeding in the hepatosplenic form of schistosomiasis mansoni is esophagogastric devascularization with splenectomy; (b) classical (proximal) splenorenal shunt should be abandoned because of the high frequency of portal-systemic encephalopathy; and (c) distal splenorenal shunt (Warren-Teixeira's technique), though better tolerated than the classical splenorenal shunt, may produce portal-systemic encephalopathy.

As far as the nonsurgical treatment of bleeding esophageal varices is concerned, it should be mentioned that BRAGHIROLLI NETO [46] demonstrated that beta-adrenergic blockade with propranolol induced a 39.1% decrease in azygos blood flow and a prospective study published by MIES et al. [47] in 1988 showed that propranolol seems to protect patients with the hepatosplenic form of schistosomiasis mansoni against gastrointestinal rebleeding, during the short period of time that precedes the definitive surgical treatment.

As far as sclerotherapy is concerned, a retrospective study by SAKAI et al. [48] showed, that eradication of the varices was achieved in near 70% of patients during a follow-up period between 48 and 132 months; sclerotherapy was effective in the control of rebleeding in 97.3% of patients in the group with previous surgery for portal hypertension and in 72.7% of those in the group without such previous surgery. Furthermore, a lower number of sclerotherapy sessions was employed per patient in the former group. These differences were statistically significant. The authors concluded that previous surgical treatment for portal hypertension in patients with schistosomiasis mansoni was of great benefit in respect of treatment of rebleeding esophageal varices by endoscopic sclerotherapy.

CORDEIRO [49], in a prospective nonrandomized elective study comparing a group receiving sclerotherapy with a control group and employing a 5-year follow-up, showed that the incidence of rebleeding was 28.1% and 44.5%, respectively, a difference not statistically significant; however, the mortality from rupture of esophageal varices was 3.1% in the sclerotherapy group and 27.7% the control group, a statistically significant difference.

Summing up, in our Department of Gastroenterology, patients with schistosomiasis mansoni and bleeding esophageal varices are treated by esophagogastric devascularization with splenectomy and, if rebleeding occurs, by sclerosis of the varices.

### 7.2 Schistosomiasis japonica

In addition to being a parasite of man, *S. japonicum* has a vast variety of reservoir hosts. In the Philipines, these hosts include dogs, cattle, water buffalo, pigs, horses, sheep, goats, wild mice, and rats, the latter being considered extremely important in maintaining local foci of transmission [1]. In the People's Republic of China, cattle are considered the most important reservoir hosts. In Japan, where *S. japonicum* was focal in nature, control efforts have been largely successful [50]. *S. japonicum* is transmitted by molluscs of the genus *Oncomelania*. The female worm produces an average of 3000 eggs daily, an oviposition ten times higher than that observed in *S. mansoni* infection. This high production of eggs may be responsible for more severe forms of liver disease.

The drug of choice for the treatment of *S. japonicum* infection is praziquantel, 20 mg/kg three times in 1 day [1].

## 8 Hydatidosis (Echinococcosis)

Hydatidosis is a human infection caused by larval stages of cestodes of the *Echinococcus* genus. The most important species from this genus is *E. granulosus*, which is responsible for the majority of human cases.

In its adult stage *E. granulosus* is found in several species of mammals of the family Canidae, especially the domestic dog (*Canis familiaris*). The larval stage (named hydatid or hydatid cyst) is usually found in herbivorous mammals, mainly sheep, cattle, and pigs. Human infection is due to oral contamination with *E. granulosus* eggs, discharged by infected dogs. When this occurs, man acts as an accidental intermediate host, developing the hydatid cyst in some viscera (Fig. 14).

Besides *E. granulosus*, other *Echinococcus* species can infect man, though with much lower frequency:

- *E. multilocularis*: adult stage in foxes of the Arctic region and larval stage in the liver of rodents of the family Crycetidae.
- *E. oligarthrus*: adult stage in the gut of mammals of the family Felidae and larval stage in the agouti, a rodent of the family Caviidae.
- *E. vogeli*: adult stage in wild dogs and larval stage in agouti and paca.

Although *E. granulosus* is considered the most important species because of its high frequency of human attack, *E. multilocularis* deserves special attention as it may produce a severe illness.

### 8.1 Clinical and Pathologic Features

The severity of the illness caused by hydatidosis depends on the size and localization of the hydatid cyst, as well as the absorption of antigenic

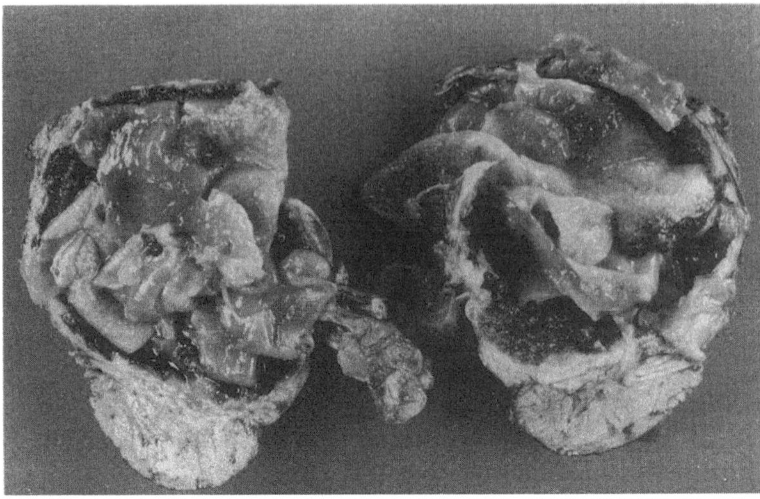

**Fig. 14.** Macroscopic appearance of a hydatid cyst showing proligerous membrane (by courtesy of the Department of Pathology, Santa Casa Medical Sciences School of São Paulo)

substances discharged by the cyst, which may be responsible for hypersensitivity reactions. Hepatic localization is observed in 60%–70% of the human cases; the symptoms usually appear when the cyst reaches 10 cm in diameter. Other localizations of hydatid cysts are: lungs (20%) kidneys (4%), muscle (4%), spleen (3%), soft tissues (3%), brain (3%) and bones (2%).

HIDALGO and BARQUET [51], reviewing 7435 human cases of abdominal hydatidosis, cited the main signs and symptoms of the disease as pain (59%), hepatomegaly (35%), palpable mass in the upper quadrant of the abdomen (25%), and jaundice (20%). Fever is a common finding. The main complications were biliary shunts (7.8%) and infection of residual cyst cavities following surgical procedures (4.4%). In an analysis of 52 patients with hepatic hydatidosis in whom cholangiography was performed during the surgery, MALLET et al. [52] detected biliocystic shunts in 50% of cases.

Human hydatidosis due to *E. multilocularis* (alveolar hydatidosis) is much more severe, with very pronounced production of cystic proligerous membrane and a neoplastic pattern of growth. Infiltration of the liver parenchyma and liberation of antigenic products, causing inflammation and necrosis are the main features of this parasitosis. Lymphatic and blood vessel invasion, giving rise to metastatic lesions of the liver and other organs, constitutes another complication.

Until recently, hydatidosis represented an important public health problem in almost all countries with a large number of sheep. However, in many developed countries well conducted campaigns achieved the control of transmission. Nowadays, hydatidosis is still a public health problem in East

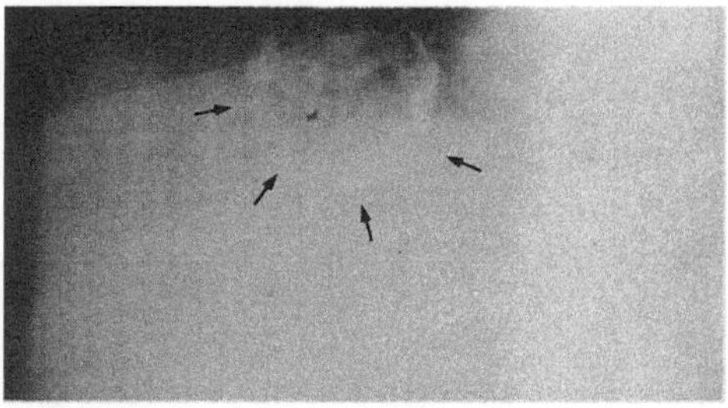

**Fig. 15.** Radiographic appearance of a calcified hydatid cyst (arrows) (by courtesy of Dr. M. Rocha)

Africa, in the Far East, in Mediterranean countries, and in some countries of South America (Chile, Argentina, Uruguay, and southern Brazil).

## 8.2 Diagnosis

As regards laboratory diagnosis, remarkable progress has been observed with immunologic tests (such as immunoelectrophoresis, immunofluorescence, hemagglutination and ELISA). Immunologic tests now represent an important method for individual and epidemiologic diagnosis of human hydatidosis. Recently, Pinel et al. [53] improved the immunologic diagnosis of this helminthiasis by using an enzyme-linked immunoelectro-diffusion assay (ELIEDA) test, which provides more specific results in cases of false-positive reactions with other tests. Furthermore, radiologic techniques (Fig. 15) such as computed tomography (Fig. 16), ultrasonography, and magnetic resonance imaging have greatly increased the possibility of characterization and localization of hydatid cysts. Good results have been obtained with the use of portable ultrasonographic equipment in field campaigns. Thus, when MacPherson et al. [54] compared serologic tests with US findings in endemic areas of Kenya, they detected more positive cases with the latter. However, in cases of intrabiliary localizations, some invasive techniques, such as endoscopic retrograde cholangiopancreatography, may be necessary for a definitive diagnosis [55].

## 8.3 Treatment

Good results in the treatment of hydatidosis, have usually been obtained with the oral use of mebendazole (50–60 mg/kg), but this treatment must be maintained for at least 6 months [56]. Surgical procedures may be used in cases of failure with anthelminthic drugs. For young hydatid cysts, Chigot et al. [57] recommend conservative surgical methods, such as cyst resection.

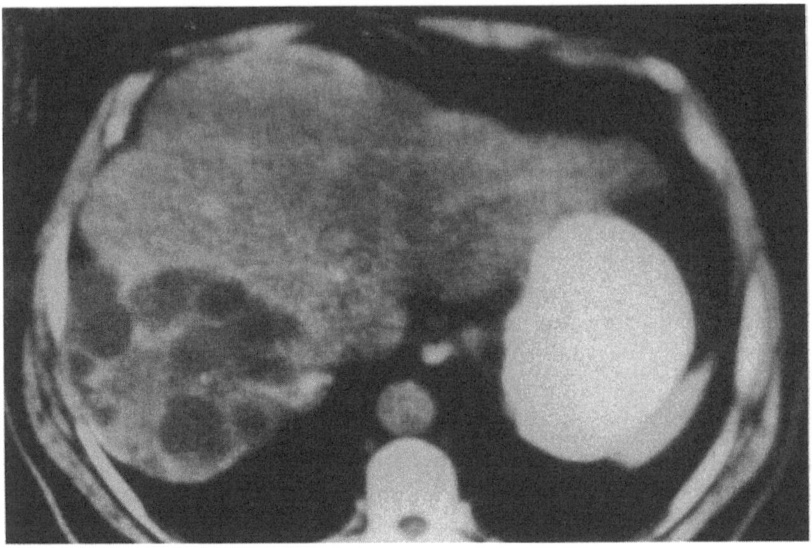

**Fig. 16.** CT scan of a liver with hydatic cyst showing proligerous vesicles (by courtesy of Dr. M. ROCHA)

When the cysts are larger and older, these authors prefer surgical procedures involving pericystectomy and, sometimes, hepatectomy.

For patients with simultaneous hepatic and pulmonary localizations of hydatid cysts, FREIXENET et al. [58] recommend initial treatment of the cysts with $H_2O_2$, followed by surgical and complete drainage. Prior treatment of the cysts also may be performed with ethanol or anthelminthic drugs, such as mebendazole. It is important, however, to avoid the instillation of formalin into hydatid cysts, in order to prevent the occurrence of biliary sclerosis [59].

The rate of post surgical recurrence of hydatid cyst is around 8%–10%. Better results may be achieved when mebendazole or albendazole is given orally for 30 days prior to surgical intervention. In HIDALGO and BARQUET'S [60] series of patients the mortality was 2.27%.

## 9 Visceral Larva Migrans (Systemic Toxocariasis)

Toxocariasis or visceral larva migrans is caused by *Toxocara canis*, a common roundworm of dogs, with a cosmopolitan distribution. Unnatural paratenic hosts, such as humans, acquire the infection by ingesting infective eggs. In these hosts, the development of the parasite is blocked in the larval stage. *T. catis*, a cat ascarid, does not play an important role in human toxocariasis.

### 9.1 Clinical and Pathologic Features

A hypereosinophilic syndrome with fever and hepatomegaly is the usual presentation. Most infections are not associated with systemic manifestations. However, severe forms are occasionally observed, particularly among small children; such cases present with fever, anorexia, muscle and joint pains, weight loss, urticarial rashes, asthma, irritability, and even convulsions. Among children, pica occurs in 90% of cases [23].

The parasite produces an extensive inflammatory process with areas of necrosis, surrounded by a dense inflammatory infiltrate composed predominantly of eosinophils. An important feature in respect of histology is the fact that the inflammatory reaction around the larvae is much larger than the organism, so that the larvae are difficult to identify without serial sectioning.

Routine laboratory tests disclose leukocytosis with hypereosinophilia, hypergammaglobulinemia, and slight elevations in serum enzymes such as alkaline phosphatase and gamma glutamyltransferase.

Serodiagnosis, based on the ELISA technique, has proved of great value.

### 9.2 Treatment

The drug used for toxocariasis is thiabendazole, 25 mg/kg twice daily for at least 5 days. An alternative is diethylcarbamazine, 2–6 mg/kg/daily for 3 weeks.

## 10 Capillariasis

*Capillaria hepatica* is a common parasite in the liver of rats. It is less frequently found in squirrels, muskrats, mice, hares, dogs, pigs, beavers, and some species of monkey [1]. When rodents, and occasionally humans, acquire the infection by eating uncooked or poorly cooked livers of rodents, the ova are passed in the feces without damage. After exposure to the air and to moisture in the soil, embryos are formed and the eggs become infective 2–6 weeks later. After ingestion by children who practice geophagia, the eggs are hatched in the cecum and free larvae migrate to the liver by way of the portal system. Bodies of adult worms can be found in liver tissue, surrounded by a granulomatous reaction which can also be elicited by ova of the parasite [23].

The clinical features are those of an acute illness which may persist for long periods. The most common manifestations are fever, hepatosplenomegaly, and eosinophilia, which occur in up to 85% of cases [61]. The hepatomegaly is massive and the eosinophil count ranges from 18% to

85%. Differential diagnosis with toxocariasis is frequently necessary. Hypochromic anemia is a consistent finding, and there may be marked hypergammaglobulinemia. The serum levels of AST, ALT, and alkaline phosphatase are frequently elevated.

### 10.1 Diagnosis

The diagnosis of capillariasis can be established only by liver biopsy, since ova are present only in the liver and are rarely found in human feces.

### 10.2 Treatment

There is no specific treatment for the disease. A good response in an acutely ill adult, treated with a combination of prednisone, pyrantel tartrate and disophenol, was reported by Pereira and França [62].

## 11 Strongyloidiasis

Strongyloidiasis is caused by the nematode *Strongyloides stercoralis* and has a high prevalence in the tropics and subtropics. It lives in the gastrointestinal tract, but in most people the infection is associated with few, if any, symptoms.

*S. stercoralis* has two modes of existence under appropriate conditions in soil. The free-living adult males and females copulate and produce rhabditiform larvae. These larvae undergo several molts and become filariform larvae, which are the infective form for humans.

Liver involvement depends upon autoinfection, a process by which filariform larvae invade the walls of the lower portions of the ileum or the colon, entering the portal system and then the lungs. Filariform larvae passed in freshly evacuated stool can also cause autoinfection upon contact with the perianal and perineal skin. In immunosuppressed patients this process of endogenous autoinfection leads to disseminated, overwhelming strongyloidiasis, also known as hyperinfection [1]. The tissue damage is caused directly by the invading worms or by secondary infection with the intestinal microorganisms [23]. In the liver the parasite may elicit a granulomatous response.

### 11.1 Diagnosis

The diagnosis of strongyloidiasis is made on the basis of the identification of the larvae, adult worms, or ova. Ova are rarely present in the feces unless diarrhea is massive, but adult worms, rhabditiform larvae, and filariform larvae may be found in feces. Duodenal aspiration gives a much higher diagnostic yield.

### 11.2 Treatment

The drug of choice is thiabendazole, 25 mg/kg twice daily for 3–5 days. The optimal duration of treatment in patients with AIDS or in other immunodeficient patients has not yet been defined.

## 12 Pentastomiasis (Porocephaliasis)

The Pentastomida are blood-sucking, endoparasitic invertebrates that live in the lungs of reptiles and birds and in the nasopharynx of mammals, usually carnivores [1].

Human pentastomiasis has mainly been reported from West Africa and the Congo basin (Zaire); snakes are implicated as vectors [63]. Autopsy records from Ibadan, Nigeria, show an *Armillifer* infestation rate of 2.2% with pentastomiasis as the third commonest cause of hepatic granulomas [64].

In more than 50% of the reported human infections, the liver is the site of involvement [65]. Necrotic granulomas are the most common lesion, eventually undergoing calcification.

## 13 Protozoal and Helminthic Diseases in the Liver and Biliary Tract in Acquired Immunodeficiency Syndrome

Liver and biliary tract abnormalities are common in patients with acquired immunodeficiency syndrome, and protozoal and helminthic parasites are frequent causes of opportunistic disease in these patients [66, 67]. Some, such as *Pneumocystis carinii*, are most commonly associated with potentially fatal pneumonia. *P. carinii* rarely affects other organs like the liver. Widespread punctate dystrophic calcifications, clustered centrally within granulomas, are revealed within the liver by computed tomography [68–70]. Other protozoa such as *Toxoplasma gondii*, involve the brain and may also be found in the liver but seem to cause little or no hepatic dysfunction. A review of clinical history and laboratory data revealed no specific risk factors or laboratory indicators associated with toxoplasmosis in AIDS [71]. Long before the AIDS epidemic, patients [72] and tissue culture experiments [73] were reported with simultaneous toxoplasmosis and cytomegalovirus (CMV) infection of individual cells. This combination has not been reported in AIDS despite the fact that both infections are common. Indeed, only 2 out of 35 patients with central nervous system toxoplasmosis and AIDS had increased aminotransferase activity in serum, and these two patients had no other evidence of liver disease [74]. Still other protozoa, such as *Cryptosporidium*, involve the gut but can also produce serious liver diseases [75, 76] (Fig. 17). *Isospora belli* [77] and Microsporidia infect the gut only, but one case of hepatitis due to Microsporidia (*Encephalitozoon cuniculi*) has been recorded [78]. Electron microscopic recognition of the organism in the liver was necessary for diagnosis in a patient who died with fever, jaundice, and hepatic necrosis. Some genera of Microsporidia have been identified as causative agents of human infections, including *Encephalitozoon cuniculi*, *Enterocytozoon bieneusi*, and *Pleitosphora sp*, which were found in AIDS patients [79]. Unrelated parasitism may occasionally be detected in the course of studying patients, e.g., lancet fluke disease (dicroceliasis) [80] and *schistosomiasis mansoni* [81]. Rhabditiform or filariform larvae can be found in the liver of patients with disseminated forms of *Strongyloides stercoralis*. This situation has rarely been reported, but since cell-mediated immunity is important to combat this organism, and since T lymphocyte function is impaired in AIDS patients, strongyloidiasis should not be overlooked in the diagnosis of opportunistic illnesses in these individuals [82].

By contrast, numerous cases have been reported with various structural abnormalities in the biliary tree in patients with CMV and *Cryptosporidium* coinfection as well as infection with either one. Enteritis was usually also

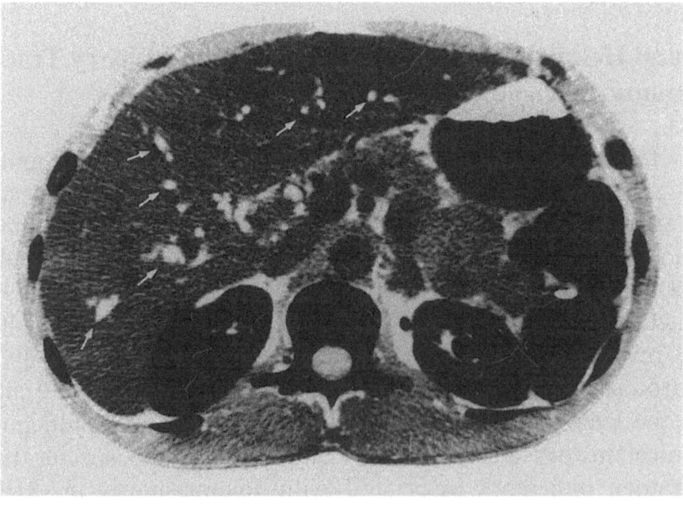

**Fig. 17.** CT scan showing dilated intrahepatic bile ducts (arrows) due to *Cryptosporidium* infection and sclerosing cholangitis in a patient with AIDS (by courtesy of Dr. M. Rocha)

present. Stenosis of the papilla of Vater [83] and of the lower portion of the common bile duct have been observed [84]. The cases of stenosis also showed evidence of irregularities of the smaller intra and extrahepatic bile ducts typical of sclerosing cholangitis [84–88]. Acalculous cholecystitis can also occur, usually with evidence of hepatitis; *Cryptosporidium* was found in the liver in such instances [89–91]. On ultrasonography one can observe thickening of the gallbladder and common bile duct wall, dilatation and irregularity of the intra and extrahepatic bile ducts with focal strictures, and increased reflectivity in the periductal regions of the liver [92–95], with a disparity between the lack of or mild symptoms and the signs related to the gallbladder and bile ducts and the ultrasonographic abnormalities [94]. Computed tomography and endoscopic retrograde cholangiopancreatography show the characteristic extra and intrahepatic bile duct lesions of sclerosing cholangitis [95]. Cholestasis may occur in AIDS in association with CMV infection [96]. Biliary tract dilatation and cholestasis with histologic features of extrahepatic biliary obstruction have been noted in infants with CMV infection with no evidence of cryptosporidial infection [97, 98]. By contrast, an immunodeficient child was reported with *Cryptosporidium* infection of the biliary tract and sclerosing cholangitis without evidence of CMV infection [99]. One patient with cryptosporidial cholecystitis underwent successful cholecystectomy with the help of postoperative enteral hyperalimentation but he succumbed to persistent cryptosporidial infection and subsequent *Pneumocystis* pneumonia [100].

Although abdominal ultrasonography and computed tomography detect ductal abnormalities, endoscopic retrograde cholangiopancreatography best shows precise ductal irregularities and serves as a guide to therapeutic intervention. Endoscopic sphincterectomy provides prompt relief of symptoms often with resolution of biochemical evidence of cholestasis [83]. Clinicians should be aware that profound biliary tract abnormalities may develop in a large number of AIDS patients. Confirmation of the anatomic abnormalities, determination of the etiology by searching for *Cryptosporidium* oocysts in the bile [93], and effective therapy may depend upon early endoscopic retrograde cholangiopancreatography [101].

## References


1. Marcial MA, Marcial-Rojas RA (1987) Parasitic diseases of the liver. In: Schiff L, Schiff ER (eds) Diseases of the liver. J.B. Lippincott, Philadelphia, pp 1171–1196
2. Sargeaunt PG (1988) Zymodemes of *Entamoeba histolytica*. In: Ravdin JI (ed) Amebiasis: human infection by *Entamoeba histolytica*. Churchill Livingstone, New York, pp 370–387
3. Mirelman D (1987) Ameba – bacterium relationship in amebiasis. Microbiol Rev 51:272–284

4. Gathiran V, Jackson TFMG (1987) A longitudinal study of asymptomatic carriers of pathogenic zymodemes of *Entamoeba histolytica*. S Afr Med J 72:669–672
5. Ravdin JI (1988) Intestinal diseases caused by *Entamoeba histolytica*. In: Ravdin JI (ed) Amebiasis: human infection by *Entamoeba histolytica*. Churchill Livingstone, New York, pp 495–510
6. Raina N, Gandhi BM, Sharma MP et al. (1987) Nutritional factors in the etiopathogenesis of amoebic liver abscess in man. J Gastroenterol Hepatol 2:351–356
7. Dandapat MC, Dora KBK (1987) Depression of jejunal IgA and peripheral T-cell counts in patients of amoebic liver abscess. Ind J Surg 49:220–224
8. Radin RD, Ralls PW, Coletti PM, Halls JM (1988) CT of amebic liver abscess. A J R 150:1297–1301
9. Ralls PW, Barnes PF, Johnson MB et al. (1987) Medical treatment of hepatic amebic abscess: rare need for percutaneous drainage. Radiology 165:805–807
10. Daher RR (1990) Doenças infecciosas e parasitárias do figado. In: Coelho JCU (ed) Aparelho digestivo. Clinica e Cirurgia, Medsi, Rio de Janeiro, pp 773–785
11. Goldman IS, Brandborg LL (1990) Parasitic diseases of the liver. In: Zakin D, Boyer TD (eds) Hepatology. A textbook of liver disease. W.B. Saunders, Philadelphia, pp 1061–1085
12. Daher RR, Almeida Netto JC, Cardisi VM (1986) Hepatic changes in malaria: study of 121 cases. Does malaria hepatitis exist? Dig Dis Sci 31:397S
13. Ramachandran S, Pereira MVF (1976) Jaundice and hepatomegaly in primary malaria. J Trop Med Hyg 79:207–210
14. Boulos M (1989) Malaria In: Amato Neto V, Baldy JLS (eds) Doenças Transmissiveis, 3rd edn. Sarvier, São Paulo, pp 585–599
15. Phillips RE, Warrell DA (1986) The pathophysiology of severe falciparum malaria. Parasitol Today 2:271–282
16. Neftel KA, Woodtly W, Śchmid M et al. (1986) Amodiaquine induced agranulocytosis and liver damage. Br Med J 292:721–723
17. Zitelli BJ, Alexander J, Taylor S et al. (1987) Fatal hepatic necrosis due to pyrimethamine sulfadoxine. Ann Intern Med 106:393–395
18. Duarte MIS, Corbett CEP (1987) Histopathological patterns of the liver involvement in visceral leishmaniasis. Rev Inst Med Trop São Paulo 29:131–136
19. Khaldi F, Bennacem B, Othman HB et al. (1990) Les formes severes d'atteinte hepatique au cours de la leishmaniose viscerale. A propos de 7 cas. Arch Fr Pediatr 47:257–260
20. Duarte MIS, Mariano ON, Corbett CE (1989) Liver parenchymal cell parasitism in human visceral leishmaniasis. Virchows Arch [A] 415:1–6
21. Chulay JD, Bryceson ADM (1983) Quantitation of amastigotes of *Leishmania donovani* in smears of splenic aspirates from patients with visceral leishmaniasis. Am J Trop Med Hyg 32:475–479
22. Ong GB (1985) Helminthic diseases of the liver and biliary tract. In: Wright R, Millward-Sadler GH, Alberti KGMM, Karran S (eds) Liver and biliary disease. Pathophysiology, diagnosis, management. Bailliere Tindall, London, pp 1523–1559
23. Gayotto LCC, Da Silva LC (in preparation) Ascariasis, *Toxocara canis* (visceral larva migrans), *Capillaria hepatica*, strongyloidiasis, and pentastomiasis. In: McIntyre M, Benhamou JP, Bircher J, Rizzetto M, Rodés J (eds) Oxford Textbook of Clinical Hepatology. Oxford University Press, Oxford.
24. Khurro MS, Zargar SA, Mahagan R et al. (1987) Sonographic appearances in biliary ascariasis. Gastroenterology 93:267–272

25. Kamath PS, Joseph DC, Chandran R et al. (1986) Biliary ascariasis: ultrasonography, endoscopic retrograde cholangiopancreatography, and biliary drainage. Gastroenterology 91:730–732
26. Jessen K, Al Mofleh I, Al Morfarreh M (1986) Endoscopic treatment of ascariasis causing acute obstructive cholangitis. Hepatogastroenterology 33:275–277
27. Gupta NM (1987) *Fasciola gigantica* in the gallbladder. Ind J Gastroenterol 6:113
28. Borey JC (1982) Fascioliasis. In: Steele (ed) CRC handbook series in zoonoses. CRM Press, Florida, pp 71–88
29. Acuna-Soto R, Braun-Roth G (1987) Bleeding ulcers in the common bile duct due to *Fasciola hepatica*. Am J Gastroenterol 82:560–562
30. Leite OHM, Higaki Y, Serpentini SLP et al. (1989) Infeccao pelo *Clonorchis sinensis* em imigrantes asiaticos no Brasil. Tratamento pelo praziquantel. Rev Inst Med Trop São Paulo 31:416–422
31. Rim HJ (1982) Clonorchiasis. In: Steele JH (ed) CRC handbook series in zoonosis. CRC Press, Florida, pp 17–32
32. Choi BI, Kim HJ, Hasi MC et al. (1989) CT findings of clonorchiasis. A J R 152:281–284
33. Pungpak S, Sornmani S, Sunthrasamai P, Vivatanasesth P (1989) Ultrasonographic study of the biliary system in opisthorchiasis patients after treatment with praziquantel. Southeast Asian J Trop Med Public Health 20:157–162
34. WHO (1985) Control de la esquistosomiasis. Informe de un Comite de expertos de la OMS. Serie de Informes Tecnicos 728. Ginebra, OMS
35. Bina JC, Prata A (1984) A evolucao natural da esquistossomose mansoni em uma area endemica. In: Aspectos peculiares da infeccao por *Schistosoma mansoni*. Edited by CEDRE – Centro de Doencas Regionais (ed). Centro Edit. Didat. U.F. Bahia, Salvador, Brazil, pp 13–33
36. Da Silva LC, Pontes JF (1965) Clinical aspects of schistosomiasis mansoni. In: Popper H, Schaffner F (eds) Progress of liver diseases. Grune & Stratton, New York, pp 243–252
37. Prata A (1982) Infection with *S. mansoni*. In: Jordan P, Webbe G (eds) Schistosomiasis. Epidemilogy, treatment and control. Heinemann Medical, London, pp 105–127
38. De Brito T, Gunji J, Camargo ME et al. (1970) Advanced kidney diseases in patients with hepatosplenic manson's schistosomiasis. Rev Inst Med Trop São Paulo 12:225–235
39. Katz N, Chaves A, Pellegrino J (1972) A simple device for quantitative stool thick smears technique in schistosomiasis mansoni. Rev Inst Med Trop São Paulo 14:397–400
40. Kanamura HY, Hoshino-Shimizu S, Camargo ME, Da Silva LC (1979) Class-specific antibodies and fluorescent staining patterns in acute and chronic forms of schistosomiasis mansoni. Am J Trop Med Hyg 28:242–248
41. Abdel-Wahab MF, Esmat G, Milad M et al. (1989) Characteristic sonographic pattern of schistosomal hepatic fibrosis. Am J Trop Med Hyg 40:72–76
42. Cerri GG, Alves VAF, Magalhaes A (1984) Hepatosplenic schistosomiasis mansoni: ultrasound manifestation. Radiology 153:777–780
43. Da Silva LC, Zeitune JMR, Rosa-Eid LMF et al. (1986) Treatment of patients with schistosomiasis mansoni: a double blind clinical trial comparing praziquantel with oxamniquine. Rev Inst Med Trop São Paulo 28:174–180
44. Da Silva LC, Strauss E, Gayotto LCC et al. (1986) A randomized trial for the study of the elective surgical treatment of portal hypertension in mansonic schistosomiasis. Ann Surg 204:148–153
45. Strauss E (1989) Hipertensao portal esquistossomotica. Analise evolutiva de intercorrencias clinicas, dados endoscopicos e laboratoriais em estudo realizado

comparando tres tipos de cirurgia. Professoral Thesis, Faculdade de Medicina de Ribeirao Preto, Universidade de Sao Paulo
46. Braghirolli Neto O (1988) Fluxo sanguineo da veia azigos na Esquistossomose hepatesplenica: Acao do Propranolol. Doctoral Thesis, Faculdade de Medicina da Universidade de Sao Paulo
47. Mies S, Pereira MB, Orlando CD et al. (1988) Propranolol na prevencao da recidiva de hemorragia digestiva em pacientes com esquistossomose hepatoesplenica. Rev Ass Med Brasil 34:24–28
48. Sakai P, Boaventura S, Ishioka S et al. (1990) Sclerotherapy of bleeding esophageal varices in schistosomiasis. Comparative study in patients with and without previous surgery for portal hypertension. Endoscopy 22:5–7
49. Cordeiro F (1990) Variceal sclerosis in schistosomotic patients – a five-year follow-up study. Gastrointest Endosc
50. Hillyer GV (1982) Schistosomiasis. In: Steele JH, Hillyer GV, Hopla CE (eds) CRC handbook series in zoonoses. CRC Press, Boca Raton, FL, pp 177–210
51. Hidalgo MP, Barquet NE (1987) Hidatidosis hepatica. Estudio de una série de 7.345 casos. Parte I: Aspectos generales, epidemiologia y diagnóstico. Rev Esp Enferm Apar Dig 71:1–6
52. Mallet B, Letrent YP, Sabiani P et al. (1987) Kyste hydatique du foie: analyse de la morbilité post-operatoire. Sem Hôp Paris 63:377–383
53. Pinel C, Fricker H, Chumpitazi B et al. (1989) The immunodiagnostic value of six serological techniques in hydatidosis. Serodiagn Immunother Infect Dis 3:231–240
54. MacPherson CNL, Romig T, Zeyhle E et al. (1987) Portable ultrasound scanner versus serology in screening for hydatic cysts in a nomadic population. Lancet II:259–261
55. Kune GA, Schellenberger R (1988) Current management of liver hydatid cysts: results of a 10-year study. Med J Aust 149:26–30
56. Bartoloni C, De Gaetano AM, Magistrelli A et al. (1989) La terapia medica con mebendazolo nella malattia cistica idatica. Minerva Med 80:205–214
57. Chigot JP, Langlois P, Teboul F et al. (1986) Le traitment des kystes hydatiques du foie. A propos de soixante-dix-sept observations. Sem Hôp Paris 62:3625–3630
58. Freixenet JL, Mestres CA, Cugat E et al. (1988) Hepaticothoracic transdiaphragmatic echinoccocosis. Ann Thorac Surg 45:426–429
59. Pain JA, Reddy PJ, Knight MJ (1988) Biliary sclerosis following formalin instillation into hydatic cysts. Br J Clin Pract 42:214–217
60. Hidalgo MP, Barquet NE (1987) Hidatidosis hepatica. Estudio de una série de 7.345 casos. Parte II: Tratamiento quirúrgico, morbimortalidad, tratamiento médico, hospitalización i implicaciones socioeconómicas. Rev Esp Enferm Apar Dig 71:103–109
61. Galvão VA (1981) Estudos sobre *Capillaria hepatica*: uma avaliação do seu papel patogênico para o homem. Mem Inst Oswaldo Cruz 76:415–433
62. Pereira VG, França LCM (1983) Successful treatment of *Capillaria hepatica* infection in an acutely ill adult. Am J Trop Med Hyg 32:1272–1274
63. Self JT, Hopps HC, Olufemi Williams A (1975) Pentastomiasis in Africans. Trop Geogr Med 27:1–13
64. Smith JA, Oladiran B, Lagundoye SB et al. (1975) Pentastomiasis and malignancy. Ann Trop Med Parasitol 69:503–512
65. Prathap K, Lau KS, Bolton JM (1969) Pentastomiasis: a common finding at autopsy among malaysian aborigines. Am J Trop Med Hyg 18:20–27
66. Schaffner F (1990) The liver in HIV infection. Progr Liver Dis 9:505–522
67. Schneiderman DJ (1988) Hepatobiliary abnormalities of AIDS. Gastroenterol Clin North Am 17:615–630
68. Feuerstein IM, Francis P, Raffeld M, Pluda J (1990) Widespread visceral calcifications in disseminated *Pneumocystis carinii* infection: CT characteristics. J Comput Assist Tomogr 14:149–151

69. Fishman EK, Magid D, Kuhlman JE (1990) *Pneumocystis carinii* involvement of the liver and spleen: CT demonstration. J Comput Assist Tomogr 14: 146–148
70. Lubat E, Megibow AJ, Balthazar EJ et al. (1990) Extrapulmonary *Pneumocystis carinii* infection in AIDS: CT findings. Radiology 174:157–160
71. Tschirhart D, Klatt EC (1988) Disseminated toxoplasmosis in the acquired immunodeficiency syndrome. Arch Pathol Lab Med 112:1237–1241
72. Demian SDE, Donnely WH Jr, Monif GRG (1973) Coexistent congenital cytomegalovirus and toxoplasmosis in a stillborn. Am J Dis Child 125:420–421
73. Gelderman AH, Grimley PM, Lunde MN et al. (1968) *Toxoplasma gondii* and cytomegalovirus: mixed infection by a parasite and a virus. Science 160: 1130–1132
74. Leport C, Raffi F, Matherson S (1988) Treatment of central nervous system toxoplasmosis with pyrimethamine (sulfadiazine combination in 35 patients with the acquired immunodeficiency syndrome). Am J Med 84:94–100
75. Dias RM, Mangini AC, Torres DM et al. (1988) Cryptosporidiosis among patients with acquired immunodeficiency syndrome (AIDS), in the county of São Paulo, Brazil. Rev Inst Med Trop São Paulo 30:310–312
76. Fernandez-Alonso J, Andrada-Becerra E, Jorda-Heras MM et al. (1987) Intestinal cryptosporidiosis with pancreato-biliary and bronchial dissemination in a female infant with AIDS. Med Clin (Barc) 19:355–358
77. Restrapo C, Macher AM, Radany EH (1987) Disseminated extraintestinal isosporiasis in a patient with acquired immunodeficiency syndrome. Am J Clin Pathol 87:536–542
78. Terada S, Reddy KR, Jeffers LJ et al. (1987) Microsporidian hepatitis in acquired immunodeficiency syndrome. Ann Intern Med 107:62–63
79. Eckert J (1989) New aspects of parasitic zoonoses. Vet Parasitol 32:37–55
80. Drabick JJ, Egan JE, Brown SL et al. (1988) Dicroceliasis (lancet fluke dicroceliasis) in an HIV seropositive man. JAMA 259:567–568
81. Hillyer GV, Climent C (1988) Acquired immunodeficiency syndrome (AIDS) and parasitic diseases in Puerto Rico. Bol Asoc Med PR 80:312–319
82. Miller SE (1988) Helminthic infections in the acquired immunodeficiency syndrome. J Electron Microsc Tech 8:133–135
83. Schneiderman DJ, Cello JP, Laing FC (1987) Papillary stenosis and sclerosing cholangitis in the acquired immunodeficiency syndrome. Ann Intern Med 106:546–549
84. Margulis SJ, Honig CL, Soave R et al. (1986) Biliary tract obstruction in the acquired immunodeficiency syndrome. Ann Intern Med 105:207–210
85. Radim DR, Cohen H, Hall JM (1987) Acalculous inflammatory disease of the biliary tree in acquired immunodeficiency syndrome: CT demonstration. J Comput Assist Tomogr 11:775–778
86. Stilman AE, Schmid R, Howe JB (1987) Acquired immunodeficiency syndrome and biliary tract disease. Ann Intern Med 106:634–635
87. Roulot D, Valla D, Brun-Vezinet F et al. (1987) Cholangitis in the acquired immunodeficiency syndrome: report of two cases and review of the literature. Gut 28:1653–1660
88. Viteri AL, Greene JF Jr (1987) Bile duct abnormalities in the acquired immune deficiency syndrome. Gastroenterology 92:2014–2018
89. Kahn DG, Garfinkle JM, Klonoff DC et al. (1987) Cryptosporidial and cytomegaloviral hepatitis and cholecystitis. Arch Pathol Lab Med 111:879–881
90. Aaron JS, Wynter CD, Kirton OC et al. (1988) Cytomegalovirus associated with acalculous cholecystitis in a patient with acquired immune deficiency syndrome. Am J Gastroenterol 83:879–881
91. Yana C, Frija J, Cyna-Gorse F et al. (1989) Radiological aspects of noncalculous inflammation of the biliary tract in AIDS. J Radiol 70:411–414

92. Grumbach K, Coleman BG, Gal AA et al. (1989) Hepatic and biliary tract abnormalities in patients with AIDS. Sonographic-pathologic correlation. J Ultrasound Med 8:247–254
93. McCarty M, Choudhri AH, Herbert M et al. (1989) Radiological features of AIDS related cholangitis. Clin Radiol 40:582–585
94. Romano AJ, van Sonnemberg E, Casola G et al. (1988) Gallbladder and bile duct abnormalities in AIDS: sonographic findings in eight patients. A J R 150:123–127
95. Dolmatch BL, Laing FC, Federle MP et al. (1987) AIDS-related cholangitis: radiographic findings in nine patients. Radiology 163:313–316
96. Jacobson MA, Cello JP, Sande MA (1988) Cholestasis and disseminated cytomegalovirus disease in patients with the acquired immunodeficiency syndrome. Am J Med 84:218–224
97. Hollman AS, Morley P, Burt AD et al. (1986) Biliary tract dilatation in acquired immune deficiency syndrome. Eur J Radiol 6:287–291
98. Lurie M, Elmalach I, Schuger L et al. (1987) Liver findings in infantile cytomegalovirus infection: similarity to extrahepatic biliary obstruction. Histopathology 11:1171–1180
99. Davis JJ, Heyman MB, Ferrell L et al. (1987) Sclerosing cholangitis associated with chronic cryptosporidiosis in a child with a congenital immunodeficiency disorder. Am J Gastroenterol 82:1196–1202
100. Moss G, Braunstein FM, Newkirk RE (1987) Postoperative enteral hyperalimentation for cryptosporidial acute cholecystitis associated with AIDS and enteritis. J Am Coll Nutr 6:351–353
101. Cello JP (1989) Acquired immunodeficiency syndrome cholangiopathy: spectrum of disease. Am J Med 86:539–546

# 18 The Liver in Pregnancy and in Systemic Diseases

M. BRUGUERA

## 1 Liver Diseases and Pregnancy

Several types of liver disease can occur during pregnancy (Table 1). Some are caused by pregnancy itself (especially those manifesting themselves during the third trimester), while others are pre-existing. The accurate diagnosis of third trimester liver disease is of great importance, as it will affect management of the patient, the newborn child and future pregnancies.

Hemodynamic changes occur during pregnancy, and these need to be carefully considered when investigating abnormalities of liver function during pregnancy. The most frequent physiological abnormalities in liver function tests in pregnant women are increased serum alkaline phosphatase activity due to placental synthesis of this enzyme, and reduced albuminemia due to hemodilution.

## 2 Liver Diseases Specific to Pregnancy

### 2.1 Recurrent Cholestasis of Pregnancy

Recurrent cholestasis of pregnancy is a cholestasis syndrome without histologic hepatic lesions that appears in the third trimester of pregnancy and disappears a few days after giving birth. It occurs with a frequency of approximately one case in every 7000–8000 pregnancies and is particularly frequent in Chile and Scandinavian countries. It has hereditary features and tends to recur in subsequent pregnancies. There is a major form with jaundice and a minor form with persistent itching without jaundice, also known as gravidic pruritus [1]. The pathogenesis is unknown, although it is related to an abnormal sensitivity to estrogens as women who have had gravidic cholestasis usually show the same symptoms after taking estrogens [2].

#### *Clinical Features*

The main symptom is generalized, mainly nocturnal, pruritus which appears before the jaundice, not infrequently (20%–30% of cases) in the first or

**Table 1.** Liver diseases and pregnancy

| |
|---|
| *Diseases specific to pregnancy* |
| Recurrent cholestasis of pregnancy |
| Acute fatty liver of pregnancy |
| Liver disease associated with eclampsia |
| – Hepatic infarction |
| – Subcapsular hematoma and liver rupture |
| – HELLP syndrome |
| Liver disease associated with gravidic hyperemesis |
| *Liver diseases occurring during pregnancy* |
| Viral hepatitis |
| Toxic hepatitis |
| Budd-Chiari syndrome |
| *Preexisting liver diseases* |
| Constitutional metabolic jaundice |
| Chronic hepatitis |
| Liver cirrhosis |
| Wilson's disease |

second trimester. Patients with jaundice may have gastrointestinal symptoms such as loss of appetite, nausea, vomiting, and discomfort in the right hypochondrium. Other symptoms are choluria and acholic feces. Steatorrhea is common and its severity is related to the degree of cholestasis [3].

Physical examination may reveal jaundice and injuries caused by scratching. Laboratory investigation shows hyperbilirubinemia, which does not usually exceed 6 mg/dl, and increased alkaline phosphatase and serum bile acids. It is common to observe a moderate increase in aminotransferases, and, exceptionally, larger increases to values in the range of viral hepatitis can be seen [4]. The prothrombin time is prolonged and can be corrected with vitamin K.

The symptoms and laboratory abnormalities disappear within 1–2 weeks of delivery. The patients have often had one or more normal pregnancies before the first episode of cholestasis. Once the patient has suffered such an attack, cholestasis recurs with greater or lesser severity in successive pregnancies. If the pruritus does not disappear after labor, primary biliary cirrhosis should be suspected.

### *Treatment*

Treatment is symptomatic and consists in eliminating the pruritus by giving cholestyramine. The pregnant patient must also be given vitamin K to prevent intracranial hemorrhage in the fetus during birth and postpartum hemorrhage in the mother. It has been pointed out that high doses of *S*-adenosyl-L-methionine may induce regression of cholestasis in these patients.

Cholestasis of pregnancy is a benign disease for the mother but causes premature births in 10%–20% of cases, with a mortality in such cases of about 40%. This has been attributed to excess bile salts in the mother, which pass through the placenta, causing prematurity and fetal distress [5]. It has been recommended that labor be induced as early as possible, once the lungs of the baby are sufficiently mature.

The mother should be warned that cholestasis will definitely recur in subsequent pregnancies and that oral contraceptives will cause the same condition.

## 2.2 Acute Fatty Liver of Pregnancy

Acute fatty liver of pregnancy (AFLP) is a disease of unknown etiology that appears in the third trimester with signs of liver failure of varying severity. The incidence of the severe form has been estimated to be one case per 13000 pregnancies [6]; the incidence of the milder forms is unknown. It is characterized histologically by microvesicular fatty change in the centrilobular areas, without inflammatory lesions or hepatocellular necrosis.

Approximately half of the cases affect primiparae and a large number of women with this syndrome have been carrying twins. It appears between weeks 28 and 40, but is more frequent after week 35.

### *Clinical Features*

The serious form of AFLP is characterized by the appearance of nausea, vomiting, headache, fatigue, retrosternal burning, and abdominal pain, particularly in the epigastrium and the right upper quadrant. After 1 or 2 weeks, or sometimes earlier, jaundice appears, which may be followed by hepatic encephalopathy and extrahepatic complications such as acute pancreatitis, renal failure, and respiratory failure. In almost half of the cases there are also signs of eclampsia such as high blood pressure and edema.

The laboratory tests usually show an increase in serum aminotransferases; in most cases the levels remain below 300 IU/liter, but on rare occasions they may increase to as high as 1000 IU/liter. Bilirubin levels are increased to a varying degree, to between 3 and 25 mg/dl. The blood film almost invariably shows a high white blood cell count with neutrophilia and thrombocytopenia. Hyperuricemia is very common. The prothrombin time is prolonged and is often associated with signs of disseminated intravascular coagulation.

In recent years, less severe forms of the disease have been recognized which are not associated with hepatic encephalopathy, liver failure, or extrahepatic complications [7].

The maternofetal mortality in the severe forms of AFLP is more than 85% but the recognition of milder forms that do not cause death has lowered the maternofetal mortality to 44%.

A definite diagnosis of AFLP requires histologic evidence of microvesicular fatty change. The liver biopsy should be performed by the transjugular route in the event of significant abnormalities in the coagulation tests. The difficulty in recognizing the fatty microvesicles justifies the use of stains for fat (oil red O) in fresh frozen tissue. The histologic examination is indispensable only when there are reasonable doubts as to the diagnosis. Some imaging methods, such as ultrasonography or computed tomography (CT), may facilitate the diagnosis by showing changes suggestive of fat deposition, such as a pattern of diffuse hyperechogenicity of the liver on the ultrasonogram or a decrease in hepatic attenuation on the CT scan.

#### *Treatment*

The experience gained in recent years suggests that an improved prognosis in AFLP is associated with early induction of delivery [8]. If attempts to induce vaginal delivery are not effective, a cesarean section should be performed. It is vital to monitor the fetus during birth. An orthotopic liver transplant has been successfully performed in a patient in coma [9]. This treatment should be considered in patients with hepatic encephalopathy, once delivery has been successfully completed.

There are no descriptions of a recurrence of the disease in patients who have survived an episode of AFLP and become pregnant again. Consequently, it is not necessary to advise patients against further pregnancies.

### 2.3 Preeclampsia and Eclampsia

Preeclampsia and eclampsia are typical complications of the last trimester of pregnancy and occur in about 5%–7% of all pregnancies. They are the major cause of maternal mortality. The condition consists of edema, proteinuria, and high blood pressure. In more serious cases, seizures, heart failure, and renal failure appear. Death occurs particularly in cases with intracerebral hemorrhage but liver involvement causes 10%–20% of eclampsia-related mortality.

#### *Clinical Features*

Although the finding of moderate abnormalities in the liver function tests not associated with symptoms is relatively common in eclampsia, the serious forms of liver involvement are rare and their appearance is not related to the severity of the toxemia.

Clinical symptoms of liver involvement are pain in the epigastrium and right upper quadrant, with fever and often jaundice. Laboratory results show a significant increase in serum aminotransferases and hyperbilirubinemia. Imaging methods may reveal focal defects corresponding to hepatic infarctions. If they are located peripherally, they may cause hematoma and spontaneous liver rupture (Fig. 1). In the latter case, hypovolemic shock develops and may be confused with an ectopic pregnancy.

Histologic examination shows fibrin deposits in the periportal hepatic sinusoids with more or less intense hepatocellular necrosis. It is postulated that these lesions are caused by intravascular coagulation in the liver as a result of segmental vasospasms. There is damage to the endothelial cells of the sinusoids, with release of thromboplastin and induction of a consumption coagulopathy [10]. Between 4% and 12% of patients with preeclampsia show abnormal results in liver function tests associated with nausea and vomiting. This syndrome has been called HELLP (from hemolysis, elevated liver tests, and low platelet count) [11] and is more frequently observed in multigravidic women.

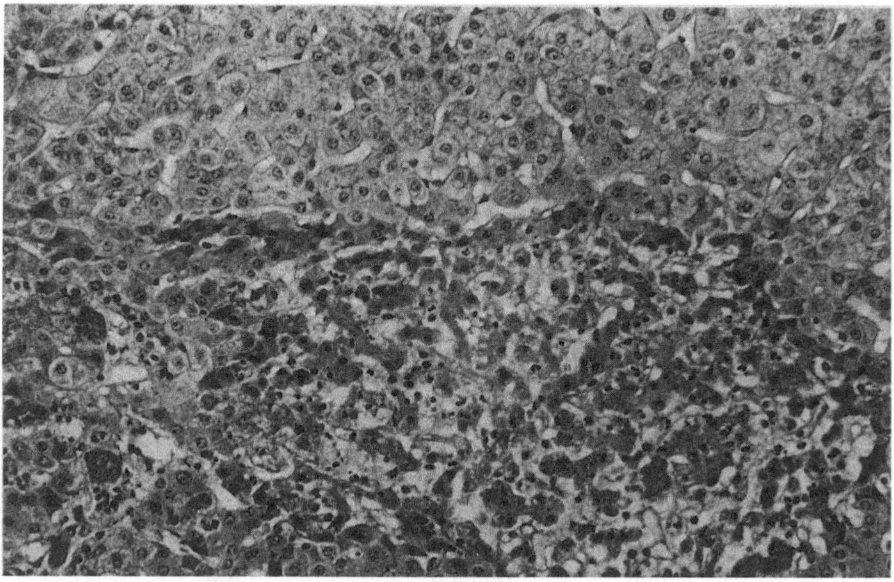

**Fig. 1.** Eclampsia. Confluent necrosis with coagulative changes of hepatic cells, fibrin deposition, and absence of inflammatory reaction. H&E, ×110

### *Treatment*

The treatment for mild forms of liver disease in patients with eclampsia is the same as that for preeclampsia. In the serious forms, delivery should be induced, as prolonging the pregnancy is associated with a greater materno-fetal mortality. Subcapsular hematomas require monitoring and blood transfusions. Surgery is indicated in those cases that do not remain hemodynamically stable. Arterial embolization has been tried with success. Rupture requires surgery.

## 2.4 Gravidic Hyperemesis

Gravidic hyperemesis is a rare disease that presents as repeated vomiting, usually in the first trimester. It is occasionally associated with slight jaundice and moderately increased serum aminotransferase levels. The histologic examination of the liver is usually normal.

# 3 Liver Diseases Occurring During Pregnancy

## 3.1 Viral Hepatitis

Viral hepatitis is the most frequent cause of liver disease during pregnancy. All forms of viral hepatitis can affect pregnant women, although Hepatitis E only occurs in the Third World. The clinical signs and their course are the same as in the nonpregnant. Hepatitis E, however, is characterized by a high mortality rate during pregnancy. The etiologic diagnosis of viral hepatitis is based on the determination of serologic markers or on the direct detection of viral genome (HBV-DNA, HCV-RNA, HDV-RNA). Clinicopathologic features that distinguish acute viral hepatitis from AFLP are shown in Table 2.

**Table 2.** Clinicopathologic features that differ in fatty liver of pregnancy (AFLP) and acute viral hepatitis (AVH)

| | AFLP | AVH |
|---|---|---|
| Serum aminotransferases | $<\times 10$ (80%) | $>\times 10$ (50%) |
| Preeclampsia | Present | Absent |
| Leukocytosis | Common | Rare |
| Intravascular coagulation | Common | Rare |
| Hypoglycemia | Common | Rare |
| Uremia | Common | Rare |
| Hyperuricemia | Common | Rare |
| Pathology | Microvesicular fat | Lobular spotty necrosis |

Viral hepatitis during pregnancy is not a cause of congenital defects in the newborn but is a cause of prematurity when it occurs in the last trimester (27% of cases) [12], without any increase being observed in the rate of miscarriage or still birth.

There is a risk of the disease being transmitted from the mother to the fetus or to the newborn child, particularly in the case of hepatitis B and D. Transmission of the hepatitis A virus is very rare due to the short duration of the viremia, and it is also very uncommon in hepatitis C.

In almost all cases in which the hepatitis B virus is replicating at the time of birth, as occurs in approximately 90% of HBeAg-positive women and in 15%–20% of anti-HBe-positive women, mother-to-child transmission of the virus takes place at the time of birth due to the neonate coming into contact with the mother's blood. Intrauterine transmission occurs in approximately 5% of cases. The risk of vertical transmission is the same in acute hepatitis as in chronic hepatitis. Infection by the hepatitis D virus only occurs in children born to mothers with a delta infection associated with active replication of the hepatitis B virus [13].

### *Prevention of Neonatal Hepatitis*

Neonatal infection by hepatitis B and D virus is usually asymptomatic, but 80%–90% of infected infants become chronic carriers of the virus and develop chronic asymptomatic hepatitis that may lead to cirrhosis and hepatocellular carcinoma.

Neonatal infection by both viruses can be avoided by passive–active immunoprophylaxis, giving hepatitis B immunoglobulin (0.5 ml i.m.) on the 1st day after birth followed by the administration of hepatitis B vaccine (10 µg i.m. per dose). Several vaccination regimens have been tested. All have been shown to be equally effective but it is recommended that the first dose be given during the 1st day after birth. The next two may be given with the mandatory vaccines (Table 3).

These measures prevent 95% of neonatal infections. The effectiveness of immunoprophylaxis of neonates born to mothers infected with hepatitis B

**Table 3.** Antenatal screening and prevention of hepatitis B virus transmission from infected mothers to newborns

1. Universal HBsAg screening of pregnant women
2. In HBsAg-positive cases:
   - Avoid procedures that entail a risk to the fetus, such as amniocentesis
   - Administration of 0.5 ml of hepatitis B immunoglobulin and 10 µg of hepatitis B vaccine to the newborn on the 1st day of life
   - The remaining two doses of vaccine should be given at months 1 and 6 (traditional schedule) or in association with the first doses of DTP-polio vaccine
   - HBsAg carrier mothers should be investigated for liver disease (serum aminotransferases) and for HBV replication (HBeAg/anti-HBe and/or HBV DNA).

or D virus justifies the systematic HBsAg screening of all pregnant women in order to detect those who may infect their child at the time of birth and to enable immunoglobulin and vaccine to be provided on the day of birth. Procedures (e.g., amniocentesis) that expose the fetus to a risk of infection should be avoided in HBsAg-positive mothers.

### 3.2 Toxic Hepatitis

The incidence of drug-induced hepatotoxicity in pregnant women is low, being similar to that observed in the rest of the population. Cases of reversible liver dysfunction associated with drugs used to stop premature labor contractions, such as terbutaline and other β-sympathomimetics, have been reported.

### 3.3 Budd-Chiari Syndrome

Although Budd-Chiari syndrome is a rare complication of pregnancy, in KHUROO and DATTA's series 16 (15%) of the 105 cases of Budd-Chiari syndrome collected in India during the period 1963–1978 were linked to pregnancy, the symptoms appearing in the 2 weeks after parturition [14]. In such cases the syndrome usually presents as an acute disease, with abdominal pain, tender hepatomegaly, and ascites. There is usually moderate hyperbilirubinemia and serum aminotransferase levels are increased. The outcome is usually fatal.

## 4 Pregnancy in Patients with Liver Disease

Pregnancies are rare in patients with liver disease since many liver diseases occur after the menopause or cause sterility if they occur at a younger age. Nevertheless, some women with liver disease may become pregnant. In general, pregnancy does not have an unfavorable effect on the liver disease, although there may be complications related to hyperestrogenism, e.g., an increase in jaundice in Dubin-Johnson's syndrome or an increase in volemia that may worsen portal hypertension and precipitate hemorrhage from ruptured esophageal varices. The latter risk makes pregnancy inadvisable in patients with liver cirrhosis, thrombosis of the splenoportal axis, or idiopathic portal hypertension.

Patients being treated with corticosteroids for autoimmune chronic active hepatitis or with D-penicillamine for Wilson's disease should not stop taking the medication if they become pregnant, owing to the risk of reactivating the liver disease [15]. Neither corticosteroids nor D-penicillamine entail any risk of teratogenesis. Patients with a liver transplant may become pregnant and they, too, should not discontinue immunosuppressive medication [16].

## 5 The Liver in Systemic Diseases

We have included under the heading of systemic diseases those that compromise several organs at the same time, such as sarcoidosis, amyloidosis, and collagen diseases, and also those that, although they initially affect only one organ, often have an impact at the systemic level, such as blood diseases, thyroid diseases, and inflammatory bowel diseases.

In some nonhepatic diseases, the liver is often directly affected, as occurs in the infiltration of the liver by blood malignancies. On other occasions complications related to the treatment of the underlying disease may appear, such as hepatitis in patients receiving multiple transfusions. In other cases, the same etiology is responsible for the liver disease and the systemic disease, as occurs in hepatitis B associated with polyarteritis nodosa. Finally, in still other diseases, liver impairment may be the primary expression of the disease, as is the case in amyloidosis and sarcoidosis.

## 6 Hematologic Diseases

### 6.1 Hodgkin's Disease

The frequency of liver involvement in Hodgkin's disease varies according to the stage of evolution of the disease: it ranges between 5% and 14% at the time of diagnosis, reaches 30% during the course of the disease, and is 60%–70% in autopsy series [17].

Liver involvement is characterized by infiltrates composed of lymphocytes, atypical histiocytes, eosinophils, and plasma cells in the portal tracts, with the occasional (although not invariable) presence of Reed-Sternberg cells (Fig. 2). Sometimes, the portal infiltrates are very large, extending toward the periportal parenchyma and forming large tumoral nodes. This is more common in the more aggressive histologic subtypes of Hodgkin's disease, such as the lymphocyte depleted and mixed cellularity forms. Spleen involvement is consistently found in cases with liver involvement.

Epithelioid granulomas are found in approximately 10% of the liver biopsies of patients with Hodgkin's disease. These should not be interpreted as indicating invasion of the liver by the disease. Nonspecific lymphoid aggregates are found in the portal tracts in one-third of the patients. Sinusoidal dilatation is almost always found in patients with systemic symptoms, such as fever or weight loss (Fig. 3) [18].

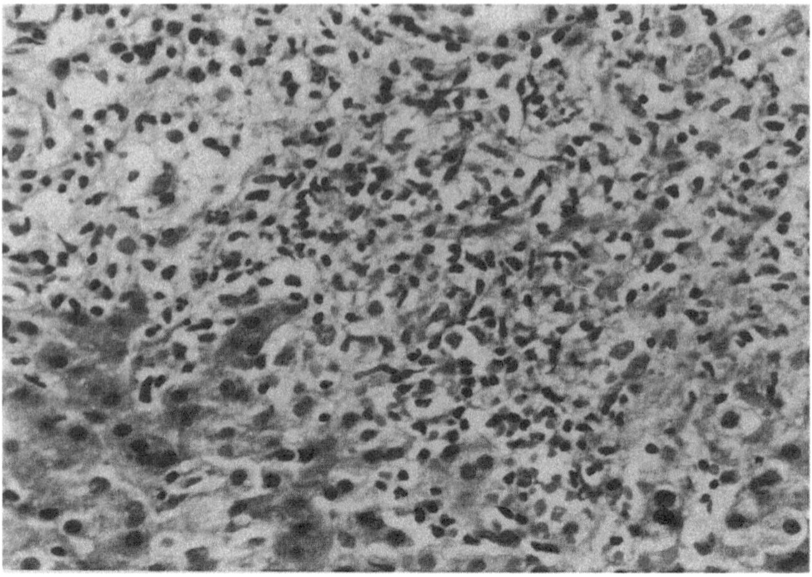

**Fig. 2.** Hodgkin's disease. Portal infiltration composed of a variety of cells, including atypical histiocytes; infiltrates are present beyond the portal tract. H&E, ×300

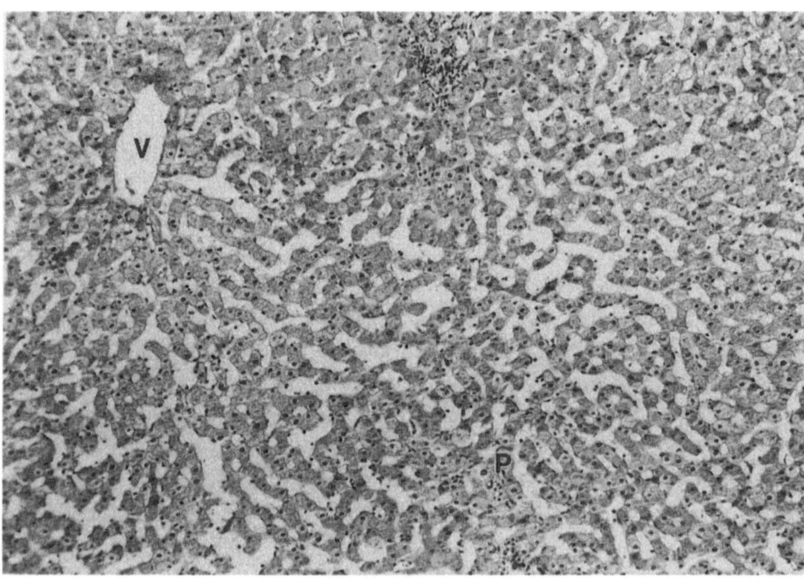


**Fig. 3.** Hodgkin's disease. Midzonal sinusoidal dilatation. No changes are seen in portal tracts (*P*) or in terminal hepatic venules (*V*) are seen. H&E, ×100

An enlarged liver is very common in patients with Hodgkin's disease but does not always indicate liver infiltration. Conversely, half of the cases with liver infiltration have no hepatomegaly. Liver function tests offer little help in assessing liver involvement in Hodgkin's disease. Most patients with liver infiltration show an increase in alkaline phosphatase, as can also be observed in patients with nonspecific histologic lesions, such as granulomas or sinusoidal dilatation. An elevated alkaline phosphatase level is observed in 80% of patients in stage IV disease and the level returns to normal values after effective chemotherapy.

In some patients, the disease initially appears as a febrile cholestasis, without any liver infiltration or bile duct obstruction being observed in the histologic examination [19]. The cause of the jaundice, which fades after successful chemotherapy, is unknown. Jaundice may also be observed in cases of extensive infiltration of the liver by the tumor (thus being an expression of a preterminal phase) and in the case of bile duct obstruction by hilar adenopathies.

Some patients with Hodgkin's disease present with pruritus, which disappears upon treatment with cholestyramine. It may be thought of as a minor form of the idiopathic cholestasis syndrome of Hodgkin's disease.

### 6.2 Non-Hodgkin's Lymphoma

The liver is one of the organs most commonly invaded in patients with non-Hodgkin's lymphomas, after the lymph glands, the spleen, and the bone marrow. Liver infiltration is more frequent in the advanced phases of the disease (60% in postmortem studies vs 20% at the time of diagnosis) and is very rare in the absence of infiltration of the spleen.

Liver involvement consists of a dense lymphoid cell infiltrate of the portal tracts which sometimes destroys blood vessels and bile ducts and is clearly separated from the parenchyma (Fig. 4). In some cases, the lymphomatous infiltrate is more extensive and replaces large areas of parenchyma, forming node-like structures. In patients in the leukemic phase, malignant cells can be identified in the sinusoids.

It is sometimes difficult to distinguish histologically a neoplastic portal infiltrate from an inflammatory infiltrate. Immunohistochemical studies, preferably on fresh frozen samples, using monoclonal antibodies against antigens of the various cell populations, may facilitate recognition of the lymphoma by demonstrating the monoclonality of the cells in the infiltrate [20].

As in Hodgkin's disease, epithelioid granulomas may be found in the liver biopsy.

In T cell lymphomas, the pattern of liver infiltration is principally sinusoidal, with concurrent infiltration of the portal tracts [21].

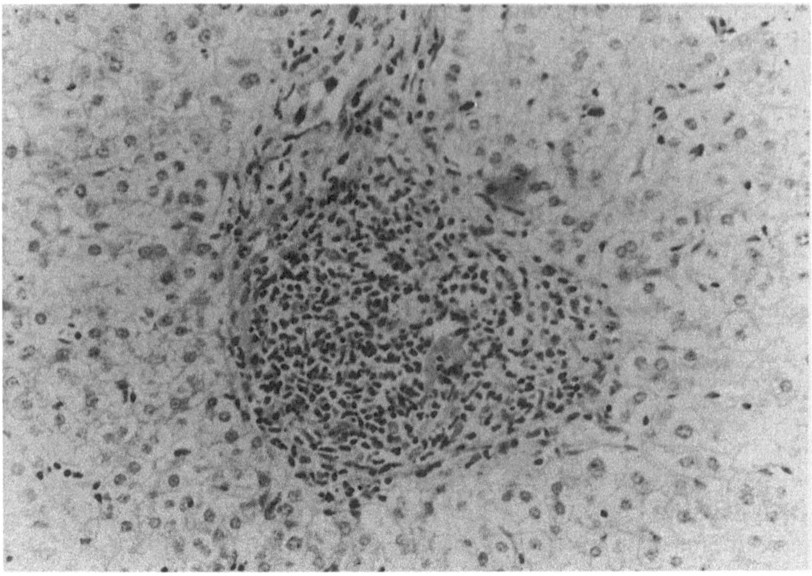

**Fig. 4.** Non-Hodgkin's lymphoma. Dense lymphocytic proliferation in a portal tract, sparing the limiting plate. H&E, ×210

In approximately half of the patients with hepatomegaly, the percutaneous liver biopsy shows liver infiltration, although this is also found in about 10% of patients without hepatomegaly.

Jaundice is a terminal event and is rarely an early finding. It may be due to compression of the common hepatic duct by hilar lymph-adenopathy. Imaging methods may suggest a liver infiltration that is indistinguishable from metastasis in cases of severe involvement with formation of large tumoral nodes.

Cases of primary liver lymphoma have been described, particularly in patients with AIDS [22].

## 6.3 Leukemias

### *Acute Leukemia*

Liver involvement is usually asymptomatic at the time of diagnosis of leukemia. The combination of abnormal liver function tests and hepatomegaly suggests leukemic infiltration of the liver, which occurs in the portal tracts in acute lymphoblastic leukemia and in the sinusoids in myeloblastic leukemia. However, other possible causes of liver damage, such as toxic or posttransfusion hepatitis, should be excluded.

Some cases of severe hepatic insufficiency simulating fulminant hepatitis, due to a massive blastic infiltration of the liver, have been described.

Patients with acute leukemia receiving chemotherapy may develop hepatosplenic candidiasis during the neutropenic recovery phase, characterized by painful hepatomegaly, fever, and increased alkaline phosphatase [23]. Grayish nodes protruding from the liver surface may be identified on laparoscopy and a characteristic "bull's-eye" image is observed on the ultrasonogram. Histologic examination is the only way to confirm the diagnosis, by demonstrating granulomatous lesions containing hyphae and spores. Blood cultures are consistently negative for fungi.

#### *Chronic Lymphoid Leukemia*

Moderate liver enlargement is a common finding in chronic lymphoid leukemia due to the presence of portal and sinusoidal infiltrates. Regenerative nodular hyperplasia has been observed in some cases and may be the cause of portal hypertension.

#### *Hairy-cell Leukemia*

Hairy-cell leukemia is a lymphoproliferative disease characterized by the proliferation of mononuclear cells that show cytoplasmic projections and exhibit a "hairy" appearance on electron microscopy. Hepatic infiltration by neoplastic cells is a consistent finding, although it is usually clinically silent. Hepatomegaly is found in 30%–40% of cases, although liver function tests are usually normal [24].

In liver biopsy specimens, the hairy cells are arranged linearly in the sinusoids. These appear to be dilated in certain areas, forming angiomatoid lesions, the central cavity of which is delimited by hairy cells (Fig. 5).

### 6.4 Polycythemia Vera

Patients in whom polycythemia is evolving toward myelofibrosis exhibit hepatosplenomegaly as a result of extramedullary hematopoiesis. In such cases, the clinical and histologic changes are identical to those observed in agnogenic myeloid metaplasia. Some patients develop Budd-Chiari syndrome or portal vein thrombosis because of blood hypercoagulability and the high platelet count.

### 6.5 Monoclonal Gammopathies

Between 25% and 40% of patients with multiple myeloma have hepatomegaly due to portal and sinusoidal infiltration by plasma cells. Rarely, large intrahepatic nodes formed by a plasmacytic infiltrate or deposits of

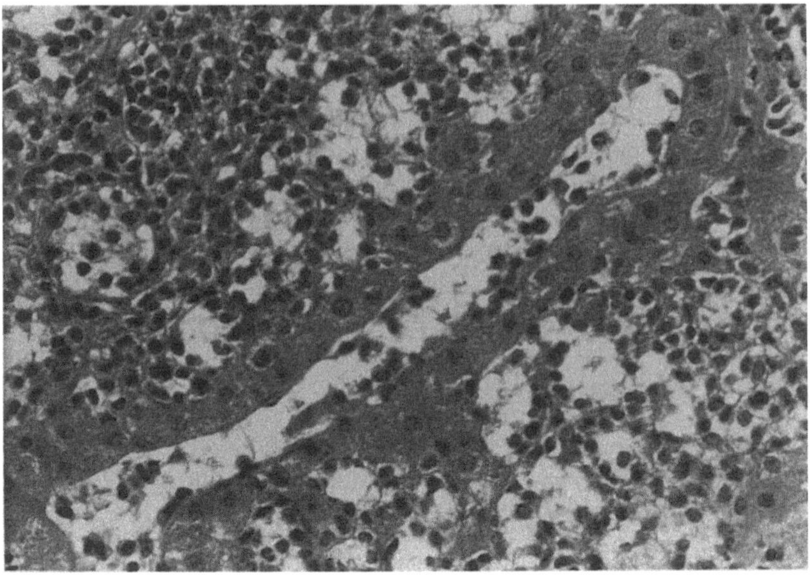

**Fig. 5.** Hairy-cell leukemia. Formation of sinusoidal angiomatous lesions lined by leukemic cells. H&E, ×340

amyloid substance are observed. Normally, these changes are symptom-free, although rare cases of jaundice caused by massive liver infiltration have been described.

## 6.6 Myeloid Metaplasia

Liver involvement is almost invariable in primary myelofibrosis. It is characterized by foci of hematopoiesis in the sinusoids and portal tracts. In early stages the nests of extramedullary hematopoiesis are located in the sinusoids, while in advanced stages they are located in the portal tracts. Immature elements of all three cell lines are usually observed, although the most consistent finding is the presence of dysplastic megakaryocytes [25] (Fig. 6). The isolated presence of megakaryocytes in the sinusoids should not be interpreted as diagnostic of myeloid metaplasia because it is also observed in some liver biopsy specimens taken from patients with Hodgkin's disease and in liver transplant patients.

In half of these patients, sinusoidal dilatation is observed; this dilatation may be attributed to zonal obstruction of the blood flow caused by foci of hematopoiesis or to damage to the sinusoid endothelial wall. In 30%–40% of cases one can also observe sinusoidal fibrosis related to the transformation of the Ito's cells in the space of Disse into fibroblasts by

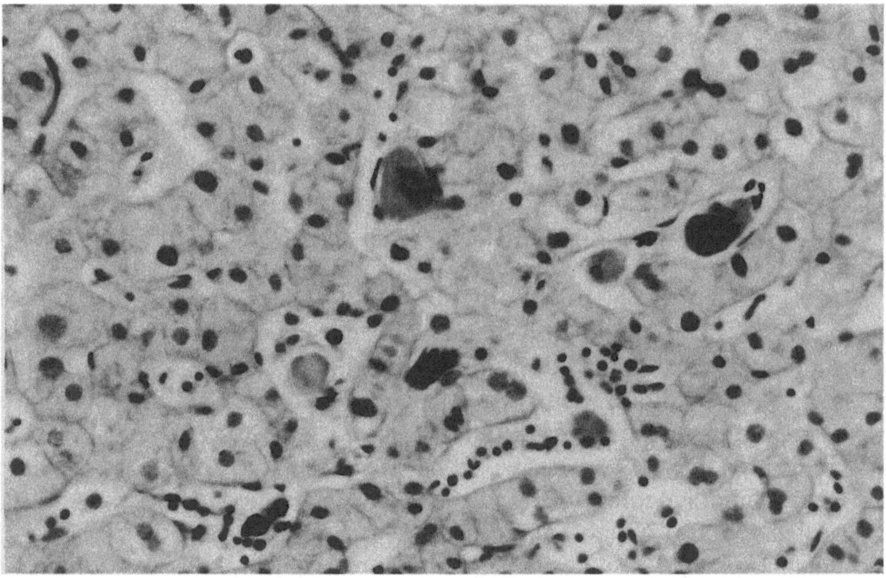

**Fig. 6.** Myeloid metaplasia. Several megakaryocytes and erythroblasts are present within dilated sinusoids. H&E, ×300

factors released by the dysplastic megakaryocytes (platelet-derived growth factor, PDGF). The sinusoidal fibrosis may play a role in the development of portal hypertension in some patients with myeloid metaplasia.

Extramedullary hematopoiesis causes hepatomegaly in 70%–80% of patients. The size of the liver correlates with the progression of the disease and with the size of the spleen. The size of the liver increases considerably after splenectomy.

Approximately 7% of these patients present with some complication of portal hypertension, such as ascites or gastrointestinal bleeding. In the remaining patients, liver involvement is asymptomatic. In 40%–60% of cases, liver function tests yield abnormal results, particularly an increase in alkaline phosphatase activity. Increased serum aminotransferase values are not typical of myeloid metaplasia and should lead one to suspect viral hepatitis, to which these patients are exposed owing to their need for blood transfusions.

The development of severe liver failure has been reported as a complication of splenectomy [26].

Patients submitted to percutaneous liver biopsy should be carefully monitored because of the risk of intraperitoneal bleeding due to platelet dysfunction.

## 6.7 Hemolytic Anemias

### *Sickle Cell Anemia*

Sickle cell anemia is a hereditary disease caused by abnormal hemoglobin which polymerizes in the red blood cells in hypoxic conditions. It causes recurrent painful veno-occlusive crises. Liver involvement is common and may be due to complications of sickle cell disease or to posttransfusion hepatitis [27].

The liver biopsy shows hyperplasia of Kupffer cells, which are full of phagocytosed sickle-shaped red blood cells and hemosiderin. The sinusoids appear dilated as a result of clusters of red blood cells. Bile thrombi and areas of cell necrosis are seen. Fatty change is common. Some patients have chronic hepatitis or cirrhosis presumably of viral etiology.

Clinically, the veno-occlusive crises are associated with acute hepatic pain that simulates acute cholecystitis as it is accompanied by fever, jaundice, leukocytosis, and a variable increase in serum bilirubin, aminotransferase, and alkaline phosphatase levels. These features typically subside within 1 or 2 weeks but in some cases display a progressive course, leading to death from liver failure.

Some patients have an extreme hyperbilirubinemia that is not associated with pain or fever and disappears spontaneously, without any sequelae, within a few weeks.

There is a high prevalence of gallstones in patients with sickle cell anemia. Consequently, the differential diagnosis of the hepatic crises from lithiasic cholecystitis is sometimes very difficult.

### *Thalassemia*

In thalassemia major there is invariably liver damage due to (a) chronic infection by hepatitis B and C virus related to the transfusion therapy or (b) secondary hemochromatosis caused more by excessive intestinal iron absorption than by the iron contained in the red blood cells transfused. The progression of hemochromatosis can be counteracted by giving desferrioxamine subcutaneously through continuous infusion pumps [28].

In thalassemia minor, mild hepatic hemosiderosis can be found, but only patients who are heterozygotic for the hemochromatosis gene actually develop hemochromatosis.

As in all hemolytic anemias, gallstones are common.

### *Paroxysmal Nocturnal Hemoglobinuria*

In paroxysmal nocturnal hemoglobinuria (PNH), a chronic hemolytic anemia, the red blood cell membrane is particularly susceptible to lysis by complement when blood pH becomes more acid during sleep. Patients with

PNH suffer from a blood hypercoagulability that favors the appearance of thrombosis. Some patients develop Budd-Chiari syndrome due to suprahepatic vein thrombosis [29].

*Other Hemolytic Anemias*

In the other congenital hemolytic anemias, such as hereditary spherocytosis and erythrocyte enzyme defects (glucose-6-phosphate dehydrogenase or pyruvate kinase), it is common to find gallstones and hepatic hemosiderosis. Infection by hepatitis virus may precipitate erythrocyte destruction in cases of glucose-6-phosphate dehydrogenase deficiency resulting in hemolytic crisis.

### 6.8 Hemophilia

Hemophilia A and hemophilia B are hereditary coagulation disorders caused by deficiency of factor VIII or factor IX, requiring replacement therapy with cryoprecipitates or concentrates of these factors prepared from pooled plasma. Acute and chronic viral hepatitis are common in these patients. More than 90% have serologic markers of hepatitis B virus, 55%–75% have anti-HCV, and 25%–50% of HBsAg carriers have anti-HDV. About 70% of hemophiliacs have abnormal liver tests and a high proportion of those who undergo liver biopsy show advanced lesions such as chronic active hepatitis or cirrhosis.

The risk of percutaneous liver biopsy is high even when it is performed after replacement therapy; the reported mortality is 1% and clinically significant hemorrhages occur in 12.5% of cases.

The likelihood of hepatitis is greater in those who have been treated regularly or in those who started therapy at a young age than in those who have received treatment on demand. The exclusion of HBsAg and anti-HCV carriers from plasma donation, the pasteurization of factor VIII, and especially the use of recombinant factor VIII will significantly reduce the incidence of hepatitis in these patients.

## 7 Connective Tissue Diseases

### 7.1 Systemic Lupus Erythematosus

The most frequent cause of liver dysfunction in systemic lupus erythematosus (SLE) is toxicity due to salicylates, which generally presents as an anicteric hepatitis with considerable increases in serum aminotransferase and alkaline phosphatase activity. It generally occurs in patients who take more than 2 g of acetylsalicylic acid daily [30].

It is not known whether SLE predisposes to aspirin toxicity or whether the greater frequency of salicylate-induced hepatitis in patients with SLE is related to the fact that these patients are often treated with high doses of this drug [31].

An asymptomatic increase in aminotransferases is observed in 10% of patients with SLE, without any reason for this abnormality except the existence of the lupus itself. In some of these patients, serum aminotransferase levels fluctuate depending on the degree of SLE activity [31].

Cases of cholestatic hepatitis associated with therapy with nonsteroidal anti-inflammatory drugs such as naproxen or sulindac have been reported.

The presence of antiphospholipid antibodies (antibodies against cardiolipin) has been associated with thrombosis of the suprahepatic veins, in the form of Budd-Chiari syndrome [32], and with veno-occlusive disease of the liver [33].

Other hepatic lesions associated with SLE have occasionally been found, such as granulomas, chronic hepatitis, and steatosis. Rare cases of primary biliary cirrhosis associated with SLE have also been reported. In some of these cases, biliary cirrhosis preceded the appearance of SLE, while in others the reverse was true. Two cases of spontaneous liver rupture have been reported.

### 7.2 Systemic Sclerosis

Liver involvement is uncommon in systemic sclerosis. Primary biliary cirrhosis (PBC) develops in less than 1% of patients with scleroderma. Most of these patients present with the clinical form called CRST (calcinosis cutis, Raynaud's phenomenon, sclerodactyly, and telangiectasia) syndrome. The association with PBC can be identified at an early stage by means of a positive mitochondrial antibody test.

### 7.3 Mixed Connective Tissue Disease

Mixed connective tissue disease (MCTD) is characterized by overlapping features of SLE, scleroderma, and polymyositis, and it is usually associated with high titers of antibodies against the ribonucleoprotein fraction of extractable nuclear antigens. Some patients end up developing SLE or scleroderma but others can only be classified as affected by MCTD.

Usually no liver changes are detected in MCTD. Marshall et al. [34] detected signs of liver disease in four patients with MCTD: active chronic hepatitis in one, steatosis in another, and passive congestion in two. Other cases of MCTD associated with active chronic hepatitis have been reported but in none has it been possible to definitely rule out a viral etiology.

### 7.4 Rheumatoid Arthritis

Abnormal liver function tests are found in 6%–10% of patients with rheumatoid arthritis (RA) – usually an increase in alkaline phosphatase and γ-glutamyltransferase activity – but they are not associated with clinical signs or with a common histologic pattern. When liver biopsies are performed in consecutive series of patients with RA, the most frequent finding (seen in 60%–70% of cases) is a nonspecific reactive hepatitis with fatty change [35]. Laffon et al. [36] have observed sinusoidal dilatation in liver biopsies from patients with RA and a mild increase in alkaline phosphatase.

The liver abnormality associated most consistently with RA is nodular regenerative hyperplasia (NRH). Seventy percent of patients with NRH have portal hypertension, which can present as ascites or as gastrointestinal bleeding due to rupture of esophageal varices. NRH has been observed particularly in patients with Felty's syndrome, which is characterized by the combination of RA, leukopenia, and splenomegaly [37]; it is very rare in uncomplicated RA. Two-thirds of patients with NRH have hepatomegaly and one-third, abnormal liver function tests. The diagnosis is achieved by means of histology but is sometimes difficult in specimens obtained by percutaneous needle biopsy (Fig. 7). Catheterization of the suprahepatic veins shows an increase in wedged suprahepatic pressure.

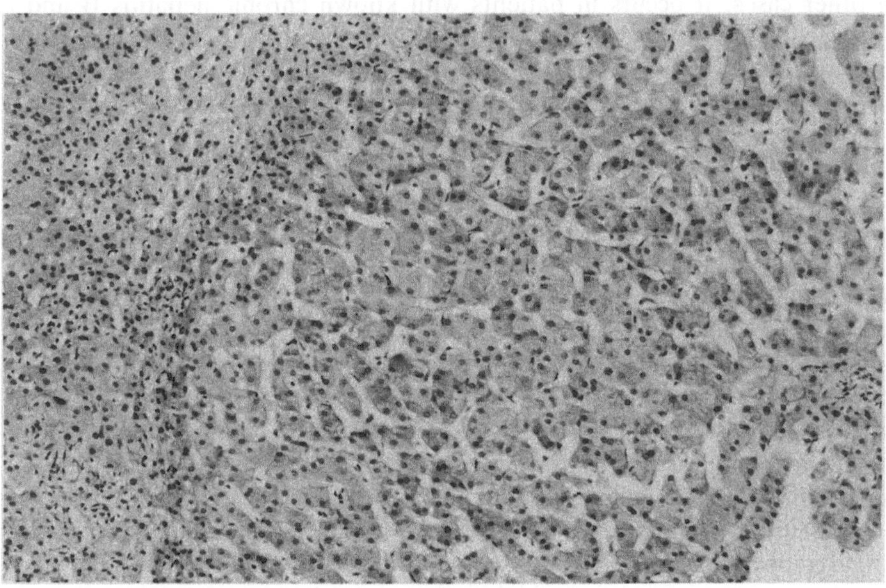

**Fig. 7.** Nodular regenerative hyperplasia. There is a well – defined nodule of hepatic cells which compresses surrounding parenchyma. H&E, ×200

Very rarely, cases of primary biliary cirrhosis and spontaneous liver rupture secondary to arteritis have been reported in patients with RA. Patients treated with nonsteroidal anti-inflammatory drugs are exposed to a risk of toxic hepatitis.

### 7.5 Polyarteritis Nodosa

Liver involvement is relatively common in polyarteritis nodosa, either because of vasculitic lesions of hepatic arteries or because of hepatitis B virus (HBV) infection, which is an important etiologic factor of this vascular condition.

The examination of the serologic markers of HBV shows HBsAg positivity in 11%–69% of cases [38], generally associated with the presence of HBeAg and HBV DNA. In some studies, viral antigens have been found by immunofluorescence in the vascular lesions and by other techniques in circulating immune complexes; this has led to the concept that HBV is involved in the genesis of the vasculitis through (a) the deposition of immune complexes in the arterial wall, (b) activation of the complement system, and (c) release of chemotactic factors that attract polynuclear leukocytes, which release lysosomal enzymes and damage the vascular wall.

In some cases, vasculitis develops at the same time as acute hepatitis B; in other cases, it occurs in patients with known chronic hepatitis B and a history of previous acute hepatitis; and, finally, some patients with polyarteritis nodosa without symptoms or a history of liver disease are found to be positive for HBsAg and yield abnormal results in the liver function tests.

Treatment with high doses of corticosteroids favors replication of the HBV and has a harmful effect on the liver disease. For this reason, for the treatment of polyarteritis nodosa associated with HBV infection an approach has been proposed that combines (a) interferon or vidarabine to inhibit viral replication, (b) plasmapheresis to deplete circulating immune complexes, and (c) short-lasting anti-inflammatory therapy with high doses of corticosteroids [39].

Vasculitic lesions in the branches of the hepatic artery are observed in more than 40% of autopsy studies from patients with polyarteritis nodosa, but such lesions are far less often clinically detectable. The vasculitic lesions induce arterial occlusion that may cause hepatic infarctions or a subcapsular hematoma, with the risk of spontaneous rupture of the liver.

Vasculitic lesions are rarely present in liver biopsy specimens. Angiography of hepatic arteries is a more useful diagnostic method as it reveals microaneurysms in a high proportion of cases. Laparoscopy may offer data of diagnostic value consisting in the formation of whitish tracts on the liver surface as an indication of inflammatory changes in the superficial arteries [40].

Occasionally, acute cholecystitis may be the initial sign of polyarteritis nodosa [41].

### 7.6 Polymyalgia Rheumatica

Abnormalities in the liver function tests, particularly increases in alkaline phosphatase, have been described in 40%–60% of patients with polymyalgia rheumatica and Horton's arteritis [42]; these changes disappear when the disease starts to regress under treatment. In some cases, granulomas are detected in the liver biopsy specimen.

## 8 Sarcoidosis

Sarcoidosis is an illness of unknown etiology and pathogenesis that is characterized by the presence of noncaseating epithelioid granulomas in numerous body tissues, particularly the lymph nodes and the lungs.

There are geographic variations in the incidence of the disease, and it is most common in Scandinavian countries. The most frequent clinical features are fever, weight loss, arthralgias, and erythema nodosum. Lytic lesions in the bones, interstitial lung infiltrates, and lymph node involvement, both in the mediastinum and in other areas, may be observed. Some patients develop ocular complications, such as iridocyclitis and uveitis. Laboratory tests frequently show hypercalcemia and increased serum angiotensin converting enzyme (ACE) levels.

The disease can only be diagnosed by histologic demonstration of granulomas, either by skin biopsy, biopsy of a mediastinal lymph node by mediastinoscopy, lung biopsy by means of a transbronchial biopsy, or liver biopsy.

### 8.1 Clinical Features of Liver Involvement

Liver granulomas are detected in 60% of patients with sarcoidosis, but they are usually asymptomatic. In 20%–25% of the cases, hepatomegaly is detected, and in half of these there is splenomegaly due to granulomatous infiltration of the spleen, portal hypertension, or both. Liver involvement is more frequent in those cases with systemic symptoms such as fever and arthralgias, those with lung and mediastinal involvement, and those with erythema nodosum.

Liver function tests are normal or mildly abnormal. Serum aminotransferase levels are slightly raised in some cases and alkaline phosphatase is increased in more than half of patients with hepatic granulomas. Hypergammaglobulinemia is a common finding. ACE levels are high in 50%–80%

of cases, but this is a nonspecific finding since ACE levels can also be high in other liver granulomatoses, such as primary biliary cirrhosis, leprosy, and miliary tuberculosis.

A small number of patients have portal hypertension or cholestasis. Portal hypertension is presinusoidal and is caused by the presence of granulomas in portal tracts [43]. In one reported case it was due to Budd-Chiari syndrome [43]. It can manifest as gastrointestinal hemorrhage due to rupture of esophageal varices or ascites.

Cholestasis is very uncommon. It may be caused by obstruction of the common bile duct due to hilar adenopathies [44], but it has more frequently been caused by a destructive lesion of the small intrahepatic bile ducts due to granulomatous infiltration of portal tracts [45]. In these cases persistent jaundice, with pruritus and increased serum alkaline phosphatase and cholesterol levels, may be present.

Cases of sarcoidosis with cholestasis have been observed in young, generally black, males, and in white middle-aged females. In the latter group it is difficult to distinguish sarcoidosis from primary biliary cirrhosis. The diagnosis of sarcoidosis is based on a negative mitochondrial antibody test and the presence of granulomas in other body tissues, although in some patients both diseases may coexist [46].

## 8.2 Hepatic Sarcoid Granulomas

The presence of sarcoid granulomas in the liver is related to the duration of the disease and to its clinical expression, since they are found in 93% of chronic sarcoidosis cases, in 70% of those associated with erythema nodosum, and in only 50% of those without erythema nodosum.

Sarcoid granulomas consist of a nodal lesion formed by a central core of epithelioid cells and one or more giant cells, mixed with lymphocytes and plasma cells (Fig. 8). The epithelioid cells are arranged on a reticulin stroma which serves as a support. They do not display caseous necrosis, and only 10% show central necrosis. The presence of ACE has been demonstrated in the cytoplasm of epithelioid cells. Occasionally, asteroid and Schaumann bodies are observed in the cytoplasm of giant multinucleated cells formed by the fusion of epithelioid cells.

The granulomas are located principally in portal and periportal areas and less frequently in the lobules. They often tend to coalesce, forming conglomerates of granulomas. The number of granulomas is very variable in a percutaneous liver biopsy specimen.

The course of hepatic granulomas is protean. Some show complete resolution and disappear without trace, while others become fibrous nodes.

Sarcoid granulomas are sometimes the only histologic change in the liver, but in some cases they are accompanied by an inflammatory reactive

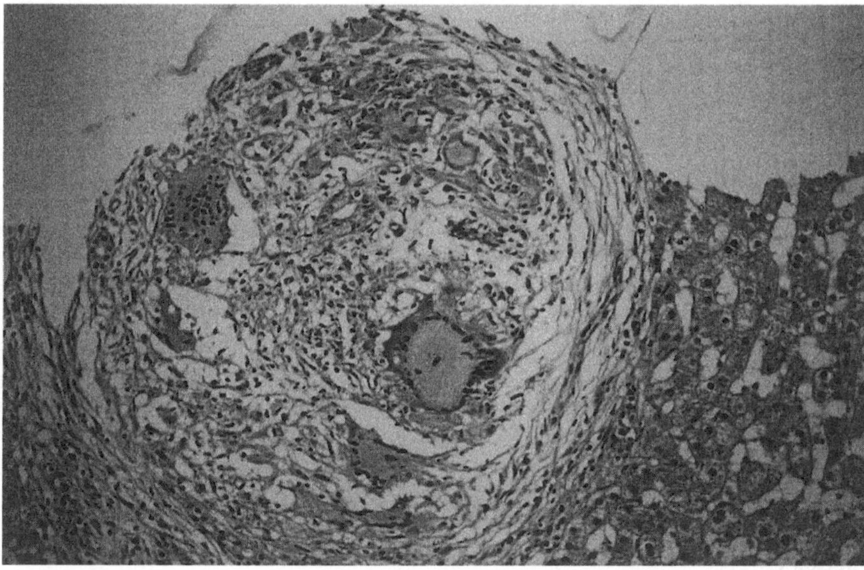

**Fig. 8.** Sarcoidosis. A large epithelioid granuloma with multinucleated giant cells surrounded by fibrosis. H&E, ×200

infiltrate in the portal tracts. In about 50% of cases, generalized or midzonal sinusoidal dilatation is observed.

There is no specific histologic feature that permits the diagnosis of sarcoidosis. Consequently, this diagnosis can only be suggested in the presence of a compatible clinical picture and when other possible causes of granulomas, such as mycobacteria, fungi, or protozoa, have been excluded by means of suitable histochemical stains.

## 9 Amyloidosis

Amyloidosis is a condition characterized by the extracellular deposition of fibrillar protein material which has a molecular configuration in the form of folded beta laminae. According to the type of protein deposited, it is classified as amyloidosis AL (immunologic) or amyloidosis AA (secondary). In the former, the amyloid substance is composed of fragments of immunoglobulin light chains, and in the latter of a protein called AA derived from a serum protein named SAA synthesized by the hepatocytes. Other types of amyloid substance are found in other types of amyloidosis which do not involve the liver (Table 4).

**Table 4.** Classification of amyloidosis

| Type | | Deposit |
|---|---|---|
| Immunologic | – Primary<br>– Associated with myeloma | AL protein |
| Nonimmunologic | – Secondary | AA protein |
| Familial | – Periodic disease | AA protein |
| | – Familial polyneuropathy | AF protein (prealbumin-like protein) |
| Localized | – Senile<br>– Endocrine tumors | AS protein (prealbumin) |
| Hemodialysis | | $\beta_2$-Microglobulin |

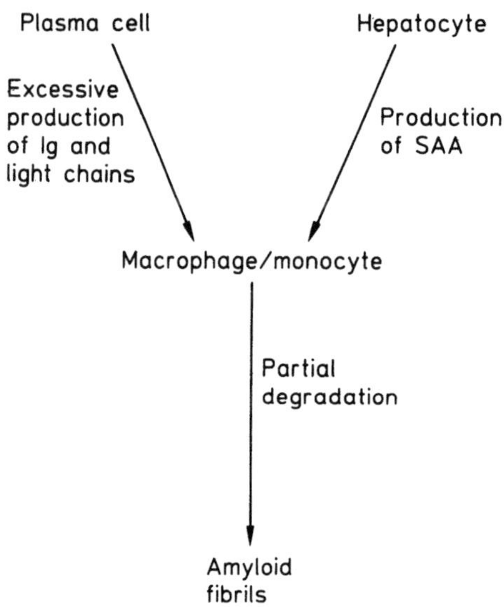


**Fig. 9.** Pathogenesis of amyloidosis

## 9.1 Pathogenesis

It is believed that a stimulus of unknown origin, or one due to a pre-existing disease, causes an increase in the rate of production of amyloid precursor (immunoglobulin light chains or SAA protein), or a modification in its structure. The phagocytic system (monocytes, macrophages) fragments these precursors and the resulting products are deposited in body tissues (Fig. 9) [47].

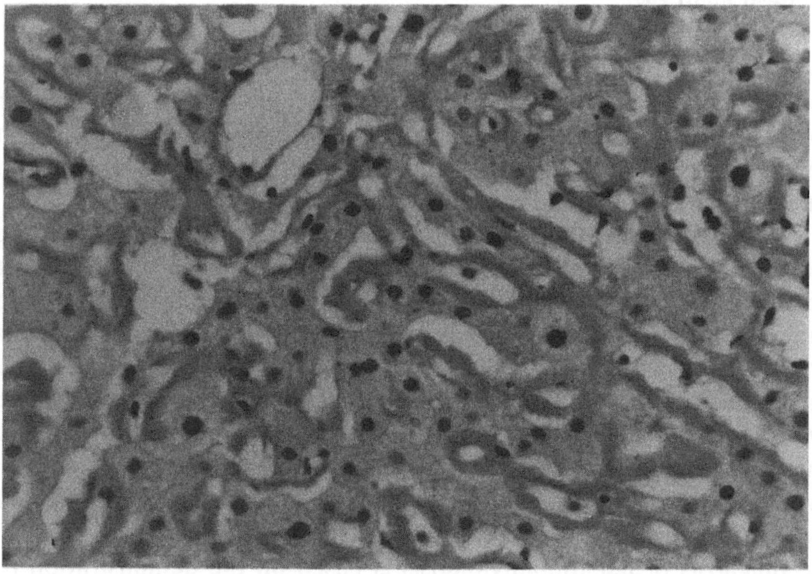

**Fig. 10.** Amyloidosis. Amyloid material lies in the sapce of Disse between the endothelial cells and hepatocytes. Congo red staining, ×300

### 9.2 Pathology

Between 75% and 90% of patients with amyloidosis, AL or AA, have deposits in the liver, which are found in the space of Disse, along the hepatic plates, and/or on the walls of arteries in the portal tracts. Although some studies have pointed out that the deposits of AL substance tend to be located in the sinusoids while the AA substance is preferentially located on the arteriolar walls [48], others have shown that there is no relationship between the type of amyloid substance and its location in the liver [49].

Amyloid substance is sometimes deposited in the form of globules 5–40 µm in diameter in the portal tracts or in the sinusoids [50]. There is no relationship between the clinical or biochemical type of the disease and this type of deposit, although it has not been found in amyloidosis associated with myeloma.

The amyloid substance has a homogeneous appearance and takes on a pink color when stained with hematoxylin and eosin and a blue or green color when stained with Masson's trichrome stain. When stained with Congo red (Fig. 10), it takes on a salmon pink color. When examined under polarized light, the amyloid substance stained with Congo red has a characteristic apple-green fluorescence.

The amyloid deposits in the sinusoids may cause atrophy of the hepatic plates and may even replace extensive areas of liver tissue. They are not associated with fibrosis or inflammatory reaction.

### 9.3 Clinical Features

Hepatic amyloidosis is usually asymptomatic. The deposits in the sinusoids may cause an increase in liver size, which may become very large. The liver function tests are normal, except for alkaline phosphatase, which is high in 60%–80% of cases, without any correlation with the degree of amyloid infiltration. Hypoalbuminemia is usually due to a nephrotic syndrome.

In exceptional cases, there is ascites and jaundice. The ascites may be secondary to hepatic amyloidosis and related to portal hypertension but it may be due to congestive heart failure or to hypoalbuminemia caused by the nephrotic syndrome. Extreme jaundice indicates a poor prognosis and is usually associated with a survival time of less than 6 months. Generally, there are no esophageal varices. Gastrointestinal hemorrhages are very rare; if they do appear, they are usually caused by amyloid infiltration and subsequent ulceration of the gastric mucosa.

Liver involvement is the cause of death in only 4%–7% of cases of amyloidosis; death is usually caused by heart and renal failure.

The diagnosis of hepatic amyloidosis is based on the demonstration of amyloid substance in the liver. However, liver biopsy is hazardous owing to an increased risk of hemorrhage (3%–5%, as opposed to 0.2% in biopsies for other indications) [51]. It is therefore preferable to confirm the presumed diagnosis of amyloidosis by histologic examination of other tissues, whose sampling is associated with a lower risk, such as rectal mucosa, gingival tissue, or abdominal fat.

The diagnosis of hepatic amyloidosis should be suspected in those patients with asymptomatic hepatomegaly who present with one or more of the items listed in Table 5.

## 10 Inflammatory Bowel Disease

Some of the hepatobiliary diseases associated with inflammatory bowel disease occur solely or predominantly in ulcerative colitis, such as primary sclerosing cholangitis and cholangiocarcinoma, while others, such as gallstones, granulomas, and hepatic amyloidosis are associated more with

**Table 5.** Clinical signs that should arouse suspicion of amyloidosis

| Signs | Frequency |
|---|---|
| Hepatomegaly disproportionate to enzyme changes | Common |
| Proteinuria | 80% |
| Hyposplenism in peripheral blood smear (Howell-Jolly bodies) | 50% |
| Hypergammaglobulinemia and monoclonal component | 30% |
| Macroglossia | 22% |
| Bilateral carpal tunnel syndrome | 20% |

Crohn's disease. It is difficult to establish the exact prevalence of each abnormality as it depends on the diagnostic means used and the patients selected for the diagnostic examination (Table 6). In autopsy series, the incidence of hepatic lesions is 75%, while abnormal liver function tests are found in 10%–50% of cases [52].

## 10.1 Primary Sclerosing Cholangitis

Primary sclerosing cholangitis (PSC) is recognized in about 1% of patients with ulcerative colitis and only very rarely in Crohn's disease. On most occasions, the symptoms of PSC appear in patients with chronic ulcerative colitis between the ages of 1 and 30 years (average 8 years), and they may arise even after complete resection of the colon has been performed. Only in one out of every ten cases does PSC present before the first symptoms of ulcerative colitis (the mean interval in such cases being 3½ years) [53].

Primary sclerosing cholangitis occurs most often in patients with general colonic involvement and its course is not related to that of ulcerative colitis. It is often asymptomatic and should be suspected in the event of a significant increase in alkaline phosphatase. Diagnosis requires endoscopic retrograde cholangiography.

The course of PSC is not affected by the therapeutic measures used in ulcerative colitis.

## 10.2 Pericholangitis

The term "pericholangitis" is applied to the inflammatory lesion of the portal tracts often observed in liver biopsy specimens from patients with ulcerative colitis. In some cases, the cellular infiltrate is arranged around the bile ducts and may be associated with a reduction in the number of bile

**Table 6.** Liver involvement in chronic inflammatory bowel disease

| | Ulcerative colitis | Crohn's disease |
|---|---|---|
| Fatty change | 30% | 30% |
| Primary sclerosing cholangitis | 5% | Rare |
| Chronic active hepatitis | 1%–2% | Rare |
| Cirrhosis | 3% | Rare |
| Bile duct carcinoma | Risk increased (tenfold) | No increased risk |
| Epithelioid granulomas | Absent | 5% |
| Amyloidosis | Absent | <1% |
| Gallstones | Normal incidence (5%) | Risk increased (15%–30%) |

ducts and cholangiolar proliferation. There is usually an increase in alkaline phosphatase and on endoscopic retrograde cholangiography the intrahepatic bile ducts have a beaded appearance identical to that observed in PSC. In such cases, the pericholangitis corresponds to sclerosing cholangitis affecting only the small intrahepatic bile ducts [54]. In other cases, the portal inflammation is asymptomatic and is not accompanied by biochemical changes; such cases must be interpreted as nonspecific reactive hepatitis.

### 10.3 Cholangiocarcinoma

Cholangiocarcinoma is usually a complication of PSC and commonly occurs in patients with ulcerative colitis, although exceptionally it has been described in association with Crohn's disease. It may appear without any prior PSC. The tumor affects particularly the extrahepatic bile duct, although cases of intrahepatic cholangiocarcinomas have been reported. Cholangiocarcinoma is difficult to recognize in patients with PSC as the x-ray images are not sufficiently discriminating.

The tumor appears a number of years after the onset of the ulcerative colitis (average: 15 years), and may do so even when a colectomy has been performed beforehand.

### 10.4 Hepatic Granulomas

Asymptomatic, nonnecrotizing, epithelioid granulomas are occasionally observed in patients with Crohn's disease. They have no prognostic significance.

### 10.5 Amyloidosis

Amyloidosis occurs with a low frequency in patients with Crohn's disease and generally involves the liver and the kidneys. The amyloid deposits appear from 1 to 21 years (average: 10 years) after the onset of symptoms of bowel disease. They may regress after excision of the inflammatory lesions, although the intraoperative morbidity and mortality are very high in these patients.

### 10.6 Other Hepatic Lesions

Fatty liver is the most common histologic lesion, in both ulcerative colitis and Crohn's disease. It consists of macrovesicular deposits in periportal hepatocytes. It is probably related to malnutrition and usually disappears without sequelae as the activity of the intestinal lesion lessens.

Between 2% and 5% of patients with inflammatory bowel disease have chronic hepatitis with or without cirrhosis. Some of the histologically diagnosed cases of chronic hepatitis may correspond to PSC, as the histologic changes observed in percutaneous liver biopsies are often similar. True cases of chronic hepatitis may be caused by infection by hepatitis B or C virus.

The therapy used for inflammatory bowel diseases, such as parenteral nutrition or sulfasalazine, may cause liver damage. Sulfasalazine-induced hepatitis is usually associated with hypersensitivity symptoms, such as fever, skin rash, or hypereosinophilia [55].

In Crohn's disease, centrilobular or diffuse sinusoidal dilatation has been observed in liver biopsies of asymptomatic patients [56].

### 10.7 Gallbladder Stones

Gallbladder stones are common in patients with Crohn's disease who present with involvement of the terminal ileum. They are attributed to oversaturation of the bile with cholesterol due to malabsorption of bile salts. They are asymptomatic in 80% of cases.

## 11 Thyroid Disease

### 11.1 Thyrotoxicosis

Liver function tests yield abnormal results in approximately 15% of cases, mainly as a mild increase in serum aminotransferase and alkaline phosphatase activity. These abnormalities revert slowly to normal after successful treatment. Patients may be misdiagnosed as having chronic hepatitis, because of the fatigue and the aforementioned mildly abnormal liver function tests. Liver biopsy is normal or shows only minor lesions.

Jaundice occurs exceptionally in severe thyrotoxicosis or in patients with cardiac failure. Three percent of patients with autoimmune chronic active hepatitis have coexistent hyperthyroidism.

### 11.2 Hypothyroidism

Hypothyroidism can be accompanied by elevated aspartate aminotransferase levels, falsely suggesting a liver lesion. This is, however, usually due to a general increase in muscle enzymes secondary to hypothyroid myopathy.

Increased alkaline phosphatase activity has been reported in some cases of subacute thyroiditis. Ascites may be erroneously taken as a sign of hepatic disease in some myxedematous patients.

## References


1. Reyes H (1982) The enigma of intrahepatic cholestasis of pregnancy: lessons from Chile. Hepatology 2:87–96
2. Schreiber AJ, Simon FR (1983) Estrogen induced cholestasis: clues to pathogenesis and treatment. Hepatology 3:607–613
3. Reyes H, Radrigan ME, Gonzalez MC et al. (1987) Steatorrhea in patients with intrahepatic cholestasis of pregnancy. Gastroenterology 93:584–590
4. Wilson JAP (1987) Intrahepatic cholestasis of pregnancy with marked elevation of transaminases in black Americans. Dig Dis Sci 32:665–668
5. Laatikainen T, Tulenheimo A (1984) Maternal serum bile acid levels and fetal distress in cholestasis of pregnancy. Int J Gynecol Obstet 22:91–94
6. Pockros PJ, Peters RL, Reynolds TB (1984) Idiopathic fatty liver of pregnancy: findings in ten cases. Medicine (Baltimore) 63:1–11
7. Riely CA, Latham PS, Romero R, Duffy TP (1987) Acute fatty liver of pregnancy. A reassessment based on observations in nine patients. Ann Intern Med 106:703–704
8. Ebert EC, Sun EA, Wright SH et al. (1984) Does early diagnosis and delivery in acute fatty liver of pregnancy lead to improvement in maternal and infant survival? Dig Dis Sci 29:453–455
9. Ockner SA, Brunt EM, Cohn SM, Krul ES, Hanto DW, Peters MG (1990) Fulminant hepatic failure caused by acute fatty liver of pregnancy treated by orthotopic liver transplantation. Hepatology 1:59–64
10. Rolfes BD, Ishak KG (1986) Liver disease in toxemia of pregnancy. Am J Gastroenterol 81:1138–1141
11. Mckenna J, Dover NL, Brame RG (1983) Preeclampsia associated with hemolysis, elevated liver enzymes and low platelets – An obstetric emergency. Obstet Gynecol 62:751–754
12. Tong MJ, Thunby M, Rakela J et al. (1981) Studies on the maternal-infant transmission of the viruses which causes acute hepatitis. Gastroenterology 80:999–1004
13. Fos E, Bruguera M, Sanchez Tapias JM (1990) Transmisión vertical del virus de la hepatitis delta. Gastroenterol Hepatol 13:54–56
14. Khuroo MS, Datta DV (1980) Budd-Chiari syndrome following pregnancy. Report of 16 cases, with roentgenologic, hemodynamic and histologic studies of the hepatic outflow tract. Am J Med 68:113–121
15. Scheinberg IH, Sternlieb I (1975) Pregnancy in penicillamine treated patients with Wilson's disease. N Engl J Med 293:1300–1302
16. Newton ER, Turksoy N, Kaplan M, Reinhold R (1988) Pregnancy and liver transplantation. Obstet Gynecol 71:499–500
17. Jaffe ES (1987) Malignant lymphomas: pathology of hepatic involvement. Semin Liver Dis 7:257–268
18. Bruguera M, Caballero T, Carreras E, Aymerich M, Rodés, J, Rozman C (1987) Hepatic sinusoidal dilatation in Hodgkin's disease. Liver 7:76–80
19. Lefkowitch J, Faikow S (1985) Hepatic Hodgkin's disease simulating cholestatic hepatitis with liver failure. Arch Pathol Lab Med 109:424–426
20. Verdi CJ, Grogan TM, Protelli R, Richter L, Rangel C (1986) Liver biopsy immunotyping to characterize lymphoid malignancies. Hepatology 6:6–13
21. Gaulard P, Zafrani ES, Mavier P et al. (1986) Peripheral T-cell lymphoma presenting as predominant liver disease: a report of three cases. Hepatology 6:864–868
22. Lopez Guillermo A, Saperas E, Campo E et al. (1987) Linfoma hepatico primario asociado a SIDA. Med Clin (Barc) 10:453–455
23. Thaler M, Pastakia B, Shawker TH, O'leary T, Pizzo PA (1988) Hepatic candidiasis in cancer patients: the evolving picture of the syndrome. Ann Intern Med 108:88–100

24. Roquet ML, Zafrani ES, Farcet JP et al. (1985) Histopathological lesions of the liver in hairy cell leukemia: a report of 14 cases. Hepatology 5:496–500
25. Pereira A, Bruguera M, Cervantes F, Rozman C (1988) Liver involvement at diagnosis of primary myelofibrosis: a clinicopathological study of twenty-two cases. Eur J Haematol 40:355–361
26. Perez Villa F, Font J, Feliu E, Campo E, Ingelmo M (1988) Insuficiencia hepatica grave postesplenectomia en una paciente con metaplasia mieloide agnogénica. Med Clin (Barc) 91:108–110
27. Omata M, Johnson CS, Tong M, Tatter D (1986) Pathological spectrum of liver disease in sickle cell disease. Dig Dis Sci 31:247–256
28. Cohen A, Witzleben C, Schwartz E (1984) Treatment of iron overload. Semin Liver Dis 4:228–238
29. Leibowitz AI, Hartman RC (1981) The Budd-Chiari syndrome and paroxysmal nocturnal haemoglobinuria. Br J Haematol 48:1–6
30. O'Gorman T, Koff RS (1977) Salycilate hepatitis. Gastroenterology 72:726–728
31. Miller MH, Urowitz MB, Gladman DD, Blendis LM (1984) The liver in systemic lupus erythematosus. Q J Med 211:401–412
32. Pomeroy C, Knodell RG, Swaim WR et al. (1984) Budd-Chiari syndrome in a patient with the lupus. Gastroenterology 86:158–161
33. Pappas SC, Malone DG, Rubin L, Hoofnagle JH, James EA (1984) Hepatic veno-occlusive disease in a patient with systemic lupus erythematosus. Arthritis Rheum 27:104–108
34. Marshall JB, Ravendrhan N, Sharp GC (1983) Liver disease in mixed connective tissue disease. Arch Intern Med 143:1817–1819
35. Webb J, Whaley K, Mc Sween RNM, Nuki G, Dick WC, Buchanan W (1975) Liver disease in rheumatoid arthritis and Sjögren's syndrome. Ann Rheum Dis 34:70–76
36. Laffon A, Moreno A, Gutierrez Bucero A, Ossorio C, Sabando P, Moreno-Otero R (1989) Hepatic sinusoidal dilatation in rheumatoid arthritis. J Clin Gastroenterol 11:653–657
37. Blendis LM, Parkinson MC, Shilkin KB, Williams R (1974) Nodular regenerative hyperplasia of the liver in Felty's syndrome. Q J Med 43:25–32
38. Le Thi Huong D, de Gennes C, Guillevin L et al. (1989) Foie et periarterite noueuse. Gastroenterol Clin Biol 13:141–148
39. Trepo C, Ouzan D, Delmont J, Tremisi J (1988) Superiorité d'un nouveau traitement étiopathogenique curateur des periarterites noueuses induites par le virus de l'hépatite B grâce à l'association corthicothérapie brève, vidarabine, échanges plasmatiques. Presse Med 17:1527–1531
40. Solis Herruzo JA, Muñoz Yagüe MT, Colina F (1979) Hallazgos laparoscopicos en la poliarteritis nodosa. Gastroenterol Hepatol 2:231–235
41. Li Volsi V, Perzin KH, Porter M (1973) Polyarteritis nodosa of the gallbladder, presenting as acute cholecystitis. Gastroenterology 65:115–123
42. Ogilvie AL, James PD, Toghill PJ (1981) Hepatic artery involvement in polymyalgia arteritica. J Clin Pathol 34:769–772
43. Valla D, Pessegueiro-Miranda H, Degott C et al. (1987) Hepatic sarcoidosis with portal hypertension. A report of seven cases with a review of the literature. Q J Med 63:531–544
44. Planas R, Pascual D, Del Castillo D et al. (1985) Colestasis extrahepática por sarcoidosis. Gastroenterol Hepatol 8:303–306
45. Bass NM, Burroughs AK, Scheuer PJ, James GD, Sherlock S (1983) Chronic intrahepatic cholestasis due to sarcoidosis. Gut 23:417–421
46. Fagan EA, Moore-Gillon JC, Turner-Warwick M (1983) Multiorgan granulomas and mitochondrial antibodies. N Engl J Med 308:572–575
47. Cohen AS, Hellen-Connors L (1987) The pathogenesis and biochemistry of amyloidosis. J Pathol 151:1–10

48. Chopra S, Rubinow A, Koff RS, Cohen AS (1984) Hepatic amyloidosis. A histopathologic analysis of primary (AL) and secondary (AS) forms. Am J Pathol 115:186–193
49. Garcia Pagan JC, Bruguera M, Rodés J (1987) Amiloidosis hepática. Estudio clinicopatológico. Gastroenterol Hepatol 10:64–68
50. Kanel GC, Uchida T, Peters RL (1981) Globular hepatic amyloid – an unusual morphological presentation. Hepatology 1:647–652
51. Gertz MA, Kyle RA (1988) Hepatic amyloidosis (primary (AL) immunoglobulin light chain): the natural history in 80 patients. Am J Med 85:73–80
52. Pariente EA (1981) Foie, voies biliaires et enterocolites cryptogenetiques. Gastroenterol Clin Biol 5:1120–1131
53. Steckman M, Drossman DA, Lesesne HR (1984) Hepatobiliary disease that precedes ulcerative colitis. J Clin Gastroenterol 6:425–428
54. Wee A. Ludwig J (1985) Pericholangitis in chronic ulcerative colitis: primary sclerosing cholangitis of the small bile ducts. Ann Intern Med 102:581–587
55. Fich A, Schwartz J, Braverman D, Zifroni A, Rachmilewitz D (1984) Sulfasalazine hepatotoxicity. Am J Gastroenterol 79:401–402
56. Capron JP, Lemay JL, Gontier MF, Dupas JL, Capron-Chivrac D, Lorriaux A (1979) Hepatic sinusoidal dilatation in Crohn's disease. Scand J Gastroenterol 14:987–992

## Suggested Reading

Bruguera M, Moreu I (1989) Sarcoidosis e hígado. In: Badrinas F, Morera J (eds). Sarcoidosis. DOYMA, Barcelona
Dao T, Davy A, Verwaerde JC, Galateau F, Valla A (1990) Amylose hépatique. Gastroenterol Clin Biol 14:534–543
Lieberman J (1985) Sarcoidosis. Grune & Stratton, Orlando, Florida
Rolfes DB, Ishak KG (1986) Liver disease in pregnancy. Histopathology 10:555–570
Rustgi VK, Hoofnagle JH (1987) Viral hepatitis during pregnancy. Semin Liver Dis 7:40–46
Schrumpf E, Fausa O, Elgjo K, Kolmannskjog F (1988) Hepatobiliary complications of inflammatory bowel disease. Semin Liver Dis 8:201–209
Weinblatt ME, Teser JRP, Gillian JH (1982) The liver in rheumatic diseases. Semin Arthritis Rheum 11:399–407

# 19 Drug-Induced Liver Diseases

D. PESSAYRE

The liver is the first organ encountered by drugs after their absorption from the gut. It is also richly endowed in enzymatic systems that metabolize foreign compounds. In the process, highly toxic intermediates may be formed. It is not surprising, therefore, that the liver should be a principal site for adverse drug reactions. Indeed, iatrogenic liver injury is a frequent cause of liver disease in elderly individuals, who are less likely than younger ones to have been exposed recently to hepatitis viruses and are more likely to take many medications simultaneously. Whereas discontinuation of the treatment usually leads to prompt recovery, pursuing it may lead to fulminant hepatitis or chronic liver lesions. Prompt recognition of an iatrogenic cause, and immediate withdrawal of the offending drug, should therefore be a major concern for physicians.

Acquiring some knowledge of drug-induced liver injury may seem a formidable task, however. Drugs may damage the liver through a variety of mechanisms and may lead to a variety of liver lesions. Indeed, it is now clear that in addition to acute hepatitis, bland cholestasis, and steatosis, drugs may also produce subacute hepatitis, chronic hepatitis, cirrhosis, rarefaction of small bile ducts, sclerosing cholangitis, vascular lesions, and hepatic tumors. As a corollary, a drug-induced etiology should be considered in almost any kind of liver disease. Also, the number of drugs which are now known to have the potential to cause liver damage has increased steadily over the years, with the introduction of new drug molecules and also with the late recognition of the hepatotoxicity of older medications such as aspirin, isoniazid, and papaverine. Currently, more than 600 drugs are thought to be potentially hepatotoxic. Finally, each drug tends to produce a particular type of liver disease. Differences concern the usual time interval between onset of treatment and onset of liver injury, the presence or not of immunoallergic and/or extrahepatic manifestations, the type of liver lesion(s), and the outcome. Clearly, the human mind cannot memorize all these data. The reader is referred to the useful book by STRICKER and SPOELSTRA [1] for such a compilation. It is important, however, to have some direct knowledge of the mechanisms responsible for drug-induced liver lesions, the types of liver lesion that may be encountered, and the main drugs producing these effects. The present chapter is an attempt to summarize this basal knowledge.

Drug-induced liver lesions are often classified into acute and chronic liver lesions [2] (Table 1). By far the most frequent liver lesion is acute hepatitis.

## 1 Mechanisms Involved in Acute Hepatitis

Acute hepatitis is often related to the formation in the liver of toxic metabolites. This formation is itself related to the primordial role of the liver in drug metabolism.

### 1.1 Role of the Liver in Drug Metabolism

Animals and man have been surrounded since ancient times by a host of foreign molecules ("xenobiotics") that differ from the normal constituents of the cells. In recent years, chemists have created thousands of new molecules that are used as drugs or end up as environmental pollutants. Such

**Table 1.** Main drug-induced liver diseases

| |
|---|
| *Acute lesions* |
| Acute hepatitis |
| Hepatocellular necrosis |
| Cholestatic hepatitis |
| Mixed hepatitis |
| Granulomatous hepatitis |
| Bland hepatocellular cholestasis |
| Steatosis |
| *Chronic lesions* |
| Subacute hepatitis, chronic hepatitis, and cirrhosis |
| Phospholipidosis and alcoholic-like liver lesions |
| Prolonged cholestasis due to rarefaction of small bile ducts |
| Sclerosing cholangitis |
| Vascular lesions |
| Lesions of hepatic artery and portal vein |
| Hepatoportal sclerosis |
| Perisinusoidal fibrosis |
| Sinusoidal dilation |
| Peliosis hepatis |
| Nodular hyperplasia |
| Veno-occlusive disease |
| Budd-Chiari syndrome |
| Hepatic tumors |
| Hepatocellular adenoma |
| Focal nodular hyperplasia |
| Hepatocellular carcinoma |
| Angiosarcoma |
| Other malignant tumors |

xenobiotics enter the body by one route or another and must be eliminated. This is easily performed for hydrophilic molecules, which can be dissolved in urine. In contrast, lipophilic compounds will not dissolve in urine and must first be transformed into hydrophilic metabolites. This transformation is mainly carried out in the liver.

Lipophilic drugs circulate in plasma bound to plasma proteins. Unlike other endothelial cells, those cells lining the hepatic sinusoids are perforated by fenestrations that allow proteins and bound drugs to enter the space of Disse and to come into direct contact with hepatocytes. After diffusion in the hepatocyte, the lipophilic drug is transformed into a soluble metabolite by a combination of oxidation(s) and/or conjugation(s). For example, a lipophilic molecule initially deprived of a group that can be conjugated may first be oxidized to a hydroxylated metabolite. This metabolite can then be conjugated with a highly polar molecule such as glucuronic acid or sulfate. The resulting hydrosoluble metabolite can leave the liver, circulate in plasma in the unbound form, be filtered by renal glomeruli, and be eliminated in urine. Other conjugates are excreted in bile.

The oxidation of drugs in the liver is mediated largely by cytochrome P-450. Cytochrome P-450 is located mainly in the endoplasmic reticulum, an organelle which can be recovered from the cells as small vesicles termed microsomes. At least 20 different human isoenzymes of cytochrome P-450 have been isolated, and several others probably remain to be identified [3].

All these isoenzymes have the same oxidizing center, namely the iron of a heme molecule. This iron is attached to the sulfur of a cysteine of the protein moiety (Fig. 1). In front of the heme iron, the protein delineates a hydrophobic binding site. After binding of the substrate to this binding site, the heme iron is reduced from the ferric to the ferrous state by introduction

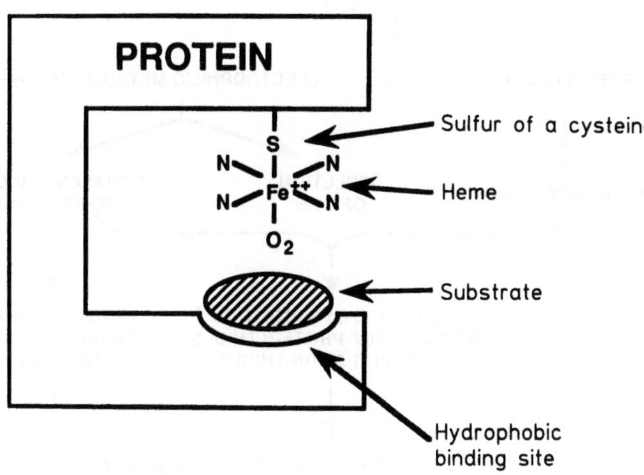


**Fig. 1.** Schematic structure of cytochrome P-450. Only the four nitrogens of the heme molecule have been drawn on this schematic representation

of an electron provided by a second microsomal enzyme, termed NADPH-cytochrome P-450 reductase. The ferrous heme iron then binds molecular oxygen. After introduction of a second electron, the oxygen molecule is split into its two constituent atoms. One of these atoms reacts with two protons to form a molecule of water. The other atom may be inserted into the drug substrate to form, for example, a hydroxylated metabolite. Oxidation by cytochrome P-450 may also lead to epoxidation, N-, S-, and O-dealkylation, N-oxidation, or, at times, desaturation.

The various isoenzymes differ in respect of their protein moiety and hydrophobic binding sites. Accordingly they have different affinities for different substrates. In addition, different isoenzymes will variously orient the same drug molecule toward the heme iron (and therefore the oxygen), so that different parts of the molecule will be oxidized. The multiplicity of the isoenzymes, the fact that each can accommodate many different substrates, and the inducibility of several isoenzymes represent a versatile system that has helped protect animals and man from xenobiotics. This system is not without drawbacks, however.

## 1.2 Formation and Inactivation of Reactive Metabolites

While many metabolites formed by cytochrome P-450 are stable entities that are more quickly eliminated and usually less toxic than the parent compound, other drugs are transformed into reactive, potentially toxic, metabolites (Fig. 2).

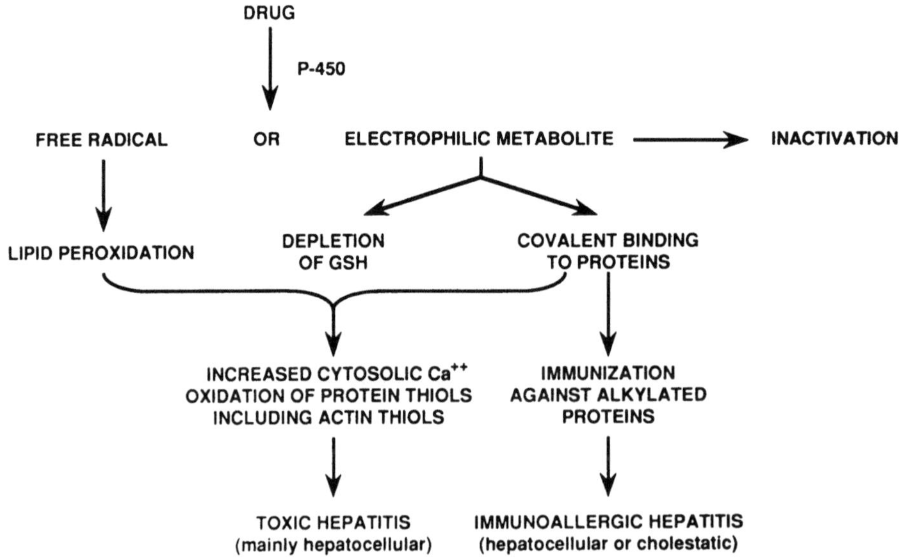


**Fig. 2.** Metabolite-mediated hepatitis

The potential toxicity of such metabolites is fortunately limited by several protective mechanisms. A first protective mechanism is the autodestruction of cytochrome P-450. Indeed, a reactive intermediate which has just been formed inside the hydrophobic pocket of cytochrome P-450 may directly attack this hemoprotein and destroy it, thereby preventing further formation of reactive species. A second protective mechanism is the transformation of a reactive metabolite into a stable metabolite. For example, the oxidation of several arenes or alkenes leads to the formation of reactive epoxides. These epoxides are transformed by epoxide hydrolases into inactive dihydrodiols. Another protective mechanism is the conjugation of reactive metabolites with hepatic glutathione, a reaction catalyzed by several glutathione-*S*-transferases. These various protective mechanisms efficiently limit the reaction of the reactive metabolites with hepatic constituents. When the formation of the reactive metabolite is important, however, some of the formed metabolite escapes inactivation and damages hepatic constituents.

### 1.3 Molecular Lesions Produced by Reactive Metabolites

Hepatotoxic metabolites may be classified into free radicals and electrophilic metabolites. Free radicals ($R^{\cdot}$) have an unpaired electron on their outer molecular orbital. They may abstract a hydrogen atom from unsaturated lipids (LH) to form a lipid radical ($L^{\cdot}$): $R^{\cdot} + LH \rightarrow RH + L^{\cdot}$. This lipid radical quickly adds molecular oxygen to form a peroxyl radical ($LOO^{\cdot}$). Unless detoxified by vitamin E, and subsequently by glutathione peroxidase, this peroxyl radical may in turn abstract a hydrogen atom from another lipid molecule, thereby propagating the process of lipid peroxidation: $\text{Lipid}_1\text{-OO}^{\cdot} + \text{Lipid}_2\text{-H} \rightarrow \text{Lipid}_1\text{-OOH} + \text{Lipid}_2^{\cdot}$.

Other free radicals (e.g., nitro anion radical, semiquinones) can react with molecular oxygen to regenerate the parent drug molecule (e.g., nitroarene, quinone) with the concomitant formation of a superoxide anion ($O_2^{\cdot-}$). The superoxide anion may in turn form other reactive oxygen species ($H_2O_2$, $^{\cdot}OH$) responsible for oxidative stress.

Most hepatotoxic reactive metabolites, however, are electrophilic metabolites. Such unstable intermediates react spontaneously with nucleophilic sites of proteins (such as the SH group of a cysteine residue, or the $\varepsilon$-$NH_2$ of a lysine moiety) to form a stable adduct, a process termed covalent binding.

### 1.4 In Situ Reaction of Reactive Metabolites

While some reactive metabolites, such as acetaldehyde, may be stable enough to leave the liver and react elsewhere, most are so highly unstable and, accordingly, short-lived that they react mainly in situ in the very organ that forms them. The abundance of cytochrome P-450 in hepatocytes and the in situ reaction of reactive metabolites explain the importance of reactive metabolites in the hepatotoxicity of drugs and chemicals. In the hepatic lobule, cytochrome P-450 predominates in the centrilobular region. These centrilobular hepatocytes therefore mainly form reactive metabolites. Because in addition centrilobular hepatocytes are relatively poor in glutathione, they are less effective in detoxifying reactive metabolites. For these two reasons, centrilobular hepatocytes are particularly susceptible to the damaging effects of reactive metabolites. These metabolites may lead to two types of hepatitis, toxic hepatitis and immunoallergic hepatitis (Fig. 2).

### 1.5 Functional Alterations Leading to Toxic Hepatitis

Lipid peroxidation may damage the endoplasmic reticulum and the plasma membrane. Extensive covalent binding to critical proteins may impair the function of enzymes, transport proteins, and structural proteins. Extensive formation of a glutathione adduct leads to the depletion of glutathione. Glutathione has three important roles in hepatocytes; consequently its depletion has severe toxicologic consequences. A first role of glutathione is to conjugate reactive metabolites. Once glutathione is depleted, the reactive metabolite which is still being formed can no longer react with glutathione and therefore remains available for binding to proteins. Depletion of glutathione allows extensive covalent binding to hepatic proteins. A second role of glutathione is to prevent lipid peroxidation through various mechanisms (reduction of lipid hydroperoxides by glutathione peroxidase and reduction of the vitamin E radical formed by the reaction of vitamin E with lipid peroxyl radicals). When glutathione is depleted, lipid peroxidation can freely develop. A third important role of glutathione is to maintain the SH groups of proteins in the reduced state. Depletion and/or oxidation of glutathione is associated with the oxidation of protein thiols into disulfides. This impairs the function of many proteins, including cytoskeletal proteins [4] and calcium translocases [5]. The molecule of actin has four reactive SH groups. Oxidation of these groups leads to the formation of macromolecular aggregates of actin which are not functional. Actin is the building block of microfilaments. Microfilaments are located under the plasma membrane and probably serve to maintain the shape of this membrane. The oxidation of actin disturbs this microfilamentous network, allowing the formation of cytoplasmic blebs. Rupture of a large bleb discharges the content of the cell in the extracellular milieu, leading to the death of the hepatocyte. A second consequence of the oxidation of protein thiols is the inactivation of calcium translocases present on the hepatocyte plasma membrane. Failure of these transporters to extrude calcium from the cell leads to a marked and sustained increase in cytosolic calcium. This will in turn activate phospholipase

$A_2$, proteases, and possibly endonucleases that will further damage the hepatocytes.

Reactive metabolites can also alter mitochondria, leading to decreased energy production. The final consequence of these various alterations is toxic liver cell necrosis.

## 1.6 Incidence of Toxic Hepatitis: Role of Acquired and Genetic Factors

A drug molecule that would produce constant or frequent hepatitis after therapeutic doses will not be introduced on the market. This fact means that toxic drug-induced hepatitis never occurs predictably after therapeutic doses. Therefore, drug-induced hepatitis can occur in only two ways: either predictably after overdoses (as in the case of paracetamol) or in an idiosyncratic fashion after therapeutic doses, which is by far the more frequent circumstance. The reasons for the susceptibility of these patients are incompletely understood. There is evidence, however, that both acquired and genetic factors may play a role in this apparent idiosyncrasy.

Induction of cytochrome P-450 may explain the susceptibility of some patients. Thus, therapeutic doses of paracetamol are usually well tolerated. In some chronic alcoholics, however, they may result in acute hepatic and renal injury. Alcohol induces cytochrome P-4502E1, which is one of the isoenzymes that transform paracetamol into a reactive metabolite. In some chronic alcoholics, the formation of the reactive metabolite may be increased sufficiently to result in toxicity at therapeutic doses. Fasting or protein malnutrition decreases hepatic glutathione. This will impair the protective effects of this tripeptide, explaining why some cases of hepatitis have been observed after therapeutic doses of paracetamol under these conditions.

A heterozygous deficiency in glutathione synthetase impairs the ability of the liver to resynthesize glutathione. This may lead to lower levels of glutathione during exposure to paracetamol, and to increased toxicity. As we will see later, genetic factors may also play an important role in the second type of drug-induced hepatitis, namely immunoallergic hepatitis.

## 1.7 Clinical Characteristics of Immunoallergic Hepatitis

The hepatitis due to many drugs exhibits features suggesting an immunoallergic mechanism. The following characteristics may help to distinguish these cases from toxic hepatitis. Immunoallergic hepatitis is usually associated with some hypersensitivity reactions such as fever, rash, or eosinophilia or even other extrahepatic immunoallergic complications such as hemolysis, immune thrombocytopenia, or interstitial nephritis. In contrast, no such association is present in toxic hepatitis. Immunoallergic hepatitis may be hepatocellular (with liver cell necrosis), cholestatic, or both, whereas toxic hepatitis is usually hepatocellular. Finally, an important feature of immunoallergic hepatitis is that it occurs much sooner after an inadvertent rechallenge (after a few hours or days of exposure) than during the first administration (often after 2 or more weeks of treatment).

## 1.8 Molecular Mechanisms Leading to Immunoallergic Hepatitis

The molecular mechanisms responsible for immunoallergic hepatitis are still poorly understood. There is evidence, however, that alkylated proteins (or peptides?) may serve as neoantigens, at least in some cases. Hepatocytes do not normally express HLA class II molecules. Kupffer cells, however, do express such molecules. During the normal cell turnover of hepatocytes, alkylated hepatocytic proteins from dead hepatocytes may be phagocytosed by macrophages and cut into alkylated peptides that may be presented on HLA class II molecules expressed on the surface of macrophages. These alkylated peptides may stimulate those helper T cells that can recognize these neoantigens, thereby initiating the immunization process, with the subsequent stimulation of cytotoxic T lymphocytes and antibody-producing B cells.

Although not expressing HLA class II molecules, hepatocytes express HLA class I molecules on their plasma membrane. These class I molecules might conceivably present alkylated peptides that might be recognized by cytotoxic T lymphocytes, although this has yet to be demonstrated. After administration of drugs transformed into reactive metabolites, there are covalently bound metabolites on plasma membrane proteins [6]. Such alkylated proteins, being exposed on the hepatocyte surface, may serve as targets for antibodies. Thus, halothane administration leads to the formation of a reactive trifluoroacyl chloride metabolite which covalently binds to the $\varepsilon$-$NH_2$ of lysine residues [7]. After exposure to halothane, trifluoroacetylated proteins are found on the plasma membrane surface of hepatocytes. In patients with severe halothane hepatitis, there are antibodies directed against these trifluoroacetylated proteins. One of these proteins is carboxylesterase. Another is probably a cytochrome P-450 isoenzyme. Indeed, cytochrome P-450 is present on the plasma membrane surface of hepatocytes [8] and serves as a neoantigen in some cases of autoimmune drug-induced hepatitis [9, 10]. In tienilic acid-induced hepatitis and in dihydralazine-induced hepatitis the patients' sera contain antimicrosomal autoantibodies termed respectively anti-$LKM_2$ and anti-LM antibodies (anti-liver kidney microsome type II and anti-liver microsome). These antibodies are specifically directed against the particular isoenzyme of cytochrome P-450 which transforms the drug into a reactive metabolite, namely cytochrome P-4502C8-10 for tienilic acid and P-4501A2 for dihydralazine. It is tempting to speculate that covalent binding of these reactive metabolites to the protein moiety of cytochrome P-450 has formed a neoantigen that has been initially responsible for the appearance of such autoantibodies.

### 1.9 Genetic Factors Involved in Immunoallergic Hepatitis

Two types of genetic factors may predispose to immunoallergic hepatitis. A first factor may be a defect in protective mechanism(s) [11–13]. This may lead to extensive alkylation of hepatic proteins by the reactive metabolite. Whereas alkylation of a few protein molecules might lead to infrequent immunization, extensive alkylation might lead to more frequent immunization. A deficiency in protective mechanisms (epoxide hydrolase, glutathione-*S*-transferase) has been suspected in immunoallergic hepatitis due to sulfonamides, phenytoin, carbamazepine, phenobarbital, amineptine, and perhaps also halothane.

A second factor may be the HLA phenotype. Different HLA molecules present different peptides so that a given HLA phenotype may favor the presentation of a given alkylated peptide, and may therefore favor immunization. An association with HLA All has been suspected in halothane-induced hepatitis and amineptine-induced hepatitis, while the HLA B8 phenotype may be more frequent in patients with hepatitis induced by oxyphenisatin, nitrofurantoin, and clometacin [14]. Because of the small numbers of patients, such associations remain only presumptive, however.

## 2 Clinicopathologic Aspects of Acute Hepatitis

Acute hepatitis is characterized by the presence in the hepatic lobule and the portal tracts of an inflammatory infiltrate, without fibrosis. This acute inflammation may be associated with liver cell necrosis ("hepatocellular necrosis"), cholestasis ("cholestatic hepatitis"), both necrosis and cholestasis ("mixed hepatitis"), or hepatic granulomas ("granulomatous hepatitis"). The most severe form is hepatocellular necrosis.

### 2.1 Hepatocellular Necrosis

The main liver lesion is hepatic necrosis, which often predominates in the centrilobular region. Necrosis is associated with an inflammatory infiltrate composed mainly of mononuclear cells and located both in the hepatic lobule and in portal tracts. Some steatosis may be present. Hepatocytic necrosis releases aminotransferases, whose activity in the serum is markedly increased.

**Table 2.** Drugs chiefly responsible for producing hepatocellular necrosis[a]

| | | |
|---|---|---|
| **Anesthesiology** | | |
| Chloroform | Ethyl ether | Isoflurane |
| Cyclopropane | Fluroxene | Methoxyflurane |
| Enflurane | *Halothane* | Trichloroethylene |
| **Oncology** | | |
| Carmustine | Estramustine | Nilutamide |
| Chlorozotocin | Flutamide | Procarbazine |
| Cyclophosphamide | Hydroxycarbamide | Streptozotocin |
| Cytarabine | Indicine *N*-oxide | Vincristine |
| Dacarbazine | Mithramycin | |
| **Cardiology** | | |
| *Dihydralazine* | Nicotinic acid | Phenprocoumon |
| Furosemide | *Papaverine* | Simvastatin |
| *Hydralazine* | Pyridinol carbamate | Suloctidil |
| *Methyldopa* | *Tienilic acid* | Verapamil |
| **Dermatology** | | |
| Etretinate | Povidone-iodine | Tannic acid |
| Methoxsalen | | |
| **Endocrinology** | | |
| Acetohexamide | Cyclofenil | Metahexamide |
| Carbutamide | Glythiazole | Propylthiouracil |
| **Hepatogastroenterology** | | |
| Calcium carbimide | Disulfiram | Trithiozine |
| Chenodeoxycholic acid | Oxyphenisatin | Salazosulfapyridine |
| **Infectious and parasitic diseases** | | |
| *p*-Aminosalicylic acid | Mebendazole | Sulfadoxine |
| *Amodiaquin* | Mepacrine | Sulfamethizole |
| Carbenicillin | Norfloxacin | *Sulfamethoxazole* |
| Clindamycin | Oxacillin | Sulfamethoxypyridazine |
| Cotrimoxazole | Piperazine | Sulfanilamide |
| *Dapsone* | *Protionamide* | Sulfapyridine |
| *Ethionamide* | *Pyrazinamide* | Sulfasuxidine |
| Hycanthone | Stibocaptate | Sulfathalidine |
| *Isoniazid* | Sulfadiazine | Sulfisoxazole |
| *Ketoconazole* | Sulfadimethoxine | Thioacetazone |
| Levamisole | | |
| **Neuropsychiatry** | | |
| Acetoxyphenacetamide | Levodopa | Pemoline |
| *Amitriptyline* | Loxapine | Phenelzine |
| Bromocriptine | Mebanazine | Pheniprazine |
| *Desipramine* | Metiapine | Phenoxyproperazine |
| Dothiepin | Methylphenidate | *Phenytoin* |
| Exifone | Nialamide | Phethenylate |
| *Imipramine* | Nomifensine | Tetrahydroaminoacridine |
| Isaxonine | Opipramol | *Valproic acid* |
| *Iproniazid* | Phenacetamide | Viloxazine |
| Lergotrile | | |
| **Nutrition and metabolism** | | |
| Fenofibrate | Gemfibrozil | Nicotinamide |

**Table 2.** *Continued*

| | | |
|---|---|---|
| **Radiology** | | |
| Iodipamide | Iopanoic acid | |
| **Rheumatology** | | |
| *Allopurinol* | Benoxaprofen | *Glafenine* |
| Aspirin | *Clometacin* | *Paracetamol* (overdosage) |
| Baclofene | *Dantrolene* | Salicylates |
| Benorylate | | |

[a] Drugs in italics are those which are more frequently implicated (either because they are widely used or because they have a marked hepatotoxic potential)

Depending on the severity of liver cell necrosis, the following presentation may be observed: (a) an asymptomatic increase in serum aminotransferases, (b) anicteric hepatitis with nausea, vomiting, abdominal pain, asthenia, anorexia, and, sometimes, hepatomegaly, (c) icteric hepatitis, (d) severe hepatitis with an increased prothrombin time, and (e) fulminant hepatitis with hepatic encephalopathy.

A diagnosis of drug-induced hepatocellular jaundice requires the immediate withdrawal of the responsible drug. Continuation of the treatment may cause either extension of liver necrosis, with the possible development of fulminant hepatitis, or the prolongation of liver cell necrosis, with the possible appearance of chronic liver lesions (see below).

The drugs chiefly responsible for hepatocellular necrosis are listed in Table 2. Only a few of them can be discussed in detail here.

### *Halothane*

Halothane is transformed by cytochrome P-450 in two ways. The reductive pathway leads to a free radical that can initiate lipid peroxidation and might be responsible for the latent, mild increase in serum aminotransferase activity observed in a sizeable percentage of recipients. The oxidative pathway leads to a trifluoroacetyl chloride intermediate which covalently binds to the $NH_2$ groups of proteins. Occasionally, immunization of recipients against these trifluoroacetylated proteins leads to the severe form of halothane-induced hepatitis. This severe form clearly has all the characteristics of an immunoallergic phenomenon [15]. It is extremely uncommon following a first exposure (1/10000) and is frequently associated with fever (75%) and eosinophilia (40%). The patient's serum contains antibodies directed against trifluoroacetylated proteins. Jaundice is more frequent after repeated exposures (7/10000) and it occurs sooner, the mean interval between exposure and onset of jaundice being 12 days after a first exposure, 7 days after a second, and 5 days after a third [15].

### *Isoniazid*

Isoniazid is first acetylated into acetylisoniazid, which is hydrolyzed into acetylhydrazine. Acetylhydrazine may be acetylated again into the nontoxic diacetylhydrazine or may be oxidized by cytochrome P-450 into the reactive acetyl radical which covalently binds to hepatic proteins and may produce a toxic type of hepatitis in some recipients [16]. Isoniazid given alone has been reported to increase serum alanine aminotransferase activity in 10% of recipients and to produce clinical hepatitis in 1% [17]. The peak incidence of hepatitis is during the 2nd month of treatment. Hypersensitivity reactions are absent. Concomitant administration of rifampicin, a microsomal enzyme inducer, increases the incidence of clinical hepatitis to 6% and hastens its occurrence, most cases beginning during the 1st month of treatment [18].

### *Paracetamol*

Paracetamol is transformed by cytochrome P-450 into a reactive quinone imine which is efficiently detoxified by glutathione. Taken at recommended doses (0.5–3 g daily), paracetamol is a safe analgesic [19]. Taken at higher doses, however, paracetamol may deplete hepatic glutathione and cause liver damage. This may occur in two circumstances. After high therapeutic doses (4–10 g daily), toxic hepatitis has occasionally been observed in alcoholics and in malnourished patients. After intentional overdoses, hepatitis is more frequent. Administration of *N*-acetylcysteine, however, liberates cysteine, allowing rapid resynthesis of glutathione and preventing severe hepatitis.

## 2.2 Cholestatic Hepatitis and Mixed Hepatitis

Cholestasis may be defined as the failure of bile to reach the duodenum. Histologically, bile pigments are deposited as bile "plugs" in caniculi or as small brownish pigments within the hepatocytes. In "cholestatic hepatitis," cholestasis is associated with an inflammatory infiltrate present mainly in the portal tracts. In "mixed hepatitis," necrosis is also present (together with cholestasis and inflammation).

Cholestatic or mixed hepatitis occurs with drugs transformed into reactive metabolites (e.g., amineptine, carbamazepine, chlorpromazine, erythromycin, imipramine, nitrofurantoin, sulfonamides). The disease is frequently associated with hypersensitivity manifestations and usually occurs earlier following a second exposure than it did on the first occasion. It is therefore tempting to speculate that it is due to immunization. The precise mechanism remains poorly understood, however. One has to speculate that the immune attack may somehow affect bile secretion and/or canalicular tight junctions in hepatocytes (canalicular cholestasis) and/or the integrity of small bile ducts in portal tracts.

In severe forms of cholestatic hepatitis, the patient is jaundiced with light stools and dark urine. Typically, pruritus is present, although it is not constant. Serum alkaline phosphatase activity and serum γ-glutamyltransferase activity are increased markedly. The activity of serum aminotransferases is increased slightly in cholestatic hepatitis and moderately in mixed hepatitis. In milder cases, there may be only pruritus or abnormalities of liver function tests.

After interruption of the drug administration, cholestatic or mixed hepatitis usually regresses. Recovery may take several months, however. In a few patients, chronic cholestasis due to rarefaction of small bile ducts may persist (see subsequent section).

The drugs that most frequently produce cholestatic or mixed hepatits are listed in Table 3. Only a few of them can be considered in some detail.

### *Amineptine*

Amineptine is a tricyclic antidepressant that is widely used in France and several other countries. It is transformed by cytochrome P-450 into a reactive metabolite and may lead during the first 3 months of treatment to mixed or cholestatic hepatitis [1]. The disease may be associated with fever and eosinophilia and recurs promptly after a rechallenge, suggesting an immunoallergic mechanism.

### *Carbamazepine*

Carbamazepine, an anticonvulsant, is transformed by cytochrome P-450 into the stable 10,11-epoxide, but also into several other (probably unstable) epoxides. Administration of carbamazepine may produce a mixed type of hepatitis within the first 6 weeks of treatment. The possible occurrence of fever, rash, eosinophilia, pancytopenia, agranulocytosis, thrombocytopenia, and lymphadenopathy, the frequent presence of hepatic granulomas, and the prompt recurrence upon rechallenge suggest an immunoallergic mechanism [20]. Lesions of cholangitis may be observed.

### *Chlorpromazine*

Chlorpromazine is transformed into reactive metabolites which occasionally lead to immunoallergic hepatitis. Jaundice due to this neuroleptic drug occurs within the first 5 weeks of therapy [15]. Pruritus is frequent. Hypersensitivity reactions such as fever, eosinophilia, or, less frequently, a skin rash are observed in up to 70% of patients. Antinuclear antibodies are found in about 40% of cases. Histologic lesions, with cholestasis and a

**Table 3.** Drugs chiefly responsible for producing mixed or cholestatic hepatitis[a]

| | | |
|---|---|---|
| **Oncology** | | |
| Aclacinomycin A | Chlorozotocin | *6-Mercaptopurine* |
| Aminoglutethimide | Chromomycin $A_3$ | Mitomycin |
| Amsacrine | Cisplatin | Streptozotocin |
| *Azathioprine* | Cytosine arabinoside | Thioguanine |
| Chlorambucil | *Cyclosporin* | |
| **Cardiology** | | |
| Ajmaline | Hydralazine | Procainamide |
| Aprindine | *Methyldopa* | Propafenone |
| Benziodarone | Mexiletin | *Quinidine* |
| Captopril | Nifedipine | Spironolactone |
| Chlorthalidone | Papaverine | *Ticlopidine* |
| Diltiazem | *Phenindione* | Verapamil |
| Disopyramide | Polythiazide | Warfarin |
| Flecainide | | |
| **Dermatology** | | |
| Isotretinoin | | |
| **Endocrinology** | | |
| Acetohexamide | Metahexamide | Thiouracil |
| Carbimazole | Methimazole | Tolazamide |
| *Chlorpropamide* | Propylthiouracil | Tolbutamide |
| Glibenclamide | Tamoxifen | |
| **Hepatogastroenterology** | | |
| Cimetidine | Penicillamine | Ranitidine |
| **Infectious and parasitic diseases** | | |
| *p*-Aminosalicylic acid | Nalidixic acid | *Sulfamethoxazole* |
| Arsphenamine | Niclofolan | *Sulfamethoxypyridazine* |
| Carbasone | *Nitrofurantoin* | *Sulfanilamide* |
| Cephalexin | Phenazopyridine | *Sulfapyridine* |
| Chloramphenicol | Quinine | *Sulfasuxidine* |
| Cotrimoxazole | Rifampicin | *Sulfathalidine* |
| *Erythromycin* | Sulfadiazine | *Thiabendazole* |
| Griseofulvin | Sulfadimethoxine | *Troleandomycin* |
| Hycanthone | Sulfadoxine | *Tryparsamide* |
| Josamycin | Sulfamethizole | |
| **Neuropsychiatry** | | |
| *Amineptine* | Fluphenazine | *Phenytoin* |
| *Amitriptyline* | Flurazepam | Prochlorperazine |
| Bromocriptine | Haloperidol | Promazine |
| *Carbamazepine* | *Imipramine* | Thioridazine |
| Chlordiazepoxide | Iprindole | Trazodone |
| *Chlorpromazine* | Isocarboxazide | Triazolam |
| *Desipramine* | Mianserin | Trifluoperazine |
| Diazepam | Phenobarbital | Zimelidine |
| **Rheumatology** | | |
| Baclofen | *Glafenine* | Phenopyrazone |
| Benoxaprofen | Gold salts | Phenylbutazone |
| Carprofen | Ibufenac | Piroxicam |
| Colchicine | Ibuprofen | Propoxyphene |
| *Diclofenac* | Indomethacin | Pyritinol |
| Diflunisal | Kebuzone | Sudoxicam |

**Table 3.** *Continued*

| | | |
|---|---|---|
| Fenbufen | Naproxen | *Sulindac* |
| Fenclozic acid | Niflumic acid | Probenecid |
| Feprazone | Oxyphenbutazone | Tolfenamic acid |
| Flurbiprofen | Penicillamine | Zoxazolamine |

[a] Drugs in italics are those which are more frequently implicated (either because they are widely used or because they have a marked hepatotoxic potential)

portal inflammatory infiltrate, are those of cholestatic hepatitis. Eosinophils are found in the liver in 25%–50% of cases, and cholangiolitis in 25%. Recovery may take several months and some cases have a chronic course (see below).

### *Erythromycin*

Erythromycin and its derivatives are transformed by cytochrome P-450 into unstable nitrosoalkane metabolites which may react with hepatic proteins and may produce immunoallergic hepatitis in some recipients [21]. Hepatitis is seen with erythromycin estolate, erythromycin propionate, and erythromycin ethylsuccinate [22]. It occurs mainly during the first 2 weeks of treatment. Associated manifestations include abominal pains (80% of patients), fever (60%), and eosinophilia (45%–80%). Hepatitis is cholestatic or mixed and usually has a good prognosis. Symptoms recur within 24–48 h after readministration of the same derivative; they may or may not recur after administration of another erythromycin derivative.

### *Nitrofurantoin*

Nitrofurantoin, a urinary tract antiseptic, is transformed into reactive metabolites. Most cases of jaundice due to nitrofurantoin occur in females, which may reflect both high use in this group and higher susceptibility [1]. Acute hepatitis occurs during the first 5 weeks of treatment. The association with fever (60%), rash (30%), and eosinophilia (70%) suggests an immunoallergic mechanism. Chronic hepatitis may also occur.

### *Sulfonamides*

Sulfonamides may be acetylated or transformed by cytochrome P-450 into a reactive metabolite. This metabolite itself may be detoxified or may covalently bind to hepatic proteins and produce an immunoallergic type of hepatitis in a few recipients. Those subjects who are poor acetylators and who have, in addition, a defect in a protective mechanism may be particularly susceptible [11]. Hepatitis due to sulfonamides usually occurs during the 1st month of treatment. It can be classified as mixed in type, although either the hepatocellular or the cholestatic component may predominate in a particular patient. Hepatitis may be accompanied by fever and rash. Hepatic granulomas may be present. The disease recurs promptly upon rechallenge.

## 2.3 Acute Granulomatous Hepatitis

A number of drugs (Table 4) may produce hepatic granulomas [23]. Small foci of epithelioid and round cells with, at times, multinucleated giant cells are present in the hepatic lobule, the portal tract, or both. Portal tract inflammation is usually present.

The presence of hepatic granulomas is thought to herald an immunoallergic disease, although the exact mechanism is still poorly understood. In some cases, the liver disease is essentially dominated by the presence of

**Table 4.** Drugs which may produce hepatic granulomas[a]

| | | |
|---|---|---|
| **Anesthesiology** | | |
| Halothane | | |
| **Oncology** | | |
| Procarbazine | | |
| **Cardiology** | | |
| Diltiazem | Phenprocoumon | *Quinidine* |
| Hydralazine | Prajmaline | Tocainide |
| Methyldopa | Procainamide | Trichlormethiazide |
| Papaverine | | |
| **Endocrinology** | | |
| Carbutamide | Glibenclamide | Tolbutamide |
| *Chlorpropamide* | | |
| **Hepatogastroenterology** | | |
| Ranitidine | Sulfasalazine | |
| **Infectious and parasitic diseases** | | |
| Bacillus Calmette-Guérin | Oxacillin | Sulfadoxine |
| Cephalexin | Penicillin | *Sulfamethoxazole* |
| Dapsone | Quinine | Sulfanilamide |
| Isoniazid | Sulfadiazine | Sulfathiazole |
| Nitrofurantoin | | |
| **Neuropsychiatry** | | |
| *Carbamazepine* | Diazepam | Nomifensine |
| Chlorpromazine | | |
| **Rheumatology** | | |
| *Allopurinol* | Gold salts | Phenazone |
| Aspirin | Oxyphenbutazone | Phenylbutazone |
| Feprazone | | |

[a] Drugs in italics are those which are more frequently implicated (either because they are widely used or because they have a marked hepatotoxic potential)

these granulomas, justifying the term "granulomatous hepatitis." Clinically, there may be pruritus and hepatomegaly. Serum alkaline phosphatase and serum $\gamma$-glutamyltransferase activity is increased, while serum aminotransferase activity is only slightly increased.

In many other cases, the presence of hepatic granulomas is discovered on the histologic slides in a patient with features of hepatocellular, cholestatic, or mixed hepatitis, as described above.

## 3 Bland Hepatocellular Cholestasis

Bland hepatocellular cholestasis is probably due to selective interference of the drug with canalicular bile secretion and/or tightness of tight junctions, without any hepatitis. Accordingly, cholestasis is the only liver lesion, without inflammation or necrosis. In the typical case, jaundice is associated with pruritus, increased serum alkaline phosphatase and $\gamma$-glutamyltransferase activity, a moderate increase in serum aminotransferase activity, and a normal biliary tree on ultrasonography. Pruritus, jaundice, or both may be absent, however.

### 3.1 Oral Contraceptives and Estrogens

Estrogens have at least three adverse effects on bile excretion. First, they are transformed into D-ring (17-β) glucuronides which exhibit an immediate and potent cholestatic effect. Second, their chronic administration increases the activity of cholesterol acylcoenzyme A acyltransferase, leading to the accumulation of cholesterol esters in plasma membrane. This may decrease membrane fluidity and inhibit $Na^+,K^+$-ATPase activity. This decreased activity may in turn reduce the uptake, and thus the canalicular secretion, of bile acids. Finally, prolonged administration of estrogens increases the permeability of tight junctions, leading to the retrodiffusion of bile components into the plasma. Jaundice due to oral contraceptives used to occur during the first 3 months of therapy and was more frequent in some countries (e.g., Chile and the Scandinavian countries) and in some families, suggesting a genetic predisposition. With the use of lower dosages of estrogens, however, jaundice due to oral contraceptives is now exceptional.

### 3.2 Anabolic/Androgenic Steroids

Anabolic/androgenic steroids with a C-17 alkyl substituent may inhibit $Na^+,K^+$-ATPase activity, selectively decrease the excretion of conjugated bilirubin into the bile canaliculi, and damage the pericanalicular microfilamentous network [24]. Jaundice due to such steroids often occurs after several months of treatment. Pruritus is uncommon, occurring in 10% of cases, and serum alkaline phosphatase activity is normal in 30%. Liver biopsy shows bilirubin casts in canaliculi and bile staining of hepatocytes. Subsidence of jaundice may require weeks or months.

## 4 Steatosis

It is convenient to distinguish two types of steatosis, microvesicular and macrovacuolar, although they may occur in association in an individual patient and although there might be transitions between the two forms.

### 4.1 Microvesicular Steatosis

The hepatocyte is occupied by many tiny lipid vesicles leaving the nucleus in a central position. An oil red O stain clearly shows the small reddish lipid vacuoles. Necrosis may be absent (as in the case of tetracycline-induced microvesicular steatosis) or present (as with valproic acid or pirprofen). Even when necrosis is abent, microvesicular steatosis, when extensive, is a serious condition. After a period of nausea, vomiting, and sometimes abdominal pain, the disease may worsen with the appearance of lethargy, hypotension, hemorrhagic episodes, and coma. Although serum aminotransferase activity and plasma bilirubin levels are not increased dramatically, the prothrombin time is nevertheless prolonged, at times markedly so. Hypoglycemia may occur. Leukocytosis is usual. Azotemia and pancreatitis may be present, contributing to the poor prognosis.

Drugs that have produced microvesicular steatosis have been shown to inhibit the mitochondrial β-oxidation of fatty acids [25–28]. Fatty acids not oxidized in the mitochondria undergo increased esterification into triglycerides and accumulate in the form of small lipid vesicles. In addition, tetracycline has been shown to inhibit the hepatic secretion of triglycerides from the liver.

Drug-induced microvesicular steatosis has been observed in the past after administration of tetracycline, Aureomycin, or minocycline in excessive doses, often by the intravenous route. This complication is not observed with the oral doses given nowadays.

Sodium valproate is a branched fatty acid used as anticonvulsant. It is desaturated by cytochrome P-450 into $\Delta_4$-valproate. This metabolite undergoes the β-oxidation process, with the formation of a reactive α,β-unsaturated ketone which inactivates β-oxidation enzymes. Administration of valproate may produce clinically silent increases in serum aminotransferase activity in 11%–67% of recipients [29]. Overt liver disease is much less common. It is seen mainly in young individuals and may be favored by the concomitant administration of phenobarbital and/or phenytoin, two microsomal enzyme inducers which increase the formation of $\Delta_4$-valproate by cytochrome P-450. Microvesicular steatosis is associated with necrosis and sometimes cirrhosis.

Pirprofen, a nonsteroidal anti-inflammatory compound with an arylpropionic structure, similarly produces a combination of necrosis and microvesicular steatosis [30]. Amineptine has produced a mild form of microvesicular steatosis in two patients.

### 4.2 Macrovacuolar Steatosis

The hepatocyte is enlarged and contains a single, large lipid droplet which displaces the nucleus to the periphery of the cells. In the absence of other liver lesions, macrovacuolar steatosis is a rather benign condition. Liver function tests may be slightly abnormal, however. The liver is sometimes enlarged and exhibits increased echogenicity on ultrasonography.

The main mechanism leading to macrovacuolar steatosis is thought to be an impaired egress of lipids from the liver [15]. Triglycerides are secreted by the liver as lipoproteins. The apoprotein moieties are synthesized in the endoplasmic reticulum and are glycosylated both here and in the Golgi apparatus. Decreased output of triglycerides may occur as a consequence of a specific biochemical lesion, as with methotrexate, which impairs protein synthesis. Glucocorticoids in high doses may also impair protein synthesis. In many other cases, decreased output of triglycerides occurs as a consequence of structural lesions of the endoplasmic reticulum, the Golgi apparatus, and perhaps the plasma membrane. This explains why macrovacuolar steatosis may be associated with hepatitis produced by a variety of drugs, such as allopurinol, halothane, isoniazid, α-methyldopa, and many others.

## 5 Subacute Hepatitis, Chronic Hepatitis, and Cirrhosis

Prolonged damage to liver cells, whatever the initial mechanism, may lead eventually to subacute hepatitis, chronic hepatitis, and even cirrhosis. Prolonged insult to the liver occurs when the drug is continued, either because the liver disease remains undetected or because its medicamentous etiology has been overlooked. In other cases, the drug has been withdrawn initially but its administration has been resumed before complete recovery. In a few cases, the liver disease continues to worsen, and chronic liver lesions may develop, despite total interruption of the treatment. This may be seen with some cationic amphiphilic drugs, such as amiodarone and perhexiline, which are stored in lysosomes and persist in the liver for several months. It also sometimes happens with drugs which, like iproniazid and tienilic acid, trigger an autoimmune response directed against normal hepatic constituents.

Three different types of liver lesion may be distinguished. *Subacute hepatitis* is characterized by lesions at different stages of evolution. Acute lesions are those of acute hepatitis, with lobular necrosis and inflammatory infiltration. They are associated with secondary lesions consisting of bridging necrosis, a term describing bands of parenchymal collapse (due to necrosis and subsequent cell drop-out) linking together two portal tracts or a portal tract and a central vein. Late lesions are suggestive of a chronic process, with portal fibrosis and, in some cases, nodular regeneration. The clinical presentation is usually severe. Jaundice may be associated with ascites, encephalopathy, hypoalbuminemia, and hypoprothrombinemia.

*Chronic hepatitis* is characterized by periportal hepatocyte necrosis (piecemeal necrosis) with portal inflammation and portal fibrosis, both of which may extend into the peripheral parenchyma. *Cirrhosis* is characterized by destruction of the lobular architecture, extensive fibrosis, and nodular regeneration. The clinical manifestations of chronic hepatitis and cirrhosis are extremely variable. In some patients, these chronic liver diseases may be discovered almost fortuitously during the investigation of slightly abnormal liver function tests. In others, the disease is heralded by jaundice, ascites, hepatic encephalopathy, hepatomegaly, or complications of portal hypertension. There may be hypoalbuminemia and hypoprothrombinemia.

Autoantibodies are frequently observed in subacute hepatitis, chronic hepatitis, and cirrhosis. Some of these antibodies, such as the antinuclear or anti-smooth muscle antibodies are not specific, being observed with several drugs, in particular clometacin, methyldopa, and papaverine. Other autoantibodies appear to be associated more specifically with a particular drug-induced liver disease. Thus, the anti-$LKM_2$ antibodies (anti-cytochrome P-4502C8-10) are observed in tienilic acid-induced hepatitis, the anti-LM antibodies (anti-cytochrome P-4501A2) in dihydralazine-induced hepatitis, and anti-M6 antimitochondrial antibodies (anti-monoamine oxidase) in iproniazid-induced hepatitis.

**Table 5.** Drugs chiefly responsible for producing subacute hepatitis, chronic hepatitis, or cirrhosis[a]

| | | |
|---|---|---|
| Acetohexamide | Glafenine | Papaverine |
| *Amiodarone* | Halothane | Paracetamol |
| Amodiaquin | *Iproniazid* | Perhexiline |
| Aspirin | Isoniazid | Propylthiouracil |
| Benzarone | Metahexamide | Suloctidil |
| Busulfan | *Methotrexate* | *Tienilic acid* |
| Chlorambucil | *Methyldopa* | Urethane |
| *Clometacin* | Nicotinic acid | Valproic acid |
| *Dantrolene* | *Nitrofurantoin* | *Vitamin A* |
| Frentizole | Oxyphenisatin | |

[a] Drugs in italics are those which are more frequently implicated (either because they are widely used or because they have a marked hepatotoxic potential)

The drugs chiefly responsible for subacute hepatitis, chronic hepatitis, and cirrhosis are listed in Table 5.

Subacute hepatitis, chronic hepatitis, and cirrhosis generally improve after withdrawal of the causative drug, with the few exceptions mentioned above. Usually, clinical manifestations disappear quickly and serum aminotransferase activity decreases markedly within the 1st month, but further improvement may be slower. Complete recovery may take several months and is inconstant. Mild liver function test abnormalities, as well as fibrosis and "inactive cirrhosis," may persist as late sequelae. Autoantibody titers tend to decline progressively.

## 6 Phospholipidosis and Alcoholic-like Liver Lesions

Hepatic phospholipidosis occurs mainly with three antianginal drugs: 4,4′-diethylaminoethoxyhexestrol, perhexiline maleate, and amiodarone [31, 32]. These cationic amphiphilic drugs accumulate within lysosomes, where they form complexes with phospholipids, and inhibit the action of lysosomal phospholipases. Phospholipids accumulate together with the drug in lysosomes which, on electron microscopy, are increased in number and size and contain reticular, lamellar, or pseudomyelinic figures. This lysosomal phospholipidosis is of little or no clinical consequence and may be extremely frequent and perhaps constant, particularly in patients treated with amiodarone.

In occasional patients, this ultrastructural phospholipidosis is associated with alcoholic-like liver lesions, including steatosis, Mallory's bodies, an inflammatory infiltrate composed of both round cells and polymorphonuclears, with fibrosis and sometimes cirrhosis. In severe forms, jaundice, ascites, and encephalopathy may be observed. Due to the persistence of the drug in its lysosomal depot, the disease may continue to worsen, and cirrhosis may develop, despite withdrawal of the offending drug. Alcohol-like liver lesions, without phospholipidosis, have also been observed after administration of diltiazem, nifedipine, and hexestrol.

## 7 Prolonged Cholestasis Due to Rarefaction of Small Bile Ducts

After an initial attack of acute, immunoallergic, cholestatis hepatitis, a few patients develop prolonged cholestasis related to rarefaction of small bile ducts. The mechanism is not established; it is tempting to speculate that it may involve an autoimmune destruction of small bile ducts.

Three different presentations may be seen [33]. In the most usual case, jaundice disappears rapidly after interruption of the treatment, but high alkaline phosphatase and $\gamma$-glutamyltransferase activities persist for more than 1 year. These abnormalities slowly regress and may eventually disappear. In rare instances, jaundice itself lasts more than 6 months before disappearing. Exceptionally, jaundice persists unabated and secondary biliary cirrhosis eventually develops.

Drugs that may produce prolonged cholestasis due to rarefaction of small bile ducts are listed in Table 6.

## 8 Sclerosing Cholangitis

Administration of 5-fluorouracil, or floxuridine, in the hepatic artery may produce strictures of intra- and extrahepatic bile ducts. These lesions affect particularly the confluence of the hepatic ducts. A toxic effect of these drugs on arterioles supplying the upper part of the common bile duct may result in ischemic lesions of the bile ducts.

## 9 Vascular Lesions

Drug-induced lesions may affect any part of the vascular tree of the liver [34].

### 9.1 Hepatic Artery and Portal Vein

Necrotizing angiitis of the hepatic artery has been observed in some subjects addicted to metamphetamine. Arterial intimal hyperplasia may occur in women on oral contraceptives and may affect the hepatic artery among other arteries. In rare instances such a lesion has led to multifocal hemorrhagic necrosis or to spontaneous rupture of the liver, but it is more commonly asymptomatic.

Thrombosis of the portal vein and its branches has been reported in women on oral contraceptives and in subjects receiving arsenical derivatives.

**Table 6.** Drugs which may produce prolonged cholestasis[a]

| | | |
|---|---|---|
| Aceprometazine | Cimetidine | Phenytoin |
| *Ajmaline* | Cyproheptadine | Prochlorperazine |
| Amitriptyline | Erythromycin | Thiabendazole |
| *Arsenical derivatives* | Haloperidol | Tiopronin |
| Barbiturate | Imipramine | Tolbutamide |
| Carbamazepine | Methyltestosterone | Troleandomycin |
| Carbutamide | Norandrostenolone | Xenalamine |
| *Chlorpromazine* | | |

[a] Drugs in italics are those which are more frequently implicated (either because they are widely used or because they have a marked hepatotoxic potential)

### 9.2 Hepatoportal Sclerosis

Hepatoportal sclerosis is characterized by portal and periportal fibrosis resulting in portal hypertension. Although its mechanism remains unknown, it is thought that it might be due to obstruction of small portal venules. This lesion may occur after administration of vitamin A, azathioprine, methotrexate, or arsenical derivatives. These drugs may also produce perisinusoidal fibrosis; indeed, both lesions are often associated in the same patient.

### 9.3 Perisinusoidal Fibrosis

In perisinusoidal fibrosis, collagen fibers are deposited within the space of Disse. The lesion may be seen on optical microscopy but is more evident on electron microscopy. It may be due to increased synthesis of collagen by activated perisinusoidal Ito cells, at least in some cases (vitamin A intoxication, methotrexate administration).

Perisinusoidal fibrosis has been reported after administration of arsenical derivatives, azathioprine, 6-mercaptopurine, methotrexate, and thorium dioxide. The usual cause, however, is vitamin A administration. Hypervitaminosis A has been reported after a wide range of daily doses (from 30000 to 1200000 units) and various lengths of treatment (from 7 weeks to 30 years) [35]. Usually, however, the disease does not become symptomatic before several years of treatment and cumulative doses exceeding $100 \times 10^6$ units. Skin lesions, in particular alopecia, are often present. Optical and electron microscopy show hyperplasia of Ito cells, which are distended by large vesicles containing vitamin A. The hepatic content of vitamin A is markedly increased, although its levels in the serum may be normal. Perisinusoidal fibrosis due to vitamin A intoxication may be associated with sinusoidal dilation, hepatoportal sclerosis, or even cirrhosis. Portal hypertension sometimes partially regresses after interruption of vitamin A administration.

### 9.4 Sinusoidal Dilation

Hepatic sinusoids are dilated despite the absence of obstruction or high pressure in the efferent vessels of the liver. Sinusoidal dilation affecting mainly periportal areas may develop during the use of oral contraceptives and regress after their withdrawal. Dilations randomly distributed in the liver have been observed in renal transplant recipients treated with both azathioprine and glucocorticoids.

### 9.5 Peliosis Hepatitis

In patients with peliosis hepatitis blood-filled cavities, bordered by hepatocytes, are randomly distributed throughout the hepatic lobule. Although it may be asymptomatic, in other cases this lesion is associated with hepatomegaly, portal hypertension, jaundice, and even hepatic failure. Peliosis hepatitis may occur after administration of anabolic/androgenic steroids, azathioprine, 6-thioguanine, vinyl chloride, and arsenical derivatives, and possibly also after oral contraceptives.

### 9.6 Nodular Hyperplasia

Nodular hyperplasia of the liver is characterized by the presence of small nodules of hepatocytes that are distributed randomly throughout the liver and are seen in the absence of fibrosis or with only mild fibrosis. The relationship of this condition with vascular lesions is suggested by the fact that it may occur in association with peliosis hepatitis or sinusoidal dilation or may follow these vascular lesions. Nodular hyperplasia has been observed after treatment with azathioprine, anabolic/androgenic steroids, oral contraceptives, and corticosteroids.

### 9.7 Veno-occlusive Disease

In veno-occlusive disease the lumina of small centrilobular (hepatic) veins are narrowed by a marked subendothelial thickening due initially to a loose, edematous connective tissue. The lesion may evolve toward complete fibrotic obstruction of the lumina. Impaired evacuation of blood from the sinusoids leads to centrilobular sinusoidal dilation and liver cell necrosis, followed eventually by centrilobular fibrosis. The most typical symptom is ascites. Other possible manifestations are abdominal pains, hepatomegaly, splenomegaly, mild jaundice, and, in severe forms, hepatic encephalopathy.

Veno-occlusive disease has been reported, mainly in Asia and Africa, after ingestion of pyrrolizidine alkaloids present in plants such as *Heliotropium*, *Senecio*, or *Crotalaria* that are used as herbal remedies. In Western countries, the main cause is chemotherapy with whole body irradiation performed in preparation for bone marrow transplantation. The condition may also occur in the absence of any irradiation in subjects receiving urethane or various thiopurine analogues such as azathioprine, 6-mercaptopurine, or 6-thioguanine.

### 9.8 Budd-Chiari Syndrome

Budd-Chiari syndrome is defined as the obstruction (usually by a thrombus) of large hepatic veins. Like veno-occlusive disease, this condition impairs the evacuation of blood from the sinusoids, resulting in centrilobular congestion, necrosis, and ultimately fibrosis. The caudate lobe is usually spared by the disease and undergoes compensatory hyperthrophy. The clinical presentation may be acute, with the abrupt onset of abdominal pain and ascites, or chronic, mimicking ascitic cirrhosis.

In women on oral contraceptives, the risk of developing Budd-Chiari syndrome is 2.5-fold that in nonusers [36]. In most cases, these women have in addition a latent myeloproliferative disorder or another thrombogenic condition, suggesting that estrogens may act mainly by exacerbating an underlying thrombogenic condition.

Budd-Chiari syndrome has also been observed in patients treated with antineoplastic agents, in particular dacarbazine.

## 10 Hepatic Tumors

### 10.1 Hepatocellular Adenoma

Hepatocellular adenoma is a benign tumor composed of normal hepatocytes separated by compressed sinusoids, but without any central vein or portal tract. The incidence of this tumor is markedly increased in women taking oral contraceptives. Comparing users and nonusers, it has been estimated that the relative risk may be 100 times higher in users after 5 years of use and 500 times higher after 7 years [37]. Hepatic adenomas are often asymptomatic, being discovered incidentally on ultrasonography. Large tumors may, however, lead to abdominal pain, hepatomegaly, and either intratumoral or intraperitoneal hemorrhages. Interruption of this type of contraception has occasionally led to slow regression of the tumor. It remains controversial whether adenomas in oral contraceptive users may degenerate into hepatocellular carcinomas.

Hepatic adenomas may also occur after administration of anabolic/androgenic steroids. In this case, it is thought that they might evolve into hepatocellular carcinomas. Isolated cases of adenoma have been reported after the administration of testosterone, clomiphene, or norethisterone.

### 10.2 Focal Nodular Hyperplasia

Focal nodular hyperplasia is a benign liver tumor characterized by a central stellate star (containing veins, arteries, bile ducts, and often inflammatory cells) surrounded by the liver cell nodule. Oral contraceptives probably do not increase the incidence of focal nodular hyperplasia, although they may perhaps increase its size and vascularity and might therefore increase the risk of an intratumoral or intraperitoneal hemorrhage.

### 10.3 Hepatocellular Carcinoma

Hepatocellular carcinoma is a malignant tumor developed from hepatocytes. The risk of developing this tumor is increased in persons receiving anabolic/androgenic steroids, and also probably in women on oral contraceptives. Two studies have estimated the risk to be 7–20 times higher in women taking oral contraceptives for 8 years or more than in nonusers [38, 39].

### 10.4 Angiosarcoma

Angiosarcoma is a malignant tumor that arises from endothelial cells. It has been observed after exposure to vinyl chloride, cupric sulfate, arsenical derivatives, and anabolic/androgenic steroids.

### 10.5 Other Malignant Tumors

Cholangiocarcinoma is a malignant tumor composed of cells resembling biliary epithelial cells. It has occasionally been observed in subjects on long-term anabolic/androgenic steroid therapy or on oral contraceptives. The causal relationship needs confirmation.

The link between the use of oral contraceptives and the occurrence of epithelioid hemangioendothelioma also remains to be confirmed.

## 11 Diagnosis

An iatrogenic cause must be considered systematically in patients presenting with any kind of liver disease. Although other etiologies may be more common, overlooking a drug-induced lesion can represent a severe medical fault.

The first step in the diagnosis consists in a patient quest to ascertain all ingested medications. In a subject claiming initially not to take any drug, one has to inquire specifically about those medications that may be thought so usual or innocuous as not to be worth mentioning, such as decoctions, oral contraceptives, aspirin, and other over-the-counter analgesics. One should also mention specifically drugs that the patient may feel embarrassed about using (or abusing), such as hypnotics, tranquilizers, antidepressants, anorectic drugs, laxatives, and diuretics. In elderly patients with uncertain memories and a long list of ever-changing medications the only solution may be to request copies of previous prescriptions, if they are available. Although prime consideration should be given to drugs taken recently before the onset of the liver disease, it should be remembered that a few drugs may continue to damage the liver after they have been withdrawn, such as perhexiline maleate, amiodarone, and vitamin A.

The second step in the diagnosis is to single out, from the list of drugs taken by the patient, those medications which are particularly likely to produce adverse drug reactions affecting the liver.

The third step consists in the comparison of the patient's condition with the type of liver disease known to be produced by each individual drug. As mentioned previously, each drug tends to imprint its seal on the liver disease it produces, the differences relating to the time of onset, the type of liver lesion and thus the clinical and biochemical manifestations, and the presence of immunoallergic and/or extrahepatic manifestations. A good fit between the patient's presentation and the liver disease known to be produced by one of the ingested drugs suggests its possible involvement. The book by STRICKER and SPOELSTRA [1] is particularly useful for such a comparison. If a drug is strongly suspected, it should be withdrawn immediately, without waiting for results of further tests. With very rare exceptions this withdrawal can be made without any difficulty, either because the treatment was not really needed or because alternative medications are available.

The fourth step in the diagnosis is to look for, and rule out, other etiologies. The patient and, if possible, his or her relatives should be carefully questioned in order to ascertain whether the patient has displayed a tendency to abuse alcohol. The disclosure of stigmata of alcoholism such as Dupuytren's contracture or parotid gland hypertrophy is suggestive of an alcohol-related disease, as are an increased mean corpuscular volume, aspartate aminotransferase values exceeding alanine aminotransferase values, and markedly raised serum $\gamma$-glutamyltransferase activity.

A subclinical drug-induced liver injury must be distinguished from the minor liver function test abnormalities that may be seen in patients with mild steatosis due to a somewhat high alcohol intake, mild obesity, or mild adult-onset diabetes. Ultrasonography suggesting steatosis and improvement after introduction of the appropriate diet (a nonalcoholic, hypocaloric, or diabetic diet, respectively) often permit the diagnosis without resorting to a liver biopsy.

Suspected drug-induced hepatocellular jaundice must be differentiated from viral hepatitis. Usual serologic tests (HBV markers, anti-HAV IgM antibodies, anti-HCV antibodies) will detect most cases of viral hepatitis although the problem of anti-HCV negative forms of HCV hepatitis and that of hepatitis E still persist. In some cases it may be necessary also to look for anti-Epstein-Barr virus and anti-cytomegalovirus IgM antibodies. Furthermore, drug-induced hepatocellular jaundice should be distinguished from the acute liver cell necrosis that may occur during an acute, reversible episode of low cardiac output. This possibility should be considered particularly in elderly subjects with impaired cardiac function, cardiac arrhythmias, or any other possible cause of a transient collapse that may have gone unnoticed. The rather rapid disappearance of a marked increase in serum aminotransferase activity, the possible association with transient azotemia, and the findings of liver histology may redress the diagnosis.

Cholestatic hepatitis must be distinguished from obstruction of the biliary tree. Ultrasonography should be performed in all cases to exclude this diagnosis.

The fifth step in the diagnosis consists in the performance of complementary investigations that may confirm the diagnosis of drug-induced hepatitis. Histologic examination of a liver specimen may often be dispensed with, although it is perfectly justified in difficult cases. This may, at times, provide confirmation of the diagnosis by showing, for example, a strictly centrilobular topography of the liver cell necrosis or the presence of eosinophils or granulomas or any other feature consistent with the diagnosis, such as Ito cell hyperplasia with vitamin A or alcoholic liver lesions with amiodarone. An ultrastructural examination may be appropriate in some circumstances, e.g., if a diagnosis of perisinusoidal fibrosis, vitamin A excess, or phospholipidosis is being considered. Looking for antibodies may also aid in diagnosis; this is particularly true for those antibodies which appear to be disease specific (anti-$LKM_2$ in tienilic acid-induced hepatitis, anti-LM in dihydralazine-induced hepatitis, anti-$M_6$ in iproniazid-induced hepatitis, and anti-trifluoroacetylated proteins in halothane-induced hepatitis).

The sixth step in the diagnosis rests on the outcome after interruption of the drug administration. Drug-induced hepatocellular jaundice often regresses within the 1st month after withdrawal, but it may be more enduring in patients with hepatitis mediated by drugs producing an autoimmune attack against normal hepatocyte structures (iproniazid, tienilic acid). Cholestatic hepatitis usually regresses after interruption of the drug administration, although recovery may take several months. In addition, prolonged cholestasis (probably due to autoimmune destruction of small bile ducts) occurs in rare cases. Pseudoalcoholic liver lesions also regress in most patients, although they occasionally continue to worsen because of the persistence of amiodarone or perhexiline maleate in the liver.

Readministration of a highly suspected drug for a diagnostic purpose is not justified ethically. When several drugs have been withdrawn, however, and only one is reasonably suspected, it may be less unethical to readminister the associated drugs. Their good tolerance will permit the hepatitis to be ascribed with certainty to the suspected drug. A definite diagnosis will ensure that the patient refrains from taking the responsible drug again, whereas uncertainty about the responsibility of the drug may entice the patient into resuming the intake of the offending drug.

## 12 Treatment and Prevention

The only therapeutic measure in most cases consists in the immediate and definitive withdrawal of the responsible drug. The efficacy of glucocorticoids in immunoallergic cases has not been demonstrated (or refuted). In fulminant hepatitis, liver transplantation may save the patient.

Clearly, the best measure would be to prevent these man-made diseases. Such prevention concerns physicians, the pharmaceutical industry, and state-run agencies. At the level of the prescribing physician, a more reasonable attitude toward prescriptions should be encouraged. In most cases of drug-induced liver lesions one has to admit that the treatment was not really needed. Clearly, physicians should try harder to resist their patients' demands for unnecessary drugs. Whenever possible, physicians should prescribe nonhepatotoxic analogues. If a frequently hepatotoxic drug has to be used, liver function tests should be carried out regularly. The pharmaceutical industry and state-run research agencies should promote renewed efforts aimed at recognizing earlier those molecules having a hepatotoxic potential, at identifying still unknown mechanisms of hepatotoxicity, at disclosing specific diagnostic procedures (which are still desperately lacking), and at devising nontoxic analogues.

## References


1. Stricker BHC, Spoelstra P (1985) Drug-induced hepatic injury. A comprehensive survey of the literature on adverse drug reactions up to January 1985. Elsevier, Amsterdam
2. Pessayre D, Larrey D (to be published) Drug-induced liver injury. In: McIntyre N, Benhamou JP, Bircher J, Rizetto M, Rodez J (eds) Oxford textbook of clinical hepatology
3. Gonzalez FJ (1990) Molecular genetics of the P-450 superfamily. Pharmacol Ther 45:1–38
4. Mirabelli F, Salis A, Marinoni V et al. (1988) Menadione-induced bleb formation in hepatocytes is associated with the oxidation of thiol groups in actin. Arch Biochem Biophys 264:261–269
5. Bellomo G, Orrenius S (1985) Altered thiol and calcium homeostasis in oxidative hepatocellular injury. Hepatology 5:876–882
6. Loeper J, Descatoire V, Amouyal G et al. (1989) Presence of covalently bound metabolites on rat hepatocyte plasma membrane proteins after administration of isaxonine, a drug leading to immunoallergic hepatitis in man. Hepatology 9: 675–678
7. Pohl LR, Kenna JG, Satoh H et al. (1989) Neoantigens associated with halothane hepatitis. Drug Metab Rev 20:203–217
8. Loeper J, Descatoire V, Maurice M et al. (1990) Presence of functional cytochrome P-450 on isolated rat hepatocyte plasma membrane. Hepatology 11:850–858
9. Beaune P, Dansette PM, Mansuy D et al. (1987) Human antimicrosome antibodies appearing in a drug induced hepatitis are directed against cytochrome P-450 hydroxylating the drug. Proc Natl Acad Sci USA 84:551–555

10. Bourdi M, Larrey D, Nataf J et al. (1990) Anti-liver endoplasmic reticulum autoantibodies are directed against human cytochrome P-450 IA2. A specific marker of dihydralazine-induced hepatitis. J Clin Invest 85:1967–1973
11. Shear NH, Spielberg SP, Grant DM et al. (1986) Differences in metabolism of sulfonamides predisposing to idiosyncratic toxicity. Ann Intern Med 105: 179–184
12. Shear NH, Spielberg SP (1988) Anticonvulsant hypersensitivity syndrome. In vitro assessment of risk. J Clin Invest 82:1826–1832
13. Larrey D, Berson A, Habersetzer F et al. (1989) Genetic predisposition to drug hepatotoxicity: role in hepatitis caused by amineptine, a tricyclic antidepressant. Hepatology 10:168–173
14. Pariente EA, Hamoud A, Goldfain D et al. (1989) Hépatites à la clométacine (Dupéran®). Etude rétrospective de 30 cas. Un modèle d'hépatite auto-immue médicamenteuse? Gastroenterol Clin Biol 13:769–774
15. Zimmerman HJ (1978) Hepatotoxicity. The adverse effects of drugs and other chemicals on the liver. Appleton-Century-Crofts, New York.
16. Timbrell JA, Mitchell JR, Snodgrass WR et al. (1980) Isoniazid hepatotoxicity: the relationship between covalent binding and metabolism in vivo. J Pharmacol Exp Ther 213:364–369
17. Black M, Mitchell JR, Zimmerman HJ et al. (1975) Isoniazid-associated hepatitis in 114 patients. Gastroenterology 69:289–302
18. Pessayre D, Bentata M, Degott C et al. (1977) Isoniazid-rifampin fulminant hepatitis. A possible consequence of the enhancement of isoniazid hepatotoxicity by enzyme induction. Gastroenterology 72:284–289
19. Prescott LF (1983) Paracetamol overdosage. Pharmacological considerations and clinical management. Drugs 25:290–314
20. Levy M, Goodman MW, Van Dyne BJ et al. (1981) Granulomatous hepatitis secondary to carbamazepine. Ann Intern Med 95:64–65
21. Pessayre D, Larrey D, Funck-Brentano C et al. (1985) Drug interactions and hepatitis produced by some macrolide antibiotics. J Antimicrob Chemother 16:181–194
22. Funck-Brentano C, Pessayre D, Benhamou JP (1983) Hépatites dues à divers dérivés de l'érythromycine. Gastroenterol Clin Biol 7:362–369
23. Ishak KG, Zimmerman HJ (1988) Drug-induced and toxic granulomatous hepatitis. Baillière's Clin Gastroenterol 2:463–479
24. Ishak KG, Zimmerman HJ (1987) Hepatotoxic effects of the anabolic/androgenic steroids. Semin Liver Dis 7:230–236
25. Kesterson JW, Granneman GR, Machinist JM (1984) The hepatotoxicity of valproic acid and its metabolites. I. Toxicologic, biochemical and histopathologic studies. Hepatology 4:1143–1152
26. Genève J, Hayat-Bonan B, Labbe G et al. (1987) Inhibition of mitochondrial β-oxidation of fatty acids by pirprofen. Role in microvesicular steatosis due to this nonsteroidal anti-inflammatory drug. J Pharmacol Exp Ther 242:1133–1137
27. Fréneaux E, Labbe G, Lettéron P et al. (1988) Inhibition of the mitochondrial oxidation of fatty acids by tetracycline in mice and man. Possible role in microvesicular steatosis induced by this antibiotic. Hepatology 8:1056–1062
28. Le Dinh T, Fréneaux E, Labbe G et al. (1988) Amineptine, a tricyclic antidepressant, inhibits the mitochondrial oxidation of fatty acids and produces microvesicular steatosis of the liver in mice. J Pharmacol Exp Ther 247:745–750
29. Zimmerman HJ, Ishak KG (1982) Valproate-induced hepatic injury. Analysis of 23 fatal cases. Hepatology 2:591–597
30. Danan G, Trunet P, Bernuau J et al. (1985) Pirprofen-induced fulminant hepatitis. Gastroenterology 89:210–213
31. Pessayre D, Bichara M, Feldmann G et al. (1979) Perhexiline maleate-induced cirrhosis. Gastroenterology 76:170–177

32. Simon JB, Manley PN, Brien JF et al. (1984) Amiodarone hepatotoxicity simulating alcoholic liver disease. N Engl J Med 311:167–172
33. Larrey D, Erlinger S (1988) Drug-induced cholestasis. Baillière's Clin Gastroenterol 2:423–451
34. Valla D, Benhamou JP (1988) Drug-induced vascular and sinusoidal lesions of the liver. Baillière's Clin Gastroenterol 2:481–500
35. Rosenbaum J, Amedée-Manesme O, Dhumeaux D (1985) Le foie et la vitamine A. Gastroenterol Clin Biol 9:255–262
36. Valla D, Le MG, Poynard T et al. (1986) Risk of hepatic vein thrombosis in relation to recent use of oral contraceptives. A case-control study. Gastroenterology 90:807–811
37. Rooks JB, Ory HW, Ishak KG et al. (1979) Epidemiology of hepatocellular adenoma. The role of contraceptive use. JAMA 242:644–648
38. Forman D, Vincent TJ, Doll DR (1986) Cancer of the liver and the use of oral contraceptives. Br Med J 292:1357–1361
39. Neuberger J, Forman D, Doll DR et al. (1986) Oral contraceptives and hepatocellular carcinoma. Br Med J 292:1355–1357

# 20 Alcoholic Liver Disease

M. Salaspuro

In the late 1940s the pathogenesis of alcoholic liver disease was regarded as being associated almost exclusively with a secondary protein and choline deficiency. Since then, however, strong evidence has emerged of a relationship between the pathogenesis of alcohol-related liver damage and the direct toxicity of ethanol, its metabolism, and its metabolites. Nevertheless, many questions still remain unanswered. Why do only a proportion of heavy drinkers or alcoholics develop liver disease? What is the basic mechanism behind the cell death caused by alcohol? What is the most important toxic factor – ethanol, its metabolism, or its metabolites? Can we indeed entirely exclude nutritional deficiency in the pathogenesis of alcoholic liver disease? All these questions, and more broadly the epidemiology of alcohol use and alcoholic liver injury, have been discussed in many recent reviews [1–14].

## 1 Epidemiologic Aspects of Alcohol Use and Alcoholic Liver Disease

### 1.1 Alcohol Consumption

Total alcohol consumption declined in almost all European countries from the 1870s to the Second World War. This was followed by a rather remarkable rise in consumption from the early 1950s to 1975 in most European countries as well as in the United States [15–17]. In particular, the preference for beer increased strikingly in Europe. In the traditional wine-drinking countries (France, Italy, Spain, and Portugal), per capita alcohol consumption has remained among the highest in the world; nevertheless, while it remained fairly constant until 1975 there has since been a significant decrease in consumption in these countries. A similar but less pronounced reduction has occurred elsewhere.

In wine-drinking countries wine is a component of every meal and a relatively inexpensive nutrient. In beer-drinking countries, by contrast, beer is consumed in leisure time and to improve social contacts outside the home. In spirit-drinking countries alcohol is used as an intoxicant. In these countries especially, the heaviest drinking 10% of the population drinks about half of all the alcohol consumed, although a very uneven distribution of drinking patterns is also observed elsewhere.

The availability of alcoholic beverages, licensing laws, and economic, cultural, and environmental conditions all influence both per capita alcohol consumption and mortality from cirrhosis. Therefore it is generally accepted that both the consumption of alcohol and the incidence of alcohol-related health problems can be regulated by means of various restrictions and tax policies.

## 1.2 Mortality and Prevalence of Alcoholic Liver Cirrhosis

Most heavy drinkers and alcoholics will develop hepatomegaly and fatty infiltration of the liver. However, only 20%–33% develop more severe liver disease, i.e., alcoholic hepatitis or liver cirrhosis. According to postmortem data the prevalence of cirrhosis in alcoholics is about 18%; in series based on liver biopsy it ranges from 17% to 30.8%.

From the 1950s onward the mortality from cirrhosis has increased considerably. For instance, in West Germany it increased from 6/100000 in 1950 to 27/100000 in 1980. Similar increases between 1950 and 1970–1980 were documented in the United Kingdom [17, 18] (Fig. 1), in most other European countries, in Australia, in the United States, and in Japan [17]. In many countries, e.g., England, alcoholic cirrhosis is now the most common form of liver disease [18].

In most cases cirrhosis of the liver remains undetected during life. Indeed, the morbidity from all types of alcoholic liver disease is much higher than the mortality, although precise and reliable data are unavailable.

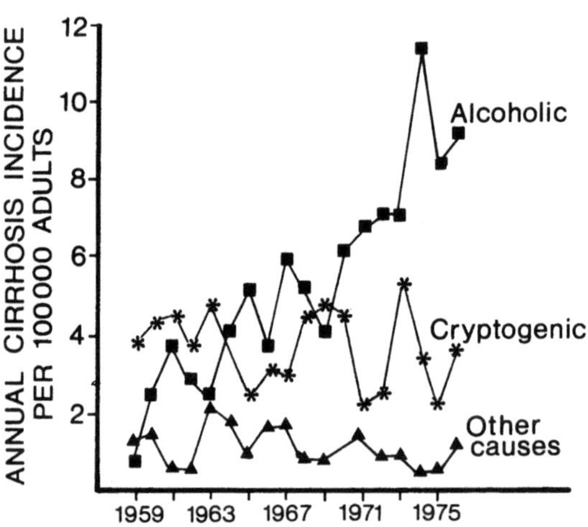


**Fig. 1.** Annual incidence of alcoholic, cryptogenic, and other types of cirrhosis in West Birmingham, 1959–1976 [SAUNDERS JB et al. (1981) 282:263]. [Reproduced with permission from MORGAN MY (1985) In: Hall P (ed) Alcoholic liver disease. Edward Arnold, London, pp 193–200]

### 1.3 Relationship Between Liver Cirrhosis and Alcohol Consumption

A close relationship between alcohol consumption and mortality due to liver cirrhosis has been demonstrated in many studies. One of the classic examples concerns the effect of wine rationing in France during the Second World War. From 1941 to 1946 alcohol consumption in France dropped drastically and this was associated with a similar decrease in mortality from cirrhosis. The subsequent rise in alcohol consumption from 1946 to 1955 resulted in an even more pronounced increase in the mortality caused by liver cirrhosis. Since 1965 alcohol consumption has decreased in parallel with a reduction in mortality from cirrhosis [16] (Fig. 2).

The development of alcoholic cirrhosis correlates with both the magnitude and the duration of alcohol consumption [1]. For males the relative risk of cirrhosis has been estimated to be six times greater at 40–60 g alcohol/day than at up to 20 g/day, and 14 times greater at 60–80 g/day [19]. The average cirrhogenous dose has been calculated to be 180 g ethanol/day consumed regularly for approximately 25 years. The probability that an individual who consumes about 210 g ethanol daily for 22 years will develop cirrhosis is 50% and this increases to 80% after 33 years [1]. In a case control study in men, the relative risk of developing cirrhosis was 1.83 for men consuming 40–59 g absolute alcohol/day when compared with those consuming less than 40 g/day. The relative risk rose to 100 for men consuming more than 80 g/day [20]. Similar trends were found in women and with regard to the risk of developing fatty liver.

There is a lot of evidence to suggest that the average cirrhogenous dose and the threshold doses are lower in females than in males [19]. There is

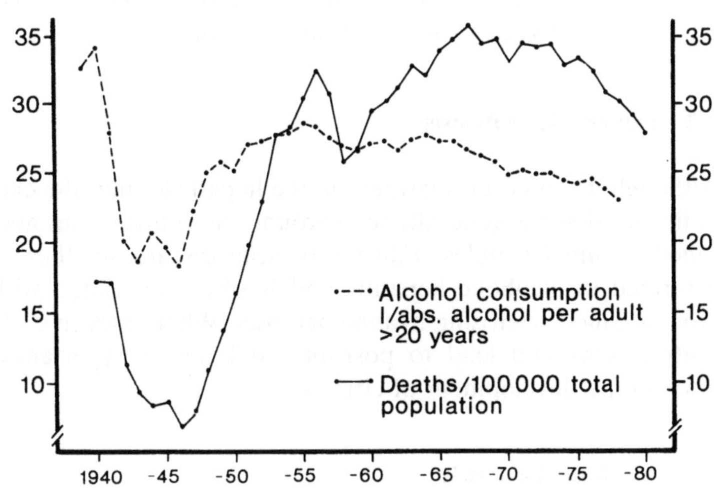


**Fig. 2.** Alcohol consumption (adults) and mortality from cirrhosis in France, 1939–1980. [Reproduced with permission from Lelbach WK (1985) In: Hall P (ed) Alcoholic liver disease. Edward Arnold, London, pp 130–166]

no valid epidemiologic or clinical evidence to suggest that drinking habits (continuous versus periodic) or the type of alcoholic beverage influence mortality from cirrhosis.

## 2 Patterns and Pathology of Alcoholic Liver Disease

The spectrum of alcoholic liver disease covers fatty liver, perivenular fibrosis, alcoholic hepatitis, and cirrhosis.

### 2.1 Fatty Liver

Fat accumulation in the liver cells is the earliest and most common response to alcohol, and alcohol is its most common cause. The normal liver weighs about 1.5 kg, whereas the alcoholic fatty liver weighs 2–2.5 kg. In rare cases massive accumulation of fat may occur, resulting in livers weighing from 4 to 6 kg. Parenchymal accumulation of lipid is seen as clear intracytoplasmic vacuoles on hematoxylin and eosin-stained sections, and as black or red globules with various Sudan stains. In massive steatosis the hepatocytes are uniformly filled by large fat droplets, the cell nucleus may be eccentrically placed, and when the cell membranes between adjacent hepatocytes rupture, fatty cysts are formed. Evidence of necrosis is usually sparse but sometimes hepatocytes are surrounded by mononuclear cells indicating a mild inflammatory response. When pronounced, these formations are called "lipogranulomas."

Ultrastructural changes consist of enlarged and distorted mitochondria with shortened cristae containing crystalline inclusions. The endoplasmic reticulum shows vacuolar dilatation and proliferation.

### 2.2 Perivenular Fibrosis

Although it can occur anywhere in the hepatic lobule, the earliest deposition of fibrous tissue is generally seen around the central veins and venules – now called terminal venules. Fibrosis or sclerosis around these veins has been described in alcoholic hepatitis and is often associated with a necrotizing process called sclerosing hyaline necrosis. When intensive, it may obliterate central veins and lead to postsinusoidal portal hypertension with ascites prior to the development of cirrhosis.

### 2.3 Alcoholic Hepatitis

The term "alcoholic hepatitis" is nowadays accepted by most pathologists and clinicians to describe the stage of disease characterized by the appearance of necrosis with an inflammatory reaction, including polymorphonuclear cells. While the incidence of fatty liver in alcoholics is very high, alcoholic hepatitis develops in only a fraction of heavy drinkers, even after decades of abuse. The long-term incidence of cirrhosis in patients with alcoholic hepatitis is nine times higher than in those with fatty liver.

Histologic characteristics of alcoholic hepatitis are ballooning and great disarray of hepatocytes (predominantly in perivenular areas), parenchymal and portal infiltration with polymorphonuclear leukocytes, varying degrees of steatosis, necrosis, fibrosis, and cholestasis. Commonly lymphocytes can be demonstrated in perivenular zones or within the parenchyma in direct contact with the plasma membranes of the hepatocytes. Mallory's alcoholic hyaline – irregular cytoplasmic bodies – can be considered as a diagnostic hallmark, but their presence is not a precondition for the diagnosis.

Ultrastructural changes in alcoholic hepatitis are similar but more severe than those seen in fatty liver. Collagenous material may be found in the space of Disse and may be associated with loss of microvilli that normally project from the hepatocyte.

Mallory's alcoholic hyaline was first defined, as the name suggests, by Mallory in 1911 as an irregular, coarse, hyaline meshwork which stains deeply with eosin. Cells containing these bodies may be surrounded by numerous polymorphonuclear leukocytes. Electron microscopically alcoholic hyaline is fibrillar, is not surrounded by a limiting membrane, and is readily distinguished from giant mitochondria. The formation of alcoholic hyaline is considered to be a manifestation of derangement of the cytoskeleton of the hepatocyte, and in addition to being present in alcoholic hepatitis it also can be seen in other liver diseases [11].

## 2.4 Cirrhosis

Macroscopically the early cirrhotic liver is golden yellow with fine uniform nodules (1–5 mm) on the surface. Traditionally this type of cirrhosis is called "micronodular" or "Laënnec's cirrhosis." The size of the liver varies, depending on the degree of fibrosis, inflammation, and steatosis, from a small, shrunken, and hard liver to a large organ weighing up to 4 kg. In later stages the size of the nodules increases to 5–50 mm and deep scars appear. This macronodular cirrhosis resembles the postnecrotic cirrhosis.

Microscopically, scar tissue distorts the normal architecture of the liver by forming bands of connective tissue joining portal and hepatic venular zones. At first, nodules are regular in size and shape. In more advanced cirrhosis nodules become larger and are frequently irregular in size and shape. The nodules eventually become "relobulized" through the formation of small hypoplastic portal tracts and excess efferent venous channels.

One of the most characteristic features of cirrhosis is the change in the hepatic blood circulation. Parivenular inflammation and fibrosis may impair outflow from the sinusoids and the regenerative nodules may compress the hepatic veins, resulting in postsinusoidal portal hypertension. In addition to fibrosis, various admixtures of fat, inflammatory reactions, and cholestasis may be seen. Histologically stainable iron deposits are common in cirrhotic livers, especially in alcoholic subjects. Quantitative measurements of hepatic iron content in these disorders have demonstrated that total iron stores are very seldom increased and never exceed 180 μmol/g (1 g/100 g). Differentiation from primary hemochromatosis can be achieved by measuring the total hepatic iron content from liver biopsies.

Hepatocellular carcinoma is a relatively frequent finding in liver cirrhosis, presumably because of improved management and prolonged survival. Pathogenetically, alcohol has traditionally been related to cirrhosis but possible carcinogenic properties of alcohol must also be considered.

## 3 Ethanol Metabolism

### 3.1 Absorption, Distribution, and Excretion of Ethanol

Ethanol is absorbed from the gastrointestinal tract by simple diffusion because of its small size and low solubility in lipids. Diffusion is rather slow from the stomach and consequently most (70%–80%) ingested ethanol is absorbed from the duodenum and upper jejunum (Fig. 3). High ethanol concentrations, similar to those of alcoholic beverages, are reached in the stomach and duodenum. In the ileum, ethanol levels are parallel to those of the vascular space. The rate of absorption is decreased by delayed gastric emptying and by the intestinal contents.

The diffusion of alcohol through the cell boundaries is a rather slow process, but the distribution of alcohol by the blood flow is very fast. In

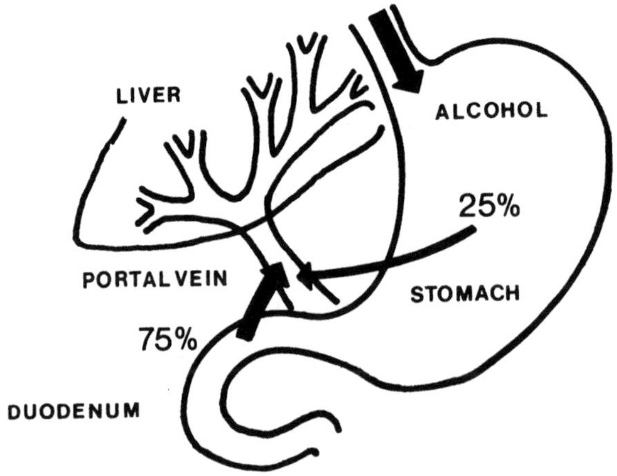


**Fig. 3.** Absorption of alcohol from stomach and upper duodenum

organs with dense vascularization and a rich blood supply, such as the brain, lungs, and liver, alcohol rapidly equilibrates with the blood. Lipids take up only 4% of the quantity of alcohol dissolved in a corresponding volume of water. Consequently, in an obese person the same amount of alcohol per unit weight gives a higher blood alcohol concentration than in a thin person. The sex differences in ethanol pharmacokinetics are due to differences in body water content. The mean apparent volume of distribution of ethanol is less in women than in men; this results in higher peak blood ethanol concentrations and greater mean areas under the ethanol concentration-time curves in women.

Most of the ethanol (90%–95%) is oxidized and excreted as carbon dioxide and water. Other routes for elimination are urine and breath. Since alcohol is not concentrated in the urine, less than 1% of ingested alcohol is removed by this route. In man under normal conditions 1%–3% can be eliminated through the lungs.

### 3.2 Elimination of Ethanol

In a normal person about 100 mg ethanol/kg body weight is eliminated in an hour (7 g alcohol per hour for a 70-kg person; 0.1 per mille per hour). This may vary owing to genetic, individual, and external factors. Most importantly, heavy alcohol consumption for years may increase the rate of ethanol elimination 30–100 percent.

### 3.3 Role of the Liver and Other Tissues

The importance of the liver in the elimination of ethanol was established in several studies in the late 1930s. It was demonstrated that perfused livers effectively remove alcohol from the perfusion medium. Ethanol oxidation was shown to be reduced in the presence of liver injury and almost totally abolished following evisceration. About two-thirds of the ethanol oxidized by liver can be recovered as acetic acid. Seventy-five percent of the oxygen normally taken up by the liver is utilized for ethanol oxidation.

Other tissues such as kidney, pancreas, intestine, and bone marrow cells can oxidize ethanol to a small extent. There is abundant alcohol dehydrogenase present in the mucosa of stomach, which results in a significant first-pass metabolism of alcohol.

### 3.4 Pathways of Ethanol Oxidation

In the liver ethanol is first oxidized within the cytosol of the hepatocyte to acetaldehyde. This is followed by the mitochondrial oxidation of acetaldehyde to acetate. Acetate produced in the liver is released into the blood and is oxidized by peripheral tissues to carbon dioxide, fatty acids, and water (Fig. 4). The main pathway for ethanol metabolism proceeds via the enzyme alcohol dehydrogenase. However, alternate pathways for ethanol oxidation, which are situated in other subcellular compartments, have been described.

### *3.4.1 Alcohol Dehydrogenase Pathway*

Alcohol dehydrogenase (ADH) catalyzes the oxidation of alcohols, including ethanol, to their corresponding aldehydes according to the following scheme:

$$CH_3CH_2OH + NAD^+ \xrightarrow{ADH} CH_3CHO + NADH + H^+$$

The activity of hepatic ADH is low during fetal life; adult levels are reached by 5 years of age in humans. In addition to the oxidation of alcohols, ADH catalyzes the oxidation of endogenous and exogenous sterols and is responsible for the ω-oxidation of fatty acids. Endogenous steroids and/or the small amounts of ethanol produced by intestinal flora may represent "physiologic" substrates for ADH.

The molecular weight of human liver ADH is 79000–83000 and each molecule contains four atoms of zinc which are vital for enzyme activity. Three major classes of ADH have been described [21]. Class I isoenzymes with low Km and high Vmax for ethanol are responsible for most of ethanol oxidation.

Various ADH forms appear in different frequencies in different racial populations. This may explain, at least in part, individual variations in the

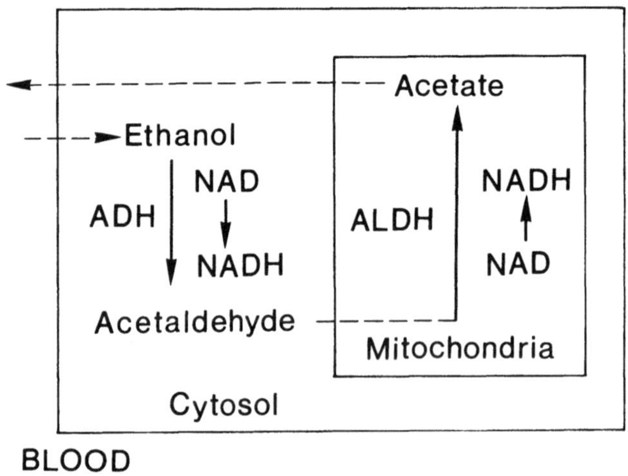


**Fig. 4.** Pathways of ethanol oxidation via hepatic alcohol and aldehyde dehydrogenase

rate of ethanol elimination. ADH phenotypes have been related to the production of acetaldehyde and to the extent of first-pass elimination of ethanol. A possible relationship between ADH genotype and the susceptibility to alcoholism or alcohol-related organ injury, however, remains to be established.

Because of the low Km of ADH (<1 mM) and because acetaldehyde is effectively removed, ethanol is eliminated from the blood at a constant rate to very low concentrations. When alcohol is oxidized to acetaldehyde via ADH, nicotinamide adenine dinucleotide (NAD) is required as a cofactor and is reduced to NADH during the reaction. Under normal conditions the rate of NADH production exceeds its rate of reoxidation, resulting in an increase in the liver NADH/NAD ratio. Most of the acute metabolic effects of ethanol are due to this major change in the intermediary metabolism of the liver.

Protein deficiency, severe liver injury, and advancing age may decrease hepatic ADH as well as the rate of ethanol elimination. The agent known to enhance ethanol elimination both in vivo and in vitro is fructose, which increases the capacity of the respiratory chain to oxidize NADH derived from the oxidation of ethanol and acetaldehyde. Corticosteroids enhance the rate of ethanol elimination by increasing the conversion of NADH to NAD as a result of enhanced gluconeogenesis.

A number of drugs have been shown to interfere with the metabolism of ethanol [22]. Of these, pyrazole and its derivatives are best characterized as ADH inhibitors. In addition to interfering with the metabolism of ethanol, they also inhibit the metabolism of other alcohols via the ADH pathway. Thus 4-methylpyrazole and other ADH inhibitors may have a role in the treatment of methanol and etylene glycol poisoning. 4-Methylpyrazole has also been used in the treatment of the alcohol–disulfiram reaction. $H_2$ blockers have structural similarities to pyrazole. Consequently some of them, such as cimetidine, may inhibit gastric ADH selectively.

### 3.4.2 *Microsomal Ethanol Oxidizing System (MEOS) and Catalase*

The existence of an independent *MEOS pathway* is now generally accepted, although its quantitative contribution to total ethanol metabolism still remains in dispute [6–8]. MEOS is located in the endoplasmic reticulum, requires NADPH and oxygen, and is relatively insensitive to catalase inhibition. The scheme of the reaction is as follows:

$$CH_3CH_2OH + NADPH^+ + H + O_2 \xrightarrow{\text{MEOS}} CH_3CHO + NADP^+ + 2H_2O$$

Chronic treatment of rats with ethanol causes a ninefold increase in a specific ethanol-inducible cytochrome P450IIE1. In addition to ethanol, it effectively oxidizes other alcohols, carbon tetrachloride, and acetaminophen. The existence of P450IIE1 isozyme with a high capacity to oxidize ethanol and other specific substrates has also been confirmed in humans. Most recent studies indicate that P450IIE1 is induced by relatively modest ethanol consumption. The P450IIE1 gene has been isolated, characterized, and localized to chromosome 7 in the rat and chromosome 10 in man.

### 3.4.3 *Catalase*

*Catalase* is a hemoprotein located in the peroxisomes of most tissues. It may play a minor role in alcohol metabolism according to the following scheme:

$$CH_3CH_2OH + H_2O_2 \xrightarrow{\text{catalase}} CH_3CHO + 2H_2O$$

$$+ \text{hypoxanthine} + H_2O + O_2 \xrightarrow{\text{xanthine oxidase}} \text{xanthine} + H_2O_2$$

Accordingly catalase is capable of oxidizing ethanol in vitro only in the presence of a hydrogen peroxide generating system. The reaction is limited by the rate of hydrogen peroxide production. It has been estimated that catalase could account for only about 2% of the in vivo rate of ethanol oxidation.

### 3.4.4 *Nonoxidative Metabolism of Ethanol*

Many human organs have been found to metabolize ethanol through a nonoxidative pathway by forming fatty acid ethyl esters [23]. Their production is related to the blood ethanol concentration and it has been suggested that the nonoxidative metabolism of ethanol might explain the tissue damage seen in organs lacking oxidative alcohol metabolism. This interesting theory is waiting confirmation and further studies.

## 3.5 Metabolism of Acetaldehyde

More than 90% of the acetaldehyde formed from ethanol is subsequently oxidized in the liver to acetate. The main enzyme of acetaldehyde oxidation is mitochondrial aldehyde dehydrogenase [5]. The enzyme has a very low Km value and a high reaction rate, which explains why, under normal circumstances, only low concentrations of acetaldehyde are found outside the liver.

Two major hepatic ALDH isoenzymes (ALDH I and II) exist in humans [24]. ALDH I with a low Km for acetaldehyde is predominantly of mitochondrial origin and ALDH II, which has a relatively higher Km, is of cytosolic origin. Interestingly, the mitochondrial isoenzyme (ALDH I) was found to be missing in about 50% of the liver specimens of Japanese. Subsequent population genetic studies showed a wide prevalence of the isoenzyme deficiency among mongoloid populations and South American

Indian tribes but not in Caucasians and Negroes [24]. The ALDH I gene locus has been assigned to the human chromosome 12. ALDH I-deficient liver extracts contain immunologically cross-reactive material with normal ALDH I, but with near loss of enzyme activity. The loss of enzyme activity is due to a change in one amino acid in the enzyme molecule. The deficiency of ALDH I in Orientals results in several metabolic and clinical consequences, which will be discussed later in this chapter.

In the oxidation of acetaldehyde to acetate, mitochondrial NAD functions as a coenzyme. Consequently, oxidation of ethanol via acetaldehyde to acetate results in the reduction of both cytosolic and mitochondrial redox states with significant secondary changes in hepatic metabolism.

### 3.6 Blood Acetaldehyde Concentrations

Blood acetaldehyde concentrations during ethanol oxidation in the peripheral blood of nonalcoholic control subjects are extremely low (0–2 μM) and are often at, or below, the limit of detection [5]. This indicates that in normal healthy individuals almost all the acetaldehyde formed during ethanol oxidation is effectively oxidized in the liver. More pronounced concentrations of acetaldehyde exist, however, in the peripheral blood of chronic alcoholics, in Orientals with inactive ALDH I, and in the presence of ALDH inhibitors.

In Orientals with ALDH I deficiency, alcohol ingestion results in marked elevations of blood acetaldehyde concentrations ranging from 10 to 50 μM. These individuals then develop facial flushing and tachycardia as a direct consequence of acetaldehyde-induced catecholamine release. Consequently homozygotic Japanese with the atypical ALDH I allele are at a much lower risk of developing alcoholic liver diseases than those with homozygotic Caucasian ALDH I.

In 1937, a sensitization reaction to alcohol caused by a tetramethylthiuram mono- and disulfide was described and the suggestion made that these compounds might be used in the treatment of alcoholism. The first animal and clinical studies using the drug disulfiram appeared more than 10 years later. Subsequently the trade name Antabuse was given to the compound, and the characteristics of the sensitization reaction were extensively studied. In 1956 calcium cyanamide and its citrated derivative, calcium carbimide (CCC, Dipsan, Temposil) were proposed for clinical use in the treatment of alcoholism.

The reaction to alcohol which occurs following use of oral antidiabetic agents of the sulfonylurea group, such as tolbutamide, carbutamide, and chlorpropamide, closely resembles the disulfiram alcohol reaction and has also been attributed to the presence of elevated blood acetaldehyde concentrations. Other compounds known to induce alcohol-sensitizing reactions include the antioxidant *n*-butyraldoxime, the antibiotic metronidazole, antianginal drugs, and cefamandole. However, the biochemical backgrounds of the reactions caused by these agents in the presence of ethanol have not been fully established.

### 3.7 Metabolism of Acetate

Acetate produced by the hepatic metabolism of ethanol is oxidized further to carbon dioxide and water by peripheral tissues. The peripheral uptake of acetate is concentration dependent. During ethanol oxidation blood acetate levels are higher in alcoholics than in nonalcoholic controls. More importantly, a highly significant positive correlation exists between blood acetate concentrations and the rate of ethanol elimination. Consequently increased blood levels of acetate in the presence of ethanol indicate metabolic tolerance to alcohol and can be used as a laboratory marker of alcoholism and heavy drinking.

### 3.8 Alterations in the Metabolism of Ethanol, Acetaldehyde, and Acetate During Chronic Alcohol Consumption

Chronic ethanol consumption results in an increased tolerance to alcohol. This is mainly due to adaptation of the central nervous system, but in addition alcoholics develop increased rates of ethanol elimination, i.e., "metabolic tolerance." This is caused by adaptive changes in the ADH pathway and by increased activity of the MEOS pathway with subsequent increases in the blood acetaldehyde and acetate concentrations.

#### *3.8.1 Changes in Ethanol Metabolism*

Most studies show that chronic alcohol consumption enhances ethanol clearance, except in the presence of significant liver damage or severe food restriction. Indeed, both experimental ethanol administration in animals and chronic alcohol abuse in man increase the rates of ethanol metabolism. Several reports show that ADH activity does not increase and may even decrease after chronic ethanol ingestion although the rate of ethanol elimination simultaneously increases.

An ethanol-induced increase in the activity of $Na^+$,$K^+$-ATPase, followed by enhanced ATP consumption, decreased phosphorylation potential, increased oxygen consumption, and increased mitochondrial NADH reoxidation rate, provides the biochemical basis for the "hypermetabolic state" of the liver, which has been suggested to be responsible for the adaptive increase in ethanol elimination. Reference has also been made to this theory as providing the rationale for the treatment of alcoholic liver disease with propylthiouracil, i.e., propylthiouracil is claimed to reduce the hepatic hypermetabolic state induced by ethanol [25].

The quantitative contribution of the MEOS pathway to the adaptive increase in ethanol elimination caused by chronic alcohol consumption is not fully established and remains controversial. Nevertheless, the microsomal system is enhanced by chronic alcohol consumption. This is associated with an increase in various constituents of the smooth endoplasmic reticulum such as phospholipids, cytochrome P-450 reductase, and cytochrome P-450.

The rate of ethanol elimination may also be influenced by the presence of alcohol-related liver injury. Cirrhotic patients with jaundice who have not taken alcohol for more than 4 weeks show decreased rates of ethanol elimination. On the other hand, ethanol elimination rates are elevated even in the presence of relatively severe liver damage, if the measurement is made in the 1st month of abstinence. Animals with chronic non-alcohol-related liver disease show decreased rates of ethanol elimination and of ADH activity. In patients with alcoholic liver injury the decreased blood ethanol clearance probably reflects decreased liver ADH activity.

### *3.8.2 Changes in Acetaldehyde Metabolism*

Chronic alcohol consumption produces three major alterations in the hepatic metabolism of ethanol and acetaldehyde which result in increases in the concentrations of acetaldehyde in both blood and tissues: (a) an increase in the rate of ethanol oxidation, (b) a reduction in the capacity of mitochondria to oxidize acetaldehyde, at least in rats, and (c) a decrease in the activity of ALDH [5].

Unusually high blood acetaldehyde levels have been found in severely intoxicated patients. These exceptionally high values are most probably caused by the increased rate of ethanol elimination at high blood ethanol concentrations and by a decrease in liver ALDH activity associated with both the liver disease and chronic alcohol consumption.

## 4 Pathogenesis of Alcoholic Liver Disease

### 4.1 Animal Models of Alcohol-Related Organ Damage

A lot of evidence supporting the direct hepatotoxicity of ethanol has been obtained from experiments involving animal models of alcohol-induced organ damage. One of the major advances has been the introduction of a technique for feeding ethanol to rats as part of a nutritionally adequate totally liquid diet (the "Lieber-DeCarli diet") [8]. However, even with the liquid diet model the rat will not consume more than 36% of total calories as ethanol. Consequently more advanced liver lesions than fatty liver cannot be produced by this diet in rats.

The alcohol intake of baboons with the liquid diet model can be increased to 50% of total calories. Furthermore baboons are phylogenetically close to man and their life span is long enough for cirrhosis to develop. In this animal model, the biochemical and morphologic alterations in the liver (even liver cirrhosis) are comparable to those seen in humans despite the fact that a complete histologic spectrum of alcoholic hepatitis as seen in man has not been produced in baboons. Some doubt has, however, recently been cast on the pathogenetic implications of the models of alcoholic liver disease in both rats [14] and baboons [26].

## 4.2 Hepatotoxic Factors Associated with Ethanol and Its Oxidation

### *4.2.1 Toxicity of Ethanol*

Ethanol, like other general anesthetics, causes physical changes in all biologic membranes, including hepatic mitochondrial and endoplasmic reticulum membranes [27]. Chronic ethanol feeding has been shown to increase the fluidity of liver plasma membranes in rats, mice, and cell cultures. This is associated with an increase in the cholesterol ester and a decrease in the vitamin A content of liver plasma membranes. These changes may, at least in part, explain the pronounced morphologic changes of the liver cells, which can be seen on scanning electron microscopy.

### *4.2.2 Ethanol-Induced Shift in the Redox State of the Liver*

The ethanol-induced increase in the NADH/NAD ratio is a sign of a major change in hepatic metabolism during ethanol oxidation. Many of the acute changes in the intermediary metabolism of the liver, including the inhibition of the tricarboxylic acid cycle and gluconeogenesis, can be explained by the

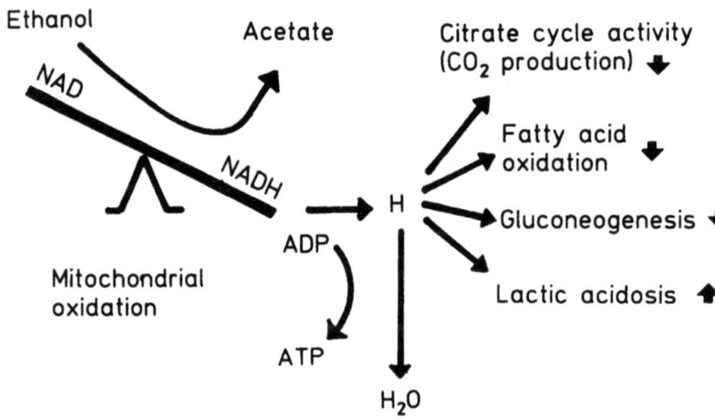


**Fig. 5.** The metabolic effects of an ethanol-induced increase in the hepatic NADH/NAD ratio

action of ethanol on the hepatic redox state (Fig. 5). The redox-related inhibition of fatty acid oxidation and the enhancement of triglyceride synthesis are the main pathogenetic mechanisms in the development of alcoholic fatty liver.

## 4.3 Pathogenesis of Alcoholic Fatty Liver

Interactions of ethanol with lipids are multiple and complex [28]. Depending on experimental conditions alcohol may (a) increase peripheral fat mobilization, (b) enhance hepatic triglyceride synthesis, (c) decrease lipid oxidation in the liver, and (d) decrease lipoprotein release.

### *4.3.1 Role of Adipose Tissue and Dietary Fat*

An acute large dose of alcohol mobilizes fat from the adipose tissue to the liver. This is mediated by catecholamines and is associated with increased serum free fatty acids. This mechanism plays a minor role in the development of fatty liver caused by chronic alcohol consumption. In this situation fatty acids accumulating in the liver resemble those of the diet. Administration of ethanol together with a high fat diet potentiates alcoholic fatty liver.

### *4.3.2 Hepatic Synthesis of Lipids*

Chronic alcohol does not stimulate the synthesis of fatty acids, but it may enhance the formation of glycerolipids as a consequence of the ethanol-induced increase in the NADH/NAD ratio. However, a decrease in the hepatic triacylglycerol-synthesizing capacity occurs during the progression of alcoholic liver injury.

### *4.3.3 Oxidation of Fatty Acids*

The inhibition of fatty acid oxidation by ethanol is also caused by the excessive generation of NADH, which suppresses the function of the citric acid cycle and the β-oxidation of fatty acids. During chronic alcohol consumption, however, the ethanol-induced shift in the redox state of the liver is attenuated and this is also associated with the attenuation of the accumulation of hepatic triglycerides.

## 4.4 Hepatotoxicity of Acetaldehyde

Acetaldehyde is both pharmacologically and chemically a very potent and reactive compound, which can be a major initiating factor in the pathogenesis of alcoholic liver damage [5–8].

In vitro acetaldehyde may form adducts – bound covalently – with phospholipids and proteins, e.g., erythrocyte membrane proteins, hemoglobin, plasma proteins, hepatic microsomal proteins, other hepatic proteins, and liver tubulin. More importantly, acetaldehyde may also bind to various proteins in vivo. The target molecule can, for instance, be the microsomal ethanol-inducible P450IIE1.

Acetaldehyde–protein adducts may serve as antigens and generate an immune response both in animals and in man. In addition they may: (a) inhibit hepatic protein secretion produced by both acute and chronic ethanol administration, (b) displace pyridoxal phosphate from its binding sites on proteins, (c) impair biologic functions of proteins, and (d) combine with tissue macromolecules and thereby cause severe tissue injury akin to many hepatotoxic drugs.

#### *4.4.1 Acetaldehyde-Induced Lipid Peroxidation*

In addition to mitochondrial aldehyde dehydrogenase, acetaldehyde may also be oxidized to acetate via xanthine oxidase. In this reaction oxygen may be metabolized to superoxide, which is a well-known lipid peroxidative agent. Normally free radicals are inactivated by glutathione. However, acetaldehyde may bind with glutathione or with cysteine, which is needed in the synthesis of glutathione. This might contribute to a reduction in liver glutathione with a secondary increase in lipid peroxidation. The ethanol-induced lipid peroxidation associated with glutathione depletion has been demonstrated both in baboons fed alcohol chronically and in human alcoholics.

### 4.5 Hepatotoxicity Associated with MEOS

Theoretically, MEOS may cause enhanced hepatotoxicity by several means [7, 8]. First, MEOS contributes to the production of the potentially hepatotoxic agent, acetaldehyde. Second, MEOS may enhance oxygen consumption, which, may potentiate hypoxia. Third, MEOS may activate hepatotoxic agents, such as carbon tetrachloride or acetaminophen. In accordance with this hypothesis, ethanol consumption in humans has been shown to be associated with an increase in the hepatotoxicity of acetaminophen. A decreased hepatic vitamin A level with some functional and structural abnormalities has been suggested to be a consequence of an ethanol-induced microsomal pathway for retinol oxidation.

### 4.6 Free Radicals and Lipid Peroxidation

Free radicals (superoxide and hydroxyl radicals) can damage via lipid peroxidation a wide range of cellular components, including proteins, nucleic acids, free amino acids, and lipoproteins. A great deal of evidence associates ethanol with lipid peroxidation, although the reliability of the currently available thiobutyric acid assay methods as an indicator of lipid peroxidation has been questioned [30].

In addition to MEOS, microsomes may oxidize ethanol by a separate pathway involving formation of hydroxyl radicals. These are also produced when acetaldehyde is oxidized to acetate via xanthine oxidase. In addition, stimulated hepatic neutrophils may generate free radicals, as discussed above. Free radicals are scavenged by superoxide dismutase and glutathione peroxidase. Chronic ethanol feeding increases glutathione turnover and the cellular requirements for glutathione. Furthermore there is an increased loss of glutathione from cells, especially from mitochondria. In chronic alcoholics there is an increase in both serum and liver lipoperoxide levels. The content of hepatic reduced glutathione is decreased, especially in patients with histologic liver necrosis. As an integral part of the enzyme glutathione peroxidase, selenium has a central role in protection against the tissue damage caused by lipid peroxides. Consequently the decrease not only in blood but also in liver selenium in patients with alcoholic liver disease may play a significant role in such damage. In addition, low vitamin E intake may potentiate hepatic lipid peroxidation.

### 4.7 Selective Perivenular Hepatotoxicity of Ethanol

Alcoholic liver injury starts and predominates in the perivenular region – zone 3 of the hepatic acinus. The enhanced injurious effect of ethanol at this site has been postulated to be due to hypoxia, resulting from ethanol-induced stimulation of hepatic oxygen consumption. The low oxygen tensions existing in perivenular zones may exaggerate the ethanol-induced redox shift in this area, a change which may contribute to the exacerbation of the damage in the perivenular area of the hepatic lobule.

The predominance of cytochrome P-450 mediated drug oxidation in perivenular hepatocytes and also the perivenular induction of P450IIE1 may contribute to the zonal distribution of alcoholic liver injury.

### 4.8 Hepatocyte Swelling

The enlargement of the liver is one of the earliest manifestations of hepatic damage produced by alcohol. It is caused by the accumulation of fat and protein in the liver. The increase in hepatic protein is associated with intrahepatocytic water retention, which results in ballooning of the hepatocytes. This hepatocyte swelling has been related to the pathogenesis of precirrhotic portal hypertension. The accumulation of exportable proteins is most probably caused by the ethanol-induced decrease in liver microtubules.

## 4.9 Alcohol and Fibrogenesis

Alcohol-induced necrosis and inflammation may trigger scarring and the development of cirrhosis. In addition, ethanol, its metabolism, and/or metabolites may have significant effects on collagen metabolism and fibrogensis [31].

The induction and proliferation of various perisinusoidal and perivenular cells have been documented in alcoholic liver injury. These mesenchymal cells, which may belong to the same cell family, include: Ito cells (fat-storing cell, lipocytes), myofibroblasts, fibroblasts, and transitional cells. Myofibroblasts were first demonstrated in cirrhotic human livers. They are actively contractile cells and produce type I, III, and IV collagen and laminin. They are predominantly present around the terminal venules and they increase in number even before the development of perivenular and pericellular fibrosis.

The basic mechanisms by which chronic alcohol consumption stimulates the mesenchymal cells to produce collagen and induces their proliferation are still largely unresolved. Possible candidates are mononuclear inflammation, acetaldehyde, and hyperlactacidemia.

Whatever its cause, the increased collagenization of the Disse space associated with the reduction of fenestrations between sinusoids and the Disse space may isolate the hepatocytes from their blood supply. Furthermore, these changes increase the vascular resistance, thereby contributing to the increased portal pressure often seen even in the early stage of liver disease.

Perivenular fibrosis is considered a predictor of the progression of fibrogenesis in patients who continue to drink [8]. Recently, perisinusoidal and pericellular accumulation of fibronectin in the perivenous area has been reported to have a definite predictive value for the development of alcoholic cirrhosis.

## 4.10 Immunologic Mechanisms, and Associated Viral Disease

So far most of the immunologic alterations as well as the changes in cellular immunity seen in patients with alcoholic liver disease have been thought to be secondary to primary hepatocellular injury [32]. Antibodies directed against ethanol-altered components of liver cells are frequently detected in the serum of patients with alcoholic liver disease. These antibodies seem to recognize a new antigen on the surface of hepatocytes, the expression of which is increased when aldehyde dehydrogenase activity is inhibited by disulfiram. These abnormal reactions – as for antibodies against acetaldehyde adducts – are also observed in patients with nonalcoholic liver disease and thus lack specificity. In theory, complement binding of acetaldehyde adduct-containing immune complexes may contribute to the perpetuation or exaggeration of liver damage.

Alcoholism and viral hepatitis can occur in the same patients, but in many patients with alcoholic cirrhosis there is no evidence of antecedent viral hepatitis. Alcoholics have an increased incidence of viral disease and hepatitis and there has been some question concerning the possible potentiation of alcohol-induced liver damage by viral disease, or of viral-induced lesions by alcohol.

### 4.11 Nutritional Factors

Although the direct hepatotoxic effect of ethanol has been indisputably proven, the role of potentiating nutritional factors has not been fully excluded [9]. If the fat content of an ethanol-containing liquid diet is decreased from 32% to 25%, hepatic triglyceride accumulation significantly decreases. Also the replacement of dietary triglycerides containing long chain fatty acids by fat-containing medium chain fatty acids markedly reduces the capacity of alcohol to produce fatty liver in rats. Excess weight is a risk factor or a predictive sign of histologic liver damage in alcoholics. At the same time there appears to be a positive correlation between fat consumption and cirrhosis mortality.

The entire spectrum of alcoholic liver disease (steatosis, mild alcoholic hepatitis, and cirrhosis) has been produced in baboons [33]. Not all investigators, however, have been able to produce fibrosis and cirrhosis in monkeys [26]. The discrepancy in the results has been related to the differences in the choline contents of the diets. It has been suggested that chronic alcohol feeding may exagerate the choline requirements of the monkeys. However, additional choline did not prevent the development of fibrosis in baboons [9].

Information about the nutritional status of alcoholics and of patients with alcoholic liver disease is equally controversial. This is largely due to the difficulties associated with reliable dietary assessments, especially in chronic alcoholics. Without doubt, however, heavy alcohol consumption has profound effects on nutrient economy and may produce nutritional imbalances in subjects eating normal diets. Using established criteria to diagnose and classify protein–calorie malnutrition, all of 248 patients with alcoholic liver disease were shown to have some evidence of malnutrition [34]. The prevalence of the malnutrition correlated closely with the severity of the liver disease, with both kwashiorkor and marasmus having an incidence of 72% in severe disease. On the other hand, malnutrition may at least partially have been secondary to the liver injury and not its cause. Only subtle nutritional alterations have been documented in several other studies.

### 4.12 Role of Enteric Bacteria

Liver damage, morphologically identical to alcohol hepatitis, often follows jejunoileal bypass surgery. As with alcoholic liver disease, histologic evidence of pericentral fibrosis in these patients identifies those at risk of developing fat necrosis and cirrhosis. These patients have successfully been treated with antibiotics, chloramphenicol, and metronidazole as well as with parenteral or enteral hyperalimentation. On this basis the pathogenesis of the liver damage associated with jejunoileal bypass has been related to bacterial overgrowth in the excluded segment.

## 5 Clinical Manifestations of Alcoholic Liver Disease

### 5.1 Alcoholic Fatty Liver

The clinical spectrum of alcoholic fatty liver extends from asymptomatic hepatomegaly to severe hepatocellular failure with cholestasis and portal hypertension. Most of the patients with pure fatty liver are virtually asymptomatic. Hepatomegaly is the commonest clinical sign, being present in 75% of patients upon physical examination. In more advanced cases hepatic tenderness, anorexia, nausea, emesis, jaundice, fluid accumulation, and even spider angiomas are present. In many of these cases associated alcoholic hepatitis may contribute to the clinical picture and laboratory findings.

The typical patient with more severe alcoholic fatty liver is young or middle aged with a history of drinking alcohol heavily for weeks or months. The liver edge may be a few centimeters below the costal margin or may extend to the iliac crest. The liver is relatively firm and its surface is smooth. Mild tenderness is common and is sometimes associated with severe epigastric or right upper quadrant pain. Severe forms of fatty liver may present a clinical picture mimicking extrahepatic obstructive jaundice, especially if associated with dark urine and acholic stools.

Typical abnormalities in laboratory tests are slightly or moderately elevated serum enzymes ($\gamma$-glutamyltransferase, GGT; aspartate aminotransferase, AST; alanine aminotransferase, ALT) and slight retention of sulfobromophthalein. The correlation between the histologic and chemical findings and the degree of hepatic steatosis is rather poor. Serum prothrombin levels are frequently low, even in mild cases. When there is associated malnutrition or malabsorption, the prothrombin time can be corrected by administration of vitamin K. Both decreased and normal serum albumin values have been reported in alcoholic fatty liver. Serum protein values should be interpreted cautiously, since they may be influenced by direct metabolic effects of alcohol as well as by nutritional factors. Unlike in more advanced alcoholic liver disease all the laboratory test abnormalities tend to return to normal within the first few days of hospitalization.

Transient anemia and albuminuria can be detected in about 25% of patients with fatty liver at the time of initial hospitalization. Albuminuria disappears within 24–72 h and its mechanism has not been resolved. Rarely, alcoholic fatty liver may be complicated by hyperlipidemia, hemolytic anemia, and jaundice (Zieve's syndrome). The syndrome consists of a combination of symptoms with a common etiology, i.e., ethanol.

## 5.2 Alcoholic Hepatitis

The spectrum of alcoholic hepatitis also ranges from mild anicteric hepatomegaly to fatal disease with jaundice, ascites, hepatic coma, and gastrointestinal hemorrhage, and with all the complications of severe hepatic insufficiency. The most frequent symptoms of the milder cases include anorexia, fatigue, intermittent fever, right epigastric pain, and hepatomegaly. In general, patients with alcoholic hepatitis are more ill than those with a simple fatty liver, and there is a correlation between (a) the severity of the histologic features of alcoholic hepatitis (hepatocellular necrosis, leukocytic infiltration, frequency of alcoholic hyaline), the degree of hepatomegaly, leukocytosis, and elevations of serum aminotransferase levels and (b) the intensity of symptoms. Patients with central hyaline sclerosis may have portal hypertension, splenomegaly, ascites, and esophageal and gastric varices, even in the absence of cirrhosis.

Characteristic laboratory findings include elevated levels of serum enzymes. GGT, AST, and ALT are elevated in all cases and alkaline phosphatase (ALP) in 80%. The incidence of abnormal laboratory values correlates with the activity of the disease. Unlike in nonalcoholic liver disease, the AST/ALT ratio and, even more clearly, the GGT/ALP ratio are increased. The increased AST/ALT ratio is due primarily to the low activity of ALT in liver and serum. The lower than expected elevation of ALT in the serum of patients with alcoholic hepatitis reflects diminished hepatic ALT activity and the lesser amounts of this enzyme which are available to leak into serum from damaged hepatocytes. Pyridoxal 5′-phosphate depletion may contribute to the decrease in ALT. An AST/ALT ratio greater than 2.0 is considered indicative of alcoholic liver disease, but this ratio may be less helpful in the presence of cirrhosis.

Serum protein changes include a decrease in serum albumin in about half of the patients, while haptoglobin and complement component 3 are usually increased and the serum transferrin concentration is relatively low. Serum IgA is usually elevated and seems to correlate with the degree of liver damage as assessed from histologic liver specimens. The depression of serum albumin and the prolongation of the prothrombin time have been shown to correlate with the severity of the histologic lesion.

Other common laboratory findings include a raised serum bilirubin level in 90% of patients. Serum bile acids are even more sensitive indicators of alcoholic liver disease. The concentration of chenodeoxycholic acid is increased, and although the correlation with the degree of liver cell necrosis is poor, bile acids may give more reliable and sensitive information than sulfobromophthalein and galactose elimination tests. Although sulfobromophthalein, galactose, indocyanine green, and antipyrine tests have been reported to be abnormal in liver disease, they lack practical discriminative value in the evaluation of initial alcoholic liver disease, fatty liver, perivenular fibrosis, and alcoholic hepatitis.

### 5.3 Alcoholic Cirrhosis

Alcoholic cirrhosis is predominantly a disease of males. It becomes symptomatic at an average age of 50 years, especially when it is not complicated by acute fatty liver or alcoholic hepatitis. Most patients are detected when they seek treatment for complications. Autopsy studies show that cirrhosis may remain unrecognized ante mortem in 40% of cirrhotic patients, and in about 20% it is discovered fortuitously on routine examination or during the evaluation of some other, unrelated, disease.

The most common signs of cirrhosis are weight loss (unless masked by ascites), weakness, and anorexia. Jaundice can be detected in about two-thirds of patients when they are first admitted to hospital. Low-grade and continuous fever is also common in decompensated cirrhosis. Jaundice and hepatomegaly are typical primary physical signs of cirrhosis. Secondary phenomena include portal hypertension with splenomegaly and ascites, encephalopathy, gastrointestinal hemorrhage from esophageal or gastric varices, and bleeding tendencies due to clotting factor abnormalities. Tertiary complications include spontaneous peritonitis caused by anaerobic bacteria and, in males, gynecomastia and a female pattern of pubic hair distribution resulting from testicular atrophy and hormonal imbalance. Other manifestations include spider angiomas, palmar erythema, parotid enlargement, and Dupuytren's contracture.

Abnormalities found on laboratory examination range from mild sulfobromophthalein retention to profound hyperbilirubinemia, hypoalbuminemia, hypoprealbuminemia, hypoprothrombinemia, and hyperglobulinemia. Frequently, IgA and also IgG and IgM are elevated. With more advanced liver injury a depression or even absence of alpha- and prebeta-lipoprotein bands can be demonstrated. This is associated with a decrease in the esterified fraction of plasma cholesterol secondary to depressed lecithin-cholesterol acyltransferase (LCAT) activity. Serum aminotransferases and alkaline phosphatase are usually only mildly elevated. Impaired glucose tolerance and an increased incidence of diabetes have been described in patients with Laënnec's cirrhosis.

## 6 Diagnosis and Differential Diagnosis of Alcoholic Liver Diseases

### 6.1 History, Clinical Signs, and Laboratory Findings

In the evaluation of the patient with either an incidental finding of pathologic laboratory values pointing to liver damage or more advanced symptomatology requiring hospitalization, the history of heavy alcohol intake for weeks or months before hospital admission is strongly suggestive of the alcoholic etiology of liver disease. For this purpose one may employ simplified screening questions such as CAGE (Table 1), which identify true alcoholics in more than 90% of cases.

No laboratory test has yet been found that has optimal sensitivity and specificity in the assessment of the alcoholic etiology of the liver disease [35, 36]. The most practical tests at present include blood or breath alcohol, elevated serum GGT level, and increased mean red blood cell volume and elevated serum carbohydrate deficient transferrin (CDT). Serum enzyme elevations can be used to detect alcoholics, but they do not differentiate alcoholic liver disease from other liver diseases.

### 6.2 Different Stages of Alcoholic Liver Disease

Laboratory tests are not much better for the differentiation of various stages of alcoholic liver disease. This is due to the great variability in the severity of both alcoholic hepatitis and fatty liver. In extreme cases both of them may simulate the clinical picture of liver cirrhosis or even extrahepatic biliary obstruction.

Serum procollagen type III peptide (PIIIP) may be helpful in monitoring fibrogenesis in alcoholic liver injury. Serum concentrations of this propeptide correlate with the degree of hepatic inflammation. The highest values are observed in patients with alcoholic hepatitis in whom numerous Mallory bodies are found. The test does not differentiate patients with simple fatty liver from those with fatty liver and early fibrosis. PIIIP does, however, discriminate between alcoholic fatty liver and alcoholic hepatitis. A modified PIIIP assay using Fab fragments has been shown to discriminate

**Table 1.** CAGE questions

1. Have you ever felt you should cut down your drinking?
2. Have people annoyed you by criticizing your drinking?
3. Have you ever felt bad or guilty about your drinking?
4. Have you ever had a drink first thing in the morning (eye opener)?

[a] The questions – if positive – should be extended to deal also with the time and frequency of the problems

between simple fatty liver and perivenular fibrosis in a significant number of patients.

### 6.3 The Role of Histology in the Differential Diagnosis

The aims of the histologic interpretation of liver biopsy specimens in alcoholic liver disease are threefold: (a) to differentiate between non-alcoholic and alcoholic liver diseases; (b) to determine the stage of alcoholic liver disease [fatty liver, early stages of fibrosis (perivenular, perisinusoidal, and pericellular), and alcoholic cirrhosis]; and (c) to evaluate the possible progression of the liver disease in serial biopsies. It is generally agreed that liver biopsy is necessary to establish the diagnosis since nonalcoholic liver disease cannot be diagnosed from the clinical data.

The determination of the stage of the alcoholic liver disease is important for both prognosis and treatment. The demonstration of perivenular fibrosis, even in the absence of more severe liver lesions, may predict the development of cirrhosis upon continued drinking. The presence of this lesion can be regarded as a warning sign which may make possible the detection of those individuals prone to develop cirrhosis.

Liver biopsy is certainly indicated when the laboratory abnormalities have persisted for 3–6 months. The frequency of subsequent biopsies can be decided individually, depending on the initial diagnosis. If the diagnosis of liver cirrhosis is certain, further biopsies are not indicated unless a complication such as hepatocellular carcinoma is suspected. In cases of fatty liver and alcoholic hepatitis, liver biopsy should be repeated within 1 or 2 years if the drinking habit cannot be controlled or the history is unreliable. Changes in laboratory patterns are crucial in making a decision.

## 7 Treatment and Prognosis of Alcoholic Liver Disease

The main goal in the management of the patient with alcoholic liver disease is abstinence from alcohol: this is the only effective way both to prevent the progression of the symptomatology and to improve the prognosis. Several studies have demonstrated that the prognosis for acute and chronic alcoholic liver disease is dramatically improved by abstinence from alcohol, while continued consumption is associated with increased morbidity and mortality. Symptomatic management of gastrointestinal and associated complications of liver injury, detoxification and treatment of alcohol withdrawal symptoms, though only the first steps in a long and arduous process of rehabilitation, are nevertheless extremely important in the long-term management of the patient. It is during this period (because of withdrawal symptoms or various medical complications) that the patient appreciates the therapeutic efforts of the physician. It is at this time that a good relationship between patient and physician can be established which eventually may determine a positive outcome in terms of control of excessive alcohol consumption and/or alcoholism.

### 7.1 Fatty Liver

Alcoholic steatosis is completely reversible in most cases. In some extremely severe cases, alcoholic fatty liver may have a fatal outcome, but as a rule even those cases needing hospitalization improve within a few days or weeks after cessation of alcohol consumption. In contrast to alcoholic hepatitis, laboratory test abnormalities rapidly return to normal levels and hepatomegaly decreases. Fat mobilization may be delayed only if steatosis has been extreme, with fatty cysts, or if it is complicated by obesity or prediabetes. Apart from alcohol withdrawal (and detoxification) and the provision of a diet with sufficient calories, vitamins, and protein, no other treatment is needed.

### 7.2 Alcoholic Hepatitis

The survival of patients with alcoholic hepatitis is dramatically improved by the discontinuation or reduction of alcohol consumption. The 7-year survival rate is 50% with continued drinking and 80% with reduced drinking. A mortality of 1.5%–17% has been found in individuals with alcoholic hepatitis ill enough to require hospitalization but well enough to permit liver biopsy.

A characteristic feature of alcoholic hepatitis is its aggravation during the initial 10 days to 2 weeks after hospitalization even though alcohol consumption has ceased. Sixty percent of the acute mortality is observed during the first 2 weeks, with a mean survival time of 16 days after admission. A fatal outcome can be anticipated in 90% of patients aged over 55 when the serum bilirubin level exceeds 25 mg/dl and the prothrombin time exceeds 5 s above control. In a Veterans Administration cooperative study on alcoholic hepatitis the overall mortality was 17% in the mild cases, 23.3% in moderate disease, and 43.8% in severe disease.

Clinical and pathologic signs of alcoholic hepatitis regress within weeks or months in most cases. A poorer short-term prognosis can be expected in patients with a prolonged prothrombin time and ascites. The long-term prognosis is unfavorably influenced by the presence of severe histologic inflammation and fibrosis in the initial liver biopsy specimen. Elevations of serum enzymes are less valuable prognostic indicators.

The general treatment of the patient with alcoholic hepatitis is the same as for alcoholic steatosis. The anorexia may be so severe as to require parenteral alimentation, including infusion of amino acids. Daily infusion of 70–85 g of amino acids has been reported to decrease mortality. Parenteral nutrition may improve morbidity (liver tests) and liver function, especially in severe alcoholic hepatitis.

Numerous pharmacologic agents have been utilized in an effort to effect a positive response in patients with alcoholic hepatitis. The most extensively tested drugs in this regard have been steroids, with at least ten randomized double-blind trials with either prednisolone or prednisone since 1971. Some controlled prospective studies reported significantly improved survival in patients with both alcoholic hepatitis and signs of encephalopathy who were treated with steroids but not in those with milder illness. Confirmatory results were obtained in four later studies. In a recent randomized study of 66 patients, methylprednisolone (39 mg/day for 28 days) significantly decreased mortality in those with severe alcoholic hepatitis [37]. So far the results suggest that methylprednisolone can be recommended in patients with severe alcoholic hepatitis manifested either by spontaneous encephalopathy or by a markedly reduced hepatic function.

Propylthiouracil (300 mg/day) has been demonstrated in a randomized trial to reduce the mortality caused by alcoholic liver disease [25]. Two other groups have not been able to confirm the positive effect of short-term therapy with propylthiouracil. D-Penicillamine, thioctic acid, (+)-cyanidanol-3, silymarin, palmitoyl-catechin, and testosterone have all been found to be ineffective in the treatment of alcohol-related liver disease.

## 7.3 Alcoholic Cirrhosis

When there is histologically proven cirrhosis, the 5-year survival rate for patients without jaundice, ascites, or hematemesis is 88.9% for abstainers and 62.8% for drinkers. The 5-year survival rates are unfavorably affected by jaundice, ascites, and hematemesis in abstainers (57.5%, 52.4%, and 35% respectively) and in drinkers (33.3%, 32.7%, and 21% respectively). The prognosis is still poor during the 1st year after the discontinuation of drinking. The survival rate of patients who live beyond the 1st year and who continue to abstain from alcohol is 86.2% for the subsequent 4 years, which is close to the expected survival for individuals of a similar age. The essential role of alcohol abstinence in the improvement of survival in patients with alcoholic cirrhosis has also been stressed in other studies.

Corticosteroids do not prolong survival of patients with alcoholic cirrhosis. Colchicine may provide a new approach for the treatment of alcoholic liver disease in the future. Prophylactic portal-systemic shunting in unselected cirrhotic patients does not improve the overall survival although the terminal event may alter from hemorrhage to hepatic failure. Recently it has been demonstrated that the survival of individuals who have undergone transplantation because of alcoholic liver disease is no different from that of those who have undergone transplantation for other forms of advanced hepatocellular disease [38].

## References


1. Lelbach WK (1976) Epidemiology of alcoholic liver disease. In: Popper H, Schaffner F (eds) Progress in liver diseases. Grune & Stratton, New York, p 494
2. Lieber CS, Salaspuro MP (1985) Alcoholic liver disease. In: Wright R, Millward-Sadler GH, Alberti KGMMM, Karran S (eds) Liver and biliary disease. Bailliere Tindall, W.B. Saunders, London, p 881
3. Hall P (1985) Alcoholic liver disease; pathobiology; epidemiology and clinical aspects. Edward Arnold, London
4. Lieber CS (1990) Interaction of ethanol with drugs, hepatotoxic agents, carcinogens and vitamins. Alcohol Alcohol 25:157–176
5. Salaspuro M, Lindros K (1985) Metabolism and toxicity of acetaldehyde. In: Seitz HK, Kommerell B (eds) Alcohol related diseases in gastroenterology. Springer, Berlin Heidelberg New York, p 106
6. Lieber CS (1988) Biochemical and molecular basis of alcohol-induced injury to liver and other tissues. N Engl J Med 319:1639–1650
7. Lieber CS (1988) Metabolic effects of ethanol and its interactions with other drugs, hepatotoxic agents, vitamins, and carcinogens: 1988 update. Semin Liver Dis 1:47–68
8. Lieber CS (1988) Pathophysiology of alcoholic liver disease. Mol Aspects Med 10:107–146
9. Lieber CS (1988) The influence of alcohol on nutritional status. Nutr Rev 46:241–254
10. Lieber CS (1989) Toxic and metabolic changes induced by ethanol. In: Goedde HW, Agarwall DP (eds) Genetics and alcoholism. Alan R. Liss, New York, p 57
11. French SW (1989) Biochemical basis for alcohol-induced liver injury. Clin Biochem 22:41–49
12. Salaspuro M (1989) The organ pathogenesis of alcoholism: liver and gastro-intestinal tract. In: Goedde HW, Agarwall DP (eds) Alcoholism: biomedical and genetic aspects. Pergamon, New York, p 133
13. Lieber CS (1990) Mechanism of ethanol induced hepatic injury. Pharmacol Ther 46:1–41
14. Derr RF, Larkin EC, Rao GA (1988) Is malnutrition necessary for the development of alcoholic fatty liver in the rat? Med Hypotheses 27:277–280
15. Sulkunen P (1976) Drinking patterns and the level of alcohol consumption; an international overview. Res Adv Alcohol Drug Probl 3:223–281
16. Lelbach WK (1985) Epidemiology of alcoholic liver disease; continental Europe. In: Hall P (ed) Alcoholic liver disease. Edward Arnold, London, p 130
17. Morgan MY (1985) Epidemiology of alcoholic liver disease; United Kingdom. In: Hall P (ed) Alcoholic liver disease. Edward Arnold, London, p 193
18. Saunders JB, Walters JRF, Davies P et al. (1981) A 20-year prospective study of cirrhosis. Br Med J 282:263–266
19. Pequignot G, Tuyns AJ, Berta JL (1978) Ascitic cirrhosis in relation to alcohol consumption. Int J Epidemiol 7:113–120
20. Coates RA, Halliday ML, Rankin JG et al. (1986) Risk of fatty infiltration or cirrhosis of the liver in relation to alcohol consumption: a case-control study. Clin Invest Med 9:26–32
21. Cotton RW, Goldman D (1988) Review of the molecular biology of the human alcohol dehydrogenase genes and gene products. Adv Alcohol Subst Abuse 7:171–182
22. Salaspuro M (1985) Inhibitors of alcohol metabolism. Acta Med Scand [Suppl] 703:219–224
23. Laposata EA, Lange LG (1986) Presence of nonoxidative ethanol metabolism in human organs commonly damaged by ethanol abuse. Q J Stud Alcohol 231:497–499

24. Goedde HW, Agarwall DP (1989) Acetaldehyde metabolism: genetic variation and physiological implications. In: Goedde HW, Agarwall DP (eds) Alcoholism: biomedical and genetic aspects. Pergamon, New York, p 21
25. Orrego H, Blake JE, Blendis LM et al. (1987) Long-term treatment of alcoholic liver disease with propylthiouracil. N Engl J Med 317:1421–1427
26. Ainley CC, Senapati A, Brown IM et al. (1988) Is alcohol hepatotoxic in the baboon? J Hepatol 7:85–92
27. Sun GY, Sun AY (1985) Ethanol and membrane lipids. Alcohol Clin Exp Res 9:164–180
28. Lieber CS, Savolainen M (1984) Ethanol and lipids. Alcohol Clin Exp Res 8:409–423
29. William AJK, Barry RE (1987) Free radical generation by neutrophils: a potential mechanism of cellular injury in acute alcoholic hepatitis. Gut 28:1157–1161
30. Dianzani MU (1985) Lipid peroxidation in ethanol poisoning: a critical consideration. Alcohol Alcohol 20:161–173
31. Hahn EG, Schuppan D (1985) Ethanol and fibrogenesis in the liver. In: Seitz HK, Kommerell B (eds) Alcohol related diseases in gastroenterology. Springer, Berlin Heidelberg New York, p 124
32. Paronetto F (1985) Ethanol and the immune system. In: Seitz HK, Kommerell B (eds) Alcohol related diseases in gastroenterology. Springer, Berlin Heidelberg New York, p 269
33. Popper H, Lieber CS (1980) Histogenesis of alcoholic fibrosis and cirrhosis in the baboon. Am J Pathol 98:695–716
34. Mendenhall CL, Anderson S, Weesner RE et al. (1984) Protein-calorie malnutrition associated with alcoholic hepatitis. Veterans Administration Cooperative Study Group on Alcoholic Hepatitis. AM J Med 76:211–222
35. Salaspuro M (1989) Characteristics of laboratory markers in alcohol-related organ damage. Scand J Gastroenterol 24:769–780
36. Salaspuro M (1987) Use of enzymes for the diagnosis of alcohol-related organ damage. Enzyme 37:87–107
37. Carithers RL Jr, Herlong HF, Diehl AN et al. (1989) Methylprednisolone therapy in patients with severe alcoholic hepatitis. Ann Intern Med 110:685–690
38. Starzl TE, Van Thiel D, Tzakis AG et al. (1988) Orthotopic liver transplantation for alcoholic cirrhosis. JAMA 260:2542–2544

# 21 Autoimmune Chronic Active Hepatitis

K.-H. Meyer zum Büschenfelde and M.P. Manns

## 1 Definition

A loss of tolerance against autologous liver tissue is regarded as the principal pathogenetic mechanism in autoimmune chronic active hepatitis (CAH). Autoimmune CAH is a chronic inflammatory disease process of unknown cause, characterized by a female predominance, a genetic predisposition, a response to immunosuppressive drug therapy, and characteristic autoantibodies. Extrahepatic autoimmune syndromes are frequently associated with autoimmune CAH (Table 1) as well as hypergammaglobulinemia.

## 2 Diagnosis and Classification

Apart from the clinical characteristics and the response to immunosuppressive drug therapy, autoantibodies are major diagnostic criteria [1, 16]. On the basis of different autoantibody specificities, at least three serologically different subgroups of autoimmune CAH can be distinguished (Table 2) [2]. Antinuclear antibodies (ANAs) characterize classical autoimmune-type "lupoid" hepatitis. In this form of autoimmune CAH, also called type I, smooth muscle antibodies (SMAs) and liver membrane antibodies (LMAs) are frequently detectable [3]. ANAs are routinely detected by indirect immunofluorescence (Fig. 1). However, they are very heterogeneous and almost all subtypes that occur in rheumatologic disorders [4] are found in "lupoid" hepatitis, including antibodies to double-stranded DNA. Classical autoimmune CAH, i.e., type I, was first described in the early 1950s in young females with hypergammaglobulinemia showing a good response to corticosteroids [5–7]. Usually the disease starts at the age of 30–40, although it may occur in childhood [8]. The female predominance is approximately 90%.

Autoimmune CAH type II is characterized serologically by liver–kidney microsomal (LKM-1) autoantibodies [9–11] (Fig. 2). In about 50% of patients, autoimmune CAH type II starts in childhood, while in the other 50% disease starts between the ages of 35 and 60. Usually, ANAs and SMAs are negative in this autoimmune liver disease [9, 10]. However, thyroid microsomal antibodies, thyroglobulin antibodies, and parietal cell

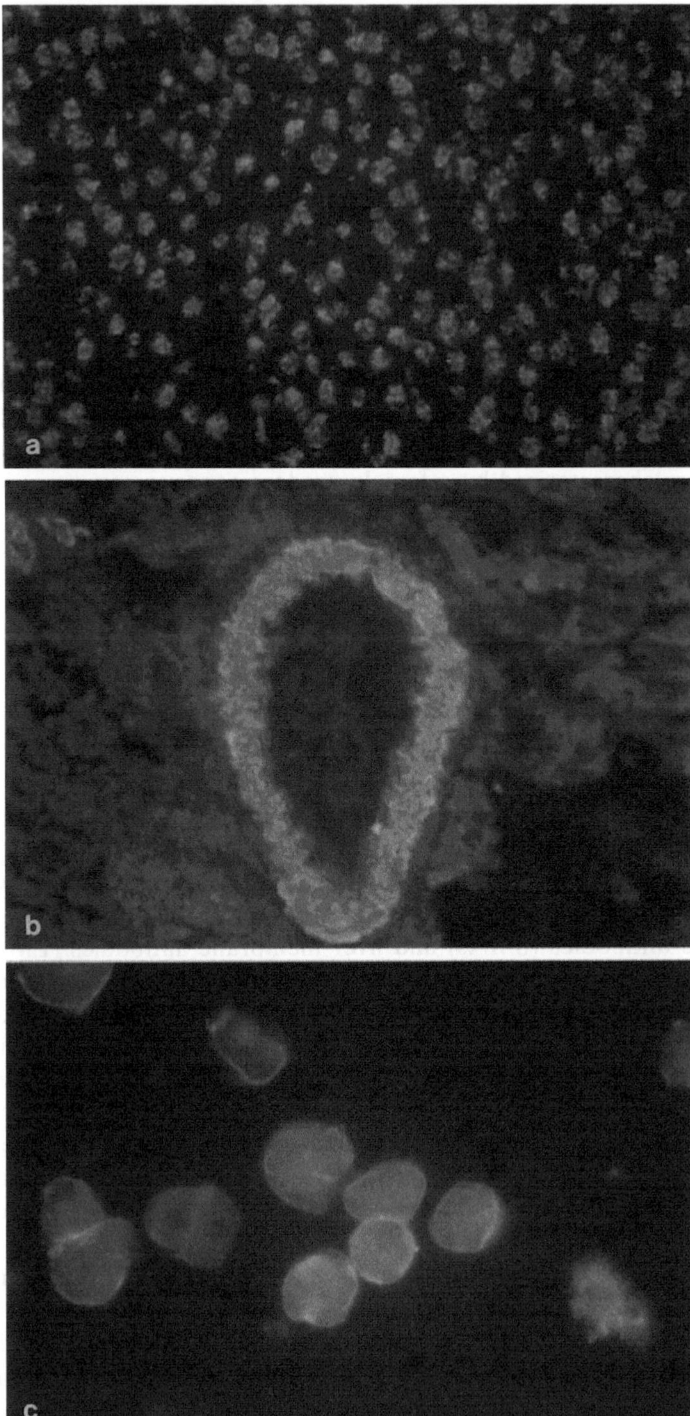


Fig. 1a–c

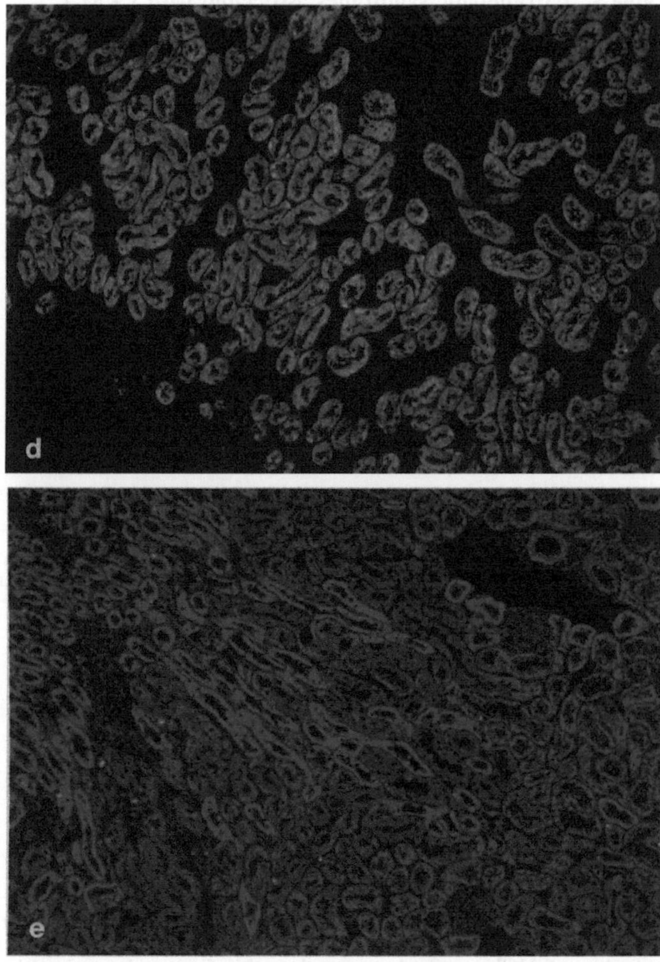

**Fig. 1a–e.** Detection of antibodies by indirect immunofluorescence: **a** antinuclear antibodies on rat liver; **b** smooth muscle antibodies on rat kidney vessels; **c** liver membrane antibodies on isolated rabbit hepatocytes; **d** liver–kidney microsomal antibodies on rat kidney; **e** antimitochondrial antibodies on rat kidney

antibodies are frequently detected. Extrahepatic syndromes are frequent in the younger patients with autoimmune CAH type II but less common in older patients [9]. Furthermore, autoimmune CAH type II is characterized by low IgA levels and hypergammaglobulinemia is less prominent. Female predominance is around 80%. The disease starts with an episode of acute hepatitis in 30%–40% of the patients. Rapid progression to cirrhosis is common. The prevalence of autoimmune CAH type II is estimated at about 5–10 cases per million population. This may differ geographically. Although autoimmune CAH type II has mainly been described in continental Europe, the disease does occur worldwide.

**Table 1.** Extrahepatic syndromes associated with LKM-1 positive CAH

| |
|---|
| Vitiligo |
| Thyroid disorders |
| Insulin-dependent diabetes |
| Autoimmune hemolytic anemia |
| Idiopathic thrombocytopenic purpura |
| Pernicious anemia |
| Rheumatoid arthritis |
| Ulcerative colitis |
| Chronic glomerulonephritis |
| Fibrosing alveolitis |
| Multiorgan vascular dysplasia |
| Celiac disease |
| Nail dystrophy |
| Alopecia |

**Table 2.** Heterogeneity of HBsAg negative CAH

| | ANA | LKM-1 | SLA | SMA | AMA | Immunosuppressive treatment | Anti-HCV (percent) |
|---|---|---|---|---|---|---|---|
| CAH non-A, non-B | – | – | – | – | – | – | 70% |
| Classical autoimmune-type ("lupoid") CAH | + | – | – | + | – | + | 7% |
| LKM-1 antibody positive CAH | – | + | – | – | – | + | 37% |
| SLA antibody positive CAH | – | – | + | +/– | +/– | + | 2% |
| SMA antibody positive CAH | – | – | – | + | – | + | n.t. |
| Primary biliary cirrhosis | – | – | – | – | + | – | 0% |

*Abbreviations*: ANA, antinuclear antibody; LKM-1, liver–kidney microsomal antibody; SLA, soluble liver antigen antibody; SMA, smooth muscle antibody; AMA, antimitochondrial antibody; anti-HCV, antibody against hepatitis C virus determined by the Ortho ELISA test and confirmed by the Chiron RIBA test; n.t., not tested

A third subgroup (type III) of autoimmune CAH is associated with anti-SLA (soluble liver antigen) autoantibodies [2]. These antibodies react with liver cytokeratins 8 and 18 [11]. In the initial study, the picture of autoimmune CAH type III was described in 23 patients [2]. Female predominance was 90% and the mean age at onset was 37 years. Hypergammaglobulinemia was evident in most patients, with a mean of 3.2 g/liter, and response to immunosuppressive treatment was good. Anti-SLA antibody titers decline during therapy in parallel with disease activity. In 25% of anti-SLA antibody positive patients no other autoantibodies are found. Therefore, this marker is important in distinguishing this subgroup o. autoimmune CAH from anti-HCV negative non-A, non-B hepatitis.

It may be that high titer SMAs directed against F-actin characterize a fourth subgroup of autoimmune CAH [8].

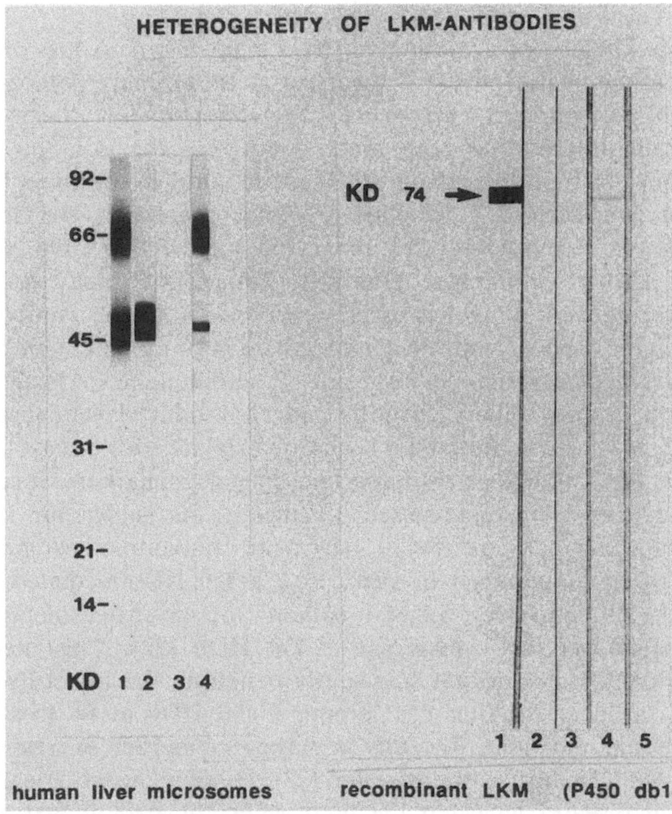


**Fig. 2.** Western blot analysis with human liver microsomes (*left*) and bacterial lysates containing recombinant LKM-1 (P-450 db1) antigen (*right*). *Lanes 1 and 4*: serum from patient with LKM-1 antibody positive liver disease reacting with LKM-1 (P-450 db1) antigen at 50 kd and an additional microsomal antigen at 64 kd. *Lane 2*: LKM variant reacting with cytochrome P-450 IA2 which recognizes a 50-kd microsomal protein but not the 74-kd recombinant LKM-1 (P-450 db1) antigen. P-450 db1 is now called P-450 IID6 according to new nomenclature agreements. *Lane 3 and 5*: control sera

## 3 Immunogenetics

Most autoimmune diseases are characterized by an immunogenetic background. In classical autoimmune-type "lupoid" hepatitis the association with the HLA haplotype A1, B8, and DRw3 is well established for Caucasians [12]. In Japan, a significant increase in DRw4 has been described [13] for autoimmune CAH type I. HLA DRw4 was also increased in the DRw3 negative population reported from Great Britain [14]. In addition, a significant increase in null alleles for complement component 4 (C4A-Q0) has been reported in autoimmune CAH type I [15]. There are no HLA data available for autoimmune CAH types II and III.

## 4 Etiology and Pathogenesis

The etiology of autoimmune CAH is unknown. A loss of tolerance against autologous liver tissue is regarded as the primary pathogenetic mechanism [16]. A number of cytotoxicity assay systems have been developed. Significant progress has been made concerning the isolation of cloned T lymphocytes from liver biopsies. Recently, antigen specificity was demonstrated for liver-derived T lymphocyte clones concerning the hepatic asialoglycoprotein receptor [17, 18] and cytochrome P-450 IID6, the major antigen of LKM-1 antibodies. However, antigen specificity for the majority of liver-derived T lymphocytes remains unknown. Antibodies against the hepatic asialoglycoprotein receptor, a liver-specific membrane component, have been described in all groups of autoimmune CAH and in some patients with primary biliary cirrhosis and viral-induced liver disease [15, 19, 20]. Titers for these antibodies seem to correlate with disease activity.

Autoantibodies are important diagnostic markers. It seems unlikely that they per se mediate tissue distruction. As shown for LKM-1 antibodies against cytochrome P-450 IID6, the autoantibodies inhibit the function of their autoantigen in vitro, i.e., P-450 IID6-mediated drug metabolism [21, 22]. However, LKM-1 patients are extensive metabolizers for drugs metabolized by cytochrome P-450 IID6 [22]. This means that LKM-1 autoantibodies do not sufficiently penetrate the intact liver cell membrane to reach and inhibit cytochrome P-450 IID6 at its location in the endoplasmic reticulum. Recently, a plasma membrane expression of cytochrome P-450 IID6 has been postulated [23]. Possibly, agents triggering autoimmune liver diseases have left the body when the patient first consults a doctor. An infectious etiology is supported by reports that autoimmune CAH has developed after well-documented viral hepatitis [24, 25]. Furthermore, measle virus-specific nucleic acid sequences were found in peripheral blood lymphocytes [26]. Autoantibodies also occur in chronic hepatitis D virus (HDV) infection. These react with antigens of basal layer and thymus cells as well as with human liver microsomes [27–29]. Furthermore, a high prevalence of hepatitis C virus antibodies (anti-HCV antibodies) has been reported for autoimmune liver diseases from various parts of the world, especially southern Europe [30–32]. The prevalence reported for anti-HCV antibodies depends on the test system applied and the geographic origin of the sera. In our experience (Table 3), a significant percentage of anti-HCV positivity is only seen for patients with LKM-1 antibody positive liver disease, i.e., autoimmune CAH type II. Of our patients, 37% are anti-HCV positive as confirmed by the Chiron recombinant immunoblot assay (RIBA) test. No significant increase compared with normal controls is seen for autoimmune CAH type I (ANA positive) and type III (anti-SLA antibody positive). Anti-HCV positivity in patients with autoimmune CAH type II is usually associated with the older patient population, when liver disease becomes clinically overt after the age of 40. These patients may have a

**Table 3.** Anti-HCV positivity in autoimmune liver diseases

| | No. | Anti-HCV+ | |
|---|---|---|---|
| | | ELISA (%) | RIBA (%) |
| Autoimmune CAH | | | |
| Total | 170 | 46 | 17 |
| ANA/SMA | 67 | 46 | 7 |
| LKM-1 | 41 | 51 | 37 |
| SLA | 62 | 42 | 2 |
| Primary biliary cirrhosis | 123 | 16 | 0 |
| Primary sclerosing cholangitis | 16 | 13 | 0 |
| Systemic lupus erythematosus | 14 | 7 | 0 |
| Extrahepatic cholestasis | 15 | 0 | n.t. |
| Inflammatory bowel disease | 6 | 0 | n.t. |
| Healthy controls | 100 | 2 | n.t. |

Abbreviations as in Table 2

**Table 4.** Microsomal autoantigens in liver diseases – 1991

| Mol. wt. (kd) | Nomenclature | Biochemical definition | Disease association |
|---|---|---|---|
| 50 | LKM-1 | P-450 db1 (IID6) | Autoimmune CAH |
| 50 | LKM-2 | P-450 meph (IIC9) | Drug-induced hepatitis (tienilic acid) |
| ? | LKM-3 | ? | Chronic hepatitis D |
| 50 | LM | P-450 IA2 | Autoimmune CAH, dihydralazine hepatitis |
| 55 | n.n. | ? | Autoimmune CAH |
| 64 | n.n. | ? | Autoimmune CAH |

n.n., not nominated

history of parenteral HCV exposure and show a milder clinical course of the disease.

Noninfectious exogenous agents, such as drugs or other environmental chemicals, may cause autoimmune liver disease. Interestingly, microsomal antibodies other than LKM-1 also react with cytochrome P-450 enzymes. They are associated with specific entities of drug-induced hepatitis. LKM-2 antibodies are induced by tienilic acid and react with cytochrome P-450 IIC9 [33]. Autoantibodies against cytochrome P-450 IA2 are found in dihydralazine-induced hepatitis [34], but also in idiopathic autoimmune CAH [35] (Table 4).

## 5 Clinical Features and Pathology

The clinical features of autoimmune CAH are fatigue, hepatosplenomegaly, and possibly jaundice. Up to one-third of patients first present with an episode of acute hepatitis. Furthermore, as already mentioned, patients with autoimmune CAH are predominantly female. In females amenorrhea is a typical early symptom. In classical autoimmune-type "lupoid" hepatitis and in autoimmune CAH type III (anti-SLA antibody positive), the mean age at onset is around 35 years. The clinical picture of autoimmune CAH is also dominated by a high frequency of extrahepatic syndromes, many of which have a presumed autoimmune background (Table 1). Most frequently, patients present with arthralgias and autoimmune thyroid diseases. Untreated patients have a rather poor prognosis (Fig. 3). However, immunosuppressive treatment does prolong survival (Fig. 3). Nowadays, diagnosis is made in earlier life.

While the clinical characteristics of classical autoimmune CAH type I and type III are very similar, clinical features for autoimmune CAH type II associated with LKM-1 antibodies are slightly different. There is also a female predominance (4:1) but hypergammaglobulinemia is less profound. Low IgA levels are typical for this syndrome. Furthermore, a bimodal age distribution is typical for autoimmune CAH type II. About 50% of the patients are children below the age of 15 while in another group of patients the disease starts at an age beyond 40 years. The young patients with LKM-1 positive autoimmune CAH, when untreated, have a poor prognosis and immunosuppressive treatment is of particular benefit to them. LKM-1 positive autoimmune CAH in adults often has a milder clinical course, and elevation of aminotransferases is less profound. On the other hand, the

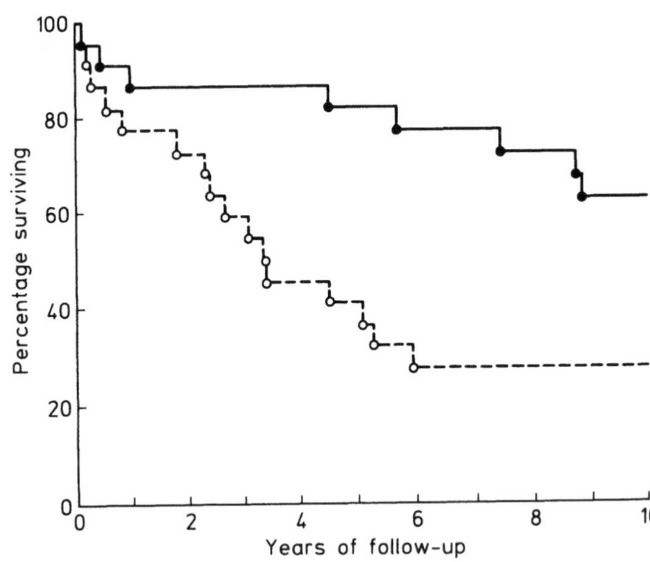


**Fig. 3.** Effect of corticosteroids on idiopathic autoimmune chronic active hepatitis compared to placebo. The life table survival curves of control (·----·) and prednisolone-treated (x——x) patients are shown. [Reproduced with permission from KIRK AP et al. (1980) Gut 21:78–83]

effect of corticosteroids is less convincing in these elderly patients. While in autoimmune CAH type II patients of the older age group detection of anti-HCVs is a common observation, anti-HCVs are usually absent in these children. The association of autoimmune CAH type II with extrahepatic clinical syndromes is well documented and is seen in at least one-third of the patients.

As regards histopathology, there are some features that are characteristic for autoimmune CAH. However, the distinction between autoimmune CAH and virus-induced liver disease cannot be made on the basis of conventional histology or by ultrastructural analysis of liver tissue. The broad spectrum of lesions ranges from chronic persistent hepatitis to acute necrotizing injury to CAH and cirrhosis. In addition, overlap syndromes between primary biliary cirrhosis and CAH have been reported. The term "plasma cell hepatitis" should be avoided since plasma cells are not a prominent feature of the cellular infiltrate in autoimmune CAH. Although pathognomonic features of autoimmune CAH have not been observed, there are characteristic alterations that can help to distinguish this type from viral hepatitis, namely: a predominant portal and periportal lymphocytic infiltration, conspicuous emperipolesis of lymphocytes, ballooning, and lytic necrosis as the leading type of hepatocyte injury in association with broad areas of collapse and an acinar arrangement of hepatocytes.

In recent years, immunoelectron microscopy has been used for an ultrastructural analysis of autoimmune CAH. Due to the availability of monoclonal antibodies, the inflammatory infiltrate has been extensively analyzed. The majority of tissue-infiltrating lymphocytes represent T cells. Furthermore, HLA antigens are expressed on hepatocytes that normally do not present these antigens on their surface. The subtyping of T lymphocytes, however, has revealed conflicting results. It seems that in autoimmune CAH the CD4/CD8 ratio is approximately 1:1, while in viral hepatitis the majority of tissue-infiltrating T lymphocytes are CD8 positive cells, i.e., they carry the cytotoxic-suppressor cell phenotype. Furthermore, in autoimmune CAH increased expression of HLA class II antigens was observed on hepatocytes adjacent to the inflammatory infiltrate. These data support the hypothesis that an aberrant HLA class II antigen expression which is frequently seen in many autoimmune disorders is involved in the presentation of autoantigens, leading to activation of CD4 positive T lymphocytes which may have cytotoxic functions.

## 6 Differential Diagnosis

Hepatitis A, B, and D virus infection can be easily diagnosed by specific viral antigens, antibodies, and the determination of viral DNA or RNA itself. The diagnosis of acute and chronic HCV infection may still provide problems, including its distinction from autoimmune liver diseases.

However, in our experience a significant percentage of anti-HCVs, confirmed by RIBA test, is only seen in the older population of patients with autoimmune CAH type II. HCV-specific RNA determination by a polymerase chain reaction assay will be necessary to provide definite clarification of this problem. Furthermore, toxic and metabolic liver diseases have to be excluded, such as Wilson's disease, $\alpha_1$-antitrypsin deficiency syndrome, and hemochromatosis. LKM-1 antibodies as markers for autoimmune CAH type II have to be distinguished from LKM-2 antibodies associated with tienilic acid-induced hepatitis, which are directed against cytochrome P-450 IIC9 [33]. These antibodies so far have only been described in France; the diuretic drug tienilic acid can only be purchased in France and the United States. There may be a diagnostic problem for autoantibodies against cytochrome P-450 IA2, since these autoantibodies have been detected not only in dihydralazine-induced hepatitis but also in idiopathic autoimmune CAH [33, 35]. An overlap syndrome between autoimmune CAH and primary biliary cirrhosis has been described [36]. Up to 20% of sera from patients with autoimmune CAH are positive for antimitochondrial antibodies (AMAs). The antigen specificity of these AMAs is the same as in primary biliary cirrhosis, i.e., the E2, E1α, and E1β subunits of pyruvate dehydrogenase complex, the E2 subunit of branched chain oxoacid dehydrogenase, and the E2 subunit of oxoglutarate dehydrogenase complex [37–39]. If ANAs or SLA antibodies (in addition to AMAs) are positive in these sera and if cholestasis is minor or absent, we regard these patients primarily as having autoimmune CAH and treat them with immunosuppression, in particular when piecemeal necrosis is evident on liver histology.

## 7 Therapy

Immunosuppressive treatment with corticosteroids alone or in combination with azathioprine prolongs survival, decreases symptoms and signs of fatigue, loss of appetite, and fever, leads to improvement in biochemical abnormalities, such as a reduction of elevated serum bilirubin and aminotransferase levels, and increases serum albumins [40, 41]. Finally, a decrease in inflammatory activity is seen in liver biopsy specimens, with development of normal liver histology [40]. Prednisolone 75 mg alone or in combination with azathioprine 2 mg/kg body weight may be used at the beginning of treatment. Corticosteroids are tapered down to 50 mg after the 1st week and then reduced by 5 mg every week until a maintenance dose of 10 mg/day is reached. In children it may be appropriate to control the disease with corticosteroids alone. Controlled treatment trials are only available for classical autoimmune-type ANA positive "lupoid" hepatitis (type I). However, on the basis of uncontrolled studies, it is justifiable to treat autoimmune CAH type II and type III with immunosuppressive drugs. If, despite all diagnostic criteria, safe distinction between autoimmune liver disease and virus-induced hepatitis C is not possible, it seems appropriate to start with immunosuppression since interferons may worsen autoimmune liver disease [41, 42]. Treatment should be continued for 2 years. After termination of therapy, a relapse may be seen in up to 60% of the patients. Unlimited immunosuppression then may be necessary, at least until the menopause.

There is no convincing evidence that alternate-day therapy with corticosteroids is superior to a daily application. In addition, there is no proof that prednisone is better than prednisolone. A theoretical advantage of prednisolone is that prednisone must be converted to prednisolone by the liver to become an active drug. However, this does not seem to be of any practical relevance. The drugs nowadays used for immunosuppression act nonspecifically. Therefore, enough treatment should be given for enough time. The goal should be to keep aminotransferase levels within twice the upper limit of normal [40].

It is uncertain whether the control of inflammatory activity by immunosuppressive drugs has a significant effect on the development of liver fibrosis and cirrhosis. It is well known that patients may develop cirrhosis despite normalization of aminotransferase levels. Today, liver transplantation offers these patients an alternative therapy for end-stage disease. Although recurrence of autoimmune CAH has been postulated in individual patients [43], the overall outcome of liver transplantation for end-stage autoimmune CAH seems very good. The immunogenetic background of the disease and the expression of HLA class II molecules on hepatocytes support a possible role of HLA class II molecules for antigen presentation in patients with autoimmune CAH. This may well be a prerequisite for proper autoantigen presentation and ultimately recurrence of autoimmune liver disease in the donor liver. It seems, logically, that donor hepatocytes expressing different HLA antigens compared to the recipient's liver cells are less vulnerable to attack by autoreactive T lymphocytes.

## References


1. Manns M (1989) Autoantibodies and antigens in liver diseases – updated. J Hepatol 9:272–280
2. Manns M, Gerken G, Kyriatsoulis A, Staritz M, Meyer zum Büschenfelde K-H (1987) Characterization of a new subgroup of autoimmune chronic active hepatitis by autoantibodies against a soluble liver antigen. Lancet I:292–294
3. Hopf U, Meyer zum Büschenfelde K-H, Arnold W (1976) Detection of a liver membrane autoantibody in HBsAg-negative chronic active hepatitis. N Engl J Med 294:578–582
4. Tan EM, Feltkamp TEW, Alarcon-Segovia D et al. (1988) Reference reagents for antinuclear antibodies. Arthritis Rheum 31:1331
5. Waldenström J (1950) Leber, Blutproteine und Nahrungseiweise. Dtsch Ges Verd Stoffw 15:113

6. Kunkel HG, Ahrens EH Jr, Eisenmenger WJ (1951) Extreme hypergammaglobulinemia in young women with liver disease of unknown etiology. J Clin Invest 30:654–659
7. Mackay IR, Taft CO, Cowling DS (1956) Lupid hepatitis. Lancet II:1323
8. Odievre AM, Maggiore G, Homberg J-C et al. (1983) Seroimmunologic classification of chronic hepatitis in 57 children. Hepatology 3:407
9. Homberg J-C, Abuaf N, Bernard O et al. (1987) Chronic active hepatitis associated with anti-liver/kidney microsome antibody type I: a second type of "autoimmune hepatitis". Hepatology 7:1333–1339
10. Manns M, Johnson EF, Griffin KJ, Tan EM, Sullivan KF (1989) The major target antigen of liver and kidney microsomal autoantibodies in idiopathic autoimmune hepatitis is cytochrome P450db1. J Clin Invest 83:1066–1072
11. Wächter B, Kyriatsoulis A, Lohse AW, Gerken G, Meyer zum Büschenfelde K-H, Manns M (1990) Characterization of liver cytokeratin as a major target antigen of anti-SLA antibodies. J Hepatol 11:232–239
12. Tait B, Mackay IR, Board P, Coggan M, Emery P, Eckardt G (1989) HLA A1, B8, DR3 extended haplotypes in autoimmune chronic active hepatitis. Gastroenterology 97:479–481
13. Zeniya M, Takahashi H, Aizawa Y, Kameda H (1990) Revaluation of liver specific protein and immunogenetic analysis on the pathogenesis of autoimmune hepatitis. Sixth International Congress of Mucosal Immunology, Tokyo, 22–27 July 1990, Abstract No. 125
14. Donaldson PT, Doherty DG, Hayllar KM et al. (to be published) Susceptibility to autoimmune chronic active hepatitis: HLA DR4 and A1-B8-DR3 are independent risk factors. Hepatology
15. Vergani D, Wells L, Larcher VF et al. (1985) Genetically determined low C4: a predisposing factor to autoimmune chronic active hepatitis. Lancet II:294–298
16. Meyer zum Büschenfelde K-H, Lohse AW, Manns M, Poralla T (1990) Autoimmunity and liver disease. Hepatology 12:354–363
17. Löhr H, Treichel U, Poralla T, Manns M, Meyer zum Büschenfelde K-H, Fleischer B (to be published) The human hepatic asialoglycoprotein receptor is a target antigen for liver infiltrating T cells in autoimmune chronic active hepatitis and primary biliary cirrhosis. Hepatology
18. Vento S, McFarlane BM, McSorley CG et al. (1988) Liver autoreactivity in acute virus A, B and non-A–non-B hepatitis. J Clin Lab Immunol 25:1–7
19. McFarlane BM, McSorley CG, Vergani D et al. (1986) Serum autoantibodies reacting with the hepatic asialoglycoprotein receptor (hepatic lectin) in acute and chronic liver disorders. J Hepatol 3:196–205
20. Treichel U, Poralla T, Hess G et al. (1990) Autoantibodies to asialoglycoprotein receptor (ASGP-R) in autoimmune-type chronic active hepatitis. Hepatology 11:606–612
21. Zanger UM, Hauri HP, Loeper J, Homberg J-C, Meyer UA (1988) Antibodies against human cytochrome P-450 db1 in autoimmune hepatitis type II. Proc Natl Acad Sci USA 27:8256–8260
22. Manns M, Zanger U, Gerken G, Sullivan KF, Meyer zum Büschenfelde K-H, Meyer UA, Eichelbaum M (1990) Patients with type II autoimmune hepatitis express functionally intact cytochrome P450 db1 that is inhibited by LKM-1 autoantibodies in vitro but not in vivo. Hepatology 12:127–132
23. Loeper J, Descatoire V, Maurice M et al. (1990) Presence of cytochrome P450 on human hepatocyte plasma membrane. Recognition by several autoantibodies. Hepatology 12:909
24. Hopf U, Möller B (1984) Die Entwicklung chronisch aktiver Hepatitiden vom autoimmunen Typ nach Hepatitis B Virusinfektion mit HBsAg-Persistenz. Z Gastroenterol 22:121–128
25. Laskus T, Slusarczyk J (1989) Autoimmune chronic active hepatitis developing after acute type B hepatitis. Dig Dis Sci 34:1294–1297

26. Robertson DAF, Zhang SL, Guy EC, Wright R (1987) Persistent measles virus genome in autoimmune chronic active hepatitis. Lancet II:9–11
27. Crivelli D, Lavarini C, Chiaberge E et al. (1983) Microsomal autoantibodies in chronic infections with HBsAg associated delta agent. Clin Exp Immunol 54:232
28. Zauli D, Fuscon M, Crespi C et al. (1984) Close correlation between basal cell layer autoantibodies and hepatitis B virus associated chronic delta infection. Hepatology 4:1103–1106
29. Amengueal MJ, Catalfana M, Pujol A et al. (1989) Autoantibodies in chronic delta virus infection recognize a common protein of 46 kD in rat forestomach basal cell layer and stellate thymic epithelial cells. Clin Exp Immunol 78:80–84
30. Esteban JI, Esteban R, Viladomiu L et al. (1989) Hepatitis C virus antibodies among risk groups in Spain. Lancet II:294–296
31. McFarlane IG, Smith HM, Johnson JP, Bray GP, Vergani D, Williams R (1990) Hepatitis C virus antibodies in chronic active hepatitis: pathogenic factor or false-positive result? Lancet I:754–757
32. Lenzi M, Ballardini G, Fusconi M et al. (1990) Type 2 autoimmune hepatitis and hepatitis C virus infection. Lancet I:258–259
33. Beaune PH, Dansette PM, Mansuy D et al. (1987) Human anti-endoplasmic reticulum autoantibodies appearing in a drug-induced hepatitis are directed against a human liver cytochrome P-450 that hydroxylates the drug. Proc Natl Acad Sci USA 84:551
34. Bourdi M, Larrey D, Nataf J et al. (1990) Anti-liver endoplasmic reticulum autoantibodies are directed against human cytochrome P-450 IA2. J Clin Invest 85:1967–1973
35. Manns MP, Griffin KJ, Quattrochi LC, Sacher M, Thaler H, Tukey RH, Johnson EF (1990) Identification of cytochrome P450IA2 as a human autoantigen. Arch Biochem Biophys 280:229–232
36. Berg PA, Wiedmann KH, Sayers T, Klöppel G, Lindner H (1980) Serological classification of chronic cholestatic liver disease by the use of two different types of antimitochondrial antibodies. Lancet I:1329
37. Mackay IR, Gershwin ME (1989) Molecular basis of mitochondrial autoreactivity in primary biliary cirrhosis. Immunol Today 10:315–318
38. Fussey SPM, Guest JR, James OFW, Bassendine MF, Yeaman SJ (1988) Identification and analysis of the major M2 autoantigens in primary biliary cirrhosis. Proc Natl Acad Sci USA 85:8654
39. Kirk AP, Jain S, Pocock S et al. (1980) Late results of the Royal Free Hospital prospective controlled trial of prednisolone therapy in hepatitis B surface antigen negative chronic active hepatitis. Gut 21:78–83
40. Maddrey WC, Combes B (to be published) Therapeutic concepts for the management of idiopathic autoimmune chronic hepatitis. Semin Liver Dis
41. Vento S, Di Perri G, Garofano T et al. (1989) Hazards of interferon therapy for HBV-seronegative chronic hepatitis. Lancet II:926
42. Ruiz-Moreno M, Rua MJ, Carreno V, Quiroga JA, Manns M, Meyer zum Büschenfelde K-H (1991) Autoimmune chronic hepatitis type 2 manifested during interferon therapy in children. J Hepatol 12:265–266
43. Neuberger J, Portmann B, Caine R et al. (1984) Recurrence of autoimmune chronic active hepatitis following orthotopic liver grafting. Transplantation 37:363–365

# 22 Primary Biliary Cirrhosis and Sclerosing Cholangitis

A. PARÉS and J. RODÉS

## A. Primary Biliary Cirrhosis

Primary biliary cirrhosis (PBC) is a chronic liver disease of unknown etiology, characterized by inflammation and progressive destruction of the small intrahepatic bile ducts that results in chronic cholestasis. The disease affects predominantly women between 40 and 60 years old. The clinical picture is the result of chronic cholestasis and comprises pruritus, jaundice, xanthomas, steatorrhea, and the complications of vitamin and mineral deficiencies [1, 2].

The first descriptions of the disease were provided by ADDISON and GULL, and subsequently by HANOT, in the last century. However, a clear comprehensive description of the disease was first given in 1950 by AHRENS et al., who adopted the term "primary biliary cirrhosis" introduced 1 year previously to distinguish biliary cirrhosis in the absence of extrahepatic biliary obstruction from that associated with obstruction of the large bile ducts. Later, in 1959, SHERLOCK proposed the term "chronic intrahepatic obstructive jaundice," and in 1965 RUBIN et al. described the histologic lesion as "nonsuppurative destructive cholangitis" [3]. Finally, in 1967, SCHEUER described the progress of liver lesions in four overlapping histologic stages, with only the last stage exhibiting true cirrhosis [4]. Therefore, the term "biliary cirrhosis" is misleading for all stages of the disease, since cirrhosis is only present in the last stage. However, this term is still used because the most suitable name which defines the morphologic lesion, "chronic destructive nonsuppurative cholangitis," is excessively long and complex.

### 1 Epidemiology

Primary biliary cirrhosis has been reported in all races and therefore in all parts of the world. The estimated prevalence in Europe is approximately 22 cases per million population, although it seems to vary considerably among different countries and within the same country in separate areas. Thus, in England the prevalence rates range from 37 to 144 cases per million inhabitants. In various regions of Spain the point prevalence ranged from

5 to 75 cases per million in 1981 [5]. Further studies indicate that the prevalence has been rising, particularly in recent years, a fact which is probably due to the increasing proportion of patients who are diagnosed. In a study covering the northern part of Sweden, a prevalence of 151 per million inhabitants was established. Although family clustering has been found, and PBC has been reported in sisters, twins, mothers, and daughters, there is no evidence that the disease is limited to certain social or ethnic population groups.

## 2 Pathology

In 1967 SCHEUER [4] proposed that the histologic lesions of PBC be classified into four stages. The earliest stage is characterized by florid bile duct lesions and the last by established biliary cirrhosis; the two intermediate stages are one of ductular proliferation and another of scarring or fibrosis. These stages are usually progressive, and in some cases an overlap between stages is present in the same histologic specimen because the lesions tend to be focal and patchy. This first staging classification was modified by LUDWIG et al., who also defined four stages: portal, periportal, septal, and cirrhotic [6].

*Stage I: Portal lesion.* This stage is characterized by inflammation and enlargement of the portal tracts with little or no periportal inflammation, features that are indistinguishable from those seen in chronic persistent hepatitis. The florid lesion consists in the presence of necrotic and ruptured septal or interlobular bile ducts (Fig. 1). They are usually surrounded by mononuclear inflammatory cells, particularly lymphocytes, large histiocytes, and plasma cells, which may break the basement membrane. Noncaseating granulomas may be seen surrounding damaged ducts. The florid lesion may also be present in histologic stages II–IV.

*Stage II: Periportal lesion.* As the lesion progresses the inflammatory cells erode the limiting plate and there is mild piecemeal necrosis of periportal hepatocytes. The lesion is similar to that observed in chronic active hepatitis. Ductular proliferation and absence or paucity of bile ducts are distinctive features of this stage.

*Stage III: Septal fibrosis.* In this stage the most prominent feature is the acellular fibrosis extending as septa from the portal tracts, with severe distortion of hepatic architecture but without regenerative nodules. There is also a marked loss of small bile ducts with conspicuous periportal cholestasis.

*Stage IV: Cirrhosis.* This stage is characterized by a macronodular cirrhosis, which is difficult to distinguish from cirrhosis from other causes, and par-

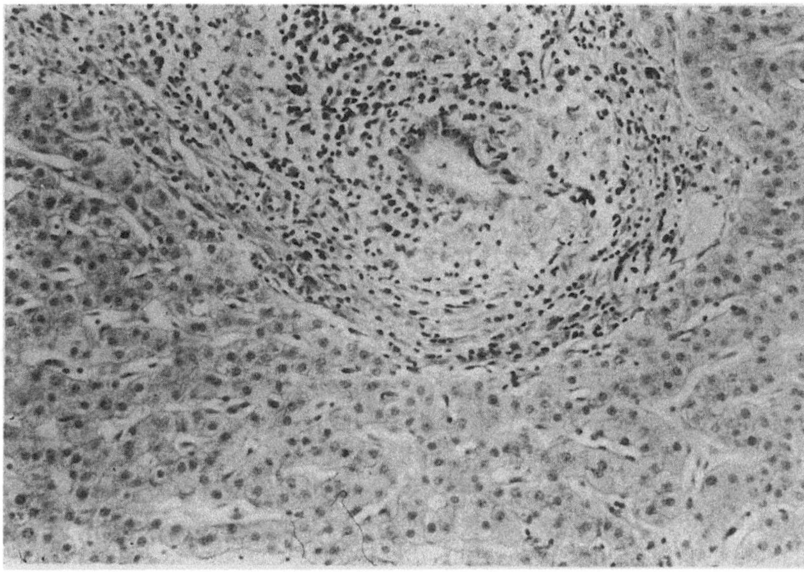

**Fig. 1.** Florid bile duct lesion of PBC, including a granuloma

ticularly from secondary biliary cirrhosis. The absence of bile ducts in portal tracts and the presence of mononuclear inflammation should suggest the diagnosis of PBC.

Besides the histologic characteristics of the four stages of PBC, other morphologic lesions may be found in liver specimens, including hyaline inclusions, which resemble Mallory bodies, and copper deposition, which is detected with specific stains. Both features are prominently distributed in hepatocytes adjacent to portal tracts, and probably they are secondary to chronic cholestasis. Nodular hyperplasia of hepatocytes has also been described in patients with early stages of PBC, and it may explain in part the presence of portal hypertension in these patients [7].

## 3 Etiology and Pathogenesis

The cause of PBC is unknown, although several etiologic agents have been proposed, including infectious, toxic, and environmental agents. Despite multiple studies, up to now there is no definite evidence that a specific infectious agent may be the precipitating mechanism that initiates the lesion of the epithelia of the bile ducts. Hepatitis A, B, and C viruses have no relationship with PBC. However, the fact that PBC sera exclusively react with specific mitochondrial antigens with molecular weights of 70 and 50 kd and with some antigens from Enterobacteriaceae of similar molecular weight suggests that an infectious agent may give rise to the ductular lesion [8].

Thus, it is possible that antimitochondrial antibodies (AMAs) in patients with PBC are induced by rough mutants of Gram-negative bacteria which may be present in the gut.

Some drugs capable of inducing cholestasis, such as phenothiazines, androgens, and contraceptive steroids, have also been related to the development of PBC. However, the association between a particular drug and PBC is very rare and consequently it could be speculated that these drugs only act by unmasking an asymptomatic preexisting disease. An etiologic role has also been suggested for some environmental toxins, but this hypothesis is only supported by one epidemiologic study which found an association between PBC and water supply.

Despite multiple studies and research on the pathogenesis of PBC, as yet there are only hypotheses for explaining the mechanisms which cause the ductular damage and the progression of the disease. However, most studies indicate that some genetic susceptibility and immunologic mechanisms may play a role in the development of PBC. Among the evidence supporting a genetic susceptibility are the familial clusterings, the increased incidence of AMAs and other immunologic abnormalities in unaffected relatives of patients with PBC, and the association with particular histocompatibility antigens. Indeed, the incidence of HLA-DRw3 [9], D4, and DR8 [10] has been found to be significantly increased in patients with PBC compared to controls. These findings are very relevant since products of the HLA-D loci are involved in the genetic regulation of the immune response, which is abnormal in patients with PBC.

There is a profusion of studies with respect to the immunologic disturbances in patients with PBC indicating that these patients have several abnormalities of humoral immunity, cell-mediated immunity, and immune regulation. Concerning the abnormalities of humoral immunity, raised serum IgM and IgG concentrations, the presence of an abnormally immunoreactive IgM, and abnormalities of the complement system, including chronic activation by the classical and the alternative pathway, have been described [1, 2, 11]. Circulating immune complexes are also present in patients with PBC, and the concentrations increase with the progression of the disease, a fact which does not support the theory that the disease is mediated by immune complexes. In addition, the material considered to be immune complexes could be the abnormal immunoreactive IgM. There are also several features of autoimmunity, particularly the presence of AMAs and other autoantibodies. However, with the exception of AMAs, these autoantibodies do not appear to be involved in the pathogenesis of PBC (the role of AMAs in the pathogenesis is also controversial).

Alterations of cell-mediated immunity and of immune regulation have also been described in PBC. The skin test anergy implies defects of cellular immunity, as well as the presence of granulomas and lymphoid aggregates in the liver and a decreased number of T cells in peripheral blood. The accumulation of cytotoxic (T8+) cells around bile ducts suggests that these

T cells may contribute to the destruction of the ductular epithelium in PBC. On the other hand, a defect in T suppressor cell function has also been observed in PBC, an abnormality which probably contributes to the autoimmune phenomena observed in this disease. However, this defect is not specific for PBC and it is more prominent as the disease progresses. Therefore, it is possible that these changes in T suppressor cell function may be secondary to the disease, and they most likely do not play a specific role in its pathogenesis.

Because of the clinical, biochemical, and histologic similarities between chronic graft-versus-host disease and PBC, it has been postulated that the T cell-mediated cytotoxicity contributes to the bile duct lesions, and that PBC may be an incomplete form of graft-versus-host disease [12]. This hypothesis is very provocative, since it has been demonstrated that bile duct cells from patients with PBC, in contrast to normal bile duct cells, express major histocompatibility antigens of class II. Consequently, it could be theorized that some external agents may induce changes in bile epithelia contributing to the expression of the class II histocompatibility antigens, and that, therefore, these modified bile ducts may be destroyed by T cells. At present, however, the issue of which features are involved in pathogenesis and which are a consequence of the disease remains unresolved, and the role of the immunologic mechanisms in the pathogenesis of PBC is thus speculative.

In summary, a complete theory to explain the pathogenesis of PBC must include a genetic predisposition which allows an external agent, infectious or toxic, to induce changes in the bile duct. As a result the class II histocompatibility antigens on bile duct cells will be aberrantly expressed and may directly elicit an autoimmune response. Accordingly the cells from the bile epithelia may be destroyed by cytotoxic T cells, resulting in the florid early lesion. The progression of the disease may be due to the effects of retained bile acids, or other substances, as a consequence of chronic cholestasis.

## 4 Clinical Features

As mentioned above, patients are usually women between 40 and 60 years old. In all series the male to female ratio is 1:9 [1, 11, 13, 14]. The clinical presentation of the disease is variable. Some cases may be diagnosed incidentally because a routine examination discloses liver or spleen enlargement or raised serum alkaline phosphatase activity (asymptomatic forms). In other patients the disease starts insidiously, as in other chronic liver diseases. The initial clinical features are similar to those observed in chronic active hepatitis or cirrhosis. In a small number of patients the disease can start during pregnancy and be confused with the idiopathic cholestasis of the last trimester, or may emerge after treatment with hormonal contraceptives.

However, the most frequent pattern of presentation is the classical form characterized by pruritus as the initial symptom, followed months to years later by jaundice. These clinical features may remain unchanged over a variable period of time, until the complete clinical spectrum of chronic cholestasis emerges (Fig. 2).

Pruritus is the most characteristic symptom in PBC, being present in 50%–70% of patients as the initial symptom. Usually, itching is first located on the palms of the hand and the feet, and as the disease progresses the pruritus affects all the body. Pruritus may be extremely distressing and may affect the patient's routine or sleeping pattern. The cause of pruritus in PBC is uncertain, but it may be related to a still unknown retained bile acid. However, pruritus does not correlate with either serum or skin concentrations of bile acids.

Jaundice may never develop, although in most patients a temporal relationship between pruritus and jaundice is often found. Jaundice usually appears within 6 months to 2 years after the onset of pruritus. Jaundice may fluctuate at first but tends to increase progressively, giving a characteristic appearance to the patient. Jaundice preceding pruritus is extremely unusual.

Besides pruritus and jaundice, most patients have some typical skin manifestations. Excoriations and skin hyperpigmentation secondary to scratching are frequently observed in the areas of severe pruritus and, therefore, patients may have an area less pigmented on their back with a butterfly wing shape. As the condition progresses the skin may become thick, hard, and rough over the fingers, ankles, and legs, probably as a consequence of chronic scratching and vitamin A deficiency. In addition,

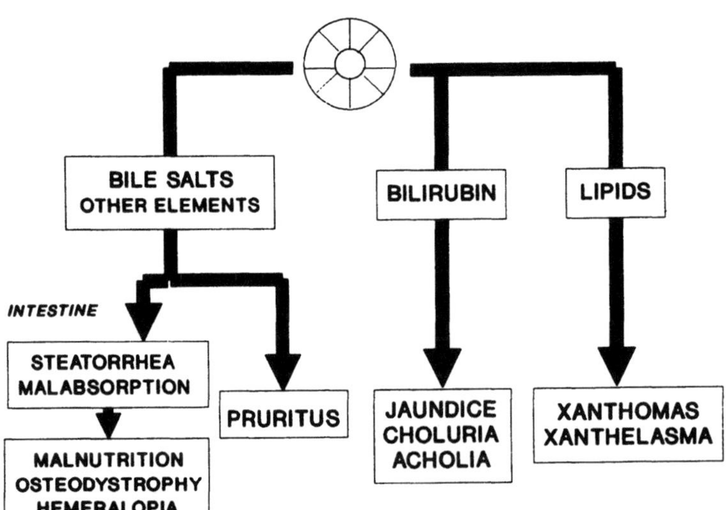


**Fig. 2.** Clinical consequences of chronic cholestasis. The inability to excrete different components in the bile determines the clinical features of chronic cholestasis

patients may develop hypertrichosis on the face and extremities. Likewise, as the disease progresses, xanthelasma and tuberous and planar xanthomas may appear, sometimes acutely. Planar xanthomas are distributed particularly on the palms, neck, trunk, and inframammary grooves, whereas tuberous xanthomas are located on the elbows, knees, and Achilles tendons. In the late stages, when liver failure is perceptible, xanthomas may disappear. Some patients may develop severe pain in their fingers and toes as a manifestation of a distressing xanthomatous peripheral neuropathy. Decreased bile secretion of copper induces its accumulation in the liver and in other tissues such as the kidneys and cornea. The deposits of copper in the cornea may explain the fact that some patients with PBC exhibit a Kayser-Fleischer corneal ring.

The physical findings are variable at the time of presentation of the disease. Most patients have hepatomegaly, which increases with the progression of the disease. A palpable spleen is less frequent initially, and if present indirectly tends to indicate the development of portal hypertension, although splenomegaly may also be due to reticuloendothelial hyperplasia. Portal hypertension of the presinusoidal type may be observed in the early stages of the disease. However, as the disease advances a sinusoidal component is added, and patients with stages III and IV of the disease have sinusoidal portal hypertension [15]. Despite the presence of portal hypertension, bleeding esophageal varices and ascites are uncommon and usually only appear as a terminal event. Likewise, hepatic encephalopathy as a sign of liver failure usually emerges a few weeks or months before death [14]. Some patients also exhibit telangiectasia that may be present as part of the CRST syndrome.

Mild steatorrhea secondary to a diminished amount of bile acid in the small intestine is common in PBC and may be present even without jaundice [16]. Steatorrhea may, however, be clinically important, reaching levels as high as 40 g of fat per day. In these cases, weight loss and muscle wasting may be prominent features. As a consequence of intestinal malabsorption, some fat-soluble vitamin levels may be low in PBC. Vitamin A deficiency is associated with intestinal malabsorption and defective mobilization from the liver. Signs of vitamin A deficiency such as night blindness are rare, although tests of dark adaptation are often abnormal. Zinc deficiency has also been reported in some patients with symptomatic vitamin A deficiency. Low serum levels of vitamin E have also been found in PBC [17], and they may cause a neuromuscular syndrome as described in children with chronic cholestasis; this neuromuscular syndrome is nevertheless extremely rare in patients with PBC. The prothrombin time may be prolonged because of poor vitamin K absorption. Vitamin D as well as calcium malabsorption may contribute to metabolic bone disease in patients with PBC.

Osteomalacia in PBC is related to vitamin D deficiency, to inadequate exposure to ultraviolet light, and to urinary loss of vitamin D. However, osteomalacia is only found in singular cases with extreme cholestasis and malnutrition. By contrast, osteoporosis is the most frequent bone disorder in PBC. The pathophysiology for osteoporosis in PBC is not well known since contradictory results have been reported with respect to the bone turnover state. However, the most recent studies indicate that osteodystrophy in PBC is characterized mainly by "low-turnover" osteoporosis, probably due to decreased osteoblast function (Fig. 3). Osteoporosis in PBC is related to the duration of the liver disease, the postmenopausal condition, and calcium malabsorption [18]. Symptoms such as backache secondary to vertebral fractures and pain over the ribs are common manifestations of advanced osteoporosis in patients with PBC.

Despite the fact that most patients with PBC exhibit clinical evidence of chronic cholestasis, approximately 13%–48% of patients are now diagnosed in the asymptomatic phase of the disease owing to better understanding of the disease along with advances in the availability and application of routine serum biochemical tests [11, 14, 19]. Such individuals are identified as a result of investigating the cause of an incidentally discovered elevation in the serum alkaline phosphatase activity. Some of these patients may, however, have signs of liver disease or portal hypertension such as liver or spleen enlargement. Another form of presentation is as an advanced hepatic disease with bleeding esophageal varices, and more rarely ascites, but with no clinical evidence of cholestasis.

Since many associated conditions have been reported in PBC, patients may exhibit a wide cohort of other clinical manifestations, depending on the nonhepatic associated disorder.

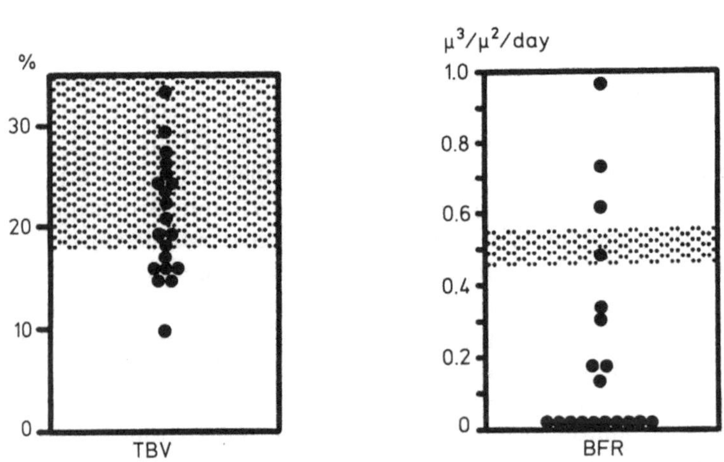


**Fig. 3.** Osteodystrophy in PBC is characterized by low bone turnover osteoporosis. The trabecular bone volume (*TBV*) and the bone formation rate (*BFR*) are decreased in patients with PBC. *Shaded areas* indicate normal values

## 5 Laboratory Tests

The laboratory abnormalities are similar to those found in other chronic cholestatic liver diseases. The serum alkaline phosphatase level is almost invariably raised and tends to reach a plateau early in the course of the disease [13, 14]. However, in rare cases that are diagnosed because of positivity of AMAs, the serum alkaline phosphatase levels may be normal [20]. Other markers of cholestasis such as the serum levels of 5′-nucleotidase and γ-glutamyltransferase are also increased. Serum bilirubin may be normal at the onset, but as the disease progresses higher levels of serum bilirubin are found.

Serum bile acid concentrations as well as the levels of serum lipids are usually increased in PBC. The pattern of serum lipids tends to change during the course of the disease. Thus, in early stages high-density lipoproteins are higher than low-density and very low-density lipoproteins, whereas patients with advanced disease have marked elevations of low-density lipoproteins and decreased high-density lipoproteins [21]. These changes are probably secondary to inhibition of hepatic lipase activity in early PBC and decreased cholesterol esterification in advanced disease.

Serum levels of aminotransferases are slightly increased and fluctuate within a narrow range. Serum albumin and prothrombin time are normal in early stages but may be altered in very advanced stages of the disease when other clinical manifestations of liver failure are found [13, 14]. Initially, globulin levels are normal, although high serum concentrations of IgM and IgG may be found by immunoelectrophoresis in almost 75% of cases. Patients may have mild to moderate normocytic and normochromic anemia. An elevated erythrocyte sedimentation rate is found in almost all patients.

### *Autoantibodies*

Antimitochondrial antibodies are present in approximately 90% of patients and represent the best established and most characteristic serologic abnormality in PBC. AMAs are a family of antibodies that react with different antigens [22]. In PBC, the most common AMA detected is anti-M2, which recognizes an antigen of the inner membrane of mitochondria and is a specific marker for the serologic diagnosis of PBC. The M2 antigen is composed of five antigenic determinants with molecular weights of 36, 43, 51, 56, and 70 kd [23]. The majority of patients with PBC react with the 70-kd antigen, which has recently been identified as the E2 component of the mitochondrial pyruvate dehydrogenase complex [24]. The 51-kd antigenic determinant also is related with the E2 component of the pyruvate dehydrogenase complex, and it is known as protein X. Three other types of AMA are also associated with PBC: anti-M4, anti-M8, and anti-M9. They react with antigens of the outer mitochondrial membrane. Anti-M4 is only found in patients who have anti-M2 and has been reported to be present in patients with histologic features of both PBC and chronic active hepatitis. Anti-M8 is also only present in patients who have anti-M2 and is associated with more rapid progression of the disease. Anti-M9 is present in anti-M2 negative and anti-M2 positive patients and seems to be present notably in patients with asymptomatic and early PBC. Anti-M9 can precede the appearance of anti-M2.

Besides AMAs, autoantibodies directed against nuclear envelope proteins which display a ring-like pattern on immunofluorescence are also very specific for PBC and may help to identify PBC patients who are AMA negative [25]. Other autoantibodies have also been found in PBC, including other antinuclear patterns [25], anti-smooth muscle, antithyroid, anti-lymphocytotoxic [26], and others.

## 6 Associated Diseases

The prevalence of presumed autoimmune disorders is very high, i.e., 70%–80%. The most frequent is Sjögren's syndrome, which is found in 33%–100% of cases when an appropriate test is performed [27]. Connective tissue and rheumatic diseases, particularly rheumatoid arthritis, dermatomyositis and polymyositis, mixed connective tissue disease, and systemic lupus erythematosus, as well as scleroderma, usually with the whole CREST syndrome, have also been described in association with PBC. Scleroderma in PBC is mild, usually being limited to sclerodactyly, although involvement of the face, arms, and legs has also been described. Most of these patients exhibit esophageal dysfunction, as do PBC patients with Sjögren's syndrome without scleroderma [28]. Therefore, the esophageal involvement as well as the pulmonary disturbances observed in PBC patients with Sjögren's syndrome could be presclerodermatous manifestations. Thus patients with PBC and Sjögren's syndrome might be prone to develop further scleroderma or scleroderma-like manifestations. Joint pain with or without inflammatory changes is present in approximately 50% of patients with PBC, and the prevalence of frank arthritis has ranged from 5% to 24% in different series [29]. The development of arthritis could be explained by the association with sicca syndrome, scleroderma, rheumatoid arthritis, and hypertrophic osteoarthropathy.

Hypothyroidism with or without signs of autoimmune thyroiditis has also been found in 18%–22% of patients with PBC [30]. Graves' disease has been reported, too. Other autoimmune conditions associated with PBC include autoimmune thrombocytopenia, cold autoimmune hemolytic anemia, IgM-associated membranous glomerulonephritis, jejunal villous atrophy resembling celiac disease, and ulcerative colitis. Besides scleroderma, other cutaneous diseases such as lichen planus, immune complex capillaritis, and bullous pemphigoid have also been described in PBC.

Pulmonary involvement including clinical and radiologic evidence of lung disease, as well as gas transfer abnormalities, has also been found in patients with PBC. The lung involvement in PBC is probably secondary to an associated connective tissue disorder such as Sjögren's syndrome [31]. In addition, bronchoalveolar lavage reveals changes similar to those of sarcoidosis. Finger clubbing and hypertrophic osteoarthropathy may be related to these pulmonary disorders, although these clinical manifestations may be found in PBC patients without lung abnormalities.

Renal tubular acidosis is present in approximately 33% of patients with PBC. It is usually subclinical and has been related to deposition of copper in the kidney, since plasma copper concentration and urinary copper excretion were significantly higher in PBC patients with renal tubular acidosis than in those without this abnormality. In addition, the decreased ability to acidify the urine after an acid load correlated with both the plasma copper concentration and the urinary copper excretion [32]. Another study also found a close relationship between cholestasis and renal tubular dysfunction, and hypouricemia and hyperuricosuria indicate more advanced tubular damage [33].

Pancreatic insufficiency, which may contribute to steatorrhea, has been reported in patients with PBC, particularly those with Sjögren's syndrome [34]. Likewise, asymptomatic gallstones, usually of the pigmented type, have been seen in 39% of cases.

Bacteriuria is frequent in patients with PBC [35]. Bacteriuria does not correlate with the severity of liver disease as assessed by serum bilirubin concentrations, and it has been postulated that urinary organisms might be invoked in the pathogenesis of PBC since a cross-reaction has been observed between *E. coli* lipopolysaccharide and HLA antigens, and because serum from patients with PBC recognizes different antigens from Enterobacteriaceae.

Although hepatocellular carcinoma used to be considered very rare in PBC, recent studies have demonstrated that the risk for developing hepatocellular carcinoma in PBC is similar to that in other types of cirrhosis. A high incidence of breast cancer has also been reported.

Pernicious anemia, multiple myeloma, progressive ophthalmoplegia, myasthenia gravis, transverse myelitis, retroperitoneal fibrosis, and restrictive and hypertrophic types of cardiomyopathy have infrequently been found in association with PBC.

## 7 Diagnosis

The diagnosis of PBC must be considered in all middle-aged women who have pruritus and elevated serum levels of alkaline phosphatase (usually more than twice the upper limit of normal). In these cases the presence of AMAs, raised levels of IgM, and a compatible liver biopsy usually establishes the diagnosis of PBC. Since the florid lesion is not present in all portal tracts, percutaneous liver biopsy is rarely diagnostic of PBC, but it usually reveals lesions compatible with the diagnosis. PBC must also be considered in women who have an unexplained high serum alkaline phospatase level with no symptoms of the disease, since asymptomatic forms are becoming more frequent. In these patients both the AMA positivity and a compatible liver biopsy confirm the diagnosis. The presence of high titers of AMAs, particularly the M2-type, and also of other antibodies such as a ring-like nuclear pattern with no anti-DNA antibodies is highly specific for PBC [25].

The biliary tract should also be evaluated in every patient by ultrasonography. In patients without AMAs or with other atypical features such as male sex, early deep jaundice, or acute presentation, it is mandatory to perform endoscopic retrograde cholangiography to demonstrate a normal pattern of intra- and extrahepatic large bile ducts. Other procedures such as computered tomography and percutaneous transhepatic cholangiography may also be performed to demonstrate a normal appearance of intrahepatic bile ducts in the early stages of PBC or a "tree-in-winter" aspect if the patient has advanced cirrhosis, and consequently to rule out mechanical biliary obstruction.

## 8 Differential Diagnosis

The differential diagnosis of PBC must take into account some biliary diseases presenting with the clinical spectrum of chronic cholestasis (Table 1), such as incomplete obstruction of the distal biliary tract as a consequence of stones, chronic pancreatitis, carcinoma of the head of the pancreas, cholangiocarcinoma, and primary sclerosing cholangitis (PSC) or other benign strictures. In these cases, ultrasonography and later endoscopic retrograde cholangiography should be sufficient to establish the diagnosis. Typically AMAs are negative, although low titers have been described in rare cases.

The other group of diseases which must be considered is cholestatic parenchymal liver diseases, particularly drug-induced cholestasis, the intrahepatic form of PSC, sarcoidosis, and some cholestatic forms of auto-

**Table 1.** Differential diagnosis of PBC

| |
|---|
| Mechanical obstruction of the biliary tract |
| Primary sclerosing cholangitis |
| Drug-induced cholestasis |
| Cholestatic chronic active hepatitis |
| Sarcoidosis |
| Adulthood idiopathic biliary ductopenia |

immune chronic active hepatitis. An idiopathic form of biliary ductopenia described recently in adults should also be considered [36]. However, in these diseases AMAs are rarely positive, and the liver biopsy usually demonstrates specific changes of each disease. The cholestatic form of chronic active hepatitis is difficult to differentiate from PBC, and it is possible that the antigen specificity of the AMAs or other autoantibodies could help in the recognition of these patients.

## 9 Natural History and Prognosis

Primary biliary cirrhosis, and particularly the asymptomatic forms, usually has a prolonged course from diagnosis. However, the course of the disease cannot be predicted in an individual patient with asymptomatic PBC, since some of these patients suddenly develop symptomatic progressive disease with severe cholestasis and liver failure whereas others remain asymptomatic for long periods [37]. The symptomatic disease usually progresses slowly, and the clinical and biochemical manifestations of cholestasis may remain unchanged for several years. During the late phase of the disease, serum bilirubin levels usually increase and clinical features of liver failure and portal hypertension may develop, particularly ascites and hepatic encephalopathy [14]. Hypoalbuminemia and prolonged prothrombin time also appear in the later phase of the disease, and there are falls in serum lipid and cholesterol levels. The other biochemical and immunologic tests tend to remain stable or display minor changes. Xanthomas and pruritus may disappear or diminish during the final phases of PBC. The histologic stage also tends to advance slowly, but some patients who die with liver failure may have no evidence of established cirrhosis.

The mean survival time from diagnosis varies between 6 and 10 years in most series [13, 14, 38], and it is longer in the most recent series published, probably because they include a larger number of patients diagnosed at earlier stages of the disease. The life expectancy of asymptomatic patients used to be considered similar to that of the general population, since no differences were observed in the first study. However, recent data indicate that a high proportion of patients develop symptoms, and therefore the actuarial survival of asymptomatic PBC is lower than that observed in general population. Indeed, in a recent series of 44 asymptomatic patients, 77% developed symptoms of liver disease. Actuarial analysis indicated that survival was comparable to that of the general population for the first 5 years and then decreased sharply [37].

Several clinical, biochemical, and histologic features have prognostic significance in PBC (Table 2), although the serum bilirubin level is the best predictor of survival [39] since this biochemical parameter appears in all mathematical models which have been developed in order to identify prognostic factors in PBC. Advanced age, low serum albumin, prolonged

**Table 2.** Prognostic features in PBC

| |
|---|
| *Clinical* |
| Age |
| Hepatomegaly |
| Edema |
| Ascites |
| Encephalopathy |
| *Biochemical* |
| Serum bilirubin |
| Serum albumin |
| Prothrombin time |
| Serum procollagen type III peptide |
| Serum hyaluronate |
| *Histologic* |
| Cirrhosis |
| Intrahepatic cholestasis |
| Granuloma |

prothrombin time, hepatomegaly, edema, ascites, encephalopathy, and centrilobular cholestasis or cirrhosis on liver biopsy are features that have been associated with a poor prognosis of PBC. These variables are included in different prognostic indices of survival in PBC [13, 14, 39–41]. In advanced cases, the development of ascites and hepatic encephalopathy as manifestations of liver failure indicates a very poor prognosis. Patients usually die within a short time, particularly if they develop encephalopathy [14]. Male sex probably also represents a poor prognostic factor because males are diagnosed in advanced stages of the disease, although in one study the actuarial survival probability was similar in men and women. Increased serum procollagen type III peptide and increased serum levels of hyaluronate are also of prognostic significance in PBC, as is the presence of granulomas in the liver. The former two parameters, as markers of liver fibrosis or fibrogenesis, are associated with a poor prognosis, whereas granulomas correlate with a good prognosis, probably because this particular lesion is more frequently seen in the early stages of PBC.

## 10 Treatment

Treatment of PBC is directed toward the relief or prevention of the effects of chronic cholestasis [1, 11, 42], and toward finding a specific treatment for the disease.

### *Treatment of Pruritus*

Pruritus is one of the most distressing symptoms in patients with PBC. Up to now, cholestyramine has been the treatment of choice for itching, given at doses not higher than 12 g per day. When response is unsatisfactory, phenobarbital given at an initial dose of 3 mg/kg body weight, and later 60–180 mg at bedtime, can be added. However, the drug may produce intolerable sedation and alters vitamin D metabolism. Other treatments such as lotions containing phenol, menthol, or camphor, as well as other procedures such as plasmapheresis, phototherapy, and the administration of some antihistaminics, rutin, androgenic steroids, lidocaine, or naloxone may ameliorate intractable pruritus.

Rifampicin, a potent microsomal inducer antibiotic, is also effective for relieving pruritus in patients with PBC. Moreover, rifampicin has better effects then phenobarbital, as was demonstrated in a randomized cross-over study in 22 patients with PBC [43]. Because of its favorable effects on biochemical cholestasis and pruritus, an additional study to assess the long-term effects of rifampicin in patients with PBC has been performed. In this study, which included 16 patients, rifampicin was given at the same doses as in the former study for a period as long as 18 months. Pruritus improved in all patients after 3 months, and the ten patients who completed 1 year of treatment were free of pruritus by this time. These beneficial effects on pruritus were associated with marked alkaline phophatase reduction, an effect that was already significant after 3 months. At 1 year, the decrease in alkaline phosphatase was as high as 40% of the baseline values. Similar effects were observed with respect to microsomal function, but no changes in aminotransferase or γ-glutamyltransferase levels were observed. Despite these effects on cholestasis two patients were withdrawn after 2 months from the beginning of the trial because they presented hepatitis due to rifampicin. No other side-effects were found.

### *Treatment of Nutritional Deficiencies*

Since most PBC patients with prolonged cholestasis have some clinical signs and symptoms as a consequence of vitamin deficiencies, parenteral or enteral administration of these vitamins is appropriate. Patients must be treated with supplements of vitamin A, vitamin E, and vitamin K. When patients have severe malnutrition or steatorrhea, supplementation of medium-chain triglycerides is given (Table 3).

**Table 3.** Treatment of nutritional deficiencies in PBC

| | |
|---|---|
| Vitamin A | 100000 IU/month, i.m. |
| Vitamin K | 10 mg/week, i.m. |
| Vitamin E | 200 mg/day, p.o. |
| Vitamin D | 25–50 μg/day, p.o. |
| Calcium gluconate 3 g/day, p.o. | |
| Medium chain triglycerides 15 ml four times/day, p.o. | |

***Treatment of Osteodystrophy***

Since osteoporosis is often present in patients with PBC, supplements of calcium and vitamin D must be given. High doses of calcium per os (as much as 3 g calcium gluconate daily) are recommended. Other regimens have been proposed such as treatment with microcrystalline hydroxyapatite. Intravenous infusions of calcium gluconate have also been used to relieve bone pain secondary to osteopenia. Osteomalacia is uncommon in PBC. However, sunbathing should be recommended and low doses of daily vitamin D given to prevent its development.

Sodium fluoride improves bone formation and increases cancellous bone mass in postmenopausal osteoporosis. Therefore, the effects of 50 mg sodium fluoride on bone mass were examined in 22 patients with PBC in a double-blind placebo-controlled trial. Bone mineral density of the lumbar spine decreased markedly in the placebo group, an effect which was already observed after 12 months. By contrast, in the fluoride group bone mineral density did not change during the 2-year period, indicating that sodium fluoride prevents bone loss in patients with PBC.

***Specific Treatments***

Several supposed specific treatments have been proposed for PBC. They can be mainly divided into two groups of drugs: The first comprises those having effects on the immunologic status, that is immunosuppressors such as corticosteroids, azathioprine, chlorambucil, cyclosporine, and methotrexate, and also other drugs that besides their anti-inflammatory effects may act upon liver fibrosis, such as penicillamine and colchicine. The other group only includes ursodeoxycholic acid, which probably acts by decreasing the levels of toxic bile acids.

*Corticosteroids* were used in patients with PBC some decades ago. Despite eventual favorable effects, they were disregarded because they increased the associated risk of osteoporosis. Nevertheless, a recent double-blind randomized pilot study comparing prednisolone and placebo in 36 patients has been reported [44]. The main results indicate that after 1 year, prednisolone significantly decreased the aminotransferase and alkaline phosphatase levels and prevented the increase in serum bilirubin. In addition, a significant decrease in serum procollagen III peptide levels was observed. Unfortunately, semiquantitative assessment of liver histology after 1 year failed to demonstrate improvement. Furthermore, bone loss was observed in patients taking corticosteroids. Thus, until this side-effect can be prevented, the use of corticosteroids in PBC should generally be avoided.

Despite the fact that the first uncontrolled trials gave rise to claims that *azathioprine* is of value in PBC, this could not be proved in the later controlled trials which enrolled larger numbers of patients. In fact, the mortality was similar in the azathioprine and placebo groups. The final analysis of the most recent study, which included an adjustment for imbalance at entry, did, however, demonstrate a favorable effect of azathioprine on survival [40]. Nevertheless, this effect was small and consequently it seems that this drug has no place in the management of PBC.

After azathioprine, attention was turned to *penicillamine*, a drug that, besides its ability to chelate copper, also inhibits collagen formation. The results of all controlled studies performed were very disappointing because no effect on the overall survival was demonstrated and because the drug produced significant side-effects [45].

*Colchicine* has also been used in PBC because of its significant anti-inflammatory and antifibrotic properties. After a pilot study of only five patients that demonstrated a significant decrease in alkaline phosphatase in all the patients, colchicine has been assessed in comparison to placebo in three randomized trials. Colchicine was usually given in doses of 1.2 mg per day. Improved liver function tests were reported in all the studies; in one survival was prolonged by the drug, and there was a trend toward increased survival in another. Despite these observations, no histologic changes were observed. However, the effects on liver function are very striking because colchicine avoids the increases in bilirubin and aminotransferases and produces a marked decrease in alkaline phosphatase levels [46]. Since colchicine has also been claimed to prolong survival in patients with cirrhosis of other etiologies, and the drug has minimal side-effects, further evaluation in more patients seems justified.

*Chlorambucil* has also been evaluated in a small prospective controlled trial [47]. Results indicate that this alkylating agent significantly decreases the mean serum bilirubin levels and that it probably retards the progression of PBC. However, 30% of patients developed bone marrow suppression. Because of the long-term toxicity of this drug, further large-scale trials have not been performed.

*Cyclosporine* has also been used in PBC because of its inhibitory effects on T helper cell function and because patients who develop hepatic rejection after liver transplantation have histologic features resembling the vanishing bile duct injury seen in patients with PBC. In a small trial cyclosporine therapy was associated with an improvement in pruritus and serum biochemical indices of the disease. Another recently published study from the Mayo Clinic, which included 29 patients, concluded that cyclosporine therapy in patients with PBC is promising but requires further evaluation [48].

The preliminary results from the as yet unpublished European multicenter double-blind randomized controlled trial, which included 349 patients with PBC, indicate that cyclosporine caused marked changes in the course of serum bilirubin levels for given values at entry. In fact bilirubin did not significantly increase in the cyclosporine group but increased in the placebo group. However, cyclosporine was associated with a high rate of arterial hypertension and increased serum creatinine levels. No significant changes were observed in the histologic evaluation. Furthermore, preliminary analysis indicated that cyclosporine did not have any effect on survival in PBC. However, it seems that cyclosporine may retard the time to death or transplantation.

Perhaps the most striking results concerning the use of immunosuppressors in PBC are those reported by Kaplan, who treated 15 patients with 15 mg *methotrexate* per week for 12–34 months [49]. Relief of symptoms and improvements in biochemical tests were observed in the nine precirrhotic patients, together with histologic improvement in some of them. In sharp contrast no effect was observed in the six cirrhotic patients. In addition methotrexate was dramatically more effective than colchicine in lowering serum alkaline phosphatase, bilirubin, and cholesterol levels. These preliminary findings are very provocative but clearly a full-scale controlled trial is warranted.

*Ursodeoxycholic acid* seems to be another promising drug for the treatment of PBC. The initial results from Poupon and co-workers indicate that 13–15 mg ursodeoxycholic acid per day was followed by marked clinical, biochemical, and histologic improvement, particularly relief of pruritus and a decrease in alkaline phosphatase [50]. Similar results have been reported by Leuschner and co-workers [51]. Treatment with 10 mg/kg ursodeoxycholic acid in ten patients with stage I and II disease over 9 months was associated with significant reductions in serum aminotransferase, alkaline phosphatase, glutamate dehydrogenase, and IgM levels, which returned to baseline values after drug suppression. No significant differences in liver histology were observed in patients receiving the drug, although there was a trend toward improvement in liver damage.

Another larger double-blind trial from Poupon and co-workers demonstrated that after 6 months of treatment with ursodeoxycholic acid, there was a marked improvement in biochemical liver tests, but it is too early to demonstrate any significant effect on survival. Other preliminary results have revealed similar effects. Further evaluation is mandatory, particularly concerning effects on liver histology and survival.

### *Liver Transplantation*

When all other treatments have been unable to prevent the progression of the disease, *liver transplantation* is currently the only definitive treatment for patients with PBC. Data from the University of Pittsburgh are very revealing since 1-year survival is currently about 75% and the actuarial curves indicate that 5-year survival is ca. 66% [52].

## B. Primary Sclerosing Cholangitis

Primary sclerosing cholangitis (PSC) is a chronic fibrotic inflammatory disease of the intra- and extrahepatic bile ducts and gallbladder. It is characterized by cholestasis, usually in association with inflammatory bowel disease, particularly ulcerative colitis. Its pathogenesis is still unknown, the prognosis is severe, and, at present, there is no specific treatment.

Primary sclerosing cholangitis was initially described by DELBET in 1924 and, before the introduction of endoscopic retrograde cholangiography in the 1970s, the diagnosis was usually established when the disease was at an advanced stage. A significant increase in its frequency has, however, now been reported [53]. While the prevalence of PSC in the general population has not yet been investigated, it may be indirectly estimated on the basis of its frequent association with ulcerative colitis: It has been reported that 70% of patients with PSC have ulcerative colitis; the prevalence of PSC in patients with ulcerative colitis ranges between 2.5% and 5.6%, and the prevalence of chronic ulcerative colitis in the general population is between 40 and 100 cases per 100000 inhabitants [54]. Therefore it can be calculated that the prevalence of PSC might be between 1 and 5 cases per 100000 inhabitants, in which case its frequency would be much higher than previously thought.

Primary sclerosing cholangitis is more frequent in males than in females, with a sex ratio of 2:1 [55–58]. This finding is in contrast to the sex ratio in chronic ulcerative colitis, which affects more women than men. Most patients are diagnosed between 25 and 50 years of age, although PSC has been observed in children.

### 1 Etiology and Pathogenesis

The cause of PSC is still unknown, although several factors may play an important role in the development of the disease [58]. Since, as has been indicated above, PSC is frequently associated with ulcerative colitis, the disease could be related to the fact that the formation of toxic bile acids or the passage of bacteria from the intestinal lumen to the portal circulation might favor inflammation of the extra- and intrahepatic biliary tree. However, this possibility seems unlikely since pylephlebitis is very uncommon in such patients and there are no differences between patients with PSC with or without inflammatory bowel disease. Furthermore, it has been recognized that PSC may develop in patients with ulcerative colitis in whom proctocolectomy has been performed several years previously.

It has been suggested, as in PBC, that the increased level of copper in hepatic tissue stimulates hepatic fibrogenesis and consequently perpetuates the disease. However, recent negative results from a controlled clinical trial with D-penicillamine do not support this hypothesis [57].

Viral infections have been considered as other factors that may play a key role in the development of PSC. Hepatitis A and B infections do not produce PSC and it is very unlikely that hepatitis C can cause inflammation of the biliary tree, although this possibility has not yet been excluded. While other viruses such as reovirus type 3 have been associated with neonatal biliary atresia and fibrosing cholangitis in primates and in children, there is as yet no evidence showing any relation between the development of PSC and reovirus type 3.

Genetic and immunologic mechanisms may be important in the pathogenesis of PSC. Occurrence among twins and other family members has been reported although its incidence is very rare. It has also been demonstrated that the frequency of HLA-B8 and D3 is higher in patients with PSC than in the general population [59]. This finding may be very relevant since it is well known that HLA-B8 and D3 are haplotypes particularly frequent in diseases whose pathogenesis is related to autoimmunity, such as chronic active hepatitis, PBC, myasthenia gravis, thyroiditis, and systemic lupus erythematosus. In addition, a strong genetic predisposition has been found in patients with PSC, since in a recent study all patients had the HLA-DRw52a antigen and about 50% had the single common haplotype: A1, B8, Cw7, DRw17, DQw2, DRw52a [60]. Furthermore, several immunologic disturbances have been demonstrated, such as abnormalities in peripheral blood lymphocyte subsets, enhanced autoreactivity of cytotoxic and suppressor T lymphocytes to class II histocompatibility antigens, and the aberrant expression of class II histocompatibility antigens of bile duct epithelium. In addition, the cells implicated in the bile duct damage are T lymphocytes. It has also been demonstrated that circulating immune complexes are increased in blood and bile, and that serum anticolon antibodies are present in patients with PSC. All these findings indicate that patients with PSC have alterations of the immune system. However, at present it is unclear whether these immunologic abnormalities are the cause or the consequence of the disease.

On the other hand, it has also been demonstrated that PSC may be present in several immunodeficiency syndromes, such as combined familial immunodeficiency, hyperimmunoglobulin M immunodeficiency, angioimmunoblastic lymphadenopathy, immunodeficiency linked to chromosome X, and acquired immune deficiency syndrome associated with cryptosporidiosis or cytomegalovirus infections. These associations suggest that normal host defensive barriers against infection are altered in these syndromes and, consequently, facilitate ascending bacterial infection of the biliary tree. Recently, it has been reported that hepatic artery infusions with 5-fluorodeoxyuridine and hepatic artery thrombosis after liver transplantation may produce extrahepatic biliary disease similar to PSC. These latter findings suggest that ischemia may also play a role in the development of PSC. In summary, it could be suggested that PSC may be considered as an infectious disease or an autoimmune liver disease precipitated by toxins or microbiologic agents in genetically predisposed subjects.

## 2 Pathology

Gross anatomy reveals a thickened and fibrosed extrahepatic biliary tree and the biliary lumen may be reduced to as little as one-eighth of its normal size [53, 61, 62]. The lesion is characterized histologically by a dense concentric fibrosis and inflammatory infiltration without involvement of the biliary mucosa (Fig. 4). Liver biopsy cannot establish the diagnosis in all cases, since the characteristic lesion of the disease is frequently not observed in the small liver specimens obtained by liver biopsy. The lesion which allows the establishment of the diagnosis of PSC is fibrous obliterative cholangitis leading to the substitution of bile ducts by solid cords of connective tissue. Usually liver biopsy shows nonspecific changes of biliary disease such as cholestasis, loss of bile ducts in the portal tracts, periportal bile duct proliferation, piecemeal necrosis, and inflammatory infiltration of the portal tracts with neutrophils and lymphocytes [58, 62]. These findings may suggest a diagnosis other than PSC such as PBC or even, in some patients, extrahepatic biliary obstruction, particularly if the pathologist examines the liver biopsy without cholangiographic information.

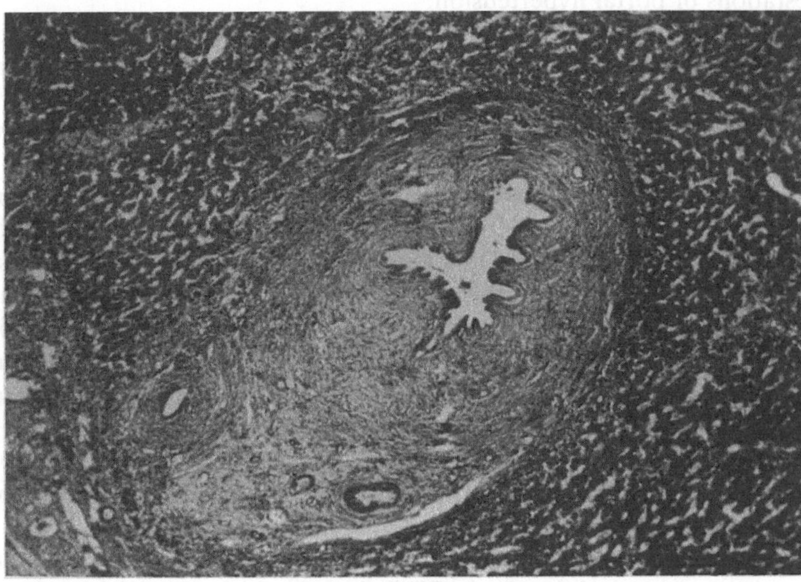

**Fig. 4.** Liver biopsy specimen from a patient with PSC, showing fibrous cholangitis

In some patients liver biopsy does not reveal any histologic evidence of large-biliary involvement but shows inflammation of the small duct in the portal tracts. These changes have beeh termed "pericholangitis." The demonstration that retrograde cholangiography in patients who only display pericholangitis shows identical radiologic lesions to those in patients with large-biliary involvement suggests that this hepatic lesion (pericholangitis) is not another clinical entity [63].

Patients with PSC have been histologically classified into four stages by Ludwig and co-workers [62]. Stage 1 is characterized by an enhancement of connective tissue with enlargement of portal tracts. In stage II connective tissue is increased in the periportal areas with minimal inflammatory changes. In stage III there is formation of fibrous septa in the hepatic parenchyma. Finally, in stage IV biliary cirrhosis develops.

## 3 Clinical Features

Clinical presentation of PSC varies from patient to patient. Some patients present fatigue, loss of body weight, abdominal pain, pruritus, and recurrent jaundice. This is the classical picture of chronic cholestasis and it is observed in about two-thirds of all patients [64]. Other patients begin with recurrent cholangitis; this is particularly often the case in those previously submitted to surgery. Some patients are diagnosed when they already have cirrhosis. In such cases diagnosis is performed as a consequence of clinical manifestations of portal hypertension.

In the last few years, asymptomatic patients with PSC have frequently been recognized, since patients with inflammatory bowel disease are now submitted to retrograde cholangiography when they have high levels of alkaline phosphatase. These patients may be asymptomatic for many years without a worsening of liver function and without jaundice [65].

Although some cases may appear normal upon physical examination, liver or spleen enlargement and jaundice are present in approximately three-quarters of patients. Dark skin and xanthomas and xanthelasmas may also be observed. Laboratory tests show raised plasma levels of alkaline phosphatase, usually three times above normal values. Plasma bilirubin levels are very variable and on rare occasions exceed 10 mg/dl. Mild elevation of aminotransferases is observed. Hypoalbuminemia is uncommon. Bilirubin and alkaline phosphatase may fluctuate during follow-up. Hepatic copper is increased in 90% of patients. High plasma levels of copper and ceruloplasmin and increased urinary copper excretion have also been observed.

In some patients antinuclear antibodies have been detected, although the titers are very low. As in PBC, increased plasma IgM levels may be present in about 50% of patients. AMAs are negative.

## 4 Cholangiographic Features

Retrograde endoscopic cholangiography is necessary to confirm and/or establish the diagnosis of PSC, since it is the only exploratory procedure capable of demonstrating in such patients the presence of short and annular strictures alternated with apparently normal or slightly dilated bile ducts. In approximately 80% of patients the intra- and extrahepatic biliary tree is affected [66], while in the remaining 20% of patients only the extrahepatic biliary tree is affected. In about 25% of the patients diverticular out-pouching may be observed. The presence of these findings is considered characteristic of PSC (Fig. 5). In a small number of patients an isolated stricture may be the only lesion of PSC [67]. The presence of this isolated stricture may induce diagnostic error since this lesion may be similar to those observed in neoplasms of the biliary tree.

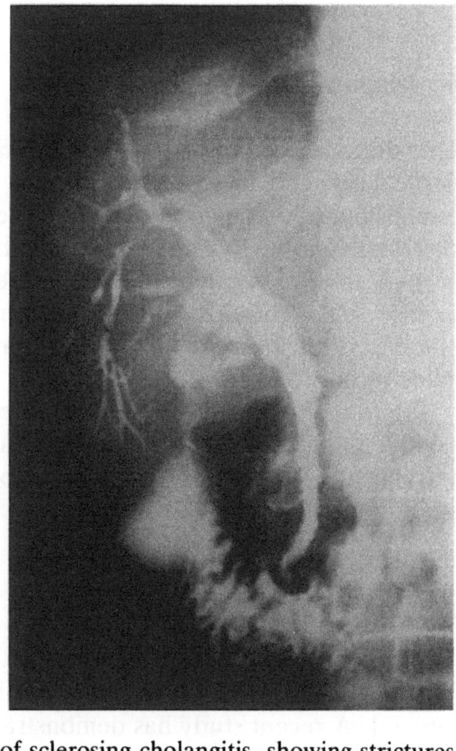

**Fig. 5.** Typical cholangiographic pattern of sclerosing cholangitis, showing strictures and ectasia of the intra- and extrahepatic ducts

## 5 Associated Diseases

Since the initial recognition of PSC associations with other inflammatory, autoimmune, and fibrosing diseases have been identified [55, 58, 64]. Chronic inflammatory bowel disease, particularly ulcerative colitis, is associated with PSC in 50%–75% of the patients. Usually the diagnosis of inflammatory bowel disease is established prior to the development of PSC, although PSC may appear after total proctocolectomy for chronic ulcerative colitis or before chronic bowel disease becomes clinically apparent. Chronic pancreatitis occurs in 7%–20% of patients with PSC [34]. Most patients, however, do not present symptoms related to pancreatic disease. There are other diseases that may be observed in patients with PSC such as thyroiditis, sarcoidosis, arthritis, celiac sprue, retroperitoneal and mediastinal fibrosis, histiocytosis X, and pseudotumor of the orbit. Patients with PSC, and particularly those in whom the disease displays a prolonged evolution, are prone to develop cholangiocarcinoma. This tumor is detected in about 10% of all the patients [68].

## 6 Diagnosis

The diagnosis of PSC is based on clinical, biochemical, histologic, and particularly cholangiographic criteria [61]. The most useful criteria for establishing the diagnosis of PSC are clinical symptoms or signs of chronic cholestasis, a high alkaline phosphatase level (three titers greater than normal value), negative AMAs, presence of chronic inflammatory bowel disease, and diffuse irregularity and narrowing of the extra- and intrahepatic bile ducts. Liver biopsy, as previously mentioned, allows the diagnosis to be made in only 30% of the cases [56].

Before the diagnosis of PSC is established other diseases should be excluded, such as PBC, sarcoidosis, autoimmune chronic active hepatitis, extrahepatic cholestasis, alcoholic hepatitis, drug-induced cholestasis, and adulthood idiopathic ductopenia.

## 7 Natural History and Prognosis

The length of survival in patients with PSC varies from 6 months to 15 years [56, 57]. A recent study has demonstrated that 75% of the patients are alive 9 years after diagnosis. These differences can be interpreted as showing that a subgroup of patients with PSC do well and that there is another subgroup of patients who have progressive disease that may be fatal unless treated by liver transplantation. Patients with asymptomatic PSC frequently develop symptoms, as observed in a series of 44 patients followed for a mean of

6 years; in fact one-third of these patients developed liver failure. In addition the prognosis of asymptomatic patients may be no different from that of symptomatic patients [65] because patients with asymptomatic PSC frequently have liver cirrhosis or clinical manifestations of portal hypertension.

## 8 Treatment

The symptomatic treatment of PSC is similar to that of PBC. On the other hand, there is no specific treatment for PSC, and all the therapeutic strategies have been directed toward increasing the biliary flow and reducing the inflammatory process which causes the biliary obstruction.

Corticosteroids have no beneficial effect on the hepatic lesion of PSC either when administered systemically [61] or when used topically in the biliary tree [69]. It has been reported in a clinical non-randomized study that the combination of prednisolone and colchicine produces an improvement in bilirubin, alkaline phosphatase, and aminotransferase levels after 1 year but not after 2 years of therapy [70].

D-Penicillamine has been evaluated in a double-blind controlled trial which included 70 patients, 39 of whom were treated initially with 250 mg/day for 4 weeks and later with 750 mg/day. There were no differences between the patients treated with D-penicillamine and those who received placebo in relation to the outcome of the disease, the survival rate, or histologic lesions. Furthermore, patients treated with D-penicillamine presented a great number of complications, some of which were serious [57].

Two patients with PSC have been treated with methotrexate with very encouraging results. The administration of 15 mg of the drug per week was associated with an improvement in standard liver function tests and the histologic lesions. None of these patients presented new episodes of cholangitis after treatment [71]. In spite of these excellent results, controlled clinical trials are required to establish the beneficial effect of methotrexate in patients with PSC.

Two other patients have been treated with azathioprine with controversial results, and other drugs with potential beneficial effects in PSC, such as cyclosporine, have still to be evaluated. Ursodeoxycholic acid may also have beneficial effects in patients with PSC. Preliminary results indicate that this bile acid may improve cholestasis in PSC, as shown in PBC, probably because ursodeoxycholic acid displaces other potential bile acids from the liver.

Patients with isolated stenosis of the extrahepatic bile ducts may be treated with dilatation or with a prosthesis placed inside the biliary tree. The development of fever and cholangitis requires antibiotic therapy. Palliative surgery in general is ill-advised since liver transplantation in terminal patients with PSC has excellent results.

Patients with PSC, like those with PBC, may benefit from hepatic transplantation. The actuarial survival of patients with PSC submitted to liver transplantation is similar to that observed in PBC patients. The probability of survival at 5 years in 75 patients who underwent liver transplantation at the University of Pittsburgh was about 73% [72]. It is important to point out that the development of cholangiocarcinoma in PSC patients influences the prognosis since, in the Pittsburgh series, the inclusion of eight patients with cholangiocarcinoma decreased the survival rate to 67%.

## References


1. Kaplan MM (1987) Primary biliary cirrhosis. N Engl J Med 316:521–528
2. Rodés J, Parés A, Bruguera M (1987) ¿Es la cirrosis biliar primaria una enfermedad generalizada de tipo autoinmune? Med Clin (Barc) 88:292–299
3. Rubin E, Schaffner F, Popper H (1965) Primary biliary cirrhosis: chronic nonsuppurative destructive cholangitis. Am J Pathol 46:387–407
4. Scheuer PJ (1967) Primary biliary cirrhosis. Proc R Soc Med 60:1257–1260
5. Triger DR, Berg P, Rodés J (1984) Epidemiology of primary biliary cirrhosis. Liver 4:195–200
6. Ludwig J, Dickson ER, MacDonald GSA (1978) Staging of chronic nonsuppurative destructive cholangitis (syndrome of primary biliary cirrhosis). Virchows Arch [A] 379:103–112
7. Nakanuma Y, Ohta G (1987) Nodular hyperplasia of the liver in primary biliary cirrhosis of early histological stages. Am J Gastroenterol 82:8–10
8. Baum H (1989) Nature of the mitochondrial antigens of primary biliary cirrhosis and their possible relationships to the etiology of the disease. Semin Liver Dis 9:117–123
9. Ercilla G, Parés A, Arriaga F et al. (1979) Primary biliary cirrhosis associated with HLA-DRw3. Tissue Antigens 14:449–454
10. Gores GJ, Moore SB, Fisher LD et al. (1987) Primary biliary cirrhosis: association with class II major histocompatibility complex antigens. Hepatology 7:889–892
11. Moreno R, Lisker M, Jones EA (1989) Primary biliary cirrhosis. Med Clin North Am 73:911–929
12. Epstein O, Thomas HC, Sherlock S (1980) Primary biliary cirrhosis is a dry gland syndrome with features of chronic graft-versus-host disease. Lancet I:1166–1168
13. Christensen E, Crowe J, Doniach D et al. (1980) Clinical pattern and course of disease in primary biliary cirrhosis based on an analysis of 236 patients. Gastroenterology 236–246
14. Parés A, Bruguera M, Rodés J (1981) Cirrosis biliar primaria. Evolución clínica y criterios de valor pronóstico. Gastroenterol Hepatol 4:76–81
15. Navasa M, Parés A, Bruguera M et al. (1987) Portal hypertension in primary biliary cirrhosis. Relationship with histological features. J Hepatol 5:292–298
16. Ros E, Garcia-Pugés A, Reixach M et al. (1984) Fat digestion and exocrine pancreatic function in primary biliary cirrhosis. Gastroenterology 87:180–187
17. Sokol RJ, Balistreri WF, Hoofnagle JH et al. (1985) Vitamin E deficiency in adults with chronic liver disease. Am J Clin Nutr 41:66–72
18. Guañabens N, Parés A, Mariñoso L et al. (1990) Factors influencing the development of metabolic bone disease in primary biliary cirrhosis. Am J Gastroenterol 85:1356–1362

19. Parés A, Bruguera M, Rodés J (1979) Cirrosis biliar primitiva asintomática. Gastroenterol Hepatol 2:126–130
20. Mitchison HC, Bassendine MF, Malcolm AJ et al. (1986) Positive antimitochondrial antibody but normal alkaline phosphatase. Is this primary biliary cirrhosis?. Hepatology 6:1279–1284
21. Jahn CE, Schaefer EJ, Toam LA et al. (1985) Lipoprotein abnormalities in primary biliary cirrhosis. Gastroenterology 89:1266–1278
22. Berg P, Klein R, Lindenborn-Fotinos J (1986) Antimitochondrial antibodies in primary biliary cirrhosis. J Hepatol 2:123–131
23. Berg P, Klein R (1989) Heterogeneity of antimitochondrial antigens. Semin Liver Dis 9:103–116
24. Yeaman SJ, Danner DJ, Multiner DJ et al. (1988) Primary biliary cirrhosis. Identification of two major M2 mitochondrial autoantigens. Lancet I:1067–1070
25. Lozano F, Parés A, Borche L et al. (1988) Autoantibodies against nuclear envelope-associated proteins in primary biliary cirrhosis. Hepatology 8:930–938
26. Parés A, Martorell J, Caballería J et al. (1985) Lymphocytotoxic antibodies in primary biliary cirrhosis. Dig Dis Sci 30:829–833
27. Alarcón-Segovia D, Diaz Jouanen E, Fishbein E (1973) Features of Sjögren's syndrome in primary biliary cirrhosis. Ann Intern Med 79:31–36
28. Parés A, Grande L, Bruix J et al. (1988) Esophageal dysfunction in primary biliary cirrhosis. J Hepatol 7:362–367
29. Guañabens N, Brancós MA, Parés A et al. (1984) Patología articular en la cirrosis biliar primaria. Gastroenterol Hepatol 7:551–555
30. Crowe JC, Christensen E, Tygstrup N et al. (1980) Primary biliary cirrhosis: the prevalence of hypothyroidism and its relation to the thyroid antibodies and sicca syndrome. Gastroenterology 76:1437–1441
31. Rodríguez-Roisin R, Parés A, Bruguera M et al. (1981) Pulmonary involvement in primary biliary cirrhosis. Thorax 36:208–212
32. Parés A, Rimola A, Bruguera M et al. (1981) Renal tubular acidosis in primary biliary cirrhosis. Gastroenterology 80:681–686
33. Izumi N, Hasumur Y, Takeuchi IJ (1983) Hypouricemia and hyperuricosuria as expressions of renal tubular damage in primary biliary cirrhosis. Hepatology 3:719–723
34. Epstein O, Chapman RWG, Lake-Bakaar G et al. (1982) The pancreas in primary biliary cirrhosis and primary sclerosing cholangitis. Gastroenterology 83:1117–1182
35. Burroughs A, Rosenstein IJ, Epstein O et al. (1984) Bacteriuria and primary biliary cirrhosis. Gut 25:133–137
36. Ludwig J, Wiesner RH, LaRusso NF (1988) Idiophatic adulthood ductopenia. A cause of chronic cholestatic liver disease and biliary cirrhosis. J Hepatol 7:193–199
37. Balasubramaniam K, Grambsch PM, Wiesner RH et al. (1990) Diminished survival in asymptomatic primary biliary cirrhosis. A prospective study. Gastroenterology 98:1567–1571
38. Roll J, Boyer JL, Barry D et al. (1983) The prognostic importance of clinical and histologic features in asymptomatic and symptomatic primary biliary cirrhosis. N Engl J Med 308:1–7
39. Shapiro JM, Smith H, Schaffner F (1979) Serum bilirubin: a prognostic factor in primary biliary cirrhosis. Gut 20:137–140
40. Christensen E, Neuberger J, Crowe J et al. (1985) Beneficial effect of azathioprine and prediction of prognosis in primary biliary cirrhosis: final results of an international trial. Gastroenterology 89:1084–1091
41. Dickson ER, Grambsch PM, Fleming TR et al. (1989) Prognosis in primary biliary cirrhosis: model for decision making. Hepatology 10:1–7
42. Warnes TW (1985) Treatment of primary biliary cirrhosis. Semin Liver Dis 5:228–240

43. Bachs L, Parés A, Elena M, Piera C, Rodés J (1989) Comparison of rifampicin with phenobarbitone for treatment of pruritus in biliary cirrhosis. Lancet I:574–576
44. Mitchison HC, Bassendine MF, Malcom AJ et al. (1989) A pilot, double-blind, controlled 1-year trial of prednisolone treatment in primary biliary cirrhosis: hepatic improvement but greater bone loss. Hepatology 10:420–429
45. Neuberger J, Christensen E, Portman B et al. (1985) Double-blind controlled trial of D-penicillamine in patients with primary biliary cirrhosis. Gut 26:114–119
46. Kaplan MM, Alling DW, Zimmerman HJ et al. (1986) Prospective trial of colchicine for primary biliary cirrhosis. N Engl J Med 315:1448–1454
47. Hoofnagle JH, Davis GL, Schafer DF et al. (1986) Randomized trial of chlorambucil for primary biliary cirrhosis. Gastroenterology 91:1327–1334
48. Minuk G, Bohne C, Burgess E et al. (1988) Pilot study of cyclosporine A in patients with symptomatic primary biliary cirrhosis. Gastroenterology 95:1356–1363
49. Kaplan MM (1989) Methotrexate treatment of chronic cholestatic liver diseases: friend or foe? Q J Med 72:757–761
50. Poupon R, Poupon RE, Calmus Y, Chretien Y, Ballet F, Darnis F (1987) Is ursodeoxycholic acid an effective treatment for primary biliary cirrhosis?. Lancet I:834–836
51. Leuschner U, Fischer H, Hubner K et al. (1989) Ursodeoxycholic acid (UDCA) treatment of primary biliary cirrhosis: clinical and histologic results of a prospective double-blind study. Gastroenterology 97:1268–1274
52. Esquivel CO, Van Thiel DH, Demetris AJ et al. (1988) Transplantation for primary biliary cirrhosis. Gastroenterology 94:1207–1216
53. Panés J, Bruguera M, Bordas JM et al. (1985) Colangitis esclerosante primaria: Una enfermedad de presentación heterogénea. Gastroenterol Hepatol 8:30–37
54. Shepard HA, Selby WS, Chapman RW et al. (1983) Ulcerative colitis and persistent liver dysfunction. Q J Med 208:503–513
55. Chapman RW, Arborg BA, Rhodes JM et al. (1980) Primary sclerosing cholangitis: a review of its clinical features, cholangiography, and hepatic histology. Gut 21:870–877
56. Wiesner RH, LaRusso NF (1980) Clinicopathologic features of the syndrome of primary sclerosing cholangitis. Gastroenterology 79:200–206
57. LaRusso NF, Wiesner RH, Ludwig J et al. (1988) Prospective trial of penicillamine in primary sclerosing cholangitis. Gastroenterology 95:1036–1042
58. Lindor KD, Wiesner RH, MacCarthy R et al. (1990) Advances in primary sclerosing cholangitis. Am J Med 89:73–80
59. Chapman RW, Varghese Z, Gaul R et al. (1983) Association of primary sclerosing cholangitis with HLA-B8. Gut 24:38–41
60. Prochazka EJ, Terasaki PI, Park MS et al. (1990) Association of primary sclerosing cholangitis with HLA-DRw52a. N Engl J Med 1842–1844
61. Wiesner RH, Ludwig J, LaRusso NF et al. (1985) Diagnosis and treatment of primary sclerosing cholangitis. Semin Liver Dis 5:241–253
62. Ludwig J, Barham SS, LaRusso NF et al. (1981) Morphological features of chronic hepatitis associated with primary sclerosing cholangitis and chronic ulcerative colitis. Hepatology 1:632–640
63. Wee A, Ludwig J (1985) Pericholangitis in chronic ulcerative colitis. Primary sclerosing cholangitis of the small bile ducts? Ann Intern Med 102:581–587
64. LaRusso NF, Wiesner RH, Ludwig J et al. (1984) Primary sclerosing cholangitis. N Engl J Med 310:899–903
65. Porayto MK, Wiesner RH, LaRusso NF et al. (1990) Patients with asymptomatic primary sclerosing cholangitis frequently have progressive disease. Gastroenterology 98:1594–1602
66. Maccarthy RL, LaRusso NF, Wiesner RH et al. (1983) Cholangiographic and pancreatographic features of primary sclerosing cholangitis. Radiology 149:39–44

67. Panés J, Bordas JM, Bruguera M et al. (1985) Localized sclerosing cholangitis? Endoscopy 17:121–122
68. Wee A, Ludwig J, Coffey RJ Jr et al. (1985) Hepatobiliary carcinoma associated with primary sclerosing cholangitis and chronic ulcerative colitis. Hum Pathol 16:719–726
69. Allison M, Burroughs AK, Noone P et al. (1986) Biliary lavage with corticosteroids in primary sclerosing cholangitis. A clinical cholangiographic and bacteriological study. J Hepatol 3:118–122
70. Leiser A, Kadish U (1986) Beneficial effect of colchicine in a case of sclerosing cholangitis. Am J Med Sci 291:416–418
71. Kaplan MM, Arora S, Pinues SH (1987) Primary sclerosing cholangitis and low dose oral pulse methotrexate: clinical and histological response. Ann Intern Med 106:231–235
72. Esquivel CD, March JW, VanThiel DH (1988) Liver transplantation for chronic cholestatic liver disease in adults and children. Gastroenterol Clin North Am 17:145–155

# 23 Wilson's Disease: Pathophysiology and Therapy

S.D. ZUCKER and J.L. GOLLAN

## 1 Introduction

Wilson's disease, or hepatolenticular degeneration, is an inherited disorder of copper metabolism, characterized by decreased biliary excretion of the metal. Copper accumulation and deposition in a variety of organ systems results in progressive tissue injury and leads inexorably to death unless appropriate therapy is initiated. Kinnear Wilson first described the familial syndrome of "progressive lenticular degeneration associated with cirrhosis of the liver" in 1912. This chapter will attempt to review the current understanding of Wilson's disease, highlighting some of he recent advances and controversies in the pathogenesis and management of this disorder.

## 2 Copper Metabolism

Copper is an essential trace element which is critical to a variety of mammalian functions, including mitochondrial energy generation, melanin formation, scavenging of oxygen radicals, and cross-linking of collagen and elastin. The ubiquitous presence of copper in nature makes acquired copper deficiency unusual. Similarly, toxic accumulation of copper also is rare due to efficient physiologic excretory mechanisms.

### 2.1 Total Body Copper and Tissue Distribution

Estimates of total body copper in normal adults range between 30 and 100 mg [1, 2]. The liver, which contains approximately 8% of total body stores [1], is the organ with the highest copper concentration, followed in decreasing order by the brain, heart, and kidneys [2]. Although levels of the metal in muscle and bone are low, these tissues contain about one-half of total body copper because of their large mass. The concentration of copper in fetal liver (mean 32 μg/g dry weight) is significantly higher than in adults [1]; however, by 3 months of age, the hepatic copper concentration declines to a level comparable to that in adults.

## 2.2 Dietary Copper and Intestinal Absorption

Although there is no recommended dietary allowance for copper, recent studies suggest that copper homeostasis is achieved with an oral intake of 0.8 mg/day [3], which is significantly lower than prior dietary recommendations. Since copper is present in most foods, it is virtually impossible to formulate a diet with a copper content below 0.5 mg/day. Typical Western diets contain approximately 1 mg copper/day. Foods with the highest copper concentrations include oysters and other shellfish, liver, nuts, chocolate, mushrooms, legumes, and cereals [4].

Intestinal copper absorption is dependent on dietary copper intake, with uptake efficiency varying from 12% on a high-copper diet to 56% on a low-copper diet [3]. Following oral administration, maximal serum copper levels are achieved within 1–2 h [5, 6], indicating that uptake occurs principally in the upper gastrointestinal tract. The absorption of dietary copper is influenced by a variety of intraluminal factors. Uptake increases in the presence of chelating agents (EDTA, oxalate), high dietary protein, L-amino acids, starch (fructose), and anions such as citrate, phosphate, and gluconate, whereas ascorbic acid, transition elements (e.g., cadmium, molybdenum, zinc), fiber, and bile salts have been found to inhibit copper absorption [4, 7].

It appears that modulation of intestinal absorption is important in copper homeostasis, although the regulatory mechanisms governing mucosal transport of copper are poorly understood. Metallothionein, a cytosolic copper-binding protein, is considered to be the principal mediator of intestinal copper absorption. This sulfhydryl-rich protein inhibits the release of copper into the portal circulation by passively binding the metal within the enterocyte, thereby blocking copper transport across the serosal surface [7]. Most of the intracellular metallothionein-bound copper is subsequently eliminated in the stool as the enterocytes exfoliate into the intestinal lumen. Thus, induction of enterocyte metallothionein is one mechanism by which copper absorption may be inhibited.

## 2.3 Hematogenous Transport of Copper

Following intestinal absorption or intravenous administration, copper is bound initially to the nonceruloplasmin fraction in plasma [6, 8], which consists primarily of serum albumin and, to a lesser extent, amino acids, particularly histidine [9]. Although amino acid-bound copper represents only a small fraction of total plasma copper, it appears to be the primary means by which the metal is transported across cell membranes, from the blood to various tissues. Albumin-bound copper is cleared rapidly by the liver ($t_{1/2} \sim 10$ min), and a significant portion is subsequently incorporated into the blue glycoprotein, ceruloplasmin. An additional high-molecular-weight protein, transcuprein, which binds approximately 7% of plasma copper, is postulated to be a nonspecific transport protein which serves a role similar to that of albumin [10].

Ceruloplasmin, the major copper-binding protein in human blood, is synthesized almost exclusively in the liver and contains ~70% of total serum copper [5]. The mean serum concentration of ceruloplasmin in adults is approximately 30 mg/dl. However, ceruloplasmin is an "acute phase reactant," so its synthetic rate increases in response to inflammation. Plasma levels also are influenced by a wide variety of humoral and hormonal agents, particularly estrogens [11]. The serum ceruloplasmin concentration is low in the human newborn, but increases to near adult levels during the first 2 years of life, coincidentally with the postnatal decline in hepatic copper concentration.

The plasma disappearance of ceruloplasmin-bound copper ($t_{1/2} \sim 12$ h) is much slower than that of albumin-bound copper [5]. Copper incorporated into the ceruloplasmin molecule is released only in the course of degradation of the protein, which occurs primarily in the hepatic lysosomes. The fact that failure of other copper-containing enzymes does not occur in patients who have undetectable levels of plasma ceruloplasmin (e.g., Wilson's disease) implies that this globulin is not an indispensable component of copper transport, and its precise biologic role remains unclear.

## 2.4 Hepatic Copper Metabolism

The liver plays a pivotal role in copper homeostasis, serving as the major site of uptake, storage, and excretion of the metal. Hepatic copper is found both in association with binding proteins, particularly metallothionein, and as a component of specific metalloenzymes (e.g., superoxide dismutase). Copper-binding proteins are presumed to be critical in the temporary storage and detoxification of copper, and also may function as donors for the synthesis of ceruloplasmin or the excretion of copper into bile.

Although copper bound to amino acids is filtered through the glomerulus, it is efficiently reabsorbed in the renal tubules so that the small amount of copper excreted in the urine (less than 70 μg daily) contributes little to the maintenance of copper balance in normal subjects. Copper homeostasis depends primarily on the biliary excretion of the metal, which ranges between 1.2 and 1.7 mg/day [12]. Biliary elimination of copper varies in response to hepatic copper load and, therefore, indirectly in response to copper intake. The immediate hepatic precursor pool(s) of biliary copper is unknown, although it is postulated that copper bound to metallothionein, located either in the cytosol or in the hepatic lysosomes, may represent the prebiliary copper compartment [13]. Since intestinal reabsorption of biliary copper is negligible [14], there appears to be no appreciable enterohepatic circulation for this metal.

## 3 Wilson's Disease

### 3.1 Genetics

Wilson's disease is a familial syndrome with an autosomal recessive mode of inheritance [15]. Recent estimates from the United States, Germany, and Japan suggest that the prevalence of the disease is approximately 1 in 30000 live births [15]. Increased rates of consanguinity, as occurs in certain isolated communities in Japan, Sardinia, and the Middle East, may lead to considerably higher incidences. Identification of a linkage between the Wilson's disease locus and the red cell enzyme esterase-D established that the gene mutation responsible for Wilson's disease is located on chromosome 13 [16]. This localization has subsequently been confirmed by studies of Middle Eastern, North American, and Sardinian families [15, 17]. Further analyses, using multipoint linkage techniques, have mapped the abnormal gene for Wilson's disease specifically to 13q14–q21 (Fig. 1) [18].

The marked variation in clinical manifestations of Wilson's disease raises the question as to whether differences exist at the molecular level. The fact that Wilson's disease is linked to chromosome 13 markers in all populations studied to date indicates that there is a single genetic locus for the disease. It has been postulated that different mutations at that locus may explain the clinical variability [15]. Indeed, there is conflicting data concerning the precise order of the genetic markers linked to the Wilson's disease locus, and it has been proposed that this region of chromosome 13 may be a "hot spot" for recombination [18]. However, detailed genetic and epidemiologic studies suggest that the variability in clinical expression observed in Wilson's disease patients is unlikely to be a consequence of allelic heterogeneity, since marked differences in presentation, age of onset, and disease course have been observed in family members who have inherited two identical mutant alleles. Hence, the phenotypic variations observed in Wilson's disease are likely due to genetic influences independent of the Wilson's disease gene, as well as cultural and environmental factors.

The rapid pace of developments involving the molecular genetics of Wilson's disease may soon provide a means for carrier detection and early diagnosis of the disorder [15]. Haplotype analysis of relatives in Sardinian families with closely linked markers has permitted precise carrier detection with less than 2% error [17]. The most likely application of genetic linkage tests will be in the screening of family members of patients afflicted with the disorder since, using conventional biochemical analyses, the preclinical diagnosis of Wilson's disease occasionally can be difficult. However, despite the advent of new genetic techniques, a confirmatory liver biopsy will probably be required before subjecting asymptomatic patients to lifelong medical therapy.

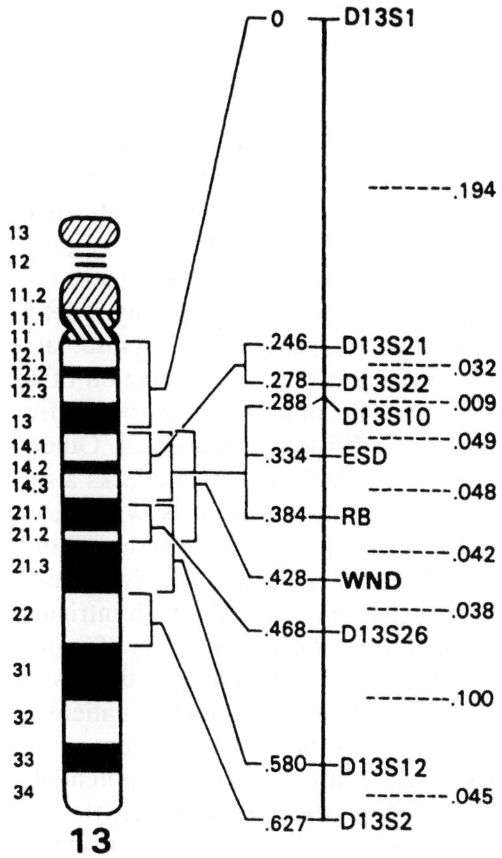


**Fig. 1.** Genetic map of chromosome 13q14–q21. The genetic distance measured cumulatively in Morgans from the D13S1 locus is indicated on the *left-hand side of the vertical solid line*. The maximum likelihood estimate of recombination (θ) between adjacent intervals is shown on the *right-hand side*. *WND* indicates the location of the Wilson's disease locus. *ESD* and *RB* represent the loci for esterase-D and the retinoblastoma gene, respectively. [Reproduced with permission from Bowcock AM et al. (1988) J Hum Genet 43:671]

### 3.2 Pathogenesis

The majority of the clinical manifestations of Wilson's disease appear to be a direct result of excessive accumulation of tissue copper. A wide variety of intracellular systems are disrupted by elevated copper concentrations, including membranes, various organelles, DNA, enzymes, and other proteins. To date, the precise biochemical defect in Wilson's disease remains undefined. Intestinal copper absorption in both heterozygotes and homozygotes with Wilson's disease does not differ from either normal subjects or cirrhotic patients, suggesting that excessive copper uptake is not the primary abnormality [14]. The prompt reversal of abnormal copper metabolism in Wilson's disease patients following orthotopic liver transplantation [19] confirms that the primary defect resides in the liver. Patients with Wilson's disease demonstrate diminished fecal elimination of copper as a result of impaired biliary excretion of the metal [13, 20], and this is believed to be the fundamental cause of copper overload in these patients.

The leading hypothesis holds that a hepatic lysosomal abnormality accounts for the diminished biliary excretion and systemic accumulation of copper [13]. Lysosomal dysfunction is thought to be the result of either enhanced retention of copper by a defective lysosomal protein or impaired transport of copper across the lysosomal membrane [21]. Alternatively, it has been proposed that the production of copper-associated protein, a peptide that is thought to protect hepatocytes from the injurious effects of copper, is impaired in Wilson's disease [22]. Others have demonstrated that the bile of patients with Wilson's disease lacks a specific copper-binding protein, which immunologically cross-reacts with ceruloplasmin and is resistant to proteolytic degradation [23]. These authors postulate that the absence of this biliary protein results in excessive intestinal reabsorption of copper excreted by the biliary system. Although intriguing, this theory does not account for the diminished biliary excretion of copper noted in Wilson's disease.

The finding that serum ceruloplasmin levels are low or absent in more than 90% of Wilson's disease patients, and that these patients have profoundly diminished incorporation of radiocopper into ceruloplasmin [24], has focused attention on the potential role of this protein in the pathogenesis of the disease. However, the primary defect does not appear to be directly related to this protein for several reasons:

1. The gene for ceruloplasmin is found on chromosome 3, while the gene for Wilson's disease has been localized to chromosome 13.
2. Some patients with Wilson's disease have normal serum ceruloplasmin levels.
3. Heterozygous individuals may have significantly reduced levels of ceruloplasmin and yet never develop toxic tissue levels of copper.
4. Serum ceruloplasmin levels do not correlate with the clinical severity of the disease.
5. Intravenous administration of purified ceruloplasmin from normal subjects to patients with Wilson's disease does not normalize copper metabolism.

Nonetheless, the strong association between ceruloplasmin deficiency and Wilson's disease raises the possibility of a potential interaction between the two genes. It has recently been shown that Wilson's disease patients have significantly lower steady-state hepatic ceruloplasmin mRNA levels compared to control patients with other hepatic diseases [25]. Hence, the low levels of serum ceruloplasmin generally observed in Wilson's disease patients may be in part due to decreased transcription of the ceruloplasmin gene. In addition, abnormalities at the translational or posttranslational level are suggested by the detection of appreciable hepatic levels of ceruloplasmin mRNA in a patient with complete absence of ceruloplasmin in the serum [25]. Since the steady-state concentrations of hepatic ceruloplasmin mRNA in the fetal and adult rat are comparable [26], it is postulated that the low level of serum ceruloplasmin in neonatal rats is due to regulation at the posttranscriptional level. These data offer support for the EPSTEIN and SHERLOCK hypothesis [27] that the hypoceruloplasminemia observed in Wilson's disease may be the result of a failure to switch from a fetal to an adult mode of ceruloplasmin gene expression.

### 3.3 Natural History

The natural history of Wilson's disease may be considered in four stages (Fig. 2) [28]. In *stage I*, patients are asymptomatic despite progressive copper accumulation in hepatocytes. Eventually, when all cytosolic copper binding sites in the liver cell become saturated, the metal is redistributed from the cytosol to the lysosomes (*stage II*). During this phase, a proportion of the metal also is released into the systemic circulation. The process of hepatic redistribution and release of copper occurs gradually in the majority (60%) of Wilson's disease patients, most of whom remain asymptomatic. However, hemolysis may result from an abrupt rise in blood levels when systemic release of hepatic copper is massive. Additionally, the sudden redistribution of hepatic copper within the hepatocyte may precipitate acute hepatic necrosis, chronic active hepatitis, or even fulminant hepatic failure. If symptomatic stage II patients survive the acute hematologic and/or hepatic insult, they may again become asymptomatic.

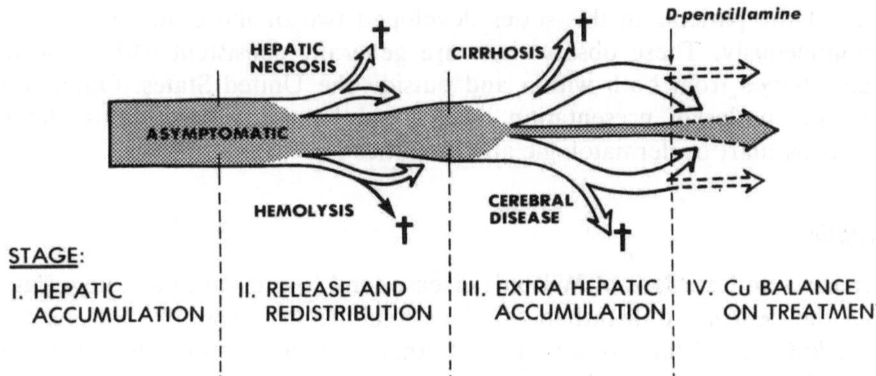


**Fig. 2.** Natural history of Wilson's disease [reproduced with permission from GOLLAN JL (1990) In: Zakim D, Boyer TD (eds) Hepatology: a textbook of liver disease, 2nd edn. W.B. Saunders, Philadelphia, p 1262]

During *stage III*, copper continues to accumulate both in the liver and in other extrahepatic organs, such as the brain, cornea, heart, and kidneys. Persistently elevated intrahepatic copper levels ultimately result in the development of progressive fibrosis and cirrhosis. The clinical presentation of Wilson's disease depends on the rate of copper accumulation in the various organs. If the cirrhosis is inactive and cerebral accumulation is slow, patients may remain asymptomatic for many years. Alternatively, the acute development of a variety of hepatic or extrahepatic manifestations may be observed. Following diagnosis, patients achieve a state of copper balance after prolonged therapy (*stage IV*) and most will become asymptomatic. Unfortunately, a few will suffer from residual hepatic and/or neurologic sequelae.

### 3.4 Clinical Features

Although the biochemical defect which leads to the accumulation of copper in Wilson's disease is present a birth, clinically apparent disease is rarely noted before the age of 6 years. Symptoms of Wilson's disease typically become manifest in older children, adolescents, and young adults; however, case reports have documented the onset as early as 4 years and as late as 58 years of age [29]. The mean age of onset varies from 12 to 23 years, depending on the location of the epidemiologic study [30, 31]. Compared with Europeans and Americans, clinical manifestations tend to develop at an earlier age in Asian populations despite a diet that is generally lower in copper content.

Wilson's disease patients typically present with hepatic and/or neurologic dysfunction. In a large series of patients [30], the initial clinical manifestations were hepatic in 42%, neurologic in 34%, psychiatric in 10%, hematologic or endocrinologic in 12%, and renal in 1%. Approximately 25% of the patients in this series developed two or more modes of onset simultaneously. These observations are generally consistent with those of other studies from both within and outside the United States. Other less common modes of presentation include ophthalmologic, musculoskeletal, cardiovascular, or dermatologic abnormalities (Table 1).

#### *Hepatic*

Hepatic manifestations of Wilson's disease tend to present at a younger age than the neurologic disturbances. Abnormalities are generally nonspecific, mimicking the features of a variety of other acute and chronic liver diseases [32]. There are three major clinical patterns of liver involvement noted in Wilson's disease patients: cirrhosis, chronic active hepatitis, and fulminant hepatic failure. Typically, the hepatic involvement is insidious in onset and, if untreated, pursues a chronic course to cirrhosis, characterized by

**Table 1.** Clinical manifestations of Wilson's disease

| | |
|---|---|
| Hepatic | – cirrhosis, chronic active hepatitis, fulminant hepatic failure |
| Gastrointestinal | – cholelithiasis, pancreatitis, spontaneous bacterial peritonitis |
| Neurologic | – extrapyramidal, cerebellar, or pseudobulbar signs, seizures |
| Psychiatric | – behavioral changes, cognitive impairment, psychosis, affective disorder |
| Hematologic | – hemolysis, hypersplenism, coagulopathy, qualitative platelet abnormalities |
| Ophthalmologic | – Kayser-Fleischer rings, sunflower cataracts |
| Renal | – renal tubular defects, diminished glomerular filtration, nephrolithiasis |
| Cardiovascular | – cardiomyopathy, arrhythmias, conduction disturbances, autonomic dysfunction |
| Musculoskeletal | – osteomalacia, osteoporosis, osteoarthritis |
| Miscellaneous | – endocrine abnormalities, azure lunulae |

progressive lassitude, fatigue, anorexia, jaundice, spider angiomas, splenomegaly, and ascites [33]. Unfortunately, all too often, Wilson's disease patients with previously unrecognized hepatic dysfunction will first present with a shrunken liver and complications of advanced cirrhosis, such as variceal hemorrhage or hepatic encephalopathy.

Less commonly (in an estimated 10%–30% of cases), patients with Wilson's disease present with clinical, biochemical, and histologic features similar to those of chronic active hepatitis [34, 35]. The diagnosis of the underlying disorder may be overlooked in these patients, since a significant percentage will have no evidence of neurologic dysfunction or Kayser-Fleischer rings on ophthalmologic examination. Serum ceruloplasmin levels also may be normal in some of these patients, despite severe hepatic disease [34]. It has been estimated that 2%–10% of patients under the age of 35 who carry the diagnosis of idiopathic chronic active hepatitis actually have Wilson's disease [35]. It is imperative that the correct diagnosis is established in these individuals since, with appropriate therapy, long-term survival can be achieved, even when cirrhosis is present.

Wilson's disease occasionally may present as fulminant hepatic failure [36, 37]. Clinically, these patients may be indistinguishable from individuals with massive viral-induced hepatic necrosis. Unfortunately, the biochemical tests used to diagnose Wilson's disease also can be abnormal in patients with other forms of fulminant hepatic failure. Features suggestive of fulminant Wilsonian hepatitis include evidence of intravascular hemolysis, splenomegaly, a relatively mild transaminitis despite massive hepatic necrosis [with aspartate aminotransferase (AST) levels much greater than alanine aminotransferase (ALT)], hyperbilirubinemia with low normal alkaline phosphatase levels, and a markedly elevated serum copper concentration [37]. A ratio of alkaline phosphatase to total serum bilirubin of less than 2.0 in association with an AST/ALT ratio of greater than 4.0 has been reported to be diagnostic of fulminant Wilsonian hepatitis [38]. Although highly suggestive, Kayser-Fleischer rings are not pathognomonic, since they are occasionally observed in other cholestatic hepatic diseases [39]. Severe coagulopathy and hypercupriuria are not useful in distinguishing Wilsonian from non-Wilsonian hepatic failure [37]. Liver biopsy may be helpful, although deranged clotting function will frequently preclude this procedure. If a biopsy specimen is obtainable, histologic evidence of cirrhosis (predominantly micronodular) in a young patient with fulminant hepatitis is suggestive of Wilson's disease, as is an elevated hepatic copper content [36]. Unfortunately, due to massive hepatic release, liver copper concentrations occasionally may be within the normal range [36].

Wilson's disease patients with acute hepatic failure tend to be young and to have a fulminant clinical course, with survival generally no longer than days to weeks unless hepatic transplantation is performed [37]. Medical treatment is frequently unsuccessful, particularly when the disorder is associated with hemolysis and consequent renal insufficiency. A prognostic index scale for patients with acute hepatic failure secondary to Wilson's disease, based on the serum bilirubin, AST, and prothrombin time at diagnosis has been developed [40]. Hepatic transplantation is recommended for cases with a calculated index of 7 or greater, since all patients with this score, studied both prospecively and retrospectively, have died within 2 months of diagnosis, despite the institution of appropriate medical therapy. Two patients, with scores of 7 and 8 (within the fatal range), underwent successful hepatic transplantation and survived [40]. However, caution should be exercised in applying this prognostic index prospectively to all patients, as there are reports of recovery from Wilsonian chronic active hepatitis with medical therapy alone, despite scores indicative of a fatal outcome [21]. Thus, even when transplantation is unavailable for patients with a poor prognostic index, it remains imperative to make the diagnosis of Wilson's disease for the purpose of aggressive medical therapy and family screening.

### *Gastrointestinal*

Wilson's disease patients have an increased incidence of both pigment and mixed cholesterol gallstones [32, 41]. Cirrhosis and hemolysis, both of which are frequent complications of Wilson's disease, predispose to the development of cholelithiasis. Hence, gallstone disease should always be considered in the differential diagnosis of abdominal pain in such patients.

There are scattered case reports of pancreatitis occurring in patients with Wilson's disease [42] and, in some cases, the pancreatitis may resolve with the initiation of D-penicillamine. Elevated pancreatic copper levels have been documented in Wilson's disease [43], and abnormal pancreatic endocrine and exocrine function has been described [44]. Other investigators, however, were unable to confirm these observations [45]. Since gallstones are a potential cause of pancreatitis in these patients, the question as to whether the underlying biochemical disorder in Wilson's disease results in direct pancreatic injury remains unresolved.

Spontaneous bacterial peritonitis has been reported in Wilson's disease patients with advanced liver disease and ascites [46]. It is speculated that D-penicillamine, with its immunosuppressive effect, may be a contributing factor.

### *Neurologic*

The neurologic features of Wilson's disease commonly appear between the ages of 12 and 30 years [47], the onset being somewhat later than for hepatic manifestations. It is unusual for neurologic dysfunction to develop prior to adolescence or after 40 years of age. Invariably, patients with neurologic abnormalities secondary to Wilson's disease exhibit Kayser-Fleischer rings on ophthalmologic examination. Initial symptoms are subtle, commonly manifesting as abnormal behavior and deteriorating school performance. Incoordination, clumsiness, tremor, dysarthria, excessive salivation, ataxia, dysphagia, and mask-like facies may subsequently develop.

Movement disorders are the predominant neurologic feature of Wilson's disease. Three distinct syndromes have been described: (a) a parkinsonian-like condition characterized by akinesia and rigidity, (b) dystonia with involuntary motions and sustained posturing, and (c) resting and intention tremors often associated with ataxia and dysarthria [47]. Despite the presence of severe motor abnormalities, cognitive function remains relatively spared [48], resulting in an extremely frustrating existence for the afflicted individual.

Wilson's disease patients have an incidence of seizures of approximately 6%, which is tenfold higher than in the general population [49]. However, there is no specific form of seizure that is characteristic of Wilson's disease. Thus, electroencephalography is not helpful in the diagnosis of Wilson's disease and, in the absence of seizures, reveals only nonspecific slow waves in those patients wih advanced neurologic or hepatic dysfunction [50].

Neurologic deterioration progresses inexorably in untreated patients, eventually resulting in the dystonia, spasticity, rigidity, and flexion contractures characteristic of end-stage Wilson's disease. The neurologic abnormalities are frequently reversible with medical therapy, the best results being achieved with early intervention. In the uncommon circumstance when an individual is left with residual extrapyramidal deficits despite adequate chelation therapy, apomorphine, a short-acting dopamine agonist, may be administered as a test to determine whether the patient might benefit from antiparkinsonian medication [51].

### *Psychiatric*

Although all untreated patients are thought to eventually develop psychiatric disturbances, these may occasionally be the predominant or presenting manifestation of Wilson's disease. Not infrequently, affected individuals are mistakenly thought to suffer from a progressive psychiatric illness and are institutionalized prior to diagnosis of the underlying metabolic disorder. It has been recommended that all psychiatric patients with signs of liver or neurologic disease, with a family history of Wilson's disease, or who are refractory to therapy should be screened for this disorder. The range of psychiatric abnormalities associated with Wilson's disease is broad and has been divided into four basic categories: behavioral, affective, schizophrenia-like, and cognitive [47]. Patients, most commonly adolescents, will demonstrate personality changes with impulsive and antisocial behavior. Psychoneuroses, major depression, schizophreniform psychosis, and organic dementia have all been described in Wilson's disease patients [52]. Psychiatric disturbances may reflect not only the biochemical manifestations of cerebral copper deposition but also the individual response to the frustration of progressive, undiagnosed neurologic decompensation.

The use of psychotherapy, along with milder tranquilizing or antidepressant drugs, is indicated when psychiatric disturbances become troublesome; however, specific therapy with D-penicillamine remains essential. Phenothiazines tend to exacerbate neurologic signs and psychiatric symptoms and, therefore, are of little value in Wilson's disease patients. Most psychiatric disturbances will resolve with medical treatment, particularly behavioral and cognitive disabilities [48]. In fact, treated Wilson's disease patients appear to function on a psychometrically normal level. Unfortunately, patients with combined neurologic and psychiatric abnormalities in whom the diagnosis of Wilson's disease was delayed, particularly those with affective disorders, may occasionally manifest persistent psychiatric dysfunction despite the initiation of therapy.

### *Hematologic*

Acute intravascular hemolysis is frequently associated with Wilson's disease and may be the presenting manifestation in as many as 15% of patients [53]. It is postulated that hemolysis results from the sudden release of copper from the liver into the blood, as evidenced by a marked rise in serum and urinary copper concentrations. The metal is subsequently taken up by the red blood cells, where it is presumed to cause oxidative damage to cell membranes and hemoglobin molecules [53]. The hemolysis of Wilson's disease is usually self-limited and typically antedates the hepatic manifestations by several years. It is recommended that all adolescents and young adults with Coombs-negative hemolytic anemia be screened for Wilson's disease. Those patients who develop hemolysis in association with acute hepatic failure have a poor prognosis, with death frequently occurring within weeks, usually as a result of hepatic or renal insufficiency [37].

Wilson's disease patients with significant hepatic dysfunction frequently exhibit an increased bleeding tendency as a result of reduced synthesis of coagulation factors and qualitative defects in platelet function [54]. Cirrhosis, with concomitant hypersplenism, is the basis for the increased incidence of thrombocytopenia and leukopenia observed in these patients.

### *Ophthalmologic*

The Kayser-Fleischer ring is a golden-brown or greenish discoloration in the limbic region of the cornea caused by copper deposition in Descemet's membrane. The rings form bilaterally, appearing initially at the superior pole of the cornea, then the inferior pole, and, ultimately, circumferentially. It is postulated that the pattern of deposition is due to the relative stagnation of corneal solvent flow in the superior pole, which facilitates the precipitation of copper [55]. The rings consist of electron-dense granules that are rich in copper and sulfur, suggesting that the metal may be bound to metallothionein. The array of colors and hues that may be observed is an optical phenomenon related to the distribution, density, and size of the copper granules, which are more numerous at the periphery of the cornea compared to the central region.

Kayser-Fleischer rings are observed in 80%–90% of individuals with *symptomatic* Wilson's disease, and are almost invariably present in those with neurologic manifestations. Even when not visible to the unaided eye, the rings may be identified by slit-lamp ophthalmoscopy or gonioscopy. However, the rings are absent in at least 60% of asymptomatic children [56] and, not uncommonly, in patients who have hepatic disease, particularly those with chronic active hepatitis [34]. Although the Kayser-Fleischer ring is a useful diagnostic sign, it is no longer considered to be pathognomonic of Wilson's disease unless accompanied by neurologic abnormalities. The rings occasionally may be seen in chronic cholestatic disorders, such as intrahepatic cholestasis of childhood, primary biliary cirrhosis, partial biliary atresia, chronic active hepatitis with cirrhosis, and cryptogenic cirrhosis [39]. The excessive deposition of copper that occurs in these conditions is most likely the result of diminished biliary excretion of the metal. However, these disorders can easily be distinguished from Wilson's disease by the clinical history, immunologic markers, serum level of ceruloplasmin, and radiocopper kinetic studies.

With adequate D-penicillamine therapy, Kayser-Fleischer rings gradually resolve over 3–5 years in 80% of patients [56], disappearing sequentially in reverse order of formation, so that the superior corneal pole is the last region to clear. There appears to be no association between the stage of the disease or the effectiveness of treatment and the rate of resolution of the rings.

Sunflower cataracts, which are a less frequent ocular manifestation of Wilson's disease [55, 57], are typically found in conjunction with Kayser-Fleischer rings. The cataract appears as a central green or golden disk in the anterior capsule of the lens, with radiating "petals" arising from the posterior capsule. Vision is generally unaffected by the cataracts, and they tend to clear more rapidly than Kayser-Fleischer rings in response to medical therapy. Sunflower cataracts, as well as Kayser-Fleischer rings, also may occur in association with copper-containing intraocular foreign bodies.

### *Renal*

A variety of renal function abnormalities are associated with Wilson's disease. Both reduced glomerular filtration and diminished renal plasma flow have been documented [58]. Renal tubular defects, which are thought to result from the toxic effect of copper on tubular cells, also have been described [59]. Proximal tubular dysfunction is manifested by aminoaciduria, glucosuria, uricosuria, hyperphosphaturia, and hypercalciuria. In addition, proteinuria, involving low-molecular-weight globulins, and peptiduria, including hydroxyproline-containing peptides, have been noted [60]. Distal renal tubular acidosis may contribute to the 16% incidence of renal calculi in Wilson's disease patients [61]. Chelation therapy generally results in a marked improvement in renal function [58], although severe renal side-effects, including nephrotic syndrome and, less frequently, a Goodpasture's-like syndrome, have been associated with D-penicillamine therapy [62].

### *Cardiovascular*

Although cardiac abnormalities have been associated with the excessive systemic accumulation of various metals, including iron (hemochromatosis), lead, and cobalt, relatively little is known about the effects of copper overload on the heart. In a prospective study of 53 Wilson's disease patients with a mean age of 21 years, electrocardiographic abnormalities were detected in 34% compared with 0% in an age-matched control group [63]. Findings included left ventricular or biventricular hypertrophy, early repolarization, ST depression, and T wave inversion. Heart rhythm and conduction disturbances, such as premature atrial and ventricular contractions, atrial fibrillation, sinoatrial block, and Mobitz type I atrioventricular block, were also noted. Since half of the patients with abnormal electrocardiograms had no prior therapy for Wilson's disease, these findings are unlikely to be related to the administration of D-penicillamine. There were three deaths among the patients during the 10-years follow-up period. two of which were cardiac related. A significant number of patients also were noted to have autonomic dysfunction, as manifested by asymptomatic orthostatic hypotension and abnormal responses to the Valsalva maneuver [63].

In a retrospective analysis of autopsy specimens from nine patients with Wilson's disease, cardiac hypertrophy was observed in five, despite a mean age of only 29 years [64]. Pathologic abnormalities included interstitial and replacement myocardial fibrosis, intramyocardial small vessel disease, and focal myocarditis. In addition, AV-nodal degeneration and premature atherosclerotic coronary artery disease were noted in one patient. Although relatively nonspecific, in the absence of other precipitating factors the occurrence of these pathologic findings in a group of young patients suggests that Wilson's disease may induce cardiac injury. The pathogenesis of the histologic cardiac abnormalities observed in Wilson's disease remains uncertain, since myocardial copper levels do not appear to correlate with the severity of the pathologic lesions or with the clinical cardiac manifestations [63, 64]. Although more data are needed, cardiac involvement should now be added to the list of clinical manifestations of Wilson's disease.

### *Musculoskeletal*

Skeletal involvement is a common feature of Wilson's disease, with more than half of patients exhibiting osteopenia on conventional radiologic examination [65]. Either osteomalacia or osteoporosis or a combination of both has been described. The former may result from renal tubular abnormalities associated with the disease. The etiology of the osteoporosis is less apparent, although it may be due in part to decreased weight-bearing secondary to neurologic disability. However, there are no pathognomonic features on radiographic examination to distinguish Wilson's disease from other causes of bone loss.

The arthropathy of Wilson's disease, observed on radiographic evaluation in three-fourths of all patients, is a degenerative process that resembles premature osteoarthritis [66]. Symptomatic joint disease, which occurs in 25%–50% of patients, usually presents late in the course of the disease, frequently after 20 years of age, although, occasionally, osteoarthritis may be the initial manifestation [67]. The arthropathy generally involves the spine and large appendicular joints, such as knees, wrists, and hips [66]. Radiologic studies reveal typical degenerative changes including osteophytes, sclerosis, subchondral pseudocysts, and bone fragmentation. Osteochondritis desiccans, chondromalacia patellae, and chondrocalcinosis also have been described. The cause of the osteoarticular changes remains speculative, with scant evidence to directly implicate copper accumulation in the pathogenesis.

### *Endocrinologic*

A variety of endocrinologic abnormalities have been described in association with Wilson's disease, including glucose intolerance [68], hypoparathyroidism [69], delayed puberty and gynecomastia in boys [30], and amenorrhea in women [70]. Detailed hormonal analyses of four female Wilson's disease patients suggest that oligomenorrhea or amenorrhea may be due to a primary disturbance of ovarian function [70].

## 3.5 Pathology

### *Hepatic*

Histologic changes are evident in liver biopsy specimens from asymptomatic Wilson's disease patients within the first decade of life [71]. The earliest changes seen on light microscopy include glycogen in the nuclei of periportal hepatocytes and moderate fatty infiltration [72], both of which are nonspecific findings. Histochemical staining of liver biopsy specimens for copper lacks sensitivity and specificity for Wilson's disease and, therefore, is of little diagnostic value [36, 73]. This is because, during the initial stages of copper accumulation, the metal is distributed diffusely in the cytoplasm and is undetectable by rhodamine or rubeanic acid stains. As the disease becomes more advanced, copper is sequestered within hepatocyte lysosomes and is detectable by routine histochemical techniques, even though the tissue concentration is actually lower than in earlier stages of the disorder.

Ultrastructural abnormalities in the liver of Wilson's disease patients may coexist with or even precede the changes observed by light microscopy. Hepatocyte mitochondria typically exhibit heterogeneity in size and shape, with increased matrix density, separation of the normally apposed inner and outer mitochondrial membranes, widened intercristal spaces, and an array of vacuolated and crystalline inclusions within the matrix (Fig. 3) [72]. In most patients, the mitochondrial changes become less pronounced or disappear after several years of therapy with D-penicillamine, indirectly supporting the notion that the abnormalities are a consequence of copper toxicity. Other ultrastructural features observed in Wilson's disease include lipid-containing lysosomes and heterogeneous, granular peroxisomes. All of these nonspecific abnormalities may actually regress as fibrosis and cirrhosis develop [72].

The rate of progression of hepatic injury in Wilson's disease patients from fatty infiltration to cirrhosis is variable, although it tends to occur by one of two general processes, either with or without significant hepatic inflammation. Some patients develop a histologic picture that is indistinguishable from chronic active hepatitis arising from other causes [34, 35]. Features include mononuclear cell infiltrates, which consist mainly of lymphocytes and plasma cells, piecemeal necrosis extending beyond the limiting plate, parenchymal collapse, bridging hepatic necrosis, and fibrosis (Fig. 4). If untreated, this histologic appearance may either evolve into macronodular cirrhosis or progress rapidly into a fulminant hepatitis which responds poorly to chelation therapy.

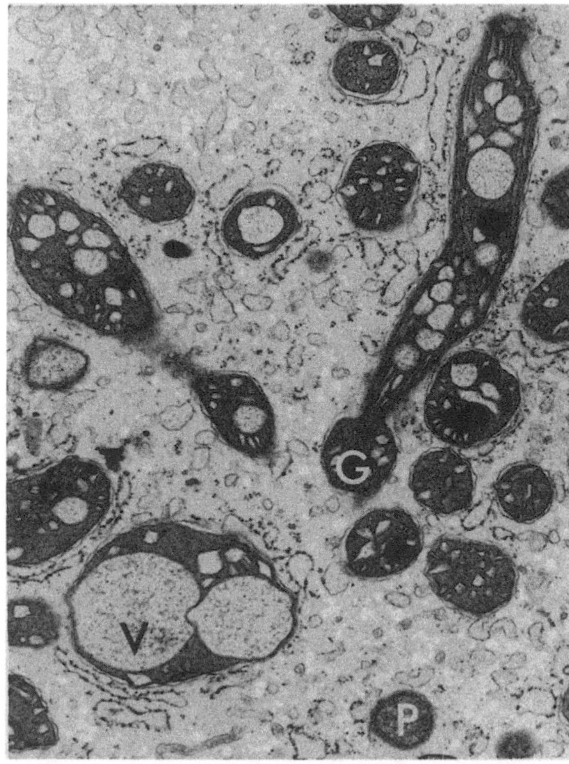


**Fig. 3.** Electron micrograph of a liver biopsy specimen from a patient with Wilson's disease. Striking pleomorphism of mitochondria is associated with abnormally arranged cristae, numerous large, electron-lucent vacuoles (*V*), and greatly enlarged mitochondrial granules (*G*). Peroxisomes (*P*) are heterogeneous with a granular matrix. On light microscopy, fatty infiltration of hepatocytes was evident. [Reproduced with permission from Sternlieb I (1972) In: Popper H, Schaffner F (eds) Progress in liver diseases, vol 4. Grune & Stratton, New York, p 511]

The progression to cirrhosis may occur in the absence of significant parenchymal inflammatory infiltrate or necrosis. The histologic pattern is a macronodular or mixed micro-macronodular cirrhosis, with fibrous septa, bile ductule proliferation, and variable septal round cell infiltration [73]. Hepatocytes at the periphery of the nodules frequently contain Mallory's hyalin. It should be noted that hepatic biopsy alone, without quantification of tissue copper levels, is insufficient to establish the diagnosis of Wilson's disease, since other hepatic conditions may exhibit similar morphologic findings [74]. In an attempt to explain the insidious progression to cirrhosis and the simultaneous occurrence of steatosis and periportal or bridging fibrosis in the absence of significant inflammation that is observed in some untreated Wilson's disease patients, it has been proposed that excess hepatic

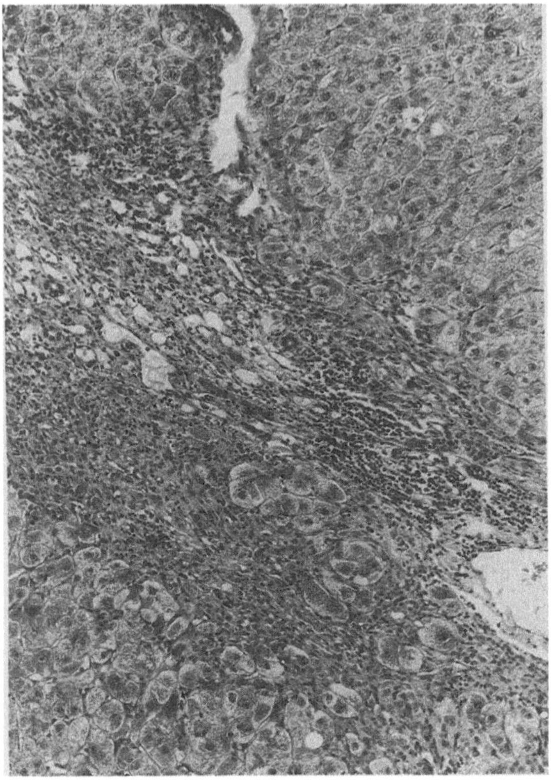

**Fig. 4.** Liver biopsy specimen from a Wilson's disease patient with the clinical appearance of chronic active hepatitis. Intense periportal mononuclear cell infiltration is present with extension beyond the limiting plate. Piecemeal necrosis is observed and there is evidence of hepatocyte swelling and fatty change. Wedge biopsy, H&E, ×150

copper may induce a discrete mobilization of mesenchymal cells and fibrogenesis [21]. This hypothesis holds that Wilsonian fulminant hepatitis and chronic active hepatitis represent complications of the underlying cirrhosis, rather than phases of progression of the hepatic injury. In support of this concept is the observation that the vast majority of Wilson's disease patients have evidence of fibrosis on liver biopsy despite widely varying levels and patterns of hepatic inflammation and injury.

In contrast to idiopathic hemochromatosis with cirrhosis, hepatocellular carcinoma is uncommon in Wilson's disease [75]. It has been proposed that this diminished risk is due to the absence of a significant inflammatory component in the pathogenesis of Wilsonian cirrhosis [21]. Animal studies offer support for the notion that copper may exert a protective effect against the development of this malignancy [75].

***Neuropathology***

Histologic studies of the central nervous system in Wilson's disease are limited to autopsy cases. Observed gross anatomic changes include degeneration and cavitation, primarily involving the putamen, globus pallidus, caudate nucleus, thalamus, and, less frequently, the brainstem and frontal cortex [76]. Little correlation has been observed between the degree of neurologic impairment and the neuropathologic findings. However, cerebral copper content does appear to correlate with the severity of both the histologic abnormalities in the brain and neurologic symptoms [76].

## 3.6 Laboratory Diagnosis

The diagnosis of Wilson's disease relies on both clinical and biochemical findings. The simplest screening evaluation includes a slit-lamp examination of the eyes, and measurement of serum ceruloplasmin and aminotransferase (ALT, AST) concentrations. If Kayser-Fleischer rings are present on ophthalmologic examination and ceruloplasmin levels are below 20 mg/dl, the diagnosis of Wilson's disease is secure. If the patient lacks corneal rings or is asymptomatic, the coexistence of a hepatic copper concentration above 250 μg/g dry weight and a low serum ceruloplasmin level is also sufficient to establish the diagnosis.

***Serum Ceruloplasmin***

The normal serum concentration of ceruloplasmin is 20–40 mg/dl. Although a decreased ceruloplasmin level per se is not diagnostic of Wilson's disease, approximately 95% of all patients and 85% of individuals presenting with hepatic manifestations of the disease have levels of this glycoprotein that are below the normal range. Hypoceruloplasminemia occasionally may occur in fulminant non-Wilsonian hepatitis, as a consequence of diminished hepatic synthetic function. Approximately one-fourth of children with chronic active hepatitis will have decreased serum ceruloplasmin levels [77]. Paradoxically, adults with this same condition virtually always appear to demonstrate normal or elevated levels [78]. Patients with nephrotic syndrome, protein-losing enteropathy, malabsorption, or severe malnutrition also may manifest low serum ceruloplasmin levels, although there is usually no diagnostic difficulty in these cases. However, confusion may arise with regard to the 10% of heterozygous carriers of the gene for Wilson's disease who manifest diminished levels of ceruloplasmin yet never develop the disease [79]. These individuals, who represent approximately 1 in 2000 persons in the general population, may present a difficult diagnostic dilemma if they fortuitously develop chronic active hepatitis or cirrhosis (of another etiology), thereby mimicking the clinical, biochemical, and histologic features of Wilson's disease.

Normal ceruloplasmin concentrations are found in up to 15% of patients with Wilson's disease and active liver involvement [34]. This is presumably due to increased hepatic synthesis and release of the glycoprotein. Elevated estrogen levels, secondary to pregnancy or exogenous administration, may increase serum ceruloplasmin concentrations [11] and, occasionally, may elevate previously low levels into the normal range.

### *Serum Copper*

In normal adults, the concentration of copper bound to serum albumin or amino acids (nonceruloplasmin copper) is 5–12 µg/dl [8]. Patients with untreated Wilson's disease have elevated concentrations of nonceruloplasmin copper, with levels as high as 50 µg/dl [8, 10]. This appears to result from the passage of excessive hepatic copper into the circulation. Total serum copper, however, typically remains below normal (less than 0.8 mg/liter) in Wilson's disease patients, since the increase in the nonceruloplasmin fraction is usually insufficient to compensate for the reduced ceruloplasmin concentrations. It is important to note that laboratories that do not perform copper assays routinely may provide inaccurate measurements of serum copper and ceruloplasmin levels. A useful method for detecting a misleading result involves calculation of the amount of ceruloplasmin copper (0.3% of the protein's weight); if this value exceeds the total serum copper concentration, the laboratory results are likely in error [21]. Although heterozygotes and treated patients with Wilson's disease have normal serum levels of nonceruloplasmin copper, the measurement of this fraction is generally unhelpful in diagnosis, since it is elevated in a variety of other parenchymal and cholestatic liver diseases [8].

### *Urinary Copper Excretion*

The urinary excretion of copper is greater than 100 µg/24 h (normal <40 µg/24 h) in most patients with symptomatic Wilson's disease. In patients with fulminant hepatic necrosis due to Wilson's disease, urinary excretion of the metal may exceed 1000 µg/24 h. Unfortunately, the measurement of urinary copper excretion is often misleading due to inaccuracies in collection and laboratory analysis, and asymptomatic Wilson's disease patients do not necessarily exhibit elevated urinary copper concentrations [21]. Urinary copper levels also may be elevated in a variety of other hepatic disorders, including cirrhosis, chronic active hepatitis, and cholestatic disorders, such as primary biliary cirrhosis [77, 78, 80]. Therefore, quantification of urinary copper should not be used as a screening test for Wilson's disease, although it may be useful as a means of confirming the diagnosis and evaluating the response to D-penicillamine therapy. The use of D-penicillamine to increase urinary copper excretion is of little diagnostic value, since it does not distinguish Wilson's disease from other types of hepatic disorder [21, 80].

### *Hepatic Copper Concentration*

In the absence of Kayser-Fleischer rings, a liver biopsy for quantitative copper determination is essential to establish the diagnosis of Wilson's disease. The biopsy needle and specimen container must be free from copper contamination. Thus, it is recommended that a disposable needle made entirely of steel or a Klatskin or Menghini needle washed in EDTA and rinsed with demineralized water should be used [21]. In addition, the syringe should contain 5% dextrose rather than saline solution. The normal hepatic copper concentration varies from 15 to 55 μg/g dry liver [81]. Virtually all untreated patients with Wilson's disease have elevated hepatic copper levels, ranging from 250 to as high as 3000 μg/g liver [71, 81]. The finding of a normal hepatic copper concentration effectively excludes the diagnosis of untreated Wilson's disease. However, an elevated liver copper level alone is insufficient to establish the diagnosis of Wilson's disease, since concentrations above 250 μg/g may be found in other chronic hepatic (mostly cholestatic) disorders, including primary biliary cirrhosis, primary sclerosing cholangitis, extrahepatic biliary obstruction or atresia, intrahepatic cholestasis of childhood, Indian childhood cirrhosis, and in vineyard sprayers inhaling copper salts [81] (Table 2). Heterozygous carriers of the Wilson's disease gene may occasionally demonstrate elevated levels of hepatic copper (rarely to 250 μg/g), but these individuals do not develop overt signs of copper toxicosis [71].

### *Incorporation of Radiocopper into Ceruloplasmin*

In rare instances where a diagnostic dilemma remains, such as when liver biopsy is contraindicated, a radiocopper loading test may be helpful [6]. Serum radioactivity is measured at 1, 2, 4, and 48 h after oral administration of the radionuclide (2 mg cupric acetate containing 0.3–0.5 mCi $^{64}Cu$, mixed in fruit juice). In healthy subjects and in patients with hepatic disorders that mimic Wilson's disease, the plasma concentrations of radiocopper rise rapidly, are maximal within 1–2 h, and then fall and rise again over the ensuing 48 h as the non-ceruloplasmin-bound radiocopper is incorporated

**Table 2.** Diseases and conditions other than Wilson's disease in which hepatic copper overload may occur

| |
|---|
| Primary biliary cirrhosis |
| Primary sclerosing cholangitis |
| Extrahepatic biliary obstruction or biliary atresia |
| Cholestatic syndromes of childhood |
| Indian childhood cirrhosis |
| Chronic active hepatitis (rare) |
| Hepatocellular carcinoma (rare) |
| Inhalation of copper salts by vineyard sprayers |

into newly synthesized ceruloplasmin in the liver and released into the circulation [6]. Wilson's disease patients, on the other hand, incorporate little or no radiocopper into nascent ceruloplasmin, even in the presence of normal ceruloplasmin concentrations [6]. Heterozygotes have a pattern of incorporation that is intermediate between that of Wilson's disease patients and healthy individuals [5].

#### *Other Laboratory Tests*

Abnormalities of somatosensory auditory and visual evoked potential conduction times have been observed in patients with Wilson's disease [82]. However, the findings are neither specific nor sensitive for the disorder. Since all patients with abnormal evoked potentials were clinically symptomatic, these specialized tests are generally unhelpful in the early diagnosis of Wilson's disease.

It has been postulated that the copper concentration of cerebrospinal fluid (CSF) may reflect CNS copper levels, since CSF contains only small quantities of protein and ceruloplasmin. In a small study of five patients with cerebral manifestations of Wilson's disease, the CSF copper concentration was consistently elevated [83]. A gradual decrease in CSF copper levels paralleled the clinical improvement in neurologic function following treatment. Although more extensive studies are required, these findings suggest that the measurement of the CSF copper concentration may find some application in the therapeutic monitoring of Wilson's disease patients with neurologic manifestations.

### 3.7 Radiologic Features

Despite rapid advances in computed tomography (CT) and magnetic resonance imaging (MRI), these radiologic modalities have little to offer in the diagnosis or evaluation of hepatic involvement in Wilson's disease. Although there are case reports of diffusely increased liver attenuation on abdominal CT scan in asymptomatic Wilson's disease patients, larger series have failed to confirm these findings [84]. A prospective evaluation of 24 patients using abdominal CT found no correlation between CT attenuation values and hepatic, urinary, or serum copper levels. In fact, all patients exhibited normal hepatic attenuation [84]. MRI also appears to be of little value in the diagnosis of early hepatic injury in Wilson's disease [85]. Ultrasonography and nuclear medicine imaging of the liver likewise have been uninformative [21, 86].

Cranial CT and MRI scans reflect the histologic abnormalities found in the brain of patients with Wilson's disease. Low attenuation regions are observed on head CT in most Wilson's disease patients with neurologic manifestations [87]. The cranial lesions observed on CT are typically bilateral and are classified into two general categories: (a) well-defined slit-like low attenuation foci involving the basal ganglia, and (b) larger regions of low attenuation in the basal ganglia, thalamus, or dentate nucleus [88]. Cerebral and cerebellar atrophy, which correlates histologically with diffuse neuronal loss, also has been described [87]. Occasionally, asymptomatic patients and those with only hepatic abnormalities also will manifest these findings on cranial CT. In these cases, the scan may provide the first indication of the underlying disorder.

Magnetic resonance imaging of the brain appears to be more sensitive than CT scanning in the detection of early lesions. In a study of 38 patients with Wilson's disease of varying duration (0–27 years) [89], 58% were found to have abnormal findings on MRI examination of the brain. Focal lesions (3–15 mm in diameter), which were hypointense on T1-weighted and hyperintense on T2-weighted images, were observed in nearly half of the patients [89]. These focal abnormalities were typically bilateral and localized to the lenticular nuclei, although involvement of the thalamic and caudate nuclei, brain stem, and white matter was also noted. Eight patients (21%) exhibited diffuse brain atrophy and widening of the ventricular system [89].

Radiologic CNS abnormalities are not, however, specific for Wilson's disease and can be observed in a variety of other conditions, including methanol and carbon monoxide poisoning, severe hypoxia, Parkinson's disease, Huntington's chorea, mitochondrial cytopathy, striatonigral degeneration, and acquired hepatocerebral degeneration. The documented reversal of cranial CT findings and neurologic dysfunction following D-penicillamine therapy or liver transplantation suggests that the presence of radiologic abnormalities is not necessarily indicative of permanent cerebral injury [87, 88]. In addition, there is no correlation between the degree of neurologic improvement and the extent or type of CT abnormality [88]. It should be noted that it is rare for a patient to exhibit abnormalities on cranial MRI scan in the absence of neurologic abnormalities, while it is not uncommon for patients with abnormal neurologic examinations to have normal MRI studies [89]. Therefore, while imaging of the brain may be supportive of the diagnosis of Wilson's disease, it is not a particularly useful screening modality.

### *Diagnostic Screening*

The approach used to diagnose Wilson's disease must be tailored to the clinical presentation. Patients with neurologic or psychiatric manifestations should undergo slit-lamp examination of the eyes and have a serum ceruloplasmin determination. The documentation of Kayser-Fleischer rings and a low serum ceruloplasmin concentration is sufficient to establish the diagnosis, which can be confirmed by the presence of increased 24-h urinary copper excretion. A liver biopsy with quantification of hepatic copper is essential if either (a) Kayser-Fleischer rings are absent (in order to rule out a possible heterozygote), or (b) ceruloplasmin levels are normal (as occurs in 5%–15% of cases).

In patients who present primarily with hepatic dysfunction, the diagnosis can be difficult, since ceruloplasmin levels may be falsely elevated and ophthalmologic findings absent. It is imperative that biochemical screening for Wilson's disease be performed in all patients under the age of 40 years who have clinical or histologic findings compatible with chronic active hepatitis, and in whom autoimmune chronic active hepatitis and hepatitis B and C have been excluded. Some authors, citing cases of Wilson's disease presenting in the fifth and even the sixth decade [29], recommend that all individuals with persistent or severe liver disease of unclear etiology, regardless of age, be screened. In patients with a high index of suspicion, a serum ceruloplasmin concentration should be obtained, urinary copper excretion measured, and a liver biopsy performed, barring any contra-indications to this procedure. If, after the above evaluation, the diagnosis remains in doubt, then radiolabeled copper studies may be necessary in occasional patients.

Since all clinical features of Wilson's disease can be prevented if the diagnosis is established before functional impairment occurs, it is imperative that all close relatives be screened [71]. Wilson's disease may be clinically silent even in the presence of significant damage in the liver, brain, and other organs. Thus, a delay in the diagnosis or in the initiation of therapy may lead to irreversible hepatic and/or neurologic injury. Unfortunately, distinguishing presymptomatic homozygote individuals from heterozygotes may occasionally be difficult. Hopefully, the application of molecular genetics with linked chromosomal markers will soon permit rapid diagnosis of the disorder and obviate the need for less accurate tests. Once the diagnosis of presymptomatic Wilson's disease is established, lifelong chelation therapy should be commenced immediately.

## 3.8 Treatment

### *Dietary Management*

Prior to the introduction of D-penicillamine by Walshe in 1956, low-copper diets were advocated for the management of Wilson's disease. However, the ubiquitous presence of copper in most foodstuffs makes stringent dietary copper restriction impractical and, therefore, low-copper diets are no longer prescribed. It is still suggested that patients avoid eating foods with a high copper content, such as liver, chocolate, nuts, mushrooms, legumes, and shellfish [4].

### *Pharmacologic Therapy*

Over the past three decades, it has been clearly demonstrated that oral *D-penicillamine* results in complete reversal or alleviation of hepatic, neurologic, and psychiatric abnormalities in most patients with Wilson's disease, and this drug remains the "gold-standard" therapy for this disorder [90]. The key to a successful outcome is early diagnosis and treatment, and clinical disease can be prevented indefinitely in asymptomatic patients, provided that they adhere to continuous maintenance therapy. Some individuals demonstrate a dramatic response within weeks of initiating D-penicillamine therapy, while others may show no clinical improvement, or even temporary deterioration, for several months.

A recent retrospective analysis [91] of serial liver biopsies in 69 patients with Wilson's disease clearly demonstrates that oral chelation therapy with D-penicillamine results in the clearance of copper from the liver. Treated patients have significantly lower levels of hepatic copper when compared with untreated individuals or with those patients who are poorly compliant with medical therapy. Most of the excess liver copper is mobilized within the initial year of therapy, with urinary copper excretion approaching 2–5 mg/day during this period [91]. After several years of treatment, urinary copper levels generally decline to 0.5–1 mg daily and, in compliant patients, hepatic copper concentrations ultimately approach normal levels.

Although the principal mode of action is ascribed to decoppering, D-penicillamine also may detoxify hepatic copper [92]. This effect is thought to be the result of the sequestration of toxic intracellular copper in an innocuous form, either by the formation of copper complexes with D-penicillamine or by the induction of metallothionein synthesis by the drug [21]. Other postulated mechanisms of action of this drug include inhibition of collagen cross-linking, suppression of inflammation, and enhancement of intracellular glutathione levels.

The usual dose of D-penicillamine is 2 g daily given orally in four divided doses before meals, although as much as 4 g/day can be administered to critically ill patients for brief periods. It is best taken on an empty stomach since food reduces its absorption. After several years of therapy, when symptoms have largely abated and a stable clinical course has been achieved, the maintenance dose of D-penicillamine may be reduced to 1 g daily. Liver function test abnormalities may persist for a year or more after the initiation of appropriate treatment. However, as laboratory values improve, a corresponding resolution of hepatic histologic and ultrastructural abnormalities (with the exception of cirrhosis) is usually observed.

A syndrome of acute neurologic deterioration occasionally has been described following the initiation of D-penicillamine therapy in Wilson's disease patients [93]. If observed, worsening of neurologic signs and symptoms tends to occur within the first 4 weeks of therapy and generally only in those patients who present with nervous system involvement. The cause of this exacerbation of neurologic manifestations remains conjectural. It has been postulated that D-penicillamine initially induces a transient rise in the levels of copper in the blood and brain as it mobilizes the substantial stores of the metal from the liver [93]. Alternatively, the drug may interact with intracellular copper, converting it into a more toxic form capable of damaging biomolecules. It is recommended that the dose of D-penicillamine be reduced to 250 mg/day in any patient who exhibits an exacerbation in neurologic dysfunction following initiation of therapy [93]. The dose should then be increased by 250 mg/day every 4–7 days until a urinary copper concentration of at least 2 mg/day is attained. Indeed, it may be prudent to introduce D-penicillamine in a low initial dose in *all* Wilson's disease patients presenting with significant neurologic impairment [47, 93]. Despite clinical deterioration, continued treatment is mandatory if there is to be subsequent improvement.

A variety of adverse effects of D-penicillamine have been recognized [62], although serious complications are infrequent. Up to 20% of Wilson's disease patients develop early side-efffects within the 1st month of therapy [21]. The most common of these is a hypersensitivity reaction consisting of fever, malaise, pruritis, rash and, occasionally, lymphadenopathy [4, 47]. These symptoms typically subside when the drug is withdrawn. Most patients can be desensitized by reintroducing D-penicillamine in low doses (250 mg/day) with steroid coverage, and gradually increasing the dose over a 1-month period [4, 47]. In rare instances, significant marrow suppression has been observed, with the development of leukopenia and thrombocytopenia [47]. This is an indication to switch the patient to an alternative medication.

Late reactions to D-penicillamine usually manifest after a year or more of therapy. The most common complication is pencillamine dermatopathy, a weakening of subcutaneous tissues due to damage to collagen and elastin, which results in excessive wrinkling and thinning of the skin, easy bruisability, and brown cutaneous papules [47]. D-Penicillamine occasionally may induce or uncover an underlying autoimmune disease in 3%–5% of Wilson's disease patients, including aphthous ulcers, dysgeusia, nephrotic syndrome, a Goodpasture's-like syndrome, myasthenia gravis, lupus erythematosus, pemphigus, neuromyotonia, agranulocytosis, or aplastic anemia. The incidence of side-effects from D-penicillamine in Wilson's disease is much lower than the 20%–30% reported when the drug is administered for other disorders such as primary biliary cirrhosis, systemic sclerosis, or rheumatoid arthritis [4, 62]. Therefore, D-penicillamine is considered effective and generally safe for use in the treatment of Wilson's disease and remains the first-line drug of choice in this disorder.

*Trientine* (triethylene tetramine dihydrochloride), 1–2 g daily administered orally in three divided doses, is an effective alternative copper chelating agent for patients who develop serious toxic reactions to D-penicillamine [94, 95]. The exact mechanism of action of this drug remains unknown. Unlike D-penicillamine, trientine causes the serum copper concentration to rise during cupruresis, suggesting that the two agents may mobilize copper from different systemic pools. Mild sideroblastic anemia is the only significant side-effect attributed to this medication during treatment for Wilson's disease [95]. Skin rash, gastrointestinal distress, and rhabdomyolysis have also been reported in patients treated with trientine for primary biliary cirrhosis [96]. Although trientine appears to cause considerably less toxicity than D-penicillamine, more experience is required before it can be recommended as primary therapy. Currently, it is indicated only in patients intolerant to D-penicillamine.

The use of oral *zinc* therapy has been advocated to decrease copper absorption in Wilson's disease [97]. It is reported that 50 mg zinc sulfate or zinc acetate administered three times per day between meals maintains neutral or negative copper balance. Zinc apparently induces the synthesis of metallothionein, which sequesters copper in the intestinal epithelial cells and prevents absorption into the portal circulation [97]. It also appears that zinc may directly exhibit a protective effect on hepatocytes by inducing the synthesis of metallothionein in the liver [98]. A common side-effect of oral zinc is gastrointestinal upset; however, major complications are rare.

Although zinc inhibits the gastrointestinal absorption of copper, neutral copper balance does not necessarily imply that a significant reduction in the copper content of the liver or brain will result. In fact, there are data suggesting that hepatic copper may continue to accrue in some Wilson's disease patients treated with zinc sulfate alone [91, 99]. Additionally, long-term follow-up studies are needed to determine whether the decoppered state is sustained with zinc therapy. Based on the data currently available, oral zinc is recommended only for the rare patient who develops intolerance to both D-penicillamine and trientine [4, 100]. If it is eventually shown to act synergistically with chelating agents, zinc may find a role as adjunctive therapy, in addition to D-penicillamine, in patients with symptomatic or progressive disease [4]. However, there is theoretical concern that zinc may complex with D-penicillamine and thereby reduce the efficacy of both medications [100].

Since the discovery that dietary molybdenum is a causative factor in the copper deficiency syndromes of ruminants, the decoppering effect of molybdenum-containing compounds has been studied extensively. Thiomolybdate apparently lowers systemic copper levels by complexing luminal copper, thereby inhibiting intestinal absorption. In addition, the portion of the drug that is systemically absorbed may bind excessive serum copper and render it unavailable for cellular uptake. Limited trials of *ammonium tetrathiomolybdate* (60–100 mg daily in two divided doses) in Wilson's disease patients in whom D-penicillamine and/or trientine was poorly tolerated or ineffective demonstrate the drug to be highly successful in lowering hepatic copper concentrations [101]. Although these results appear promising, thiomolybdate has caused bone marrow suppression in two patients [102]. Thus, further testing is imperative before the use of this drug can be recommended.

### 3.9 Long-term Management

Wilson's disease patients require careful supervision during the first several months of therapy to ensure adequate copper excretion and to monitor for the potential development of early adverse reactions to D-penicillamine. It is suggested that a physical examination be performed and 24-h urinary copper excretion, complete blood count, and routine urinalysis checked on a weekly basis for the first 4–6 weeks following the initiation of chelation therapy [47]. Bimonthly evaluations are then recommended for the 1st year, followed by at least yearly examinations thereafter. When patients with Wilson's disease are maintained on an appropriate therapeutic regimen, they exhibit a progressive fall in the urinary excretion of copper and the serum ceruloplasmin and free serum copper concentrations with time. Adequate therapy will result in a free serum copper level (the difference between total serum copper and ceruloplasmin-copper) of less than 0.1 mg/liter, and a 24-h urinary copper excretion below 0.5 mg [47]. The persistence of abnormal laboratory tests, or the redevelopment of increased copper levels following an initial decline, suggests either subtherapeutic dosing or patient noncompliance. Six to 12 months of uninterrupted therapy may be necessary before significant clinical improvement is observed [21].

Lifelong chelation therapy, *without interruption*, is required in all Wilson's disease patients. Cessation of therapy may result in rapid and irreversible hepatic and neurologic deterioration [95, 103]. In a study of 11 patients who discontinued treatment, eight patients died of fulminant hepatitis after an average survival of only 2.6 years [103]. Thus, it is essential that trientine be administered to any patient who is unable to continue D-penicillamine due to adverse effects, since it has been clearly documented that trientine is effective in preventing the rapid clinical deterioration which frequently follows the discontinuation of D-penicillamine therapy [95].

Successful pregnancy has been achieved in treated, asymptomatic patients with Wilson's disease. D-Penicillamine, in a dose of 1 g/day, does not appear to pose any undue risk to the fetus and, therefore, should be continued throughout pregnancy in order to protect the mother from relapse [104, 105]. In addition, no adverse effects of trientine have been noted in the limited experience with this agent in pregnancy [106].

Major surgery is poorly tolerated by patients with Wilson's disease and, therefore, should be undertaken only when absolutely essential. Surgical decompression of portal hypertension is reserved for those patients with recurrent or uncontrolled variceal bleeding that is unresponsive to standard conservative measures, including endoscopic sclerotherapy or variceal banding. Surgical intervention in such patients carries a high mortality and may precipitate neurologic deterioration. When surgery is necessary, the dose of D-penicillamine should be reduced for 1–2 weeks postoperatively, since the drug inhibits collagen cross-linking and potentially may interfere with wound healing.

### *Liver Transplantation*

Despite numerous advances in medical therapy, significant death rates are still observed in specific subsets of patients with Wilson's disease. These patients, in whom orthotopic liver transplantation has proven most successful, include individuals with acute fulminant hepatic failure associated with hemolysis and hypercupremia (either as the initial presentation or due to poor compliance with medical therapy) and patients with advanced cirrhosis and hepatic insufficiency unresponsive to an adequate trial of chelation therapy and supportive measures [95, 107]. In the absence of severe hepatic disease, liver transplantation generally is not recommended for the management of refractory extrahepatic manifestations, such as neurologic deterioration [21]. To date, approximately 50 patients with Wilson's disease have undergone hepatic transplantation [21] and, in the largest published series, 13 of 18 patients (72%) were alive with a follow-up time of 1–6 years [19]. Transplant recipients uniformly exhibit complete reversal of the underlying defects in copper metabolism [19]. In some transplant patients, improvement in neurologic and cranial CT abnormalities has been noted [88, 108]. Postdilution hemofiltration has been proposed as an adjunctive measure to stabilize Wilson's disease patients with severe hepatic dysfunction while awaiting liver transplantation [109].

## 4 Summary

Wilson's disease remains a complex and challenging disorder with regard to the pathophysiology, diagnosis, and management. The pathogenesis remains obscure, although researchers gradually are elucidating the biochemical and genetic basis of the disease. A high index of suspicion is required, since early diagnosis and treatment is the most effective form of therapy. Aggressive screening should be performed in all close relatives. "It is in the detection of . . . [Wilson's] disease in the asymptomatic siblings that the best of all medicine, preventive medicine, can be practiced. The disease can be diagnosed before illness occurs, and the development of all clinical manifestations can be prevented" [110].

## References


1. Bloomer LC, Lee GR (1978) Normal hepatic copper metabolism. In: Powell LW (ed) Metals and liver. Marcel Dekker, New York, pp 179–239
2. Saltzman BE, Gross SB, Yeager DW et al. (1990) Total body burdens and tissue concentrations of lead, cadmium, copper, zinc, and ash in 55 human cadavers. Environment Res 52:126–145
3. Turnlund JR, Keyes WR, Anderson HL et al. (1989) Copper absorption and retention in young men at three levels of dietary copper by use of the stable isotope $^{65}$Cu. Am J Clin Nutr 49: 870–878
4. Lipsky MA, Gollan JL (1987) Treatment of Wilson's disease: In D-penicillamine we trust – What about zinc? Hepatology 7:593–595
5. Sternlieb I, Morell AG, Tucker WD et al. (1961) The incorporation of copper into ceruloplasmin in vivo: studies with copper$^{64}$ and copper$^{67}$. J Clin Invest 40:1834–1840
6. Sternlieb I, Scheinberg IH (1979) The role of radiocopper in the diagnosis of Wilson's disease. Gastroenterology 77:138–142
7. Cousins RJ (1985) Absorption, transport, and hepatic metabolism of copper and zinc: special reference to metallothionein and ceruloplasmin. Physiol Rev 65:238–309
8. Frommer DJ (1976) Direct measurement of serum non-ceruloplasmin copper in liver disease. Clin Chim Acta 68:303–307
9. Neumann PZ, Sass-Kortsak A (1967) The state of copper in human serum. Evidence for an amino-acid bound fraction. J Clin Invest 46:646–658
10. Barrow L, Tanner MS (1988) Copper distribution among serum proteins in pediatric liver disorders and malignancies. Eur J Clin Invest 18:555–560
11. German JL, Bearn AG (1961) Effects of estrogens on copper metabolism in Wilson's disease. J Clin Invest 40:445–453
12. Van Berge Henegouwen GP, Tangedahl TN, Hoffmann AF et al. (1977) Biliary secretion of copper in healthy man: quantitation by an intestinal perfusion technique. Gastroenterology 72:1228–1231
13. Sternlieb I, Van den Hamer CJA, Morell AG et al. (1973) Lysosomal defects of hepatic copper excretion in Wilson's disease. Gastroenterology 64:99–105
14. Strickland GT, Beckner WM, Leu ML (1972) Absorption of copper in homozygotes and heterozygotes for Wilson's disease and controls: isotope tracer studies with $^{67}$Cu and $^{64}$Cu. Clin Sci 43:617–625
15. Frydman M (1990) Genetic aspects of Wilson's disease. J Gastroenterol Hepatol 5:483–490
16. Frydman M, Bonne-Tamir B, Farrer LA et al. (1985) Assignment of the gene for Wilson's disease to chromosome 13: linkage to the esterase D locus. Proc Natl Acad Sci USA 82:1819–1821
17. Figus A, Lampis R, Devoto M et al. (1989) Carrier detection and early diagnosis of Wilson's disease by restriction fragment length polymorphism analysis. J Med Genet 26:78–82
18. Bowcock AM, Farrer LA, Hebert JM et al. (1988) Eight closely linked loci place the Wilson disease locus within 13q14–q21. Am J Human Genet 43:664–674
19. Esquivel CO, Marino IR, Fioravanti V et al. (1988) Liver transplantation for metabolic disease of the liver. Gastroenterol Clin North Am 17:167–175
20. Frommer DJ (1974) Defective biliary excretion of copper in Wilson's disease. Gut 15:125–129
21. Sternlieb I (1990) Perspectives on Wilson's disease. Hepatology 12:1234–1239
22. Evans J, Newman SP, Sherlock S (1980) Observations on copper-associated protein in childhood liver disease. Gut 21:970–976
23. Iyengar V, Brewer GJ, Dick RD et al. (1988) Studies of cholecystokinin-stimulated biliary secretions reveal a high molecular weight copper-binding

substance in normal subjects that is absent in patients with Wilson's disease. J Lab Clin Med 111:267–274
24. Vierling JM, Shrager R, Rumble WF et al. (1978) Incorporation of radiocopper into ceruloplasmin in normal subjects and in patients with primary biliary cirrhosis and Wilson's disease. Gastroenterology 74:652–660
25. Czaja MJ, Weiner FR, Schwarzenberg SJ et al. (1987) Molecular studies of ceruloplasmin deficiency in Wilson's disease. J Clin Invest 80:1200–1204
26. Barrow L, Tanner MS, Critchley DR (1989) Expression of the caeruloplasmin gene in the adult and neonatal rat liver. Clin Sci 77:259–263
27. Epstein O, Sherlock S (1981) Is Wilson's disease caused by a controller gene mutation resulting in perpetuation of the fetal mode of copper metabolism? Lancet I:303–305
28. Cartwright GE, Lee GR (1974) The pathogenesis and evolution of Wilson's disease. Epatologia 20:51–56
29. Danks DM, Metz G, Sewell R et al. (1990) Wilson's disease in adults with cirrhosis but no neurological abnormalities. Br Med J 301:331–332
30. Sternlieb I, Scheinberg IH (1985) Wilson's disease. In: Wright R, Alberti KGM, Karran S et al. (eds) Liver and biliary disease. Bailliere Tindall, London, pp 949–961
31. Strickland GT, Frommer D, Leu ML et al. (1973) Wilson's disease in the United Kingdom and Taiwan. Q J Med 42:619–638
32. Walshe JM (1989) Wilson's disease presenting with features of hepatic dysfunction: a clinical analysis of eighty-seven patients. Q J Med 70:253–263
33. Sternlieb I (1975) The development of cirrhosis in Wilson's disease. Clin Gastroenterol 4:367–379
34. Scott J, Gollan JL, Samourian S et al. (1978) Wilson's disease presenting as chronic active hepatitis. Gastroenterology 74:645–651
35. Sternlieb I, Scheinberg IH (1972) Chronic hepatitis as a first manifestation of Wilson's disease. Ann Intern Med 76:59–64
36. Davies SE, Williams R, Portmann B (1989) Hepatic morphology and histochemistry of Wilson's disease presenting as fulminant hepatic failure: a study of 11 cases. Histopathology 15:385–394
37. McCullough AJ, Fleming CR, Thistle JL et al. (1983) Diagnosis of Wilson's disease presenting as fulminant hepatic failure. Gastroenterology 84:161–167
38. Berman DH, Leventhal RI, Gavaler JS et al. (1989) Rapid clinical identification of fulminant Wilson's disease from other causes of fulminant hepatic failure using readily available laboratory tests (abstr). Hepatology 10:574
39. Frommer D, Morris J, Sherlock S et al. (1977) Kayser-Fleischer-like rings in patients without Wilson's disease. Gastroenterology 72:1331–1335
40. Nazer H, Ede RJ, Mowat AP et al. (1986) Wilson's disease: clinical presentation and use of prognostic index. Gut 27:1377–1381
41. Rosenfeld N, Grand RJ, Watkins JB et al. (1978) Cholelithiasis and Wilson's disease. Pediatrics 92:210–213
42. Weizman Z, Picard E, Barki Y et al. (1988) Case report: Wilson's disease associated with pancreatitis. J Pediatr Gastroenterol Nutr 7:931–933
43. Leu ML, Strickland GT, Yeh SJ (1971) Tissue copper, zinc, and manganese levels in Wilson's disease: studies with the use of neutron activation analysis. J Lab Clin Med 77:438–444
44. Dreiling DA, Grateron H (1983) Studies in pancreatic secretion. VIII. Pancreatic function in patients with Wilson's disease. J Mt Sinai Hosp 50:335–337
45. Lankisch PG, Kaboth U, Koop H (1978) Pankreasbeteiligung bei Morbus Wilson? Klin Wochenschr 56:969–971
46. Person J, Anderson DS, Brower RA (1987) Spontaneous bacterial peritonitis in Wilson's disease. Am J Gastroenterol 82:66–68

47. Marsden CD (1987) Wilson's disease (editorial). Q J Med 65:959–966
48. Lang C, Muller D, Claus D et al. (1990) Neuropsychological findings in treated Wilson's disease. Acta Neurol Scand 81:75–81
49. Dening TR, Berrios GE, Walshe JM (1988) Wilson's disease and epilepsy. Brain 111:1139–1155
50. Westmoreland BF, Goldstein NP, Klass DW (1974) Wilson's disease. Electroencephalographic and evoked potential studies. Mayo Clin Proc 49:401–404
51. Frankel JP, Hughes A, Lees AJ et al. (1989) Use of apomorphine to test for dopamine responsiveness in Wilson's disease (letter). Lancet II:801–802
52. Goldstein NP, Ewert JC, Randall RV et al. (1968) Psychiatric aspects of Wilson's disease (hepatolenticular degeneration): results of psychometric tests during long term therapy. Am J Psychiatr 124:1555–1561
53. Deiss A, Lee GR, Cartwright GE (1970) Hemolytic anemia in Wilson's disease. Ann Intern Med 73:413–418
54. Owen CA, Goldstein NP, Bowie EJ (1976) Platelet function and coagulation in patients with Wilson's disease. Arch Intern Med 136:148–152
55. Wiebers DO, Hollenhorst RW, Goldstein NP (1977) The ophthalmologic manifestations of Wilson's disease. Mayo Clin Proc 52:409–416
56. Lobner A, Lobner J, Bachmann H et al. (1986) The Kayser-Fleischer ring during long-term treatment in Wilson's disease (hepatolenticular degeneration): a follow-up study. Graefes Arch Clin Exp Ophthalmol 224:152–155
57. Cairns JE, Williams HP, Walshe JM (1969) "Sunflower cataract" in Wilson's disease. Br J Med 3:95–96
58. Leu ML, Strickland GT, Gutman RA (1970) Renal function in Wilson's disease: response to penicillamine therapy. Am J Med Sci 260:381–398
59. Fulop M, Sternlieb I, Scheinberg IH (1968) Defective urinary acidification in Wilson's disease. Ann Intern Med 68:770–777
60. Asatoor AM, Milne MD, Walshe JM (1976) Urinary excretion of peptides and of hydroxyproline in Wilson's disease. Clin Sci Mol Med 51:369–378
61. Wiebers DO, Wilson DM, McLeod RA et al. (1979) Renal stones in Wilson's disease. Am J Med 67:249–254
62. Steen VD, Blair S, Medsger TA (1986) The toxicity of D-penicillamine in systemic sclerosis. Ann Intern Med 104:699–705
63. Kuan P (1987) Cardiac Wilson's disease. Chest 91:579–583
64. Factor SM, Cho S, Sternlieb I et al. (1982) The cardiomyopathy of Wilson's disease: myocardial alterations in nine cases. Virchows Arch 397:301–311
65. Mindelzun R, Elkin M, Scheinberg IH et al. (1970) Skeletal changes in Wilson's disease: a radiological study. Radiology 94:127–132
66. Menerey KA, Eider W, Brewer GJ et al. (1988) The arthropathy of Wilson's disease: clinical and pathologic features. J Rheumatol 15:331–337
67. Lugassy G, Michaeli J, Oren R (1988) Wilson's disease presenting as isolated arthritis of the hip (letter). Arthritis Rheum 31:573–575
68. Johansen K, Gregersen G (1972) Glucose intolerance in Wilson's disease. Arch Intern Med 129:587–590
69. Carpenter TO, Carnes DL, Anast CS (1983) Hypoparathyroidism in Wilson's disease. N Engl J Med 309:873–877
70. Kaushansky A, Frydman M, Kaufman H et al. (1987) Endocrine studies of the ovulatory disturbances in Wilson's disease (hepatolenticular degeneration). Fertil Steril 47:270–273
71. Sternlieb I, Scheinberg IH (1968) Prevention of Wilson's disease in asymptomatic patients. N Engl J Med 278:352–359
72. Sternlieb I (1968) Mitochondrial and fatty changes in hepatocytes of patients with Wilson's disease. Gastroenterology 55:354–367
73. Stromeyer FW, Ishak HG (1980) Histology of the liver in Wilson's disease. A study of 34 cases. Am J Clin Pathol 73:12–24

74. Geubel AP, Gregoire V, Rahier J et al. (1988) Hypoceruloplasminemia and ultrastructural changes resembling Wilson's disease in non-alcoholic liver steatosis: a clinical and pathological study of five cases. Liver 8:299–306
75. Wilkinson ML, Portmann B, Williams R (1983) Wilson's disease and hepatocellular carcinoma: possible protective role of copper. Gut 24:767–771
76. Horoupian DS, Sternlieb I, Scheinberg IH (1988) Neuropathological findings in penicillamine-treated patients with Wilson's disease. Clin Neuropathol 7:62–67
77. Perman JA, Werlin SL, Grand RJ et al. (1979) Laboratory measures of copper metabolism in the differentiation of chronic active hepatitis and Wilson's disease in children. J Pediatr 94:564–568
78. LaRusso NF, Summerskill WHJ, McCall JT (1976) Abnormalities of chemical tests for copper metabolism in chronic active liver disease: differentiation from Wilson's disease. Gastroenterology 70:653–655
79. Spechler SJ, Koff RS (1980) Wilson's disease: diagnostic difficulties in the patient with chronic hepatitis and hypoceruloplasminemia. Gastroenterology 78:803–806
80. Frommer DJ (1981) Urinary copper excretion and hepatic copper concentrations in liver disease. Digestion 21:169–178
81. Smallwood RA, Williams HA, Rosenoer VM et al. (1968) Liver-copper levels in liver disease: studies using neutron activation analysis. Lancet II:1310–1313
82. Grimm G, Oder W, Prayer L et al. (1990) Evoked potentials in assessment and follow-up of patients with Wilson's disease. Lancet 336:963–964
83. Weisner B, Hartard C, Dieu C (1987) CSF copper concentration: a new parameter for diagnosis and monitoring therapy of Wilson's disease with cerebral manifestations. J Neurol Sci 79:229–237
84. Dixon AK, Walshe JM (1984) Computed tomography of the liver in Wilson's disease. J Comput Assist Tomogr 8:46–49
85. Lawler GA, Pennock JM, Steiner RE et al. (1983) Nuclear magnetic resonance (NMR) imaging in Wilson's disease. J Comput Assist Tomogr 7:1–8
86. Gainey MA, Faerber EN (1985) Disparate hepatic imaging with technetium-99m sulfur colloid and disofenin in Wilson's disease. J Nucl Med 26:368–372
87. Williams JB, Walshe JM (1981) Wilson's disease: an analysis of the computerized tomographic appearances found in 60 patients and the changes in response to treatment with chelating agents. Brain 104:735–752
88. Rothfus WE, Hirsch WL, Malatack JJ et al. (1988) Case report: improvement of cerebral CT abnormalities following liver transplantation in a patient with Wilson's disease. J Comput Assist Tomogr 12:138–140
89. Prayer L, Wimberger D, Kramer J et al. (1990) Cranial MRI in Wilson's disease. Neuroradiology 32:211–214
90. Sternlieb I, Scheinberg IH (1964) Penicillamine therapy in hepatolenticular degeneration. JAMA 189:748–754
91. Gibbs K, Walshe JM (1990) Liver copper concentration in Wilson's disease: effect of treatment with "anti-copper" agents. J Gastroenterol Hepatol 5:420–424
92. Scheinberg IH, Sternlieb I, Schilsky M et al. (1987) Penicillamine may detoxify copper in Wilson's disease (letter). Lancet II:95
93. Brewer GJ, Terry CA, Aisen AM et al. (1987) Worsening of neurologic syndrome in patients with Wilson's disease with initial penicillamine therapy. Arch Neurol 44:490–493
94. Walshe JM (1982) Treatment of Wilson's disease with trientine (triethylene tetramine) dihydrochloride. Lancet I:643–647
95. Scheinberg IH, Jaffe ME, Sternlieb I (1987) The use of trientine in preventing the effects of interrupting penicillamine therapy in Wilson's disease. N Engl J Med 317:209–213
96. Epstein O, Sherlock S (1980) Triethylene tetramine dihydrochloride toxicity in primary biliary cirrhosis. Gastroenterology 78:1442–1445

97. Brewer GJ, Hill GM, Prasad AS et al. (1983) Oral zinc therapy for Wilson's disease. Ann Intern Med 99:314–320
98. Schilsky ML, Blank RR, Czaja MJ et al. (1989) Hepatocellular copper toxicity and its attenuation by zinc. J Clin Invest 84:1562–1568
99. Stremmel W, Strohmeyer G (1988) Oral zinc therapy is not always effective for treatment of Wilson's disease (abstr). Hepatology 8:1335
100. Scheinberg IH, Sternlieb I (1988) The efficacy of oral zinc therapy as an alternative to penicillamine for Wilson's disease (letter). N Engl J Med 318:323
101. Walshe JM (1986) Tetrathiomolybdate ($MoS_4$) as an anti-copper agent in man. In: Scheinberg IH, Walshe JM (eds) Orphan diseases and orphan drugs. Manchester University Press, Manchester, pp 76–85
102. Harper PL, Walshe JM (1986) Reversible pancytopenia secondary to treatment with tetrathiomolybdate. Br J Haematol 64:851–853
103. Walshe JM, Dixon AK (1986) Dangers of non-compliance in Wilson's disease. Lancet I:845–847
104. Scheinberg IH, Sternlieb I (1975) Pregnancy in penicillamine-treated patients with Wilson's disease. N Engl J Med 293:1300–1302
105. Walshe JM (1977) Pregnancy in Wilson's disease. Q J Med 46:73–83
106. Walshe JM (1986) The management of pregnancy in Wilson's disease treated with trientine. Q J Med 58:81–87
107. Sternlieb I (1988) Wilson's disease: transplantation when all else has failed. Hepatology 8:975–976
108. Polson RJ, Rolles K, Calne RY et al. (1987) Reversal of severe neurologic manifestations of Wilson's disease following orthotopic liver transplantation. Q J Med 64:685–691
109. Rakela J, Kurtz SB, McCarthy JT et al. (1988) Postdilution hemofiltration in the management of acute hepatic failure: a pilot study. Mayo Clin Proc 63:113–118
110. Cartwright GE (1978) Diagnosis of treatable Wilson's disease. N Engl J Med 298:1347–1350

# 24 Haemochromatosis

L.W. Powell, K.M. Summers and J.W. Halliday

## 1 Normal Iron Metabolism

The body of a healthy adult male normally contains about 90 mmol (5 g) of iron. Of this, approximately 80% is present in compounds such as haemoglobin, myoglobin and tissue enzymes, while the remainder (about 1 g) represents a store which is located largely in the reticuloendothelial system. One-third of these iron stores are in the liver. Storage iron exists in two forms: firstly, in the large iron storage protein, ferritin, and secondly as haemosiderin, a poorly defined molecule which consists of mixed iron and protein aggregates derived from ferritin. There is recent evidence that the structure of the iron cores in haemosiderin differs in different types of iron overload, e.g., in thalassaemia and haemochromatosis.

Ferritin has both a protective and a reserve function. A protective role is required because free iron is toxic and daily losses are small (see below). Iron stored as ferritin and haemosiderin is accessible for haemoglobin production although iron mobilisation is a relatively slow process, particularly from haemosiderin; this may be related to the structure of the iron "cores". In normal subjects approximately 18 µmol (1 mg) of iron enters and leaves the storage compartment each day.

There is increasing evidence that different structural and metabolic forms of ferritin occur in different tissues and even within the same tissue. Each tissue has a characteristic isoferritin profile that alters in different physiological and pathological states, especially iron overload and malignancy. While the functional significance of these isoferritins is unclear, their existence appears to be due to two different subunits designated H and L, which differ in molecular weight, immunological reactivity and amino acid composition.

Ferritin also circulates in small amounts in serum. Normal values range from 20 to 250 µg per litre. The concentration varies according to age and gender, being generally higher in males. The concentration is also elevated in some disease states not related to increased iron loading, including inflammatory states, alcoholic liver disease, malignant hepatoma and leukaemia. However, the origin and function of serum ferritin remains one of the enigmas of iron metabolism.

The recent studies of AISEN and co-workers have shown that Kupffer cells synthesise and release ferritin after ingestion of red cells, although the carbohydrate and iron content of this ferritin apparently differs from that of serum ferritin [1, 2]. Ferritin released from Kupffer cells may then be taken up by the recently described ferritin receptor on hepatocyte membranes.

### 1.1 Iron Absorption

Iron absorption is regulated via poorly understood mechanisms to maintain body iron stores at optimal levels. In the normal subject absorption is greater than normal when the stores are depleted and diminished when stores are increased.

Iron is absorbed both as haem and as non-haem iron. In an average Western diet non-haem iron accounts for over 90% of total iron. Highly refined foods commonly used in Western countries contain approximately 90 μmol (5 mg) iron per 1000 calories. Normal males consuming 3000 calories per day would therefore obtain, at most, 270 μmol (15 mg) iron per day, of which 9–27 μmol (0.5–1.5 mg) would be absorbed. It is thus apparent that the possible range of absorption from the normal diet is quite narrow, extending from less than 9 μmol (0.5 mg) daily in the iron-replete subject to approximately 72 μmol (4 mg) in the iron-deficient subject. The availability of dietary iron may be modified by other factors, including drugs such as cholestyramine and tetracyclines which decrease iron absorption.

There is no physiological mechanism for excretion of excess iron; hence normal iron balance is maintained by regulation of iron absorption by the intestine but the mechanism is unknown. The most important factor in the physiological regulation of mucosal iron absorption is the total body iron content. The available data suggest that the ultimate control of iron uptake and transport by the intestine lies primarily within the intestinal cell itself and that this is influenced by other factors such as the degree of erythropoiesis, but the presence of circulating "messengers" cannot be discounted.

Much interest is currently focussed on the possible role of membrane receptors for transferrin, ferritin and their iron complexes. Evidence now points to the fact that the transferrin receptor does not play a role in the absorption of iron. The recent discovery of an iron-responsive element (IRE) in the untranslated regions of the mRNAs for both the transferrin receptor and ferritin suggested the possibility that a protein binding to this sequence might be involved in iron storage and perhaps absorption. A 90-kd cytoplasmic protein binds to RNA sequences corresponding to the IREs from both ferritin and transferrin receptor transcripts, simultaneously altering ferritin translation and protecting the transferrin receptor in RNA from an endonuclease when cytoplasmic iron concentration is low; this results in reduced ferritin synthesis and increased expression of the transferrin receptor [3, 4]. The reverse applies with cellular iron overload. The gene for the IRE-binding protein has been mapped to human chromosome 9, in contrast to the chromosome 6 location of the haemochromatosis gene.

Re-examination of intestinal iron-binding proteins has recently been of interest. Several newly identified iron-binding proteins in the intestine have been described. PETERS et al. [5–7] have identified a basolateral membrane-binding site for recently absorbed iron which shows increased binding in vivo following chronic hypoxia, a state which is known to be associated with increased iron absorption. This binding site can donate its iron to apotransferrin via a low molecular iron chelate and it may be involved in the transfer step in intestinal absorption of iron. CONRAD et al. [8] have reported two further iron-binding compounds of 57 and 520 kd. They suggest that these newly identified proteins, which are immunologically distinct from transferrin and ferritin, may be important in the regulation of iron absorption in the small intestinal mucosa. STREMMEL et al. (personal communication) have found evidence for a facilitated transport mechanism mediated by a 54-kd iron-binding protein located in the microvillous membranes.

Further genetic and biochemical investigation of all of these proteins will be necessary to establish their role in iron absorption and a possible abnormality in haemochromatosis. Whether this defect is resident within the intestinal mucosal cell or is related to an unidentified corporeal factor which signals the gut to increase or decrease iron absorption remains to be elucidated.

### 1.2 Iron Delivery to Tissues

The interaction between transferrin and the erythroid cell involves three main steps: the binding of the iron–transferrin complex to specific cell receptors and the internalisation of the protein–receptor complex through the cell membrane, followed by the release of iron within the cell. Within the reticulocyte, transferrin concentrates in lysosome-like organelles in close proximity to the Golgi apparatus, where an intravesicular acid pH facilitates the removal of iron from transferrin. This receptor-mediated endocytotic process delivers iron to an intracellular chelatable iron pool which can be utilised and incorporated with enzymes or stored as ferritin.

### 1.3 Iron Excretion

The obligatory daily iron losses are of the order of 18 μmol (1 mg) in adult males. Approximately two-thirds of this is lost via the gut and most of the remainder in the urine and skin. These obligatory losses are reduced by about half in iron deficiency and may rise to figures of up to three times normal in states of iron overload. In the female, additional losses are incurred through menstruation and pregnancy. The mean normal menstrual losses, when expressed in terms of daily iron balance, are approximately 9 μmol (0.5 mg), although there is much variation. During pregnancy the requirement is even greater. It has been calculated that approximately 18 mmol (1 g) of iron is needed for each pregnancy. This is equivalent to an average daily requirement of between 90 and 110 μmol (between 5 and 6 mg) throughout the last two trimesters. Urinary losses of iron are about 1.8 μmol (0.1 mg) per day. The wide variation in iron intake, iron losses and requirements among various groups in a community and between different populations causes considerable difficulty in planning programmes for fortification with iron in order to eliminate iron deficiency without exacerbating iron overload.

### *Pathogenesis of Iron Overload*

An absolute increase in total body iron content may arise in several different ways:

1. In haemochromatosis, the outstanding example of a regulatory abnormality in iron storage, the absorption of iron is inappropriately high, permitting the accumulation of 270–900 mmol (15–50 g) of body iron over a period of 25–50 years. With increasing body iron stores, absorption decreases towards the level found in the normal individual. However, this amount is still greater than that absorbed by an individual without this disorder who has a similar iron load, a point of some diagnostic significance. When iron is removed by phlebotomy, absorption regains its former high level. The cause of the abnormal iron absorption in haemochromatosis has not been identified. Current interest focusses on possible abnormal gene expression in the liver or the intestine.
2. Disorders of erythropoiesis are also associated with increased iron absorption. However, gross iron overload is usually restricted to those conditions with ineffective erythropoiesis, as in thalassaemia major and hereditary sideroblastic anaemia (see below).
3. The association of liver disease and various degrees of iron overload has been recognised for over a century and, indeed, has resulted in much controversy as to its distinction from haemochromatosis, as discussed earlier. The precise pathogenesis of the increased iron storage is still uncertain. However, liver disease associated with excess iron storage is usually complicated by factors such as ineffective erythropoiesis, folate deficiency or haemolytic anaemia. However, it is important to emphasise that subjects with alcoholic liver disease associated with gross

iron overload are usually homozygous for the HLA-linked iron-loading gene.

4. Whether significant iron overload can be produced in the normal individual by prolonged oral iron intake is still unclear. However, if the oral intake is massive and sufficient to overcome mucosal regulation, iron overload will result. The massive iron overload previously seen in South African blacks was attributable to a gross increase in dietary iron and ethanol, resulting from brewing Kaffir beer in large iron pots. Several reports have concluded that the syndrome of haemochromatosis had occurred in white subjects following medicinal iron intake totalling more than 18 mol (1000 g) over many years. Obviously such reported cases may have carried the gene for haemochromatosis. Elucidation of this problem awaits the successful identification of the gene responsible for haemochromatosis.
5. Parenteral iron administration also results in iron overload. Since iron excretion is limited to about 3.6 μmol (2 mg) per day, iron overload is easily produced by repeated blood transfusions or injections of iron preparations. Parenterally administered iron undergoes reticolo-endothelial RE processing before its iron becomes available to other body tissues and usually results in predominantly RE haemosiderosis. Cellular dysfunction and tissue injury appear to be related more closely to parenchymal iron loading.

## 1.4 Iron Toxicity

Until recently the evidence that excess tissue iron is responsible for fibrosis and cellular injury was circumstantial and based largely on clinical observations. These include the histological development of fibrosis and collagen deposition in areas associated with dense parenchymal cell iron deposits and the impressive clinical, biochemical and histological improvement which follows iron removal. Many recent studies have shown conclusively that excess iron is accompanied by increased lipid peroxidation.

There is now convincing evidence that the presence of iron in parenchymal cells over many years is an important aetiological factor in determining tissue damage, although a causal relation between iron-induced lipid peroxidation and fibrosis has not been firmly established. However, other metals and undefined genetic factors may also be important in individual cases in determining the extent of hepatic damage and which particular organs are affected, as, for example, in relation to the development of diabetes mellitus and, particularly the arthropathy (chondrocalcinosis) which is encountered in about 25% of patients (see later) but which appears to bear no relation to the iron overload.

## 2 Definitions and Classification

Haemochromatosis is an iron-storage disease in which an inappropriate, increase in intestinal iron absorption results in deposition of iron with eventual tissue damage and functional impairment of the organs involved, especially the liver, pancreas, heart and pituitary. In 1889, von Recklinghausen named the iron-storage pigment "haemosiderin" and the disease "haemochromatosis" because he believed that the pigment was derived from the blood. The terms "haemosiderosis" and "siderosis" are often used to describe the presence of stainable iron in tissues, but quantitative measurement of tissue iron is necessary for accurate assessment of body iron status (see below). Haemochromatosis implies progressive iron overload leading to fibrosis and organ failure. The essential feature is an increase in total body iron with predominantly parenchymal cell deposition. The inappropriate iron absorption may result from a genetically determined error of iron metabolism (primary genetic or hereditary haemochromatosis) in which the basic metabolic defect leading to the increased iron absorption is unknown, or the inappropriate iron absorption may result from ineffective erythropoiesis (secondary, acquired or erythropoietic haemochromatosis). Excessive body iron stores have also been described in association with a high dietary intake of iron and with some forms of liver disease, e.g., after portal-systemic shunting. Although there is debate about the definitions, it seems logical to use the following terminology: (a) "genetic" or "hereditary haemochromatosis" – the inherited disease now known to be associated with an abnormal gene tightly linked to the A locus of the HLA complex on chromosome 6 [9]; (b) "acquired haemochromatosis" – iron overload with tissue injury arising as a result of another disease, usually an iron-loading anaemia such as thalassaemia or sideroblastic anaemia in which increased erythropoiesis is present. In the acquired iron-loading disorders massive iron deposits in parenchymal tissues can lead to the same clinical and pathological features that are seen in genetic haemochromatosis. However, it is very unusual to see iron stores of this magnitude in cases of dietary iron excess or liver disease and in the rare cases reported in the literature the presence of genetic haemochromatosis cannot be excluded. Increasingly, genetic haemochromatosis is being diagnosed during its early stages when the iron overload is of lesser degree and organ damage is slight or absent. At this stage, the condition is best referred to as "early or precirrhotic haemochromatosis".

## 3 Primary (Genetic) Haemochromatosis

### 3.1 Definition and Prevalence

By definition, the term "genetic" or "hereditary haemochromatosis" should be used for those patients in whom there is evidence of familial, HLA-linked parenchymal iron loading. In practice the diagnosis is a presumptive one if no definite family history is available, since there is no genetic or phenotypic marker for the disease other than iron loading. HLA antigen studies are useful in identifying subjects at risk within a family, but are not helpful in diagnosing the disease, particularly in the index case (see later).

It is now established that haemochromatosis is inherited as an autosomal-recessive trait (see later) and that the susceptibility locus is tightly linked to the HLA-A locus of the histocompatibility antigen complex on chromosome 6. Numerous recent genetic studies have allowed estimates of the prevalence of the disease to be revised. The gene frequency has been calculated to be approximately 1 in 20 and the calculated homozygote frequency about 1 in 400. Thus, contrary to earlier beliefs, it is clear that haemochromatosis is amongst the most common genetic disorders in Western countries, with a gene carrier rate of 1 in 10, i.e., higher than that of cystic fibrosis and phenylketonuria.

However, expression of the disease is modified by several factors, especially blood loss associated with menstruation and pregnancy in women. The clinical expression of disease is observed five to ten times more frequently in males than in females. Nearly 70% of patients develop their first symptoms between the ages of 40 and 60 [10]. The disease is rarely clinically evident below the age of 20, although with family screening asymptomatic subjects with iron overload can be identified, including young menstruating women.

### 3.2 Genetic Aspects

Sheldon [11] proposed that haemochromatosis results from an inherited error of iron metabolism which leads to progressive body iron loading. This has been confirmed by the demonstration of a strong linkage between the disease locus and certain histocompatibility loci on chromosome 6. Simon initially reported an increased frequency of HLA-A3, B14 and A3, B7 haplotypes. These findings have since been confirmed and extended by numerous other groups, particularly in England, Salt Lake City [12] and Australia [13, 14]. In the latter studies there was a stronger association of haemochromatosis with HLA-A3 and B7 than with B14. The increase in HLA-B7 probably reflects the linkage disequilibrium between HLA-B7 and A3 in these populations since there is no association with B7 when the effect of A3 is removed.

Several large genetic studies have now been performed in which the pattern of inheritance within a particular family has been traced by HLA typing of first-degree relatives of the proband. Affected siblings of the proband usually have two HLA haplotypes identical to those of the proband and are presumed to be homozygous for the iron-loading gene. Unaffected siblings have either one HLA haplotype identical to the proband (i.e., heterozygous) or neither haplotype identical (homozygous normal). Such studies have confirmed inheritance as an autosomal-recessive trait [9, 15–17]. Furthermore the distribution of haplotypes identical to those of the proband among affected siblings fits the criterion proposed by THOMSON and BODMER [18] for a recessively inherited disease coded by an HLA-linked susceptibility gene with a frequency of at least 0.05. In Australia, the majority of relatives predicted by HLA typing to be homozygous exhibit full clinical and biochemical expression of the disease, although this clearly depends on iron intake and physiological blood loss. In a recent study by POWELL et al. [19], 47 of 50 homozygous relatives as determined by HLA studies expressed the disease either at first assessment or during a follow-up period of up to 8 years. In contrast, heterozygotes may demonstrate minor biochemical abnormalities of iron status but rarely develop a progressive increase in body iron stores of the order seen in homozygotes [15, 19]. In rare "heterozygotes" who appear to develop progressive iron overload, a chromosomal recombination resulting in misclassification of homozygotes as heterozygotes is likely [15, 20, 21]. In addition, the high carrier frequency means that putative heterozygous offspring of an affected individual may be homozygous due to homozygous–heterozygous mating. It should be emphasised, however, that the degree of penetrance of the disease in putative homozygous subjects (determined by HLA typing) appears to be variable. For example, the gene appears less penetrant in Utah than Queensland (KUSHNER, personal communication). This may be due to genetic heterogeneity or to environmental factors.

The calculated gene frequency and homozygote and heterozygote frequencies for the disease are approximately 5%, 0.3% and 10% respectively [22]. Haemochromatosis is thus probably the most common disease inherited as an autosomal-recessive trait. However, it is noteworthy that the figures apply to populations of European origin. Haemochromatosis is quite rare amongst other population groups, notably in Asia and the Middle East, and it is of interest that the HLA-A3 locus is relatively uncommon in these areas. SIMON et al. [9, 17] have proposed that haemochromatosis is basically a disease of Celtic peoples, arising from a new mutation in an ancestral Celtic group, because a review of the relevant literature reveals a similarity in geographical distribution of case reports and the current settlements of Celtic peoples. The disease locus lies close to the HLA-A locus on chromosome 6 and the disease may have risen to high frequencies because of a selective effect on the MHC region, because of advantageous interaction with specific HLA alleles or because of a selective advantage to the disease gene itself [23].

### 3.3 Pathogenesis

The various hypotheses that have been advanced for the underlying metabolic defect in this disease have included: (a) a lysosomal abnormality or an abnormal avidity of liver and other tissues for iron [24]; (b) abnormal kinetics of the iron–transferrin complex or of the transferrin receptor [14, 25]; (c) aberrant reticuloendothelial function [15]; (d) abnormal luminal factors, including abnormalities in pancreatic and gastric secretions [26], and (e) abnormal mucosal cell function [27]. However, despite extensive studies, no consistent defects in luminal secretions, in the intestinal mucosal cell, in the RE system or in the transferrin molecule or its ability to bind iron have been demonstrated [28–30].

The elucidation of the basic metabolic defect must presumably await the cloning and sequencing of the HLA-A-linked gene on the short arm of chromosome 6, a task that should soon be achieved. The fact that the only iron-loading gene so far documented is tightly linked to the HLA loci and displays linkage disequilibrium with HLA-A alleles suggests that abnormalities of a key protein coded at a single locus result in overt haemochromatosis. However, a clear understanding of the function of the disease gene is hampered by the observation that the expression of the disease phenotype and the age of symptomatic onset can be highly variable even within the one family. This suggests that not only may some individuals carry a mutation causing a more severe form of the disease, but also that the interaction of the haemochromatosis gene with other genes may be variable. A number of genes have been considered potential candidates for the HC gene on the basis of their function. Modern genetic techniques such as genetic linkage analysis, in situ hybridisation, and somatic cell hybrid deletion mapping panel analysis have demonstrated that most of them can be excluded on the basis of incorrect chromosomal location (Table 1). The most promising candidate genes at the present time would appear to be those for iron-regulatory element (HRE)-(IRE) binding proteins, one of which is involved in the coordinated regulation of synthesis of ferritin and transferrin receptor. However, the IRE-binding protein gene expressed in hepatocytes maps to chromosome 9 [31]. It is possible that there is an intestinal cell-specific protein similar to the IRE-binding protein. A mutation in its gene could explain the observed reduction in ferritin-H in duodenal epithelial cells in patients with haemochromatosis [32, 33]. Another candidate is the gene for the ferritin receptor [32–34] but this gene has not yet been identified. Little is known about the tissue expression or

**Table 1.** Summary of candidate genes for haemochromatosis

| Candidate | Function | Location | Comment |
|---|---|---|---|
| HLA-A | Immune response | 6p 21.3 | Known recombinants |
| Transferrin | Iron transport | 3q | Wrong chromosome |
| Transferrin receptor | Transferrin into cells | 3q | Wrong chromosome |
| Ferritin L* | Iron storage | 19, 20, X | Wrong chromosomes |
| Ferritin H** | Iron storage | Many chromosomes, including 6p12–21.3 | Wrong region of 6p |
| IRE-binding protein | Regulation of transferrin receptor Ferritin synthesis | 9 | Wrong chromosome but similar proteins possible |
| Ferritin receptor | Ferritin into cells | | Little available information |

[a] Ferritin light (L)** and heavy (H)** subunits

the chromosomal location of the 53-kd hepatic membrane ferritin receptor [35–37].

The available evidence thus suggests that iron absorption is inappropriately high at an early stage in haemochromatosis as a result of increased iron transfer across the intestinal mucosal cell. It is not known whether this is due to a primary intestinal cell defect, to a generalised metabolic defect or to an abnormality in reticuloendothelial cell function which secondarily affects mucosal iron absorption. Thus, whatever the fundamental error or errors in iron metabolism in patients with haemochromatosis, there seems little doubt that the control of iron absorption is involved and that the disorder causes an increase in iron absorption from the diet and a gradual accumulation of iron over many years.

### 3.4 Pathology

In the fully established disease, the total iron content of the body is usually between 360 and 720 mmol (20 and 40 g) [11]. Iron deposits are heaviest in the liver and pancreas, in which the iron concentration is 50–100 times normal. The iron content of other organs is also elevated from 5 to 25 times normal, particularly in the endocrine glands, cardiac muscle and skin. A notable exception is the testis, the iron content of which is relatively low despite the fact that impaired gonadal function is a characteristic and early feature of the disease. The gonadal atrophy is due to iron deposition in the pituitary.

The detailed pathological findings in the disease have been described elsewhere [11]. The most characteristic and diagnostically the most important findings are seen in the liver. This is usually greatly enlarged, weighing over 2000 g. The cut surface has a striking reddish-brown colour and is firm in consistency. Histologically, the two outstanding features are extensive pigmentation and fibrosis. The appearances are best appreciated in autopsy or wedge-biopsy specimens. They show a characteristic pattern of fibrosis and iron deposition with dense fibrous septa forming a network surrounding groups of lobules ("holly-leaf" pattern) somewhat analogous to that seen in chronic biliary disease. A fully established cirrhosis with nodularity develops comparatively late in the disease. The haemosiderin deposits characteristically appear first in the periportal parenchyma, being found within lysosomes in the pericanalicular cytoplasm of the hepatocytes. Later, they are distributed widely throughout the lobules as well as in biliary duct epithelium, Kupffer cells and connective tissue. Cell necrosis and inflammation are usually absent and the parenchymal cells otherwise appear normal. In alcoholic subjects features of alcoholic liver disease may be superimposed on the above appearances and these may make the differentiation from alcoholic liver disease on histological grounds alone difficult unless a wedge biopsy of the liver is available. However, it is now known that alcoholic liver disease itself does not lead to iron overload of the degree seen in haemochromatosis and the distinction can be made readily by measuring the hepatic iron concentration [38, 39].

In patients with haemochromatosis secondary to erythropoietic disorders such as thalassaemia, haemosiderin deposits are much more prominent in Kupffer and other sinusoidal cells but in other respects the appearance of the liver closely resembles that in the genetic form of the disease.

Microscopic examination of the pancreas usually shows heavy deposits of haemosiderin in the acinar cells and, to a lesser extent, in the islets of Langerhans, with the number of islets diminished. Haemosiderin is also found in the heart muscle fibres in nearly all cases of well-established haemochromatosis but fibrosis is rare. Haemosiderin is also deposited in the conducting fibres of the atrioventricular node, as opposed to the sinoatrial node, and is presumably responsible for the cardiac arrhythmias which occur in this disease. The pituitary, adrenal, thyroid and parathyroid glands frequently contain extensive haemosiderin deposits, although evidence of functional impairment is usually confined to the pituitary. The epidermis of the skin is atrophic with increased melanin in the cells of the basal layer. The characteristic metallic grey hue results from increased melanin (with or without iron) in the dermis. Increased iron deposition in the skin is variable and tends to occur around the sweat glands.

### 3.5 Clinical Features

For many years the disease is latent as body iron stores increase progressively and the course depends on a number of factors, including sex of the subject, dietary intake of iron and physiological (menstrual) blood loss. The overt clinical manifestations occur from five to ten times more frequently in men than in women. The less common incidence of overt disease in women is explained in part by blood loss during the reproductive years and in part by lower dietary iron intake. The majority of *symptomatic* patients present in the fourth or fifth decade, or less commonly in the second or third decade, when the disease is commonly associated with endocrine or cardiac manifestations. POWELL, MORTIMER and HARRIS analysed the symptoms and signs at presentation of an unselected group of symptomatic patients with haemochromatosis compared with those seen in other forms of cirrhosis. In the majority of patients the classical triad described by SHELDON [11] (pigmentation of the skin, hepatomegaly and diabetes mellitus) was present. The major differences between the clinical features of patients with haemochromatosis and other forms of cirrhosis were the relatively high incidence of gonadal atrophy, skin pigmentation and hepatomegaly, and the relatively prolonged and benign course of the liver disease. Indeed, more than 50% of patients had no symptoms other than lethargy and loss of libido, and no physical signs other than hepatomegaly, skin pigmentation and testicular atrophy. Furthermore, over half the patients had little or no laboratory evidence of functional liver impairment in spite of the presence of cirrhosis [40]. Thus, haemochromatosis should be considered in any patient with skin pigmentation and an enlarged firm liver, especially in males if testicular atrophy is present. Carbohydrate intolerance occurs in up to 80% of patients with idiopathic haemochromatosis, but overt diabetes mellitus presents in only 60%. This is multifactorial in origin, with contributions from hepatic cirrhosis, pancreatic islet cell damage from iron and the inheritance of a gene for susceptibility to idiopathic diabetes mellitus. This contrasts with other forms of hepatic cirrhosis in which carbohydrate intolerance is due to insulin insensitivity. Clinically, the diabetes of haemochromatosis may be mild or severe and is occasionally insulin resistant. Degenerative complications such as retinopathy, nephropathy and peripheral neuropathy occur as in idiopathic diabetes mellitis. Evidence of endocrine involvement in addition to decreased gonadal function is occasionally seen, most commonly as hypopituitarism. Haemosiderin is almost invariably found in the pituitary gland [11] and deficiency of other pituitary hormones has been demonstrated in this disease. Hypoparathyroidism, hypothyroidism and Addison's disease have also been described but are exceedingly rare.

Cardiac manifestations occur in about 15% of patients and characteristically take the form of arrhythmias or progressively severe heart failure. Symptoms of congestive heart failure may develop quite rapidly with progression to death if untreated. In our experience, this occurs not infrequently in subjects ingesting large doses of ascorbic acid. The heart is diffusely enlarged and such cases may be misdiagnosed as idiopathic cardiomyopathy if other overt manifestations are absent. A variety of cardiac arrhythmias may be present, especially supraventricular and paroxysmal tachyarrhythmias. However, with the widespread use of phlebotomy therapy, these complications appear to be much less common than 30 years ago.

A recently described and characteristic feature in some 25%–50% of cases is the presence of an arthropathy characterised by the deposition of calcium pyrophosphate and iron in the synovium – *chondrocalcinosis*. Both small and large joints are involved, predominantly the first and second metacarpophalangeal and knee joints, with pain, swelling and limitation of movement. There is a correlation between the degree of chondrocalcinosis and the severity of the joint disease, but the exact relationship of the iron deposition to the arthritis is unclear. Symptoms and progress of the arthropathy are not related to the degree of iron loading and the course of the disease is not influenced by phlebotomy therapy.

Osteoporosis and vertebral collapse have also been described, frequently in association with ascorbic acid depletion, presumably because of the oxidative effects of body iron. However, this complication appears to be confined almost exclusively to the black of southern Africa. Primary liver cell cancer is increasing as a complication of haemochromatosis and this is presumably related to the increase in life span as a result of more effective therapy for the disease. In some instances the viruses of hepatitis B or C may be involved. Hepatic cirrhosis appears to be an important prerequisite for the development of malignant hepatoma and this complication is almost unknown in precirrhotic cases that are adequately treated. This has obvious important implications for the early diagnosis of the disease.

### 3.6 Precirrhotic (Early or Presymptomatic) Haemochromatosis

There is increasing evidence that iron plays a major role in producing tissue damage and that early detection and treatment of the disease prolongs life and may delay or prevent irreversible complications [40]. For this reason, and because cirrhosis represents a critical and largely irreversible stage in the development of haemochromatosis, the physician who diagnoses the disease has a responsibility to inform all the patient's blood relatives and to see that they are screened for the disease. There is therefore much interest in non-invasive methods for detecting the early precirrhotic stage of the disease (see below) and also in the natural history of the disease. There is now good evidence that iron deposition precedes fibrosis and other evidence of tissue injury [13, 15, 40]. Experimental observations in the rat using the carbonyl iron model are also consistent with this sequence [10–12]. Importantly, cirrhosis does not develop from this disease if it is diagnosed in the precirrhotic stage and if adequate venesection therapy is instituted Furthermore, primary hepatocellular cancer is almost unknown if precirrhotic cases are adequately treated. The rare reported cases may have had large macronodules. Increasingly, early cases are diagnosed after finding an elevated serum iron unexpectedly on biochemical analysis. This should lead to measurement of transferrin saturation and serum ferritin levels. The high prevalence of the gene for this disease in populations of European origin and the easy prevention of complications probably warrant inclusion of measurement of the serum iron levels (if not the transferrin saturation) in standard health checks [41].

### 3.7 Diagnosis and Differential Diagnosis

The diagnosis of symptomatic haemochromatosis is usually made on the basis of the above clinical features with or without a positive family history together with laboratory investigations indicative of excessive iron stores and tissue damage. These include an elevated serum iron level >30 μmol/litre (>170 μg/100 ml) associated with an elevation of percentage transferrin saturation (greater than 60%) and an elevated serum ferritin concentration.

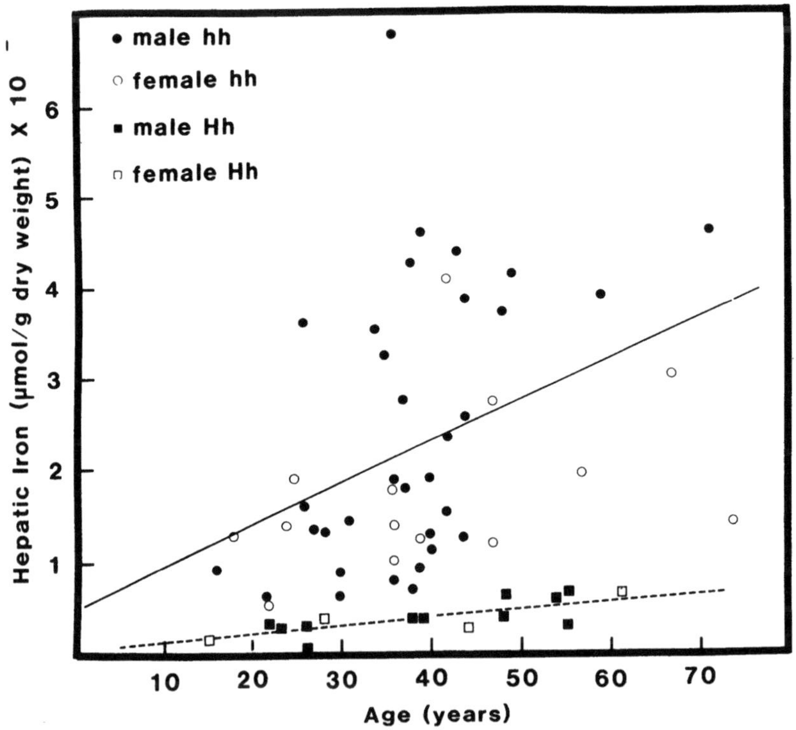


**Fig. 1.** Age-related rise in hepatic iron concentration in subjects with haemochromatosis. *hh*, homozygous; *Hh*, heterozygous. [Reproduced with permission from Summers KM et al. (1990) Hepatology 12:20–25]

Hepatic biopsy is very important in defining the extent of tissue damage as well as in allowing both histochemical assessment of tissue iron and measurement of a hepatic iron concentration. In the absence of causes of secondary iron overload the ultimate diagnosis rests on the demonstration of increased body iron stores. Therefore, an attempt should be made to quantify the degree of iron excess. Reliance is best placed on chemical analysis of tissue obtained by biopsy or at necropsy and also retrospectively on the amount of iron removed by phlebotomy [42–46]. In patients with symptomatic haemochromatosis the hepatic iron concentration is usually in excess of 180 μmol/g (1 g/100 g) dry weight. Furthermore, because of the age-related rise in hepatic iron in haemochromatosis homozygotes (Fig. 1), calculation of a hepatic iron index (hepatic iron/age) allows distinction between early homozygotes and heterozygotes [38, 39] (Fig. 2). Presymptomatic homozygotes usually have values for hepatic iron concentration more than twice normal (i.e., >60 μM/g dw) and a hepatic iron index greater than 2. Tests involving measurement of urinary iron excretion after injection of chelating agents are cumbersome and have now largely been replaced by the above. Computed tomography, squid biomagnetometry and magnetic measurement of hepatic iron have been investigated as non-invasive tests for the detection of iron overload. CT shows increased density of the liver due to iron deposition. Dual-energy scanning is necessary and the lower limits for accurate assessment of liver iron are debatable. Magnetic resonance can also detect increased tissue iron but it is costly and the relatively poor sensitivity at lower iron concentrations limits its value. If the techniques are simplified and become widely available, they could be useful non-invasive screening tests, but liver biopsy will remain the gold standard for determining the histological pattern and degree of hepatic injury. The most satisfactory non-invasive screening tests for *precirrhotic haemochromatosis* at present are the transferrin saturation and the serum ferritin concentration. Since each has limitations both are usually performed. With parenchymal iron overload the transferrin saturation is usually greater than 50% and the serum ferritin rises above the normal range when the hepatic iron stores are about twice normal. Recent population studies have suggested that in otherwise healthy persons, a fasting serum transferrin saturation greater than 62% strongly suggests homozygoslty for haemochromatosis. However, two points should be noted. Firstly, the serum ferritin level may be elevated out of proportion to body iron stores when there is hepatocellular necrosis, especially in alcoholic liver disease. Secondly, some rare families have been reported in which the serum ferritin concentration has been normal in relatives despite unequivocal increase in body iron stores. The reason for this is uncertain and it would appear to be an exceptional situation. The serum ferritin concentration usually rises in proportion to total body iron stores until it reaches levels of 1000 ng/ml or more [16]. A recent population survey has indicated that, at least in some populations, levels up to 250 ng/ml in females and 400 ng/ml in males may

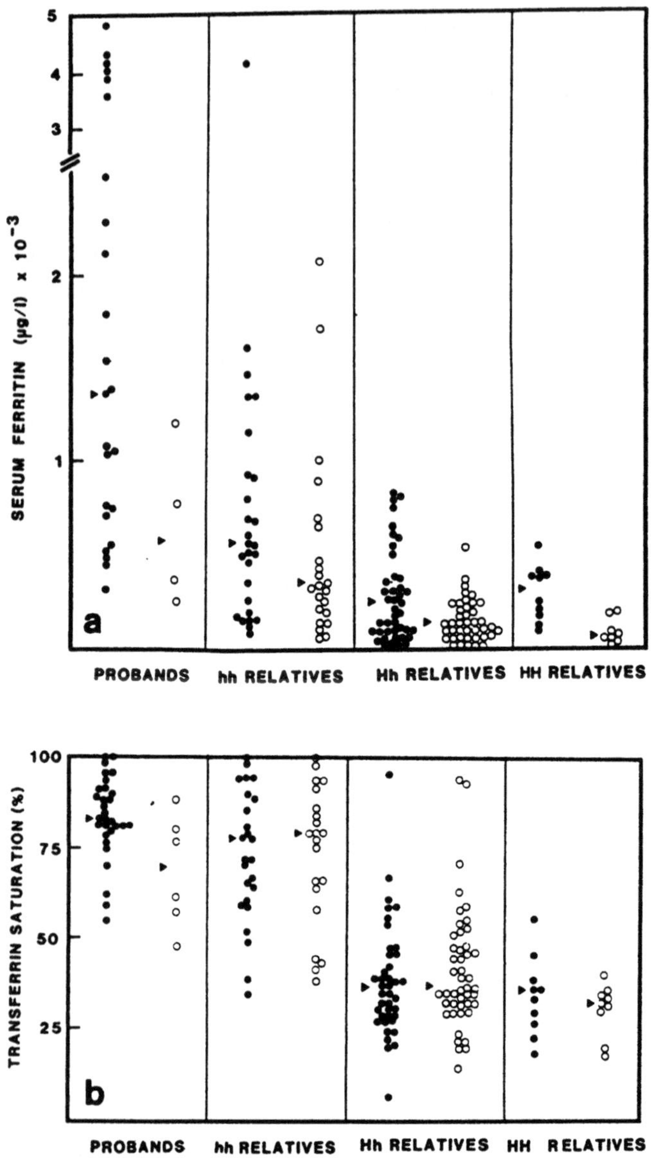


**Fig. 2a–d.** Iron indices in probands and relatives: **a** serum ferritin concentration; **b** serum transferrin

be present with normal iron stores [41]. Representative values for serum ferritin, transferrin saturation, hepatic iron and hepatic iron index in probands and relatives are given in Fig. 2.

Since the HC locus is tightly linked to the HLA-A locus on chromosome 6, HLA typing is helpful in determining the probability of a sibling being a putative homozygote or heterozygote [19, 42, 43]. Thus, siblings sharing two

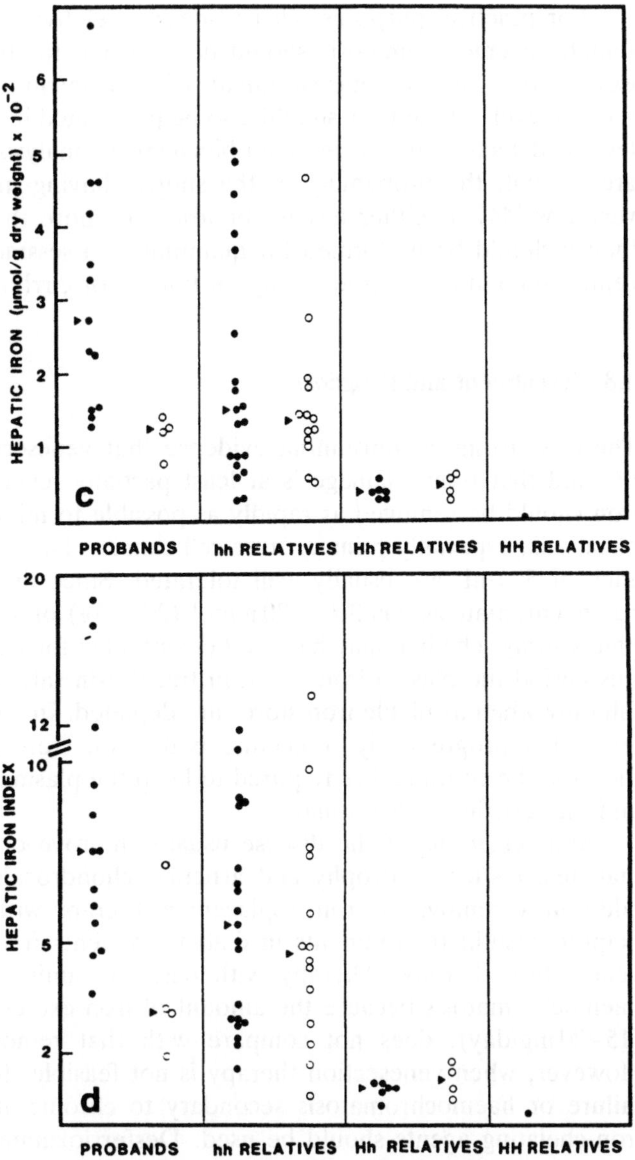


**Fig. 2.** **c** Hepatic iron concentration (HIC); **d** hepatic iron index (HIC divided by age). [Reproduced with permission from POWELL LW et al. (1990) Gastroenterology 98:1625–1632]

HLA haplotypes with a patient (putative homozygotes) are at high risk of having or developing iron overload and should be checked on a regular basis for the disease.

For practical purposes, all first-degree relatives of patients with symptomatic haemochromatosis should be screened for the disease by physical examination and by measurement of transferrin saturation and serum ferritin level. These tests should also be performed if an elevated serum iron level is detected unexpectedly on biochemical analysis. If both these indices are normal, the probability of the subject having increased iron stores is very low [44]. If either test is abnormal on more than one occasion, liver biopsy should be performed for quantitative assessment of tissue iron concentration and the degree, if any, of fibrosis or cirrhosis.

### 3.8 Treatment and Prognosis

There is strong circumstantial evidence that venesection therapy prolongs life and that tissue damage is at least partially reversible [45]. The excess iron should be removed as rapidly as possible to minimise the risk of complications, especially primary liver cell cancer. Twice-weekly phlebotomies, each of 500 ml, are usually well tolerated. Since the average patient with haemochromatosis has 360–720 mmol (20–40 g) of stored iron, the weekly phlebotomy schedule may have to be continued for up to 2–3 years. During this period the plasma iron and iron transferrin saturation remain high and fall only when available iron stores are depleted. In contrast, plasma ferritin levels fall progressively, reflecting body iron stores. Venesection should therefore be continued as required to keep the plasma transferrin saturation and the ferritin levels normal.

Manifestations of the disease usually improve or disappear except for diabetes, testicular atrophy and articular chondrocalcinosis. Therefore, in addition to removal of iron, replacement therapy with testosterone may be helpful. Insulin requirements in diabetic patients frequently decrease after venesection therapy. Therapy with desferrioxamine is not practicable in haemochromatosis because the amount of iron excreted, 270–360 µmol/day (15–20 mg/day), does not compare with that removed by venesections. However, when venesection therapy is not feasible, for example in cardiac failure or haemochromatosis secondary to chronic anaemia, therapy with iron-chelating agents should be used. Desferrioxamine can be given intravenously in glucose-saline following each transfusion (e.g., 1 g 8 hourly) and up to 18 mmol (1 g) of iron may be excreted over 2–3 days during such therapy. Long-term therapy can be instituted with subcutaneous infusions overnight twice or thrice weekly.

The prognosis of haemochromatosis appears to depend on the amount and rapidity of parenchymal iron loading and the presence of associated liver disease of other aetiology. The mean survival after diagnosis in 1935 was 4.4 years [46] when treatment was limited to supportive measures for diabetes, liver disease and cardiac failure. At that time, 14% of patients developed primary liver cell cancer. In contrast, of patients treated by phlebotomy at the present time, 89% survive for at least 5 years from the time of diagnosis [47] although the incidence of primary hepatocellular cancer is increased to 25%–30% with longer survival [48]. The disease appears to be preventable in individuals whose tissues are overloaded with iron but not yet damaged, as long as the excess iron is removed and future accumulation of iron prevented [15, 44] and it is now established that the prognosis for life in precirrhotic subjects so treated does not differ from the general population [49]. Malignant hepatoma develops only very rarely if the disease is treated in the precirrhotic phase [50] and two large studies have shown no increase in other forms of internal malignancy in the disease [48, 49]. Thus, especially in relatives of patients and in those patients with early disease, the complications and course of haemochromatosis appear to be entirely preventable.

## 4 Secondary (Acquired) Haemochromatosis

### 4.1 Haemochromatosis Associated with Chronic Anaemias ("Erythropoietic Haemochromatosis")

Increased erythropoiesis in the human or induced experimentally in animals results in increased iron absorption. In the human, such increased iron absorption occurs primarily in those forms of haemolytic anaemia associated with ineffective erythropoiesis, as in hereditary siderobiastic anaemia and thalassasemia major. Where haemochromatosis has been described in association with other disorders such as chronic refractory anaemias and congenital spherocytosis, it is likely that such patients carried the gene for haemochromatosis. Diseases associated with ineffective erythropoiesis and increased iron absorption lead to predominantly parenchymal iron loading, whereas in those whose iron load has been acquired primarily parenterally, there is predominantly RE cell involvement. Fibrosis and functional impairment of the affected organs, although uncommon overall, are seen more often in the former group. The full clinicopathological syndrome of haemochromatosis, including cardiac failure, diabetes mellitus and hypopituitarism, has been described in such patients.

Treatment is rather unsatisfactory at present. Cautious phlebotomy, pyridoxine and chelating agents may be tried. Intensive regular chelation therapy with desferrioxamine has been shown in a controlled trial to be effective in reducing the iron load and delaying the onset of hepatic fibrosis. The development of more effective oral chelating agents is eagerly awaited for this group of patients. At present, desferrioxamine remains the most effective form of chelation therapy. It should be given by slow subcutaneous or intravenous infusion and the subject should be ascorbic acid replete. However, excess ascorbate should be avoided since this may aggravate iron toxicity.

### 4.2 Cirrhosis with Subsequent Secondary Iron Overload

As discussed above, it has long been recognised that patients with hepatic cirrhosis may secondarily develop increased stainable hepatic iron [51]. However, the increase in body iron stores is usually small (2–3 g). The problem has now been greatly clarified by the recognition of the HLA-related genetic disease (discussed previously) and may be summarised as follows:

1. A proportion of patients with hepatic cirrhosis accumulate iron secondarily, but rarely do the body iron stores or hepatic iron concentrations reach levels comparable with those seen in patients with haemochromatosis [48, 52, 53]. When gross iron overload is encountered in association with cirrhosis, one is usually dealing with the genetic disease.

2. The factors that have been implicated as contributing to increased iron absorption and iron accumulation in patients with cirrhosis of the liver are:
a) Increased oral iron intake in alcoholic beverages or iron tablets
b) Stimulation of absorption of inorganic iron by alcohol
c) Pancreatic insufficiency
d) Folic acid deficiency
e) Portacaval shunt surgery

These factors and the relevant literature have been discussed in depth elsewhere [13, 40].

3. There is an increased incidence of alcoholism in patients with idiopathic haemochromatosis, varying from between 25% and 50% of patients. The reason for this is still unclear. However, systematic comparisons of alcoholic and non-alcoholic subjects with haemochromatosis as defined above have shown no significant difference between the two groups with respect to the clinical and pathological features or to the degree of iron overload, except for the presence of active hepatocellular disease in some alcoholic patients. A detailed study of the pathology of the liver in haemochromatosis revealed that the hepatic findings were the same in alcoholic and non-alcoholic patients, except that in about 25% of the alcoholic patients there were changes of alcoholic liver disease superimposed on the underlying haemochromatosis. This is, of course, an incidence of alcoholic liver disease very similar to that reported amongst heavy drinkers in the general population.

Thus the available data suggest that the majority of alcoholic subjects with haemochromatosis possess the basic genetic defect of iron metabolism and that the iron accumulation and liver injury have been accelerated by alcoholism.

4. Persons who are heterozygous for the haemochromatosis allele rarely, if ever, develop a progressive increase in body iron stores even with alcoholism or prolonged intake of dietary iron [15, 44].

5. While phlebotomy therapy is indicated in patients with primary idiopathic haemochromatosis, whether alcoholic or non-alcoholic, it has no therapeutic role in the alcoholic cirrhotic with increased iron stores [46].

### 4.3 Dietary Iron Overload

Gross iron overload resulting from excess absorption of dietary iron is very rare in all populations that have been studied with the single exception of the blacks of southern Africa, among whom it was previously common (so-called Bantu-type haemochromatosis). The disease in that population has been extensively reviewed and will not be discussed further. In whites, the situation in which haemochromatosis has been described solely as a result of secondary iron accumulation from dietary sources is the patient with alcoholic cirrhosis who is mildly anaemic, usually due to folic acid and not iron deficiency, and who is prescribed oral iron supplements. However, it is a rare condition and the possibility that such subjects carry the gene for haemochromatosis cannot be excluded.

The prolonged ingestion of pharmacological doses of iron may lead to excessive iron accumulation but an association with the gene for haemochromatosis cannot be excluded until a gene probe becomes available for use in such patients.

### References


1. Kondo H, Saito K, Grasso JP, Aisen P (1988) Iron metabolism in the erythrophagocytosing Kupffer cell. Hepatology 8:32–38
2. Sibille J-C, Kondo H, Aisen P (1988) Interactions between isolated hepatocytes and Kupffer cells in iron metabolism. A possible role for ferritin as an iron carrier protein. Hepatology 8:296–301
3. Casey JL, Hentze MW, Koeller DM, Caughman SW, Roualt TA, Klausner RD, Harford JB (1988) Iron-responsive elements: regulatory DNA sequences that control mRNA levels and translation. Science 240:924–928
4. Leibold FA, Munro HN (1988) Cytoplasmic protein binds in vitro to a highly conserved sequence in the 51 untranslated region of ferritin heavy and light subunit mRNA's. Proc Natl Acad Sci USA 85:2171–2175
5. Osterloh KRS, Simpson RJ, Snape S, Peters TJ (1987) Intestinal iron absorption and mucosal transferrin in rats subjected to hypoxia Blut 55:421–431
6. Simpson RJ, Moore R, Peters TJ (1988) Significance of nonesterified fatty acids in iron uptake by intestinal brush-border membrane vesicles. Biochim Biophys Acta 941:39–47
7. Peters TJ (1989) Mechanisms of cellular iron uptake and release. Proceedings of the second international haemochromatosis conference, Gold Coast, Australia, 1989, p 35
8. Conrad ME, Umbreit JN, Moore EG, Peterson RDA, Jones MBA (1990) A newly identified iron binding protein in duodenal mucosa of rats. J Biol Chem 265:5273–5279
9. Simon M, Brissot P (1988) The genetics of haemochromatosis. J Hepatology 6:116–124

10. Williams R, Scheuer PJ, Sherlock S (1962) The inheritance of idiopathic haemochromatosis. A clinical and liver biopsy study of 16 families. Q J Med 31:249–265
11. Sheldon JH (1935) Haemochromatosis. Oxford University Press, London
12. Cartwright GE, Edwards CO, Skoinick M (1979) Letter to edltors: genetics of hemochromatosis. N Engl J Med 301:1291–1292
13. Bassett ML, Halliday JW, Powell LW (1984) Genetic haemochromatosis. Semin Liver Dis 4:217–227
14. Summers KM, Tam KS, Halliday JW, Powell LW (1989) HLA determinants in an Australian population of haemochromatosis patients and their families. Am J Hum Genet 45:41–48
15. Bassett ML, Halliday JW, Powell LW (1981) HLA typing in idiopathic haemochromatosis: distinction between homozygotes and heterozygotes with biochemical expression. Hepatology 1:120–126
16. Edwards CO, Carroll M, Bray P, Cartwright GE (1977) Hereditary hemochromatosis. N Engl J Med 297:7–13
17. Simon M, Alexandre J-L, Fauchet R et al. (1980) The genetics of hemochromatosis. Prog Med Genet 4:135–168
18. Thomson G, Bodmer W (1977) The genetic analysis of HLA and disease associations. In: Dausset J, Svejgaard A (eds) HLA and disease. Williams and Wilkins, Baltimore, pp 84–93
19. Powell LW, Summers K, Board PG, Axelsen E, Webb S, Halliday JW (1990) Expression of haemochromatosis in homozygous subjects: implications for early diagnosis and prevention. Gastroenterology 98:1625–1632
20. Simon M, Alexandre JL, Bourel M et al. (1977) Heredity of idiopathic haemochromatosis: a study of 106 families. Clin Genet 11:327–341
21. Powell LW, Ferluga J, Halliday JW, Bassett ML, Kohonen-Corish MK, Serjeantson S (1987) Genetic hemochromatosis and HLA linkage. Hum Genet 77:55–56
22. Edwards CQ, Griffin LM, Goldgar D, Drummond C, Skoinick MH, Kushner JP (1988) Prevalence of hemochromatosis among 11,065 presumably healthy blood donors. N Engl J Med 318:1355–1362
23. Skoinick M (1989) Evaluation of the HLA region of chromosome G and linkage disequilibrium: relevance to the genetics of haemochromatosis. Proceedings of the second international haemochromatosis conference, Gold Coast, Australia, 1989, p 2
24. Peters TJ, Seymour CA (1976) Acid hydrolase activities and lysosomal integrity in liver biopsies from patients with iron overload. Clin Sci Mol Med 50:75–78
25. Sciot R, Paterson AC, Van Den Oord JJ, Desmet VJ (1987) Lack of hepatic transferrin receptor expression in hemochromatosis. Hepatology 7:831–837
26. Powell LW, Campbell CB, Wilson E (1970) Intestinal mucosal uptake of iron and iron retention in idiopathic haemochromatosis as evidence of a mucosal abnormality. Gut 11:727–731
27. Whittaker P, Skikne BS, Covell AM, Flowers C, Cooke A, Lynch SL, Cook JD (1989) Duodenal iron proteins in idiopathic haemochromatosis. J Clin Invest 83:261–268
28. Anderson GJ, Powell LW, Halliday JW (1990) Transferrin receptor distribution and regulation in the rat small intestine: effect of iron stores and erythropoiesis, Gastroenterology 98:576–585
29. Young SP, Aisen P (1981) Transferrin receptors and the uptake and release of iron by isolated hepatocytes. Hepatology 1:114
30. Zak O, Aisen P (1989) Differences between the two iron-binding sites of rabbit transferrin in donating iron rabbit reticulocytes. Proceedings of IXth international conference on proteins of iron transport and storage, Brisbane, 1989, p 91

31. Klausner RD (1988) From receptors to genes – insights from molecular iron metabolism. Clin Res 36:494–500
32. Francanzani AL, Fargion S, Romeno R, Piperno A, Arosio P, Fiorelli G (1989) Immunohistochemical evidence for a lack of ferritin in duodenal absorptive epithelial cells in idiopathic haemochromatosis. Gastroenterology 96:1071–1078
33. Summers KM, Tam KS, Bartley PB, Halliday JW, Powell LW (1989) Exclusion of the chromosome 6 ferritin sequence as a candidate for the haemochromatosis gene. Proceedings of the XIIIth annual scientific meeting of the human genetics society of Australasia, Alice Springs, Australia, July 1989
34. Aisen P, Sibille JC, Osterloh K, Kondo H (1989) The role of ferritin in iron release and uptake by hepatic cells. Proceedings of IXth international conference on proteins of iron transport and storage, Brisbane, p 27
35. Adams PC, Powell LW, Halliday JW (1988) Isolation of a human hepatic ferritin receptor. Hepatology 8:719–721
36. Mack U, Powell LW, Halliday JW (1983) Detection and isolation of a hepatic membrane receptor for ferritin. J Biol Chem 258:4672–4675
37. Mack U, Storey EL, Powell LW, Halliday JW (1985) Characterization of the binding of ferritin to the rat liver ferritin receptor. Biochem Biophys Acta 843:164–170
38. Bassett ML, Halliday JW, Powell LW (1986) Value of hepatic iron measurements in early hemochromatosis and determination of the critical iron level associated with fibrosis. Hepatology 6:24–29
39. Summers KM, Halliday JW, Powell LW (1990) Identification of homozygous haemochromatosis subjects by measurement of hepatic iron index. Hepatology 12:20–25
40. Bothwell TH, Charlton RW, Cook JD, Finch CA (1979) Iron metabolism in man. Blackwell Scientific, Oxford
41. Leggett BA, Brown NN, Bryant SJ, Powell LW, Halliday JW (1990) Factors affecting the concentration of ferritin in serum in a healthy Australian population. Clin Chem 36:1350–1355
42. Bassett ML, Halliday JW, Powell LW (1979) Early detection of idiopathic haemochromatosis, relative value of serum-ferritin and HLA typing. Lancet II:4–7
43. Bassett ML, Doran TJ, Halliday JW et al. (1982) Idiopathic haemochromatosis: demonstration of homozygous-heterozygous mating by HLA typing of families. Hum Genet 60:352–357
44. Bassett ML, Halliday JW, Ferris RA, Powell LW (1984) Diagnosis of haemochromatosis in young subjects: predictive accuracy of serum iron, transferrin saturation and serum ferritin. Gastroenterology 87:628–633
45. Williams R, Smith PM, Spicer EJF et al. (1969) Venesection therapy in idiopathic haemochromatosis. O J Med 38:1–16
46. Grace ND, Powell LW (1974) Iron storage disorders of the liver. Gastroenterology 64:1257–1283
47. Finch SC, Finch CA (1955) Idiopathic hemochromatosis, an iron storage disease. A. Iron metabolism in hemochromatosis. Medicine (Baltimore) 34:381
48. Bradbear RA, Bain C, Siskind V et al. (1985) Cohort study of internal malignancy in genetic hemochromatosis and other nonalcoholic liver diseases. JNCI 74:81–84
49. Niederau C, Fisher R, Sonnenberg A, Stremmel W, Trammpisch HJ, Strohmeyer G (1985) Survival and causes of death in cirrhotic and non-cirrhotic patients with primary hemochromatosis. N Engl J Med 313:1256–1262
50. Powell LW, Kerr JFR (1975) The pathology of the liver in hemochromatosis. In: Joacim H (ed) Pathobiology annual. Appleton-Century-Crofts, New York, pp. 317–337

51. Powell LW (1965) Iron storage in relatives of patients with haemochromatosis and in relatives of patients with alcoholic cirrhosis and haemosiderosis. A comparative study of 27 families. O J Med 34:427–442
52. Simon M, Bourel M, Genetet B et al. (1977) Idiopathic hemochromatosis and iron overload in alcoholic liver disease: differentiation by HLA phenotype. Gastroenterology 73:655–658
53. Zimmerman HJ, Chomet B, Kulesch MH, McWhorter CA (1961) Hepatic hemosiderin deposits. Incidence in 558 biopsies from patients with and without intrinsic hepatic disease. Arch Intern Med 197:494–503

# 25 $\alpha_1$-Antitrypsin Deficiency

J.M. ZOZAYA and J. PRIETO

## 1 Structure and Function of $\alpha_1$-Antitrypsin

$\alpha_1$-Antitrypsin (AAT), also referred to as $\alpha_1$-protease inhibitor, is the main antiprotease of human serum. It belongs to the class of proteins known as serpins (serine protease inhibitors). Because trypsin was the first serine protease tested, the inhibitor was termed $\alpha_1$-antitrypsin. However, the major function of AAT is to inhibit the powerful neutrophil elastase. Other serine proteases, such as cathepsin G, chymotrypsin, plasmin, thrombin, factor Xa, and kallikrein, are also inhibited by AAT, although less efficiently [1, 2].

$\alpha_1$-Antitrypsin is a 52-kd glycoprotein synthesized in hepatocytes. It consists of a folded polypeptide chain of 394 amino acids (the full sequence is known) and three carbohydrate side chains, which represent 12% of the total molecular weight and are composed of *N*-acetylglucosamine, mannose, galactose, and sialic acid [3].

With a molecular mass smaller than albumin, AAT readily diffuses throughout the interstitial fluids, being found in low concentrations in nasal secretions, saliva, tears, cerebrospinal fluid, bronchial secretions, duodenal fluid, maternal milk, and amniotic fluid [4]. Normal serum levels vary between 150 and 350 mg/dl [2] and there are no differences in relation to either age or sex. Because AAT is an acute phase reactant, serum concentration increases in inflammatory processes and in patients with malignancies. Serum levels are also elevated in pregnancy, in females taking oral contraceptives, and in patients with cirrhosis, especially in the presence of cholestasis [5].

The plasma half-life of AAT is short, between 4 and 6 days [6, 7]. Because of this, there is a rapid decline in its serum concentration in cases of fulminant liver failure [5].

## 2 Genetics and $\alpha_1$-Antitrypsin Variants

$\alpha_1$-Antitrypsin is coded for by a gene of 122 kb located on chromosome 14 [8]. This gene, which shows pleomorphism, comprises seven exons and six introns. The two AAT genes of each individual (one on each chromosome 14) are codominantly expressed. Therefore, in a given individual, the AAT

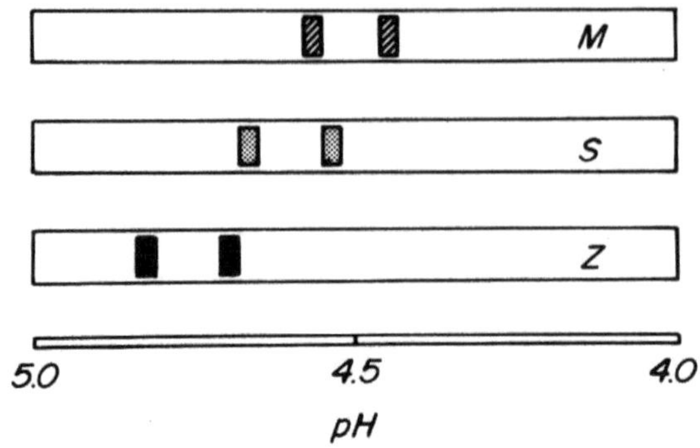


**Fig. 1.** Isoelectric focusing of serum at pH 4.0–5.0. Major bands represent normal (*M*) and deficient (*S, Z*) AAT variants

phenotype is the result of the independent expression of the two parental alleles.

$\alpha_1$-Antitrypsin is a highly pleomorphic protein, as evidenced in studies using agarose gel electrophoresis [9] and, more recently, isoelectric focusing in polyacrylamide gel [10]. With the latter technique, more than 70 AAT variants have been identified. Molecular biology methods have shown that the variants of clinical importance have arisen from mutations in exons of the AAT gene.

Since AAT synthesis depends on two alleles, each person can express either one or two AAT variants, depending on his/her being homozygous or heterozygous for the AAT gene. Each variant gives rise to two major (and three minor) bands in isoelectric focusing. These bands result from post-transcriptional changes in the protein encoded by the corresponding allele. The different AAT phenotypes present in the population are collectively named the Pi system (Pi stands for protease inhibitor).

Variants of AAT have been assigned letters of the alphabet according to their mobility in isoelectric focusing. The common variant is called M ("medium" mobility). Slow-moving variants are named by late letters in the alphabet (S, Z). Earlier letters of the alphabet (B, F) are used to identify fast-moving forms (Fig. 1).

Variants are categorized as "normal," "deficient," or "null," based on their rate of secretion and contribution to AAT serum levels (Table 1). The normal variant is the common M variant, which in fact consists of a family of subtypes [M1 ($Val^{213}$), M1 ($Ala^{213}$), $M_2$, $M_3$]. M1 ($Val^{213}$) is the commonest allele in the population and serves as the classic AAT protein sequence. M1 ($Ala^{213}$), which also possesses a high allelic frequency, can only be identified by DNA sequencing, since it has the same mobility as M1 ($Val^{213}$) in isoelectric focusing [2].

The two most important deficient variants are Z and S [2, 3]. The Z variant results from a single amino acid substitution in position 342

**Table 1.** Serum levels and allelic frequency of AAT variants

| | Serum levels[a] (mg/dl) | Allelic frequency[b] |
|---|---|---|
| *Normal variants* | | |
| $M_1$ ($Ala^{213}$) | 150–350 | 0.20 |
| $M_1$ ($Val^{213}$) | 150–350 | 0.45 |
| $M_2$ | 150–350 | 0.15 |
| $M_3$ | 150–350 | 0.10 |
| *Deficient variants* | | |
| S | 100–200 | 0.03–0.10 |
| Z | 15–50 | 0.01–0.02 |
| *Null variants* | 0 | <0.001 |

[a] In homozygous persons
[b] In white persons from the United States and Europe (data from BRANTLEY et al. [2])

(glutamine to lysine) due to a change in the codon GAG to AAG. In the S variant, there is a substitution of glutamine for valine in position 264 because of mutation in the codon GAA to GTA. The allelic frequency of the Z variant ranges between 0.01 and 0.026 in white individuals from the United States and Europe. The S variant is commoner than the Z variant, with an allelic frequency of 0.02–0.03 in whites from the United States and higher in some European countries (reaching 0.15 in the Iberian Peninsula). Unlike the white population of Europe and North America, where the major AAT variants are not very rare, African and Asian races are more exclusively of the MM phenotype [2, 11].

The Z type is the classic AAT deficiency variant. The prevalence of ZZ homozygotes varies from 1 in 1700 in Sweden [12] to 1 in 5000 in North America [13]. ZZ homozygotes have AAT serum levels ranging between 15 and 50 mg/dl instead of the normal values of 150–350 mg/dl.

In the ZZ homozygote there is normal transcription of the AAT gene. The Z protein, however, folds abnormally in the lumen of the rough endoplasmic reticulum, producing aggregates which fail to undergo the final processing of their carbohydrate side chains. This causes a failure in the transport, such that only 15% of newly synthesized Z polypeptide is secreted into the plasma while the remaining 85% is retained in the endoplasmic reticulum of hepatocytes, forming microscopically visible globoid inclusions [13]. This abnormality in cellular transport of the Z variant, resulting in intracellular accumulation of the aggregated Z protein, is the main reason for reduced serum AAT levels found in ZZ homozygotes.

In contrast with the Z mutation, the S mutation is not associated with intracellular accumulation of AAT. The subtle structural change of the S variant renders this protein less stable and, thus, more susceptible to intracellular proteolysis [1, 3]. As a consequence, serum AAT levels in SS homozygotes are approximately 50% of the normal values.

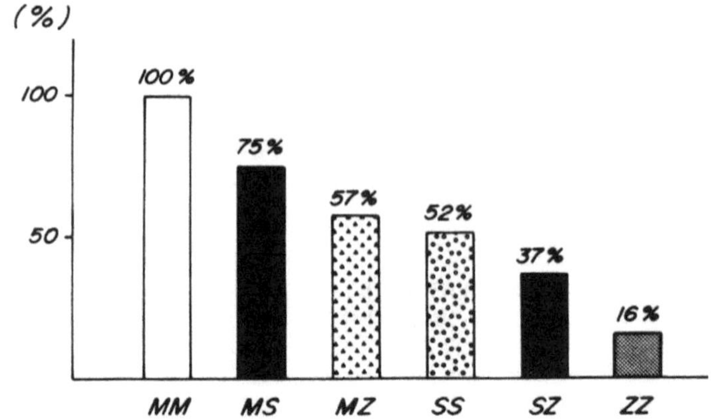


**Fig. 2.** Percentage of the normal AAT serum concentration corresponding to different Pi phenotypes

The "null" variants (Pi null or Pi-) constitute a very rare group of AAT alleles that are unable to direct the synthesis of mRNA. In subjects homozygous for the null alleles, AAT is undetectable in serum [14].

Figure 2 depicts the six possible phenotypes derived from the M, S, and Z variants and the serum AAT levels of each variant expressed as a percentage of the normal values.

## 3 $\alpha_1$-Antitrypsin Deficiency and Liver Disease

In 1963, Laurell and Eriksson [15] noted a relationship between low serum levels of AAT and the development of emphysema. Since then, a vast number of observations have implicated AAT deficiency in the pathogenesis of chronic obstructive lung disease [16].

The first report of liver damage in patients with AAT deficiency was by Sharp et al. in 1969 [17]. Many studies thereafter confirmed an association between ZZ homozygosity and the development of various forms of liver disease, including neonatal cholestasis, cirrhosis, and primary liver cancer. It is now recognized that significant hepatic disease occurs in 10%–20% of Pi ZZ individuals [12], with males more commonly affected than females. Liver and lung disease may coexist in the same patient.

The earliest and most frequent hepatic disturbance is neonatal cholestasis [18–20]. This condition, which affects 10% of Pi ZZ infants [19], must be differentiated from biliary atresia and other diseases, infectious or metabolic, causing neonatal hepatitis. The clinical picture is characterized by jaundice, pale stools, failure to gain weight, and biochemical signs of cholestasis, appearing between the 2nd and 8th weeks of life. Neonatal cholestasis may resolve or may progress to juvenile cirrhosis, particularly in infants with prolonged cholestatic jaundice. Progression to cirrhosis was observed in 21% of cases in the study by Sverger [12] and in 53% in the report by Ghishan and Greene [20]. Asymptomatic Pi ZZ children may present with abnormal liver function tests and/or hepatomegaly. The long-term prognosis of these cases remains to be established.

In adults, a relationship between Pi ZZ phenotype and the development of cirrhosis has been established [21]. In a study from Sweden [22] comprising 246 AAT-deficient subjects, 29 had evidence of liver damage, 24 with biopsy-proven cirrhosis. The risk of presenting significant liver disease is higher in men than in women and becomes greater with increasing age [22–24]. A history of neonatal hepatitis may be obtained in adult patients with cirrhosis [25]. The liver disease associated with AAT deficiency frequently has a long asymptomatic stage, followed by a relatively short symptomatic phase, usually with manifestations of portal hypertension. Once in this advanced stage, the condition often leads to death within a few years.

Partial AAT deficiency of the types Pi MZ and Pi SZ has also been related to the presence of chronic hepatitis and cirrhosis in adulthood [24, 26–28]. Heterozygotes for the Z variant, however, develop significant liver damage at more advanced ages than homozygotes [24]. Thus, AAT deficiency should be considered as a potential cause of chronic hepatitis and should be excluded in all patients with cryptogenic cirrhosis.

The prevalence of primary liver cancer is considerably increased in cirrhotic patients with AAT deficiency, both in homozygotes and in heterozygotes for the Z variant [21, 29–31]. The pathogenesis of this association is unknown. The risk is greater in males. Hormonal and exogenous factors may play a contributory role in the carcinogenic process.

### 3.1 Histopathology

Hepatocytes from homozygous ZZ patients contain eosinophilic cytoplasmic globules which are visible with hematoxylin and eosin staining and which localize preferentially in the periportal zone (Fig. 3). These globules, which range from 1 µm to 10 µm in diameter, exhibit a characteristic positive periodic acid-Schiff (PAS) staining after diastase treatment. Electron microscopy shows that they correspond to amorphous material contained mainly in dilated rough endoplasmic reticulum [32]. Globular inclusion bodies are composed of aggregated AAT protein and are stained positively by AAT-antiserum with immunofluorescence or immunoperoxidase techniques [32, 33].

In neonatal cholestasis, different types of lesions can be seen [32, 33]. Cholestasis is a predominant finding. Giant cell transformation of hepatocytes is less conspicuous than in other forms of neonatal hepatitis. Fibrosis can be present, either forming bridges or being limited to the portal area.

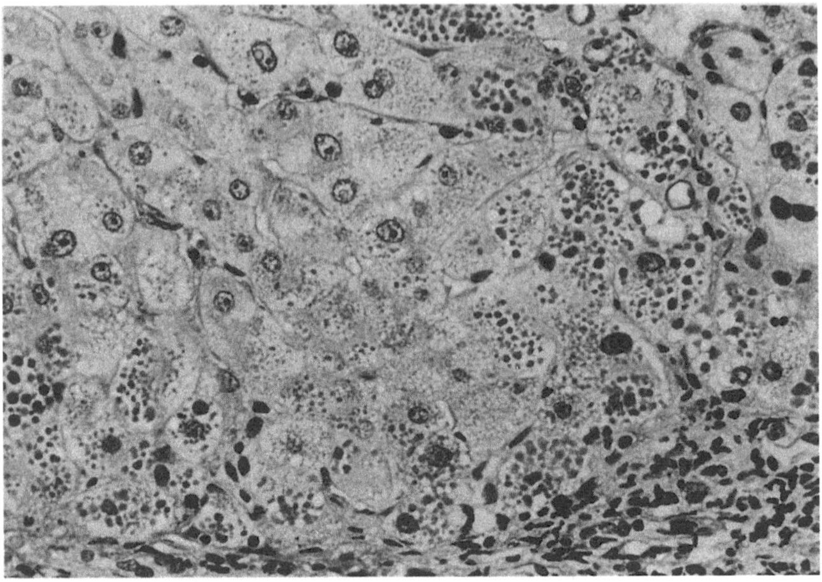

**Fig. 3.** AAT deficiency. Many liver cells contain numerous PAS-positive globules of different sizes. Hepatocytes near the fibrous septum contain larger and more numerous globules. PAS, ×400

Ductular hypoplasia or proliferation may be observed. It has been suggested that intense fibrosis and ductular proliferation are markers of poor prognosis [34].

In children and adults, cirrhosis may be of the macro- or micronodular variety.

### 3.2 Pathogenesis

In AAT deficiency, liver disease is restricted to subjects expressing the Z variant. Although it occurs primarily in ZZ homozygotes, it can also be present in MZ and SZ heterozygotes.

There is still debate as to the mechanism responsible for the associated liver damage. Two main theories have been advanced. The first proposes that liver damage is a consequence of the plasma deficiency of AAT that renders the liver cell more susceptible to the unopposed action of proteolytic enzymes [35]. The second view is based on the morphologic observation that in type Z homozygotes and heterozygotes there is an accumulation of AAT in hepatocytes forming cytoplasmic globules. This blockage in the transport of the Z variant is proposed to enhance lysosomal activity and proteolytic processes within the cell with ensuing hepatocellular damage and death [3]. The absence of liver disease in the rare Pi null homozygotes, which lack

AAT in serum but do not have accumulation of AAT globules in liver cells [14], supports the second view or "engorgement" hypothesis. However, the fact that AAT-deficient males are at higher risk of developing cirrhosis and the observation that some emphysematous Pi ZZ individuals possess cytoplasmic AAT globules in hepatocytes without accompanying liver damage suggest that additional hormonal, metabolic, or environmental factors are needed for liver disease to occur.

### 3.3 Diagnosis

The existence of AAT deficiency should be systematically excluded in all cases of neonatal cholestasis, as well as in cases of liver cirrhosis in children. AAT deficiency has also to be considered in the elucidation of the etiology of liver cirrhosis in adulthood, particularly if liver disease is associated with pulmonary emphysema. This diagnosis should be suspected if in the electrophoresis of serum there is a clear reduction of the $\alpha_1$-globulin band, of which AAT is the main component. Low serum levels of AAT can be confirmed using radial immunodiffusion or nephelometry methods. If AAT levels are diminished, the phenotype of AAT should be established by polyacrylamide gel isoelectric focusing. Family studies can then be performed.

Histologically, the diagnosis depends on finding cytoplasmic PAS positive globules in periportal hepatocytes. Immunofluorescence techniques, using AAT antiserum, are more sensitive in the detection of AAT globules than ordinary PAS staining [25].

### 3.4 Treatment

The emphysema of AAT deficiency is believed to result from insufficient serum levels of the antiprotease to protect against the destructive action of neutrophil elastase on alveolar structures. Taking this into consideration, the logical approach to therapy in this condition is to reduce the release of the elastase by avoiding smoking and to replace the missing inhibitor by intravenous administration of AAT derived from human plasma or obtained by recombinant technology [7]. However, the liver lesion associated with AAT deficiency may have a different pathogenesis. As mentioned above, it may result more from accumulation of AAT protein in liver cells than from reduced plasma antiprotease levels. If this is the case, plasma replacement therapy is unnecessary and attempts to increase serum levels of AAT with stimulants of its synthesis, such as danazol (a testosterone-like compound without androgenic properties), would be potentially dangerous [1].

Liver transplantation is the only rational approach to the treatment of the liver disease associated with AAT deficiency. This therapeutic modality has been carried out successfully in patients with advanced hepatic disease

[36]. The procedure corrects the metabolic disorder in such a way that, after transplantation, the phenotype of the recipient becomes that of the donor and AAT levels are restored to normal [36]. In adults, however, the advanced age of many individuals and the occasional presence of pulmonary emphysema limit the applicability of this therapeutic option [24].

## References


1. Carrell RW (1986) $\alpha_1$-Antitrypsin: molecular pathology, leucocytes and tissue damage. J Clin Invest 78:1427–1431
2. Brantly M, Nukiwa T, Crystal RG (1988) Molecular basis of $\alpha_1$-antitrypsin deficiency. Am J Med 84[Suppl 6A]:13–28
3. Carrell RW, Jeppsson JO, Laurell CB et al. (1982) Structure and variations of human $\alpha_1$-antitrypsin. Nature 298:329–334
4. Talamo RC (1975) Basic and clinical aspects of the $\alpha_1$-antitrypsin. Pediatrics 56:91–99
5. Sharp HL (1976) The current of $\alpha_1$-antitrypsin, a protease inhibitor in gastrointestinal disease. Gastroenterology 70:611–621
6. Makino S, Reed CE (1970) Distribution and elimination of exogenous $\alpha_1$-antitrypsin. J Lab Clin Med 75:742–746
7. Wewers MD, Casolaro MA, Sellers SE et al. (1987) Replacement therapy for $\alpha_1$-antitrypsin deficiency associated with emphysema. N Engl J Med 316:1055–1062
8. Darlington GJ, Astrin KH, Muirhead SP et al. (1982) Assignment of human $\alpha_1$-antitrypsin to chromosome 14 by somatic cell hybrid analysis. Proc Natl Acad Sci USA 79:870–873
9. Fagerhol MK, Braend M (1965) Serum prealbumen: polymorphism in man. Science 149:986–987
10. Hoffmann JJML, van den Broek WGM (1977) Application of isoelectric focusing in $\alpha_1$-antitrypsin phenotyping. Clin Chim Acta 75:233–242
11. Pierce JA, Eradio B, Dew TA (1975) Antitrypsin phenotypes in St. Louis. JAMA 231:609–612
12. Sveger T (1976) Liver disease in $\alpha_1$-antitrypsin deficiency detected by screening of 200 000 infants. N Engl J Med 294:1316–1321
13. O'Brien ML, Buist NRM, Murphey WH (1978) Neonatal screening for $\alpha_1$-antitrypsin deficiency. J Pediatr 92:1006–1010
14. Talamo RC, Langley CE, Reed CE et al. (1973) $\alpha_1$-Antitrypsin deficiency: a variant with no detectable alpha-1-antitrypsin. Science 181:70–71
15. Laurell CB, Eriksson S (1963) The electrophoretic $\alpha_1$-globulin pattern of serum in $\alpha_1$-antitrypsin deficiency. Scand J Clin Lab Invest 15:132–140
16. Hutchison DCS (1988) Natural history of $\alpha_1$-protease inhibitor deficiency. Am J Med 84[Suppl 6A]:3–12
17. Sharp HL, Bridges RA, Krivit W et al. (1969) Cirrhosis associated with $\alpha_1$-antitrypsin deficiency: a previously unrecognized inherited disorder. J Lab Clin Med 73:934–939
18. Porter CA, Mowat AP, Cook PJL et al. (1972) $\alpha_1$-Antitrypsin deficiency and neonatal hepatitis. Br Med J 3:435–439
19. Sveger T (1978) $\alpha_1$-Antitrypsin deficiency and early childhood. Pediatrics 62:22–25
20. Ghishan FK, Greene HL (1988) Liver disease in children with Pi ZZ $\alpha_1$-antitrypsin deficiency. Hepatology 8:307–310
21. Berg NO, Eriksson S (1972) Liver disease in adults with $\alpha_1$-antitrypsin deficiency. N Engl J Med 287:1264–1267

22. Larsson C (1978) Natural history and life expectancy in severe $\alpha_1$-antitrypsin deficiency Pi Z. Acta Med Scand 204:345–356
23. Cox DW, Smyth S (1983) Risk for liver disease in adults with $\alpha_1$-antitrypsin deficiency. Am J Med 74:221–227
24. Rakela J, Goldschmiedt M, Ludwig J (1987) Late manifestation of chronic liver disease in adults with $\alpha_1$-antitrypsin deficiency. Dig Dis Sci 32:1359–1362
25. Fisher RL, Taylor L, Sherlock S (1976) $\alpha_1$-Antitrypsin deficiency in liver disease: the extent of the problem. Gastroenterology 71:646–651
26. Campra JL, Graig JR, Peters RL et al. (1973) Cirrhosis associated with partial deficiency of $\alpha_1$-antitrypsin in an adult. Ann Intern Med 78:233–238
27. Hodges JR, Millward-Saaler GH, Barbatis C et al. (1981) Heterozygous MZ $\alpha_1$-antitrypsin deficiency in adults with chronic hepatitis and cryptogenic cirrhosis. N Engl J Med 304:557–560
28. Aliaga L, Sauras MA, Prieto J et al. (1988) Deficit de alfa-1-antitripsina. Alteraciones hepáticas asociadas a fenotipos diferentes del ZZ. Gastroenterol Hepatol 2:54–57
29. Eriksson S, Carlson J, Velez R (1986) Risk of cirrhosis and primary liver cancer in $\alpha_1$-antitrypsin deficiency. N Engl J Med 314:736–739
30. Rawlings W, Moss J, Cooper HS et al. (1974) Hepatocellular carcinoma and partial deficiency of $\alpha_1$-antitrypsin (MZ). Ann Intern Med 81:771–773
31. Carlson J, Eriksson S (1985) Chronic cryptogenic liver disease and malignant hepatoma in intermediate $\alpha_1$-antitrypsin deficiency identified by a Pi Z-specific monoclonal antibody. Scand J Gastroenterol 20:835–842
32. Ishak KG, Sharp HL (1987) Metabolic errors and liver disease. In: MacSween RNM, Anthony PP, Scheuer PJ (eds) Pathology of the liver. Churchill-Livingstone, Edinburgh, pp 118–123
33. Scheuer PJ (1988) Liver disease in childhood and heredofamilial disorders. In: Scheuer PJ (ed) Liver biopsy interpretation. Bailliere-Tindall, London, pp 196–197
34. Hadchouel M, Gautier M (1976) Histopathologic study of the liver in the early cholestatic phase of $\alpha_1$-antitrypsin deficiency. J Pediatr 89:211–215
35. Udall JN, Bloch KJ, Walker WA (1982) Transport of proteases across neonatal intestine and development of liver disease in infants with $\alpha_1$-antitrypsin deficiency. Lancet I:1441–1443
36. Hood JM, Koep LJ, Peters RL et al. (1980) Liver transplantation for advanced liver disease with $\alpha_1$-antitrypsin deficiency. N Engl J Med 302:272–275

# 26 The Porphyrias

J. Prieto and J. Camps

## 1 Introduction

The porphyrias represent a group of diseases which have in common an alteration in one of the steps of the biosynthesis of heme. Porphyrinogens and porphyrins are intermediates in this pathway. Heme or Fe-protoporphyrin IX is produced in all cells, but principally in the liver and bone marrow. In the liver it combines with apoproteins to form cytochrome P-450 and other heme proteins. In the bone marrow it binds to the globin moiety, giving rise to hemoglobin. Free porphyrins lack physiologic functions and in humans they are normally produced in only very low amounts as by-products of the biosynthesis of heme.

Defects in heme biosynthesis may be inherited or acquired, and each type of porphyria has a characteristic pattern of overproduction and hyper-excretion of porphyrins or porphyrin precursors.

## 2 Porphyrins and Porphyrinogens (Fig. 1)

Porphyrins are cyclic structures formed by four pyrrole rings. Carbon atoms 1–8 (Fisher numeration) have side chains attached to them. These side chains are four acetate and four propionate groups in uroporphyrin, four methyl and four propionate in coproporphyrin, and four methyl, two propionate, and two vinyl in protoporphyrin. Water solubility depends on the number of carboxyl substituents. Uroporphyrin, which possesses eight carboxyl groups, is water soluble and is excreted in urine when produced in excess. Coproporphyrin has four carboxyl substituents; it is soluble both in water and in ether and it can be found both in bile and in urine. Because protoporphyrin has only two carboxyl groups, it is scarcely hydrosoluble and is predominantly excreted in bile.

Since both uroporphyrin and coproporphyrin have two different types of side chain, these compounds have four possible isomers of which isomers I and III are present in nature and only isomer III is found in the heme biosynthetic pathway. Protoporphyrin has three different substituents and 15 possible isomers, isomer IX being the only one found in nature.

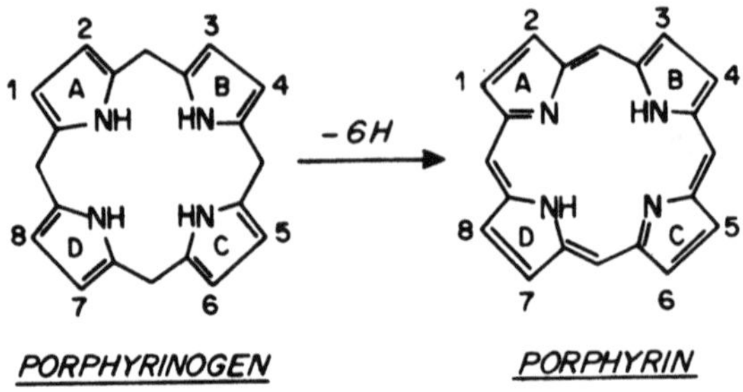


| | Substituents | | | | | | | |
|---|---|---|---|---|---|---|---|---|
| Carbon number | 1 | 2 | 3 | 4 | 5 | 6 | 7 | 8 |
| Uroporphyrinogen III | Ac | Pr | Ac | Pr | Ac | Pr | Pr | A |
| Uroporphyrinogen I | Ac | Pr | Ac | Pr | Ac | Pr | Ac | Pr |
| Coproporphyrinogen III | Met | Pr | Met | Pr | Met | Pr | Pr | Met |
| Coproporphyrinogen I | Met | Pr | Met | Pr | Met | Pr | Met | Pr |
| Protoporphyrin IX | Met | Vin | Met | Vin | Met | Pr | Pr | Met |

Ac = acetate , Pr = propionate , Met = methyl , Vin = Vinyl

**Fig. 1.** The biochemical structure of porphyrin and its precursors

The porphyrinogens, which are the reduced congeners of porphyrins, constitute the true tetrapyrrole intermediates of the heme biosynthetic pathway until the formation of protoporphyrin. Porphyrins result from the irreversible oxidation of porphyrinogens, a process that takes place spontaneously in urine and bile, but that can also occur intracellularly when porphyrinogens accumulate in excess.

Porphyrins absorb light at around 400 nm (Soret band) and emit intense red fluorescence. The gain in energy is transmitted to oxygen, resulting in the generation of oxygen free radicals that can induce tissue damage and complement activation [1]. This is the basis of the photosensitivity observed in different types of porphyria.

## 3 The Heme Biosynthetic Pathway (Fig. 2)

The first reaction of this pathway is the fusion of one molecule of glycine with one of succinyl-CoA to form δ-aminolevulinic acid (ALA). This reaction is catalyzed by the mitochondrial enzyme ALA synthase, which has a short life span and is considered to be the rate-controlling enzyme in heme biosynthesis [2]. The synthesis of ALA synthase and its activity in hepato-

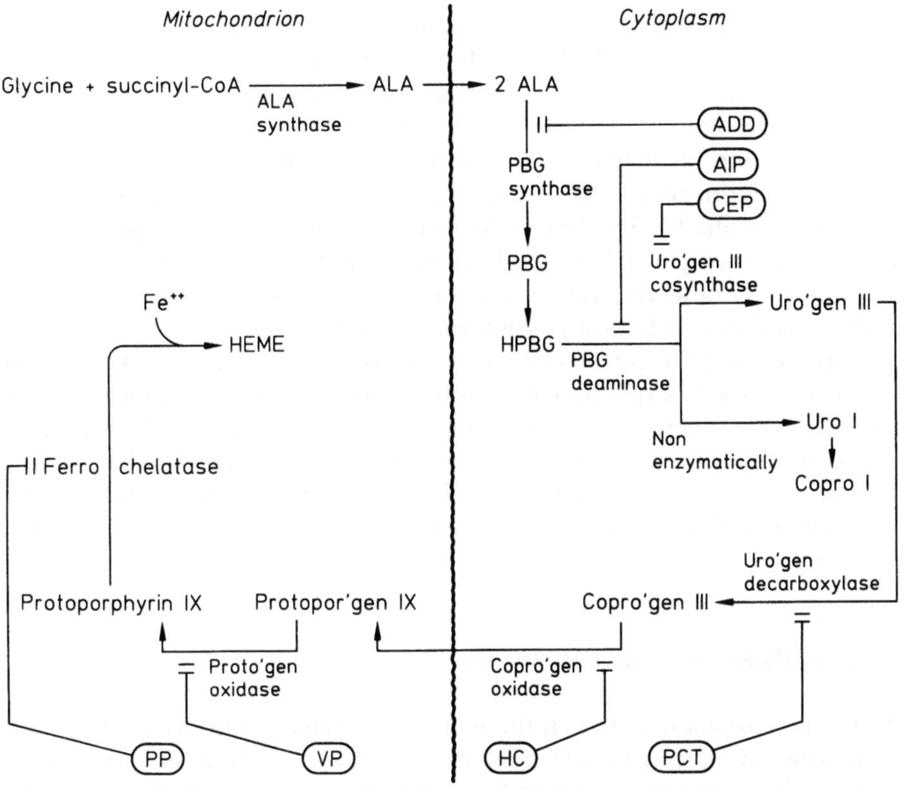


**Fig. 2.** The heme biosynthetic pathway. The enzymatic defect of each type of porphyria is represented. *AIP*, acute intermittent porphyria; *ADD*, δ-aminolevulinic acid dehydrase (PBG synthase) deficiency; *CEP*, congenital erythropoietic porphyria; *HC*, hereditary coproporphyria; *PCT*, porphyria cutanea tarda; *PP*, protoporphyria; *VP*, variegate porphyria

cytes is inhibited by heme, the end product of the pathway. It has been postulated that heme not only exists in hepatocytes as an integral part of heme proteins but also as a free heme regulatory pool. Changes in this pool influence ALA synthase activity and therefore the rate of the heme biosynthetic pathway. Agents that block heme formation or induce cytochrome P-450 synthesis reduce the heme regulatory pool and increase the concentration of ALA synthase and its activity. In contrast with the liver, in erythroid cells ALA synthase does not appear to play a significant role in the control of heme synthesis.

Two molecules of ALA condense in the cytoplasm to form the monopyrrole porphobilinogen (PBG). This reaction is mediated by the enzyme PBG synthase (also named ALA dehydrase). Four molecules of PBG join to yield uroporphyrinogen, a cyclic tetrapyrrole. This transformation takes place in two steps. The first is catalyzed by the enzyme PBG deaminase, which generates a linear tetrapyrrole named hydroxymethylbilane.

The second step consists in the cyclization of this compound, which can take place spontaneously, with the resulting formation of uroporphyrinogen I, or through the action of the enzyme uroporphyrinogen III cosynthase, generating uroporphyrinogen III. Uroporphyrinogens undergo stepwise decarboxylation mediated by the enzyme uroporphyrinogen decarboxylase. Thus, porphyrinogens with seven, six, five, and four carboxyl groups are formed sequentially. The last of these compounds is coproporphyrinogen. Coproporphyrinogen III is used in the synthesis of heme. Coproporphyrinogen I, however, represents the last metabolite of the "aberrant" pathway and has no known physiologic functions.

Coproporphyrinogen oxidase acts on coproporphyrinogen III to yield the two carboxyl porphyrinogen, protoporphyrinogen IX. In this reaction the metabolic pathway of heme formation reenters the mitochondrion, where protoporphyrinogen oxidase catalyzes the oxidation of protoporphyrinogen to protoporphyrin IX. Finally ferrochelatase facilitates the incorporation of iron in the protoporphyrin ring, yielding Fe-protoporphyrin IX or heme.

## 4 Classification of the Porphyrias

A specific enzymatic defect in the heme biosynthetic pathway accompanies each form of porphyria and explains its specific pattern of biochemical abnormalities. The expression of the defect may occur mainly in the liver, in erythroid cells, or in both. Therefore, three main types of porphyria can be distinguished, depending on the site of accumulation of the excess of porphyrins, or porphyrin precursors, formed as a result of the enzymatic blockade. These three types are erythropoietic, hepatic, and erythrohepatic porphyria (Table 1).

**Table 1.** Classification of the porphyrias

| |
|---|
| *Erythropoietic* |
| Congenital erythropoietic porphyria (autosomal recessive; very rare) |
| Erythropoietic coproporphyria (exceedingly rare) |
| *Hepatic* |
| a) With acute neurovisceral attacks |
| Acute intermittent porphyria (autosomal dominant) |
| ALA dehydrase deficiency (autosomal recessive; very rare) |
| Hereditary coproporphyria (autosomal dominant) |
| Variegate porphyria (autosomal dominant; frequent in S. Africa) |
| b) Without acute neurovisceral attacks |
| Porphyria cutanea tarda (autosomal dominant or sporadic; common) |
| *Erythrohepatic* |
| Protoporphyria (autosomal dominant with variable penetrance) |

Two forms of erythropoietic porphyria are known: the rare Günther disease or congenital erythropoietic porphyria and the extremely uncommon erythropoietic coproporphyria. The former is due to a decreased activity of uroporphyrinogen III cosynthase and is inherited in an autosomal recessive fashion. This disease manifests in infancy as hemolysis and cutaneous photosensitivity causing facial mutilation. Increased urinary excretion of uroporphyrin I, overproduced in erythroid cells, and fluorescent normoblasts in the bone marrow are also found. In two patients in whom cDNA from uroporphyrinogen III cosynthase was analyzed, a point mutation in codon 53 was discovered which led to replacement of proline by leucine [3]. Erythropoietic porphyrias are not considered further in this chapter.

Hepatic porphyrias are characterized by increased production of heme precursors in liver cells and can be subdivided into two main categories, according to clinical and biochemical features (Table 1). The first main subdivision of the hepatic porphyrias comprises those entities which can present acute neurovisceral attacks as a consequence of enhanced production of the porphyrin precursors ALA and PBG. These entities are acute intermittent porphyria, ALA dehydrase deficiency, hereditary coproporphyria, and variegate porphyria. The second subdivision of hepatic porphyrias comprises conditions without acute neurovisceral attacks. The only representative of this subgroup is porphyria cutanea tarda.

The third type of porphyrias are the erythrohepatic porphyrias, which have as a defining feature the combination of porphyrin overproduction in erythroid cells and porphyrin deposition in liver parenchyma. The representative of this category is protoporphyria.

The porphyrias can also be classified according to the inherited or acquired nature of the basic enzymatic defect. With the sole exception of porphyria cutanea tarda, which can be acquired or inherited, the rest of these porphyrias are inherited as mendelian autosomal dominant or recessive traits (Table 1).

Finally, porphyric patients can be categorized according to the phenotypic expressiveness of the enzymatic abnormality that causes the porphyric condition. Thus, there are carriers of the enzymatic deficiency who do not show hyperexcretion of heme precursors, others overproduce porphyrins or porphyrin precursors but do not express the disease clinically and are referred to as having "latent porphyria", and finally others display both the clinical and the biochemical features of the disease and are said to have "manifest porphyria".

## 5 Hepatic Porphyrias with Acute Neurovisceral Attacks

As mentioned above, this group includes acute intermittent porphyria, hereditary coproporphyria, variegate porphyria, and ALA dehydrase deficiency. The last condition will not be considered in detail since it is a very uncommon process, with only three cases having been described up until 1988 [4]. Its clinical features are similar to those of acute intermittent porphyria, from which it differs in the pattern of urinary excretion of porphyrin precursors (increased ALA and PBG in acute intermittent porphyria and a selective increase in ALA in ALA dehydrase deficiency).

## 5.1 Acute Intermittent Porphyria

Acute intermittent porphyria (AIP) is due to a defect in PBG deaminase, inherited as an autosomal dominant trait. AIP is genetically a heterogeneous disease, since it can stem from different types of mutations. Thus, while some patients exhibit reduced PBG deaminase concentration (91% of gene carriers), others show a normal concentration but reduced enzyme activity (9% of carriers) [5]. The structural gene encoding PBG deaminase has been localized at the long arm of chromosome 11 [6] and seems to be transcribed from two different promoters, to produce erythroid and nonerythroid mRNAs that differ at their 5′ ends. This explains why some AIP carriers have normal PBG deaminase activity in red cells, but reduced activity in the liver [7].

### *Clinical Findings and Pathogenesis*

The main clinical feature of AIP is the acute neurovisceral attack [2, 8]. These acute episodes may be very difficult to differentiate from acute intra-abdominal processes. Patients complain of abdominal pain, frequently accompanied by nausea, vomiting, and constipation but not by physical signs of peritoneal irritation. On occasions the pain is felt in the back, chest, or thighs. Radiography may reveal bowel dilatation. Signs of autonomic dysfunction such as mydriasis, sinus tachycardia, hypertension, sweating, and loss of sphincter control are often present. The degree of tachycardia is a good index of the severity of the attack and of its evolution. Neurologic and neuropsychiatric manifestations are common and may represent the clue to the correct diagnosis. Seizures, motor neuropathy (with or without cranial nerve involvement), and respiratory failure are among the neurologic features of acute porphyric attacks. Memory and concentration difficulties, anxiety, and depression are not infrequent in acute episodes and in certain cases they may become chronic. In fact, carriers of AIP are more prevalent in psychiatric communities than in the general population [9].

Acute neurovisceral attacks are associated with overproduction and increased urinary excretion of PBG and ALA as a result of the enzymatic blockade in the conversion of PBG to hydroxymethylbilane. This block is also responsible for the increased ALA synthase activity observed in the liver of patients with active AIP [10]. As a general rule, in AIP urinary levels of PBG exceed those of ALA. PBG polymerizes in urine exposed to sunlight, yielding porphobilin, which causes a characteristic darkening of the urine on standing. No structural changes are observed in the liver in these patients.

Different theories have been advanced to explain the mechanism of pain and neurodysfunction in AIP. While some authors propose that neurologic symptoms are due to reduced heme availability in the nervous system, others maintain that ALA and PBG have a neurotoxic role. The hypothesis of the neurotoxicity of ALA is favored by the observation that neurodysfunction occurs in lead poisoning and in ALA dehydrase deficiency [11], conditions in which ALA is formed in higher amounts than PBG.

### *Precipitants of the Attacks*

Inducers of cytochrome P-450, such as barbiturates or hydantoins, deplete the intracellular heme regulatory pool and increase ALA synthase activity, hence having the potential to precipitate acute porphyric attacks. On the other hand, endogenous steroids such as estrogens may stimulate ALA synthase activity directly [12] and this would explain why attacks appear almost exclusively after puberty and are more frequent in the premenstrual period [2, 13]. Fasting is another factor that may exacerbate AIP, while, in contrast, glucose attenuates ALA synthase induction [14].

### *Detection of Carriers*

In the general population, AIP carriers are more prevalent (around 5 per 100000) than patients with manifest disease. In fact, it has been estimated that less than 20% of those who inherit the enzyme deficiency will have symptoms [15]. Detection of asymptomatic carriers is therefore important to avoid exposure to precipitating factors, thus preventing potentially lethal porphyric attacks. Screening tests for PBG such as the Watson-Schwartz or the Hoesch test (both based on the reaction of PBG with Ehrlich's reagent) are not sensitive enough outside the acute episode. More sensitive liquid chromatography techniques may be used to quantify urinary PBG levels, which are elevated in many AIP patients during quiescent periods. Urinanalysis, however, may be normal in some carriers [16]. In these cases the determination of PBG deaminase activity in erythrocytes is one of the most specific and sensitive tests available [17]. Since a minority of carriers may have normal PBG deaminase in erythrocytes (although reduced in the liver), it has been recommended that ALA synthase be measured in leukocytes together with PBG deaminase in red blood cells [18]. Increased values of the former and/or reduced activity of the latter suggest the disease. Recently, specific mutations of the PBG deaminase gene have been described in patients with AIP [19]. Hybridization analysis using the specific oligonucleotide probes, after in vitro amplification of genomic DNA, offers the possibility of detecting asymptomatic carriers of the mutation in affected families.

### *Management*

Management of acute attacks of porphyria [20] necessitates admission to hospital, since serious complications may develop within a short time. First, it is important to eliminate drugs that could be inducers of the attack (see Table 2). Glucose must be given to reverse the fasting state which develops as a consequence of anorexia and vomiting. The recommended dose is between 300 and 400 g in 24 h. It can be administered intravenously with a central catheter using hypertonic solutions to avoid dilutional hypo-

**Table 2.** Common drugs considered to be safe or unsafe in acute porphyrias[a]

| Safe | Unsafe |
|---|---|
| Acetaminophen | Aminoglutethimide |
| Acyclovir | Barbiturates |
| Allopurinol | Carbamazepine |
| Aminoglycosides | Clonidine |
| Amitriptyline | Danazol |
| Aspirin | Diclophenac |
| Atropine | Diphenylhydantoin |
| Bromides | Ergot preparations |
| Colchicine | Erythromycin |
| Dicumarol | Estrogens |
| Digoxin | Glutethimide |
| Epinephrine | Griseofulvin |
| Glucocorticoids | Hydralazine |
| Heparin | Meprobamate |
| Ibuprofen | Methyldopa |
| Insulin | Nalidixic acid |
| Lithium | Novobiocin |
| Methylphenidate | Pentazocine |
| Naproxen | Phenylbutazone |
| Narcotic analgesics | Progestins |
| Neostigmine | Pyrazinamide |
| Penicillamine | Rifampicin |
| Penicillin and derivatives | Spironolactone |
| Phenothiazines | Succinimides |
| Procaine | Sulfonamide antibiotics |
| Propranolol (β-blockers) | Tolbutamide |
| Succinylcholine | Trimethadione |
| Tetracycline | Valproic acid |
| Thiouracil | |
| Thyroxine | |
| Tubocurarine | |
| Vitamins B and C | |

[a] For a more complete list see ref. 2

natremia. This treatment alone brings about remission in some cases. It is advisable to begin treatment with hematin if there is no response to glucose administration in 48 h. This product, derived from heme, increases the intracellular pool of heme and reduces ALA synthase activity. Hematin (4 mg/kg body weight) is infused intravenously in 100–200 ml of isotonic saline for 30–45 min. This dose may be repeated in 4 days.

In sedation chlorpromazine is a useful drug. In a recent study [21] inhibition of luteinizing hormone and follicle-stimulating hormone secretion with gonadotropin-releasing hormone analogues succeeded in preventing premenstrual exacerbations of AIP.

## 5.2 Other Acute Porphyrias: Hereditary Coproporphyria and Variegate Porphyria

Hereditary coproporphyria (HC) and variegate porphyria (VP) are inherited in an autosomal dominant fashion. They share with AIP the occurrence of acute neurovisceral attacks precipitated by similar factors and with identical clinical features (abdominal, neurologic, and psychiatric symptoms). During these episodes, there is in both HC and VP, as in AIP, overproduction and increased urinary excretion of ALA and PBG. In addition to acute attacks, HC and VP are characterized by the presence of cutaneous photosensitivity. This manifestation, which is absent in AIP, results from excessive production of formed porphyrins.

In HC the enzyme primarily affected is coproporphyrinogen oxidase [22]. As a consequence, coproporphyrin III accumulates in the liver and is excreted in high amounts in bile, and consequently in feces. In VP there is a deficiency of protoporphyrinogen oxidase [23]. This defect is responsible for overproduction of protoporphyrin and to a lesser extent of coproporphyrin, which are excreted in excess in feces. Therefore these two entities, which have many clinical similarities, may be distinguished by the different pattern of fecal excretion of porphyrins, coproporphyrin being the predominant compound excreted in HC and protoporphyrin in VP (Table 3).

Since copro- and protoporphyrin are directly transported from hepatocytes into the bile, the amounts of these substrates which are available for the corresponding deficient oxidase may not suffice to ensure adequate heme synthesis in situations of augmented demand for heme formation (e.g., induction of cytochrome P-450). In these situations depletion of the heme pool would induce ALA synthase and acute attacks might supervene.

Accumulation of porphyrins in liver cells makes liver biopsies fluoresce when exposed to near-ultraviolet light. However, no other consistent liver changes are observed in either of the two conditions [24, 25]. Deposition of porphyrins in the skin, by contrast, causes photosensitivity in 30%–80% of the patients, manifested by vesiculous eruptions, skin fragility, hypo- or hyperpigmentation, and hypertrichosis in areas exposed to sunlight.

**Table 3.** Pattern of porphyrin and porphyrin precursor excretion in urine and/or feces in the hepatic and erythrohepatic porphyrias

| | Urine | Feces |
|---|---|---|
| Acute intermittent porphyria | ALA, PBG | |
| ALA dehydrase deficiency | ALA | |
| Hereditary coproporphyria[a] | COPRO | COPRO |
| Variegate porphyria[a] | | COPRO; PROTO |
| Porphyria cutanea tarda | URO; 7, 6, 5, and 4 COOH-P | URO; COPRO |
| Protoporphyria[b] | | PROTO |

ALA, δ-aminolevulinic acid; PBG, porphobilinogen; COPRO, coproporphyrin; PROTO, protoporphyrin; URO, uroporphyrin; 7, 6, 5, and 4 COOH-P, hepta, hexa, penta, and tetra carboxyporphyrins

[a] In acute episodes there are elevations of ALA and PBG in urine

[b] There is an associated increase in PROTO in red cells; in this condition COPRO increases in urine if hepatobiliary disease develops

Treatment of the acute attack should be along the same lines as in AIP. In patients who present photosensitivity, β-carotene may be beneficial [26]. This compound inactivates free radicals, thus blocking the initiation of the inflammatory reaction. Topical sunscreens should also be used.

## 6 Hepatic Porphyrias without Acute Neurovisceral Attacks

This group encompasses only one entity: porphyria cutanea tarda. This disorder is characterized by cutaneous photosensitivity, liver damage of variable intensity, and absence of acute porphyric crises.

### 6.1 Porphyria Cutanea Tarda

Porphyria cutanea tarda (PCT), the most common alteration of porphyrin metabolism in the Western world, was first described by Waldeström in 1937 [27]. The basic metabolic defect is a reduced activity of hepatic uroporphyrinogen decarboxylase (UROD), the enzyme which catalyzes the stepwise decarboxylation of the octocarboxylic uroporphyrinogen to the tetracarboxylic coproporphyrinogen. As a consequence uroporphyrin and to a lesser extent hepta-, hexa- and pentacarboxylporphyrins accumulate in the liver and are excreted in excess in urine (Table 3). Fecal excretion of uroporphyrin and coproporphyrin may also be increased. Decarboxylation of pentacarboxylporphyrin by coproporphyrinogen decarboxylase yields dehydroisocoproporphyrin, which can be found in the feces of patients with PCT.

### *Heterogenicity of PCT*

Porphyria cutanea tarda is not a single disorder but a group of conditions which share a decreased activity of hepatic UROD.

A disturbance of porphyrin metabolism similar to that observed in patients with PCT can be induced experimentally in rats by administration of chemicals, such as hexachlorobenzene, that inhibit hepatic UROD. Between 1955 and 1959 approximately 4000 people in southeast Anatolia developed severe PCT due to the ingestion of hexachlorobenzene, which had been used as a fungicide added to wheat seedlings [28]. Nowadays, cases of toxic PCT are very rarely encountered.

The two main types of PCT are the so-called familial and sporadic forms.

Familial PCT is inherited in an autosomal dominant fashion. It is characterized by a parallel reduction in the activity and concentration of UROD to half of normal values. This defect is encountered in both liver cells and erythrocytes [29–31]. The homozygous condition of the familial PCT defect is the very rare hepatoerythropoietic porphyria, in which UROD levels are 5%–10% of normal values [32].

Familial PCT itself is not a homogeneous disease. In some pedigrees a point mutation in the UROD gene causing single amino acid substitution and reduced half-life of the enzyme has been described [33]. Recently, a few families have been identified in which UROD activity in erythrocytes was found to be normal, suggesting that autosomal genes not at the UROD locus, but influencing the activity of this enzyme in liver cells, may be important in the development of PCT [34].

In sporadic PCT, the more common of the two forms, UROD activity is normal in erythrocytes but diminished in hepatocytes during clinically active periods. In these periods, the reduction in hepatic UROD activity is not accompanied by a decrease in the immunoreactive levels of the enzyme. During clinical remission hepatic UROD activity returns to normal or near normal levels [29]. In familial PCT, by contrast, the remission does not normalize UROD activity [29].

### *Pathogenesis*

In both sporadic and familial PCT, the clinical expression of the disease depends on acquired factors that block or further depress UROD activity. In agreement with this concept is the observation that in familial PCT the majority of individuals with reduced UROD levels do not have clinically apparent disease [35].

Formation of free radicals in liver cells is a process which has been shown to inactivate UROD [36]. In fact, the porphyrogenic effect of hexachlorobenzene is simultaneous with and parallel to its ability to induce free radical formation and subsequent lipid peroxidation in the liver [37].

Thus, it is thought that free radical-forming agents may unmask PCT. For these agents to induce the disease, it would be necessary to have either low basal levels of UROD in the liver (as occurs in familial PCT) or a defect in the metabolic mechanisms that neutralize UROD-inactivating factors (as may be the case in sporadic PCT).

The three main acquired factors incriminated in the overt expression of PCT are iron, alcohol, and estrogens.

Iron appears to play a significant role in the pathogenesis of PCT. Moderate siderosis is frequently found in this disease [38], and reduction of liver storage iron by phlebotomy leads to remission [39] which can be reversed by oral iron administration [40]. Iron can inhibit UROD directly and also indirectly through its ability to facilitate the formation of oxygen free radicals [36]. An oxidative reaction mediated by iron in the active center of UROD might be responsible for its inactivation. However, iron by itself does not cause PCT, since this condition is not observed in association with conditions involving marked iron overload such as idiopathic hemochromatosis. As mentioned above, it is believed that a concurrent defect in UROD or in mechanisms preventing its inactivation (production of cellular antioxidants?) might be necessary for the expression of the disease. On the other hand, the cause of hepatic siderosis in PCT is a matter of debate. The finding of a higher prevalence of hemochromatosis-linked HLA antigens in PCT than in the general population has suggested that hepatic siderosis might be due to the associated inheritance of a hemochromatosis allele [41].

Alcohol is an additional factor which has been implicated in the exacerbation of PCT. Excessive alcohol consumption is very often present in patients with this disease. Alcohol has been shown to inhibit UROD [42] and to facilitate iron absorption [43]. Estrogen administration for carcinoma of the prostate, or for contraceptive purposes, has also been reported to precipitate or aggravate PCT [2]. The mechanism of the porphyrogenic effect of estrogens is imperfectly understood. Many nonspecific insults to the liver might affect UROD activity, partly through the formation of free radicals. Thus, PCT has been observed to be associated with a variety of liver conditions, viral infections, metabolic disturbances, and systemic diseases, including hepatitis B [44], AIDS [45], uremia [46], diabetes mellitus [47], and lupus erythematosus [48].

### *Clinical Findings*

The mean age of presentation is around 40 years in sporadic PCT and somewhat earlier in the familial type. The two forms of the disease share the same clinical picture [49]. The dominant finding is the presence of cutaneous lesions in sun-exposed areas, including the dorsum of hands, the face, and arms. Skin fragility is increased in these regions, where well-defined erosions, crusts, and small atrophic scars can be observed (Fig. 3a). Hyper- or hypopigmentation of the skin with a mottled distribution may be present.

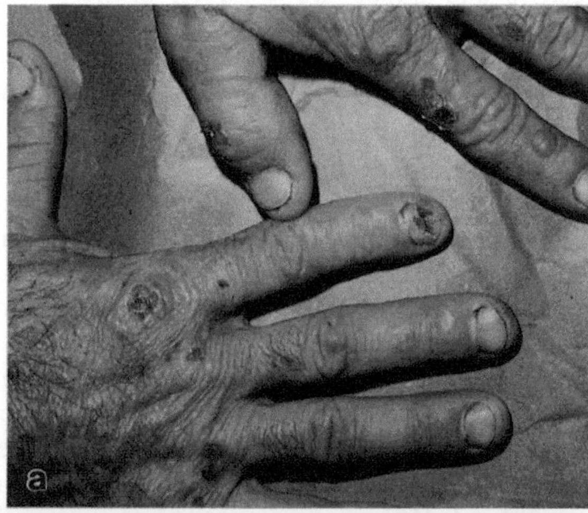

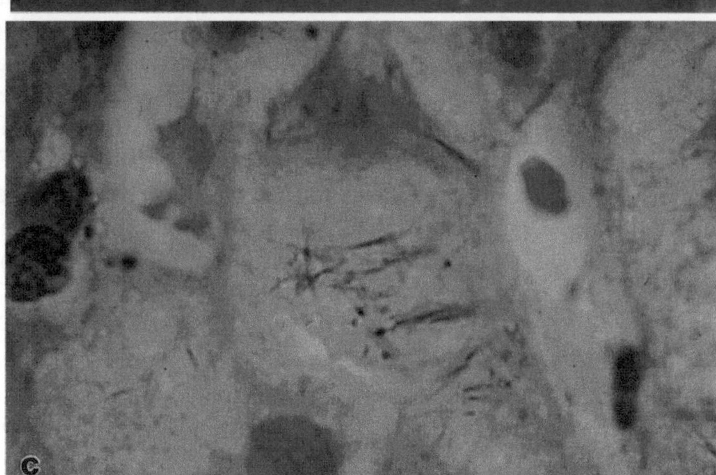

**Fig. 3a–c.** Porphyria cutanea tarda. **a** Cutaneous lesions on the dorsum of the hands. Vesicles, crusts, atrophic scarring, and erosions can be seen. **b** Red fluorescence of hepatic tissue under ultraviolet light. **c** Needle-like cytoplasmic inclusions of porphyrins in hepatocytes

Vesicles and bullae are common primary lesions occurring after minor trauma. Many patients are unaware of the association between sun exposure and development of new skin lesions. Facial hypertrichosis is frequently noticeable. Hair may grow in periorbital regions, between eyebrows, and between eyebrows and the scalp at the temples. Sclerodermoid plaques may develop on the face and hands.

The presence of increased levels of uroporphyrin (isomer I) and heptacarboxylporphyrin (isomer III) in urine, and of isocoproporphyrin in feces, is the biochemical hallmark of PCT. The majority of patients (about 60%) show slight or moderate elevation of aminotransferases, while alkaline phosphatase and $\gamma$-glutamyltransferase are less often increased. Values of aspartate aminotransferase are higher in those patients in whom alcohol ingestion is an associated factor [49]. Hypersideremia and hepatic siderosis are frequently found in PCT [50, 51]; however, iron stores are only moderately increased in this disease, not surpassing two to three times normal levels [52].

Liver damage is of variable intensity [53–55]. Many patients exhibit nonspecific changes, including fatty infiltration, mild portal or periportal inflammation, focal necrosis, and slight fibrosis. In some cases liver histology is normal, but others show chronic active hepatitis or cirrhosis. Because of the high uroporphyrin content, liver biopsy exhibits red fluorescence when illuminated with ultraviolet lamp (Fig. 3b). Needle-like cytoplasmic inclusions may be observed when precautions are taken to avoid dissolution of these hydrosoluble structures (Fig. 3c).

The pathogenesis of the liver lesion in PCT remains obscure. The wide spectrum of liver damage observed suggests that accumulated porphyrins may not have a direct hepatotoxic action. Chronic alcohol ingestion increases the likelihood of hepatocellular injury, but liver disease is also found in the absence of ethanol consumption [56, 57]. Iron is unlikely to be the only factor, since iron overload is not marked and liver damage can be observed without accompanying siderosis [58]. Serum antibodies directed against porphyric hepatocytes, but not against normal hepatocytes, have been detected in patients with PCT and significant liver disease [53]. This finding has suggested that porphyrins might act as haptens in the induction of an immune response against hepatocellular constituents. Finally, it must be considered that in some cases the liver lesion (of unrelated cause) might be the primary event and PCT secondary to hepatocellular injury (that would result in UROD inactivation in susceptible individuals).

### *Treatment*

The therapeutic approach consists essentially in the avoidance of ethanol and estrogens, combined with phlebotomies and administration of low doses of chloroquine.

Phlebotomies, by mobilizing parenchymal iron, reduce urinary porphyrin levels and induce clinical remission [59]. Usually 450 ml of blood is withdrawn for each phlebotomy, and approximately 12 phlebotomies are performed to remove 3–4 g of iron. Initially blood extractions may be carried out every week, and later every other week or monthly. Treatment should be individualized and guided by the hemoglobin level and by the concentration of serum ferritin. Phlebotomies must be interrupted if hemoglobin falls to 11 g/dl or if biochemical remission is achieved. This frequently occurs when iron stores are depleted (serum ferritin less than 10 ng/ml).

Phlebotomy is contraindicated in anemic patients or in those with cardiopulmonary disorders. In these cases, the administration of low doses of chloroquine (250 mg twice a week) is of benefit [60]. Chloroquine forms soluble complexes with porphyrins and facilitates urinary excretion of these compounds. However, at higher doses chloroquine may induce an acute exacerbation of the liver lesion. In the black population the deficiency of glucose-6-phosphate dehydrogenase should be excluded to avoid chloroquine-induced hemolytic crises. Periodic ophthalmologic examination is advisable in long-term treatments.

## 7 Erythrohepatic Porphyria or Protoporphyria

Protoporphyria is a relatively common form of porphyria, second only to PCT in frequency. Formerly it was included among erythropoietic porphyrias, but now it is more appropriately considered as erythrohepatic [61]. Protoporphyria is inherited in an autosomal dominant fashion, and results from a deficiency of the enzyme ferrochelatase [62]. Many carriers are asymptomatic. Its main clinical manifestation is cutaneous photosensitivity. However, the liver is frequently involved, and at times the liver lesion is rapidly progressive.

### *Biochemistry and Pathogenesis*

Biochemically the ferrochelatase defect results in increased concentrations of protoporphyrin in erythrocytes, plasma, bile, and feces. Unlike several other forms of porphyria, urinary porphyrin levels are not elevated. Protoporphyrin is scarcely water soluble and therefore it is not excreted in urine. Thus, it is the liver which is the organ responsible for its excretion from the body. Although in some cases the liver may contribute to the overproduction of protoporphyrin, in the majority of patients the main sources of the excess of protoporphyrin are the normoblasts in the bone marrow and the newly released reticulocytes [63, 64].

An increase in free intraerythrocytic protoporphyrin is also observed in ferropenia. In this condition, however, protoporphyrin in excess is chelated with zinc, while this does not happen in protoporphyria owing to the defective function of ferrochelatase. While zinc protoporphyrin remains inside the red cells, free protoporphyrin diffuses to plasma and is taken up by liver cells for its secretion into bile [65, 66].

In protoporphyria the decreased ferrochelatase activity is present in all tissues and, although hepatic ALA synthase activity has been found to be increased [67], acute porphyric attacks do not occur, probably because of a compensatory elevation in the activity of PBG deaminase [65].

Photoexcitation of free protoporphyrin in the skin leads to the generation of reactive oxygen species [68] and to the activation of complement [69]. These processes appear to be related to the dermatologic manifestations of this disease. In some patients with protoporphyria, a marked accumulation of protoporphyrin takes place in the liver. This occurs when the biliary excretion of protoporphyrin is lower than the load of this substance presented to the liver [70]. In these circumstances, solid deposits of protoporphyrin are formed within hepatocytes, in Kupffer cells, and in small biliary ducts. Deposits in liver cells induce cell damage and in bile canaliculi cause cholestasis. Cholestasis, by reducing biliary excretion of protoporphyrin, initiates a vicious circle which tends to increase red cell and plasma levels of protoporphyrin and to facilitate a progressive deposition of this substance in the liver. This mechanism explains why in some cases fatal hepatic failure supervenes only some months after initial detection of abnormal liver function tests.

### *Clinical Findings*

The most frequently reported symptom is a burning or stinging sensation in the skin followed by erythema or edema, soon after exposure to sunlight. This occurs mainly on the face and arms, and also may happen upon exposure to artificial lights. The symptoms abate in fall and winter, and may consist only in subjective sensations without objective cutaneous lesions. This may result in the incorrect diagnosis of psychogenic pruritus. Chronic dermatologic changes are milder and less common than those of PCT. Bullae, skin fragility, hypertrichosis, and hyperpigmentation are unusual in protoporphyria. However, petechiae, vesicles, and crusting may develop after sun exposure.

Liver involvement occurs in protoporphyria more frequently than has previously been reported. When present, the liver lesion may show variable degrees of severity. In some patients it is manifested by slight changes in biochemical liver function tests. Other cases show hepatic fibrosis or cirrhosis. In a minority of patients, progressive cholestasis and fatal hepatic failure develop within a relatively short time. In a recent study comprising 55 patients, impaired liver function was found in 35%, cirrhosis was present in 13%, and two patients (aged 20 and 22 years) died from fatal liver disease [61].

Patients with advanced liver disease may exhibit hepatomegaly, signs of portal hypertension, jaundice, and encephalopathy. Laboratory tests reveal hypoalbuminemia, variable hyperbilirubinemia, and moderate increases in aminotransferases and alkaline phosphatase. In these patients the liver is nodular due to cirrhosis and black in color due to massive deposits of a dark brown pigment in hepatocytes, Kupffer cells, and biliary canaliculi [70, 71]. These pigment deposits, which are composed of protoporphyrin, exhibit a characteristic birefringence when viewed under polarized light. The fibrous septa separating nodules contain numerous lymphocytes, monocytes, and proliferating ductules. Liver tissue displays red fluorescence under Wood's light.

In cases of less advanced liver damage, lobular structure is preserved but enlarged portal triads show mild fibrosis, mononuclear infiltration, and ductular proliferation. The same birefringent intracanalicular deposits are evident, although less numerous. Subtle liver changes are found in many patients. The risk of progression to cirrhosis in these cases has not been established. In patients with normal liver histology, fine ultrastructural changes can be observed, indicating that the liver is involved even in early stages of the disease [72].

Gallstones with a high content of protoporphyrin are found in about 10% of patients [68]. Most of these stones produce symptoms at an unusually early age.

The diagnosis of protoporphyria is based on clinical suspicion in a patient complaining of photosensitivity. It is confirmed by the determination of free protoporphyrin in feces, plasma, and red cells. The presence of protoporphyrin in both plasma and erythrocytes is specific to protoporphyria. In this condition, fluorescence of peripheral reticulocytes is a simple study which suggests the diagnosis.

### *Treatment*

Avoidance of sun exposure and the use of topical sunscreens should be advised. β-Carotene administration (oral doses of 120–180 mg daily) may afford systemic photoprotection, probably by neutralizing oxygen free radicals [2, 68]. Vitamin E has proved to be less effective against photosensitivity than β-carotene.

In treating and preventing protoporphyria hepatopathy, four goals should be pursued: firstly to identify those subjects at risk of developing significant liver damage; secondly, to reduce protoporphyrin production; thirdly, to improve biliary secretion of protoporphyrin; finally, to interrupt the enterohepatic circulation of protoporphyrin [70].

Since the course of the liver lesion is very insidious until decompensation occurs, any patient with abnormal liver function tests should be biopsied and closely observed. When liver damage is significant, protoporphyrin decreases in bile and feces and increases further in plasma and red cells. These biochemical changes are, however, found in fairly advanced liver disease. Perhaps early preventive treatment should be instituted in those patients with high biliary and fecal protoporphyrin output, since this reflects a higher load to the liver and probably a greater risk of developing parenchymal damage [70]. Recently, it has been proposed that increased urinary coproporphyrin (mainly isomer I) might be a sensitive and early marker of liver involvement in protoporphyria and therefore an indication for active treatment [61]. Coproporphyrinuria is a consequence of cholestasis since this process, even when mild, reduces coproporphyrin secretion into bile, facilitating its urinary excretion.

To reduce protoporphyrin synthesis different approaches have been used. Hematin administration has been shown to be effective in suppressing protoporphyrin overproduction, both in the liver and in bone marrow. This effect was associated with an improvement in liver function tests in some patients [73]. Similarly, an amelioration of cholestasis was obtained in selected cases through the combination of plasma exchange and blood transfusions [74]. The former alleviates the protoporphyrin load to the liver, while the latter reduces protoporphyrin production by restraining erythropoiesis.

Since ferropenia enhances protoporphyrin synthesis, intensive iron therapy has been tried in some patients. Although this treatment was found to be effective in isolated cases [75], in others it induced an exacerbation of the dermatopathy and an increase in plasma protoporphyrin levels [76].

Choleretic bile salts, such as chenodeoxycholic acid, facilitate bile excretion of protoporphyrin [77] and appear to stimulate its conversion to heme [78]. Thus, the use of these substances is an attractive therapeutic option, which should be further evaluated. On the other hand, cholestyramine and activated charcoal can both bind protoporphyrin in the intestinal lumen. They can be given to patients with liver damage or high biliary output of protoporphyrin to interrupt the enterohepatic circulation of this compound [79, 80].

Orthotopic liver transplantation has been successfully performed in patients with advanced protoporphyric hepatopathy [81]. The new liver, however, continues to bear the burden of protoporphyrin overload, and it is therefore susceptible to porphyrin-induced damage. Although bone marrow transplantation should be considered, its indication meets with considerable pitfalls because on the one hand patients with advanced protoporphyric liver damage are bad candidates and on the other hand prediction of the risk of developing significant hepatopathy is uncertain in subjects with normal livers [70].

## 8 Secondary Porphyrinuria

In patients with alcoholic liver disease and in cirrhotic patients in general, there is an alteration of porphyrin metabolism, characterized by the finding of a modest elevation of urinary coproporphyrin [82]. The mechanism of this augmented porphyrinuria appears to be the defective biliary excretion of coproporphyrin in patients with hepatobiliary disorders, which leads to a compensatory increase in the urinary excretion of this compound. Secondary porphyrinuria is also observed in aplastic and hemolytic anemia, in Hodgkin's disease, and in heavy metal toxicity, among other conditions [83]. Rotor's syndrome is an additional example of secondary coproporphyrinuria [84]. In Dubin-Johnson syndrome, total urinary coproporphyrin excretion is normal, but the ratio of isomer I to isomer III is markedly increased [85].

### References


1. Lim HW, Pérez HD, Goldstein IM et al. (1981) Complement-derived chemotactic activity is generated in human serum containing uroporphyrin after irradiation with 450 nm light. J Clin Invest 67:1072–1077
2. Kappas A, Sassa S, Galbraith RA et al. (1989) The porphyrias. In: Scriver CR, Beaudet AL, Sly WS, Valle D (eds) The metabolic basis of inherited disease. McGraw-Hill, New York, pp 1305–1365
3. Deybach JC, de Verneuil H, Boulechfar S et al. (1990) Point mutations in the uroporphyrinogen III synthase gene in congenital erythropoietic porphyria (Gunther's disease). Blood 75:1763–1765
4. Thunell S, Holmberg L, Lundgren J (1987) Aminolevulinate dehydratase porphyria in infancy. A clinical and biochemical study. J Clin Chem Clin Biochem 25:5–10
5. Lannfelt L, Wetterberg L, Gellerfors P et al. (1989) Mutations in acute intermittent porphyria detected by ELISA measurement of porphobilinogen deaminase. J Clin Chem Clin Biochem 27:857–862
6. Wang AL, Arredondo-Vega FX, Giampietro PF et al. (1981) Regional gene assignments for human porphobilinogen deaminase and esterase A4 on chromosome 11. Proc Natl Acad Sci USA 78:5734–5738
7. Grandchamp B, de Verneuil H, Beaumont C et al. (1987) Tissue-specific expression of porphobilinogen deaminase: two isoenzymes from a single gene. Eur J Biochem 162:105–110
8. Moore MR, McColl KE, Fitzsimons EJ et al. (1990) The porphyrias. Blood Rev 4:88–96
9. Tishler PV, Woodward B, O'Connor J et al. (1985) High prevalence of intermittent acute porphyria in a psychiatric patient population. Am J Psychiatry 142:1430–1436
10. Strand LJ, Felsher BF, Redeker AG et al. (1970) Heme biosynthesis in intermittent acute porphyria. Decreased hepatic conversion of porphobilinogen to porphyrins and increased delta aminolevulinic acid synthetase activity. Proc Natl Acad Sci USA 67:1315–1320
11. Mercelis R, Hassoun A, Verstraeten L et al. (1990) Porphyric neuropathy and hereditary delta-aminolevulinic acid dehydratase deficiency in an adult. J Neurol Sci 95:39–47
12. Javitt NB, Rifkind AB, Kappas A (1973) Porphyrin-heme pathway: regulation by intermediates in bile acid synthesis. Science 182:841–843

13. Anderson KE, Spitz IM, Bardin CW et al. (1990) A gonadotropin releasing hormone analogue prevents cyclical attacks of porphyria. Arch Intern Med 150:1469–1474
14. Bonkowsky HL, Magnussen CR, Collins AR et al. (1976) Comparative effects of glycerol and dextrose on porphyrin precursor excretion in acute intermittent porphyria. Metabolism 25:405–414
15. Llewellyn DH, Elder GH, Kalsheker NA et al. (1987) DNA polymorphism of human porphobilinogen deaminase gene in acute intermittent porphyria. Lancet II:706–708
16. Meyer UA (1973) Intermittent acute porphyria: clinical and biochemical studies of disordered heme biosynthesis. Enzyme 16:334–340
17. Pierach CA, Weimer MK, Cardinal RA et al. (1987) Red blood cell porphobilinogen deaminase in the evaluation of acute intermittent porphyria. JAMA 257:60–61
18. Goldberg A (1985) Molecular genetics of acute intermittent porphyria. Br Med J 291:499–500
19. Grandchamp B, Picat C, Mignotte V et al. (1989) Tissue-specific splicing mutation in acute intermittent porphyria. Proc Natl Acad Sci USA 86:661–664
20. Devars du Mayne JF, Deybach JC, Phung L et al. (1986) Crises aiguës de porphyries hépatiques. Traitement par l'hématine. Cinq observations. Presse Med 15:1673–1676
21. Anderson KE, Spitz IM, Bardin CW et al. (1990) A gonadotropin releasing hormone analogue prevents cyclical attacks of porphyria. Arch Intern Med 150:1469–1474
22. Goldberg A, Rimington C, Lochhead A (1967) Hereditary coproporphyria. Lancet I:632–636
23. Brenner DA, Bloomer JR (1980) The enzymatic defect in variegate porphyria: studies with human cultured skin fibroblasts. N Engl J Med 302:765–769
24. Roberts DT, Brodie MJ, Moore MR et al. (1977) Hereditary coproporphyria presenting with photosensitivity induced by the contraceptive pill. Br J Dermatol 96:549–554
25. Campbell JAH (1963) The pathology of South African genetic porphyria. S Afr J Lab Clin Med 9:197–203
26. Eales L (1978) The effects of canthaxanthin on the photocutaneous manifestations of porphyria. S Afr Med J 54:1050–1052
27. Waldenström J (1937) Studien über Porphyrie. Acta Med Scand 82 [Suppl]:1
28. Gocmen A, Peters HA, Cripps DJ et al. (1989) Hexachlorobenzene episode in Turkey. Biomed Environ Sci 2:36–43
29. Elder GH, Urquhart AJ, Enriquez de Salamanca R et al. (1985) Immunoreactive uroporphyrinogen decarboxylase in the liver in porphyria cutanea tarda. Lancet II:229–232
30. Elder GH, Sheppard DM, Tovey JA et al. (1983) Immunoreactive uroporphyrinogen decarboxylase in porphyria cutanea tarda. Lancet I:1301–1304
31. De Verneuil H, Beaumont C, Deybach J-C et al. (1984) Enzymatic and immunological studies of uroporphyrinogen decarboxylase in familial porphyria cutanea tarda and hepatoerythropoietic porphyria. Am J Hum Genet 36:613–622
32. Lazaro P, de Salamanca RE, Elder GH et al. (1984) Is hepatoerythropoietic porphyria a homozygotic form of porphyria cutanea tarda? Inheritance of uroporphyrinogen decarboxylase deficiency in a Spanish family. Br J Dermatol 110:613–617
33. Garey JR, Hansen JL, Harrison LM et al. (1989) A point mutation in the coding region of uroporphyrinogen decarboxylase associated with familial porphyria cutanea tarda. Blood 73:892–895

34. Elder GH, Roberts AG, de Salamanca RE (1989) Genetics and pathogenesis of human uroporphyrinogen decarboxylase defects. Clin Biochem 22:163–168
35. De Verneuil H, Aitken G, Nordmann Y (1978) Familial and sporadic porphyria cutanea: two different diseases. Hum Genet 44:145–151
36. Mukerji SK, Pimstone NR, Burns M (1984) Dual mechanism of inhibition of rat liver uroporphyrinogen decarboxylase activity by ferrous iron: its potential role in the genesis of porphyria cutanea tarda. Gastroenterology 87:1248–1254
37. Visser O, van den Berg JW, Edixhoven-Bosdijk A et al. (1989) Development of hexachlorobenzene porphyria in rats: time sequence and relationship with lipid peroxidation. Food Chem Toxicol 27:317–321
38. Kushner JP, Edwards CQ, Dadone MM et al. (1985) Heterozygosity for HLA-linked hemochromatosis as a likely cause of the hepatic siderosis associated with sporadic porphyria cutanea tarda. Gastroenterology 88:1232–1238
39. Elder GH, Lee GB, Tovey JA (1978) Decreased activity of hepatic uroporphyrinogen decarboxylase in sporadic porphyria cutanea tarda. N Engl J Med 299:274–278
40. Lundvall O (1971) The effect of replenishment of iron stores after phlebotomy therapy in porphyria cutanea tarda. Acta Med Scand 189:51–63
41. Edwards CQ, Griffen LM, Goldgar DE et al. (1989) HLA-linked hemochromatosis alleles in sporadic porphyria cutanea tarda. Gastroenterology 97:972–981
42. McColl KEL, Moore MR, Thompson GG et al. (1981) Abnormal haem biosynthesis in chronic alcoholics. Eur J Clin Invest 11:461–468
43. Felsher BF, Kushner JP (1977) Hepatic siderosis and porphyria cutanea tarda: relation of iron excess to the metabolic defect. Semin Hematol 14:243–251
44. Rocchi E, Gibertini P, Cassanelli M et al. (1986) Hepatitis B virus infection in porphyria cutanea tarda. Liver 6:153–157
45. Wissel PS, Sordillo P, Anderson KE et al. (1987) Porphyria cutanea tarda associated with the acquired immune deficiency syndrome. Am J Hematol 25:107–113
46. Disler P, Day R, Burman N et al. (1982) Treatment of hemodialysis-related porphyria cutanea tarda with plasma exchange. Am J Med 72:989–993
47. Rook A, Champion RH (1960) Porphyria cutanea tarda and diabetes. Br Med J I:860–861
48. Clemmensen O, Thomsen K (1982) Porphyria cutanea tarda and systemic lupus erythematosus. Arch Dermatol 118:160–162
49. Grossman ME, Bickers DR, Poh-Fitzpatrick MB et al. (1979) Porphyria cutanea tarda. Clinical features and laboratory findings in 40 patients. Am J Med 67:277–286
50. Felsher BF, Jones ML, Redeker AG (1973) Iron and hepatic uroporphyrin synthesis: relation in porphyria cutanea tarda. JAMA 226:663–665
51. Lundvall O, Weinfeld A, Lundin P (1970) Iron storage in porphyria cutanea tarda. Acta Med Scand 188:37–53
52. Turnbull A, Baker H, Vernon-Roberts B et al. (1973) Iron metabolism in porphyria cutanea tarda and in erythropoietic protoporphyria. Q J Med 166:341–355
53. Baravalle E, Prieto J (1983) Serum antibodies against porphyric hepatocytes in patients with porphyria cutanea tarda and liver disease. Gastroenterology 84:1483–1491
54. Cortés JM, Oliva H, Paradina FJ et al. (1980) The pathology of the liver in porphyria cutanea tarda. Histopathology 4:471–485
55. Doss M, Look D, Hennings H (1970) Chronic hepatic porphyria in chronic aggressive hepatitis. Klin Wochenschr 49:52–54
56. Elder GH, Gray CH, Nicholson DC (1972) The porphyrias: a review. J Clin Pathol 25:1013–1033

57. Welland FH, Carlsen RA (1969) Porphyria cutanea tarda in an 8-year-old boy. Arch Dermatol 99:451–454
58. Chlumska A, Chlumsky J, Malina L (1980) Liver changes in porphyria cutanea tarda patients treated with chloroquine. Br J Dermatol 102:261–266
59. Ippen H (1977) Treatment of porphyria cutanea tarda by phlebotomy. Semin Hematol 14:253–259
60. Enriquez de Salamanca R, Muñoz JJ, Valls V (1990) Tratamiento de las porfirias. Inf Ter Sist Nac Salud 14:197–214
61. Doss MO, Frank M (1989) Hepatobiliary implications and complications in protoporphyria, a 20-year study. Clin Biochem 22:223–229
62. Bonkowsky HL, Bloomer JR, Ebert PS et al. (1975) Heme synthetase deficiency in human protoporphyria. Demonstration of the defect in liver and cultured skin fibroblasts. J Clin Invest 56:1139–1148
63. Schwartz S, Johnson JA, Stephenson BD et al. (1971) Erythropoietic defects in protoporphyria: a study of factors involved in labelling of porphyrins and bile pigments from ALA-$^{3}$H and glycine-$^{14}$C. J Lab Clin Med 78:411–434
64. Lamon JM, Poh-Fitzpatrick MB, Lamola AA (1980) Hepatic protoporphyrin production in human protoporphyria: effects of intravenous hematin and analysis of erythrocyte protoporphyrin distribution. Gastroenterology 79:115–125
65. Bonkovsky HL (1990) Porphyrin and heme metabolism and the porphyrias. In: Zakim D, Boyer TD (eds) Hepatology. A textbook of liver disease, 2nd edn. W.B. Saunders, Philadelphia, pp 378–424
66. Piomelli S, Lamola AA, Poh-Fitzpatrick MB et al. (1975) Erythropoietic protoporphyria and lead intoxication: the molecular basis for difference in cutaneous photosensitivity. I. Different rates of disappearance of protoporphyrin from the erythrocytes, both in vivo and in vitro. J Clin Invest 56:1519–1527
67. Cripps DJ, McEachern WN (1971) Hepatic and erythropoietic protoporphyria. Arch Pathol 91:497–505
68. DeLeo VA, Poh-Fitzpatrick M, Mathews-Roth M et al. (1976) Erythropoietic protoporphyria: 10 years' experience. Am J Med 69:8–22
69. Lim HW, Pérez HD, Poh-Fitzpatrick M et al. (1981) Generation of chemotactic activity in serum from patients with erythropoietic protoporphyria and porphyria cutanea tarda. N Engl J Med 304:212–216
70. Bloomer JR (1988) The liver in protoporphyria. Hepatology 8:402–407
71. Bloomer JR, Phillips MJ, Davidson DL et al. (1975) Hepatic disease in erythropoietic protoporphyria. Am J Med 58:869–882
72. Rademakers LH, Cleton MI, Kooijman C et al. (1990) Early involvement of hepatic parenchymal cells in erythrohepatic protoporphyria? An ultrastructural study of patients with and without overt liver disease and the effect of chenodeoxycholic acid treatment. Hepatology 11:449–457
73. Bloomer JR, Pierach CA (1982) Effect of hematin administration to patients with protoporphyria and liver disease. Hepatology 2:817–821
74. Van Wisk HJ, Van Hattum J, Baart de la Faille H et al. (1988) Blood exchange and transfusion therapy for acute cholestasis in protoporphyria. Dig Dis Sci 33:1621–1625
75. Gordeuk VR, Brittenham GM, Hawkins CW et al. (1986) Iron therapy for hepatic dysfunction in erythropoietic protoporphyria. Ann Intern Med 105:27–31
76. Milligan A, Graham-Brown RAC, Sarkany I et al. (1988) Erythropoietic protoporphyria exacerbated by oral iron therapy. Br J Dermatol 119:63–66
77. Poh-Fitzpatrick MB, Sklar JA, Goldsman C (1983) Protoporphyria hepatopathy. Effects of cholic acid ingestion in murine griseofulvin-induced protoporphyria. J Clin Invest 72:1449–1458
78. Van Hattum J, Baart de la Faille H, Van den Berg JWO et al. (1986) Chenodeoxycholic acid therapy in erythrohepatic protoporphyria. J Hepatol 3:407–412

79. McCullough AJ, Barron D, Mullen KD et al. (1988) Fecal protoporphyrin excretion in erythropoietic protoporphyria: effect of cholestyramine and bile acid feeding. Gastroenterology 94:177–181
80. Pimstone NR, Mukerji S, Chow H et al. (1986) Oral charcoal therapy for protoporphyria cirrhosis. Hepatology 6:1176
81. Bloomer JR, Weimer MK, Bossenmaier IC et al. (1989) Liver transplantation in a patient with protoporphyria. Gastroenterology 97:188–194
82. Aziz MA, Schwartz S, Watson CJ (1964) Studies of coproporphyrin. VIII. Reinvestigation of the isomer distribution in jaundice and liver diseases. J Lab Clin Med 63:596–604
83. Tschudy DP, Lamon JM (1980) Porphyrin metabolism and the porphyrias. In: Bondy PK, Rosenberg (eds) LE (eds) Metabolic control and disease. W.B. Saunders, Philadelphia, pp 939–1007
84. Wolkoff AW, Wolpert E, Pascasio FN et al. (1976) Rotor's syndrome: a distinct inheritable pathophysiologic entity. Am J Med 60:172–179
85. Koskelo P, Toivonen I, Aldercreutz H (1967) Urinary coproporphyrin isomer distribution in the Dubin-Johnson syndrome. Clin Chem 13:1006–1009

# 27 Pediatric Metabolic Liver Diseases

A.P. MOWAT

## 1 Inborn Errors of Metabolism Associated with Disordered Liver Function or Hepatomegaly

This chapter aims to assist the clinician in the recognition, diagnosis and treatment of selected inborn errors of metabolism in which hepatomegaly and/or disturbed liver function and structure form part of a clinical syndrome. The emphasis will be on disorders for which effective treatment is available or in which hepatic complications cause prominent or presenting symptoms. Many highlight the liver's key role in metabolism [1] while glycogen storage diseases and disorders of fat oxidation highlight its capacity to provide energy required by other tissues. Numerically important metabolic disorders such as $\alpha_1$-antitrypsin deficiency and Wilson's disease are considered elsewhere (see Chaps. 25 and 23). Modes of presentation include neonatal ascites, hepatitis syndrome in infancy (Table 1), cirrhosis (Table 2), neurological dysfunction and hepatosplenomegaly. All conditions discussed are inherited in an autosomal recessive fashion unless otherwise stated. In the majority prenatal diagnosis is now possible. Specialist texts should be consulted for further biochemical, metabolic, genetic [2, 3] or clinical [4] information. With gene therapy in man a reality, hepatic targeting of functioning genes in experimental animals already achieved [5] and

**Table 1.** Inherited disorders associated with hepatitis syndrome in infancy

| |
|---|
| Galactosaemia |
| Fructosaemia |
| Tyrosinaemia |
| $\alpha_1$-Antitrypsin deficiency |
| Cystic fibrosis |
| Niemann-Pick disease type II |
| Gaucher's disease |
| Wolman's disease |
| Zellweger syndrome |
| Erythrophagocytic reticulosis |
| Neonatal haemochromatosis |
| Defects in synthesis of primary bile acids |
| Infantile polycystic disease and related syndromes |

**Table 2.** Genetic disorders associated with cirrhosis

| | |
|---|---|
| Wilson's disease | Gaucher's disease |
| Galactosaemia | Wolman's disease |
| Fructosaemia | Abetalipoproteinaemia |
| Glycogen storage disease type IV | Defects in fatty acid oxidation |
| Glycogen storage disease type III | Sickle cell disease |
| Hurler's syndrome | Thalassaemia |
| Cystic fibrosis | Hepatic porphyria |
| $\alpha_1$-Antitrypsin deficiency | Haemochromatosis, idiopathic |
| Tyrosinaemia | Haemochromatosis, secondary |
| Cystinosis | Zellweger syndrome |
| Ornithine carbamyl transferase deficiency | Defects in primary bile salt synthesis |
| Niemann-Pick disease type II | Shwachmann's syndrome |
| Cholesterol ester storage disease | |

the determination of the DNA sequence of the human genome an achievable goal, the next decade will see exciting developments in the understanding of the pathophysiology and treatment of inherited metabolic disease. Already bone marrow [5a] or liver transplantation [16] has revolutionised the outlook for patients with some metabolic disorders.

## 2 Congenital or Neonatal Ascites

Intrauterine, congenital or neonatal ascites may be a presenting feature of metabolic disorders. It has been reported in association with sialidosis, $GM_1$ gangliosidosis, Gaucher's disease. Wolman's disease, Salla disease and Niemann-Pick disease type IIA. The cause of the ascites is obscure. It may respond to restriction of fluid and salt intake or spironolactone. In severe cases death may occur in the 1st month of life from pulmonary hypoplasia and ventilatory insufficiency [6].

## 3 Glycogen Storage Diseases

Glycogen storage diseases (GSDs) (Fig. 1) are disorders in which the concentration and/or molecular structure of glycogen is abnormal in any tissue of the body. The estimated frequency is 1 in 50000 births. Liver and skeletal muscle are the tissues most severely affected but heart, kidney, bones and brain may be involved. Each disease arises from a deficiency of an enzyme or a transporter involved in the degradation of glycogen by phosphorolysis or hydrolysis. The type and severity of the deficiency define the GSD and determine the biochemical and pathological features, including the long-term prognosis and treatment. This chapter will concentrate on those types in which hepatomegaly is a prominent clinical sign, namely types I, III, IV

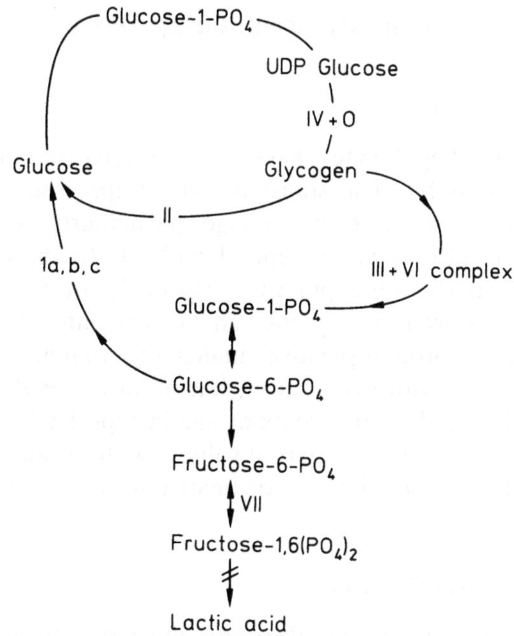


**Fig. 1.** Metabolic pathway of glycogen–glucose–fructose. Shown are the main products and the site of action of enzymes deficient in GSDs: o = glycogen synthase; 1a,b,c = glucose-6-phosphatase; II = acid α-glucosidase; III = amylo-1,6-glucosidase; IV = amylo-1,4:1,6-glucan transferase; VI complex = phosphorylase and various phosphorylase kinases; VII = fructose-1,6-bis-phosphatase. This step is reversed by phosphofructokinase. Lactic acid is produced from glucose via pyruvate by anaerobic metabolism but is produced more readily from fructose

and VI. A wide spectrum of clinical severity can occur within each type. Type I is now recognised [7, 8] as having five variants (a, b, c, d and IaSP). Seven different genetic variants of type VI, phosphorylase kinase deficiency, have been identified [9]. Some were previously categorised as types IX–XII. One in which only liver, leucocytes, and erythrocytes are affected, muscle being spared, is inherited in an X-linked fashion.

## 3.1 Biochemistry

Glycogen is formed from glucose postprandially. Hepatic glycogen is broken down during periods of fasting to maintain a supply of glucose to other organs, the blood glucose level being kept within a narrow range. Muscle glycogen is used locally as a glycolytic fuel. Many metabolic steps are involved in glycogen breakdown. The essential features of hepatic involvement are hepatomegaly and the effects of intermittent glucose "starvation" in other tissues.

## 4 Hepatic Glycogen Storage Diseases

### *Pathology*

The hepatocytes have pale cytoplasm being distended by glycogen and excess fat. The sinusoids are compressed. There may be increased fibrosis and rarely cirrhotic change, particularly in type III GSD, but these changes can also occur in types I and VI. In these types adenomata develop particularly after puberty, especially in types I and III. These appear to be slow growing but can be associated with massive bleeding and rarely α-fetoprotein-positive malignant change. Focal glomerulonephritis associated with proteinuria, haematuria, renal calculi and renal failure may be detected from 8 years of age in type I GSD. In type IV GSD the abnormal glycogen is only partial soluble with diastase and there is severe fibrosis with death from cirrhosis or heart failure usually by 3 years of age.

### *Clinical Features*

Glycogen storage disorders must be considered in any infant or child who presents with hepatomegaly, or with cardiac, muscular or neurological dysfunction. Symptoms often start at birth or soon afterwards. The large liver, which may extend to the iliac crest, is typically smooth with only minimal increase in firmness. If hypoglycaemia is severe or persistent, convulsions and mental retardation may occur. Adiposity with particularly fat cheeks and trunk but with poor muscle bulk in the limbs is a striking feature. From the age of 6 months short stature is prominent. The hepatomegaly becomes less prominent throughout childhood, especially in type III disease. By adolescence the liver may not be palpably enlarged.

In type Ia GSD acidosis, vomiting and diarrhoea are major problems in some patients. Xanthoma may develop in association with high serum triglycerides and cholesterol. Gouty tophi with high uric acid may occur. Metabolic disorders other than the high serum uric acid become less troublesome with increasing age but renal problems and adenoma become more frequent. Type 1b and c are similar but recurrent neutropenia makes the patient very susceptible to bacterial infection.

The features in type III disease are similar to those in type 1 except that growth retardation is less and muscle involvement, including cardiac muscle, is more prominent. Cardiac failure and sudden death may occur. Cirrhosis may develop.

Type IV disease is characterised by cirrhosis with or without evidence of cardiac or cranial involvement. Survival to 8 years of age is exceptional [10].

Type VI is a heterogeneous disorder comprising at least seven different genetic defects. In general the features are milder than types I and III with normal serum lactate and uric acid. Puberty is not delayed.

### *Biochemical Abnormalities*

Hypoglycaemia on fasting is a feature of nearly all GSDs. Hyperlipidaemia is marked in types I and II and to a lesser extent in all other hepatic forms. Lactic acid and pyruvic acid are frequently elevated in type I in the fasting state. Uric acid may be raised. Raised serum transaminases are found in over 50% of patients with types 1 and 3.

### *Diagnosis*

The diagnosis of GSD is suspected on the basis of the clinical findings. Hypoglycaemia on fasting is important supporting evidence. Glucagon given intravenously in a dose of $0.7\,mg/m^2$ normally produces a rise in blood glucose of more than 35 mg/100 ml in the first hour. The rise in blood sugar is less in GSD types I and III (in the fasting state). In GSD type VI the response is often decreased but not invariably so. False-positive and -negative results occur with all types.

More specific investigations of glycogen metabolism are required for accurate diagnosis. In GSD types III and VI erythrocyte glycogen is increased. Specific enzyme defects may be demonstrated in leucocytes in types II, III, IV and VI. If these investigations are not diagnostic, percutaneous liver biopsy (essential in GSD types I), and possibly muscle biopsy, is indicated to obtain tissues for enzymatic or biochemical studies [11].

### *Treatment*

The aim of treatment is to maintain the blood sugar within the normal range [12]. This minimises secondary metabolic problems and produces a normal growth rate. Small feeds 2–3 hourly or continuous nasogastric feeding at night to provide constant glucose absorption, increased at times of excessive utilisation, is the mainstay of management. The diet must contain sufficient calories and other nutrients. The intensity of treatment obviously will vary with the severity of the disorder and to some extent with the specific enzymatic defect.

In type I disease a high glucose/glucose polymer intake with continuous nasogastric feeding during sleep affords optimum control. There is a hazard in that patients treated in this fashion become extremely carbohydrate dependent and have severe, even fatal, hypoglycaemic features at blood sugar concentrations which had previously been well tolerated, the brain having acquired the ability to utilise the high serum lactic acid. It is essential therefore to guarantee a continuous supply of glucose, particularly during intercurrent infections with additional CHO before vigorous exercise. An alternative is to give cold, uncooked corn starch in a dose of 2 g/kg at 4- to 6-h intervals. Because it is slowly digested it may maintain the blood sugar within the normal range for up to 6 h. It may produce diarrhoea, particularly in infants. Galactose and fructose are omitted from the diet in type I GSD since they aggravate lactic acidaemia.

It is uncertain what effect the management has on increased intrahepatic fibrosis or the development of adenoma or hepatocellular carcinoma [13] or on renal complications [14]. Anecdotal reports suggest that adenomas do regress with strict dietary management. Allopurinol may occasionally be required for control of hyperuricaemia. Bicarbonate may be required for acidosis.

In type III GSD frequent feeds of a high protein diet, with protein providing 25% of the calories and carbohydrates 50%–55% (partly in the form of corn starch), will correct hypoglycaemia, growth retardation and myopathic symptoms and reduce liver size. It is not clear whether diet influences intrahepatic fibrosis. Severe disease may need nasogastric feeding.

Type VI GSD requires similar but less rigorous treatment to type 1. Galactose and fructose are permitted. Cold, uncooked corn starch is a useful carbohydrate source.

Liver transplantation corrects the disorder [15, 16]. It should be considered in infants with very severe disease or in adults with malignant disease confined to the liver. Its role in those with adenomata, which may be stable for up to 5 years, has not been defined.

## 5 Transferase Deficiency Galactosaemia: Galactose-1-phosphate Uridyl Transferase Deficiency

Galactose-1-phosphate uridyl transferase deficiency (GAL-1-PUTD), a severe form of galactosaemia, is characterised by an almost complete inability to metabolise galactose to carbon dioxide. The deficiency is lifelong. Exposure to galactose causes a severe toxicity syndrome comprising inanition, vomiting, diarrhoea, liver disease, failure to thrive, cataracts and mental retardation. Several variants have been described in which up to 10% of normal enzymatic activity is found in the liver and such patients may be able to metabolise limited amounts of galactose. The reported incidence is from 1 in 18000 to 1 in 180000 births. The gene locus is chromosome 9p13.

### *Hepatic Pathology and Pathogenesis of Hepatic Lesion*

Marked fatty change, periportal cholangiolar proliferation and pseudoacinar formation followed by 6 weeks of age by increasing fibrosis leads to cirrhosis by 3–6 months of age if galactose intake continues. The exact mechanism of hepatic toxicity is unknown. Galactose-1-phosphate accumulates intracellularly, restricting the availability of phosphate for high-energy bonds. Adenosine 5′-triphosphate (ATP), guanosine 5′-triphosphate and cytidine 5′-triphosphate concentrations are reduced with severe metabolic derangement of the brain, liver and kidney. GAL-1-PUTD causes hypoglycaemia by decreasing glucose release from glycogen and inhibiting enzymes involved in gluconeogenesis. The high galactose-1-phosphate levels lead by alternate pathways to the production of potentially toxic galactitol, galactonate and galactonolactone. There is no evidence of galactosamine accumulation.

### *Clinical Features*

Death from septicaemia within a day or two of ingesting milk occurs in the most severe forms. In less severely affected infants a marked unconjugated hyperbilirubinaemia with haemolysis occurs on the 2nd or 3rd day, followed within 1–3 days by a conjugated hyperbilirubinaemia with clinical and biochemical evidence of fulminant liver failure with hepatomegaly, bleeding diathesis, ascites and renal tubular dysfunction. Increased intracranial pressure may be a presenting feature. The most common presentation is with prolonged neonatal jaundice with failure to thrive, vomiting and a less severe hepatitis. The mildest cases present with mental retardation and cataracts and are found to have hepatomegaly and abnormal biochemical tests of liver function. Cataracts may be seen on slit-lamp examination at as early as 5 days. Irreversible brain damage may occur from the effects of hyperbilirubinaemia or from galactosaemia.

### *Laboratory Investigations*

Liver function tests are deranged, the blood galactose is elevated and there may be hyperchloraemic acidosis with albuminuria and hyperaminoaciduria. Hypoglycaemia is rare. Galactosuria may be detected for a short period after a galactose load.

### *Diagnosis*

A presumptive diagnosis may be made if the urine contains reducing substances which are negative on testing with glucose oxidase. It is essential to confirm the diagnosis by demonstrating absent enzymatic activity in red blood cells since galactosuria is a frequent finding in infants with other forms of liver disease. Transfused red blood cells may give false normal values for up to 3 months.

### *Treatment and Prognosis*

As soon as the diagnosis is suspected a galactose-free diet is commenced. Patients with severely deranged liver function and hyperbilirubinaemia require exchange transfusion. Following institution of the diet there should be a rapid improvement in the infant's condition. Infants with severe metabolic derangement when treatment is started may die within a few days. The majority do improve and have no subsequent hepatic problems. A few patients with very advanced cirrhosis may decompensate in childhood or early adult life. They become candidates for liver transplantation. Hepatocellular carcinoma may develop. The diet is maintained for life. Dietary control is considered optimum if the erythrocyte galactose-1-phosphate is consistently below 3 mg/dl.

Even with excellent control, children frequently have lower IQs than their healthy siblings and require intensive teaching to overcome difficulties with language, visual perception and abstract thinking [17]. Hypotonia, tremor, ataxia and mental retardation may develop in late childhood. It was been postulated that some of the neurological problems stem from intrauterine brain damage from maternal galactose crossing the placenta. Thus galactose restriction in carrier "at risk" pregnancies has been advised although there is no evidence of its efficacy.

Hypergonadotrophic hypogonadism with infertility has been reported in females even with "good" dietary control from birth. The incidence of ovarian dysfunction and neurodevelopmental abnormalities is similar in those diagnosed because of clinical problems or as a result of screening [17].

Prenatal diagnosis by measurement of GAL-1-PUT enzymatic activity in cultured amniocytes or chorionic villus biopsy is available.

## 6 Epimerase Deficiency Galactosaemia

The majority of patients with epimerase deficiency galactosaemia are asymptomatic, being discovered during neonatal screening programs which detect high blood galactose. In these UDP-galactose-4-epimerase deficiency is limited to red blood cells. In a few families a generalised deficiency has been found, giving the features of transferase deficiency galactosaemia. Dietary therapy aims to provide sufficient galactose to avoid toxicity but enough for essential galactoprotein and galactolipid synthesis.

## 7 Fructosaemia

Fructose is widely distributed, with the free monosaccharide and the glucose–fructose disaccharide, sucrose, being important sources of dietary carbohydrate. Fructose is absorbed at half the rate of other monosaccharides and rapidly metabolised in the liver, small intestine and kidney. It is synthesised in vivo from glucose via sorbitol.

Two clinically important defects in fructose metabolism have been characterised (Fig. 2).

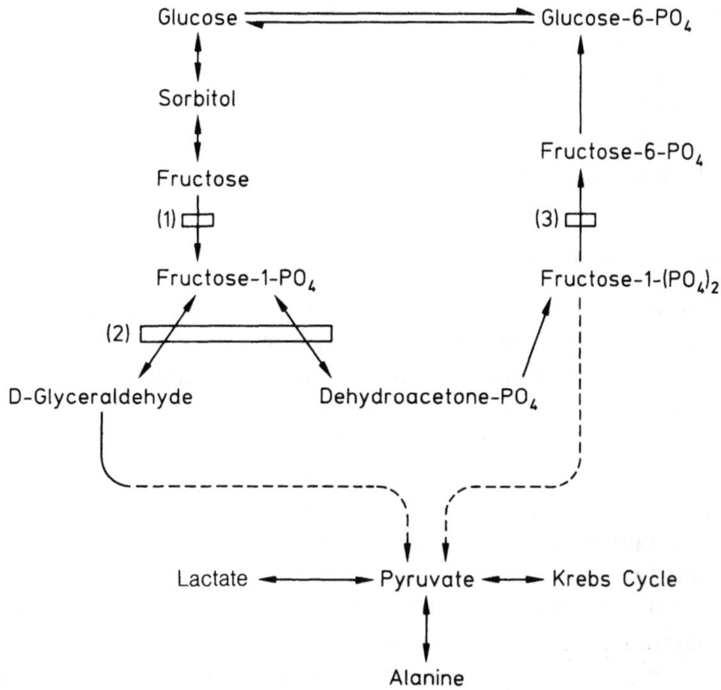


**Fig. 2.** The main metabolic pathways of fructose and its interaction with glucose, pyruvate, alanine and the Krebs cycle. The three defects in fructose metabolism are indicated by the rectangles. (*1*) Fructokinase (EC. 7.1.3) catalyses the phosphorylation of fructose to fructose-1-phosphate. (*2*) Fructoaldolase (fructose-1, 6-bisphosphate aldolase, aldolase, EC. 4.1.2.13) reversibly splits fructose-1-phosphate into D-glyceraldehyde and dihydroxyacetone phosphate. (*3*) Fructose-1,6-bisphosphatase (EC. 3.1.3.11) splits fructose-1-diphosphate to fructose-6-phosphate. The reaction is irreversible but the opposite conversion can be accomplished by an equally irreversible phosphofructokinase

## 7.1 Hereditary Fructose Intolerance

Hereditary fructose intolerance is characterised by an absence of, or severely reduced, activity of fructose-1-phosphate aldolase B in liver, renal cortex and small intestinal mucosa. More than one genotype may be involved. Exposure to fructose causes vomiting, hepatic and renal dysfunction, neurological abnormalities and behaviour difficulties. The incidence has been estimated at 1:20000 in Switzerland. The disorder is probably underdiagnosed elsewhere.

### *Hepatic Pathology*

There may be complete hepatic necrosis. In the typical case biopsied after fructose withdrawal there is diffuse steatosis with necrosis of a few hepatocytes, some of which may show giant cell transformation. If fructose ingestion continues, periportal and intralobular fibrosis progresses to cirrhosis. Ultrastructural studies show polymorphic cytoplasmic inclusions in both hepatocytes and Kupffer cells. The pathological effects are all secondary to the accumulation of fructose-1-phosphate and ATP depletion. The latter causes high serum $Mg^{2+}$ and uric acid.

### *Clinical Features*

Symptoms start as soon as fructose is ingested. Classically this occurs when breast milk is substituted by a milk containing fructose, sucrose or honey or on weaning. Vomiting is a particularly prominent feature. Poor feeding, failure to thrive, hepatomegaly and spontaneous bleeding are almost universally present in cases presenting in infancy. Many such infants also have pallor, jaundice, drowsiness, irritability, tremor with jerky limb movements and oedema. They may be critically ill with the syndrome of acute liver and renal failure. Convulsions may complicate hypoglycaemia, which is typically short-lived. Death may occur.

Older infants and children may show a marked aversion to fructose-containing food but this is slowly learned and continuous exposure to fructose causes hepatomegaly, abdominal distension and features suggesting a chronic hepatitis, storage disorder or cirrhosis. Behaviour may be very disturbed and development slow. Inadvertent ingestion of large doses of fructose causes acute symptoms such as drowsiness and vomiting and may precipitate fulminant hepatic failure. Thus, fructose intolerance presents as a disorder of extreme variability, particularly in early infancy. Differential diagnosis includes pyloric stenosis, hiatus hernia, food intolerance, galactosaemia and other metabolic disorders affecting the liver.

### *Laboratory Findings*

Raised serum transaminases, prolonged prothrombin time, hyperaminoacidaemia, hyperuricacidaemia, hypoalbuminaemia and jaundice occur in the majority of cases. Hypoglycaemia, if present, may be transient. Anaemia, acanthocytosis and thrombocytopenia are frequently present. Serum phosphate and potassium are low. A lactic acidosis is usual. Fructosuria, proteinuria, hyperaminoaciduria and organic aciduria are often found.

### *Diagnosis*

The diagnosis is suggested by the above clinical features in an infant or child with a history of fructose intake. A detailed dietary history is therefore essential. Withdrawal of fructose from the diet causes regression of vomiting almost immediately and thereafter a gradual improvement in the other features unless fulminant liver and/or renal failure has occurred. The diagnosis is subsequently confirmed by demonstrating low enzymatic activity in liver or intestinal mucosal biopsy.

### *Treatment and Prognosis*

A fructose-, sucrose- and sorbitol-free diet must be maintained for life. Vitamin C supplements are required. For acute liver failure exchange transfusions, plasma and blood infusions and intravenous glucose may be essential. With the institution of a fructose-free diet hepatomegaly gradually regresses and liver function tests return to normal. The hepatic steatosis diminishes but never completely clears. Patients or their parents should state their intolerance to fructose on any hospital admission since fructose given in infusion solutions or enterally may cause fatal fulminant hepatic failure.

The structure of the gene and its localisation (chromosome 9q13–32) and the mutation has been defined in four patients, suggesting that antenatal diagnosis should soon be possible. Subsequent siblings should be regarded as suffering from fructosaemia until the diagnosis has been excluded.

## 7.2 Fructose-1,6-diphosphatase Deficiency

Fructose-1,6-diphosphatase deficiency is characterised by an absence of fructose-1,6-diphosphatase in liver, jejunum and kidney. Exposure to fructose severely impairs gluconeogenesis with hypoglycaemia and ketosis.

### *Hepatic Pathology*

The liver is enlarged. Light microscopy shows fatty infiltration without any increase in fibrosis.

### *Clinical Features*

Patients often present in infancy following fructose ingestion. In the newborn there is hypoglycaemia with irritability, convulsions and apnoea or hyperventilation due to severe acidosis. Hypotonia and hepatomegaly are prominent. In older children these may be the main features between exacerbations which are precipitated by fasting, vomiting usually during intercurrent infections or fructose or sucrose ingestion. A similar pattern of features as in the newborn with hypoglycaemia and ketosis may develop. There is no aversion to fructose-containing foods. Vomiting is unusual.

### *Laboratory Features*

Hypoglycaemia associated with increased lactate, ketones and amino acids in the blood and urine are the characteristic abnormalities, although ketosis may occur without hypoglycaemia. Liver and renal function tests are normal.

### *Diagnosis*

Diagnosis may be suspected on the basis of the history, the severe hypoglycaemia and ketoacidosis. The main differential diagnoses are other defects of gluconeogenesis. Diagnosis is confirmed by demonstrating the specific enzymatic deficiency in a liver biopsy specimen.

### *Treatment and Prognosis*

Dietary fructose and sucrose are severely reduced. Acute exacerbations are controlled by intravenous glucose and bicarbonate. Fasting must be avoided. If vomiting occurs, intravenous glucose should be given. Hepatomegaly and hypotonia gradually regress and normal growth and development should occur if there has been no brain damage due to hypoglycaemia. In the majority of case reports the mode of inheritance appears to be autosomal recessive but two families have been reported with parents and children affected. Antenatal diagnosis is at present not possible.

## 8 Tyrosinaemia

Hypertyrosinaemia may occur secondarily to acute and chronic liver disease. Neonatal tyrosinaemia is thought to be due to a relative deficiency of *p*-hydroxyphenylpyruvate oxidase. This transient abnormality causes lethargy, poor feeding and jaundice, disordered liver function or hepatomegaly. It may be followed by mental retardation in premature infants. The protein intake should be reduced to 2–3 g/kg daily. Some infants respond to ascorbic acid 100 mg, four times daily.

Two genetically determined forms of hypertyrosinaemia are currently recognised. Type II, associated with deficiency of hepatic aminotransferase, is not associated with liver disease.

### 8.1 Tyrosinaemia Type I (Fumaryl Acetoacetate Hydrolase Deficiency)

Hereditary tyrosinaemia is due to an inherited defect of fumaryl acetoacetate hydrolase. It is characterised by progressive hepatocellular damage, renal tubular dysfunction, hypophosphataemic rickets and excretion of two tyrosine metabolites, succinylacetone or succinyl acetoacetate at concentrations more than 100 times normal.

### *Pathology*

The liver is large. Hepatocytes show intense fatty infiltration and hepatocellular necrosis in the acute stage. There is gradually increasing intrahepatic fibrosis which progresses to cirrhosis with prominent regeneration nodules. Hepatoma develops in up to 33% of cases surviving beyond 2 years of age.

### *Clinical Features*

The disorder exists in an acute and a chronic form. The acute presents in the first weeks or months of life with failure to thrive, vomiting, diarrhoea, a cabbage-like odour, hepatomegaly, oedema, ascites, splenomegaly and a bleeding diathesis with melena and epistaxis. Jaundice occurs in about one-third of patients. Death from liver failure occurs usually by 8 months of age, with only 10% surviving beyond 12 months.

The chronic form may continue from the acute or present between 6 months and 17 years of age with features of cirrhosis, hypophosphataemic rickets and/or renal tubular dysfunction. The Fanconi syndrome may be severe and complicated by glomerular failure. Hypoglycaemia occurs in both forms of the illness. Episodes of acute abdominal pain, polyneuropathy and hypertension with intermittent porphyria-like biochemical abnormalities occur in up to one-third. Death from hepatic failure with or without tumour formation or renal failure usually occurs in the first decade. Both acute and chronic forms may occur in the same family. The diagnosis should be considered in any child with cirrhosis or rickets.

### *Laboratory Investigations*

Standard biochemical tests of liver function are abnormal with decreased albumin and cholesterol concentrations and prolonged prothrombin time. There may be a normochromic anaemia with leucocytosis. Serum α-fetoprotein is raised to 1–100 times the upper limit of normal. There may be severe hypoglycaemia and hypophosphataemia. Both acidosis and alkalosis may occur. Haematuria, glycosuria and a generalised hyperaminoaciduria is present.

Plasma tyrosine and phenylalanine are increased with high methionine in the acute form. There is always excessive urinary excretion of other products of tyrosine degradation, including δ-aminolaevulinic acid and catecholamines. Red cell glutathione and plasma cysteine are decreased.

### *Diagnosis*

Excessive serum and urinary concentrations of succinylacetone are diagnostic. Fumaryl acetoacetate hydrolase deficiency can be demonstrated in fibroblast cultures.

***Treatment and Prognosis***

Dietary restriction of phenylalanine, tyrosine and methionine and controlling the effects of renal tubular damage are the mainstays of treatment. Tyrosine levels should be between 0.5 and 1 mg/dl. Diet must be continued for life. Rickets is controlled by phosphate and vitamin D supplements. Hypoglycaemia, hypopotassaemia, acidosis, alkalosis, ascites and bleeding may all require symptomatic management. These measures improve well-being and promote growth for a time but it has yet to be shown that they delay the inevitable progression to liver failure or the development of hepatocellular carcinoma. Liver transplantation must be considered for patients with the acute form in the second 6 months of life if there is growth arrest or other signs of deteriorating liver function. For the chronic form liver transplantation should be considered in the 3rd year of life because detection of tumour formation by scanning or rise in α-fetoprotein concentration before metastases develop is unreliable. Combined liver and renal transplantation may be necessary if there is a severe Fanconi syndrome or glomerular failure.

Features of tyrosinaemia but with normal succinyl acetoacetate and fumaryl acetoacetate hydrolase have been described in one patient with maleylacetoacetate isomerase deficiency and in two siblings with elevated polyunsaturated fats, optic atrophy and exocrine pancreatic hypoplasia.

## 9 Urea Cycle Disorders

The function of the urea cycle is to convert nitrogen not required for biosynthetic purposes into urea and thus avoid neurotoxicity due to ammonium and glutamine accumulation. The cycle is also responsible for the synthesis of arginine, which becomes an essential amino acid in all defects of the cycle except arginase deficiency. Six enzymatic reactions are involved. They function almost exclusively in the liver. Substrates are formed in muscle, kidney, intestine and liver.

### 9.1 Main Urea Cycle Defects

Four well-documented diseases are each caused by defective functioning of one of four enzymes involved in the urea cycle, namely deficiencies of carbamyl phosphate synthetase (CPSD), ornithine transcarbamylase (OTCD), argininosuccinic acid synthetase (ASD) and argininosuccinase (ALD). The symptoms and signs of all four are induced by the accumulation of precursors of urea, ammonia and glutamine and are sufficiently similar to be considered together. All show considerable genetic and phenotypic variability with a continuous spectrum of clinical expression. The treatment differs with the disorder and its severity. OTCD deficiency is inherited as an X-linked disorder.

### *Clinical Features of CPSD, OTCD, ASD and ALD*

Symptoms may start with a lethal episode in the neonatal period or be delayed until late childhood or adult life. Even with late onset, irreversible hyperammonaemic coma may rapidly develop. Hepatomegaly and raised transaminases indicate hepatic involvement.

The most dramatic presentation is at 2–3 days of age. After appearing normal for 24–48 h, these neonates develop progressive lethargy, hypothermia and hyperventilation. The chest x-ray is clear and there is a respiratory alkalosis. Without appropriate intervention cardiorespiratory arrest may occur. Increased intracranial pressure may be evident. Severe hepatomegaly occurs in ALD. Pulmonary, intracranial and gastrointestinal haemorrhage may occur as a terminal event. There may be a history of consanguinity or neonatal deaths in the sibship or close male relatives.

In those cases without neonatal onset, symptoms may appear in later infancy, early childhood or even adult life. The onset may be related to intercurrent infection or high protein meal or may occur for no obvious reason. Classical features are vomiting and neurological dysfunction, which may take the form of lethargy, irritability, agitation, combative behaviour, drowsiness, disorientation, bizarre conduct, slurred speech, ataxia and coma. Seizures may occur. There may be features of increased intracranial pressure. There may be delayed physical growth and physical development. Characteristically these symptoms occur in an episodic fashion. The patient may select a relatively low protein intake. ALD and ASD may be associated with trichorrhexis nodosa.

### *Pathology*

The principal abnormalities at autopsy are cerebral, cerebellar and basal ganglia degeneration and atrophy. In experimental animals the initial changes in hyperammonaemia are in astrocytes, which show swelling with pleomorphic mitochondria. These occur before there any changes in neurones or their processes. The changes may be mediated by glutamine, which is formed from ammonium in astrocytes. Glutamine levels in cerebrospinal fluid may be between 10 and 12 times higher than normal in hyperammonaemic coma. Serum glutamine levels may increase prior to the onset of coma. Because astrocyte processes are intimately related to cerebral capillaries and venules, it is believed that the astrocyte-induced changes in cerebral blood flow cause cerebral oedema and many secondary biochemical and pathological abnormalities.

The liver is usually reported as being normal or showing a minimal increase in fat and glycogen with no other histological abnormality. Patients with CPSD or OCTD may have mild hepatic necrosis and portal inflammation. Portal fibrosis has been reported in OTCD and ALD; it is usually mild but may be severe with possible cirrhosis.

### *Laboratory Findings*

Hyperammonaemia without acidosis and/or ketosis is a characteristic feature of defects of the urea cycle. The extent of these biochemical changes varies with the severity of the lesion and with protein intake. Abnormalities are aggravated by intercurrent infection, operations and anaesthesia. Glutamine, alanine and aspartate concentrations in the serum may also be elevated. Urea concentration in blood and urinary urea excretion are normal, urea being produced by accumulation of substrate proximal to the block and from arginine (except in arginase deficiency). Serum aminotrasferase concentrations are usually high during acute episodes and may remain elevated between attacks.

### *Diagnosis*

Depending on the site of the metabolic lesion, ornithine, citrulline and arginosuccinic acid concentrations may be high or low. Citrulline levels exceed 1000 μM/litre in AS, are between 100 and 300 in ALD and are very low or undetectable in OTCD and CPSD (normal 10–20 μM/litre) in cases with neonatal onset. With the late-onset forms of OTCD and CPSD there may be no diagnostic amino acid abnormality. Arginosuccinic acid concentration is high in ALD.

Orotic aciduria increases from diversion of carbamyl phosphate to pyrimidine in OTCD, ASD and ALD. The diagnosis may be confirmed, after the patient's clinical condition has been stabilised, by measuring the specific enzymatic activity in a percutaneous liver biopsy in CPSD and OTCD or in fibroblasts in the others.

*If hyperammonaemia is recognised* the main differential diagnosis in the newborn period is transient hyperammonaemia of the newborn, which occurs in premature infants, and pyruvate dehydrogenase deficiency or glutaric acidaemia type II occurring in full-term infants, both with onset usually in the first 24 h of life. With onset after 24 h the absence of acidosis excludes methylmalonic acidaemia but propionic acidaemia may occasionally occur without acidosis.

With the late-onset forms a wider differential diagnosis must be considered. This includes an increasing range of organic aciduria, e.g., fatty acid acyl CoA dehydrogenase deficiencies and isovaleric acidaemia. Lysinuric protein intolerance must also be considered. Acute hepatic necrosis or Reye's syndrome is to be suspected if there is a prolonged prothrombin time or hypoglycaemia.

In achieving a diagnosis it is often essential to obtain at presentation plasma and urine specimens in which to measure plasma pH, bicarbonate, amino acids, urinary orotic acid and organic acids by gas chromatography–mass spectroscopy.

### *Treatment*

The aim of treatment is to allow normal growth and development while avoiding or rapidly controlling episodes of encephalopathy. The immediate objectives are to reduce concentrations of ammonia and glutamine to normal, to decrease the need for urea formation and to prevent arginine deficiency. Such treatment can only be achieved with rigorous dietetic control with careful monitoring of the concentrations of serum amino acids and ammonia. A normal plasma glutamine may be the best single indication of effective treatment since serum concentrations increase before ammonium levels. Urinary orotic acid excretion should be normal in OTCD heterozygotes.

Exact details of management will vary from case to case. The mainstay of chronic management is to provide just sufficient protein for growth and development and to promote excretion of waste nitrogen by alternate pathways. It may be necessary to restrict protein intake to essential amino acids only. Keto analogues of amino acids have been used in an effort to decrease further the protein load but are bitter and poorly tolerated. Sufficient calories must be provided in the form of carbohydrates. Two agents which cause increased urinary nitrogen excretion are helpful in controlling acute hyperammonaemic crisis and in preventing hyperammonaemia. Sodium benzoate combines with glycine to form hippurate and phenylacetate combines with glutamate to form phenylacetylglutamine, both conjugates being excreted in the urine. The latter is the more efficient pathway provided the capacity of the liver and kidney to form phenylacetylglutamine is not exceeded. Both agents are potentially toxic and have to be used with care, particularly in the presence of renal failure.

It is important to appreciate that as growth slows protein accretion declines, causing a decrease in protein tolerance.

Acute exacerbations with hyperammonaemic coma occur unpredictably as well as with intercurrent infections, surgery or anaesthesia. These are treated with infusions of glucose, arginine and (except in ALD) benzoate and phenylacetate, with removal of ammonia by haemodialysis or exchange transfusion and with ventilatory support if necessary.

With such management even severe cases may survive through the 1st year of life. Therapy is highly effective in ASD but in ALD brain damage may occur. With neonatal-onset OTCD and CPSD many are mentally retarded. Cases of later onset have a better prognosis. In patients in whom dietary management proves ineffective liver transplantation should be considered.

### 9.2 Arginase Deficiency

Arginase deficiency is a rare disorder characterised by progressive spastic paraplegia, seizures and mental retardation. There is hyperammonaemia, hyperargininaemia, diaminoaciduria and orotic aciduria. Treatment with a reduced amino acid intake and diversion of nitrogen from urea genesis by sodium benzoate and phenylacetate may be beneficial.

### 9.3 *N*-Acetylglutamate Synthetase Deficiency

*N*-Acetylglutamate synthetase deficiency was described in a single asymptomatic neonate with hyperammonaemia. Two siblings had died in the neonatal period. Treatment with carbamylglutamate controlled the hyperammonaemia.

### 9.4 Genetic Counselling for Urea Cycle Defects

Where enzyme deficiency can be detected in fibroblasts, antenatal diagnosis by amniocentesis has been achieved. Techniques for identification of distinct restriction fragment length polymorphisms have been employed in the diagnosis of CPSD, OTCD and arginase deficiency. Fetal liver biopsy for enzyme analysis has been performed in some families at risk of OCTD.

## 10 Rare Disorders with Hyperammonaemia and Disturbed Amino Acid Metabolism

### 10.1 Familial Protein Intolerance (Lysinuric Protein Intolerance)

Familial protein intolerance appears to be due to a genetically determined defect in the transport of basic amino acids, lysine and arginine. There is both a defect in absorption and increased renal losses. The enzymatic abnormality underlying this defect has not been identified. There is a secondary failure of the urea cycle due to lack of essential substrate amino acids. Pathological changes are limited to the liver, in which there is some lymphocyte and macrophage infiltrate in the portal tract with increased fibrosis. In older patients this progresses to early cirrhosis.

Clinical features are vomiting and diarrhoea, which start when protein intake increases when breast feeding is supplemented. An aversion to protein-rich foods develops around the age of 1 year. There is growth failure, hepatomegaly and splenomegaly, hypotonia and sparse hair. The limbs are very thin, the torso relatively stocky with adequate subcutaneous fat. There may be mental retardation. With high protein intakes there may be psychotic behaviour, abdominal pain and coma. Osteoporosis occurs due to lysine deficiency. Interstitial pneumonia may develop.

The blood ammonia is normal when fasting but increases to above normal with moderate amounts of protein. Urinary orotic acid is high reflecting urea cycle failure. The blood urea is typically low. Serum lysine, argine and ornithine are low while alanine and citrulline are high. There is excessive lysine and arginine in the urine.

Treatment consists of a low protein intake (<1.5 g/kg in children, <0.8 g/kg in adults), with 2.5–8.5 g (14–48 mmol) as citrulline. The citrulline guarantees adequate urea cycle intermediates for urea formation. Hyperammonaemic crises require treatment with protein withdrawal and intravenous glucose.

### 10.2 Hyperornithinaemia, Hyperammonaemia, Homocitrullinuria Syndrome

An enlarged liver with bizarre elongated mitochondria containing crystalloid structures has been described in patients with hyperornithinaemia, hyperammonaemia, homocitrullinuria syndrome. The underlying defect(s) has not been identified. There is thought to be a defect in transport of ornithine into mitochondria. The syndrome, which has a wide range of clinical severity, is characterised by intermittent postprandial hyperammonaemia and mental retardation. Symptoms may start in the neonatal period or in adult life. Treatment is by dietary protein restriction.

## 11 Defects in Pyruvate Metabolism Causing Lactic Acidosis

### 11.1 Pyruvate Carboxylase Deficiency

Pyruvate carboxylase is an intramitochondrial enzyme with a key regulatory role in gluconeogenesis in the liver. In astrocytes it stimulates glutamine and γ-aminobutyric acid synthesis while in neurones it stimulates myelin formation. It is totally acetyl CoA dependent. The deficiency may be limited to the brain, causing Leigh's disease with lactic acidaemia, but if generalised it also causes hyperammonaemia, with high citrulline, lysine, alanine and proline. The liver is enlarged with lipid accumulation in hepatocytes, hyperplasia of the endoplasmic reticulum and abnormal mitochondria. Death by 3 months of age is usual.

### 11.2 Phosphoenolpyruvate Carboxykinase Deficiency

Phosphoenolpyruvate carboxykinase converts oxaloacetic acid formed from pyruvate to phosphoenolpyruvate from which glucose is formed. In the deficiency state lactic acidosis, hypotonia and failure to thrive are associated with hepatomegaly and disordered liver function. Death by 1 year of age is usual.

Unfortunately there is as yet no treatment for these disorder.

## 12 Disorders with Hyperammonaemia and Massive Fat Accumulation in Hepatocytes

### 12.1 Methylmalonic Acidaemia

Methylmalonic acidaemia is characterised by a deficiency of a mitochondrial matrix enzyme methylmalonyl coenzyme A (CoA) mutase which catalyses the conversion of methylmalonyl CoA to succinyl CoA. Adenosylcobalamine is an essential co-factor. Many different biochemical abnormalities may cause inherited methylmalonic acidaemia.

Lethargy, failure to thrive, vomiting, acidosis (usually with ketosis), hypotonia, mental retardation, anaemia, leucopenia and thrombocytopenia are major manifestations. There is an increased susceptibility to infection. Hepatic features are rapid changes in liver size due to microvesicular fatty infiltration, hyperammonaemia and raised transaminases. Symptoms start in the 1st week of life in the majority but in some mutations occur after 1 year of age. The diagnosis is suspected on the basis of the clinical features and the presence of ketosis and acidosis. It is established by demonstrating the typical urinary methylmalonic excretion and confirmed by specific enzyme determination in fibroblasts. There are at least seven different biochemical forms whose response to parenteral cobalamin supplements and protein restriction varies from survival in health through 20 years of age to early death. Those with early onset usually fare badly. Prenatal diagnosis by methylmalonic determination in amniotic fluid or enzyme levels in amniotic cells has been accomplished.

## 13 Defects in Fatty Acid β-Oxidation

### 13.1 Acyl-CoA Dehydrogenase Deficiencies

Fatty acid oxidation in mitochondria is a major energy source during fasting. Acyl-CoA dehydrogenases are responsible for initiating a complex cycle of oxidative reactions which remove two carbon atoms from fatty acid acyl-CoA esters which have formed in the cytoplasm and traverse the mitochondrial membrane as carnitine esters. Acetyl-CoA is produced and the chain-shortened acyl-CoA re-enters the oxidation cycle. Electron transfer flavoproteins are necessary to complete this process, transferring electrons to the electron transport chain.

In the last decade a series of disorders of the fatty acid β-oxidation pathway have been described (Fig. 3). Three forms of acyl-CoA dehydrogenase deficiency have been described with different but overlapping chain length specificities. These are respectively long chain (LCAD), medium chain (MCAD) and short chain (SCAD). Deficiency of the flavoproteins involve all three chain lengths. MCAD is the most common. Fatty acids proximal to the metabolic block accumulate and are excreted in the urine as their acylcarnitine derivatives. Excretion may be episodic.

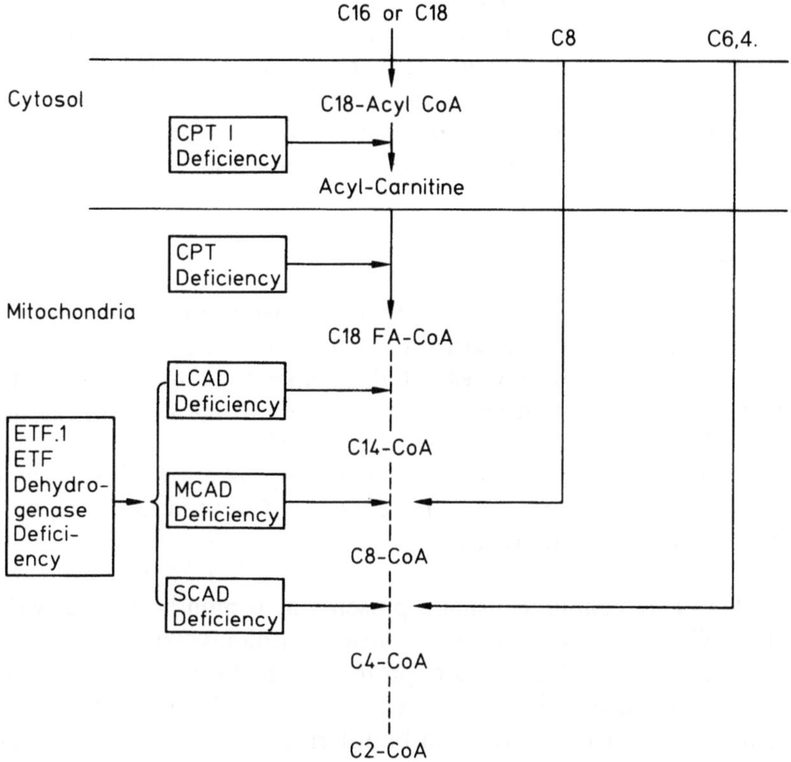


**Fig. 3.** Diagrammatic representation of the metabolism of free fatty acids of different chain lengths as they pass from the plasma to the mitochondria. Sites of defects of β-oxidation within the mitochondria are illustrated. *CPT I*, carnitine palmitoyl transferase I; *ETF*, electron transfer fluoroprotein

### *Clinical Features*

The clinical features are episodic. The onset is usually between 2 and 48 months of age, when the feeding frequency has decreased sufficiently for the infant to utilise fat stores between feeds. The child often presents with an episode of vomiting and lethargy followed by coma. Precipitating factors are infection and starvation. The blood sugar is low and there is a prompt response to intravenous 10% dextrose unless cerebral oedema has developed. There may be a previous history of recurrent episodes of coma, convulsions or Reye's syndrome. There may be a family history of sudden infant death syndrome or Reye's syndrome.

Hepatic features include rapid changes in liver size due to microvesicular or macrovesicular fatty infiltration, raised serum transaminase and blood ammonium. The prothrombin time may be prolonged. Urinary ketones are inappropriately low. Plasma carnitine is also low.

The diagnosis is suspected when acylcarnitine derivatives specific for the metabolic block are detected as dicarboxylic acids by gas-liquid chromatography–mass spectroscopy. It has to be emphasised that the excretion may only occur when the patient is symptomatic. The diagnosis is confirmed by specific enzyme studies in fibroblasts.

### *Treatment*

*MCAD.* Acute episodes require treatment with intravenous glucose and the management of coma associated with increased intracranial pressure. To prevent recurrences it is essential to take food more frequently than 8 hourly. The dietary fat should be restricted to 20% of the calorie requirements. Dietary supplements with medium chain triglycerides or intravenous fat emulsions must be avoided. Sodium valproate is contraindicated since it may further inhibit mitochondrial function. Carnitine supplements 25 mg/kg three or four times daily help.

*LCAD.* This condition usually presents at 6 months of age with features like MCAD, but in addition a chronic cardiomyopathy, muscle weakness and developmental delay are prominent features. The serum creatinine phosphokinase is raised. The treatment is similar to that for MCAD but medium chain triglycerides can be tolerated. Nasogastric tube feeding may be required because of hypotonia.

*SCAD.* The clinical features of this very rare condition are similar to those of LCAD. The management is as of MCAD.

Infants with a defect in the *flavoprotein electron transfer* cycle have similar features to LCAD but respond to riboflavin in a dose of 100 mg twice daily and a low fat intake. Carnitine may worsen the disorder.

### 13.2 Carnitine Palmitoyl Transferase Deficiency

Palmitoyl CoA combines with carnitine in the presence of carnitine palmitoyl transferase (CPT), allowing palmitoyl carnitine to traverse the mitochondrial membrane. CPT 1 deficiency is characterised by fasting hypoglycaemia, moderate hepatomegaly and massive lipid accumulation in hepatocytes. Free fatty acids are high. There are no ketones. Total hepatic carnitine concentration is normal. CPT activity in liver and fibroblasts is undetectable. The onset is in the 1st year of life. Dietary supplements with nutrient triglycerides correct the metabolic consequences of this deficiency state.

### 13.3 Systemic Carnitine Deficiency

Systemic carnitine deficiency is characterised by low serum, urinary and tissue carnitine. It is associated with episodic hepatic and cerebral dysfunction, underdeveloped muscles and sometimes cardiomyopathy. Carnitine is synthesised predominantly in the liver. It is not known whether carnitine deficiency results from a failure in synthesis and/or a failure in transport. Secondary carnitine insufficiency, which occurs in many organic acidurias but is usually associated with an increased or normal excretion of acyl carnitine, is more common.

Hepatic features during acute exacerbations are those of Reye's syndrome with markedly elevated transaminases and blood ammonia and hypoglycaemia, but with macrovesicular lipid accumulation in the hepatocytes. There is no ketosis but dicarboxylic acid excretion is increased. Diagnosis is indicated by a low free carnitine and decreased acyl carnitine concentrations in plasma and urine. Diagnosis is confirmed by a low carnitine concentration in liver and muscle tissue after some months of carnitine supplementation. Symptomatic episodes can be prevented by carnitine administration in a dose sufficient to prevent dicarboxylic aciduria. A dose of 1–4 g/day is usually required. Biotin 0.5 mg daily is also helpful.

## 14 Abetalipoproteinaemia

Abetalipoproteinaemia is a genetic disorder in which the major defect is absence of plasma β-lipoprotein and complete inability to produce chylomicrons and very low density lipoproteins. The underlying mechanisms may vary in different kindreds. Severe malabsorption and tocopherol deficiency are responsible for the clinical features.

Liver function tests and liver histology are usually normal although lipid droplets may be seen in hepatocytes. Cirrhosis has been reported by the age of 30 months but seems to be related to treatment with medium chain triglycerides.

### *Clinical Features*

The disease is characterized by steatorrhoea, starting in the first months of life, progressive ataxia, and retinitis pigmentosa becoming detectable after the 5th years of life. Patients surviving until adult life may be severely physically and mentally handicapped unless they receive adequate vitamin E.

### *Diagnosis*

The diagnosis may be suggested by the finding of acanthocytosis in a fresh, wet, peripheral blood film. Serum cholesterol phospholipid and triglyceride levels are extremely low. Electrophoretic demonstration of lack of β-lipoprotein confirms the diagnosis.

### *Treatment*

A low fat diet eliminates the steatorrhoea. Massive doses of vitamin E prevent the neurological changes. Vitamin A and K supplements may also be required.

## 15 Bile Salt Metabolism

The *major* pathway of primary bile acid synthesis together with the main intermediates and key *enzymes* in its early part is shown in Fig. 4. The microsomal cholesterol 7α-hydroxylase responsible for the first reaction is subjected to a negative feedback regulation by primary bile acids, chenodeoxycholic acid and cholic acid, reabsorbed from the gut. In the adult it is considered that side chain oxidation and hydroxylation which reduces the steroid from a $C_{27}$ sterol to a $C_{24}$ bile acid occurs only after the nucleus has been modified.

In an *alternative* pathway 7α-hydroxy-4-cholesten-3-one may undergo 26 hydroxylation to form 7α,26-dihydroxy-4-cholesten-3-one, which can be metabolised to chenodeoxycholic acid. In another alternative pathway for side chain oxidation 5β-cholestane-3α,7α,12α-triol may be 25-hydroxylated by a microsomal 25-hydroxylase to yield 5β-cholestane-3α,7α,12α,25-tetrol. This compound may be metabolised to cholic acid. This pathway is particularly active when there is a defect in 26-hydroxylation, as occurs in the cerebrotendinous xanthomatosis. All of the above reactions occur in liver mitochondria but the final steps after 26-hydroxylation occur in peroxisomes and are thus defective in Zellweger syndrome.

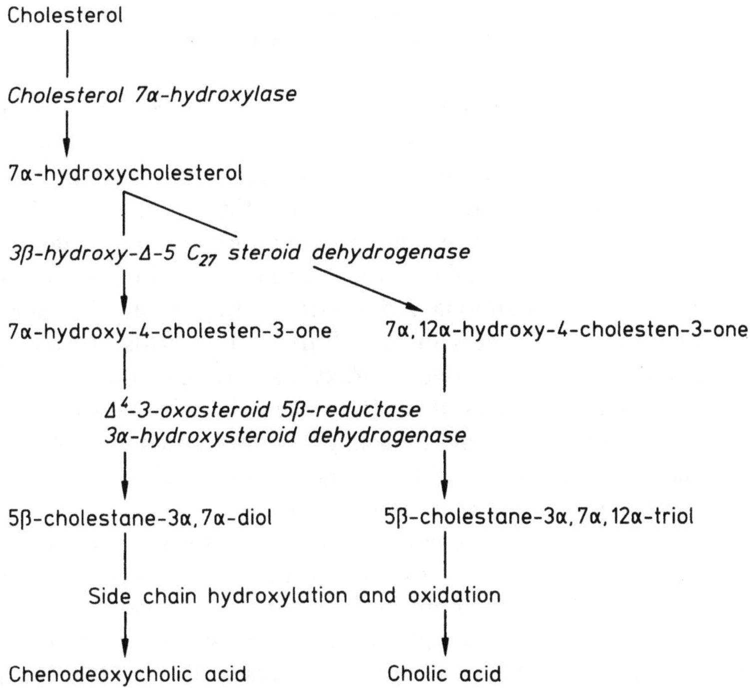


**Fig. 4.** Diagrammatic representation of the major pathway of primary bile acid synthesis

## 16 Defects in Bile Acid Synthesis

1. A specific defect in bile acid metabolism with the formation of trihydroxycholestanoic acid was described in two male siblings who died by 2 years of age with intrahepatic disease, including bile duct hypoplasia. A defect in side chain oxidation is considered responsible.

2. Abnormal bile salt metabolites and no primary bile acids were described in one of three affected siblings with cirrhosis, suggesting a defect of 3β-hydroxy-Δ-5 $C_{27}$ steroid dehydrogenase, the enzyme responsible for the second step in the pathway illustrated above. The severity of liver disease improved with the administration of chenodeoxycholic acid [18].

3. Three children in one family with an excess of 3-oxo-$\Delta^4$ bile acids and high plasma concentration of chenodeoxycholic acid were considered to have a deficiency of $\Delta^4$-3-oxosteroid 5β-reductase. Severe hepatitis syndrome in early infancy was present in two probands. Liver disease improved with ursodeoxycholic acid [19]. It should be noted that 3-oxo-$\Delta^4$ bile acids may be present in excess in other forms of liver disease [18].

4. In Zellweger syndrome abnormal bile salts are found as part of a generalised defect in peroxisomal β-oxidation affecting the cholesterol side chain (see below).

## 16.1 Cerebrotendinous Xanthomatosis (Hepatic Mitochondrial 26-Hydroxylase Deficiency)

Cerebrotendinous xanthomatosis is a rare recessively inherited disorder initially classified as a lipid storage disease. It is a particularly interesting defect in that oral therapy with a primary bile acid prevents excessive production of bile acid precursors and thus controls the disorder. The major clinical features are tendon xanthomas, cataracts, dementia, pyramidal paresis and cerebellar ataxia. Premature atherosclerosis, endocrine hypofunction and pulmonary dysfunction may occur. The onset is usually between 10 and 20 years of age. Primary bile acids are not formed from cholesterol due to defective hydroxylation of C26 on the cholesterol side chain. Enzymatic reactions early in the bile acid pathway are depressed, causing overproduction of bile acid precursors which are synthesised into the bile alcohol cholestanol. Cholestanol replaces cholesterol in the central nervous system and peripheral nerve myelin.

Hepatocytes contain golden-brown pigment which on electronmicroscopy is seen as amorphous electron–dense material. Diagnosis is based on the clinical features and is confirmed by a plasma cholestanol level of greater than 1 mg/dl (between 3 and 15 times normal). Long-term treatment with chenodeoxycholic acid, 75 mg/day reverses the metabolic abnormality, arrests progression of the disease and may cause reversal of dementia and peripheral neuropathy.

## 16.2 Peroxisomal Disorders

### *Zellweger Syndrome (Cerebro-hepato-renal Syndrome)*

Zellweger syndrome, an autosomal recessive condition, is characterised by absence of peroxisomes and defective function of peroxisomal enzymes. It is the most common of the peroxisomal disorders, which are estimated to occur with a frequency of 1 in 25 000 to 1 in 50 000 births. It is a multisystem disorder with profound abnormalities of neuronal migration and brain structure, hepatic malfunction, renal cortical cysts, abnormal calcification, retinal degeneration and multiple congenital anomalies [20, 21]. Diagnostic biochemical abnormalities include greatly diminished levels of plasmalogens, defects in bile acid synthesis with an increase in dihydroxy- and trihydroxycoprostanic acid, defective oxidation and abnormal accumulation of very long chain fatty acids and of phytanic acid and increased pipecolic acid (a product of lysine degeneration).

The recognition of milder incomplete forms with features shared with other disorders of peroxisomes will create diagnostic difficulty until the underlying pathogenesis is clarified. At present it is not clear whether Zellweger syndrome arises from a structural defect in assembly of the peroxisomal membrane or a deficient receptor system necessary for the incorporation of enzymes into the membrane. Both phenotypic and genetic heterogeneity are reported. These disorders illustrate the metabolic role of peroxisomes and demonstrate the deleterious effect on hepatic function and structure which accompanies diffuse defects in peroxisomal metabolism.

### *Hepatic Pathology*

The histology of the liver varies from near normal to diffusely fibrotic or micronodular cirrhosis depending on the age of the patient. There is excessive hepatic iron in the first 8 weeks of life. In neonates in whom the biopsy looks normal there is frequently an irregular relationship between portal tracts and central veins. In the first month of life abnormalities are absent or may consist of mild portal or perilobular fibrosis, cholestasis, intrahepatic bile duct hypoplasia or proliferation, giant cell transformation and fatty metamorphosis. By 8–10 weeks of age fibrosis is severe with distortion of the architecture, and micronodular cirrhosis is established by 20 weeks of age. Ultrastructural studies show absence of peroxisomes and distorted mitochondria.

### *Clinical Features*

Patients with "classical" Zellweger syndrome manifest profound hypotonia, hyporeflexia, a typical craniofacial dysmorphism and severe psychomotor retardation, sometimes complicated by blindness and deafness. The forehead is prominent with shallow orbital ridges, epicanthic folds and a broad nasal bridge. The sutures are abnormally open and the fontanelle large. There is micrognathia and the external ear is abnormal. Poor sucking and feeding difficulties are almost universal. Corneal clouding, cataract, glaucoma and nystagmus are frequently described. Hepatomegaly is present at birth in approximately 40% of cases but develops in the 1st month in the majority. Sixty percent are jaundiced after 1 week of age. Cirrhosis has been documented in 40% of reported cases.

### *Laboratory Investigations*

Standard biochemical tests of liver function are abnormal. There may be hypoglycaemia, prolonged prothrombin time and high serum iron levels. X-rays show calcific stippling of the patella, acetabulum or greater trochanter. Increased pipecolic acid is found in serum and urine after 4 weeks of age. There is increased urinary excretion of dicarboxylic acids. Diagnostic investigations are given in the introduction.

5β-cholestane-3α,7α,12α-triol is oxidised to 3α,7α,12α,trihydroxy-5β-cholestanoic acid, 5β-cholestane-3α,7α-diol to 3α,7α,dihydroxy-5β-cholestanoic acid. These are not metabolised to cholic acid or desoxycholic acid but accumulate and undergo either side chain elongation to form $C_{29}$ bile acids or nuclear changes.

### *Treatment*

There is no effective treatment. The administration of ether lipids and reduction of long chain fat and phytanic acid intake normalises some of the biochemical abnormalities but has no clinical effects. Clofibrate, which markedly increases the number of peroxisomes in mammalian liver, does not induce them or influence bile acid metabolism.

### *Prenatal Diagnosis*

The following biochemical studies initially developed on fibroblasts from patients have now been used to establish a prenatal diagnosis using amniocytes:

1. A more than fivefold increase in very long chain fatty acid concentrations
2. Defective dihydroxyacetone phosphate acyl transferase (first step in plasmalogen formation)
3. A reduced ratio of 1,4C-hexadecanol to 1-*O*-(9,10-3H) hexadecyl glycerol incorporation in plasmalogens (the former is reduced in Zellweger syndrome).

### *Hepatic Aspects of Other Peroxisomal Disorders*

Increased hepatic fibrosis occurs in *neonatal onset adrenoleucodystrophy*, a disorder with a few peroxisomes and similar but less severe phenotype than Zellweger syndrome. The function of at least five different peroxisomal enzymes is impaired. There is impaired cortisol response to ACTH. Neonatal jaundice, hepatomegaly, abnormal biochemical tests of liver function and cirrhosis have been reported in *juvenile Refsum disease*, another disorder of peroxisomal biogenesis with similar but less severe phenotypic features than Zellweger syndrome. Cholesterol and lipoprotein concentrations are often low. In a third somewhat similar relatively mild disorder, *hyperpipecolic acidaemia*, hepatomegaly and cirrhosis have been reported.

## 17 Disorders of Lysosomal Enzymes

Almost all disorders of lysosomal enzymes are caused by the deficiency of a specific enzyme required for the degradation of complex macromolecules. Diagnosis (post- and prenatal) is by specific enzyme assay on leucocytes, fibroblasts or chorionic villi. The exceptions are I-cell disease and pseudo-Hurler polydystrophy, in which lysosomal enzymes are normally synthesised

**Table 3.** Disorders of lysosomal enzymes

| Disorders | Age of onset | Multisystem involvement | Splenomegaly |
|---|---|---|---|
| Mucopolysaccharidosis | ½–3 yr | ++++ | + |
| Multiple sulphatase deficiencies | 1 yr | +++ | + |
| I-cell disease | Neonatal | +++ | ± |
| Pseudo-Hurler polydystrophy | 2–4 yr | +++ | − |
| Glycoprotein storage diseases | Neonatal to adult | ++ | + |
| Gangliosidoses | Neonatal to 10 yr | ++ | ± |
| Lipid storage disorders (see text) | Neonatal to adult | + | + |

but are secreted into the extracellular matrix rather than being targeted to lysosomes. Undegraded molecules accumulate in the cytoplasm in these two disorders as opposed to lysosomes in the others. Cellular, tissue or organ dysfunction results. Hepatomegaly (usually with splenomegaly), abnormal facies, progressive mental deterioration, corneal clouding, ophthalmological abnormalities, skeletal changes, cardiac dysfunction, lung involvement and vacuolated lymphocytes manifest to varying degrees should prompt consideration of these conditions. The genetic basis of the considerable heterogeneity within each disorder is gradually being unravelled. Features of the main groups of such disorders are given in Table 3. There is considerable overlap. The more common lipid disorders with prominent hepatic features are considered in the text. Treatment is supportive. Early bone marrow transplantation from a compatible donor may have a role in Gaucher's, Hurler's and Niemann-Pick type I disease.

## 18 Lipid Storage Disorders

### 18.1 Definition

Lipid storage disorders are disorders in which fatty acids, cholesterol or complex lipids are abnormally stored. Although hepatomegaly and/or splenomegaly is a prominent feature in lipid storage disorders, gastrointestinal symptoms and hepatic dysfunction are of little clinical significance in the majority of cases compared with features due to nervous system involvement. These disorders do require consideration in the differential diagnosis of hepatomegaly and/or splenomegaly.

## 18.2 Sphingomyelin–Cholesterol Lipidosis (The Niemann-Pick Group of Diseases)

The Niemann-Pick group of diseases are characterised by abnormal storage of sphingomyelin, cholesterol and complex glycolipids which are seen as large "foam" cells in the reticuloendothelial system. In type I sphingomyelinase activity is less than 10% of normal. In type II sphingomyelinase activity is normal in solid tissues. It may be normal or decreased by as much as 80% in cultured fibroblasts. In vitro cholesterol esterification is decreased. Both types are divided into acute (A), subacute (S) and chronic (C) forms. The clinical features common to all forms are hepatosplenomegaly and central nervous system involvement.

Type IIA and S usually present as a hepatitis syndrome in early infancy. Approximately 30% of patients die of liver disease in infancy. In the remainder features of hepatitis regress, liver function tests return to normal but modest hepatomegaly or splenomegaly persists. There may be progression to cirrhosis but symptomatic liver disease is rare.

The diagnosis is established by the sphingomyelinase activity the presence of storage typical Sudan black positive cells in bone marrow and in nerve cells in a rectal biopsy in type II disease. In cultured fibroblasts decreased in vitro cholesterol esterification can be demonstrated.

## 18.3 Sulphatide Lipidosis

Metachromatic leucodystrophy is caused by the accumulation of galactosyl sulphatide due to deficiency of arylsulphatase A (EC 3.1.6.1). Tissues with an excretory function such as bile duct cells contain metachromatic material but such material is also found in periportal hepatocytes and Kupffer cells. The gallbladder is particularly affected, being small, fibrotic with polypoid masses and non-functioning. There are usually no clinical features of hepatobiliary involvement.

## 18.4 Acid Esterase Deficiency

### *Wolman's Disease*

Wolman's disease is due to a total deficiency of lysosomal acid esterase resulting in an accumulation of cholesterol esters and triglycerides in many organs, particularly the liver and the intestinal mucosa. The liver is large, firm and yellow in colour. The parenchymal cells are engorged by membrane-lined vacuoles of different size. Foamy histiocytes with similar vacuoles are found in clumps, both in the portal areas and between parenchymal cells. There is an increase in portal fibrosis and cirrhosis may develop. The disease commonly presents in the first few weeks of life with vomiting, abdominal distension, diarrhoea, hepatosplenomegaly, steatorrhoea and failure to thrive.

Standard tests of liver function are abnormal. Radiology will show adrenal calcification in more than 90% of cases. There is decreased adrenal endocrine activity. The diagnosis is confirmed by the low esterase concentration in leucocytes. Prenatal diagnosis in amniocytes has been accomplished. There is no specific treatment. Bone marrow transplantation corrected metabolic features in one patient who died of aspergillosis 80 days after grafting.

The clinical course is of progressive deterioration with anaemia, massive hepatosplenomegaly and death usually by 6 months of age. In some cases there is very severe liver involvement with jaundice prior to death.

### *Hepatic Cholesterol Ester Storage Disease*

Hepatic cholesterol ester storage disease is associated with a partial deficiency of acid esterase activity in the liver to values between 10% and 30% of normal. The liver shows similar lipid accumulation, with 50% of cases having increased fibrosis.

The clinical presentation is usually asymptomatic hepatomegaly noticed at a median age of 3 years (range: birth to 23 years). One-third of patients develop splenomegaly, and variceal bleeding has been recorded. Hypertriglyceridaemia and hypercholesterolaemia are found in the majority. Standard biochemical tests of liver function are usually mildly abnormal. The long-term prognosis is uncertain, but death from liver failure has occurred at 18 years of age and one patient underwent liver transplantation for hepatic failure at 14 years of age. Suppression of cholesterol and apolipoprotein B synthesis by HMG-CoA reductase inhibitors (simvastatin) may be beneficial.

## 18.5 Gaucher's Disease (Glucosylceramide Lipidosis)

Gaucher's disease, in which glucosylceramide accumulates because of deficiency of glucocerebrosidase, is the most prevalent lysosomal storage disease. It takes three main forms:

*Type 1* is a chronic non-neuropathic disorder starting at any time between birth and old age with very variable but frequently slow progression.
*Type 2* (acute neuropathic) starts in the first 6 months of life and leads to a neurological death by the age of 2 years.
*Type 3* (subacute neuropathic) presents with visceral features but neurological features develop usually in the first 5 years of life and are gradually progressive thereafter. Death usually occurs in the third decade.

*Hepatic Pathology*. Groups of Gaucher cells – large, multinucleated cells with a reticular pale-staining cytoplasm – surround the central hepatic veins and obstruct the sinusoids. The liver architecture is often deranged and hepatic fibrosis may be severe. This may be complicated by portal hypertension and ascites in all three types of the disease. Chronic active hepatitis has been described. Death from liver failure is rare.

Liver function tests are frequently abnormal but there is no specific pattern. Hypersplenism eventually occurs in nearly all patients with type 1 or type 3 disease. It may be aggravated by an associated haemolytic anaemia or by displacement of erythrocyte precursors from the bone marrow by Gaucher's cells. Bone marrow transplantation from an HLA-matched sibling immediately following splenectomy produces some regression in the clinical features, with a decrease in bone pain and a reduction in liver size, but intrahepatic fibrosis may progress.

## 19 Mucopolysaccharidosis

Mucopolysaccharides are complex structures containing amino acids, amino sugars, uronic acids and sulphates. The mucopolysaccharidoses are a group of disorders caused by deficiency of lysosomal enzymes needed for their degradation. They may be excreted in the urine. Ten distinct enzyme deficiencies have been identified. There is both considerable overlap between the various disorders and considerable range in severity. The hepatic presentation is hepatosplenomegaly. Hunter's syndrome is inherited in an X-linked fashion.

### *"Mucopolysaccharidosis"-like Conditions*

I-cell disease and pseudo-Hurler polydystrophy are mucolipidoses that have many clinical features in common with the mucopolysaccharidoses; splenomegaly, however, is minimal. They are not true lysosomal storage diseases, arising as they do from abnormal lysosomal enzyme transport which produces abnormal inclusions in cytoplasm. Diagnosis is established by the clinical features and high serum concentration of lysosomal enzymes. There is no treatment. Prenatal diagnosis is possible.

### *Disorders of Glycoprotein Degradation*

Glycoproteins comprise oligosaccharide chains covalently linked to serine, threonine or asparagine in a peptide backbone. They too share many features of mucopolysaccharidoses. Vacuolation can usually be found in lymphocytes.

## 20 Progressive Neuronal Degeneration of Childhood with Liver Disease

This familial disorder is characterised by a distinctive pattern of cortical neuronal loss and of pathological change in the liver. The metabolic basis is unknown. There is fatty infiltration, hepatocellular necrosis, bridging fibrosis and cirrhosis. There is cortical atrophy affecting particularly the occipital area. Neuronal loss and astrocytosis are associated with pigment-laden macrophages which give a distinctive dark-brown discolouration to the cortical ribbon. The liver shows a subacute hepatitis comprising massive fatty degeneration, hepatocyte loss, bile duct proliferation, bridging necrosis and cirrhosis. Twenty-four cases have been reported from 16 kindreds, suggesting an autosomal recessive inherited metabolic defect.

Early development is normal but between 1 month and 3 years of age developmental arrest, intractable epilepsy, vomiting or failure to thrive develop. Long-track and cranial nerve signs may appear. Typical high-voltage slow waves with polyspikes are seen on EEG. The visual evoked response is absent or disorganised. The majority die of status epilepticus by 3 years of age.

Abnormal biochemical tests of liver function are recorded from 4–80 months of age. There are usually no early clinical features of liver involvement. Death from liver failure occurs at 4–8 years of age.

## 21 Indian Childhood Cirrhosis

Indian childhood cirrhosis is a familial disorder which may be genetically determined although environmental factors such as a large copper intake appear to be responsible for disease expression, if not causation [22].

The cirrhosis, which occurs almost exclusively in the Indian subcontinent, is characterised by necrosis of hepatocytes which contain Mallory's hyalin and orcein-staining coarse granular material representing copper-associated protein. The liver copper concentration is very high. There is marked pericellular collagen deposition and a distinct lack of regeneration nodules except in chronic cases. Symptoms start between 6 and 48 (median 18) months of age. The disorder begins insidiously in more than 75% of cases with irritability, anorexia and hepatomegaly. Slight jaundice heralds the onset of decompensated cirrhosis with all its complications. The remainder present with features of acute or subacute icteric hepatitis. Over 80% are dead within 6 months. Less than 5% are alive in good health 1–2 years later. If exposure to excessive dietary copper, mainly in boiled buffalo milk stored in copper-containing vessels, can be prevented, the disease may be eliminated. Penicillamine in a dose of 20 mg/kg daily gives a 50% survival if given to patients before the onset of ascites or jaundice.

## 22 Familial Erythrophagocytic Lymphohistiocytosis

Familial erythrophagocytic lymphohistiocytosis appears to be inherited in an autosomal recessive fashion. The metabolic basis is unknown. It is characterised by progressive visceral, central nervous system and bone marrow infiltration with lymphocytes and large erythrophagocytic histiocytes. The clinical features are fever, irritability, pallor, oedema, hepatosplenomegaly, jaundice, and skin rash, usually starting in the 1st year of life. Pancytopenia, liver dysfunction, coagulopathy with prevalent hypofibrinogenaemia, a lymphohistiocytic meningitis and hypertriglyceridaemia are the main laboratory abnormalities. The diagnosis is established by demonstration of erythrophagocytic histiocytes in bone marrow or of cells in the cerebrospinal fluid, or by liver or brain biopsy. The main differential diagnosis is virus-associated haemophagocytic syndrome. Treatment with epipodophyllotoxin, steroids and intrathecal methotrexate with cranial irradiation may prevent a fatal outcome.

## 23 Cystic Fibrosis

Cystic fibrosis, the most common lethal genetic disorder in Caucasian populations, is due to defective expression of a transmembrane conductance regulator which controls $Cl^-$ channel activation in the apical membrane of epithelial cells and maintains an intracellular negative potential. These two functions are necessary for bile production in canaliculi. It is presumed that this abnormality affects the biliary pole of the hepatocyte and/or bile duct cells. In other tissues the effect is impaired $Cl^-$ reabsorption and increased sodium and chloride concentrations in secretions [23]. The abnormally tenacious viscid secretion of mucus-producing glands is secondary. More than 60 different mutations have been found in the CF gene. An unexplained feature of the condition is the variable severity of pathological change in different organs. Principal changes occur in the respiratory system, intestine and pancreas. Affected males are usually sterile due to absence of the vas deferens. Nasal polyps are common. Heat prostration due to salt loss occurs in warm environments. The course of the disease is very variable from patient to patient. The prognosis is largely determined by the degree of pulmonary involvement. With earlier diagnosis, the introduction of comprehensive treatment of pulmonary problems prior to the onset of irreversible lung damage and better nutritional care, there has been a steadily improving prognosis in the last 40 years. Why particular subjects with cystic fibrosis develop hepatobiliary complications remains unknown.

### *Hepatic Pathology*

The most characteristic hepatic lesion is focal biliary fibrosis ("cirrhosis"). Amorphous eosinophilic PAS-positive diastase-resistant material blocks bile ducts and causes oedema, chronic inflammatory cell infiltrate, bile duct proliferation and increased fibrosis in portal tracts. Such lesions are present in 10% of infants of less than 3 months but occur in 27% of older children. Over a period of months or years the lesions of focal biliary fibrosis extend, coalesce and cause atrophy of the hepatic parenchyma. Ultimately regenerative nodules encircled by fibrous tissue develop, giving a true cirrhosis and all its sequelae. Biliary abnormalities take the form of micro gallbladder, which is present in up to a third. Gallstones occur in as many as 12%. Cholecystitis may develop. Biliary excretion scans shows a high incidence of impaired bile flow, in some instances attributable to a narrowing of the biliary system as it passes through the pancreas. Sclerosing cholangitis and cholangiocarcinoma may develop. To what extent these abnormalities are interrelated is unclear. Fatty infiltration of the liver is a very usual finding.

The very variable frequency of cirrhosis in different centres suggests environmental factors may have a role in causing symptomatic liver disease. The possible pathological factors or mechanisms contributing to liver disease in cystic fibrosis include impaired bile formation secondary to the $Cl^-$ channel defect, bile duct obstruction by viscid mucus, structural abnormalities in the biliary system, secondary changes in bile salt metabolism, inappropriate immune responses to liver membrane antigens and liver injury from microbial products, nutritional factors and drugs.

### *Clinical Features*

Rare clinical syndromes include prolonged conjugated hyperbilirubinaemia in infancy presenting as a hepatitis syndrome sometimes difficult to distinguish from biliary atresia and massive hepatic steatosis in early infancy which reverses as nutrition improves. Neither predisposes to chronic liver disease. Gallstones and cholecystitis may cause symptoms.

The most serious effect of hepatic involvements is a slowly progressive cirrhosis which usually is detected as asymptomatic hepatosplenomegaly or because of complications of portal hypertension such as variceal haemorrhage, hypersplenism and splenic pain. The incidence appears to increase with age, cirrhosis being reported in 0.5%–8% of children and 5%–20% of adults. In a study of 506 cystic fibrosis subjects under 30 years of age, 7 (1.4%) had bled from varices, 24 (4.7%) had clinical evidence of liver disease and 50 (10.3%) had abnormal biochemical tests of liver function. In another study 57 (24%) of 233 patients over 15 years of age had evidence of liver disease. The presence of liver disease is unrelated to the nature of the gene mutation [24].

***Treatment***

The treatment is aimed at improving nutrition, particularly deficiency of fat-soluble vitamins, controlling sepsis and the management of portal hypertension. There is no specific treatment for the liver disease although preliminary reports indicated that ursodeoxycholic acid given orally in a dose of 15–25 mg/kg per day improves standard biochemical tests of liver function and biliary excretion [25]. It does not improve galactose utilisation and its effect on long-term prognosis is unknown. Cholestasis in infancy may resolve spontaneously but may require irrigation of the biliary system if it is occluded by inspissated material. Complications of cirrhosis are managed as in other conditions. Hepatic encephalopathy is possibly less frequent after portosystemic shunts in this disorder than in other forms of cirrhosis but can still occur and injection sclerotherapy is the treatment of choice for bleeding varices. Surgery may be required for symptomatic gallstones. Bile drainage through the gallbladder has been advocated for patients with distal bile duct obstruction, and the short-term results have been encouraging [26]. Liver transplantation has also been performed with surprisingly little deterioration in the pulmonary status [16].

## References


1. Arias IM, Jakoby WB, Popper H, Schachter D, Shafritz DA (1987) The liver: biology and pathobiology, 2nd edn. Raven, New York
2. Scriver CR, Beaudet AL, Sly WS, Valle D (eds) (1989) The metabolic basis of inherited disorders, 6th edn. McGraw-Hill, New York
3. Schaub J, Van Hoof F, Vis HL (eds) (1991) Inborn errors of metabolism. Raven, New York
4. Mowat AP (1987) Liver disorders in childhood, 2nd edn. Butterworths, London
5. Wu GY, Wilson JM, Wu CH (1988) Targeting genes: delivery and expression of a foreign gene driven by an albumen promoter in vivo. Hepatology 8:1251

5a. Hobbs JR (1989) Correction of Certain Genetic Diseases by Transplantation Cogent. London

6. Maconochie IK, Chong S, Mieli-Vergani G et al. (1989) Fetal ascites: an usual presentation of Niemann-Pick disease type C. Arch Dis Child 10:1391–1393
7. Burchell A, Waddell ID (1990) Diagnosis of a novel glycogen storage disease: type 1aSP. J Inherited Metab Dis 13:247–249
8. Burchell A, Jung RT, Lang CC et al. (1987) Diagnosis of type 1a and type 1c glycogen storage diseases in adults. Lancet II:1059–1062
9. van den Berg IET, Berger R (1990) Phosphorylase b kinase deficiency in man: a review. J Inherited Metab Dis 13:442–451
10. Green HL, Brown BI, McClenathan DT et al. (1988) A new variant of type IV glycogenosis: deficiency of branching enzymatic activity without apparent progressive liver disease. Hepatology 8:302–306
11. Shin YS (1990) The diagnosis of glycogen storage disease. J Inherited Metab Dis 13:419–434
12. Fernandes J, Leonard JV, Moses SW et al. (1988) Glycogen storage disease: recommendations for treatment. Eur J Pediatr 147:226–228
13. Smit GPA, Fernandes J, Leonard JV et al. (1990) The long-term outcome of patients with glycogen storage disease. J Inherited Metab Dis 13:411–418

14. Chen YT, Coleman RA, Scheinman JI et al. (1988) Renal disease in type 1 glycogen storage disease. N Engl J Med 18:7–11
15. Mowat AP (1987) Liver disorders in childhood: the indicatons for liver replacement in parenchymal and metabolic diseases. Transplant Proc 19:3236–3241
16. Cohen A, O'Grady J, Mowat AP, Williams R (1989) Liver transplantation for metabolic disorders. Bailliere's Clinical Gastroenterology 3:767–786
17. Waggoner DD, Buist N, Donnell D (1990) Long-term prognosis in galactosaemia: results of a survey of 350 cases. J Inherited Metab Dis 13:802–818
18. Ichimiya H, Nazer H, Gunasekaren T et al. (1990) Treatment of chronic liver disease caused by 3v-hydroxy-$\Delta$-$C_{27}$-steroid dehydrogenase deficiency with chenodeoxycholic acid. Arch Dis Child 65:112–114
19. Setchell KDR, Suchy FJ, Welsh MB et al. (1988) $\Delta^4$-3-oxosteroid 5beta-reductase deficiency described in identical twins with neonatal hepatitis. A new inborn error of metabolism. J Clin Invest 82:2148–2157
20. Wilson GN, Holmes RD, Hajra AK (1988) Peroxisomal disorders: clinical commentary and future prospects. Am J Med Genet 30:771–792
21. Wanders RJA, van Roermund CWT, Schutgens RBH et al. (1990) The inborn errors of peroxisomal beta-oxidation: a review. J Inherited Metab Dis 13:411–errors of peroxisomal beta-oxidation: a review. J Inherited Metab Dis 13:4–36
22. Tanner MS, Bhave SA, Pradhan A et al. (1987) Clinical trials of *d*-penicillamine in Indian childhood cirrhosis. Arch Dis Child 62:1118–1124
23. Rich DR, Anderson MP, Gregory RJ et al. (1990) Expression of transmembrane conductance regulator corrects defective chloride channel regulation in cystic fibrosis airway epithelial cells. Nature 347:358–363
24. Duthie A, Doherty DG, Williams C et al. (submitted for publication) Genotype analysis for F508, G551D, R553X mutations in children and young adults with cystic fibrosis with and without liver disease.
25. Colombo C, Setchell KDR, Poda M et al. (1990) Effects of ursodeoxycholic acid therapy for liver disease associated with cystic fibrosis. J Pediatr 117:482–489
25a. Scott-Jupp R, Lama M, Tanner MS (1991) Prevalence of Liver Disease in cystic fibrosis. Arch Dis Child 66:698–701
26. Lloyd-Still JD (1990) Cystic fibrosis, Crohns's disease, biliary abnormalities and cancer. J Pediatr Gastroenterol Nutr 11:434–437

# 28 Disordered Embryogenesis of the Hepatobiliary Tract

P. Van Eyken and V. Desmet

## 1 Introduction

This chapter starts with a brief overview of the current state of knowledge of the normal development of the biliary tree and a short discussion of the "ductal plate malformation." Because of their rarity and/or lack of clinical importance, anatomic anomalies of the bile ducts are only briefly touched upon. Atresia of extrahepatic bile ducts and paucity of intrahepatic bile ducts are more extensively discussed since they are important causes of neonatal jaundice. The final section deals with cystic and dysplastic lesions.

## 2 Normal Development of the Bile Ducts and the Ductal Plate Malformation

### 2.1 Normal Development of the Extra- and Intrahepatic Bile Ducts

During development, the liver primordium arises as a bud of cells (the hepatic diverticulum) growing from the cranioventral edge of the junction of the yolk sac with the foregut [18, 30, 64]. In man and in the mouse, the hepatic diverticulum consists of a pars caudalis or cystica and a pars cranialis or hepatica [30, 64, 67]. The latter gives off cords of liver precursor cells that grow into the mesenchyme of the septum transversum. It is generally assumed that the liver sinusoids develop from the capillary network between the vitelline veins present in this septum. The connective tissue of the liver presumably originates from the mesenchymal cells of the septum transversum [18, 30]. A portion of the cephalic end of the diverticulum is reduced to a small tubular structure, the common hepatic duct [64]. Both hepatic ducts and possibly part of the cystic duct are also derived from this part of the diverticulum [67]. The caudal part of the hepatic diverticulum develops into the gallbladder, (part of) the cystic duct, and the common bile duct [64].

The development of the intrahepatic bile ducts takes place in close association with the branches of the portal vein. Their origin has been debated for decades. Three main theories have been proposed: (a) an ingrowth of branches of the extrahepatic bile ducts ("ductal" hypothesis);

(b) a derivation of bile duct cells from primitive hepatocytes around portal vein branches ("hepatocytogenic" theory), and (c) a combination of both [for more extensive discussion see 30]. Recently, the use of immunohistochemical staining techniques, especially for cytokeratin-type intermediate filaments and cell surface markers, and cell culture experiments have led to new insights into the cell lineage relationships in developing liver [20, 45, 73]. It appears that the early embryonic liver is composed of at least bipotential progenitor cells which can develop into liver parenchymal cells or intrahepatic bile duct cells [20, 45, 73]. The latter develop from that layer of progenitor cells located around the portal vein branches. First, a layer of cells adjacent to the mesenchyme surrounding the portal vein radicles gradually acquires characteristics of bile duct cells. This layer is duplicated over a variable segment of its perimeter, giving rise to a partly duplicated cylinder surrounding the portal vein branches. This structure is termed the ductal plate [16, 17, 26, 30] (Fig. 1). Ductal plates are subsequently remodeled. Segments dilate and form tubular structures which are – from about 12 weeks of gestation onward – gradually incorporated into the mesenchyme of the portal tracts. The development as well as the remodeling of the ductal plate starts around large portal vein branches close to the porta hepatis and gradually proceeds throughout the liver. This implies that portal tracts only gradually acquire an individual bile duct tube. It is important to

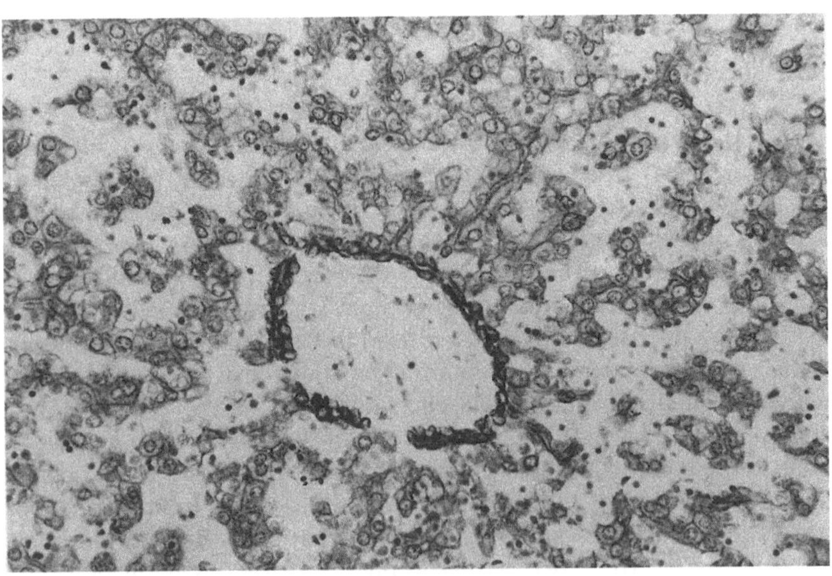

**Fig. 1.** Paraffin section of fetal human liver stained for cytokeratin-type intermediate filaments. A partly duplicated layer of cells surrounding a portal vein branch is more strongly immunoreactive than the adjacent epithelial cells. This structure corresponds to the ductal plate. Indirect immunoperoxidase using monoclonal antibody CAM 5.2 reactive with cytokeratins 8, 18, and 19, counterstained with Harris' hematoxylin, ×400

note that both in the rat and in the human the development of the intrahepatic biliary tree is not fully terminated at birth [73].

Several fundamental problems pertaining to the development of the biliary tree remain. The factors inducing the progenitor cells to develop into ductal plate cells/bile duct cells are unknown at present. It is very likely that the extracellular matrix plays a fundamental role in this process. It is still not clear how the continuity between the different segments of the biliary tree is maintained or established. In the mouse, bile ducts were reported to be initially discontinuous but subsequently to become confluent [67]. During normal bile duct development, apparently an excess of normal structure is formed that subsequently disappears during the "remodeling phase" of the ductal plate. The factors regulating this process are completely unknown.

### 2.2 The Ductal Plate Malformation

In 1976, JØRGENSEN described a peculiar bile duct lesion characterized in histologic sections by what appeared to be a surprisingly large number of longitudinally cut bile duct profiles [30]. Using three-dimensional reconstructions and stereologic principles, he was able to demonstrate that this ductal population was a mixture of geometric shapes ranging from circular cylinders to very flat elliptical cylinders or two plates of ductal epithelium around a plate-shaped lumen [30]. The bile duct profiles seemed to partially or totally ensheath vessels. JØRGENSEN noted the resemblance of these bile duct profiles to the embryonic ductal plate. He coined this lesion the "ductal plate malformation." It was proposed that it results from an arrest of or a wrong remodeling of the normal ductal plate [16, 17, 30].

Although originally described in infantile polycystic disease and congenital hepatic fibrosis [30], it later became apparent that the ductal plate malformation is also a component of other cholangiopathies, including extra- and intrahepatic bile duct atresia, Meyenburg's complexes, Caroli's disease, and a number of syndromes such as Meckel's syndrome and Ivemark's syndrome [16, 17]. The presence of (incompletely remodeled) ductal plates in these disorders may yield information as to the time of onset of a disease process. It is conceivable that a destructive process affecting the intrahepatic bile ducts at an early stage of their formation will result in involution of "immature" ducts, still in ductal plate arrangement. Disease processes operative at later stages of development or in postnatal life will result in involution of bile ducts with a "mature" appearance [16, 17].

## 3 Anatomic Anomalies of the Bile Ducts

Anatomic variations and abnormalities of the biliary tree are important for radiologists and biliary and transplant surgeons [55, 66]. "Variations" are not uncommon and have no pathologic significance [55]. They can be demonstrated by radiographic techniques. "Abnormalities" are pathologically significant deviations from the normal pattern [55]. In a large series of operative cholangiograms, such abnormalities were found in 18.4% of cases [55].

### 3.1 Agenesis of the Common Bile Duct; Agenesis of the Extrahepatic Bile Ducts

Markle reported a case of agenesis of the common bile duct, in which the common hepatic duct emptied into the gallbladder. Bile was drained through a long cystic duct emptying into the duodenum [47]. Schwartz et al. [61] recently reported four cases of agenesis of the proximal extrahepatic bile ducts and one case of total absence of extrahepatic bile ducts and gallbladder. There was no fibrous remnant at the porta hepatis. Patients had an early onset of jaundice. Liver transplantation is believed to be the treatment of choice.

### 3.2 "Aberrant" and "Accessory' Bile Ducts

Accessory hepatic ducts have also been described which pass beyond the porta hepatis and terminate in other segments of the extrahepatic bile duct system [55]. The extra duct is usually the right hepatic [66].

The so-called aberrant hepatic duct corresponds to a dorsocaudal branch draining into the common hepatic duct or even the cystic duct [55].

Cholecystohepatic ducts are worth mentioning because failure to recognize them at cholecystectomy can lead to complications such as biliary fistula or bile peritonitis [27].

### 3.3 Bile Duct Duplication

Bile duct duplication is exceptionally rare [19, 27]. The condition does not cause clinical symptoms unless complications like obstruction or infection occur [27]. The diagnosis is usually made during surgical intervention for presumed cholangitis or choledochal cyst [19].

### 3.4 Congenital Bronchobiliary Fistula

Congenital bronchobiliary fistula is a very rare malformation which leads to aspiration pneumonia and atelectasis in infancy [27].

### 3.5 Spontaneous Perforation of the Common Bile Duct

Spontaneous perforation of the common bile duct is a rare but highly specific entity occurring between birth and 3 months [19]. The perforation is situated at the junction of the cystic duct and the common bile duct [19, 27]. The etiology is unknown. A congenital weakness of the bile duct wall at this site, mucous plugs, gallstones, and even viral infection have all been implicated [19, 27, 65]. The condition usually manifests itself with fluctuating jaundice, acholic stools, and dark urine or with general symptoms of weight loss, irritability, or vomiting. Clinical examination reveals abdominal distention due to bile ascites [19]. There are usually no signs of peritonitis. Liver enzyme tests are normal but there is a rise in serum levels of bilirubin [19]. The presence of fluid with a high concentration of bilirubin on paracentesis suggests the diagnosis [19]. Intravenous cholangiography or scanning with rose bengal sodium iodine 131 can also be used to establish the diagnosis. Treatment of this condition is surgical and the prognosis is excellent.

### 3.6 Bile Duct Hypoplasia

In bile duct hypoplasia, the extrahepatic biliary ducts are grossly visible and are radiographically patent but they are exceedingly small [19, 59]. It is not a single specific disease entity. Hypoplasia of the extrahepatic bile ducts may be associated with intrahepatic cholestasis of any cause. In "low flow" states such as $\alpha_1$-antitrypsin deficiency, the disorder may represent a form of "disuse atrophy." Small and thready extrahepatic bile ducts have also been reported in the setting of atresia of the extrahepatic bile ducts, choledochal cyst, and in some patients with Alagille's syndrome [19, 32, 59]. The "hypoplasia" may progress to a complete obliteration of the bile duct lumen, suggesting that this disease may represent an intermediate stage in the development of extrahepatic bile duct atresia [19]. In such cases, histologic examination reveals inflammatory and degenerative lesions of the bile duct epithelium, i.e., changes indistinguishable from those observed in the fibrous remnants of extrahepatic bile duct atresia [19]. The diagnosis of bile duct hypoplasia is usually made during exploratory laparotomy for jaundice in infancy [19, 59]. Patients with persistent hypoplasia may gradually progress to cirrhosis, analogous to the development of cirrhosis in adults with narrowed extrahepatic bile ducts [19]. Treatment of bile duct hypoplasia depends upon the underlying hepatobiliary disorder. In patients with hypoplasia progressing toward total obstruction, hepatic portoenterostomy should be considered [19]. The small diameter of the biliary radicles may present a problem at the time of orthotopic liver transplantation [59].

### 3.7 Anomalies of the Gallbladder and Cystic Duct

Anomalies of the gallbladder include absence of the gallbladder, double and bilobed gallbladder, and left-sided, folded, and intrahepatic gallbladder. These conditions are discussed more extensively by Sherlock [66]. They are usually of no clinical significance.

In 20% of subjects, the cystic duct does not join the common hepatic duct directly but instead runs parallel to it for some distance and occasionally makes a spiral turn around it. This variation is obviously important for the biliary surgeon.

## 4 Atresia of Extrahepatic Bile Ducts

### 4.1 Definition

Extrahepatic bile duct atresia (EHBDA) is defined as "the lack of a lumen in part or all of the extrahepatic biliary tract, causing complete obstruction to bile flow" [19]. The disorder occurs in various anatomic variants and has classically been divided into a "correctable" and a "noncorrectable" group [19, 59, 62]. In the former category, comprising less than 10% of all patients with EHBDA, only limited segments of the extrahepatic bile ducts are atretic. After resection of the obliterated segment, the preserved proximal parts of the extrahepatic bile duct system can be reimplanted into the duodenum. In the vast majority of cases, however, there are no cystically dilated ducts in the porta hepatis that can be used for reanastomosis. These cases were thus truly "incorrectable" until Kasai introduced the portoenterostomy procedure (see Sect. 4.6).

### 4.2 Incidence

Extrahepatic bile duct atresia occurs in 1/10000 to 1/13000 live births [62]. This incidence is similar all over the world. Girls are more frequently affected than boys. Familial cases have been reported, but there is no specific mode of inheritance. Associated malformations such as the polysplenia syndrome are present in 11% of patients [62].

### 4.3 Clinical Features and Diagnostic Workup

Neonatal cholestasis can be caused by a vast number of extra- and intrahepatic disorders and presents a challenging problem to clinicians and pathologists alike. Several schemes for the diagnostic workup for conjugated hyperbilirubinemia in infancy have been proposed. It is imperative to secure the diagnosis of EHBDA as rapidly as possible because succesful surgery becomes increasingly unlikely with increasing patient age [19, 59]. It is important to differentiate EHBDA from neonatal hepatitis because the prognosis and management of the two disorders differ considerably. Unfortunately, there is no pathognomonic clinical symptom or sign that distinguishes EHBDA from other causes of neonatal cholestasis. Still, clinical features may aid in the differential diagnosis [19]. EHBDA occurs more frequently in girls, usually with a normal birth weight. Familial cases are rare. Neonatal hepatitis, in contrast, is more common in boys, and a familial incidence is noted in 15%–20% of cases. Associated polysplenia syndrome suggests EHBDA [62]. Neonatal jaundice persists in 34% of patients with EHBDA, but in 66% a jaundice-free interval of about 2 weeks separates the physiologic and pathologic icterus [62]. In neonatal hepatitis, pathologic jaundice immediately follows the physiologic hyperbilirubinemia. In EHBDA, stools are consistently acholic and urine is dark. In intrahepatic cholestasis, stools may be acholic but incompletely or intermittently decolored stools rule out EHBDA. Pruritus may become severe and skin xanthomas appear [65]. Prolonged steatorrhea can result in osteomalacia ("biliary rickets").

Various laboratory tests and imaging techniques used to differentiate extrahepatic from intrahepatic cholestasis and for checking the patency of the extrahepatic bile ducts are reviewed extensively by SUNARYO and WATKINS [69]. The reported usefulness of determining the ratio of chenodeoxycholic acid to cholic acid in serum has been questioned. Quantitative determination of lipoprotein-X in serum before and after a 10-day course of cholestyramine has also been proposed as a screening method for EHBDA. A vitamin E absorption test – apart from assessing the need for parenteral vitamin E supplementation – is unlikely to be helpful. Duodenal intubation and visual examination of the duodenal fluid collected over 24 h has been recommended as an easy and inexpensive test for determining complete cholestasis. The test can be repeated after injection of cholecystokinin [62]. A negative result is not informative but a positive one rules out EHBDA. Endoscopic retrograde cholangiopancreatography is technically difficult in infants and may be hazardous. It has not yet found wide application in the diagnosis of EHBDA. Percutaneous transhepatic cholangiography, on the other hand, is easier to perform in children. Flow of contrast medium into the duodenum excludes EHBDA. The value of measurements of the excretion of rose bengal sodium iodine 131 is much debated. Hepatobiliary scintigraphy using $^{99m}$Tc-IDA is probably useful to differentiate EHBDA from other causes of neonatal jaundice. Ultrasonography is a safe and noninvasive procedure. A decrease in gallbladder size following feeding virtually precludes the diagnosis of EHBDA [19, 59].

There has been some debate concerning the value of liver biopsy in confirming the diagnosis of EHBDA and in the differential diagnosis of this disease from neonatal giant cell hepatitis [19]. In recent years, however, the diagnostic accuracy of liver biopsy is reported to be greater than 90% [19].

The biopsy should be sufficiently large and should contain at least six portal tracts [62]. Due attention should be paid to portal tract changes, including ductular proliferation and bile duct damage. The pathologist should be aware of the dynamic nature of the disease process and the changes in histopathologic appearance with time (see Sect. 4.4).

Whenever clinical, laboratory, and imaging studies as well as liver biopsy are inconclusive, an operative exploration with cholangiogram is the next logical step in the diagnostic evaluation [59].

## 4.4 Pathology

### *Pathology of the Extrahepatic Bile Ducts*

Macroscopically, it is useful to distinguish between "correctable" and "noncorrectable" types of EHBDA (see definition). With the introduction of the Kasai procedure, the resected extrahepatic biliary tree became available for microscopic examination. Confirmation of EHBDA at the microscopic level requires complete fibrous obliteration of at least a segment of the extrahepatic biliary tree. The remaining parts usually reveal remnants of lumina and a variable inflammatory infiltrate. Several types of lesion have been described [12, 22, 49]. The lesion referred to as Gautier type I corresponds to the absence of any lumen lined by biliary epithelium. The histologic picture described as Gautier type II is made up of a number of epithelium-lined tubular structures, randomly distributed or grouped in clusters. The epithelial lining shows signs of damage and an inflammatory infiltrate is usually present. In some specimens, described as Gautier type III, a central structure corresponding to an altered bile duct is seen (Fig. 2). The lumen contains a loose connective tissue meshwork, cellular debris, or a bile concrement. The histologic lesions described above are interpreted as the reflection of a dynamic process leading to progressive obliteration of the extrahepatic bile ducts [19]. Necrosis of the epithelial lining and inflammatory infiltration are also seen distal to completely obliterated segments, indicating that they are not events secondary to distal obstruction. Numerous attempts have been made to correlate the number, size, or area of bile ducts present at the porta hepatis with postoperative bile flow [19].

### *Pathology of the Liver and the Intrahepatic Bile Ducts*

It is useful to distinguish between "classical" EHBDA and EHBDA associated with either hyperplasia or hypoplasia of intrahepatic bile ducts. The latter entity is discussed in Sect. 5.3.

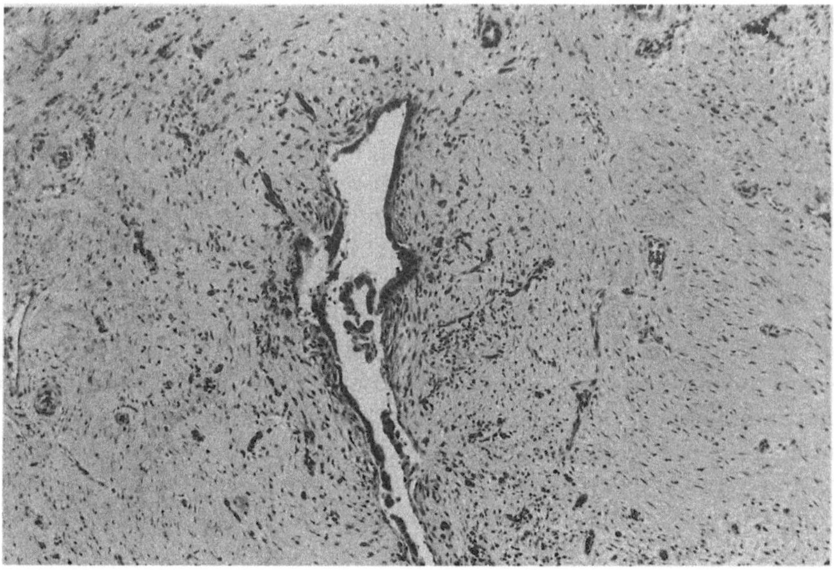

**Fig. 2.** EHBDA, Gautier type III fibrous remnant. Note the centrally located altered bile duct with irregularities of the lining cells and partial sloughing of epithelium. The bile duct structure is surrounded by fibrous tissue containing scattered inflammatory cells. H&E, ×160

*Classical EHBDA*

It is extremely important for the pathologist to be aware of the dynamic nature of the disease process. A liver biopsy can only be considered a "snapshot" of a dynamic lesion [19]. Its value in the diagnosis and differential diagnosis of EHBDA has already been discussed. There is also some controversy with regards to the "optimal timing" of a liver biopsy. Because the ductular proliferation, considered to be typical of EHBDA (see below), takes some time to develop, SCHWEIZER and MÜLLER proposed postponing liver biopsy until the 6th week of life [62]. However, the variability both in speed of development of the ductular reaction and in its extent makes the existence of such an arbitrarily defined optimal time unlikely. The "optimal time" for a given patient may rather depend on clinical judgment and on the experience of the physician [19]. If a biopsy taken too early does not provide a definitive answer, a second (later) biopsy is mandatory.

A comprehensive discussion of the pathology of EHBDA is given by SCHWEIZER and MÜLLER [62]. These authors divide the disease into successive stages, the timing of which can only be approximate. Biopsy findings in the earliest stage (1–4 weeks) are nonspecific and consist of bilirubinostasis with intra- and intercellular bile thrombi. The amount of bilirubin in Kupffer cells increases with the duration of the cholestasis. Hepatocellular degeneration and necrosis may be seen as well as parenchymal giant cells. There is no inflammatory infiltrate. Some degree of extramedullary hematopoiesis may persist. In the second stage of the disease (4–7 weeks), the changes "diagnostic of EHBDA" gradually develop. They consist of edema of the portal tracts with concomitant ductular proliferation. The ductular structures are typically located at the interface between the connective tissue and the parenchyma ("marginal bile duct proliferation") and are accompanied by neutrophils and lymphocytes. The portal bile ducts also show lesions which can be characterized as inflammatory destruction (Fig. 3). The interlobular bile ducts are permeated by inflammatory cells and the epithelium shows an increased acidophilia, vacuolation, flattening, or frank necrosis. These lesions are strikingly similar to those observed in the extrahepatic bile duct remnants and may lead to progressive disappearance of intrahepatic bile ducts. The third stage (7–8 weeks) is characterized by progressive development of portal and periportal fibrosis and periportal extension of the ductular proliferation. The edema of the portal tracts subsides and the inflammatory infiltrate becomes less dense. Ductules may contain bile concrements. The biliary epithelium shows signs of biliary reabsorption. Bilirubinostasis persists. The lobular parenchyma still reveals no inflammatory infiltration. After about the 10th week, the extending periportal fibrosis leads to establishment of portoportal fibrous connections. Both the density of the portal

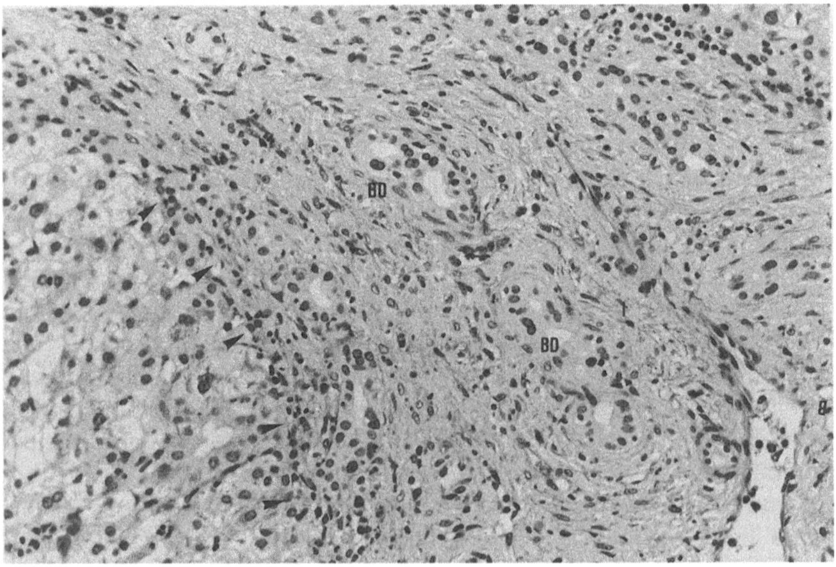


**Fig. 3.** "Classical" EHBDA. Part of a portal tract is shown with an increased number of ductular structures at the interface between the connective tissue and the liver parenchyma (*arrowheads*). Note the presence of polymorphs close to the ductules. The interlobular bile ducts (*BD*) show signs of damage with pyknotic nuclei and presence of a few lymphocytes between the epithelial cells. H&E, ×400

inflammatory infiltrate and the number of ductular structures decrease. The interlobular bile ducts show "fibrous cholangitis." Concentric periductal fibrosis develops and leads to progressive atrophy of the biliary epithelium. This degree of "biliary" fibrosis implies that the infant is beyond the optimal stage for hepatoportoenterostomy. In the final stage of the disease (beyond the 12th week) biliary fibrosis further develops into biliary cirrhosis. At that time, surgery is contraindicated.

A few points merit special comment. It is important to realize that not only the increase in ductular structures or ductular proliferation is an important histologic hallmark of EHBDA but also the lesions of the intrahepatic bile ducts [19, 24, 28]. The latter present a spectrum ranging from vacuolation and flattening of the lining cells to nuclear pyknosis, condensation of cells, and frank necrosis. These lesions probably represent an intrahepatic component of the "basic disease process" affecting the extrahepatic bile ducts and can lead to disappearance of interlobular bile ducts [19, 24, 28]. EHBDA thus also qualifies as a "disappearing bile duct" disease. Another striking observation is the hypoplastic appearance of the portal vein branches in the sclerosing portal tracts [19]. Also in later biopsies of children with EHBDA, fusion between large preterminal portal tracts may be observed, suggesting that there is a lack of outgrowth of the finer ramifications of the portal tracts [19].

### *EHBDA with Hyperplasia of Intrahepatic Bile Ducts*

In 1984, Schweizer and Müller made the important observation that in 7 of 69 studied patients, EHBDA was associated with "hyperplasia" of intrahepatic bile ducts [62]. The latter lesion is also known as cholangiodysplastische Pseudozirrhose, cholangiodysplasia of the hyperplastic type, fibroangioadénomatose, or congenital hepatic fibrosis [19]. The "hyperplastic ductules" as described by Schweizer and Müller correspond in fact to incompletely remodeled ductal plates, i.e., ductal plate malformations. Thorough examination of 41 biopsies of children with EHBDA revealed ductal plate malformations in ten (ca. 25%) [19] (Fig. 4). In several specimens two or even three layers of bile ducts in ductal plate arrangement were seen surrounding vessels, suggesting that repetitive "waves" of ductal plate formation had occurred. This probably represents a fetal type of ductular reaction in response to distal obstruction. Histologic features of such "early severe" cases further include absence of extramedullary hematopoiesis and of parenchymal giant cell transformation, excess of hepatic artery branches, and small-sized portal vein branches [19]. A recent study by Raweily et al. confirmed the presence of ductal plate-like structures in 21.6% of cases of EHBDA [56]. The "immature" ducts show the same necroinflammatory or degenerative lesions as the mature ducts in classical EHBDA. In the "early severe" cases, the basic disease process thus leads to involution and eventual disappearance of ducts in ductal plate arrangement. The presence of the

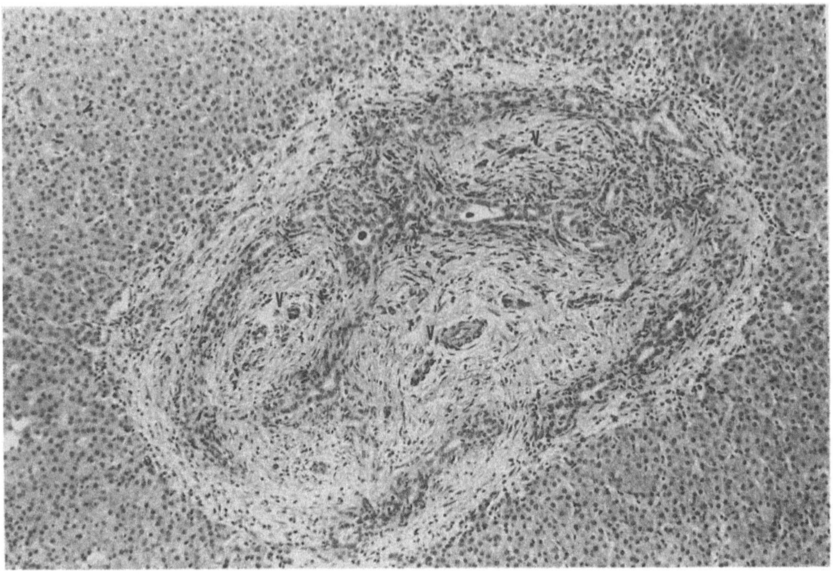

**Fig. 4.** "Early severe" EHBDA. Three central connective tissue cores containing a vessel (*V*) are surrounded by a double layer of biliary epithelium in ductal plate configuration. H&E, ×160

ductal plate malformation suggests that in these cases the disease process had an early (fetal/antenatal) onset.

### 4.5 Etiology and Pathogenesis

The etiology and pathogenesis of the disease are unknown. Several infectious agents, including cytomegalovirus and reovirus type 3, have been implicated but definite proof of an infectious etiology is lacking. The hypothesis of a primary ischemic insult with subsequent fibrous obliteration of the bile ducts derives some support from animal experiments but hard evidence that this mechanism is also operative in the human disease is lacking. Reflux of pancreatic juice into the biliary tree and angiofibromatosis have also been proposed as pathogenetic mechanisms. An exogenous toxic origin has so far not been substantiated. As to a suggested endogenous toxic origin, the hypothesis that abnormal or unusual bile acids are pathogenetically important merits further investigation.

## 4.6 Treatment

### *Hepatic Portoenterostomy*

#### *The Kasai Procedure*

If left untreated, EHBDA leads to death before the age of 2 years [18]. In cases of "correctable" EHBDA, the proximal ductal structures are patent and selective reconstruction can be undertaken [59]. The introduction of the Kasai procedure [37] or hepatic portoenterostomy has changed the treatment of "noncorrectable" EHBDA. This procedure is based on the concept that – at least in the early stage of the disease – bile ducts proximal to the fibrous mass at the porta hepatis are still patent. The fibrous mass of obliterated ducts is transected parallel to the liver surface [59]. The intestine is then anastomosed to the inferior hepatic surface [59]. Several modifications of the original Kasai procedure have been developed, mainly to prevent postoperative cholangitis [19]. In the 25% of patients with an atretic common hepatic duct but with patent cystic duct, gallbladder, and common bile duct, hepatic portocholecystostomy is the procedure of choice [19].

#### *Determinants of Success*

The age of the infant at the time of operative correction is the most significant prognostic factor [59]. Ideally, the operation should be performed within 60 days after birth, in which case excretion of bile is obtained in more than 80% of patients [19, 59, 63]. Unfortunately, bile flow does not equate with cure (see below). Operative results also depend on a precise dissection and adequate transection of the porta hepatis, prevention of postoperative cholangitis, absence of significant alterations of the intrahepatic bile ducts, and the experience of the surgeon [59, 63]. The degree of hepatic fibrosis also bears a close relationship to the prognosis but this parameter is linked to the age of the patient. The amount of bile flow and bile acid excretion also correlate with the overall functional result of the portoenterostomy [59]. Numerous attempts have been made to correlate the size of the ductal remnants with postoperative flow of bile. Data, however, are conflicting, and for discussion of this confused issue the reader is referred to Desmet and Callea [19].

#### *Postoperative Complications*

Postoperative cholangitis is beyond doubt the most common and also most devastating complication [59]. It has a reported incidence of 30%–60% in most long-term survivors and usually responds to medical treatment [59]. The modifications of the Kasai procedure devised to reduce the incidence of cholangitis have met with relatively little success [19]. Portal hypertension is another major complication. Its severity and reported incidence vary [see ref. 19]. In surgical reports, it is usually ascribed to progressive development of liver fibrosis and cirrhosis following repeated episodes of cholangitis. There is, however, growing suspicion that the most serious long-term complications are due to a relentless progression of the basic disease process (see below). Other complications include nutritional (fat-soluble vitamins) and growth deficiencies, delayed development, osteomalacia and osteoporosis, and social and psychiatric difficulties [18].

It has become increasingly clear that a successful portoenterostomy is not tantamount to cure. Real cure is limited to a small minority of patients. Most reports on long-term follow-up after a Kasai procedure [reviewed in ref. 19] mention some abnormalities in liver enzyme and bile salt levels, hepatomegaly, splenomegaly, or portal hypertension [19]. The main beneficial effect of the Kasai procedure is the relief of the bile duct obstruction, which if left untreated would rapidly lead to biliary cirrhosis [19]. The portoenterostomy procedure, however, does not influence the intrahepatic component of the basic disease process, as is apparent from the following section.

*Liver Alterations After Hepatic Portoenterostomy*

The histologic findings in liver biopsies of patients who have undergone a successful Kasai procedure will be briefly discussed and an attempt will be made at interpreting these changes. "Successful" is defined as an adequate postoperative flow of bile, disappearance of jaundice, and a generally good condition of the patient [19].

Development of bile duct cysts and bile duct dilatation is mostly seen after unsuccessful portoenterostomy. An improvement of liver histology comprising a decrease in ductular and parenchymal cholestasis, inflammation, and fibrosis is exceptional. Most patients show progressive liver damage, which can take several histologic appearances. Some liver biopsies show only a mild periportal fibrosis, without appreciable inflammatory infiltration. A minimal degree of cholangiolitis usually persists and special immunohistochemical stains reveal a latent cholestasis. Occasional portal tracts lack an interlobular bile duct. When pronounced, the periportal fibrosis leads to an accentuation of the lobular pattern of the liver, a histologic picture reminiscent of the pig's liver. A second histologic pattern is characterized by periportal fibrosis and an increased number of bile ducts often in ductal plate arrangement. The bile duct epithelium shows signs of damage compatible with ongoing duct destruction. There is usually a minimal degree of cholangiolitis. Immunohistochemical stains again reveal a smoldering cholestasis. Portal vein branches are often strikingly hypoplastic. It is important to note that all patients will this pattern on follow-up biopsy had ductal plate malformations in the initial biopsy ("early severe" cases, cf. above). This histologic pattern is referred to as "congenital hepatic fibrosis-like." A third pattern corresponds to secondary biliary fibrosis and cirrhosis. It is not always easy to discern between fibrosis and cirrhosis on small biopsy specimens. In the stage of biliary fibrosis, portoportal fibrous septa predominate and the parenchyma appears as garland-shaped masses in between. The development of portocentral fibrous septa and nodular parenchymal regeneration mark the transition to true cirrhosis. Portal vein branches appear hypoplastic but there may be an increased number of dilated lymphatics. In some cases, bile ducts are lacking altogether ("acholangic biliary fibrosis/cirrhosis"). In other cases, the lack of interlobular bile ducts is not complete and the biliary epithelium shows signs of involution and necrobiosis. The involuting ducts may have a normal shape or a ductal plate configuration. There is no bilirubinostasis but there is cholangiolitis and accumulation of stainable copper. Some patients who were jaundice-free for several years may suddenly become icteric. Biopsies taken at that time show signs of active biliary disease superimposed on one of the three patterns described above (although rarely on the periportal fibrosis pattern). Signs of active disease comprise an unsharp borderline between the portal connective tissue and the parenchyma due to biliary piecemeal necrosis, bilirubinostasis, and even feathery degeneration of hepatocytes. Portal tracts may still contain an interlobular bile duct, either a mature one or one in ductal plate configuration, which shows involutive changes.

The liver lesions observed after portoenterostomy can best be explained by the following hypothesis. EHBDA is a progressive inflammatory destructive process affecting both the extra- and intrahepatic bile ducts [19, 24, 39]. Even a successful portoenterostomy does not cure the intrahepatic component of the disease. The latter progresses at variable speed but may also heal spontaneously at any time. In a small minority, the disease process heals spontaneously and the liver biopsy shows improvement. In the majority of patients the disease is progressive. In some, it heals with only minor sequelae in the form of periportal fibrosis. As has been discussed, initial liver biopsies of "early severe" cases show extensive fibrosis and ductal plate malformations. When, after portoenterostomy, further destruction of bile ducts ceases, liver histology will be characterized by fibrosis and numerous ducts in ductal plate configuration, i.e., a pattern strongly reminiscent of congenital hepatic fibrosis. The histologic picture is further determined by the degree of remodeling of the ductal plates. If the destruction of both mature ducts and ductal plates progresses relentlessly, a liver biopsy will finally reveal periportal fibrosis or frank cirrhotic transformation with ductopenia. This pattern corresponds to acholangic biliary fibrosis or cirrhosis. In some patients, clinical deterioration is accompanied by or may even be preceded by histologic signs of active biliary disease. The cause of this clinical deterioration is not clear.

In summary, the histologic changes observed after successful portoenterostomy are determined to a large extent by the progression of the basic disease process and the degree of (or lack of) remodeling of ductal plates.

As has been discussed, the presence of the latter probably relates to an earlier, antenatal onset of the disease and to a fetal type of ductular reaction.

#### *Liver Transplantation*

Hepatic portoenterostomy is still considered the treatment of choice for EHBDA by some authors [18, 63]. Even if the procedure is not successful, it might still buy the patient some time until a more appropriate age is reached or an organ has become available. Orthotopic liver transplantation is the only alternative for patients who have had unsuccessful attempts at achieving biliary drainage [59]. In fact, this constitutes the most common indication for hepatic transplantation in childhood [59]. Previous surgical procedures at the porta hepatis do of course cause technical problems at the time of transplantation. Surgeons feel, however, that operative efforts to achieve or reestablish bile drainage should not be withheld from suitable candidates [59]. Liver transplantation is the only treatment modality that actually removes the diseased organ and replaces it with a healthy one [19]. The observation that even after a successful Kasai procedure, the intrahepatic disease is usually progressive combined with the gradual improvement in survival after liver transplantation may change the surgeon's view on the optimal treatment in the future.

## 5 Paucity of Intrahepatic (Interlobular) Bile Ducts

Paucity of intrahepatic (interlobular) bile ducts is also known as atresia of intrahepatic bile ducts, intrahepatic biliary hypoplasia, hypoplasia of interlobular bile ducts, ductular paucity, or ductular hypoplasia [18]. It consists of a reduced ratio in the number of interlobular bile ducts to the number of portal tracts. The normal ratio is between 0.9 and 1.8. "Paucity" is histologically defined as a ratio less than 0.5 [2] (Fig. 5). Paucity of intrahepatic bile ducts may be associated with other extrahepatic anomalies or may be an isolated defect. The former variety corresponds to Alagille's syndrome. The latter is referred to as nonsyndromatic paucity of intrahepatic bile ducts.

### 5.1 Syndromatic Paucity of Intrahepatic Bile Ducts (Alagille's Syndrome, Arteriohepatic Dysplasia)

#### *Definition and Clinical Features*

Observations of a cholestatic disorder in children associated with a diminution of the number of intrahepatic bile ducts date from the 1950s [57]. The syndromatic type of paucity of intrahepatic bile ducts was recognized as a distinct disorder by Alagille et al. in 1975 [3]. The five major features of

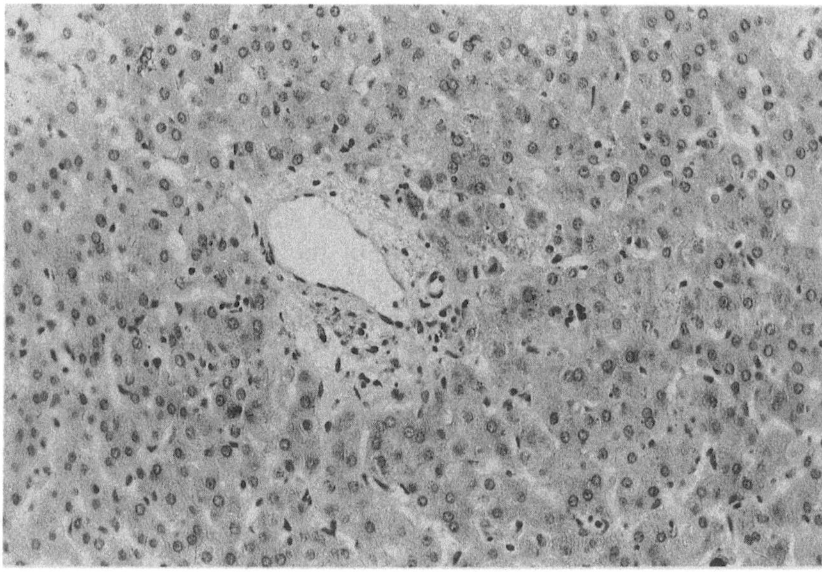

**Fig. 5.** Paucity of intrahepatic bile ducts. The portal tract shown contains a portal vein and a branch of the hepatic artery but no interlobular bile duct. H&E, ×400

**Table 1.** Major features of Alagille's syndrome

| |
|---|
| Peculiar facies |
| Chronic cholestasis |
| Butterfly-like vertebral arch defects |
| Posterior embryotoxon |
| Peripheral pulmonary artery hypoplasia or stenosis either isolated or associated with complex cardiovascular abnormalities |

Based on ALAGILLE D et al. (1987) J Pediatr 110:195–200

this syndrome are listed in Table 1. In the "complete" syndrome all five features are present [2]. However, patients with the complete syndrome are outnumbered by those showing only four or even three major features ("partial" syndrome) [2]. Alagille's syndrome is seen worldwide and is the most common form of familial intrahepatic cholestasis [57]. It is probably inherited in an autosomal dominant pattern with variable expression and penetrance [57, 58, 65].

Affected infants are often of low birth weight relative to gestational age [57]. Most cases present in the first 3 months of life with jaundice, dark urine, and pale stools [2, 57]. However, jaundice may develop between the 4th month and 3rd year of life [57]. Other cases are discovered during evaluation of congenital heart disease [2, 57]. Failure to thrive, pruritus, and spontaneous bleeding due to vitamin K malabsorption are other possible modes of presentation [15]. Pruritus is usually noted when the infant is able to scratch, by 4–6 months of age [2, 57]. Modest to moderate hepatosplenomegaly is usually found. Patients often demonstrate xanthomas, which are usually progressive from 4 years of age onward [2, 57, 65]. The peculiar facies consists of a prominent forehead, moderate hypertelorism with deep-set eyes, a small chin pointed anteriorly, and a saddle or straight nose [2, 3]. This facial appearance may be difficult to recognize in early infancy [15]. Moreover, the specificity of the facies has been questioned [15, 19, 57]. Most affected patients have a cardiac murmur. A posterior embryotoxon is found on slit lamp examination in a large proportion of patients [2]. It also occurs in 8%–10% of the normal population [2, 57]. Retinal pigmentary changes, cataracts, and high myopia with retinal detachment may also occur [57]. Vertebral arch defects are present in 87% of patients [2]. Other bone and joint abnormalities include an abnormally narrow interpedicular distance, shortened distal phalanges, a short ulna, and even arthropathy [2, 57]. Neurologic abnormalities are also found. Areflexia is presumably part of the vitamin E deficiency syndrome. Mental retardation was reported by Alagille et al. in 16% of cases [2]. Many patients have a high-pitched voice in the absence of laryngeal abnormalities [2]. Renal involvement was documented in 17–23 patients studied [2]. The histologic abnormality consisted of mesangiolipidosis. A tubulointerstitial nephropathy has also been reported [57].

Laboratory tests reflect an "obstructive" picture. Serum levels of bile acids, alkaline phosphatase, 5′-nucleotidase, γ-glutamyltransferase, and bilirubin are elevated. The hyperlipidemia which is characteristic of the syndrome becomes apparent only in late infancy or early childhood [15].

### *Pathology*

The pathologic hallmark of the disease is a decreased ratio of the number of interlobular bile ducts as defined above. A sufficient number of portal tracts should be evaluated. Some authors advocate the use of surgical wedge biopsies [3]. Others claim that the diagnosis can be established using needle biopsies, provided that they comprise at least six portal tracts [62]. The portal areas lacking a bile duct usually appear hypoplastic as a whole [18, 19]. The total number of portal tracts per $mm^2$ is reduced in patients with paucity of intrahepatic bile ducts as compared with normal controls [19].

A few important points are worth mentioning. It has become clear that in Alagille's syndrome, bile ducts are not congenitally absent. In a series of six patients reported by Dahms et al. [14], three had normal numbers of interlobular bile ducts in biopsies taken during the first 6 months of life. However, paucity developed later in life. This fact, together with the finding of destructive inflammatory changes of the bile ducts in the same study, indicates a progressive destruction of bile duct branches. This also implies that a histopathologic diagnosis of paucity of bile ducts may be impossible during the first months of life and emphasizes the need for clinicopathologic dialogue [15, 19]. Caution has also been raised as to the interpretation of bile duct to portal space ratios in infants. KAHN et al. have clearly demonstrated that this ratio increases with post-conceptional age [34]. This is not surprising in view of the gradual incorporation of bile ducts into the portal connective tissue (see Sect. 2.1). Bile duct to portal space ratios less than 0.9 are therefore physiologic prior to 38 weeks postconception. Since it is not always easy to identify a bile duct in a tissue section, staining for cytokeratins or tissue polypeptide antigen may be of great help to the pathologist.

Biopsies taken early in life reveal bilirubinostasis, occasional giant cell transformation of parenchymal cells, slight periportal fibrosis, and portal lymphocytic infiltration [14, 32]. Bilirubinostasis and inflammation gradually resolve. Fibrosis may persist but may also increase or decrease [15, 32]. There is usually a mild increase in stainable copper. According to DAHMS et al. [14] ductular proliferation is a highly unusual feature. Others, however, state that it may be seen during the phase of inflammatory destruction [19]. When ductular proliferation is prominent, it renders the histologic differential diagnosis with extrahepatic bile duct atresia very difficult. The extrahepatic bile ducts in cases of Alagille's syndrome have been reported to be hypoplastic (see Sect. 3.6).

### *Pathogenesis*

The etiology and pathogenesis are unknown. As discussed in the previous section, there appears to be a destructive inflammatory process affecting the intrahepatic bile ducts. An electron microscopic study suggested a block in bile secretion at the level of the Golgi apparatus and explained the paucity by "disuse atrophy" [72]. These findings were only partly confirmed by WITZLEBEN et al. [76]. Any proposed etiologic mechanism should also account for the extrahepatic abnormalities of this syndrome [57]. The resemblance of the latter to the lesions produced by intrauterine infections such as rubella and cytomegalovirus has been noted [57]. The reported presence of a chromosomal anomaly del (20p) in patients with Alagille's syndrome may be highly relevant to the pathogenesis [18].

### *Evolution*

It is usually stated that Alagille's syndrome runs a benign clinical course [1, 65]. Early hepatic mortality is low and is considerably less than that of nonsyndromatic paucity of interlobular bile ducts [15]. DÉPRETTERE et al. have stressed the fact that the morbidity throughout childhood attributable to liver disease is considerable [15]. In their series of 27 cases, 85% had major complications due to malabsorption of fat-soluble vitamins, or intractable pruritus with excoriation and insomnia. The severity of the cardiac abnormalities obviously influences the prognosis [2]. The long-term prognosis is still debated. Jaundice can decrease progressively from about 5 years of age but biochemical signs of cholestasis persist [2]. Xanthomas may disappear along with a decrease in serum cholesterol levels and pruritus may improve [2, 57]. Growth can normalize after recovery from malnutrition. Normal pregnancy is possible. At present it is impossible to predict which patients will eventually develop liver cirrhosis. Liver failure or portal hypertension accounted for only 4 out of 21 deaths in a series of 80 cases reported by ALAGILLE [2]. Hepatocellular carcinoma may be a complication but is infrequent [57, 65].

### *Treatment*

Treatment consists of low-fat diets with medium chain triglyceride supplementation and administration of fat-soluble vitamin supplements. Hypercaloric diets may be needed in cases of severe malnutrition. Phenobarbital or cholestyramine can reduce the pruritus but does not affect the course of the cholestasis [2].

## 5.2 Nonsyndromatic Paucity of Intrahepatic Bile Ducts

### *Definition and Clinical Features*

This heterogeneous group includes patients with a biopsy-proven "paucity of interlobular bile ducts" but lacking the features of Alagille's syndrome as discussed in the previous section. It occurs in various clinical settings (Table 2). In the majority of cases, no specific underlying condition is identified

**Table 2.** Non-syndromatic paucity of intrahepatic bile ducts: clinical settings

| | Reference |
|---|---|
| Congenital rubella | 33 |
| $\alpha_1$-Antitrypsin deficiency | 33 |
| Down's syndrome | 33 |
| Cystic fibrosis | 33 |
| Choledochal cyst | 33 |
| Lymphedema | 33 |
| Trihydroxycoprostanic acidemia | 33 |
| Hypopituitarism | 33 |
| Ivemark's syndrome | 33 |
| Cytomegalovirus infection | 33 |
| Congenital syphilis | 18 |
| Trisomy 17–18 | 62 |
| 45 X (Turner's syndrome) | 27 |
| "Idiopathic" | 33 |

("idiopathic" nonsyndromatic paucity). Presenting signs and symptoms vary according to the underlying disease. The majority of infants are premature and of low birth weight [33, 57]. In full-term infants, clinical jaundice is usually noted between 5 and 8 weeks of age [33]. Stools are acholic. Serum levels of conjugated bilirubin are elevated. Serum cholesterol levels are usually normal [33].

### *Pathology*

The histologic criteria for diagnosing "paucity" are mentioned at the beginning of Sect. 5. In a study of 17 cases of nonsyndromatic paucity of interlobular bile ducts, liver biopsy taken before 90 days of age revealed paucity of interlobular bile ducts, fibrosis, and bilirubinostasis [33]. Giant cell transformation, extramedullary hematopoiesis, and perisinusoidal fibrosis were also noted in a variable proportion of cases. Late changes (defined as changes occurring after 90 days of age) comprised duct paucity and persistent periportal fibrosis [33]. Bilirubinostasis decreases with age. The established paucity of bile ducts and the fibrous expansion of the portal tracts in biopsies taken early in life contrast with the liver biopsy findings in Alagille's syndrome [33]. Biopsies taken early in life (i.e., before 90 days) may allow for a morphologic differential diagnosis between syndromatic and nonsyndromatic bile duct paucity [33]. Ductular proliferation – when present – is an unfavorable histologic sign heralding deterioration of liver function [33]. It is not clear whether the recently described entity "idiopathic adulthood ductopenia" may correspond to a nonsyndromatic paucity of interlobular bile ducts manifesting itself in adulthood [44].

### *Pathogenesis*

Light and electron microscopy provided evidence for a primary ductal insult with bile duct destruction, undulation, and breaks in the basal lamina and infiltration of the epithelium by lymphocytes [33]. The precise factors triggering this process are unknown.

### *Evolution*

Since the nonsyndromatic group is a heterogeneous one, it is not surprising that the prognosis appears to be quite variable. ALAGILLE reported cirrhosis and death in 10 out of 18 patients [1]. In the series of 17 patients reported by KAHN et al., four died between 3 weeks and 11 months but only one death was related to primary liver failure [33]. Two patients had regenerative nodules in their livers but were anicteric. It has been proposed that two subgroups of nonsyndromatic paucity of intrahepatic bile ducts exist: one that runs a benign course and one with progressive disease [33].

### 5.3 Combined Extra- and Intrahepatic Bile Duct Atresia

This topic is discussed extensively by DESMET and CALLEA [19]. SCHWEIZER and MÜLLER noted this association in more than 10% of cases of extrahepatic bile duct atresia [62]. It is intriguing that in those cases, liver biopsy reportedly revealed ductular proliferation only in portal tracts containing an interlobular bile duct [62]. This suggests that the absence of a genuine interlobular bile duct prevents the development of a ductular reaction. This again would imply that if a needle biopsy contains only ductless portal tracts, an associated extrahepatic bile duct atresia cannot be diagnosed. In the series of KAHN et al., one child with nonsyndromatic paucity of interlobular bile ducts developed extrahepatic bile duct atresia [33]. Alagille's syndrome may also affect the extrahepatic bile duct but this lesion represents hypoplasia rather than genuine atresia (see Sect. 3.6). Given the progressive disappearance of bile ducts in Alagille's syndrome (see Sect. 5.1), the diagnosis of combined extrahepatic bile duct atresia and Alagille's syndrome is probably impossible on biopsies taken early in life. The problem of the association of both diseases is further compounded by the fact that the destructive inflammatory process in extrahepatic bile duct atresia also affects the intrahepatic bile ducts and may lead to their disappearance [19].

Recently, a sclerosing cholangitis with neonatal onset has been described [6]. This disease appears clinically similar to extrahepatic bile duct atresia and nonsyndromatic paucity of intrahepatic bile ducts. It may represent a near-miss atresia [19]. It has been suggested that extra- and intrahepatic bile duct atresia and neonatal sclerosing cholangitis are expressions of a disease process starting in pre- or early postnatal life and affecting the extra- and intrahepatic bile ducts in varying proportions and with varying degrees of severity [6]. Further research into the relationships – if any – between these three disorders is indicated.

## 6 Cystic and Dysplastic Lesions

With the exception of solitary cyst, the diseases discussed in this section have a number of features in common [66, 68]. They often occur in combinations, the most striking of which is the association of congenital hepatic fibrosis with Caroli's disease [68]. Association with cystic renal changes is common. The basic liver lesion is the ductal plate malformation affecting bile ducts of large or small caliber or both. Most of the disorders discussed carry a risk of development of cancer. It has therefore been proposed that the fibropolycystic diseases are members of one family [66, 68]. However, a number of problems and controversies remain. The terminology for these disorders is confusing. As pointed out by WITZLEBEN, a number of terms are currently being used, whether accurately or inaccurately, as synonyms for all or specific disease entities [75]. Controversy still exists as to the exact nature of the associated renal pathology. The mode of inheritance of some of the fibropolycystic diseases is still debated. It is therefore likely that some diseases discussed in this section will be better delineated in the future and that their classification may change as insight into their pathogenesis increases.

### 6.1 Solitary (Nonparasitic) Cyst

Solitary cysts are distinctly uncommon and have no association with cysts in other viscera [75]. The widespread use of ultrasonography, however, has led to an increased detection rate [66, 75]. Solitary cysts have been reported to occur at all ages [75]. They may be present at birth but it is not clear whether all cases should be considered congenital [75]. The majority of solitary cysts are asymptomatic [66, 75]. Symptomatic solitary cysts usually present in the fourth and fifth decades of life with increased abdominal girth [75]. Other symptoms include weakness, nausea, and vomiting. Usually a mass is palpable in the right upper quadrant [75]. Complications are hemorrhage, infection, and perforation [75]. Laboratory tests are usually normal. The cyst can be demonstrated by ultrasonography or computed tomography. If more than one cyst is present, one of the polycystic diseases has to be excluded [75]. Solitary cysts involve the right lobe of the liver more frequently than the left one [27, 75]. There is a broad variation in diameter. Ninety-five percent of all cysts are unilocular [27]. Microscopically, the outermost layer of the cyst wall consists of loose fibrous tissue containing blood vessels, nerves, and bile ducts. The middle layer is a compact layer of fibrous tissue. The inner layer consists of less dense fibrous tissue and often has an epithelial lining [27, 75]. The latter is usually a single layer of flat cuboidal or columnar epithelium but ciliated, pseudostratified colummar epithelium and even squamous epithelium have been described. As a rule, there are no connections with bile ducts, vessels, or lymphatics [27, 75]. The pathogenesis of solitary cysts is not clear and may not be the same for all cysts [75]. Solitary cysts are a benign condition and the patient should be reassured [66]. Development of carcinoma in a cyst is extremely rare [75]. Surgical intervention is only indicated when complications such as hemorrhage or rupture occur. Prognosis is excellent.

Ciliated hepatic foregut cysts are solitary, unilocular, rather small cysts lined by a pseudostratified columnar epithelium with mucous cells. They are believed to arise from the embryonic foregut and to differentiate toward bronchial structures in the liver [70].

## 6.2 Autosomal Dominant Polycystic Disease ("Adult Polycystic Disease")

The existence of a purely hepatic type of polycystic disease, i.e., multiple non-communicating cysts of bile ducts without associated renal cysts, has been postulated [35] but awaits further confirmation. This section deals only with the well-known entity of autosomal dominant or "adult" polycystic disease. This is one of the most common genetic disorders and the most common heritable renal disease, affecting about 1 in 1000 persons [74]. It is inherited as an autosomal dominant trait with nearly complete penetrance [74]. Recognizable hepatic cysts are found in 29% of cases [75]. There is, however, evidence that the prevalence of hepatic cysts increases with age and may even approach 75%–90% [74]. About 10% of patients have pancreatic cysts and fewer than 5% have cysts in the spleen [74]. Clinical presentation is usually in the third or fourth decade with renal failure occurring some 10 years later [74]. Rarely, the disorder may present in infancy or childhood [9, 74, 75]. Patients complain of abdominal pain caused by palpably enlarged kidneys [74]. There may be gross or microscopic hematuria. Hypertension is usually present. The liver may be enlarged and nodules may be felt on palpation [66]. Occasionally, the cysts may cause portal venous obstruction and esophageal varices [66]. Rarely a large cyst may cause mechanical bile duct obstruction [75]. Hepatic function is excellent. Serum alkaline phosphatase and $\gamma$-glutamyltransferase levels may be increased [66]. The hepatic cysts show no association with the severity of the renal disease.

The clinical diagnosis of autosomal dominant polycystic disease is usually not difficult. In doubtful cases, a positive family history is extremely helpful. The hepatic cysts can be demonstrated using ultrasonography or CT scan.

The renal cysts are cylindrical, fusiform, or spherical dilatations of or outpouchings from preexistent renal tubules and may involve any level of the nephron or collecting duct system [74]. For a detailed discussion of the renal pathology, the reader is referred to WELLING and GRANTHAM [74]. Hepatic cysts are often numerous and scattered throughout the liver but they may be restricted to a single lobe [74] (Fig. 6). They vary in size and are lined by biliary epithelium. They do not communicate with the biliary system [75]. The cyst fluid resembles the bile salt-independent fraction of bile and is thought to result from secretion by the lining epithelium [66, 74]. The cysts often coexist with Meyenburg's complexes (see below) and supposedly arise from progressive dilatation of the latter [23, 35]. GRUNFELD et al. reported liver lesions closely resembling congenital hepatic fibrosis, i.e., ductal plate malformations, in 60% of cases of autosomal dominant polycystic disease but the significance of this finding is as yet unclear [23, 75].

Prognosis is largely determined by the degree of renal involvement [66]. Renal failure eventually occurs in about half of the patients at risk [74].

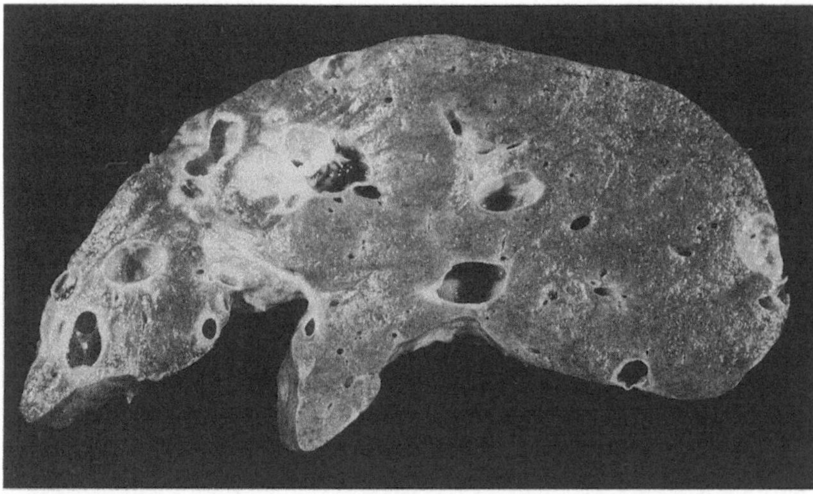

**Fig. 6.** Macroscopic appearance of the liver in adult polycystic disease. Several variably sized cysts are scattered throughout both lobes. (By courtesy of Dr. P. Moerman)

Treatment is generally supportive. End-stage renal disease is treated with hemodialysis or renal transplantation. The increased survival of patients with autosomal dominant polycystic disease has revealed that hepatic complications may not be as insignificant as was previously thought. In a study by GRUNFELD et al., 10.5% of deaths in patients with adult polycystic disease were ascribed to hepatic complications [23]. The latter include infection of cysts, cholangiocarcinoma, and portal hypertension. Patients with symptoms resulting from a pressure effect of the cysts may benefit from unroofing of cysts with drainage into the peritoneal cavity [75]. Highly symptomatic polycystic liver disease may be treated with a combined hepatic resection–fenestration procedure [53].

### 6.3 Meyenburg's Complexes (Microhamartomas)

Meyenburg's complexes are considered to be part of the spectrum of autosomal dominant polycystic disease [27, 35]. They usually measure less than 0.5 cm in diameter and are scattered in both lobes. Microscopically, Meyenburg's complexes have a round to irregular shape and are usually found in a periportal location. They consist of ducts, often with an irregular shape and dilated lumen, embedded in a collagenous stroma (Fig. 7). This configuration basically corresponds to the ductal plate malformation [16, 17]. The ducts are lined by a low columnar or cuboidal epithelium and may contain amorphous material or inspissated bile. Meyenburg's complexes are usually discovered incidentally and do not cause symptoms [60].

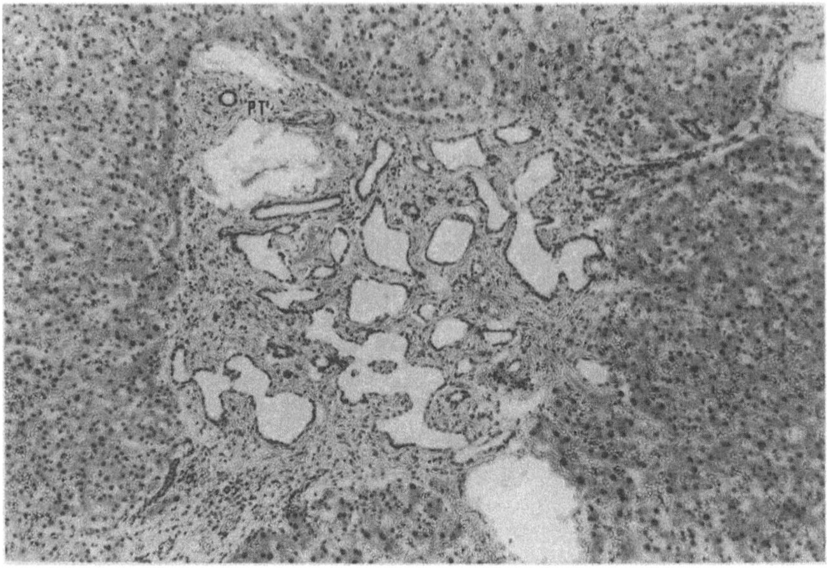


**Fig. 7.** Meyenburg's complex. The lesion is located close to a portal tract (*PT*) and consists of irregularly dilated bile duct structures lined by cuboidal epithelium and embedded in a fibrous stroma. H&E, ×160

## 6.4 Autosomal Recessive or "Infantile" Polycystic Disease and Congenital Hepatic Fibrosis

It is not yet clear whether these are two separate entities or different presentations of the same disorder [27, 40, 74, 75]. In both congenital hepatic fibrosis and infantile polycystic disease, the basic liver lesion corresponds to the ductal plate malformation.

### *Infantile Polycystic Disease*

Infantile polycystic disease is a rare disorder, inherited as an autosomal recessive trait and occurring once in 6000–14000 live births [75]. BLYTH and OCKENDEN discerned four groups according to the clinical presentation: perinatal, neonatal, infantile, and juvenile [9]. In their series, clinical presentation was always the same within a single affected family and it was suggested that the four groups represented separate genetic entities [9]. This hypothesis, however, seems no longer tenable [5, 40, 74, 75]. The disease usually manifests itself at birth with grossly enlarged kidneys causing abdominal distention [9, 74]. Newborns usually die within the first few days of life [9, 30, 74]. The immediate cause of death is probably pulmonary insufficiency [74]. Patients who survive the newborn period have a variable clinical course. Renomegaly may or may not be present. Renal size may decrease from the age of 1–2 years [74]. Renal function may be nearly normal and glomerular filtration rate may remain adequate or may progressively decrease over a variable period of time, leading to renal failure [13]. Hypertension is an important complication and may lead to heart failure [42, 74, 75]. In the "juvenile" form of the disease, renal involvement is usually minimal but patients may present with complications of portal hypertension. Liver function tests are normal. An enlarged liver and spleen may be palpable. Some authors suggested that this form corresponds to congenital hepatic fibrosis [40]. In patients presenting at or around birth, diagnosis is usually not difficult. Antenatal diagnosis is possible using ultrasonography. The latter technique is also the most useful for screening purposes and usually allows a firm diagnosis [74]. Computed tomography and excretory urography can also be used.

The gross appearance of the kidneys depends on the extent and duration of the disease. For a detailed discussion of the renal pathology, the reader is referred to WELLING and GRANTHAM [74]. In children dying in the newborn period, both kidneys are grossly enlarged and contain innumerable, radially oriented cysts (Fig. 8). Microscopically, the latter correspond to cylindrically dilated terminal branches of collecting ducts. In patients who survive the newborn period, the extent of the cystic involvement is less and cysts tend to be more irregularly distributed [9]. The liver may be enlarged and firm. Occasionally, small cysts are visible macroscopically [27]. The amount of fibrosis is variable. Portal tracts show fibrous extensions that may lead to formation of portoportal fibrous linkages [9, 27, 30]. The portal tracts contain an increased number of bile ducts that often appear to be sectioned longitudinally to an unusual extent [9, 30]. Stereologic anaylsis has shown that the ductal population is a mixture of different tubular shapes ranging from circular cylinders to flat elliptical cylinders or two plates of epithelium around a plate-shaped lumen [30]. As has been discussed, this lesion corresponds to the ductal plate malformation [30] (Fig. 9). The liver parenchyma shows no alterations. It is not yet clear whether the liver lesion is evolving and whether fibrosis may increase with age [8, 30, 40]. Morphometric analysis has demonstrated that the liver lesions in the perinatal, neonatal, and infantile forms of the disease are the same but differ from those in the juvenile form [40]. The main difference consisted in a greater degree of fibrosis in the latter [40]. Infantile polycystic disease may be associated with nonobstructive dilatations of the intrahepatic biliary tree ("Caroli's disease") [46, 52].

The etiology of the disease is unknown. As has already been discussed, prognosis is variable. Therapy is supportive. In case of renal failure, dialysis may be required and renal transplantation may be considered [74]. Portal hypertension may necessitate portocaval or splenorenal shunting [74]. Cases with associated Caroli's disease may be complicated by cholangitis.

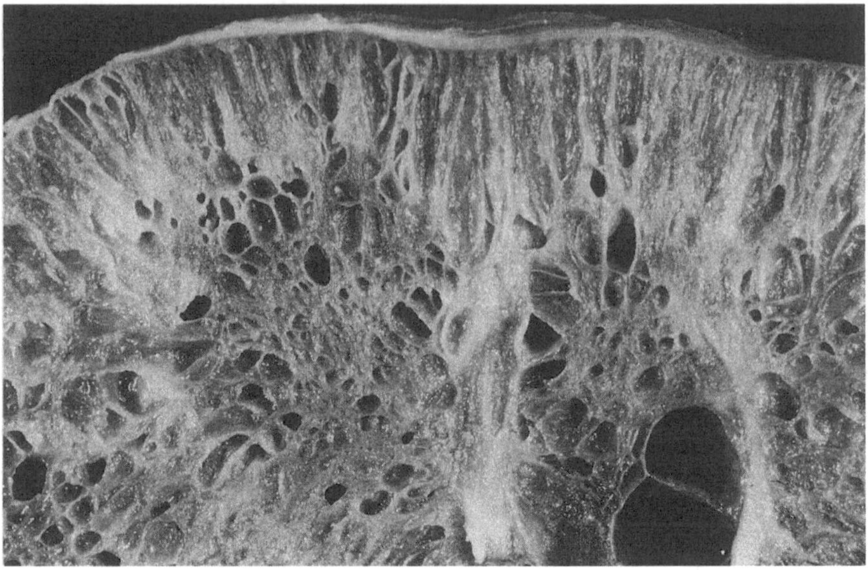

**Fig. 8.** Infantile polycystic disease. A cut section of the kidney reveals the typical radially oriented cysts. (By courtesy of Dr. P. Moerman)

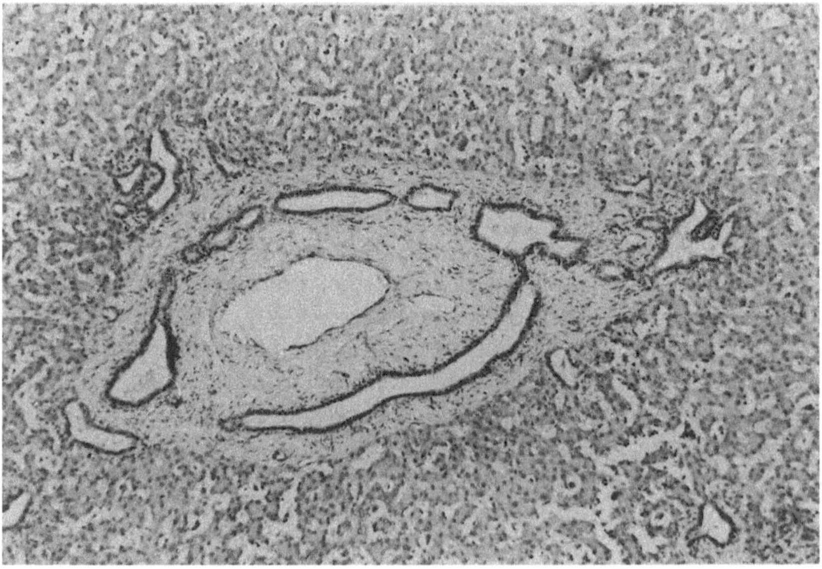

**Fig. 9.** Microscopic appearance of the liver in infantile polycystic disease. A portal tract contains bile duct structures arranged around a central vessel in a ductal plate-like arrangement. Compare to the normal ductal plate shown in Fig. 1. H&E, ×160

### *Congenital Hepatic Fibrosis*

The term "congenital hepatic fibrosis" was coined by KERR et al. [38]. The disorder is probably inherited in an autosomal recessive way [66]. It has been suggested that congenital hepatic fibrosis is part of the spectrum of infantile polycystic disease since the liver lesions are morphometrically identical to those of the "juvenile" form of infantile polycystic disease [40]. Other authors state that congenital hepatic fibrosis is not a single clinical entity but may be part of a spectrum of diseases including infantile polycystic disease, Caroli's disease, and adult polycystic disease [8, 51]. It may also occur as an isolated finding. Congenital hepatic fibrosis as described by KERR et al. is typically diagnosed at between 3 and 10 years of age [38, 66]. The patient presents with hemorrhage from esophageal varices. In a variable proportion of cases, congenital hepatic fibrosis is associated with non-obstructive dilatation of intrahepatic bile ducts (Caroli's disease) [68]. In those children, cholangitis may be a feature [5, 21, 66, 68]. The liver is enlarged and exceptionally firm [38]. An enlarged spleen is usually palpable [38]. ALVAREZ et al. reported liver function tests to be normal [5] but SUMMERFIELD et al. noted modestly elevated levels of serum aspartate aminotransferase and alkaline phosphatase in 50% of their patients [68]. Thrombocytopenia may be present and is caused by hypersplenism [5]. Portal venography demonstrates collateral circulation and a normal or distorted intrahepatic portal venous system [38]. Duplication of intrahepatic venous channels has been reported in cases of congenital hepatic fibrosis with portal hypertension [5, 54]. Ultrasonography shows bright areas of sound reflectivity caused by the dense fibrous strands [66] and can at the same time be used to evaluate the kidneys [5]. Kidney abnormalities are present in most patients [5, 8, 38] but some controversy exists as to their exact nature. In most patients, the renal lesion is consistent with infantile polycystic disease although LANDING has claimed that morphometric differences exist between the two types of renal lesion [41]. Congenital hepatic fibrosis may be associated with nephronophthisis (medullary cystic disease) [77] and exceptionally even with adult polycystic disease of the kidneys [51, 66]. Cases with no apparent renal involvement are rare and it is possible that cystic renal changes may develop later in life [5, 38]. Although hepatosplenomegaly, normal liver function tests, and kidney abnormalities strongly suggest congenital hepatic fibrosis [5], definite diagnosis requires a liver biopsy. The architecture of the liver is probably best evaluated on surgical specimens [38, 66]. Histologically, there is a variable degree of periportal fibrosis [27, 38]. The liver parenchyma appears as garland-shaped masses in between portoportal fibrous septa (Fig. 10). Numerous bile ducts of various sizes are scattered in the fibrous tissue and are usually located at the interface between the latter and the liver parenchyma. The basic lesion again corresponds to the ductal plate malformation [30]. The ducts may contain mucinous material or inspissated bile [38]. Portal vein radicles have

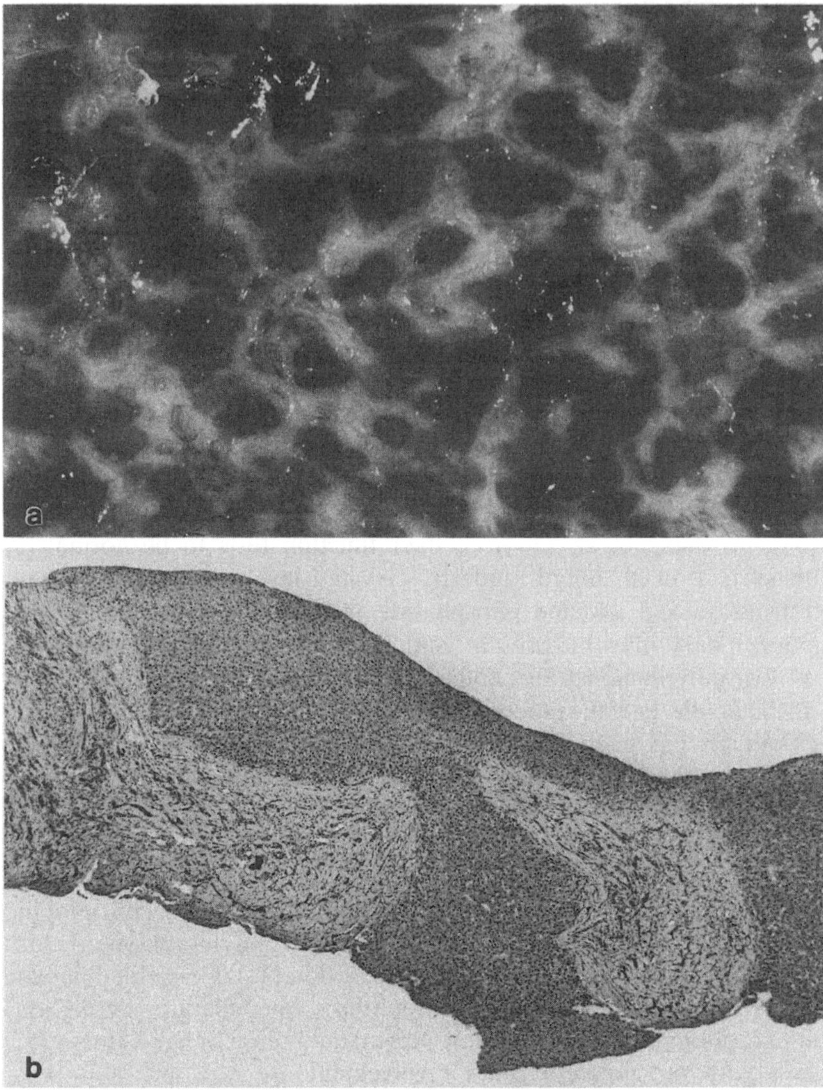


**Fig. 10.** **a** Gross appearance of the liver in congenital hepatic fibrosis. Pale areas of fibrosis surround garland-shaped masses of parenchyma. (By courtesy of Dr. P. Moerman). **b** Microscopic appearance. Broad fibrous areas contain numerous bile duct structures. The intervening parenchyma appears essentially normal. H&E, ×64

been reported to be scanty [38]. The liver parenchyma appears normal and cholestasis is not a feature, except when cholangitis occurs. In these cases, numerous neutrophils are present in the portal tracts [27]. Progression of fibrosis may occur with age [8]. Factors responsible for the evolving morphology of congenital hepatic fibrosis include localized intrahepatic biliary obstruction and biliary sepsis with suppuration [8]. The etiology of the disorder is unknown. It is striking that the overall histologic picture of congenital hepatic fibrosis resembles a biliary type of fibrosis but with presence of ductal plates. Some liver specimens obtained after successful portoenterostomy (see Sect. 4) show a histologic picture strongly resembling congenital hepatic fibrosis. This observation raises the question of whether congenital hepatic fibrosis may represent an "abortive" form of extrahepatic bile duct atresia with an onset early in fetal life (i.e., when ductal plates are still present), leading to a biliary type of fibrosis with ductal plate malformations.

The portal hypertension requires medical measures. If patients avoid aspirin, they may have many years free from bleeding [48]. Since no hepatic parenchymal disease is present, patients with congenital hepatic fibrosis are ideal candidates for portal-systemic shunting. In one series, the mean age at surgery was 9 years 3 months [5]. The type of shunt has to be selected so that it will not impair a renal transplantation – if such an operation is indeed foreseeable [5]. The natural history of congenital hepatic fibrosis is still poorly understood [48]. In the series of ALVAREZ, no further impairment of hepatic function was detected [5]. Hepatocellular carcinoma and cholangiocarcinoma may be a complication [66].

### 6.5 Congenital Intrahepatic Biliary Dilatation, Communicating Cavernous Ectasia of the Intrahepatic Bile Ducts, "Caroli's Disease"

This disorder was first described by CAROLI in 1958 [11]. The originally described entity consisted of segmental cystic dilatation of intraheptic bile ducts in the absence of portal fibroiss [10, 11]. This form, also referred to as the "simple" form, is exceedingly rare [29, 75]. Subsequently, Caroli described a second, "periportal fibrosis associated" type characterized by gross alterations of the liver architecture and "hyperplasia of small dilated biliary branches with an angiomatous appearance" [10]. It is still debated whether this latter type really corresponds to congenital hepatic fibrosis associated with dilatation of the intrahepatic bile ducts [75]. WITZLEBEN proposes that the term "Caroli's disease" be used only to designate the rare "simple" form.

The exact mode of inheritance is unknown [66] but an autosomal recessive pattern has been suggested [10, 29]. Both "simple" and "periportal fibrosis associated" types usually present in childhood or early adult life [10, 66]. The "simple" form is characterized by episodes of fever. Jaundice is not a feature and there is no hepatosplenomegaly or evidence of portal hypertension [10]. The more common "periportal fibrosis associated" form can present with abdominal pain, fever with Gram-negative septicemia, or bleeding from esophageal varices. Hepatosplenomegaly is usually found [10]. Ultrasonography and computed tomography may be very helpful

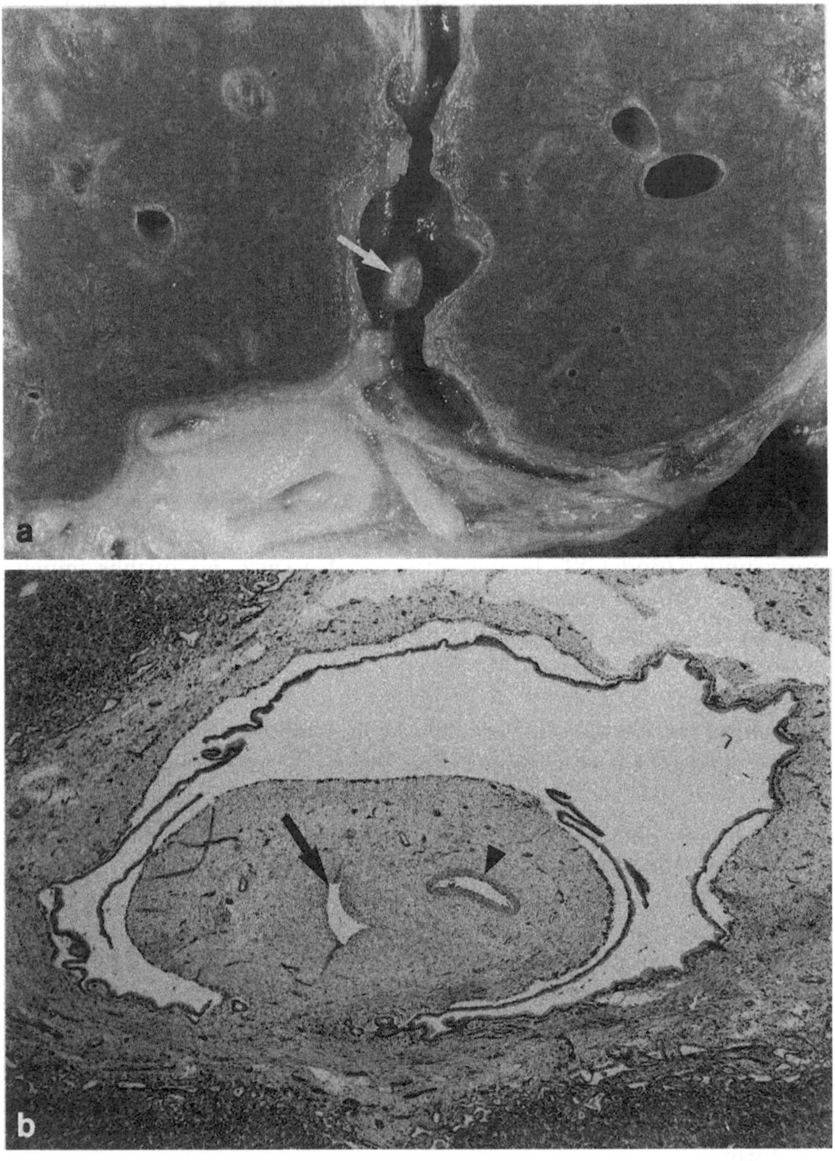


**Fig. 11a–c.** Caroli's disease. **a** Macroscopic view of a cystically dilated bile duct with a polypoid wall protrusion containing cross-sectioned vessels (*arrow*). **b** Microscopic study of the central fibrous core reveals a central (portal) vein (*arrow*) and accompanying (hepatic) artery (*arrowhead*)

in demonstrating the cystic bile duct dilatations [46, 66]. Endoscopic or percutaneous cholangiography are diagnostic [66]. Liver function tests are generally normal except during episodes of obstructive jaundice [10, 27].

The condition usually involves the entire liver but may be segmental or lobar [10, 27]. The cystic dilatations are round to lanceolate and vary in size

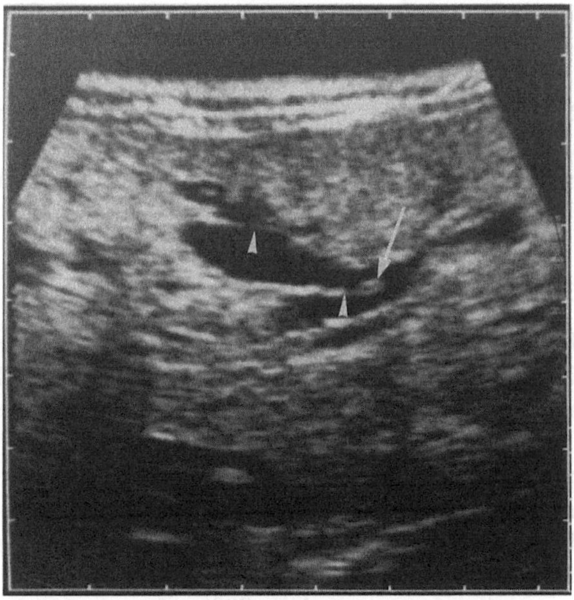

**Fig. 11c.** Ultrasonogram (10 MHz) shows irregularly dilated bile ducts and complete and incomplete bridging of the ductal walls (*arrowheads*). A small portal branch is seen at the end of an incomplete bridge (*arrow*). Reproduced with permission from Marchal G. et al. (1986) Radiology 158:507–511]

from 10 to 45 mm. They may be separated by stretches of essentially normal ducts [10, 27]. Friable bilirubin calculi may be present in the lumen. Nakanuma et al. have described bulbar protrusions of the duct wall into the lumen and bridge formation of the duct wall across the lumen [52]. Both features can be detected using ultrasonography [46] (Fig. 11). Microscopically, the ducts are lined by normal appearing biliary epithelium. The latter may be focally ulcerated or hyperplastic. The wall shows variable degrees of inflammation and fibrosis and may contain abundant mucous glands. During bouts of cholangitis, pus can be seen in the lumen [27]. In the "periportal fibrosis associated" form, there is periportal fibrosis, portoportal fibrous septa, and an increased number of bile ducts, sometimes in ductal plate configuration [46].

Cystic dilatation of the intrahepatic bile ducts may be associated with renal disease. Caroli states that the renal changes are usually those of renal tubule ectasia (medullary sponge kidney) but lesions consistent with infantile and even adult polycystic disease have also been described [10, 29, 46, 52].

Cholangitis is treated with antibiotics. Rare cases with lobar involvement are amenable to partial hepatic resection [10]. The prognosis is poor [10, 66]. Cholangiocarcinoma may be a complication [66].

## 6.6 Congenital Bile Duct Cysts (Choledochal Cyst, Congenital Cystic Dilatation of the Common Bile Duct)

The incidence of congenital bile duct cysts, a nonheritable condition, shows striking geographic differences [59, 75]. For reasons unknown, choledochal cysts are much more common in Japan than in Western countries [59, 75]. Females are more frequently affected than males.

### *Classification*

The disorder may occur in multiple anatomic variants and several classification systems have been proposed [4, 25, 43, 71]. The recent classification by TODANI et al. [71] takes into account that cysts need not to be limited to the common bile duct but may occur in any segment of the extrahepatic biliary tree. Moreover, they may be associated with cystic dilatations of the intrahepatic bile ducts. TODANI et al. therefore use the term "congenital bile duct cysts." Their classification comprises five types (Table 3) and also has clinical relevance (see Sect. 7.7). Type I is by far the most common variant, accounting for more than 90% of cases in the United States [59]. The relationship (or identity?) of types IV A and V to Caroli's disease is not clear [27, 59, 71].

### *Clinical Features*

The condition may present at any age but symptoms, signs, and clinical course are markedly different in infants as compared to older patients [59]. The infantile form is part of the clinical spectrum of conjugated hyperbilirubinemia in infancy and has to be differentiated from extrahepatic bile duct atresia [59]. In this form, distal ductal atresia is frequently seen [59]. Patients are usually in the first few months of life and the majority have jaundice and acholic stools [59]. Hepatomegaly and a palpable abdominal mass are often present. Other symptoms include pain, vomiting, and failure to thrive [59]. The clinical course is frequently complicated. Cholangitis,

**Table 3.** Classification of congenital bile duct cysts according to TODANI et al. [71]

| | |
|---|---|
| Type I | "Common type" |
| | a) Choledochal cyst |
| | b) Segmental dilatation |
| | c) Diffuse or cylindrical dilatation |
| Type II | Diverticulum |
| Type III | Choledochocele |
| Type IV | A. Multiple cysts (intra- and extrahepatic) |
| | B. Multiple cysts (extrahepatic only) |
| Type V | Intrahepatic bile duct cysts (single or multiple) |

cirrhosis, and portal hypertension may develop. The adult or noninfantile form (patients beyond the age of 2 years) most commonly presents with pain [59]. Intermittent jaundice and recurrent cholangitis may occur. The classic triad of pain, jaundice, and a palpable abdominal mass is only present in about 25% of cases [78]. The noninfantile form runs a milder clinical course than the infantile one [59].

### *Diagnosis*

Ultrasonography is the best screening technique and some cases have even been diagnosed in utero [59, 75, 78]. Radionuclide scintigraphy and percutaneous transhepatic cholangiography are also useful [59, 78]. The definitive diagnosis and classification are made by intraoperative cholangiography at the time of surgical intervention. It is imperative to delineate the anatomy of both extra- and intrahepatic bile ducts.

### *Etiology and Pathogenesis*

The etiology and pathogenesis of congenital bile duct cysts represent a confusing issue, and it is not clear whether all variants share the same etiology [75]. One hypothesis holds that choledochal cysts are the result of "maldevelopment" resulting in an inherent abnormality of the ductal wall [59]. A theory proposed by Babbit et al. [7] holds that the cysts are actually the result of an acquired injury due to an anomalous arrangement of the distal pancreaticobiliary tree. The latter is referred to as a long "common channel" formed when the common bile duct joins the pancreatic duct well above the duodenum. The role of a stenotic distal common channel and of the reflux of pancreatic juice into the bile duct is much debated [59]. Congenital and acquired factors may also operate in concert to produce cystic dilatations [59]. It has also been suggested that choledochal cysts presenting in infancy may be the result of an obliterative inflammatory process of the distal common bile duct, analogous to extrahepatic bile duct atresia [39, 59].

### *Pathology*

The cysts vary greatly in size. They have a fibrous wall. Often an epithelial lining is lacking but islets of cylindrical or columnar epithelium may still be present [27, 75]. The wall may be thickened by inflammation and fibrosis and may be bile stained. Occasional smooth muscle fibers are seen [27].

### *Complications*

Complications are reported to occur in 16.5% of cases [78]. Stone formation is the most frequent one [78]. Development of carcinoma is the second and most dreaded long-term complication, occurring in 4.2%–8% of cases [75, 78]. Tumors only rarely develop before 20 years of age [59]. The typical malignancy is an adenocarcinoma but squamous cell carcinoma, undifferentiated carcinoma, and adenoacanthoma have also been reported [71, 78]. Tumors may arise in various parts of the pancreaticobiliary system, including the liver, gallbladder, and pancreas, but cancer arising in the cyst accounts for the large majority of cases [78]. The high incidence of carcinoma goes unexplained but it has led surgeons to abandon nonresection procedures in favor of resection (see below). Tumors, however, may still develop after resection of the cyst [31, 75]. Other complications include obstruction, cholangitis, and, rarely, perforation [75, 78].

### *Treatment and Prognosis*

The treatment of choledochal cyst is surgical [31, 59, 75]. It is imperative that the precise anatomy of the intra- and extrahepatic bile ducts is documented because treatment varies according to the type of cyst. For a more detailed discussion of the various surgical procedures, the reader is referred to excellent reviews [59, 71, 78]. For type I cysts, excision of the cyst and reconstruction of the biliary tree using a Roux-en-Y hepaticojejunostomy or an interposed jejunal segment is currently preferred over internal drainage [59, 78]. With modern surgical and anesthetic techniques, mortality and morbidity should be low and success rates high [31, 59].

## 6.7 Various Syndromes

In a number of syndromes, the basic liver lesion corresponds to the ductal plate malformation. Meckel's syndrome is an autosomal recessively inherited condition. Its three main features comprise postaxial hexadactyly, occipital encephalocele, and multicystic renal dysplasia not associated with urinary tract obstruction [50]. Jeune's syndrome or thoracic asphyxiating dystrophy is also inherited as an autosomal recessive trait and consists of dwarfism, pulmonary hypoplasia, retinal lesions, and cystic disease of the kidneys [40]. Ivemark's syndrome is a familial dysplasia of kidneys, liver, and pancreas [75]. In the vaginal atresia syndrome, tuberous sclerosis, and the Ellis-van Creveld syndrome (chondroectodermal dysplasia), liver lesions consistent with the ductal plate malformation have been described [40, 75]. Morphometric analysis has revealed that some differences may exist between the ductal plate malformation as seen in some of the above syndromes and that seen in autosomal recessive polycystic disease [40].

## References


1. Alagille D (1979) Cholestasis in the first three months of life. Prog Liver Dis 6:471–485
2. Alagille D, Estrada A, Hadchouel M, Gautier M, Odièvre M, Dommergues JP (1987) Syndromic paucity of interlobular bile ducts (Alagille syndrome or arteriohepatic dysplasia): review of 80 cases. J Pediatr 110:195–200
3. Alagille D, Odièvre M, Gautier M, Dommergues JP (1975) Hepatic ductular hypoplasia associated with characteristic facies, vertebral malformations, retarded physical, mental and sexual development and cardiac murmur. J Pediatr 86:63–71
4. Alonso Lej F, Rever WB, Pessagno DJ (1959) Congenital choledochal cyst, with a report of two and an analysis of 94 cases. Surg Gynecol Obstet 108:1–30
5. Alvarez F, Bernard O, Brunelle F, Hadchouel M, Leblanc A, Odièvre M, Alagille D (1981) Congenital hepatic fibrosis in children. J Pediatr 99:370–375
6. Amedee-Manesme O, Bernard O, Brunelle F et al. (1987) Sclerosing cholangitis with neonatal onset. J Pediatr 111:225–229
7. Babbitt DP, Starshak RJ, Clemett AR (1973) Choledochal cyst: a concept of etiology Am J Radiol 119:57–62
8. Bernstein J, Stickler GB, Neel IV (1988) Congenital hepatic fibrosis: evolving morphology. APMIS [Suppl] 4:17–26
9. Blyth H, Ockenden BG (1971) Polycystic disease of kidneys and liver presenting in childhood. J Med Genet 8:257–284
10. Caroli J (1973) Diseases of the intrahepatic biliary tree. Clin Gastroenterol 2:147–161
11. Caroli J Soupault R, Kassakowski J (1958) La dilatation polykystique congénitale des voies biliaires intra-hépatiques: essai de classification. Sem Hop Paris 34:128–135
12. Chandra RS, Altman RP (1978) Ductal remnants in extrahepatic biliary atresia. A histopathological study with clinical correlations. J Pediatr 93:196–200
13. Cole BR, Conley SB, Stapleton FB (1987) Polycystic kidney disease in the first year of life. J Pediatr 111:693–699
14. Dahms BB, Petrelli M, Wyllie R et al. (1982) Arteriohepatic dysplasia in infancy and childhood: a longitudinal study of six patients. Hepatology 2:350–358
15. Deprettere A, Portmann B, Mowat AP (1987) Syndromic paucity of the intrahepatic bile ducts. Diagnostic difficulty; severe morbidity throughout early childhood. J Pediatr Gastroenterol Nutr 6:865–871
16. Desmet VJ (1985) Intrahepatic bile ducts under the lens. J Hepatol 1:445–559
17. Desmet VJ (1987) Cholangiopathies: past, present and future. Semin Liver Dis 7:67–76
18. Desmet VJ (to be published) Embryology. In: McIntyre N, Benhamou J-P, Bircher J, Rizzetto M, Rodes J (eds) The Oxford textbook of clinical hepatology. Oxford University Press, Oxford
19. Desmet VJ, Callea F (1990) Cholestatic syndromes of infancy and childhood. In: Zakim D, Boyer TD (eds) Hepatology. A textbook of liver disease, vol 2, 2nd edn. W.B. Saunders, Philadelphia, pp 1355–1385
20. Desmet VJ, Van Eyken P, Sciot R (1990) Cytokeratins for probing cell lineage relationships in developing liver. Hepatology 12:1249–1251
21. Fauvert R, Benhamou J (1974) Congenital hepatic fibrosis. In: Schaffner F, Sherlock S, Leevy CM (eds) The liver and its diseases. Georg Thieme, Stuttgart, pp 283–288
22. Gautier M, Jehan P, Odièvre M (1976) Histologic study of biliary fibrous remnants in 48 cases of extra-hepatic biliary atresia: correlation with postoperative bile flow restoration. J Pediatr 89:704–709
23. Grunfeld J-P, Albouze G, Junger P (1985) Liver changes and complications in adult polycystic kidney disease. Adv Nephrol 14:1

24. Haas JE (1978) Bile duct and liver pathology in biliary atresia. World J Surg 2:561–569
25. Hadad AR, Estbrook KC, Campbell FT, Morris WO (1976) Congenital dilatation of the bile ducts. Am J Surg 132:799–804
26. Hammar JA (1926) Über die erste Entstehung der nicht kapillaren intrahepatischen Gallengänge beim Menschen. Z. Mikrosk Anat Forsch 5:59–89
27. Ishak KG, Sharp HL (1987) Developmental abnormality and liver disease in childhood. In: MacSween RNM, Anthony PP, Scheuer PJ (eds) Pathology of the liver, 2nd edn. Churchill Livingstone, Edinburgh, pp 66–98
28. Ito I, Nagaya M, Nünomi N, Ishiguro X, Ando H, Iio K (1987) Intrahepatic bile ducts in biliary atresia.. In Ohi R (ed) Biliary atresia. Professional Postgraduate Services, Tokyo, pp 62–68
29. Jordon D, Harpaz N, Thung SN (1989) Caroli's disease and adult polycystic kidney disease: a rarely recognized association. Liver 9:30–35
30. Jørgensen MJ (1976) The ductal plate malformation. A study of the intrahepatic bile duct lesion in infantile polycystic desease and congenital hepatic fibrosis. Acta Pathol Microbiol Scand [Suppl] 257:1–88
31. Joseph VT (1990) Surgical techniques and long-term results in the treatment of choledochal cyst. J Pediatr Surg 25:782–787
32. Kahn EI, Daum F, Markowitz J et al. (1983) Arteriohepatic dysplasia II. Hepatobiliary morphology. Hepatology 3:77–84
33. Kahn E, Daum F, Markowitz J, Teichberg S, Duffy L, Harper R, Aiges H (1986) Nonsyndromatic paucity of interlobular bile ducts: light and electron microscopic evaluation of sequential liver biopsies in early childhood. Hepatology 6:890–901
34. Kahn E, Markowitz J, Aiges H, Daum F (1989) Human ontogeny of the bile duct to portal space ratio. Hepatology 10:21–23
35. Karhunen PJ (1986) Adult polycystic liver disease and biliary microhamartomas (Von Meyenburg's complexes). Acta Pathol Microbiol Immunol Scand [A] 94:397–400
36. Kasai M (1974) Treatment of biliary atresia with special reference to hepatic portoenterostomy and its modifications. Prog Pediatr Surg 6:5–52
37. Kasai M, Kimura S, Asakura S, Suzuki H, Taira Y, Ohashi E (1968) Surgical treatment of biliary atresia. J Pediatr Surg 3:665–675
38. Kerr DNS, Harrison CV, Sherlock S, Milnes Walker R (1961) Congenital hepatic fibrosis. Q J Med 30:91–117
39. Landing BH (1974) Considerations on the pathogenesis of neonatal hepatitis, biliary atresia and choledochal cyst. The concept of infantile obstructive cholangiopathy. Prog Pediatr Surg 6:113–139
40. Landing BH, Wells TR, Claireaux AE (1980) Morphometric analysis of liver lesions in cystic diseases of childhood. Hum Pathol 11:549–560
41. Landing B, Wells T, Helczynski L (1988) Some problems in the meaning of terms as exemplified by tubulointerstitial and medullary cystic diseases of the kidneys (cystic diseases of liver and kidneys.) In: Rosenberg H, Bernstein J (eds) Perspectives in pediatric pathology, vol 12. S. Karger, Basel, pp 20–43
42. Lieberman E, Salinas-Madrigal L, Gwinn JL, Brennan LP, Fine RN, Landing BH (1971) Infantile polycystic disease of the kidneys and liver. Clinical, pathological and radiological correlations and comparison with congenital hepatic fibrosis. Medicine 50:277–318
43. Longmire WP, Mandiola SA, Gordon HE (1971) Congenital cystic disease of the liver and biliary system. Ann Surg 174:711–724
44. Ludwig J, Wiesner RH, La Russo NF (1988) Idiopathic adulthood ductopenia. A cause of chronic cholestatic liver disease and biliary cirrhosis. J Hepatol 7:193–199
45. Marceau N (1990) Cell lineages and differentiation programs in epidermal, urothelial and hepatic tissues and their neoplasms. Lab Invest 63:4–20

46. Marchal GJ, Desmet VJ, Proesmans WC, Moerman PL, Van Roost WW, Van Holsbeeck MT, Baert AL (1986) Caroli desease: high frequency US and pathologic fingings. Radiology 158:507–511
47. Markle GB (1981) Agenesis of the common bile duct. Arch Surg 116:350–352
48. Mieli-Vergani G (1990) Congenital hepatic fibrosis. Ital J Gastroenterol 22:306–307
49. Miyano T, Surugo K, Tsuchiya H (1977) A histopathological study of the remnant of extrahepatic bile duct in so-called uncorrectable biliary atresia. J Pediatr Surg 12:19–25
50. Moerman P, Verbeken E, Fryns JP, Goddeeris P, Lauwerijns JM (1982) The Meckel syndrome. Pathological and cytogenetic observations in eight cases. Hum Genet 62:240–245
51. Murray-Lyon IM, Ockenden BG, Williams R (1973) Congenital hepatic fibrosis – is it a single clinical entity? Gastroenterology 64:653–656
52. Nakanuma Y, Terada T, Ohta G, Kurachi M, Matsubora F (1982) Caroli's disease in congenital hepatic fibrosis and infantile polycystic disease. Liver 2:346–354
53. Newman KO, Torres VE, Rakela J, Nagorney DM (1990) Treatment of highly symptomatic polycystic liver disease. Preliminary experience with a combined resection fenestration procedure. Ann Surg 212:30–37
54. Odièvre M, Chaumont P, Montagne JPh, Alagille D (1977) Anomalies of the intrahepatic portal venous system in congenital hepatic fibrosis. Radiology 122:427–430
55. Puente SG, Bannura GC (1983) Radiological anatomy of the biliary tract. Variations and congenital abnormalities. World J Surg 7:271–276
56. Raweily EA, Gibson AAM, Burt AD (1990) Abnormalities of intrahepatic bile ducts in extrahepatic biliary atresia. Histopathology 17:521–527
57. Riely CA (1987) Familial intrahepatic cholestatic syndromes. Semin Liver Dis 7:119–133
58. Riely CA, Cotlier E, Jensen PS, Klatskin G (1979) Arteriohepatic dysplasia: a benign syndrome of intrahepatic cholestasis with multiple organ involvement. Ann Intern Med 91:520–527
59. Ryckman FC, Noseworthy J (1987) Neonatal cholestatic conditions requiring surgical reconstruction. Semin Liver Dis 7:134–154
60. Scheuer PJ (1988) Liver disease in childhood and heredofamilial disorders. In: Scheuer PJ (ed) Liver biopsy interpretation, 4th edn. Bailliere Tindall, London, pp 186–206
61. Schwartz MZ, Hall RJ, Reubner B, Lilly JR, Brogen T, Toyama WM (1990) Agenesis of the extrahepatic bile ducts: report of five cases. J Pediatr Surg 25:805–807
62. Schweizer P, Müller G (1984) Gallengangsatresie. Cholestase-Syndrome im Neugeborenen- und Säuglingsalter. Hippokrates, Stuttgart, pp 1–118
63. Schweizer P (1988) Long-term results and prognosis after hepatic portoenterostomy for the treatment of biliary atresia. In: Waldschmidt J, Charissis G, Schier F (eds) Cholestasis in neonates. W. Zuckschwerdt, Munich, pp 88–94
64. Severn CB (1972) A morphological study of the development of the human liver. II. Establishment of liver parenchyma, extrahepatic ducts and associated venous channels. Am J Anat 133:85–108
65. Sherlock S (1989) The liver in infancy and childhood. In Sherlock S (ed) Diseases of the liver and biliary system, 8th edn. Blackwell Scientific, Oxford, pp 501–522
66. Sherlock S (1989) Cysts and congenital biliary abnormalities. In: Sherlock S (ed) Diseases of the liver and biliary system, 8th edn. Blackwell Scientific, Oxford, pp 639–654
67. Shiojiri N, Katayama H (1987) Secondary joining of the bile ducts during the hepatogenesis of the mouse embryo. Anat Embryol 177:153–163

68. Summerfield JA, Nagafuchi Y, Sherlock S, Cadafalch J, Scheuer PJ (1986) Hepatobiliary fibropolycystic disease: a clinical and histological review of 51 patients. J Hepatol 2:141–156
69. Sunaryo FP, Watkins JB (1983) Evaluation of diagnostic techniques for extrahepatic biliary atresia. In: Daum F (ed) Extrahepatic biliary atresia. Marcel Dekker, New York, pp 11–22
70. Terada T, Nakanuma Y, Kono N, Ueda K, Kadoya M, Matsui O (1990) Ciliated hepatic foregut cyst. A mucus histochemical, immunohistochemical and ultrastructural study in three cases in comparison with normal bronchi and intrahepatic bile ducts. Am J Surg Pathol 14:356–363
71. Todani T, Watanabe Y, Narusue M, Tabuchi K, Okajima K (1977) Congential bile duct cysts. Classification, operative procedures and review of thirty-seven cases including cancer arising from choledochal cyst. Am J Surg 134:263–269
72. Valencia-Mayoral P, Weber J, Cutz E (1984) Possible defect in the bile secretory apparatus in arteriohepatic dysplasia (Alagille's syndrome). A review with observations on the ultrastructure of the liver. Hepatology 4:691–698
73. Van Eyken P (1990) Phenotypic modulation of hepatocytes: a cytokeratin-immunohistochemical study. PhD Thesis, Katholieke Universiteit Leuven. Acco, Leuven, pp 1–185
74. Welling LW, Grantham JJ (1989) Cystic diseases of the kidney. In: Tisher CC, Brenner BM (eds) Renal pathology with clinical and functional correlations. J.B. Lippincott, Philadelphia, pp 1233–1275
75. Witzleben CL (1990) Cystic diseases of the liver. In: Zakim D, Boyer TD (eds) Hepatology. A textbook of liver disease, vol 2, 2nd edn. W.B. Saunders, Philadelphia, pp 1395–1411
76. Witzleben CL, Finegold M, Piccoli DA, Treem WR (1987) Bile canalicular morphometry in arteriohepatic dysplasia. Hepatology 7:1262–1266
77. Witzleben CL, Sharp A (1982) "Nephronophtisis–congenital hepatic fibrosis". An additional hepatorenal disorder. Hum Pathol 13:728–733
78. Yamaguchi M (1980) Congenital choledochal cyst. Analysis of 1433 patients in the Japanese literature. Am J Surg 140:653–657

# 29 Fatty Liver Disease and Nutritional Liver Damage

J. Prieto, J.M. Zozaya, and F. Conchillo

## 1 Introduction

Located at the junction of the portal and systemic circulation, the liver plays an important role in the regulation of intermediary metabolism. The liver receives nutrients from the intestine and peripheral tissues; it is able to store glucose as glycogen, to esterify fatty acids, and to synthesize fatty acids and cholesterol. It can transform carbohydrates into fat, amino acids into glucose (gluconeogenesis), and acetyl-CoA into ketone bodies. The liver synthesizes proteins, such as albumin, lipoproteins, and clotting factors; it releases glucose to the blood and exports lipids to the periphery, packed as lipoproteins. Oxidation of free fatty acids and amino acids takes place in the liver and this organ is also the main site of urea formation from ammonia.

This intense metabolic activity entails a considerable expenditure of energy (20% of the total energy consumed by the resting individual) [1]. This explains the alterations that occur in the liver parenchyma as a result of derangements in the body's nutritional status. Thus, the liver is damaged when calorie intake is excessive (obesity), when protein-deficient diets are consumed (kwashiorkor), when nutrients are delivered unphysiologically (total parenteral nutrition), and in the presence of endocrinologic disorders influencing intermediary metabolism (diabetes). Usually, all these disturbances manifest as fatty liver disease.

## 2 Fat Metabolism and Fatty Liver

Fatty liver is defined by morphologists as an accumulation of fat within hepatocytes. Although this definition covers many different metabolic products, triglycerides are by far the most common material encountered. Thus, the expression "fatty liver" without any additional qualifications indicates triglyceride fatty liver. In most cases, triglycerides accumulate in the nonstructural part of the cytoplasm. Only in one case, so-called Wolman's disease, is the deposit intralysosomal. This condition, which is due to congenital lack of lysosomal acid lipase, is, however, very rare [2].

## 2.1 Fat Metabolism

Triglyceride synthesis (lipogenesis) takes place by esterification of fatty acids with glycerol-3-phosphate, a product of the glycolytic pathway. As depicted in Fig. 1, there is an active fatty acid cycle involving the gut, liver, adipocytes, and other peripheral tissues. Fatty acids may enter the liver cell from the blood or may be synthesized intracellularly [1]. The basic building block for fatty acid formation is acetyl-CoA, the common product of the metabolism of glucose, amino acids, and fatty acids. Fatty acids imported into the liver cell may proceed from intestinal absorption of dietary fat or from lipolysis of triglycerides stored in adipocytes. In the first case, they may enter directly into the portal circulation bound to albumin (if they are of less than 10 carbon atoms) or alternatively, and more importantly, they are incorporated as triglycerides in chylomicrons secreted by the enterocytes into the lymph. Chylomicrons are delipidated by lipoprotein lipase, an enzyme located on the endothelium of capillaries of adipocytes and other peripheral tissues. Lipoprotein lipase hydrolyzes triglycerides, making fatty acids available for cells. The resulting chylomicron remnants are taken up efficiently by liver cells [3]. In muscle and other peripheral tissues, fatty

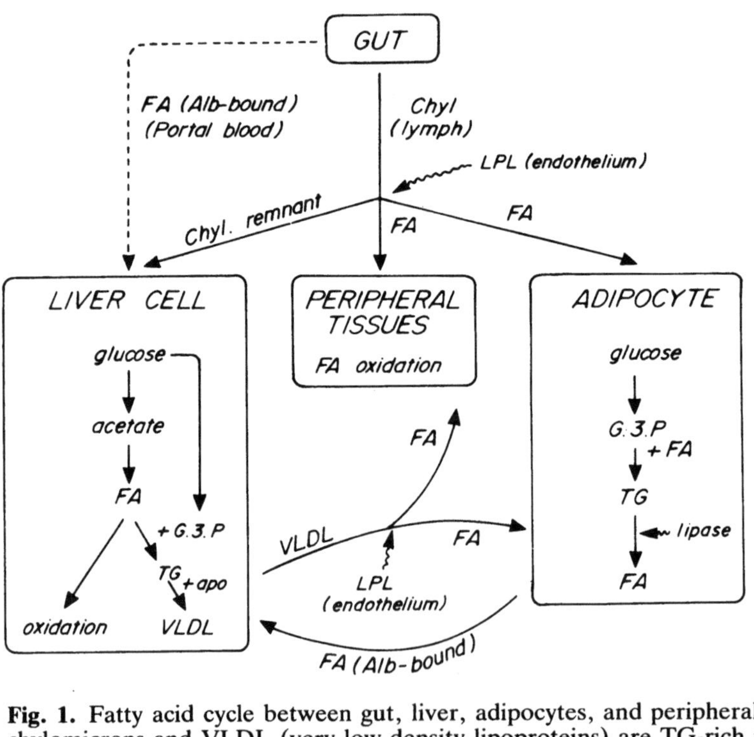


**Fig. 1.** Fatty acid cycle between gut, liver, adipocytes, and peripheral tissues. Both chylomicrons and VLDL (very low-density lipoproteins) are TG-rich particles. *Alb*, albumin; *apo*, apolipoproteins; *FA*, fatty acid; *G-3-P*, glycerol-3-phospate; *chyl*, chylomicrons; *LPL*, lipoprotein lipase; *TG*, triglycerides

acids can be used as a source of energy. In adipocytes during the fed state, fatty acids are esterified to form triglycerides and used as storage of energy. Lipogenesis is favored by insulin. Fatty acids can be released from adipocytes by the action of a hormone-sensitive local lipase which is modulated by the intracellular levels of cyclic AMP [2]. Hormones, such as cortisol, glucagon, epinephrine, norepinephrine, and ACTH, stimulate lipolysis. Released fatty acids are transported in the blood complexed to albumin. In this way, they reach different organs and an important fraction is captured by hepatocytes. Fatty acids entering the liver cells or synthesized in these cells can undergo mitochondrial β-oxidation to produce energy or serve to esterify cholesterol or to be included in other complex lipids. Importantly, they can be used together with glycerol-3-phosphate to form triglycerides. Triglyceride is mobilized from the liver as very low-density lipoproteins (VLDL). Lipoproteins are composed of lipid and associated proteins called apoproteins [3]. The lipid moiety of lipoproteins is synthesized in the smooth endoplasmic reticulum, whereas apoproteins are produced by ribosomes in the rough endoplasmic reticulum. At the junction of smooth and rough endoplasmic reticulum, lipid and apoproteins are assembled into VLDL [4]. Vesicles containing VLDL are transported to the Golgi apparatus and then to the plasma membrane, where the newly formed VLDL is discharged to the Disse's space, from which they then enter the general circulation. In the intracellular transport of VLDL, microtubules are believed to play a significant role [4]. In the peripheral circulation, VLDL particles, like chylomicrons, suffer the action of lipoprotein lipase, which releases free fatty acids to be used by peripheral tissues or stored in adipocytes as triglycerides. VLDL remnants give rise to low-density lipoproteins (LDL) which are cleared by internalization in cells possessing LDL receptors, such as hepatocytes.

## 2.2 Mechanisms Causing Fatty Liver

The liver's capacity to remove fatty acids from the blood and synthesize triglycerides far exceeds its capacity for oxidizing fatty acids and exporting triglycerides as VLDL. Thus, fatty liver develops when there is a disproportion between triglyceride synthesis and secretion [2]. Different mechanisms can be responsible for this imbalance (Table 1). Increased triglyceride synthesis occurs when there is an excessive supply of fatty acids to the liver from intestinal sources or from adipose tissue. Thus, diets containing excess triglycerides or conditions associated with increased fatty acid mobilization from adipocytes can lead to fat accumulation in liver cells. These conditions include obesity, diabetes, steroid therapy, and situations involving physical stress, as in fever. In obesity, both the enlarged mass of fat deposits and the accompanying insulin resistance contribute to increased fatty acid release from adipose tissue. There is, however, no

**Table 1.** Fatty liver: mechanisms

| | |
|---|---|
| A. Increased triglyceride synthesis | |
| 1. Excessive fatty acid influx in liver cells | |
| a) From intestine: hyperlipidemic diets | |
| b) From parenteral nutrition | |
| c) From adipose tissue: | obesity |
| | diabetes |
| | steroid therapy |
| | fever |
| 2. Increased availability of precursors for fatty acid synthesis | |
| a) Hypercaloric, carbohydrate-rich diets | |
| b) Alcohol | |
| 3. Reduced fatty acid oxidation | |
| a) Mitochondrial damage: | sodium valproate |
| | Reye's syndrome |
| b) Acyl-CoA dehydrogenase deficiency | |
| B. Diminished triglyceride secretion | |
| 1. Reduced protein synthesis | |
| a) Protein malnutrition: | kwashiorkor |
| | intestinal bypass |
| | gastrointestinal disease |
| b) Metabolic cell damage: | tyrosinemia |
| | Wilson's disease |
| c) Toxic cell damage: | tetracycline |
| | $CCl_4$ |
| | puromycin |
| | asparaginase |
| 2. Microtubular dysfunction | alcohol |
| C. Cryptogenic | |

relationship between the degree of obesity and the intensity of hepatic steatosis, indicating that additional factors might be implicated in this process [5]. It has been suggested that defects in protein synthesis and/or the packaging of VLDL, as a result of protein–calorie imbalance (diets with high carbohydrate content with relative protein and choline deficiency), could play a role in the genesis of fatty liver in some obese subjects. Fatty liver may also result from consumption of hypercaloric, carbohydrate-rich diets, which increase the availability of precursors for triglyceride synthesis in the liver cells.

Fatty liver is not uncommon in type II (adult-onset) diabetes, a condition usually associated with obesity and insulin resistance [6]. In contrast, steatosis is rarely observed in type I (juvenile-onset) diabetes, except when ketosis develops as a result of poor control of the disease. In this situation, insulin deficiency favors lipolysis and therefore hepatic steatosis.

Alcohol is one of the most common causes of fatty liver. This drug affects many steps in lipid metabolism [2, 7]. Ethanol increases acetate levels in hepatocytes and augments the ratio of NADH to NAD. These changes contribute to increased fatty acid synthesis and reduced fatty acid oxidation. Additionally alcohol enhances lipolysis in adipose tissue and impairs lipoprotein secretion by liver cells. All these factors induce hepatic fat accumulation.

Mitochondrial damage, as is observed in valproate toxicity or in Reye's syndrome, may also cause fatty liver by depressing fatty acid oxidation. In these cases, a microvesicular pattern of fat deposition is frequently encountered.

Fatty liver can also stem from disturbances in VLDL assembly or secretion. This occurs in cases of impaired protein synthesis due to metabolic cell damage (e.g., tyrosinemia) or toxic liver cell injury (e.g., due to tetracycline, $CCl_4$, or asparaginase). Reduction in protein synthesis leading to fatty liver is also observed in cases of protein malnutrition, as in the kwashiorkor syndrome and in intestinal bypass surgery.

Finally, there is a group of subjects who exhibit liver steatosis without any obvious cause. These individuals may be prediabetics or may present some, as yet undefined, metabolic abnormality.

### 2.3 Pathology, Clinical Findings, and Therapy

Histologically, two types of hepatic steatosis are recognized: macrovesicular and microvesicular fat deposition (Fig. 2). The former is the most common and it is characterized by large lipid droplets displacing peripherally the cell nucleus. This is the type observed in obesity, alcoholism, diabetes, and malnutrition. Microvesicular fat consists of small droplets of lipid surrounding central nuclei. This pattern of fat accumulation is seen in Reye's syndrome, acute fatty liver of pregnancy, toxicity due to tetracycline or valproate, toxic shock syndrome, delta hepatitis in South America and Central Africa, metabolic disorders affecting mitochondrial fatty acid oxidation, and certain alcoholic patients after acute/massive ethanol ingestion [2, 8].

In many cases, fatty liver causes few or no subjective clinical symptoms. Occasionally, it may cause discomfort at the right upper abdomen. The liver is usually palpable. Liver function tests are either normal or may detect slight elevations of $\gamma$-glutamyltransferase and serum aminotransferases. Decreased parenchymal density is found in magnetic resonance and computed tomographic studies. Increased echogenicity is seen by ultrasonography. In some instances, these imaging techniques demonstrate focal fatty liver instead of widespread fatty change.

Treatment of fatty liver should be oriented toward correcting the underlying disorder. Thus, diet, weight reduction, control of diabetes, or withdrawal of the offending drug should be considered in their respective cases. There is no solid evidence in humans that benefit may be gained from so-called hepatoprotective agents or lipotropic factors.

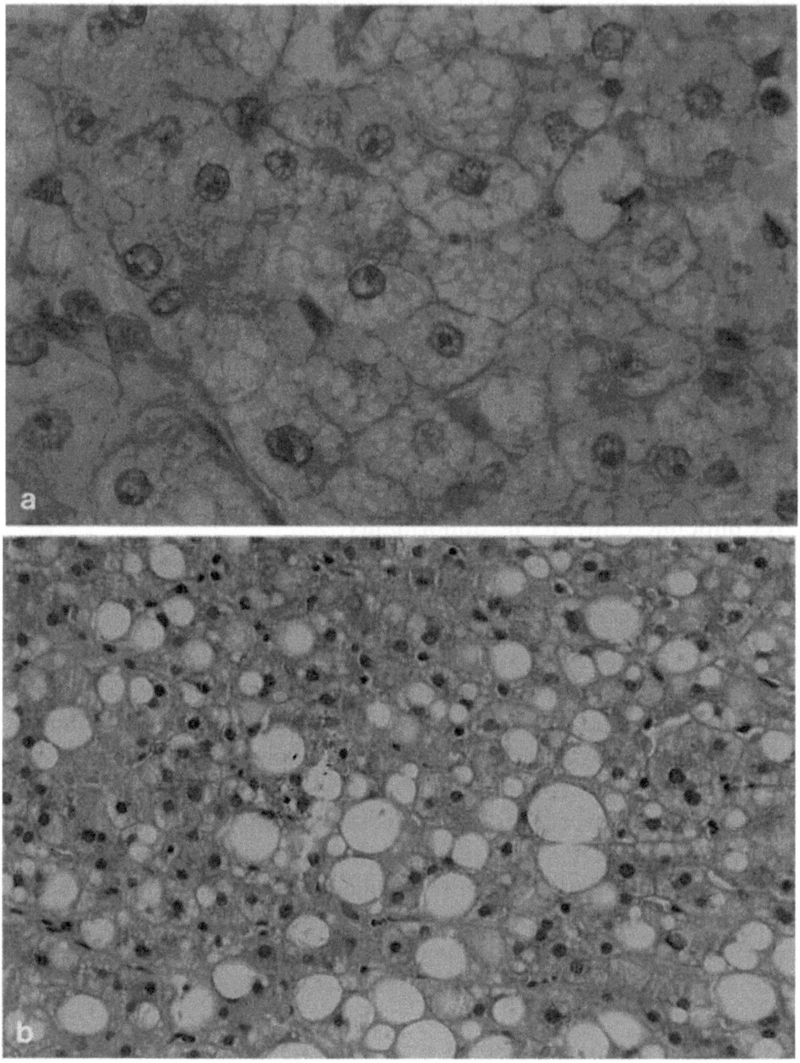

**Fig. 2. a** Microvesicular fatty liver (tetracycline). ×1000. **b** Macrovesicular fatty liver. ×100

## 3 Reye's Syndrome

The original report by REYE et al. of encephalopathy and fatty degeneration of viscera dates from 1963 and since then thousands of cases have been studied all over the world [9]. The syndrome is characterized by an acute encephalopathy without cerebrospinal fluid pleocytosis in association with marked liver dysfunction. Serum aminotransferases and blood ammonia are elevated ($\geqslant 3 \times$ normal) and the liver shows widespread microvesicular steatosis.

Reye's syndrome may affect both sexes. It mainly occurs at between 6 and 11 years of age although the condition has now been recognized at every age from birth to adulthood [10]. When untreated its course is very severe, with a 30% mortality.

The characteristic clinical picture is usually preceded by an influenza-like illness. Although a variety of viral infections have been associated with the development of the syndrome, influenza B and varicella-zoster have been the agents most frequently implicated [11]. Often the child is recovering from the viral illness when hyperemesis ensues. Vomiting introduces the second or encephalopathic phase of the process.

Indeed, when confronted with a delirious or comatose child, if there is a history of recent viral infection followed days later by pernicious vomiting, Reye's syndrome is the favored diagnosis. The stage of encephalopathy at the time of admission correlates with survival [10, 12]. In stage 0 there is absence of neurologic manifestations, in stage I the patient is confused and lethargic, in stage II the patient shows an agitated delirium or a stuporous state or light coma, in stage III there is coma with decerebrate posturing, and in stage IV there is absence of brain stem function with flaccidity, circulatory collapse, and dilated and nonreactive pupils.

The encephalopathy is due to cerebral edema and is the essential prognostic factor since in survivors the liver returns to normal [11]. It has been shown that blood ammonia higher than 400 μg/dl. is indicative of a bad prognosis [13]. It is conceivable that both the cerebral disorder and the elevation in blood ammonia stem from multivisceral mitochondrial damage [14]. In fact, brain mitochondria show ultrastructural changes similar to those in the liver [15].

A large array of biochemical abnormalities has been described in Reye's syndrome. These include increased serum aminotransferase levels, hypoproteinemia, hypoglycemia, hyperammonemia, organic acidemia, and reduced carbon dioxide. Serum cholesterol, VLDL, and various clotting factors are low [10]. In tissues there is a universal decrease in mitochondrial enzymes, including ornithine transcarbamylase, carbamylphosphate synthase, the pyruvate dehydrogenase complex, pyruvate carboxylase, succinate dehydrogenase, and cytochrome oxidase [10] (Fig. 3). The pathologic changes in the liver consist of microvesicular steatosis, distortion of mitochondria, absence of glycogen, peroxisomal proliferation, and depletion of Golgi membranes [10].

Recently some epidemiologic evidence has emerged relating Reye's syndrome to the use of aspirin. In the United States there has in recent years been a marked decline in the use of aspirin among children, which has been accompanied by a dramatic decline in the incidence of Reye's syndrome [16]. Similar observations have been reported in Britain [17].

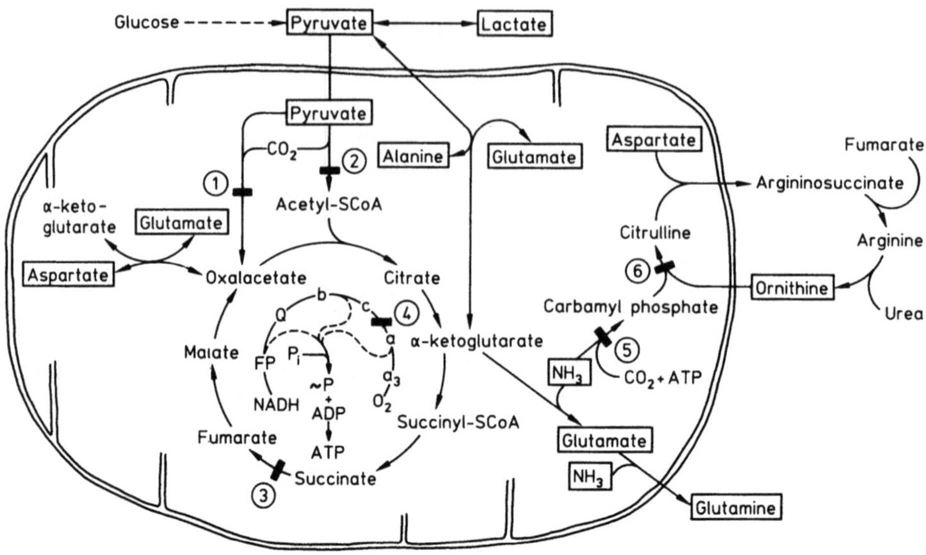


**Fig. 3.** Integrated mitochondrial metabolic functions. Enzymatic blockades present in Reye's syndrome are depicted. [Reproduced with permission from DE VIVO D (1987) In: KELLEY VC (ed) Practice of pediatrics, vol 9. Harper and Row, Philadelphia, pp 1–8]

Management of diseased children should be carried out in an intensive care unit with monitoring of vital signs, water–electrolyte balance, blood glucose, renal function, coagulation profile, serum aminotransferases, amylase, lactate, blood gases, and pH. Endotracheal intubation should be placed (stages II–IV) to ensure proper ventilation. Patients should receive intravenous glucose in a 25%–30% solution. Vitamin K is administered i.v. 1 mg every 24 h. Monitoring of intracranial pressure is advisable in those who have progressed to stage III. Mannitol (1 g/kg) and glycerol (1 g/kg) can be given intravenously at a frequency (every 4–8 h) related to the severity of the illness to lower the intracranial pressure [10, 18]. Intracranial pressure should be maintained below 20 torr. The fatality rate at present has fallen below 20% [18].

## 4 Fatty Liver Hepatitis (Nonalcoholic Steatohepatitis)

In some patients, fatty liver may progress to a more severe form of liver disease known as "nonalcoholic steatohepatitis" or simply "fatty liver hepatitis" [19]. Histologically this condition is characterized by macrovesicular fat deposition, presence of Mallory bodies in zone 3, intra-acinar neutrophil infiltration, and pericentral necrosis and fibrosis, constituting a picture indistinguishable from alcoholic hepatitis. Although in the past these lesions have been attributed to covert alcoholism, it has become clear during

**Table 2.** Fatty liver hepatitis (nonalcoholic steatohepatitis)

| | | |
|---|---|---|
| 1. | Obesity | |
| 2. | Diabetes | |
| 3. | Jejunoileal bypass | |
| 4. | Drugs: | Estrogen therapy |
| | | Amiodarone |
| | | Perhexiline maleate |
| 5. | Weber-Christian disease | |

the last few years that fatty liver hepatitis can occur in a variety of clinical settings unrelated to alcohol (Table 2). Nonalcoholic steatonecrosis has been described in obesity, in diabetes, after intestinal bypass surgery for morbid obesity, in nonsuppurative panniculitis, and in subjects receiving high doses of synthetic estrogens [20–24]. Drugs, such as amiodarone and perhexiline maleate, have also been associated with a histologic lesion resembling alcoholic hepatitis. In amiodarone and perhexiline toxicity, there is in addition to steatonecrosis an accumulation of lysosomal phospholipid in hepatocytes that causes the appearance of numerous round "lamellar materials" on electron microscopy. This peculiar drug-induced lesion has been called "phospholipid fatty liver" [25].

Nonalcoholic steatohepatitis is a relatively uncommon process, usually of benign evolution, although it can in some cases progress to cirrhosis. Numerous studies have underlined its strong association with female gender, obesity, hyperlipidemia, and diabetes mellitus [20, 23, 24]. Obese and diabetic patients developing this condition should undergo liver biopsy electively to evaluate incidentally detected hepatomegaly and/or abnormal liver tests. This establishes a difference from alcoholic hepatitis, where the majority of patients appear systemically ill at the time of liver biopsy [20]. In nonalcoholic steatohepatitis, clinical symptoms are mild or absent and aminotransferase levels are slightly to moderately elevated. Serum bilirubin, albumin, and prothrombin time are often normal, in contrast to the significant alteration in these parameters commonly found in alcoholic hepatitis. Thus, the two forms of steatohepatitis – alcoholic and nonalcoholic – differ clinically and biochemically but present a similar histologic pattern [20, 23, 24]. On the whole, however, the histology tends to show more inflammation and fibrosis and less macrovesicular fat deposition in the alcoholic form than in the nonalcoholic. In nonalcoholic cases progression of the liver lesion is very slow, although cirrhosis may develop in spite of the control of blood sugar and successful weight reduction. It is likely that the observed increase in cirrhosis among diabetics is at least partly the result of fatty liver hepatitis [26]. Nonalcoholic steatohepatitis should be recognized as a possible cause of "cryptogenic cirrhosis" [23].

The pathogenesis of fatty liver hepatitis is unknown. It may be related to the cytotoxic potential of fatty acids. These substances are highly reactive and can damage biologic membranes [2, 23]. It is believed that increased levels of free fatty acids resulting from enhanced lipolysis might be responsible for liver cell injury in obesity or diabetes.

Intestinal bypass surgery for morbid obesity induces rapid weight loss and causes serious liver disease in about 15% of patients. Of these, some die from hepatic failure and some develop cirrhosis. Pathogenetic factors include accelerated lipolysis, bacterial toxins, and protein malnutrition. Metronidazole and parenteral therapy with amino acid mixtures are of benefit [27].

## 5 Nutritional Liver Injury

### 5.1 Kwashiorkor and Marasmus

Marasmus results from diets deficient in total calorie intake. Kwashiorkor develops at the time of weaning and originates from diets with a protein–calorie imbalance, that is, carbohydrate-rich diets with a very low protein content. Kwashiorkor, but not marasmus, causes fatty liver [28]. Marasmus, on rare occasions, may cause peliosis hepatis [29].

Kwashiorkor is characterized by a typical syndrome which includes hair abnormalities, edema, growth failure, wasting of muscles, irritability, psychomotor retardation, anemia, and hypoalbuminemia. In the liver, there is fatty change and mitochondrial damage. Occasionally, there is inflammation and fibrosis that may be related to additional hepatotoxic factors or exposure to viruses. Kwashiorkor is a condition of tropical areas.

### 5.2 Total Parenteral Nutrition

Different hepatobiliary abnormalities have been described in association with total parenteral nutrition (TPN) [30]. Asymptomatic biochemical changes and hepatic steatosis are the most common pathologic findings. Fatty liver is probably related to the infusion of large amounts of glucose which stimulates acetyl CoA decarboxylase activity, the regulatory enzyme of fatty acid synthesis. Some patients who receive long-term TPN develop florid nonalcoholic steatohepatitis. Intrahepatic cholestasis occurs commonly after 2 or 3 weeks of TPN and is more frequently observed in infants. Usually it is a transitory disturbance that subsides after discontinuation of TPN. In a few cases, liver function tests remain abnormal and liver biopsy shows portal fibrosis and periportal inflammation. The pathogenesis of intrahepatic cholestasis is likely multifactorial and includes altered enterohepatic circulation of bile salts due to the "enterically fasted" state, bacterial overgrowth in the small intestine, increased lithocholic acid production, portal endotoxemia, nutritional deficiencies, and in some cases systemic infections. Biliary sludge, cholelithiasis, and acalculous cholecystitis are common complications of TPN both in children and in adults. Gallbladder stasis resulting from lack of enteral nutrition facilitates stone formation. Concentration of bile in the gallbladder causes bilirubin saturation and precipitation of calcium bilirubinate crystals.

Patients subjected to TPN and developing cholestasis should receive, after exclusion of other causes, a trial of metronidazole and, if possible, small lipid and protein meals, or cholecystokinin, to stimulate bile flow.

## References


1. Seifter S, Englard S (1988) Energy metabolism. In: Arias IM, Jakoby WB, Popper H et al. (eds) The liver: biology and pathobiology, 2nd edn. Raven, New York, p 279
2. Dianzani MU (1979) Reactions of the liver to injury: fatty liver. In: Farber E, Fisher MM (eds) Toxic injury of the liver, part A. Marcel Dekker, New York, p 281
3. Hoeg JM, Brewer HB Jr (1986) Human lipoprotein metabolism and the liver. Prog Liver Dis 8:51–64
4. Glickman RM, Sabesin SM (1988) Lipoprotein metabolism. In: Arias IM, Jakoby WB, Popper H et al. (eds) The liver: biology and pathobiology, 2nd edn. Raven, New York, p 331
5. Faloon WW (1988) Hepatobiliary effects of obesity and weight-reducing surgery. Semin Liver Dis 8:229–236
6. Van Thiel DH (1986) Diabetes mellitus and hepatobiliary disease. Curr Concepts Gastroenterol 4:4–13
7. Weiner FR, Czaja MJ, Zern MA (1988) Ethanol and the liver. In: Arias IM, Jakoby WB, Popper H et al. (eds) The liver: biology and pathology, 2nd edn. Raven, New York, p 1169
8. Hautekeete ML, Degot C, Benhamou JP (1990) Microvesicular steatosis of the liver. Acta Clin Belg 45:311–326
9. Reye RDK, Morgan G, Baral J (1963) Encephalopathy and fatty degeneration of viscera: a disease entity in childhood. Lancet II:749–752
10. De Vivo D (1987) Reye syndrome. In: Kelley VC (ed) Practice of pediatrics, vol 9. Harper and Row, Philadelphia, pp 1–8
11. Bellman MH, Hall SM (1983) Aetiology of Reye's syndrome. Arch Dis Child 58:670–672
12. DeLong GR, Glick TH (1982) Encephalopathy of Reye's syndrome: a review of pathogenetic hypotheses. Pediatrics 70:997–1000
13. Chi CS, Law KL, Wong TT, Su GY, Lin N (1990) Continuous monitoring of intracranial pressure in Reye syndrome. Five years experience. Acta Pediatr Jpn 32:426–434
14. De Vivo DC (1978) Reye syndrome: A metabolic response to an acute mitochondiral insult? Neurology 28:105–108
15. Partin JS, McAdams AJ, McLaurin RL et al. (1979) Brain ultrastructure in Reye's syndrome; acute injury and repair. In: Crocker JFS (ed) Reye's syndrome II. Grune & Stratton, New York, pp 237–249
16. Hurwitz ES (1989) Reye's syndrome. Epidemiol Rev 11:249–253
17. Porter JD, Robinson PH, Glasglow JF et al. (1990) Trends in the incidence of Reye's syndrome and the use of aspirin. Arch Dis Child 65:826–829
18. Wulur H, Kho LK (1990) Treatment of Reye syndrome at Sumber Waras Hospital. Acta Pediatr Jpn 32:435–442

19. Ludwig J, Viggiano TR, McGill DB et al. (1980) Nonalcoholic steatohepatitis. Mayo Clinic experiences with a hitherto unnamed disease. Mayo Clin Proc 55:434–438
20. Diehl AM, Goodman Z, Ishak KG (1988) Alcohollike liver disease in nonalcoholics. Gastroenterology 95:1056–1062
21. Snodgrass PJ (1970) Obesity, small bowel bypass and liver disease. N Engl J Med 282:870–871
22. Seki K, Minami Y, Nishikawa M et al. (1983) Nonalcoholic steatohepatitis induced by massive doses of synthetic estrogen. Gastroenterol Jpn 18:232–240
23. Powell EE, Graham W, Cooksley E et al. (1990) The natural history of nonalcoholic steatohepatitis: a follow-up study of forty-two patients for up to 21 years. Hepatology 11:74–80
24. Nagore N, Scheuer PJ (1988) The pathologic of diabetic hepatitis. J Pathol 156:155–160
25. Oda T, Shikata T, Naito C et al. (1970) Phospholipid fatty liver: a report of three cases with a new type of fatty liver. J Exp Med 40:127–140
26. Stone BG, Van Thiel DH (1985) Diabetes mellitus and the liver. Semin Liver Dis 5:8–28
27. Balistreri WF, Bive KE (1990) Hepatobiliary consequences of parenteral alimentation. In: Popper H, Shaffner F (eds) Progress in liver diseases IX. W.B. Saunders, Philadelphia, p 567
28. Quigley EMM, Zetterman RK (1988) Hepatobiliary complications of malabsorption and malnutrition. Semin Liver Dis 8:218–228
29. Simon DM, Krause R, Galambos JT (1988) Peliosis hepatis in a patient with marasmus. Gastroenterology 95:805–809
30. Klein S, Nealon WH (1988) Hepatobiliary abnormalities associated with total parenteral nutrition. Semin Liver Dis 8:237–246

## Suggested Reading

Balistreri WF, Bive KE (1990) Hepatobiliary consequences of parenteral alimentation. In: Popper H, Shaffner F (eds) Progress in liver diseases IX. W.B. Saunders, Philadelphia, p 567

Shaffner F, Thaler H (1986) Nonalcoholic fatty liver disease. In: Popper H, Shaffer F (eds) Progress in liver diseases VIII. Grune & Stratton, New York, p 283

# 30 Circulatory Disorders and Vascular Disease Affecting the Liver

P.A. McCormick and A.K. Burroughs

## 1 Effects of Liver Disease on the Systemic Circulation

Cirrhosis is associated with a hyperdynamic circulatory state. This is manifested by increased cardiac output with a decreased arterial blood pressure and peripheral vascular resistance. Cirrhotic patients tend to have faster heart rates and lower blood pressures than controls and in general have warm, vasodilated peripheries [1]. The cardiac output is related to the severity of the liver disease [2]. As liver function and clinical status improve, the cardiac output returns towards normal. It is now believed that peripheral arterial vasodilatation, particularly in the splanchnic circulation, is the initiating factor in these haemodynamic disturbances [3]. The mechanisms causing this arterial vasodilatation are not clearly understood. It has been suggested that hyperglucagonaemia is an important cause but this is still controversial. Peripheral arterial vasodilatation is believed to lead to a reduction in "central blood volume", causing functional hypovolaemia [4], although in cirrhosis total plasma volume is increased. Vasoconstrictor hormones such as renin, angiotensin, catecholamines, and antidiuretic hormone are secreted in response to this functional hypovolaemia and the sympathetico-adrenal axis is activated, causing renal salt and water retention and ultimately leading to the formation of ascites [3]. There are also abnormalities in regional haemodynamics: renal (discussed in Chap. 12), hepatic and splanchnic (discussed in Chap. 11) and in the pulmonary circuit.

## 2 Effects of Liver Disease on the Pulmonary Circulation

### 2.1 Hepatopulmonary Syndrome

Hypoxemia is a frequent complication in patients with severe cirrhosis, which may be due to intrapulmonary shunting, ventilation–perfusion mismatch or a diffusion–perfusion defect [5]. Hypoxemia is probably due to a combination of all three factors. It has also been described in idiopathic portal hypertension in which liver function is well preserved. The term "diffusion–perfusion defect" has been coined to describe hypoxemia due to shunt blood flow through small intrapulmonary vascular dilatations (IPVDs). As many of these IPVDs are in close proximity to alveoli, breathing 100% oxygen may significantly raise the arterial $pO_2$, in contrast to a classical right-to-left shunt. It was thought that significant hypoxemia was a contraindication to liver transplantation. However, it now appears that liver transplantation may reverse the ventilation–perfusion mismatch and the diffusion–perfusion defect and that the hepatopulmonary syndrome may be a functional disorder similar to the hepatorenal syndrome [6].

### 2.2 Pulmonary Hypertension

Pulmonary hypertension is a rare condition in the general population. However, it appears to occur with increased frequency in patients with liver disease [7]. Patients may present with dyspnoea on exertion, or signs of right heart failure. It occurs particularly in patients following portacaval shunting for portal hypertension but has also been reported in patients with portal vein thrombosis without underlying liver disease. The prevalence in patients with cirrhosis may be as high as 2% [8]. Minor degrees of pulmonary hypertension may be reversed by liver transplantation. However, symptomatic pulmonary hypertension is regarded as a contraindication to liver transplantation but can be treated by combined heart–lung and liver transplantation. Pharmacological treatment is disappointing and in general the prognosis is poor.

## 3 Cardiomyopathy Associated with Cirrhosis

Although there is a background of a hyperkinetic circulation, some cirrhotics have subclinical or clinical impairment of ventricular contractility [9]. The vast majority of reports describe abnormalities in alcoholic cirrhotics, and thus it is difficult to separate the known cardiomyopathic effect of alcohol from cirrhosis per se. True beri-beri cardiomyopathy secondary to thiamine deficiency due to malnutrition is very rare. A wide spectrum of abnormalities may be observed from echocardiographic evidence of ventricular dysfunction in asymptomatic patients with chronic liver disease (which may only be present following exercise or pharmacological stress) to end-stage low output dilated cardiomyopathy. The peripheral vasodilatation and reduced systemic vascular resistance probably mask the signs of left ventricular failure for a time [10]. This may explain why the combination of alcoholic cirrhosis and clinical cardiomyopathy is rare.

Autopsy reports show a similar frequency of abnormal cardiac findings in alcoholic and non-alcoholic cirrhosis [11]. However, clinical cardiomyopathy in non-alcoholic cirrhosis has not been described in the absence of primary cardiac causes. Mechanisms for cardiomyopathy may be related to jaundice, which exerts cardiodepressant effects, raised serum catecholamine concentrations (raised in cirrhosis), which may have a role in the development of cardiomyopathy, and the induction of a high output failure state secondary to the hyperkinetic circulation.

Treatment of cardiomyopathy is difficult and follows cardiological management principles – digoxin is ineffective. In alcoholic cardiomyopathy abstinence may improve ventricular function or slow down the rate of deterioration, but there is little evidence to substantiate this.

## 4 The Effect of Ascites on Cardiac Function

Massive ascites will lead to underestimation of cardiac output based on the standard height/weight tables to derive surface area. There may be hydrostatic pressure on the diaphragm with a decrease in cardiac transmural filling pressure due to increased intrathoracic and intrapleural pressure [12]. The right ventricle has been shown to be compressed in echocardiographic studies [13]. Paracentesis for relief of ascites transiently improves cardiac output [13]. Conversely, peritoneovenous shunting can greatly increase cardiac output as there is increased venous return, but a readjustment occurs by 2 months with a return to baseline values [14]. Small pericardial effusions detected on echocardiography may be frequently found in patients with massive ascites but very rarely do they impair cardiac function [15].

## 5 Endocarditis and Pericarditis

The defects in chemotaxis, opsonisation and phagocytosis lead to an increased prevalence of bacteraemia in cirrhosis, and an increased incidence of endocarditis may be expected. In the series of SNYDER et al., consisting of 41 151 hospital admissions, 0.34% of cirrhotics versus 0.1% of non-cirrhotics had endocarditis [16]. Drug addicts with or without liver disease have an increased incidence of right-sided endocarditis, which has also been reported as a complication of peritoneovenous shunting. Although sclerotherapy of varices causes bacteraemia, endocarditis has only been reported in those patients with heart valve defects. Routine antibiotic prophylaxis is not needed. Fibrinous pericarditis has been found with acute renal failure due to hepatorenal syndrome. In a recent autopsy study, 9% of alcoholic cirrhotics had fibrinous pericarditis compared to no patients with non-alcoholic cirrhosis: alcoholics may have a predisposition to develop this complication [17].

## 6 Atherosclerosis and Arterial Hypertension

Autopsy studies demonstrate a lower prevalence of coronary atherosclerosis and myocardial infarction [18]. Alcohol in modest daily amounts may decrease the risk of ischaemic coronary events. Arterial hypertension is seen in cirrhotics, but may improve with worsening liver disease due to the systemic hypotension and peripheral vasodilatation which accompany worsening liver function. The relationship between the complex lipoprotein changes seen in cirrhosis and the risk of atheroma or coronary events has not been well studied.

## 7 Arteriohepatic Dysplasia Syndrome

Arteriohepatic dysplasia syndrome (Alagille's syndrome) is a congenital syndrome which consists of unusual facies, vertebral anomalies, intrahepatic biliary atresia, and congenital cardiac abnormalities, the commonest of which is pulmonary stenosis. Congenital hepatic fibrosis has on rare occasions been associated with congenital cardiac defects.

## 8 Hereditary Haemorrhagic Telangiectasia

Also known as Rendu-Osler-Weber disease, hereditary haemorrhagic telangiectasia, an autosomal-dominant congenital syndrome, is a disease of vascular structure. Telangiectases are characteristically present on the lips, face and tongue. Hepatosplenomegaly occurs in 50% of patients and some have portal hypertension. In the liver there may be telangiectases with or without fibrosis or cirrhosis, cirrhosis alone, and/or arteriovenous fistulae. High output cardiac failure may occur due to the shunting in the liver.

## 9 Arterioportal Fistulae

Arterioportal fistulae may be congenital, associated with other arterio-venous malformations due to trauma, a sequela of liver biopsy, secondary to hepatocellular tumours, due to rupture of an aneurysm of the hepatic artery (usually following sepsis), or associated with hereditary haemorrhagic telangectasia. If small they are of no consequence. Large fistulae can lead to high output heart failure and portal hypertension. Embolisation of the arterial side or ligation of the hepatic artery can cure the condition.

## 10 Heart Failure [19]

Hepatomegaly with or without abnormalities in liver function is frequently found in patients with congestive cardiac failure. With chronic heart failure the hepatic abnormalities are usually minor. Occasionally, especially with acute heart failure, they may be sufficiently marked to suggest primary hepatic disease and divert attention from the underlying cardiac problem [20]. The liver function test abnormalities are caused by a combination of congestion and low cardiac output. Congestion causes hepatomegaly and the combination of congestion and low cardiac output results in liver cell hypoxia. Arterial hypoxia is correlated with centrilobular necrosis in patients with heart failure. High aminotransferase values are correlated with centrilobular necrosis, which usually, but not always, follows an acute decrease in cardiac output; prothrombin times can be grossly prolonged [21].

### 10.1 Pathology

In patients dying of congestive heart failure the liver is dark and enlarged. Cut sections show a typical "nutmeg" appearance [22]. This is because the congested centri-acinar zones, around the hepatic veins, appear darker than the surrounding mid zones and periportal areas. The centrilobular zones are the most sensitive to hypoxia and in severe prolonged heart failure they are affected by necrosis [23]. This is followed by fibrosis around the central veins leading to the condition described as cardiac sclerosis. In some cases bridging fibrosis may develop, connecting central veins to central veins and portal tracts, and occasionally a true cirrhosis develops – the rare condition "cardiac cirrhosis" [24].

### 10.2 Symptoms and Signs

Hepatomegaly is very common in patients with congestive cardiac failure [25]. Usually this is asymptomatic but it may cause right upper quadrant discomfort and may be associated with nausea and vomiting. If there is moderate tricuspid regurgitation the liver may be pulsatile. Splenomegaly, ascites and jaundice are less common physical signs although they have been reported in approximately 20% of patients with liver involvement in cardiac failure. However, the presence of splenomegaly, ascites or jaundice should prompt a search for other causes of liver disease before the diagnosis of liver disease due to heart failure is accepted. Constrictive pericarditis should always be excluded by echocardiography. It may be necessary to await resolution of these signs following successful treatment of heart failure before ascribing them definitively to cardiac disease.

### 10.3 Liver Function Tests

Increased levels of serum bilirubin, aminotransferases, lactic dehydrogenase, and alkaline phosphatase are frequently found in patients with heart failure [26]. The serum bilirubin concentration rarely exceeds 85 μmol/litre and is usually less than 50 μmol/litre. Aminotransferase concentrations depend on the rapidity and severity of heart failure. In severe, acute heart failure very high levels (>1000 u/litre) may be seen, whereas only mild elevations, usually less than 100 u/litre are seen in chronic heart failure. Elevations of serum alkaline phosphatase are generally modest. The prothrombin time is frequently slightly prolonged, and does not respond to vitamin K, whereas the serum albumin may be mildly reduced in 30%–50% of patients. Prothrombin time and albumin abnormalities usually resolve over several weeks following treatment of heart failure, whereas bilirubin and aminotransferase values resolve within a week.

## 11 Hepatic Abnormalities in Other Cardiac Diseases

### 11.1 Acute Myocardial Infarction [27]

Hepatomegaly and abnormal liver function tests may be seen in patients with acute myocardial infarction complicated by cardiogenic shock or congestive cardiac failure. In uncomplicated myocardial infarction there may be a transient rise in plasma unconjugated bilirubin concentration.

### 11.2 Shock Liver [23, 28]

Severe hypotension due to any cause can cause shock liver. The duration of the liver insult is important as shock liver in the majority of patients usually occurs following a period of 24 h with hypotension. The most frequent manifestation is a dramatic rise in aminotransferase concentrations (1000–10 000 u/litre), with lesser derangements in other liver function tests. These may also occur with shorter periods of hypotension and are usually very transient. Occasionally shock liver can result in a picture of fulminant liver failure with jaundice and hepatic encephalopathy; this has been seen in children following cardiac surgery who have very low cardiac outputs. More frequently the evidence of liver injury in shock liver is solely biochemical and may be overshadowed by abnormalities in other organ systems. The prognosis is dependent on the prognosis of the underlying cause of hypotension [29].

### 11.3 Constrictive Pericarditis

Constrictive pericarditis is a rare condition, but when it occurs it frequently causes hepatic abnormalities including hepatomegaly, splenomegaly and ascites. In view of the prominence of the hepatic signs, and the sometimes subtle nature of the cardiac signs, the diagnosis may not be suspected and is difficult to make at the bedside. In particular it may be confused with the Budd-Chiari syndrome [30]. It should always be considered in the differential diagnosis and looked for by echocardiography. A low blood pressure, a small volume pulse, a paradoxical rise during inspiration of the jugular venous pulse, and signs of a low cardiac output state may alert the clinician to the cardiac origin of the hepatic signs.

### 11.4 Valvular Heart Disease

Hepatic abnormalities may occur in any valvular heart condition associated with congestive cardiac failure or a low cardiac output state. The most frequent valvular heart conditions encountered with clinical evidence of hepatic abnormalities are tricuspid incompetence and severe aortic stenosis. Tricuspid incompetence typically leads to an enlarged pulsatile liver which is attenuated in the presence of significant hepatic fibrosis as for other hepatic pulsations.

## 12 Cardiac Surgery

Jaundice is still a frequent complication of cardiopulmonary bypass surgery, occurring in up to 20% even in recent series. The pathogenesis is unclear and is probably multifactorial: age, bypass time, pre-operative cardiac status, sepsis, blood transfusion, hypothermia and shock appear to be risk factors. It has a poor prognosis with approximately 25% hospital mortality.

Children may develop a "shock" liver picture with low cardiac output states following surgery.

There has been a high incidence of non-A, non-B hepatitis (mostly confirmed as hepatitis C) following cardiac surgery. New tests for the detection of hepatitis C should greatly lessen this complication.

## 13 Hepatic Infarction

The liver is relatively protected from vascular injury because it has a dual blood supply. It receives arterial blood from the hepatic artery and portal venous blood from the portal vein. The normal liver blood flow is about

1000–1200 ml/min. In the fasting state it receives about 40% of this blood supply from the hepatic artery and the rest from the portal vein. Following a meal portal vein blood flow increases and hepatic arterial flow declines. There is thus a reciprocal relationship between hepatic arterial and portal venous blood flows [31]. This reciprocal relationship seems to be regulated at the level of the hepatic artery as the liver is unable to alter portal vein blood flow. Because of this vascular supply the normal liver can survive either portal vein occlusion or hepatic arterial thrombosis. However, infarction may occur in hypertensive disease of pregnancy (see Chap. 18), in association with vasculitis or arteritis, or due to septic emboli. Presentation is with epigastric or right upper quadrant pain, nausea, vomiting and fever. Jaundice is rare. A contrast-enhanced CAT scan is the most useful investigation.

Although the liver has two routes for blood inflow, most of the liver blood supply exits via the main hepatic veins with only a small portion of the caudate lobe draining directly into the vena cava through multiple small veins. The liver is thus vulnerable to obstruction of its venous outflow tract.

## 14 Budd-Chiari Syndrome

Budd-Chiari syndrome is due to obstruction of the major hepatic veins [32]. In the Western world the principal cause of this is venous thrombosis, most commonly due to an underlying thrombogenic disorder. This may be overt as in polycythaemia rubra vera or essential thrombocythaemia but may be latent and can only be diagnosed using special techniques to detect spontaneous erythroid colony production [33]. Other thrombogenic conditions causing Budd-Chiari syndrome include paroxysmal nocturnal haemoglobinuria, pregnancy, oral contraceptive use, Behçet's disease, deficiencies of antithrombin III, protein S or protein C or the presence of antiphospholipid antibodies in systemic lupus erythematosus (lupus anticoagulant) [34]. Malignant neoplasms of the kidney, adrenal gland, liver or vena cava, trauma, parasitic infections of the liver, inflammatory bowel disease and nodular regenerative hyperplasia may be associated with or cause Budd-Chiari syndrome. In the Far East and in southern Africa, Budd-Chiari syndrome is associated with suprahepatic inferior vena caval webs [35]. These webs characteristically obstruct the inferior vena cava just below the junction with the right atrium. They may extend into the hepatic veins or further down the vena cava, occasionally obliterating the entire inferior vena cava. The aetiology of the webs is unclear. They may be congenital but they may represent organisation of thrombus following hepatic vein thrombosis. In South Africa there is a well-established association between vena caval webs and the subsequent development of hepatocellular carcinomas [35]. Recently webs in the hepatic veins have been described, presenting with resistant ascites and responding to balloon

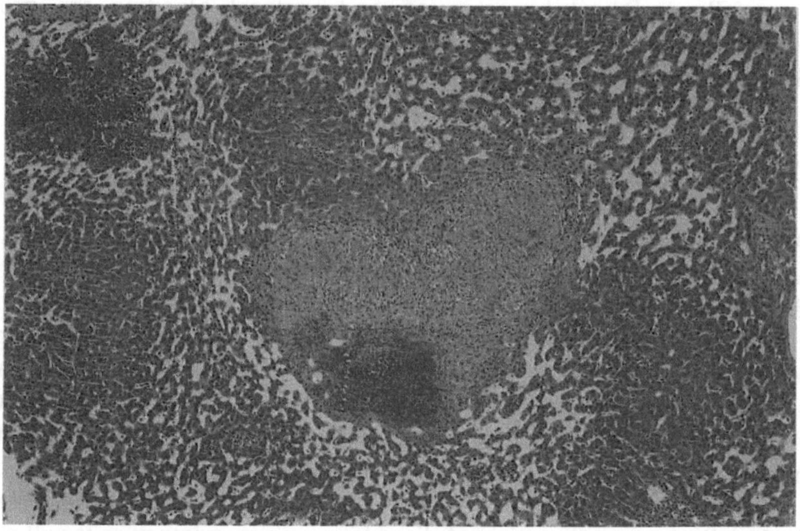

**Fig. 1.** Budd-Chiari syndrome. Necrosis and congestion are seen in the centrolobular area

dilatation [36]. Thrombosis in the hepatic veins is associated with inferior vena cava thrombosis in up to 20% of cases and in the portal vein in up to 10% of patients.

An important aspect is that thrombosis is asynchronous in many cases. Thus in the drainage field of previously thrombosed hepatic veins there may be fibrosis and atrophy of hepatocytes, whereas in recently thrombosed veins there is congestion and necrosis (Fig. 1). In about half the patients, the caudate lobe develops compensatory hypertrophy as it has a direct drainage into the inferior vena cava.

### 14.1 Clinical Features

The rapidity and extent of the hepatic vein thrombosis determines the mode of presentation [32]. In approximately 5% of cases it presents with fulminant hepatic failure with an acute onset of abdominal pain, hepatic encephalopathy, jaundice and renal failure. There are marked increases in aminotransferase values. Death usually occurs within 2 weeks without surgical intervention. More often there is subacute presentation with abdominal pain, jaundice and ascites developing over a few weeks. The most common presentation is with progressive ascites over a few months, with mild or no jaundice and mild disturbance in liver function. Intractable ascites is the main problem in these patients. Necrosis occurs around the hepatic vein radicles where the congestion is worse. Progressive liver damage with fibrosis and cirrhosis occurs and these patients may ultimately develop liver failure. Portal hypertension and variceal bleeding are prominent features across the spectrum of Budd-Chiari syndrome and are treated in the same way as in cirrhotics.

## 14.2 Diagnosis

Ascitic fluid protein content is very high. Ultrasonography, particularly with Doppler, is usually sufficient to confirm a diagnosis. Venography of the inferior vena cava and hepatic veins with pressure measurements is essential. It allows the identification of webs and the degree of compression of the inferior vena cava by the caudate lobe, and the measurement of inferior vena caval pressures above and below the liver. The portal vein should be visualised on superior mesenteric angiography. Percutaneous transhepatic venography may also be used to visualise the hepatic veins. Venographic and pressure studies are cardinal for planning surgery including liver transplantation. A liver biopsy is mandatory as it will show the degree of fibrosis and necrosis and help to estimate how much reversible liver injury exists. A plugged live biopsy is a useful technique in patients with disturbed coagulation and with occluded hepatic veins not amenable to transjugular liver biopsy.

## 14.3 Treatment

For patients presenting with fulminant hepatic failure, immediate liver transplantation is the best treatment available. There is probably too much necrosis for regeneration to occur. The benefit of fibrinolytic therapy in this situation is not well studied owing to the few cases reported.

With less acute presentations, all patients should be anticoagulated to prevent progression of thrombosis. Very few patients have been documented to have spontaneous regression of their disease. The optimal treatment depends on the presence or absence of fibrosis on liver biopsy, the site of the thrombosis, the results of pressure studies in the vena cava above and below the liver, and the interval from onset of symptoms to presentation.

Shunt procedures should be performed in those without hepatic fibrosis; these patients usually present within 3 months of onset of symptoms [37]. The type of shunt, infrahepatic or suprahepatic (Table 1), depends on the pressure gradient in the inferior vena cava across the liver. If there is a high vena caval gradient (>20 mmHg) across the liver or thrombosis in the inferior vena cava then suprahepatic shunts should be performed – usually a meso-atrial shunt. Alternatively portacaval or mesocaval shunts should be fashioned. The hypertrophied caudate lobe usually makes portacaval shunt surgery difficult. Interposition mesocaval shunts are the commonest shunt

**Table 1.** Shunts and surgery for Budd-Chiari syndrome

| *Infrahepatic shunts* | *Suprahepatic shunts* |
|---|---|
| Side-to-side portacaval | Meso-atrial |
| Interposition portacaval | Porto-atrial |
| Mesocaval | Azygo-atrial |
| Mesocaval + spring stent in the inferior vena cava | Meso-innominate |
| | Iliac–mesenteric–atrial |
| *If SVC obstruction – innominate–atrial shunt* | |
| *Transcaval posterocranial resection* | |
| *Splenopneumopexy* | |

SVC, superior vena cava

performed and do not interfere too much with liver transplantation should this become necessary. Other forms of surgery have been tried (Table 1) but these are probably contraindicated as they would make liver transplantation impossible. Patients should be anticoagulated. Fibrosis may still develop and progress following shunt surgery.

If fibrosis is present at the time of diagnosis then patients have usually presented late. In this case liver failure usually supervenes following shunting, so that liver transplantation is the treatment of choice [38]. Anticoagulation must be continued after transplantation.

Webs can be successfully balloon dilated, but the liver disease may progress due to involvement of smaller, more distal venous radicles.

## 15 Hepatic Veno-occlusive Disease

Hepatic veno-occlusive disease is a non-thrombotic obliteration of the small hepatic veins. It was originally described in Jamaican children with a history of ingesting "bush teas" containing toxic pyrrolizidine alkaloids [39] and has been described in association with other herbal preparations [40], heroin [41] and irradiation [42]. Now it is most commonly seen following bone marrow transplantation and is thought to reflect cytotoxic drug-induced injury to the endothelium of the small hepatic venules. Patients typically present with jaundice, tender hepatomegaly and ascites. The prognosis is poor [42]; a few cases have been treated successfully with portasystemic shunting. Azathioprine in renal transplant patients may lead to hepatic veno-occlusive disease and is often associated with nodular regenerative hyperplasia [42].

## 16 Peliosis Hepatis

Peliosis hepatis is characterised by blood-filled cavities bordered by hepatocytes and randomly distributed throughout the lobule. It may be asymptomatic or there may be hepatomegaly, portal hypertension or haemoperitoneum. Liver function tests are only mildly deranged. Androgenic steroids, azathioprine, oral contraceptives, Hodgkin's disease and rheumatoid arthritis have been associated with peliosis hepatis. Pathogenesis is unknown. Diagnosis is made by liver biopsy.

## 17 Systemic Vasculitis

A number of systemic diseases associated with systemic vasculitis may affect the liver. These include the collagen vascular diseases. Those which most commonly affect the liver are mentioned below. It is important to note that the liver abnormalities may not necessarily be due to vasculitis in these patients and other causes such as drug-induced liver disease should always be considered.

### 17.1 Polyarteritis Nodosa and Giant Cell Arteritis

There is a high incidence of hepatitis B virus infection in polyarteritis nodosa [43]. Involvement of the hepatic vessels in polyarteritis nodosa is frequently found at postmortem examination, but hepatic symptoms are rare in life. Polyarteritis nodosa is one of the most common causes of hepatic infarction and may also cause hepatomegaly or jaundice in a minority of cases [44]. Rupture of intra- or extrahepatic arterial aneurysms may occur. Giant cell arteritis may affect the liver and abnormal liver function tests (usually alkaline phosphatase and aminotransferase elevations) are common in this condition [45]. Granulomas may be seen on liver biopsy.

### 17.2 Systemic Lupus Erythematosus

Hepatomegaly and elevated aminotransferase levels are not uncommon in patients with systemic lupus erythematosus (SLE) [46]. Fatty liver is the commonest lesion seen on liver biopsy. Enzyme elevations may be partially due to the drugs used to treat SLE, in particular aspirin. Patients with SLE who also have circulating antiphospholipid antibodies are predisposed to venous thrombosis, and cases of Budd-Chiari syndrome have been described [47].

### 17.3 Rheumatoid Arthritis

Minor abnormalities in liver function tests are frequent in patients with rheumatoid arthritis. In large series of liver biopsies histological abnormalities are common but significant liver disease is rare [48]. Again, many of the changes may be partly due to drug therapy. Nodular regenerative hyperplasia is frequently associated with rheumatoid arthritis.

## 18 Nodular Regenerative Hyperplasia

Nodular regenerative hyperplasia is characterised by the presence of hepatocellular nodules throughout the liver in the absence of fibrosis. The main manifestation is portal hypertension and it is a major cause of non-cirrhotic portal hypertension. A large series has reported a prevalence of 2.6% in autopsy livers but this rises to 5.6% in patients over 80 years of age [49]. The pathogenesis is thought to involve thrombosis or obliteration of small portal vein radicals leading to atrophy of the area of liver they supply, and hypertrophy (nodule formation) of the surrounding liver with intact vascular supply. Obliteration of portal vein radicals leads to the development of portal hypertension with splenomegaly and less commonly ascites. Liver function tests usually show a raised alkaline phosphatase. Jaundice is rare. Bleeding from oesophageal varices varices may be the presenting feature [50]. Nodular regenerative hyperplasia has been described in a number of conditions [49, 51] (Table 2) the most frequent association being with Felty's syndrome, which is the triad of rheumatoid arthritis, splenomegaly and leucopenia. It is being increasingly recognised as a complication following bone marrow transplantation [52] and may be confused with hepatic venoocclusive disease. It has also been recognised in association with Budd-Chiari syndrome [53]. Wanless [49] has described nodular regenerative hyperplasia as the "hepatic analogue of arterial and arteriolar nephrosclerosis".

**Table 2.** Nodular regenerative hyperplasia – associations

| |
|---|
| Rheumatoid arthritis ± Felty's syndrome |
| Polymyalgia rheumatica |
| CREST syndrome |
| Systemic lupus erythematosus |
| Bone marrow transplantation |
| Early primary biliary cirrhosis |
| Mineral oil deposition |
| Mixed cryoglobulinaemia |
| Monoclonal gammopathy |
| Advanced age (>80 years) |
| Massive tumour infiltration |
| Cardiac disease |
| Budd-Chiari syndrome |
| Pulmonary disease with right heart failure |
| Systemic amyloidosis |
| Hereditary haemorrhagic telangiectasia |

## 19 Non-cirrhotic Portal Fibrosis; Idiopathic Portal Hypertension

Non-cirrhotic portal fibrosis is a clinicopathological entity in which portal hypertension and portal fibrosis are present. Liver histology demonstrates obstruction of portal venules. Some drugs which cause perisinusoidal fibrosis have also been implicated in non-cirrhotic portal fibrosis: vitamin A, azathioprine, chronic arsenic ingestion and methotrexate.

Idiopathic portal hypertension is the term used in Japan for a similar clinicopathological entity to non-cirrhotic portal fibrosis (India) and hepatoportal sclerosis (North America). It is also thought to have a vascular aetiology and is similarly characterised by well-preserved liver function, portal hypertension with a large spleen and bleeding varices. Narrowing, obliteration, subintimal thickening, thromboemboli and phlebosclerosis of the portal venous radicles, elastosis and sclerosis of the portal venous radicles and portal tracts, thickening of hepatic veins and atrophy of liver parenchyma have been described by various groups [54]. The changes in the small portal venous radicles have been implicated in the development of portal hypertension. Recently detailed morphology of the hepatic microcirculation has shown that inlet venules of the portal venous tree into the sinusoids, located close to the limiting plate in the portal tracts, were reduced in idiopathic portal hypertension [55].

## References


1. Murray JF, Dawson AM, Sherlock S (1958) Circulatory changes in chronic liver diseases. Am J Med 24:358–367
2. Braillon A, Cales P, Valla D et al. (1986) Influence of the degree of liver failure on systemic splanchnic haemodynamics and on the response to propranolol in patients with cirrhosis. Gut 27:1204–1209
3. Schrier RW, Arroyo V, Bernardi M, Epstein M, Henriksen JH, Rodes J (1988) Reripheral arterial vasodilation hypothesis: a proposal for the initiation of renal sodium and water retention in cirrhosis. Hepatology 8:1151–1157
4. Henriksen JH, Bendtsen F, Sorensen TIA, Stadeager C, Ring-Larsen H (1989) Reduced central blood volume in cirrhosis. Gastroenterology 97:1506–1513
5. Krowka MJ (1990) Hepatopulmonary syndrome: an evolving perspective in the era of liver transplantation. Hepatology 11:138–142
6. Eriksson LS, Soderman C, Ericzon BG, Eleborg L, Wahren J, Hedensteirna G (1990) Normalization of ventilation/perfusion relationships after liver transplantation in patients with decompensated cirrhosis: evidence for a hepatopulmonary syndrome. Hepatology 12:1350–1357
7. McDonnell PJ, Toye PA, Hutchins GM (1983) Primary pulmonary hypertension and cirrhosis: are they related? Am Rev Respir Dis 127:437–441
8. Hadengue A, Benhayoun MK, Lebrec D, Benhamou JP (1991) Pulmonary hypertension complicating portal hypertension: prevalence and relation to splanchnic hemodynamics. Gastroenterology 100:520–528
9. Lunzer M, Newman SP, Bernard AG et al. (1975) Impaired cardiovascular responsiveness in liver disease. Lancet II:382–385
10. Kelbaek H, Erikson J, Brynjolf I et al. (1984) Cardiac performance in patients with asymptomatic alcoholic cirrhosis of the liver. Am J Cardiol 54:852–855

11. Lunseth JH, Olmstead EG, Forks G et al. (1958) A study of heart disease in 180 hospitalized patients dying with portal cirrhosis. Arch Intern Med 102:405–413
12. Guazzi M, Polese A, Magrini F et al. (1975) Negative influences of ascites on the cardiac function of cirrhotic patients. Am J Med 59:165–171
13. Panos MZ, Moore K, Vlavianos P et al. (1990) Single total paracentesis for tense ascites: sequential hemodynamic changes and right atrial size. Hepatology 11:662–667
14. Blendis LM, Greig PD, Langer B et al. (1981) Renal and hemodynamic effects of the periteovenous shunt. Long term effects. Gastroenterology 80:119–125
15. Shah A, Variyam E (1988) Pericardial effusion and left ventricular dysfunction associated with ascites secondary to hepatic cirrhosis. Arch Intern Med 148:585–588
16. Synder N, Atterbury CE, Pinto-Correia J, Conn H (1977) Increased concurrence of cirrhosis and bacterial endocarditis. Gastroenterology 73:1107–1113
17. Yang SS, Kanel G (1989) Fibrinous pericarditis in alcoholic liver disease. J Clin Gastroenterol 11:53–55
18. Grant WC, Wasserman F, Rodernsky PL et al. (1959) The incidence of myocardial infarction in portal cirrhosis. Ann Intern Med 51:774–779
19. Dunn GD, Hayes P, Breen KJ, Schenker S (1973) The liver in congestive heart failure: a review. Am J Med Sci 265:174–189
20. Hoffman BJ, Pate MB, Marsh WH, Lee WM (1990) Cardiomyopathy unrecognized as a cause of hepatic failure. J Clin Gastroenterol 12:306–309
21. Henrion J, Luwaert R, Colin L et al. (1990) Hepatite hypoxique. Etude prospective clinique et hemodynamique de 45 episodes. Gastroenterol Clin Biol 14:836–841
22. Sherlock S (1957) The liver in heart failure: relation of anatomical, functional and circulatory changes. Br Heart J 13:273–293
23. Lefkowich JH, Mendez L (1986) Morphological features of hepatic injury in cardiac disease and shock. J Hepatol 2:313–327
24. Garvin CF (1943) Cardiac cirrhosis. Am J Med Sci 205:515–518
25. White TJ, Leevy CM, Brusca AM, Gnassi AM (1955) The liver in congestive heart failure. Am Heart J 49:250–257
26. Kubo SH, Walter BA, John DHA, Clark M, Cody RJ (1987) Liver function abnormalities in chronic heart failure: influence of systemic hemodynamics. Arch Intern Med 147:1227–1230
27. Das G, Nussbaum HE, Leff WA (1974) Hepatic function in acute myocardial infarction. JAMA 230:1558–1560
28. Ellenberg M, Osserman KE (1951) The role of shock in the production of central liver cell necrosis. Am J Med 11:170–178
29. Hickman PE, Potter JM (1990) Mortality associated with ischaemic hepatitis. Aust NZ J Med 20:32–34
30. Solano FX, Young E, Talamo TS, Dekker A (1986) Constrictive pericarditis mimicking Budd-Chiari syndrome. Am J Med 80:113–115
31. Lautt WW, Greenway CV (1987) Conceptual review of the hepatic vascular bed. Hepatology 7:952–963
32. Klein AS, Cameron JL (1990) Diagnosis and management of the Budd-Chiari syndrome. Am J Surg 160:128–133
33. Valla D, Casadevall N, Lacombe C et al. (1985) Primary myeloproliferative disorder and hepatic vein thrombosis. A prospective study of erythroid colony formation in vitro in 20 patients with Budd-Chiari syndrome. Ann Intern Med 103:329–334
34. Asherson RA, Thompson RPH, McLachlan N et al. (1989) Visceral arterial occlusions, Budd-Chiari syndrome, recurrent fetal loss and the "lupus anticoagulant" in systemic lupus erythematosus. J Rheumatol 16:219–224
35. Simson IW (1982) Membranous obstruction of the inferior vena cava and hepatocellular carcinoma in South Africa. Gastroenterology 82:171–178

36. Vickers CR, West RJ, Hubscher SG, Elias E (1989) Hepatic vein webs and resistant ascites. J Hepatol 8:287–293
37. Orloff MJ, Girard B (1989) Long term results of treatment of Budd Chiari syndrome by side to side portocaval shunt. Surg Gynecol Obstet 168:33–41
38. Campbell DA, Rolles K, Jamieson N et al. (1988) Hepatic transplantation with perioperative and long term anticoagulation as treatment for Budd-Chiari syndrome. Surg Gynecol Obstet 166:511–518
39. Bras G, Jelliffe Stuart KL (1954) Veno-occlusive disease of the liver with non-portal type of cirrhosis, occurring in Jamaica. Arch Pathol 57:285–300
40. Valla D, Benhamou J-P (1988) Drug induced vascular and sinusoidal lesions of the liver. Bailliere's Clin Gastroenterol 2:481–500
41. Trigueiro de Araujo MS, Gerard F, Chossegros P et al. (1990) Vascular hepatotoxicity related to heroin addiction. Virchows Arch [A] 417:497–503
42. Wolford JL, McDonald GB (1988) A problem-oriented aproach to intestinal and liver disease after marrow transplantation. J Clin Gastroenterol 10:419–433
43. Gocke DJ, Hsu K, Morgan C et al. (1970) Association between polyarteritis and Australia antigen. Lancet II:1149–1153
44. Mowrey FH, Lundberg EA (1954) The clinical manifestations of essential polyangitis (periarteritis nodosa) with emphasis on the hepatic manifestations. Ann Intern Med 40:1145–1164
45. Dickson ER, Maldonado JE, Sheps SG (1973) Systemic giant-cell arteritis with polymyalgia rheumatica (Reversible abnormalities of liver function). JAMA 224: 1496–1498
46. Runyon BA, La Brecque DR, Anuras S (1980) The spectrum of liver disease in systemic lupus erythematosus. Am J Med 69:187–194
47. Terabayashi H, Okuda K, Nomura F, Ohnishi K, Wong P (1986) Transformation of inferior vena caval thrombosis to membranous obstruction in a patient with the lupus anticoagulant. Gastroenterology 91:219–224
48. Rau R, Pfenninger K, Boni A (1975) Liver function tests and liver biopsies in patients with rheumatoid arthritis (abstr). Ann Rheum Dis 34:198–199
49. Wanless IR (1990) Micronodular transformation (nodular regenerative hyperplasia) of the liver: a report of 64 cases among 2500 autopsies and a new classification of benign hepatocellular nodules. Hepatology 11:787–797
50. Naber AHJ, Haelstvan U, Yap SH (1991) Nodular regenerative hyperplasia of the liver: an important cause of portal hypertension in the non-cirrhotic patients. J Hepatol 12:94–99
51. Nakanuma Y (1990) Nodular regenerative hyperplasia of the liver: retrospective survey in autopsy series. J Clin Gastroenterol 12:460–465
52. Snover DC, Weisdorf S, Bloomer J, McGlvar P, Weisdorf D (1989) Nodular regenerative hyperplasia of the liver following bone marrow transplantation. Hepatology 9:443–448
53. De Sousa JMM, Portmann B, Williams R (1991) Nodular regenerative hyperplasia of the liver and the Budd-Chiari syndrome. J Hepatol 12:28–35
54. Okuda K, Nakashima T, Okudaira M et al. (1982) Liver pathology of idiopathic portal hypertension. Comparison with non-cirrhotic portal fibrosis of India. Liver 2:176–192
55. Terada T, Hoso M, Nakanuma Y (1989) Microvasculature in the small portal tracts in idiopathic portal hypertension. A morphological companion with other hepatic diseases. Virchows Archiv [A] 415:61–67

# 31 Acute Hepatic Failure

S.W. SCHALM, R.J. DE KNEGT, H.J. METSELAAR,
and B. VAN DEN BERG

Acute hepatic failure is generally defined as the development of hepatic encephalopathy in an individual with no evidence of previous liver disease. The majority of cases are due to virus- or drug-induced hepatic necrosis. The clinical features are characterized by progressive mental impairment, often rapidly advancing to coma and death by decerebration, cardiovascular or respiratory failure, and the occurrence of other liver failure-associated syndromes, such as renal failure, gastrointestinal bleeding, and sepsis. Despite progress in intensive care regimens the mortality of patients with coma is still about 80%. The introduction of various artificial liver support systems has not improved survival. However, the survival rate for patients with acute liver failure undergoing liver transplantation is now more than 50%. Therefore, the availability of liver transplantation has altered the approach to patients presenting with acute liver failure and a new issue in the current management of acute liver failure is the decision "to transplant or not to transplant."

## 1 Nomenclature

Many terms have been used to describe the syndrome of acute hepatic failure or a subvariety thereof (Table 1). The boundaries of the syndrome of acute hepatic failure are unclear with regard to both the definition of *acute* and the definition of *hepatic failure*. With regard to the time span between the onset of jaundice in a previously asymptomatic person and the appearance of encephalopathy, the term *acute* is appropriate for the period of 0–8 weeks. The term *fulminant*, originally proposed by TREY and DAVIDSON [1], should be restricted to those with very rapid onset (time span between jaundice-encephalopathy less than 2 weeks). Recently the entity of "late-onset hepatic failure" has been described, with etiologic, histologic, and prognostic features similar to those of acute hepatic failure [2]. In "late-onset" hepatic failure the duration of illness prior to encephalopathy is more prolonged, but as in patients with acute hepatic failure, there is no evidence of previous liver disease. The term "late onset" does not delineate clearly from chronic liver disease; since in hepatology chronic disease starts at 6

**Table 1.** Terms used to describe the syndrome of acute hepatic failure or a subvariety thereof

| | |
|---|---|
| Acute liver failure | Subacute atrophy of the liver |
| Acute hepatic failure | Subchronic atrophy of the liver |
| Severe acute hepatic failure | Subacute hepatitis |
| Fulminant hepatic failure | Subacute hepatic necrosis |
| Severe fulminant hepatic failure | Subacute fulminant hepatic failure |
| Subfulminant hepatic failure | Late-onset hepatic failure |

months (=26 weeks), the term subacute is to be preferred for the period of 9–26 weeks [3].

With regard to the appearance of encephalopathy in a person with severe liver dysfunction (coagulation factors less than 50%), the term *hepatic failure* or *liver failure* is appropriate. Terminology based on pathology, i.e., atrophy, hepatitis, or hepatic necrosis, should not be used for a clinical syndrome. The term *hepatic failure* should only be used if the encephalopathy is in all likelihood due to the liver dysfunction, and other causes (sedative use, nonhepatic metabolic abnormalities like hypoxia, and focal neurologic disease) have been excluded [4].

The current terminology of acute hepatic failure and its subvarieties is given in Table 2.

## 2 Etiology

The most common cause of acute hepatic failure is viral hepatitis. Hepatitis B virus is the major etiologic agent [5–7], since about 1% of cases of acute viral hepatitis B progress to a fulminant course. Hepatitis D virus, concurrent with acute hepatitis B-positive disease, has an even higher incidence of acute hepatic failure [8], but is less prevalent. Hepatitis A virus is uncommonly associated with acute hepatic failure [5–7], but the high prevalence of hepatitis A infection accounts for the fact that acute hepatic failure due to hepatitis A is not exceptional. Hepatitis E virus carries a high risk of acute liver failure in pregnant women [9]. Hepatitis C virus is an unlikely cause, since among 500 patients with posttransfusion hepatits C no case of acute hepatic failure was observed [5].

Herpes simplex virus [10] and varicella-zoster virus [11] occasionally produce massive liver cell necrosis. No convincingly documented cases of acute hepatic failure due to other hepatotropic viruses such as cytomegalovirus and Epstein-Barr virus have been reported [5].

Drug toxicity accounts for the other important etiologic group; it is of either the predictable or the idiosyncratic type. The number of drugs capable of producing liver cell necrosis is very large [12]. In some countries (e.g., the United Kingdom), paracetamol overdose is implicated in 50% of cases of acute hepatic failure [13]; in other countries the responsible drugs

**Table 2.** New terminology for acute hepatic failure and subvarieties thereof

| Name | Interval between onset of jaundice and appearance of encephalopathy |
|---|---|
| Acute hepatic failure | 0–8 weeks |
| Fulminant hepatic failure | 0–2 weeks |
| Subacute hepatic failure | 9–26 weeks |

are isoniazid [14], antidepressants [15], nonsteroidal anti-inflammatory drugs (NSAIDs) [16], and halothane [17]. The combination of isoniazid or antidepressants with enzyme inducers (rifampicin) enhances the hepatotoxicity. The hepatotoxicity of NSAIDs is low; however, the number of patients taking these drugs is very high and therefore acute hepatic failure due to such drugs is not uncommon. Repeated administration of halothane within several months increases the risk of acute hepatic failure.

*Amanita* mushroom poisoning is a rare cause of severe hepatitis in continental Europe; carbon tetrachloride is highly toxic to the liver, but no longer a common cause of acute liver failure since its industrial use has been prohibited.

Ischemic liver cell necrosis can be the consequence of an acute diminution in cardiac output and may in some cases result in acute hepatic failure [18]; vascular obstruction of the hepatic veins (Budd-Chiari syndrome) is a very uncommon cause [19]. Acute hepatic failure may develop after liver transplantation; the main causes are inadequate preservation of the donor liver, acute graft rejection, and liver ischemia due to hepatic artery thrombosis with or without portal vein or hepatic vein thrombosis. Hyperthermia due to heatstroke or phencyclidine intoxication can also result in massive ischemic liver cell necrosis.

Acute hepatic failure without typical extensive liver cell necrosis occurs occasionally by way of massive infiltration of malignant cells [20, 21] (histocytosis, leukemia, lymphoma, metastatic breast carcinoma) or microvesicular steatosis. The main causes of microvesicular steatosis are acute fatty liver of pregnancy [22], Reye's syndrome [23], and valproic acid toxicity [24].

The syndrome of acute hepatic failure may occur in those with previously asymptomatic chronic liver disease. Acute hepatic failure can be the first manifestation of Wilson's disease [25] and is then commonly associated with intravascular hemolysis. Chronic hepatitis B carriers can develop acute hepatic failure due to superinfection with hepatitis D virus [26] or due to hepatitis B virus reactivation, sometimes preceded by antineoplastic or immunosuppressive therapy [27].

Twenty to forty percent of cases of acute hepatic failure have been attributed to non-A, non-B hepatitis. With the discovery of the two hepatitis viruses C and E, doubts about the viral origin is emerging. Autoimmune chronic active hepatitis can mimic acute hepatitis and some patients, particularly those with the subacute form, may have immunologically mediated massive liver cell necrosis [28]; such patients have high serum levels of γ-globulin or immune complexes (C1q binding).

## 3 Clinical Features

The characteristics of the syndrome of acute hepatic failure can be described under three headings: hepatic encephalopathy, the liver in acute hepatic failure, and extrahepatic complications other than encephalopathy.

### 3.1 Hepatic Encephalopathy

Hepatic encephalopathy is a neuropsychiatric picture of stimulation of the reticular system of the brain, followed by alteration of consciousness and terminal depression of brain stem function. Clinically, the syndrome consists of personality changes, impairment of mental function, motor abnormalities, depression of consciousness, and neuro-ophthalmologic changes [29]. Early signs are changes in personality, antisocial behavior, inability to maintain sphincter control, slowness of mentation, disordered sleep rhythm, slurred speech, and flapping tremor [1]. In later stages the patient is disoriented in time, place, and person, his speech is incoherent, and he sleeps most of the time; thereafter coma sets in. With progression of the depth of coma, the picture is that of decerebrate rigidity with extension and hyperpronation of the arms, extension of the legs, and plantar flexor responses. Convulsions may occur. In most cases hyperventilation is marked. Dysconjugate eye movements are common; pupillary reflexes persist until very late. Elevated intracranial pressure often develops due to cerebral edema and is best monitored by unilateral or bilateral changes in pupillary responses. As intracranial pressure continues to increase, trismus and opisthotonos occur, followed by respiratory arrest and terminal depression of brain stem coning [30]. Respiratory arrest and circulatory failure with hypotension and arrhythmias are also manifestations of severely depressed brain stem function without cerebral edema.

The stage of hepatic encephalopathy is usually graded according to the level of consciousness. A simplified classification is given in Table 3. Terminology in the past has been confusing, but there is now general agreement that hepatic encephalopathy grade 4 is coma. The depth of coma can best be assessed by one of the available coma scales [31, 32]. The outline of the assessment is shown in Table 4.

Hepatic encephalopathy is reflected in biochemical changes in the cerebrospinal fluid (CSF). CSF glutamine is characteristically elevated in hepatic encephalopathy and a reasonable correlation between the grade

**Table 3.** Stages of hepatic encephalopathy

| Grade | Clinical features |
|---|---|
| 1 | Slowing of mentation |
| 2 | Confusion, euphoria, inappropriate behavior, or drowsiness |
| 3 | Permanent somnolence |
| 4 | Coma |

**Table 4.** A clinical coma profile for bedside use

| |
|---|
| Reaction to acoustic stimuli |
| Reaction to pain |
| Pupil size |
| Pupil response to light |
| Position of bulbi |
| Oculovestibular responses |

of encephalopathy and CSF glutamine levels has been described [33]. In addition, elevations of catecholamines (dopamine, norepinephrine, epinephrine), other amines and derivatives (serotonin, tyramine, histamine), and amino acids (methionine, phenylalanine, tyrosine, tryptophan) have been described [34, 35]. Repeated sampling of CSF is difficult in patients with acute hepatic failure because of the bleeding tendency, and biochemical monitoring of CSF has not been used to monitor hepatic encephalopathy.

The electroencephalogram is often used to assess the clinical state objectively. In the normal individual the EEG predominantly depicts an alpha rhythm. With progression of the encephalopathy, the frequency of the rhythm decreases (theta rhythm, then delta rhythm) and the amplitude increases. When coma sets in, triphasic waves are often noticed. With the progression of coma the frequency shows little change but the amplitude decreases again [36]. Spectral analysis of the EEG [37] makes tracings more accessible for clinicians and adds to the objectivity of the measurements.

In general the EEG correlates well with the clinical state, although in early stages it may be more severely abnormal than the clinical picture suggests and later may continue to be abnormal for some time in recovering patients despite the patient's level of consciousness being normal.

### 3.2 The Liver in Acute Hepatic Failure

The patient is characteristically in a good nutritional state and lacks signs of chronic liver disease such as spider nevi or splenomegaly. Jaundice is usually present, but neuropsychiatric changes may develop before jaundice. Ascites is absent in acute hepatic failure, but may occur in the subacute form. Serum bilirubin is elevated and is mainly conjugated in type. The serum aminotransferases are almost always markedly elevated early in the syndrome; levels tend to fall as the patient's condition worsens. Serum albumin is usually normal initially. Serum α-fetoprotein is often elevated as a consequence of hepatocyte regeneration [38, 39]. Coagulation factors are depressed and reflect residual hepatic function [40, 41]. Plasma ammonia, when measured by an enzymatic method, is elevated; serum urea is low but increases later with progressive renal failure.

Clearance of both galactose and antipyrine is subnormal [42, 43]. Endotoxinemia is often detected as a possible consequence of reduced reticuloendothelial function [44].

The liver is usually small. Computed tomography shows a reduced liver volume. At laparoscopy the liver exhibits in the majority of cases focal areas of collapse, whereas other areas still have preserved liver tissue. In a minority of cases the necrosis is diffuse, affecting both lobes equally [45]. Microscopic examination of the liver in acute and subacute hepatic failure shows either extensive hepatocyte necrosis with or without inflammatory reaction or, rarely, microvesicular steatosis or infiltration with malignant cells.

The pathologic variant together with the etiology of the liver disease is of importance for estimating the potential for regeneration of the diseased liver (Table 5).

The etiology of the liver disease is assessed by searching for virologic markers and a history of drug or toxin ingestion complemented by screening for uncommon diseases. Acute hepatitis A should be diagnosed by serum IgM-anti HAV. Hepatitis B surface antigen (HBsAg) as well as IgM-anti HBc should be measured as in 20% of cases of hepatitis B HBsAg has already been cleared [3]. In those positive for hepatitis B, anti HDV should be measured. Fulminant Wilson's disease can be diagnosed indirectly by a low level of alkaline phosphatase in relation to a high bilirubin and a high level of aspartate aminotransferase in comparison to low levels of alanine aminotransferase [46]; a high urinary copper excretion is direct proof of the disease. Autoimmune hepatitis is characterized by a high serum IgG or C1q binding assay. If there are appropriate indications, blood or urine is checked for drug or toxin levels.

**Table 5.** Pathobiologic variants in acute hepatic failure

| Variant | Regeneration |
|---|---|
| Total hepatic necrosis | Impossible |
| Partial hepatic necrosis | Possible |
| Cause of liver disease persistent | Unlikely |
| Cause of liver disease eliminated | Likely |

### 3.3 Extrahepatic Complications Other than Encephalopathy

Common complications in acute hepatic failure are hypoglycemia, electrolyte and acid-base disturbances, renal failure, gastrointestinal hemorrhage, infection, pancreatitis, and respiratory and circulatory failure. The complications are discussed in more detail in relation to the management of acute hepatic failure.

## 4 Prognosis

Prognosis is related to the residual functioning liver cell mass, the persistence of the cause of the liver disease, the extent of liver regeneration, and the occurrence of complications. Prognosis of acute hepatic failure has traditionally been estimated by the stage of hepatic encephalopathy, since the survival rate was 66% in patients with encephalopathy grade 2 or less, 42% in those with grade 3, and 18% in those with grade 4 (95% confidence limits 12%–21%) [1]. Current experience [47, 48] indicates that the grade of encephalopathy alone is a too imprecise indicator of survival; the difference in death rate between encephalopathy grade 3 and grade 4 has decreased to 16%, probably due to improved management of cerebral edema.

A further means of estimating residual liver function might be provided by the level of coagulation factors. Factors V and VII are in theory the tests of choice, because their plasma half-lives are short (24 and 4 h respectively). Factor V levels less than 15%–20% indicate the likelihood of survival to be less than 10% [47], while the prothrombin time (measuring factors II, V, VII, and X) was of prognostic value in another large series [48]. Coagulation factor assays are poorly standardized at present, but the use of well-defined international reference reagents and units may eliminate current discrepancies [49].

Prognosis is considerably better for patients without persistence of the cause of the liver disease, such as paracetamol intoxication, hepatitis A, and hepatitis B, than for idiosyncratic drug reactions (halothane) or cryptogenic acute hepatic failure (previously called non-A, non-B hepatitis) [50]. Virus replication in fulminant hepatitis A or B is usually terminated by massive liver necrosis; prognosis of fulminant hepatitis B with persistent virus replication is poor [3].

The extent of liver regeneration can be monitored by measuring the levels of $\alpha_1$-fetoprotein [38, 39]; in one study [51] survival was 64% in patients with >60 μg/ml and 0% below this limit. Patients older than 30–45 years are thought to have diminished hepatic regeneration and survival is poor [52].

The occurrence of extrahepatic complications or the coexistence of other disease has an important effect on prognosis, with survival of 11% in patients with complications versus 36% in those without complications [52].

Several factors therefore provide prognostic information in acute hepatic failure. Improved prognostic evaluation is to be expected when a combination of independent factors is used.

## 5 Medical Treatment

### 5.1 General

Patients with acute liver failure should be admitted to a unit experienced in 24-h monitoring of vital functions: grade of encephalopathy, temperature, blood pressure, heart rate, respiratory rate, urinary output, and fluid balance. A large-bore catheter is introduced via the arm and positioned in the superior caval vein. Comatose patients should also receive a nasogastric tube and a urinary catheter. Equipment for endotracheal intubation should be present at the bedside. All attending personnel in contact with the patient must be aware of the nature of the disease and consequently the importance of personal hygiene; they should have been vaccinated against hepatitis B.

### 5.2 Hepatic Encephalopathy and Cerebral Edema

The grade of hepatic encephalopathy must be assessed every 6–12 h. In patients with grade 4 encephalopathy (coma), a coma scale should be scored in addition every 2–4 h. Daily objective measurement of encephalopathy by means of spectral analysis of the EEG [37] is advocated.

Since nitrogenous substances arising from the gastrointestinal tract are considered of importance in the pathogenesis of hepatic encephalopathy, bowel cleansing is advised to diminish the production of gastrointestinal toxins. One or two lactulose enemas (300 ml lactulose 50% and 1000 ml water) are given for complete bowel evacuation; maintenance therapy consists of oral lactulose 15–30 ml 6-hourly. In the presence of gaseous distention, magnesium sulfate 15 g can be given.

Flumazenil, a benzodiazepine receptor blocker, may diminish the grade of encephalopathy [53]; the effect is marked in patients having used benzodiazepines, but not detectable in those with "pure" hepatic encephalopathy [4].

Cerebral edema is a major complication, occurring in about 50% of patients. Control of blood pressure (mean: 80–100 mmHg) and partial carbon dioxide pressure (3.3–4.6 kPa) may prevent rises in intracranial pressure and thereby aggravation of cerebral edema. Clinical signs of cerebral edema include increased muscle tone in the arms and legs, which gradually progresses to full decerebrate posturing with hyperpronation and adduction of the arms. Hyperventilation is marked; the pupils are

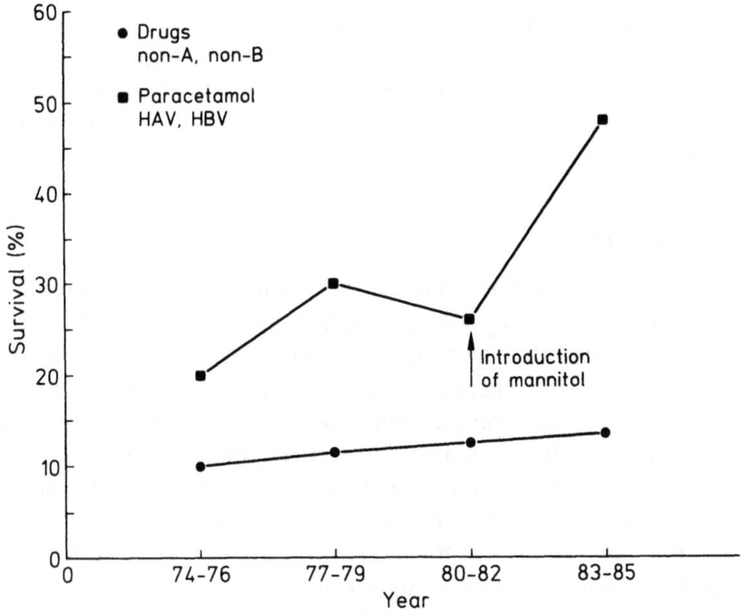


**Fig. 1.** Survival rates for patients with acute hepatic failure before and after the introduction of mannitol for the management of cerebral edema [reproduced with permission from WILLIAMS R (1986) Semin Liver Dis 6: Foreword]

dilated and react unequally or sluggishly to light [30]. Continuous monitoring of intracranial pressure by means of a subarachnoid screw should be considered [54].

Bolus infusions of mannitol (0.5 g/kg body weight) can normalize intracranial pressure [55]. Repeated infusions of mannitol may increase serum osmolarity, especially in patients with impaired renal function; monitoring of serum osmolarity in patients receiving mannitol infusions is therefore mandatory. The survival rates for patients with acute hepatic failure before and after the introduction of mannitol for the management of cerebral edema are shown in Fig. 1. Corticosteroids are of no value in the management of cerebral edema of acute hepatic failure [55].

Sedatives should be avoided in patients with acute liver failure as they aggravate the encephalopathy. However, the management of some patients can be virtually impossible without sedation; in such cases lorazepam or oxazepam is the drug of choice.

## 5.3 Liver Therapy

### *Elimination of the Cause*

Etiologic therapy in acute hepatic failure has yielded few positive results. Anti HBs immunoglobulin in fulminant hepatitis B is of no benefit [56], and corticosteroids may even be of negative value [57]. Recently, efficacy of acyclovir in herpetic fulminant hepatitis and of high dose *d*-penicillamine in wilsonian fulminant hepatic failure [58] has been reported. Elimination of the cause of the liver disease might therefore be beneficial if achieved quickly.

#### *Liver Support*

Artificial liver support systems for acute hepatic failure are directed to restoration of the physiologic "milieu intérieur" and the removal of putative toxins, thereby normalizing cerebral function as well as allowing the diseased liver to regenerate. Hemodialysis, exchange transfusion, cross-circulation, extracorporeal liver perfusion, hemofiltration, and charcoal hemoperfusion have all been tested for their enhancement of survival in acute hepatic failure. Since single cases with a favorable outcome are more likely to be published, only reports describing more than two patients were used for meta-analysis. Of the artificial liver support systems, only charcoal hemoperfusion showed a significant improvement in survival (Fig. 2). Patients with charcoal hemoperfusion also received treatment for cerebral edema, which in itself may affect survival [55]. When charcoal hemoperfusion was subjected to controlled evaluation, no clinical benefit could be demonstrated [50].

The daily blood flow through artificial liver support systems (about 50–100 liters) is usually less than 5% of the normal daily liver blood flow (2160 liters) and the clearance capacity is less than that of the normal liver. In view of the limitations on the capacity of thse systems and the results reported for acute hepatic failure, artificial liver support systems are rarely if ever indicated. The prevention and treatment of cerebral edema, hypoglycemia, metabolic disturbances, hemorrhage, infection, renal failure, and respiratory and circulatory failure, together with standard high care measures, should form the basic therapeutic approach.

### 5.4 Prevention and Treatment of Complications

#### *Nutrition and Metabolic Disturbances*

The nutritional status is normal in most patients with acute liver failure. To provide a basic amount of calories, at least 200 g of carbohydrates (800 kcal) should be administered per 24 h, preferably by continuous parenteral administration of 20% glucose (1 liter/24 h). Blood glucose levels should be measured every 2–4 h, as hypoglycemia may occur spontaneously [59] or as a result of sudden discontinuation of intravenous glucose infusion (plasma insulin levels are high). For additional nutrition, the enteral route can be used; in the case of gastric retention total parenteral nutrition should be

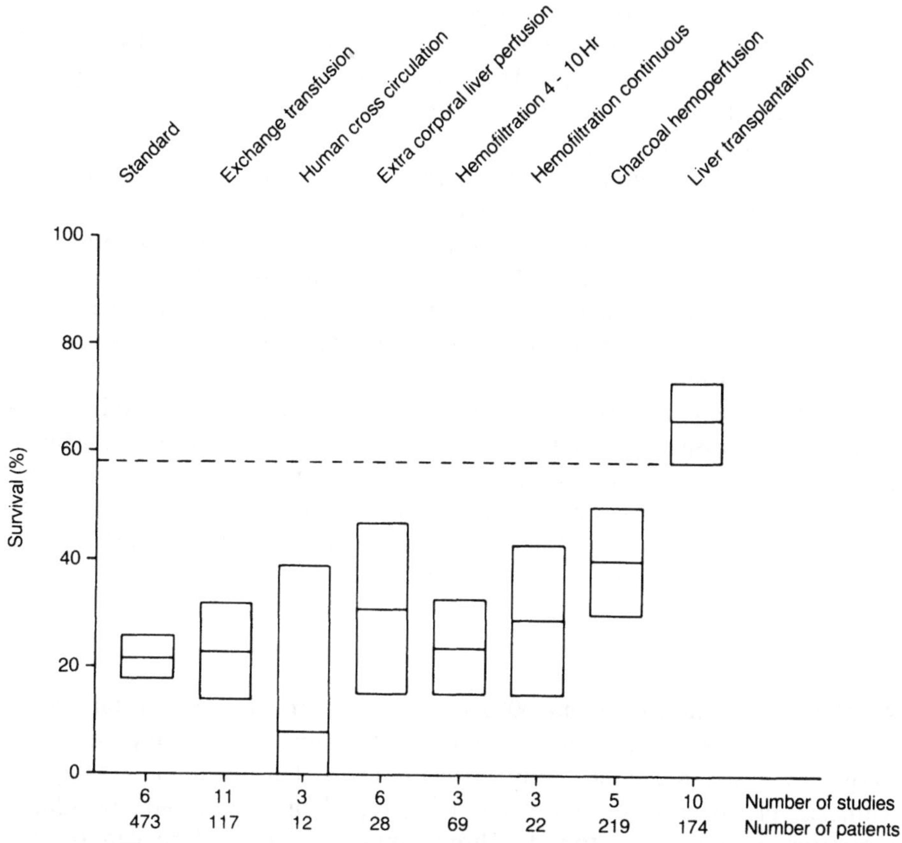


**Fig. 2.** Survival rate for patients with acute hepatic failure on artificial liver support systems and undergoing liver transplantation. Data based on literature review (up to 1 January 1990) of reports describing three or more patients [reproduced with permission from DE KNEGT RJ, SCHALM SW (1991) Neth J Med 38:131–141]

given. The use of special amino acid mixtures with enrichment of branched chain amino acids [60] or the keto analogues of essential amino acids [61] appears attractive, but clinical benefit has not been proven. After 1–3 days 40–60 g of protein is given to prevent progressive depletion of body proteins. Human albumin can be administered intravenously when hypoalbuminemia (<34 g/liter) is present together with signs of fluid retention; the benefits of such infusions are doubtful in the presence of capillary hyperpermeability.

Major disturbances in electrolytes and acid-base homeostasis are frequently observed. Plasma sodium levels tend to be low, due to impaired renal free water excretion [62]. Correction should be by fluid restriction, and not by administration of hypertonic sodium chloride (unless there is clear evidence of sodium loss from the body). In the terminal stage hyponatremia can result from impaired active transport of sodium across cell membranes.

Hypokalemia may result from poor intake, vomiting, urinary loss, and parenteral glucose administration. Body stores may be depleted by as much as 500 mmol [63]. Metabolic alkalosis follows potassium deficiency and enhances the alkalosis associated with hyperventilation; toxicity of ammonia may then be increased [64]. Potassium chloride supplements must be given, sometimes both parenterally and enterally. If urinary output is normal, more than 100 mmol daily is often needed.

Serum zinc and magnesium, often low in chronic liver failure, are usually normal in acute hepatic failure. Serum calcium tends to be low and may reflect pancreatitis and hypoalbuminemia; additional calcium may be needed. Hypophosphatemia can be prevented by addition of phosphate to the glucose infusion.

Metabolic acidosis due to hyperlactatemia is probably caused by anaerobic metabolism in patients with very low systemic vascular resistance and low tissue oxygen extraction [65]. Sodium bicarbonate infusion must be given with caution, to avoid metabolic alkalosis and possibly aggravation of encephalopathy. In some instances only hemodialysis will effectively rectify hyperkalemia, hyponatremia, or metabolic acidosis.

### *Renal Failure*

Renal failure occurs in about 50% of the cases and in most instances no histopathologic substrate can be found [66]. Renal failure may be precipitated by gastrointestinal hemorrhage or sepsis. Due to impaired hepatic synthesis, blood urea levels are low initially; when renal failure develops, a progressive uremia is found. Three types of renal failure can be encountered: (a) prerenal azotemia due to dehydration, (b) acute tubular necrosis, and (c) functional renal failure. In prerenal uremia a low urinary sodium concentration is found; prerenal uremia responds well to expansion of plasma volume. In acute tubular necrosis there is oliguria together with a high urinary sodium concentration. Functional renal failure is found most frequently, characterized by a low urinary sodium concentration, no proteinuria, and a failure to respond to volume expansion. The cause of this functional renal failure is unknown. The intense renal vasoconstriction is the result of local hormonal factors within the kidney or of an extrarenal circulating vasoconstrictor substance. Candidate factors include endotoxin, norepinephrine, angiotensin II, prostaglandin $E_2$, and thromboxane $A_2$ [67].

Fluid intake should be matched to fluid output. When renal failure progresses, hemodialysis or high volume continuous hemofiltration must be actively pursued.

### *Hemorrhage*

Severe bleeding occurs in 20%–40% of the patients and is lethal in most instances [68]. The most common site of bleeding is gastrointestinal, mainly from gastric mucosal erosions. The other principal sites of bleeding include nasopharynx, lungs, and skin puncture sites. In addition to low levels of clotting factors, thrombocytopenia (<70000 × $10^9$/liter) is often present in patients having major episodes of bleeding.

Preventive measures include avoidance of active aspiration of the stomach and the use of an $H_2$ receptor blocker [69]. The prophylactic administration of fresh frozen plasma in patients without bleeding was not found to reduce morbidity or mortality [70]; the administration of clotting factor concentrate can be disastrous owing to induction of intravascular coagulation [71]. Invasive procedures are an indication for administration of fresh frozen plasma and platelet transfusion in cases of thrombocytopenia.

Management of upper gastrointestinal bleeding includes endoscopy for location of the bleeding site together with local therapy when possible. Blood losses should be replaced either by transfusion of fresh blood or by a combination of packed erythrocytes, fresh frozen plasma, and platelet concentrate. Tranexamic acid 1 g twice daily may be given in cases of fibrinolysis.

### *Infections*

Infections are common in acute liver failure, and they contribute significantly to death: bacteremia has been reported in 12%–36% of the patients and is thought to have contributed to death in one-third of these cases [72]. Bacteremia is often clinically latent or manifested by deterioration of encephalopathy or renal function. Fungal infections such as candidiasis and aspergillosis are increasingly being recognized.

Selective intestinal decontamination to prevent infections arising from the gastrointestinal tract can be achieved with the administration of poorly absorbable antibiotics against aerobic Gram-negative rods and fungi [73]. This selective decontamination does not interfere with the anaerobic bacterial gut flora or the metabolism of lactulose. Further prevention of infections, mainly bacteremia, pneumonia, and urinary tract infections, can only come from meticulous nursing care. Basic monitoring consists in repetitive cultures of blood, urine, sputum, and all insertion sites of various catheters, in addition to daily physical examination, leukocyte count, urine sediment analysis, and chest x-ray. When bacterial infection is strongly suspected, broad-spectrum antibiotics should be given intravenously. In patients with acute liver failure, complement synthesis, opsonization capacity, and neutrophil adherence [74] are diminished. Plasma therapy may improve opsonization, but no clinical benefit has been demonstrated.

### *Circulatory Disturbances*

In acute liver failure a hyperdynamic circulation is present. There is an inappropriate systemic vasodilatation with compensatory increase in cardiac output; blood pressure is usually low and heart rate high.

The pathogenesis is undefined. Prostacyclin, bradykinin, substance P, and atrial natriuretic peptide have all been implicated, but clear evidence of their involvement is lacking. Recently, increased synthesis of nitric oxide, a potent vasodilator, has been suggested with endotoxin and cytokines as persistent inducers of nitric oxide synthetase in vessel walls [75].

The development of edema is usually associated with a reduction in colloid osmotic pressure due to decreasing plasma albumin levels. However, capillary hyperpermeability may also be of importance. Volume expansion with crystalloids seldom has any effect on blood pressure; response to catecholamines such as norepinephrine is about normal [76]. Overt circulatory failure (severe hypotension with or without bradycardia) can also develop from the depressed brain function itself in the later stages of grade 4 encephalopathy; prognosis is then very poor.

### *Respiratory Disturbances*

Hyperventilation is a common feature and leads to respiratory alkalosis. The hyperventilation results from stimulation of the medullary vital centers. In advanced coma, depression of brain stem function leads to hypoventilation and ultimately respiratory arrest. The hyperdynamic circulation may be associated with increased pulmonary shunting and cause hypoxemia [77]. Hypoxemia can also result from pneumonia due to aspiration of saliva and gastric contents or to bleeding. In the event of infection, chest x-rays reveal interstitial and alveolar patterns, but these patterns are also found in cases of pulmonary edema associated with overhydration or the adult respiratory distress syndrome (ARDS). Insertion of a Swan-Ganz catheter may be helpful to differentiate.

At the first sign of an impaired "gag" reflex in comatose patients, endotracheal intubation should be performed for prevention of aspiration. Endotracheal intubation facilitates endobronchial suctioning. Modern ventilators enable the patients to breathe spontaneously through the ventilation circuit. Positive end-expiratory pressure should be used in the case of ARDS, but with caution as positive end-expiratory pressure may increase intracranial pressure [77].

### *Pancreatitis*

Pancreatitis is frequent in patients dying with acute liver failure [78]. At autopsy acute hemorrhagic and necrotic pancreatitis is observed, whereas symptoms during life can be minimal. The exact cause of pancreatitis remains unknown; it is regarded – like the respiratory distress syndrome and stress ulceration of the gastrointestinal tract – as part of a multiple organ failure syndrome. Monitoring of serum and urinary amylase levels should performed, but neither prevention nor therapy is currently possible.

## 6 Liver Transplantation for Acute Hepatic Failure

Despite the improvements in intensive care medicine, the prognosis for many patients with acute liver failure remains poor. Recently orthotopic liver transplantation has improved survival. By January 1990, 174 cases of liver transplantation for acute liver failure had been published by ten transplantation centers presenting three or more patients [references cited in 79]. Survival for these patients was 66% (95% confidence interval, 58%–73%), which can be considered a clinically significant improvement over conservative treatment (Fig. 2). Neither the etiology nor the age of the transplanted patient appeared to have any influence on the outcome.

A major cause of death related to liver transplantation for acute liver failure is decerebration, either during or in the first 6h following transplantation. Some patients develop a chronic neuropsychiatric disorder after liver transplantation. These sequelae are the consequence of severe metabolic encephalopathy and/or cerebral edema.

Recurrence of the disease in the transplanted liver is not very common. It is interesting to note that patients with acute liver failure from hepatitis B infection who undergo liver transplantation can recover without recurrent disease. Most centers give anti HBs immunoglobin prophylaxis before, during, and after transplantation [80].

Before a decision to perform liver transplantation is made, contraindications should be considered. Irreversible neurologic damage, as reflected by unreactive pupils, absent brain stem reflexes, or absent cerebral electric activity on electroencephalography, is an absolute contraindication to liver transplantation. Moreover, uncontrollable extrahepatic sepsis, extrahepatic malignancy, and other severe diseases that markedly affect life expectancy are other absolute contraindications.

Clinical staging of acute hepatic failure should then follow, based on the degree of encephalopathy and the residual functioning liver cell mass as indicated by factor V levels (Table 6). Patients with stage 1 should receive medical therapy, while patients with stage 4 should undergo liver transplantation; for patients with stage 2 or 3 there is a need for further clinical decision making.

For the decision to transplant in acute hepatic failure stage 2 or 3, the pathobiology should be considered (Table 5), since the pathologic variant,

**Table 6.** Stages of acute hepatic failure

| Stage | Coma | Factor V/prothrombin |
|---|---|---|
| 1 | Absent | >15% |
| 2 | Absent | <15% |
| 3 | Present | >15% |
| 4 | Present | <15% |

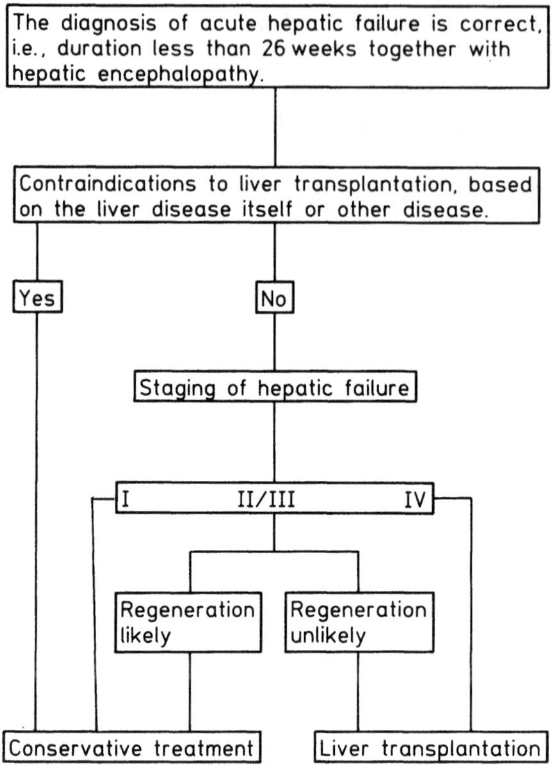


**Fig. 3.** Flow diagram for use in determining whether or not to perform liver transplantation in patients with acute hepatic failure

together with the etiology of the liver disease, determines the potential for regeneration of the diseased liver. The diagnosis of the pathobiology should therefore be considered crucial for the decision to perform liver transplantation. Thus in the case of total hepatic necrosis, regeneration of the liver is impossible and liver transplantation is indicated, whereas in the case of partial hepatic necrosis (liver reserve >40%) spontaneous liver regeneration should be awaited. However, liver transplantation is still indicated when the etiology predicts irreversible liver disease.

The strategies for the treatment of acute and subacute hepatic failure are summarized in a flow diagram (Fig. 3).

Although orthotopic liver transplantation results in improved survival of patients with acute hepatic failure, one of the main disadvantages is the lifelong requirement for immunosuppression with its associated clinical care and complications. Another approach is, in theory, a temporary graft which offers metabolic support while the diseased liver has a chance to regenerate. Once regeneration has occurred, immunosuppression can be discontinued and the graft will atrophy. Such an approach, called auxiliary heterotopic liver transplantation, has been successfully completed recently [81].

Only time will tell whether heterotopic liver transplantation, orthotopic liver transplantation, or a new form of medical therapy will ultimately become the standard treatment for acute hepatic failure.

## References


1. Trey C, Davidson C (1970) The management of fulminant hepatic failure. In: Popper H, Schaffner F (eds) Progress in liver disease, vol 3. Grune & Stratton, New York, pp 292–298
2. Gimson AES, O'Grady J, Ede RJ, Portmann B, Williams R (1986) Late onset hepatic failure: clinical, serological and histological features. Hepatology 6:288–294
3. Bernuau J, Rueff B, Benhamou JP (1986) Fulminant and subfulminant liver failure: definitions and causes. Semin Liver Dis 6:97–106
4. Van der Rijt CCD, Schalm SW, Meulstee J, Stijnen T (to be published) Flumazenil therapy for hepatic encephalopathy: a double-blind cross-over study. Hepatology
5. Acute Hepatic Failure Study Group (1979) Etiology and prognosis in fulminant hepatitis (abstr). Gastroenterology 77:A33
6. Papaevangelou G, Tassopouos N, Roumeliotoy-Karayannis A et al. (1984) Etiology of fulminant viral hepatitis in Greece. Hepatology 4:369–372
7. Gimson AES, White YS, Eddleston ALWF et al. (1983) Clinical and prognostic differences in fulminant hepatitis type A, B and non-A, non-B. Gut 24:1194–1198
8. Smedile A, Farci P, Verme G et al. (1982) Influence of delta infection on severity of hepatitis B. Lancet II:945–947
9. Borhammanesh F, Haghighi P, Hekmat K et al. (1973) Viral hepatitis during pregnancy. Severity and effect on gestation. Gastroenterology 64:304–312
10. Francis TI, Osuntokun BO, Seligman SJ et al. (1972) Fulminant hepatitis due to herpes hominis in an adult human. Am J Gastroenterol 57:329–332
11. Morishita K, Kodo H, Asana S et al. (1985) Fulminant varicella hepatitis following bone marrow transplantation. JAMA 252:511
12. Stricker BHC, Spoelstra P (1985) Drug-induced hepatic injury. Amsterdam, Elsevier
13. O'Grady JG, Williams R (1986) Management of acute liver failure. Schweiz Med Wochenschr 116:541–544
14. Pessayre D, Bentata M, Degott C et al. (1977) Isoniazid-rifampin fulminant hepatitis. A possible consequence of the enhancement of isoniazid hepatotoxicity by enzyme induction.Gastroenterology 72:284–289
15. Powell WJ, Koch-Weser J, Williams RA (1968) Lethal hepatic necrosis after therapy with imipramine and desipramine. JAMA 205:642–645
16. Babany G, Pessayre D (1984) Hépatitis dues aux nouveaux anti-flammatoires non stéroidiens. Gastroenterol Clin Biol 8:523–529
17. Carney FMT, Van Dyke RA (1972) Halothane hepatitis: a critical review. Anesth Analg 51:135–160
18. Nouel O, Henrion J, Bernuau J et al. (1980) Fulminant hepatic failure due to transient circulatory failure in patients with chronic heart disease. Dig Dis Sci 25:49–52
19. Sandle GI, Layton M, Record CO, Cowan WK (1980) Fulminant hepatic failure due to Budd-Chiari syndrome. Lancet I:1199
20. Harrison HB, Middleton HM III, Crosby JH, Dasher MN (1981) Fulminant hepatic failure: an unusual presentation of metastatic liver disease. Gastroenterology 80:820–825

21. Zafrani ES, Leclercq B, Vernant JP et al. (1983) Massive blastic infiltration of the liver: a cause of fulminant hepatic failure. Hepatology 3:428–432
22. Davies MH, Wilkinson SP, Hanid MA et al. (1980) Acute liver disease with encephalopathy and renal failure in late pregnancy and the early puerperium. A study of fourteen cases. Br J Obstet Gynaecol 87:1005–1014
23. Reye RDK, Morgan G, Baral J (1963) Encephalopathy and fatty degeneration of the viscera: a disease entity in childhood. Lancet II:249–252
24. Zimmerman HJ, Ishak KG (1982) Valproate-induced hepatic injury: analyses of 23 fatal cases. Hepatology 2:591–597
25. Roche-Sicot J, Benhamou JP (1977) Acute intravascular hemolysis and acute liver failure associated as a first manifestation of Wilson's disease. Ann Intern Med 86:301–303
26. De Cock KM, Govindarajan S, Redeker AG (1984) Fulminant delta hepatitis in chronic hepatitis B infection. JAMA 252:2746–2748
27. Galbraith RM, Eddleston ALWF, Williams R et al. (1975) Fulminant hepatic failure in leukemia and choriocarcinoma related to withdrawal of cytotoxic drug therapy. Lancet II:528–530
28. Bernuau J, Valli C, Boyer N et al. (1985) Fulminant hepatic failure due to autoimmune hepatitis (abstr). J Hepatol [Suppl] 2:S193
29. Duffy TE, Plum T (1982) Hepatic encephalopathy. In: Arias I, Popper H, Schachter D, Shafritz DA (eds) The liver: biology and pathology. Raven, New York, pp 693–713
30. Ede RE, Williams R (1986) Hepatic encephalopathy and cerebral edema. Semin Liver Dis 6:107–118
31. Bates D, Caronna JJ, Cartlidge NEF et al. (1977) Prospective study of nontraumatic coma: methods and results in 310 patients. Ann Neurol 2:211–220
32. Marosi MJ, Gerstenbrand F, Luef GJ, Zimmerman S, Schmutzhard E (1991) Realiability and accuracy of the Glasgow Coma Scale. Lancet 337:1042
33. Houvani BT, Hamlin EM, Reynolds TB (1971) Cerebrospinal fluid glutamine as a measure of hepatic encephalopathy. Arch Intern Med 127:1033-1036
34. Borg J, Warter JM, Schlienger JL (1982) Neurotransmitter modifications in human cerebrospinal fluid and serum during hepatic encephalopathy. J Neurol Sci 57:343
35. Casino A, Cangiano C, Fiaccadori F et al. (1982) Plasma and cerebrospinal fluid amino acid patterns in hepatic encephalopathy. Dig Dis Sci 27:828
36. Kennedy J, Parbhoo SP, MacGillivray B et al. (1973) Effect of extracorporeal liver perfusion on the electroencephalogram of patients in coma due to acute liver failure. Q J Med 42:549
37. Van der Rijt CCD, Schalm SW, De Groot GH, De Vlieger M (1984) Objective measurement of hepatic encephalopathy by means of automated E.E.G. analysis. Electroencephalogr Clin Neurophysiol 57:423–426
38. Karvountzis GG, Redeker AG (1974) Relation of alpha-fetoprotein in acute hepatitis to severity and prognosis. Ann Intern Med 80:156–160
39. Bloomer JR, Waldmann TA, Mclntire KR, Klatskin G (1977) Serum alpha-fetoprotein in patients with massive hepatic necrosis. Gastroenterology 72:479–482
40. Dymock IW, Tucker JS, Woolf LF et al. (1975) Coagulation studies as a prognostic index in acute liver failure. Br J Haematol 29:385–395
41. Koller F (1973) Theory and experience behind the use of coagulation tests in diagnosis and prognosis of liver disease. Scan J Gastroent 8 (Suppl 19):51–61
42. Ramsoe K, Andreasen PB, Ranek L (1980) Functioning liver mass in uncomplicated and fulminant acute hepatitis. Scand J Gastroenterol 15:65–72
43. Tygstrup N, Ranek L (1986) Assessment of prognosis in fulminant hepatic failure. Semin Liver Dis 6:129–137
44. Wilkinson SP, Arroyo V, Gazzard BG et al. (1974) Relation of renal impairment and haemorrhagic function in fulminant hepatic failure. Lancet I:522–524

45. De Knegt RJ, Schalm SW, Van den Berg B, Ten Kate FWJ (1986) Causes of death in fulminant hepatic failure. A guide to future management. Neth J Med 29:235–241
46. Berman DH, Leventhal RI, Gavaler JS, Cadoff EM, van Thiel DH (1991) Clinical differentiation of fulminant wilsonian hepatitis from other causes of hepatic failure. Gastroenterology 100:1129–1134
47. Bernuau J, Goudeau A, Poynard T et al. (1986) Multivariate analysis of prognostic factors in fulminant hepatitis B. Hepatology 4:648–654
48. O'Grady JG, Alexander GJM, Hayllar KM, Williams R (1989) Early indicators of prognosis in fulminant hepatic failure. Gastroenterology 97:439–445
49. Munoz SJ (1991) Prothrombin time in fulminant hepatic failure. Gastroenterology 100:1480–1489
50. O'Grady JG. Gimson AES, O'Brian CJ, Hughes RD, Williams R (1988) Controlled trials of charcoal hemoperfusion and prognostic factors in fulminant hepatic failure. Gastroenterology 94:1186–1192
51. Pastore G, Dentico P, Angarano G et al. (1981) Hepatitis B virus markers, alpha-fetoprotein and survival in fulminant viral hepatitis. J Med Virol 7:97–103
52. Trey C, Lipworth L, Davidson CS (1970) Parameters influencing survival in the first 318 patients reported to the fulminant hepatic failure surveillance study. Gastroenterology 58:306
53. Grimm G, Katzenschlager R, Schneeweiss B et al. (1988) Improvement of hepatic encephalopathy treated with flumazenil. Lancet II:1392–1394
54. Munoz SJ, Robinson M, Northrup B et al. (1991) Elevated intracranial pressure and computed tomography of the brain in fulminant hepatocellular failure. Hepatology 13:209–212
55. Canalese J, Gimson AES, Davis C, Mellon PJ, Davis M, Williams R (1982) Controlled trial of dexamethasone and mannitol for the cerebral edema of fulminant hepatic failure. Gut 23:625–629
56. Acute Hepatic Failure Study Group (1977) Failure of specific immunotherapy in fulminant type B hepatitis. Ann Intern Med 86:272–277
57. EASL Study Group (1979) Randomized trial of steroid therapy in acute liver failure. Gut 20:620
58. Durand F, Bernuau J, Samuel D, Saliba F, Shouval D, Benhamou JP (1990) Severe acute Wilson's disease: an indication for emergency administration of high doses of D-penicillamine (abstr). J Hepatol II [Suppl]:S20
59. Samson RI, Trey C, Timme AJ, Saunders SJ (1967) Fulminant hepatitis with recurrent hypoglycaemia and haemorrhage. Gastroenterology 54:291–300
60. Wahren J, Denis J, Desurmont P et al. (1983) Is intravenous administration of branched chain amino acids effective in the treatment of hepatic encephalopathy: a multicenter study. Hepatology 3:475
61. Maddrey WC, Weber FL, Coulter AW et al. (1976) The effects of keto analogues of essential amino acids on portal systemic encephalopathy. Gastroenterology 71:190–195
62. Wilkinson SP, Arroyo VA, Moodie H et al. (1976) Abnormalities of sodium excretion and other disorders of renal function in fulminant hepatic failure. Gut 17:501–505
63. Casey TH, Summerskill WHJ, Orvis AL (1965) Body and serum potassium in liver disease in relationship to hepatic function of associated factors. Gastroenterology 48:198–207
64. Stabenau JR, Warren KS, Rall DP (1959) The role of pH gradient in the distribution of ammonia between blood and cerebro-spinal fluid, brain and muscle. J Clin Invest 38:373–383
65. Bihari DJ, Gimson AES, Lindridge J, Williams R (1985) Lactic acidosis in fulminant hepatic failure. Some aspects of pathogenesis and prognosis. J Hepatol 1:405–416

66. Ring-Larsen H, Palazzo U (1981) Renal failure in fulminant hepatic failure and terminal cirrhosis: a comparison between incidence, type and prognosis. Gut 22:585–591
67. Bihari DJ, Gimson AES, Williams R (1986) Cardiovascular, pulmonary and renal complications of fulminant hepatic failure. Semin Liver Dis 6:119–128
68. Nusinovici V, Crubille C, Opolon P, Touboul JP, Darnis F, Caroli J (1977) Hepatites fulminantes avec coma. Revue de 137 cas. I. Complications. Gastroenterol Clin Biol 1:861–873
69. Macdougall BRD, Williams R (1978) $H_2$-receptor antagonists in the prevention of acute upper gastrointestinal hemorrhage in fulminant hepatic failure. A controlled trial. Gastroenterology 74:464–465
70. Gazzard BG, Henderson JM, Williams R (1975) Early changes in coagulation following a paracetamol overdose and a controlled trial of fresh frozen plasma therapy. Gut 16:617–620
71. Gazzard BG, Lewis ML, Ash G et al. (1974) Coagulation factor concentrate in the treatment of the haemorrhagic diathesis of fulminant hepatic failure. Gut 15:993–998
72. Wyke RJ, Canalese JC, Gimson AES, Williams R (1982) Bacteraemia in patients with fulminant hepatic failure. Liver 2:45–52
73. Salmeron JM, Tito L, Rimola A et al. (to be published) Selective intestinal decontamination in the prevention of bacterial infection in patients with acute liver failure. J Hepatol
74. Altin M, Rajkovic JA, Hughis RD et al. (1983) Neutrophil adherence in chronic liver disease and fulminant hepatic failure. Gut 24:746
75. Vallance P, Moncada S (1991) Hyperdynamic circulation in cirrhosis: a role for nitric oxide? Lancet 337:776–778
76. Trewby P, Williams R (1978) Pathofysiology of hypotension in patients with fulminant hepatic failure. Gastroenterology 74:859–865
77. Trewby PN, Ponzetto A, Gerin JL (1978) Incidence and pathophysiology of pulmonary edema in fulminant liver failure. Gastroenterology 74:859
78. Achord JL (1968) Acute pancreatitis with infectious hepatitis. JAMA 205:129
79. De Knegt RJ, Schalm SW (1991) Fulminant hepatic failure: to transplant or not to transplant? Neth J Med 38:131–141
80. Samuel D, Bismuth A, Mathieu D et al. (1991) Passive immunoprophylaxis after liver transplantation in HBs-Ag-positive patients. Lancet 337:813–815
81. Metselaar HJ, Hesselink EJ, de Rave S et al. (1990) Recovery of failing liver after auxiliary heterotopic transplantation. Lancet II:1156–1157

# 32 Tumors of the Liver and Biliary Tract

M. Colombo, O. Beloqui, and B. Sangro

Various benign or malignant tumors may arise within the liver (Table 1). Benign tumors are rare conditions. However, since the advent and widespread use of the new imaging techniques, they have been increasingly diagnosed. In contrast, primary liver malignancies, particularly hepatocellular carcinoma, are a major health issue because of their high prevalence worldwide.

## 1 Malignant Liver Tumors of Adulthood

### 1.1 Hepatocellular Carcinoma

***Introduction***

Hepatocellular carcinoma (HCC) is a highly malignant tumor with an extremely poor prognosis and an estimated incidence of at least 250000 cases per year. It represents 4% of all malignant tumors and is the seventh most common cancer in man worldwide [1]. Years ago, HCC was recognized only after it had reached an advanced clinical stage, which led to the misconception that HCC is a rapidly growing, devastating tumor. More recently, an important contribution to the understanding of the natural history of this tumor has been made by the prospective studies of cohorts of patients with cirrhosis who are at risk for developing HCC. These studies have clearly established that HCC is often an asymptomatic and slowly expanding tumor, whose natural history in many instances is an extension of that of the underlying cirrhosis [2]. In contrast with a plethora of data on HCC in patients with cirrhosis, there is insufficient information about HCC developing in noncirrhotic livers. One serious gap is the lack of knowledge of the risk factors for this type of tumor, which has impeded prospective cohort studies of high-risk patients.

***Epidemiology***

The geographic distribution of HCC has been reported in terms of (a) relative frequency, i.e., the percentage of this type of cancer within a series

**Table 1.** Histologic classification of tumors and tumor-like lesions of the liver.

| | Benign | Malignant |
|---|---|---|
| *Epithelial* | | |
| Hepatocellular | Hepatocellular adenoma | Hepatocellular carcinoma |
| | Nodular regenerative hyperplasia | |
| | Focal nodular hyperplasia | |
| Cholangiocellular | Bile duct adenoma | Cholangiocarcinoma |
| | Biliary cystadenoma | Squamous carcinoma |
| | Biliary papillomatosis | Biliary cystadenocarcinoma |
| | Biliary microhamartomas | |
| *Nonepithelial* | | |
| Vascular | Hemangioma | |
| | Infantile hemangioendothelioma | Epithelioid hemangioendothelioma |
| | Lymphangiomatosis | Angiosarcoma |
| | Peliosis hepatis | Kaposi's sarcoma |
| Nonvascular | Lipomatous tumors | Fibrosarcoma |
| | Fibroma | Leiomyosarcoma |
| | Leiomyoma | Embryonal rhabdomyosarcoma |
| *Mixed* | Mesenchymal hamartoma | Undifferentiated sarcoma |
| | Benign teratoma | Hepatoblastoma |
| *Miscellaneous* | Inflammatory pseudotumor | |
| | Adrenal rest tumor | |
| | Pancreatic heterotopia | |

of cancer patients, (b) age-adjusted incidence rates, and (c) mortality [3]. For extensive areas of the world that correspond to the regions with the highest risk for liver cancer, the information is based on a limited number of cancer registries. From this limited information, however, HCC appears to be one of the most common malignant tumors in sub-Saharan Africa, the South Pacific, and Asia, and it is also relatively frequent in the Mediterranean Basin. By contrast, it is relatively rare in northern Europe, North America, and Australia (Table 2).

Time-trend analyses can be performed in respect of those countries for which incidence data for HCC are available over at least two different periods. Preliminary evidence indicates that the frequency of HCC is increasing in North America, north European countries, and Japan, and is decreasing in some populations of South Africa [3]. One important point that must be kept in mind when considering these epidemiologic studies is that it is uncertain whether increases in tumor rates are true or artifactual, i.e., due to increased sensitivity of diagnostic tools.

**Table 2.** Worldwide incidence of hepatocellular carcinoma per 100000 inhabitants, as reported by cancer registries

| | *Age-adjusted incidence rates* | |
|---|---|---|
| | *Males* | *Females* |
| *Africa* | | |
| Mozambique | 112.9 | 30.8 |
| Zimbabwe | 64.6 | 25.6 |
| Senegal | 25.6 | 9.0 |
| *Asia* | | |
| China | 31.7 | 9.1 |
| Japan | 11.9 | 2.9 |
| Indonesia | 9.5 | 2.8 |
| India | 4.7 | 1.6 |
| *Europe* | | |
| Romania | 11.8 | 7.9 |
| Switzerland | 9.7 | 1.3 |
| Poland | 8.3 | 4.9 |
| Italy | 6.9 | 2.7 |
| Spain | 6.9 | 5.1 |
| France | 4.9 | 0.7 |
| United Kingdom | 2.1 | 0.8 |
| *North America* | | |
| United States | 2.0–18.1 | 1.0–3.6 |
| Canada | 1.3–6.9 | 0.5–3.7 |
| *South America* | | |
| Argentina | 9.9 | 5.8 |
| Brazil | 3.8 | 3.8 |
| *Oceania* | | |
| Australia | 1.1 | 0.4 |
| New Zealand | 8.7 | 2.5 |

### *Risk Factors*

Chemicals, hormones, viruses, metabolic diseases, and cirrhosis have all been identified as risk factors for HCC. These factors, in turn, are likely to be modulated by such characteristics as the patient's age, sex, and race. In all populations, independently of the risk, the incidence of HCC increases progressively with age, with a tendency to level off in the older groups [3]. In the high-incidence areas there is a shift toward the younger age groups, as compared to intermediate- and low-risk areas.

Males are more prone to develop HCC than females [3]. In high-risk areas, the male to female ratio is around 4–8:1, whereas the male predominance is less marked in the low-risk populations of America and Europe. Despite many studies, it is still unclear whether the male predominance reflects increased susceptibility to the tumor or higher exposure to the environmental factors associated with HCC.

Studies of migrants provided unequivocal evidence that the risk of HCC in some ethnic groups largely depends on the population's exposure to certain environmental factors. The rates of HCC are lower for the Chinese, Japanese, and Filipino populations who were born in the United States than for those who emigrated there. The latter, in turn, have lower rates than those living in their home countries [3]. The better standards of hygiene in the United States as compared to Asian countries, which result in reduced exposure to alimentary carcinogens, and diminished intrafamilial spread of hepatitis B virus (HBV) are likely explanations.

Aflatoxin, alcohol, and tobacco-related compounds are potentially carcinogenic [4]. Humans can be exposed to the mycotoxins produced by *Aspergillus flavus* and *Aspergillus parasiticus* fungi through the ingestion of contaminated foodstuffs or of products from animals fed with aflatoxin-contaminated cereals. There is strong evidence of a carcinogenic effect of aflatoxin in many animal species but the evidence that it has a carcinogenic role in humans is only epidemiologic and is not conclusive, mainly because of the lack of appropriate methods to assess past exposure of individuals. Confusion also derives from the interplay of different environmental oncogenic factors (hepatitis viruses and alcohol) which are not homogeneously distributed in the various geographic areas.

Ethanol has not been shown experimentally to be mutagenic or carcinogenic, but there is sufficient epidemiologic evidence of an association between alcohol abuse and HCC [3, 4]. In general, alcohol has a moderate effect (relative risk: 1.5–3.0). In areas in which the prevalence of HBV carriers is low, alcohol may be an important risk factor for HCC since it is the most common cause of cirrhosis, which will evolve to HCC in some cases.

The association between tobacco smoking and HCC is uncertain [3, 4]. Most of the evidence available on this association is based on case control studies, which, however, have yielded conflicting results. While four such studies have provided evidence of an association between tobacco and HCC, especially in HBsAg-negative patients who are long-term and heavy smokers, six others have failed to identify any relationship. Important methodologic problems in the designs of the studies concerning the evaluation of the joint effects of tobacco, alcohol, and hepatitis viruses might explain some of the discrepancies.

The evidence for an etiologic role of sex hormones (in particular oral contraceptives) in the development of HCC is also inconclusive [3, 4]. An increase in the risk of HCC was observed primarily in long-term users of oral contraceptives, in the absence of other factors known to be associated with liver cancer. Recent increments in the incidence of HCC and in HCC-associated mortality have paralleled the increasing prevalence of oral contraceptive use in some countries in which the background rates of HCC are low, e.g., England, Wales, Sweden, and West Germany, although this has not been observed in other low-risk populations (e.g., the United States,

Australia, and the Netherlands). The results of a large collaborative study sponsored by the WHO also militate against a role of oral contraceptives in HCC. This study demonstrated that there was no association between oral contraceptives and HCC in women living in areas in which HBV was endemic or in women who were short-term users [5].

In contrast there is convincing evidence that persistent infection with HBV is an important causative factor in HCC. This evidence is based upon epidemiologic studies and animal experiments indicating that the association between HBV and HCC is strong and specific. In a prospective study of 22707 Chinese men in Taiwan, BEASLEY [6] reported that the incidence of the tumor in the HBsAg-positive population was 473/100000 persons per year, compared to only 4.6 in the HBsAg-negative individuals (relative risk = 102). Another important piece of evidence connecting HCC to HBV comes from the study of either naturally or experimentally infected woodchucks (reviewed by YANG et al. [7]). One hundred percent of captive animals infected at birth with woodchuck hepatitis virus and maintained in captivity develop HCC after 17–36 weeks of persistent infection. Different types of evidence also connect HCC with the RNA hepatitis C virus (HCV) (reviewed by TABOR) [8]. Sequential development of cirrhosis and HCC has been observed in patients with transfusion-associated hepatitis. Recently, a high prevalence of serum antibody to HCV has been observed in patients with HCC [9]. Although these findings establish a strong link between chronic HCV infection and neoplastic transformation, it is unlikely that HCV plays a direct role in HCC, since no reverse transcriptase activity has been found in infected liver tissue.

Hepatocellular carcinoma has also developed in patients with rare metabolic conditions: patients with porphyria cutanea tarda, hereditary hemochromatosis, tyrosinemia, hypercitrullinemia, or $\alpha_1$-antitrypsin deficiency are considered to be at high risk [10]. Patients with glycogenosis (types 1 and 3), Wilson's disease, or hereditary fructose intolerance may also develop HCC, but are at substantially lower risk.

The above analysis of the risk factors associated with HCC clearly indicates that patients with cirrhosis are a risk population for HCC. This agrees with the epidemiologic observations that 30%–40% of patients who die of cirrhosis are found at autopsy to have HCC, and that 90% of patients with HCC have associated cirrhosis [11]. More recently, close follow-up studies of cirrhotic patients with highly sensitive and specific diagnostic methods such as real-time ultrasonography (US) have led to recognition of the tumor at an early stage. The significance of the association of HCC and cirrhosis is still obscure: HCC could be either the inevitable consequence of long-standing hepatic disease or an independent response to a hepatic insult common to HCC and cirrhosis.

### *Pathogenesis*

Classical studies by Farber and co-workers in rat hepatocarcinogenesis models have led to the hypothesis that liver cancer develops in a stepwise manner, through the phases of initiation, promotion, and progression [7]. According to this hypothesis, the fundamental mechanism of hepatocellular carcinogenesis is clonal expansion of transformed normal liver cells. During the long period of cancer development, the transformed liver cells become more basophilic, indicating active growth, followed by the appearance of focal proliferations of *nodules* of altered hepatocytes. The appearance of additional altered foci of cells or *nodules within nodules* has been taken as evidence of carcinogenic progression within nodules.

In addition to this proposed stepwise cellular pathway to HCC, recent evidence strongly suggests that the predominant cellular pathway to HCC begins with proliferation of a population of stem cells called *oval cells* [7]. In the experimental animal, electron microscopic and autoradiographic studies were able to show that oval cells, which originate in the portal tracts, are the first cells to proliferate 1–3 days after carcinogen treatment and that these cells have the potential to differentiate into basophilic, albumin-producing hepatocytes as well as bile duct cells. Useful models for investigating these pathways to HCC are the animals infected with hepadnaviruses, i.e., woodchuck, Peking duck, and ground-squirrel. When infected persistently, these animals are exposed continuously to both a carcinogenic agent, the hepadnavirus, and a mitogenic stimulus, the accompanying chronic hepatitis generated by a limited immune response, which places them at very high risk for HCC. In such studies, oval cells and necrotic inflammation were always observed in the precancerous stages preceding and accompanying the development of the tumor. No single mechanism has been proposed for hepadnavirus-induced oncogenesis. Most data speak against the existence of a viral transforming oncogene. The persistence of virus integration in animals and in man may cause genetic alterations and epigenetic phenomena [7]. The unstable nature of cellular DNA, into which hepadnavirus is integrated, may cause such chromosome alterations as deletion, inverted duplications, and translocations, which are found in HCC. More specific mechanisms of genetic damage (insertional mutagenesis) have also been observed in man, in whom virus integration has created new genes with potential regulatory properties. The gradual accumulation of these mutations in the cellular genome causes a cell to become predisposed to malignant transformation.

The interpretation of the pathogenesis of HCC in livers in which no viral insertions are found is more complex. In these instances, hepadnaviruses may cause cellular DNA mutations which are no longer linked to viral DNA, by a "hit and run mechanism." Like many other DNA viruses, most hepadnaviruses have transactivational potential in the X region of their genome, indicating that proteins encoded by these genes are able to influence the expression of cellular nuclear proto-oncogenes, which in turn influence the growth and differentiation of infected hepatocytes. A second transcriptional transactivator has very recently been identified in the pre S2/S region of an integrated HBV-DNA which was cloned from an HCC.

### *Macroscopic and Microscopic Classification*

The macroscopic descriptions of liver cancer in clinical cases are divided into nodular, massive, and diffuse (Eggel's classification) [12] (Fig. 1). Histologically, HCC can be divided into four types: trabecular, pseudoglandular, compact, and scirrhous. The trabecular type is composed of tissue strands of various thickness, with the cells being separated by blood-filled sinusoids. The pseudoglandular type is composed of gland-like structures of varying sizes. The compact tumor has a basically trabecular structure but the tumor cells proliferate to yield solid and medullary structures, with modest amounts of stroma. The scirrhous type consists of strands of tumor cells surrounded by large amounts of fibrous interstitial tissue. HCC is also defined cytologically as (a) pleomorphic (when there is marked variation in both cellular and nuclear size and in the shape and staining of the nuclei) and (b) clear cell (when the tumor is composed of cells with clear cytoplasm). Finally, the degree of atypia of the tumor cells is classified according to Edmonson and Steiner's criteria: grade 1, highly differentiated tumor cells resembling normal hepatocytes; grade 2, slight but definite atypism; grade 3, prominent nuclear atypism and pleomorphism, with the appearance of multinucleated giant cells; grade 4, uniformly composed of anaplastic tumor cells with very scanty cytoplasm. It is not uncommon for two or more of the above histologic and cytologic characteristics to be present in the same tumor. It is therefore recommended that the predominant histologic type and degree of cellular atypia be indicated.

### *Natural History*

The time lag between exposure to carcinogenic factors and tumor development can vary from a few years to many decades. In many patients, HCC grows slowly within the liver, without causing any significant clinical signs or symptoms; thus patients with a small HCC may only occasionally complain of abdominal pain or malaise. Signs and symptoms of more advanced disease include hepatosplenomegaly, jaundice, ascites, weight loss, and fever. In South African patients, HCC may present with hepatosplenomegaly and jaundice as a result of its accelerated growth rate. Hemoperitoneum, caused by spontaneous rupture of the tumor, is a rare event in Caucasians but occurs more frequently in Orientals and Africans. Several endocrine and paraneoplastic manifestations may accompany the development of HCC. Erythrocytosis, probably due to increased erythropoietic

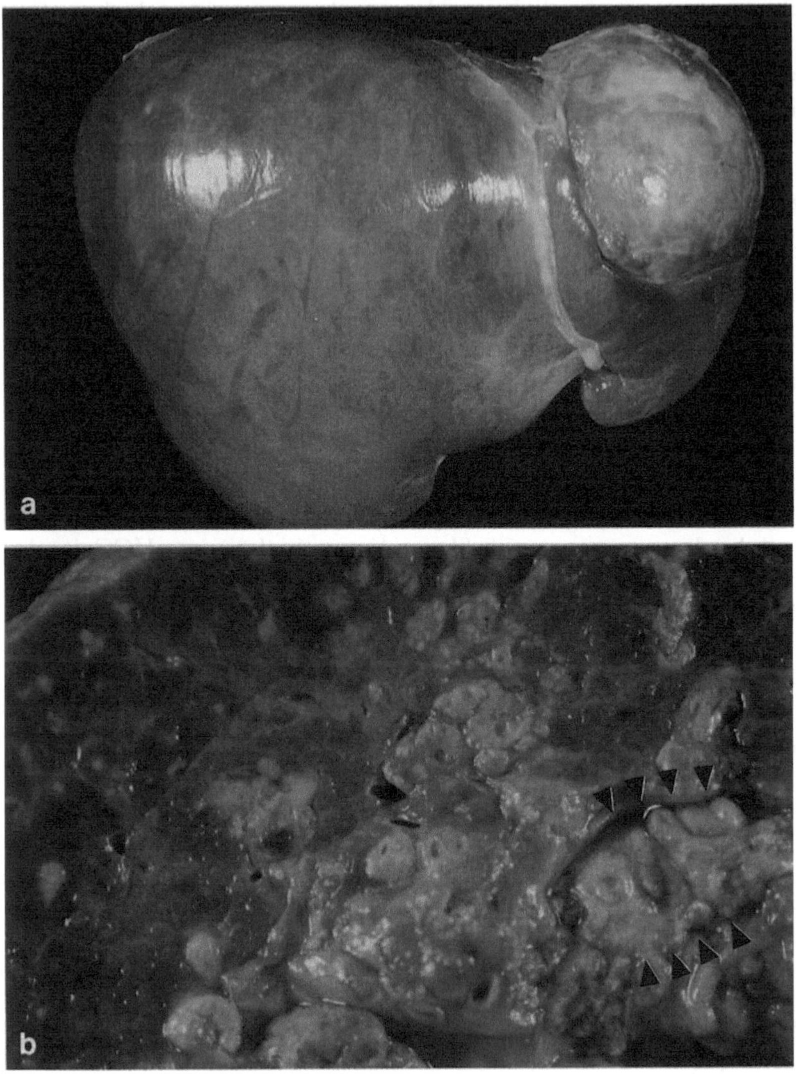


**Fig. 1. a** Macroscopic aspect of a liver cell cancer. **b** Massive hepatocellular carcinoma. Tumoral portal vein thrombosis is signaled by *arrowheads*

production, occurs in between 5% and 10% of cases. Episodes of hypoglycemia are not uncommon and are attributable to production by the tumor of a large molecular weight pro-IGFII (pro-insulin-like growth factor II), and, in the terminal stages of the disease, to increased demand for glucose by the tumor. Symptomatic hypercalcemia is most uncommon and is usually associated with either bone metastases or ectopic parathormone secretion. Thyrotoxicosis and Cushing's disease have been described.

Whether HCC originates from one or more than one clone of transformed liver cells is a matter of controversy. The finding of solitary HCC nodes in variable proportions of patients subjected to routine periodic follow-up examinations with US suggests that in many patients HCC may have a long-lasting subclinical incubation period during which it may grow as a solitary mass [13]. There are important regional differences in the growth patterns of HCC. The so-called encapsulated expanding type is frequent in Oriental, Italian, and French patients with small tumors, whereas it is rarely found in North America and South Africa. This type of tumor is often a relatively well-differentiated variety and is associated with cirrhosis. Whether the fibrous tissue surrounding the tumor node is a true capsule or condensed cirrhotic stroma is controversial. In a minority of the patients, the small HCC has tended to grow either by replacing the adjacent hepatic parenchyma or mixed with it. The presence of one or another histologic growth pattern is clinically important since it may influence the prognosis after resection.

The growth rate of a symptomatic HCC varies greatly. When expressed as tumor volume doubling time, the tumor growth rate ranges from 1 to 19 months, with a median of 4, and this may be correlated directly with the patient's survival time [14]. It is not clear why the growth rates of HCC vary so greatly from patient to patient. Sequential studies of untreated patients have shown different growth kinetics of single HCC nodes. Some tumors have constant rates of growth during follow-up, while others either have a declining growth rate in the late phase of follow-up or, after an initial phase of no growth, increase exponentially in volume [15]. Thus, the wide range in tumor volume doubling times that has been reported in the literature reflects the existence of different patterns of tumor growth.

The US patterns of HCC may change as tumor size increases [16]. During tumor growth, the low echo-pattern which is characteristic of smaller tumors may be progressively replaced by a high or mixed echo pattern. The latter are rather common in advanced tumor disease, i.e., when the tumor has grown massively [14].

In many patients, serum levels of α-fetoprotein (AFP) seem to parallel tumor growth. Obviously this is true only for AFP-secreting tumors, which represent 30%–71% of all HCCs. In massive HCCs, the serum levels of AFP often exceed the cut-off value of 400 ng/ml. In some patients with cirrhosis, the pattern of serum AFP during follow-up may predict when HCC will develop.

Hepatocellular carcinoma may spread outside the liver, but only in the late phase of the disease metastases may become clinically evident. The most common sites of extrahepatic metastases are lung, adrenals, and skeleton.

The survival times for patients with HCC are correlated inversely with the degree of hepatic replacement by the tumor and the severity of the liver impairment. Prospective study of Oriental and Italian patients with cirrhosis and early detected HCC has further demonstrated the prolonged, slow growth of HCC in these racial groups. In fact, the survival of 22 Japanese patients with cirrhosis and minute (less than 3 cm) HCCs was 91% at 1 year, 55% at 2 years, and 13% at 3 years [14]. The survival of 12 corresponding Italian patients with Child's A cirrhosis ranged from 7 to 36 months, with a 2-year survival of 44% [15].

Cancer is considered to be the cause of death in patients with HCC who die with advanced tumor or from cachexia and deterioration in general condition without developing rapidly progressive jaundice. In a series of 659 patients with HCC, hepatic failure and gastrointestinal bleeding were the leading causes of death (39% and 23% respectively) whereas cancer was the cause of death in only 70 (18%) [16]. In studies on untreated patients with HCC who had been followed prospectively, hepatic failure and hemorrhage were the leading causes of death [14, 15].

Numerous epidemiologic, laboratory, and clinical parameters have been shown to be of prognostic value in patients with HCC. It is unanimously agreed that liver function tests alone or in combination with ascites and encephalopathy are the best prognostic indicators for these patients. The predictive value of such variables as sex, age, serum AFP, and alcohol consumption is a matter of debate. Male sex and advanced age have been found by some to be correlated with a poor prognosis. There is also debate as to whether the histologic features of HCC are of prognostic value. Other studies have demonstrated correlations between patient survival and cytologic grading of the tumor, and between tumor volume doubling time and patient survival.

### *Fibrolamellar Carcinoma*

Fibrolamellar carcinoma develops in young people (5–35 years) of either sex and is not associated with cirrhosis. Histologically, clumps of tumor cells are interspersed with bands of mature fibrous tissue. Serum AFP is frequently normal and markers of serum hepatitis are rarely detected. Prognosis is slightly better than for other forms of HCC.

### *Diagnosis*

Real-time US plus thin-needle liver biopsy is the more sensitive and specific diagnostic method for HCC, having an estimated accuracy of 90% [17]. The few false-negative results with this procedure are mainly due to very small tumors (less than 1 cm in diameter) and initial neoplastic changes of the liver cells which can be recognized only by very experienced pathologists. In the absence of a liver biopsy, HCC can be diagnosed with confidence only in those patients who with cirrhosis have a liver mass on US and serum levels of AFP greater than 400 ng/ml. The diagnostic accuracy of serum AFP alone is poor, since this serum marker rarely exceeds the diagnostic level of 400 ng/ml in patients with small tumors and is within the normal range in 25% of all cases of HCC. In patients with small HCCs and severe coagulopathy, tumor cells for diagnosis can also be obtained by needle aspiration. This approach is safe, since very thin needles are used, but gives numerous false-positive and false-negative results. Computed tomography (CT) is less sensitive than US for detecting tumors less than 2 cm in diameter, but has the advantage of screening for secondaries in the regional lymph nodes, spleen, and liver vessels. Selective hepatic arteriography with Lipiodol is a very sensitive technique for detecting microfoci of tumor cells which would escape detection with US. The diagnostic utility of magnetic resonance imaging (MRI) in this area is still under investigation.

*Early Diagnosis.* The early diagnosis of HCC is made possible by the existence of individuals with recognizable risk factors for this tumor, and by such characteristics of the disease as the long phase of incubation and its tendency to grow as a solitary mass in the liver. Although strategies of HCC screening should be modified according to the local epidemiologic situation, there are general rules for the design of such studies. These rules take into account whether populations of individuals or groups of patients are being investigated. In population-based studies only a few individuals have identifiable risk factors, most of them are asymptomatic, and the screening intervals are standardized. This is not the case for clinic-based studies, in which participants may have more than one risk factor for HCC, most are symptomatic, and the screening intervals are not standardized. Recently, in a consensus development conference held in Anchorage (Alaska) [18], chronic HBsAg carriers, carriers with cirrhosis or a family history of HCC, and patients with rare metabolic diseases were identified as high-risk patients for HCC and, therefore, as candidates for periodic screening. It was recommended that healthy carriers of HBsAg have yearly determinations of serum AFP, and that patients with cirrhosis be screened every 6 months by abdominal US and determination of serum AFP. In a prospective study carried out in Alaskan natives, 16 tumors were identified in a population of 1400 HBsAg carriers who had been tested annually for serum AFP [18]. In a prospective study of 236 Chinese patients with cirrhosis, 20 patients with HCC were identified by US; some of these cases were detected at a stage early enough for successful hepatic resection to be performed [17]. However, even in the face of this evidence that screening high-risk individuals may increase the yield of potentially operable tumors, no firm conclusion has yet been reached that such policies reduce the mortality due to HCC. The theoretical reasons for this include the high rate of tumor recurrence after hepatic resection, the high rate of second primary tumors in the liver, and the coexistence of cirrhosis, which may reduce the number of patients eligible for surgery and increase postoperative mortality.

### *Treatment*

There is no evidence that mortality from HCC can be reduced by any of the available treatments. Hepatic resection is the primary therapeutic option, although it is often restricted by the coexistence of cirrhosis and the degree of liver replacement by the tumor. Up to 50% of selected cirrhotic patients with small HCCs have survived 3 years after hepatic resection, although many of them have signs of recurrence of the disease [19]. Survival rates are better for patients with encapsulated tumors than for patients with infiltrating HCCs. The rate of survival was 20%–40% for patients with HCC who had been treated by orthotopic liver transplantation, although the subgroup of patients with tumors detected by chance had a longer life expectancy [20]. Doxorubicin and its analogues given at 75–100 $mg/m^2$ of body surface area every 3 weeks have had only palliative effects in a minority of patients [21]. The efficacy of such therapeutic approaches as transcatheter-arterial chemoembolization and percutaneous ethanol injection is under evaluation.

### *Prevention*

The only realistic way to reduce mortality due to HCC is prevention. Eradication of the HBV carrier state is now feasible by mass vaccination programs, and some have already been started in endemic areas. It is not yet possible to adopt a similar strategy to control the spread of HCV, another leading cause of cirrhosis, but this will be feasible as soon as a vaccine is developed. Educational programs and new regulations can help to decrease alcoholism, which accounts for one-third of all cases of cirrhosis worldwide. Contamination by mycotoxins can be reduced by improved agricultural methods and better storage and transport of cereals.

## 1.2 Cholangiocarcinoma

Carcinomas arising from the bile ducts can be classified into three groups according to their location: (a) carcinoma of the intrahepatic bile ductules or *peripheral cholangiocarcinoma*; (b) carcinoma of the major intrahepatic bile ducts or *hilar cholangiocarcinoma* (Fig. 2); and (c) carcinoma of the extrahepatic bile duct or *bile duct carcinoma*. Differentiation is often difficult, especially between peripheral and hilar cholangiocarcinoma (CC). The peripheral to hilar CC ratio is about 2:1, except in the case of Thorotrast-related CC, in which peripheral CC is more frequent than the hilar type.

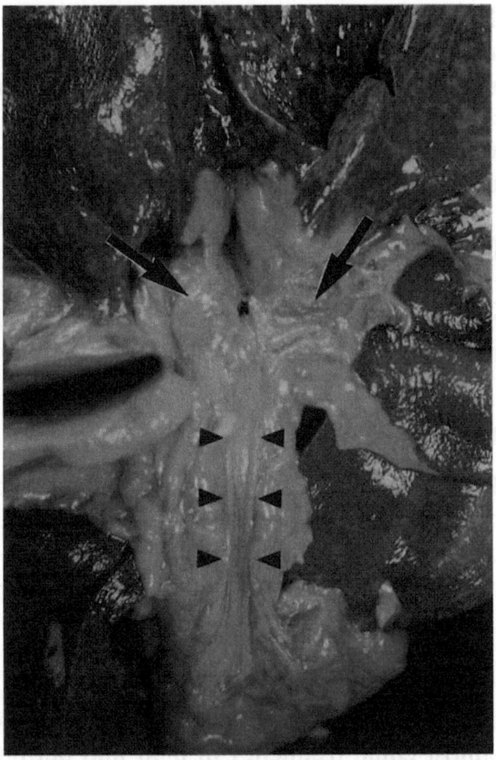

**Fig. 2.** Cholangiocarcinoma. The common bile duct is identified by *arrowheads* and tumoral tissue by *arrows*

### *Epidemiology and Pathogenesis*

Cholangiocarcinoma accounts for some 10%–20% of all primary liver cancers. The CC to HCC ratio is somewhat higher in Western Europe and the United States than in Africa and Asia, probably because of the high incidence of HCC in the latter [22]. CC usually appears in the 5th to 7th decades of life, with hilar tumors presenting at slightly younger ages. No sex predominance has been consistently found in either type of CC.

Thorotrast, a colloidal solution of thorium dioxide used as a contrast medium for x-ray examination in the 1930s and 1940s, is a well-known cause of CC (usually of the peripheral type, as mentioned above). Chronic infestation by *Clonorchis sinensis* and *Opisthorchis viverrini* is very common in the Far East and an epidemiologic association between infestation by these parasites and CC has been shown. However, there is no conclusive evidence of a direct causal relationship. CC is a well-recognized complication of the fibropolycystic diseases of the liver and other developmental abnormalities of the biliary tract [23]. In such cases, malignant transformation may appear anywhere in the intra- or extrahepatic bile ducts.

Hepatolithiasis is being increasingly found in Asian patients with CC. It has thus been argued that persistent inflammation of the bile duct epithelium might contribute to the development of this tumor. In fact, the papillary and adenomatous changes frequently seen in the nontumoral bile ducts may represent preneoplastic disorders. CC might also complicate sclerosing cholangitis through a similar mechanism.

The molecular biology of CC is far from being understood. Nevertheless, some oncogenes known to participate in normal liver tissue growth and differentiation have been found to be expressed in CC [24]. Additionally, *ras* oncogene point mutations have been shown in CC but not in other liver malignancies [25].

### *Pathology*

Four types of CC can be distinguished macroscopically: nodular, infiltrative, diffuse, and periductular [22]. The nodular type is well demarcated and usually solitary. The infiltrative type is ill-defined and multiple intrahepatic metastases are rather common. The diffuse type consists of small nodules uniformly scattered throughout the liver. Finally, in the periductular type, tumor proliferates along the extrahepatic bile duct and mass formation is minimal despite extensive parenchymal infiltration. This type is almost exclusive to hilar CC whereas the nodular and infiltrative types occur with almost equal frequency in hilar and peripheral CC.

Microscopically, CC usually appears as a differentiated tubular adenocarcinoma, but it may show papillary structures or be poorly differentiated. The cells are cuboidal or columnar, usually with clear cytoplasm and small nuclei that contain abundant chromatin granules [1]. The nucleolus is not so prominent as in HCC. Mucin secretion may be abundant. No marked differences are found between hilar and peripheral tumors. Adenosquamous, squamous, and mucoepidermoid carcinomas are considered to be specific but rare forms of CC. Immunohistochemically, most tumors stain positively for CEA and CA 19.9.

### *Natural History and Diagnosis*

Cholangiocarcinoma is usually clinically silent for long periods, even though malaise, anorexia, and weight loss may be reported retrospectively. Abdominal pain, jaundice, ascites, and an abdominal mass are the most frequent symptoms in peripheral tumors. The clinical appearance of hilar CC and bile duct carcinoma is almost invariably that of progressive obstructive jaundice.

Cholangiocarcinoma shows a strong tendency toward early locoregional spread, with lymph nodes in the hilar, peripancreatic, and periaortic areas being the most common site of extrahepatic metastatic disease. Hematogenous metastases to the peritoneum, lung, adrenal glands, intraperitoneal organs, and bone may also be observed during later stages. Death supervenes after an average of 7 months as a result of liver failure, infection, gastrointestinal bleeding, or cachexia. Survival without therapy is shorter in patients with hilar tumors.

At the time of presentation, laboratory studies often disclose varying degrees of cholestasis in peripheral CC. Serum CEA and CA 19.9 are frequently elevated but AFP is nearly always within normal limits. Peripheral CC tends to be homogeneously hyperechoic on US, hypodense on CT, and hypovascular on angiography, but none of these features is specific. The true sensitivity of imaging procedures has not been established because of the low overall incidence of the tumor.

Hilar CC and bile duct cancer display the biochemical picture of obstructive jaundice. US usually shows dilated intrahepatic ducts and CT may disclose a small hilar mass and/or a thickening of the common duct. Endoscopic retrograde and percutaneous transhepatic cholangiography allows accurate localization of the stricture. Percutaneous transhepatic cholangiography also provides valuable information for determining resectability and surgical approaches and may make possible temporary external drainage until a definitive therapeutic decision has been made. Several benign strictures, however, may mimic hilar CC and bile duct cancer; this is particularly true of sclerosing cholangitis, which poses the main diagnostic dilemma. It has recently been shown that brush cytology taken at the time of either endoscopic or percutaneous cholangiography may help to confirm malignancy, yielding a specificity of 100% and an overall sensitivity of 50%–60% [26, 27]. Sensitivity can be further improved with repeated brushings.

### *Treatment and Prognosis*

Despite some recent therapeutic advances, the prognosis of CC remains dismal. Surgical resection offers the only chance of cure but is seldom attemptable. In general, the more distally the tumor is located in the biliary tract, the greater the chance will be of accomplishing successful excision and so improving the outcome. Since many patients are not eligible for surgery, attention has increasingly focused on palliative forms of therapy.

#### *Surgical Resection*

Radical resections of peripheral CC are seldom performed, and results are far from encouraging: resectability ranges from 15% to 30%, and there are only anecdotal reports of long-term survivors. Nevertheless, resection increases survival when compared with no treatment.

The surgical approach to hilar CC is moving toward a more aggressive attitude. The resectability rate is ca. 20% and is gradually increasing as new resection modalities are developed. Operative mortality is 10%–20% for radical hepatic resections and close to 0% for local resections. In a retrospective assessment of 499 resections for hilar CC between 1980 and 1989, the 3- and 5-year survival rates were found to be 24% and 13%, respectively [28]. In the same study, radical liver resections compared favorably with local resections in terms of long-term survival, probably because complete tumor removal was achieved more frequently when radical resections were performed. In a prospective study, median survival was 25 months for patients dying after radical resection (most of them because of tumor recurrence) [29]. From the above data, it can be concluded that radical resection of hilar CC, although frequently unsuccessful in the long run, provides the best outcome. Therefore, every patient should be carefully assessed for resection before other palliative procedures, such as internal biliary drainage, are adopted.

As for extrahepatic bile duct carcinoma, resectability rises to 40%–50% and long-term survival after resection is better than in patients with hilar tumors (with reported 3- and 5-year survival rates of 44% and 28%, respectively) [30].

The results of liver transplantation in patients with hilar or peripheral CC not amenable to partial hepatectomy have been disappointing. Tumor recurrence either in the grafted liver or at distant sites is the rule, in spite of extensive preoperative searching for disseminated disease. This probably reflects the strong tendency of CC toward early dissemination as well as the permissive effect of immunosuppressive therapy. The 3-month survival rate is about 50% and overall survival ranges from 1 to 1.5 years [31].

### *Palliative Procedures*

Most patients with hilar CC are not eligible for resection. Since death commonly results from liver failure or ascending infection, biliary decompression by means of surgical bypass or transtumoral intubation may improve the short-term prognosis. In most instances, internal biliary drainage using an endoprosthesis can be successfully accomplished either endoscopically or percutaneously. However, it carries a significant early mortality (15%–40%, mainly because of infection), and median survival after the procedure is about 6 months [32]. On the other hand, palliative biliary–enteric anastomosis provides a mean survival or only 7 months and carries an operative mortality of 40% [33]. Liver atrophy due to long-standing obstruction should be ruled out since it makes palliative procedures useless.

The outcome of palliative intubational or surgical procedures for inoperable bile duct carcinoma is very much the same as for hilar CC.

### *Radiotherapy and Chemotherapy*

Neither radiotherapy nor chemotherapy is regarded as effective for the treatment of peripheral CC, although partial tumor responses may be eventually achieved. Internal or external irradiation together with endoprosthesis placement has been used for palliation of unresectable hilar CC. No conclusive benefit has been proved so far, but some long-term survivors have been reported and further studies should be encouraged. The paucity of information available on adjuvant chemotherapy for hilar CC precludes any conclusions as to its value.

### 1.3 Squamous Carcinoma

Adenosquamous and pure squamous cell carcinomas of the liver are extremely rare. Very few cases have been reported in adults (age range 44–85 years) of either sex. Since they may contain adenomatous and squamous elements, terms such as *adenosquamous carcinoma*, *adenoacanthoma*, or *mucoepidermoid carcinoma* have been used. Being considered a subtype of cholangiocarcinoma, they may arise from congenital hepatic cysts. Fever and abdominal pain, related to cholangitis, are the most prominent symptoms. A single cystic mass may be seen on CT. Prognosis is poor, with a median survival of 4.5 months (range 1–17 months), because of widespread metastases. There is no effective treatment, although radiotherapy may prolong survival [34].

### 1.4 Epithelioid Hemangioendothelioma

The term *epithelioid hemangioendothelioma* (EHE) was first proposed in 1982 by WEISS and ENZINGER [35] in soft tissue tumors because tumor cells resembled epithelial cells. Although hepatic metastases have been reported, liver involvement usually occurs as a primary tumor. Since the original report in 1984 by ISHAK et al. [36] of a series of 32 cases involving the liver, several new cases have been described.

The age at presentation ranges from the second to the eight decade, with an average of 45 years. Women are more commonly affected than men (2:1). Upper abdominal pain, weight loss, weakness, anorexia, nausea, vomiting, and jaundice are the most prominent clinical signs, although some patients remain asymptomatic. Increased white blood cell count and elevated serum alkaline phosphatase activity are common laboratory abnormalities [36]. AFP is normal. A relationship between oral contraceptive use and hepatic EHE has been suggested [37].

Lesions are generally multiple, involving both lobes of the liver. Plain radiographs of the abdomen frequently reveal multiple calcific densities. US studies show well-defined hypoechoic nodules which apear as areas of low attenuation on CT scans. Multiple "filling defects" appear on liver scintigrams. Selective hepatic arteriograms disclose hypovascular masses with mild neovascularity [38]. As the lesions become larger, a diffuse mass of low attenuation may be seen on CT scans. Since none of the above findings are suggestive of a vascular tumor, guided liver biopsy is essential for diagnosis.

Microscopically, two types of cells are recognized: dendritic and epithelioid. They infiltrate the parenchyma along the sinusoids and intrahepatic veins and form vessels within an abundant fibrous matrix, which may undergo calcification. Histopathologic diagnosis is frequently difficult; the presence of cytoplasmic inclusions reminiscent of Weibel-Palade bodies, a marker of normal endothelial cells, and the demonstration of factor VIII-related antigen in neoplastic cells are essential for confirmation of the vascular nature of the tumor [36].

Prognosis is unpredictable and extrahepatic metastases are frequent. Most patients experience long survival, but fatal, rapidly progressive disease may occur. Since chemotherapy is not effective, hepatic resection or orthotopic liver transplantation might be considered [37–39]. The efficacy of transcatheter arterial embolization has yet to be proven.

### 1.5 Angiosarcoma

Although angiosarcoma is the most frequent malignant mesenchymal tumor of the liver, few cases are diagnosed each year. In the United States 168 cases were identified during the period 1964–1974 [40]. The tumor affects middle-aged adults, with a male to female ratio of 4:1 [41].

The multicenter survey cited above [40] shows that in the vast majority (75%) of hepatic angiosarcomas the cause is unknown. In 42 out of 168 cases, the development of the tumor was related to toxic exposure to thorium dioxide (20 cases), vinyl chloride (12 cases), inorganic arsenic (6 cases), and androgenic anabolic steroids (4 cases). Latent periods between exposure and the appearance of the tumor are usually long; the length of the latent period depends on the iatrogenic agent and may vary from 6 to 36 years [42]. The carcinogenic capacity of vinyl chloride is supported by experimental evidence. In addition, vinyl chloride workers show an increased risk of developing acro-osteolysis, scleroderma-like lesions, and Raynaud's syndrome[43]. Moreover, most of the agents cited above have also been related to the production of sinusoidal dilatation, peliosis hepatis, and perisinusoidal fibrosis with portal hypertension [43, 44]. Other agents such as radium, external radiation, copper sulfate, estrogens, oral contraceptives, and phenelzine have also been incriminated in the pathogenesis of angiosarcoma [42, 44].

According to Ishak [42], presenting complaints are abdominal pain, anorexia, nausea, weight loss, fever, hepatomegaly, or ascites in 62% of patients, hemoperitoneum due to rupture of the tumor in 15%, splenomegaly in 5%, and pulmonary or skeletal metastases in 9%. The patient is often jaundiced. Thrombocytopenia (mostly due to platelet entrapment within the tumor), altered sulfobromophthalein retention, elevated serum alkaline phosphatase, and prolonged prothrombin time are usually present [41, 42]. Splenomegaly, secondary to portal hypertension, is a common finding. Plain radiographs of the abdomen may show tumor calcification or hepatosplenic radiopaque deposits of thorium dioxide in Thorotrast-related cases. Although isotope or CT scans may disclose the tumor within the liver, arteriography is the most valuable technique for diagnosis. Main hepatic arteries are of normal size; the tumor shows a characteristic circumferential stain at the periphery, which persists for seconds, while the central area remains radiolucent [41, 45]. Percutaneous biopsy or fine-needle aspiration cytology is contraindicated because of the vascular nature of the tumor and the risk of massive bleeding.

The tumor is usually multicentric and macroscopically appears as large, blood-filled cysts. In drug-related angiosarcomas, the premalignant stage is characterized by hyperplasia of hepatocytes and endothelial cells, sinusoidal dilatation, and perisinusoidal fibrosis. Later on, the neoplastic overgrowth of spindle-shaped, sinusoidal cells leads to the formation of solid nodules that undergo cavitation and hemorrhage [46].

Angiosarcoma is rapidly fatal, death occurring within a few months. Effective treatment is not available, although hepatic resection, when possible, or chemotherapy may prolong survival [41]. Orthotopic liver transplantation in five cases has been unsuccessful [31].

### 1.6 Kaposi's Sarcoma

The clinical presentation of Kaposi's sarcoma (KS) ranges from the indolent skin lesion affecting the lower extremities of elderly men of Mediterranean origin, to the aggressive systemic form seen in African adolescents, patients receiving immunosuppressive therapy, and AIDS cases. Liver involvement usually occurs in the course of multivisceral dissemination of the disease [47].

Kaposi's sarcoma is the most common intrahepatic neoplasm in AIDS, being found in 14%–37% of postmortems on patients who have died of AIDS [48]. There are no specific symptoms, and the majority of the cases of hepatic KS are diagnosed at the time of autopsy. Abdominal pain and/or hepatomegaly may be present. Liver function tests are normal or show anicteric cholestasis [48, 49]. The appearance of liver KS on US, CT, and scintigraphy is nonspecific [50]. Nevertheless, in a patient with known KS of other sites, liver involvement is to be strongly suspected if hyperechoic areas are present on US. Baseline CT shows hypodense nodules with contrast enhancement on delayed scans [51]. Guided liver biopsy does not always confirm the diagnosis [50]. Histopathologically, multiple lesions are present within the liver; they are mainly found in the portal areas and resemble those seen in other sites.

Since KS of the liver generally appears in the disseminated form of the disease, the treatment of choice is chemotherapy. Nevertheless, in patients with AIDS, liver involvement by KS does not in itself modify the overall prognosis of the underlying disease [47].

### 1.7 Fibrosarcoma

Fibrosarcoma of the liver is a rare tumor predominantly found in adult males. There are no specific symptoms, although severe hypoglycemia is present in a small number of cases. Since the tumor is usually large at the time of diagnosis, an abdominal mass may be palpable on examination. Intratumoral necrosis and hemorrhage are frequently found, although hemoperitoneum is rare. Microscopically, the tumor is characterized by spindle-shaped cells with collagen fibers showing a herring-bone pattern [42]. Vimentin is positive and, on electron microscopy, cells are rich in rough endoplasmic reticulum without a basement membrane [52]. Prognosis is poor but surgical resection and/or radiotherapy may improve survival [42].

### 1.8 Leiomyosarcoma

A few cases of primary leiomyosarcoma of the liver have been reported. Adult women are more frequently affected. The presenting symptoms are nonspecific. The tumor usually arises as a solitary mass with a gross and microscopic appearance resembling similar tumors from other sites. The poor natural prognosis may improve after surgical resection [42].

### 1.9 Malignant Fibrous Histiocytoma

Malignant fibrous histiocytoma of the liver is an extremely rare tumor of adulthood. Abdominal discomfort may be the presenting symptom. Single or multiple lesions may be present. The tumor is usually large (more than 6 cm in diameter) at the time of diagnosis. The broad range of histologic patterns makes it difficult to establish its origin (histiocytes, fibroblasts, undifferentiated mesenchymal cells). Prognosis is poor in most patients [53].

### 1.10 Lymphoma

Although liver involvement in stage IV lymphomas is the rule, primary lymphomas of the liver are not frequent. They affect adults of any age, with a male predominance of 2:1. AIDS patients show an increased risk for this malignancy [50]. Pain in the right upper quadrant, malaise, fever, and night sweats are the presenting symptoms. The tumor may appear as a solitary mass, although multiple masses and diffuse types have been reported. In most cases, the tumor is a large cell non-Hodgkin's lymphoma, usually of the B type. After hepatic resection and/or polychemotherapy, complete remission has been achieved in some cases [54].

## 2 Benign Liver Tumors of Adulthood

### 2.1 Hepatocellular Adenoma

A rarity until the advent of oral contraceptives in 1960, hepatocellular adenoma (HCA) is still an uncommon tumor that usually appears as a solitary nodule larger than 5 cm in diameter, although multiple and smaller lesions may be observed. The vast majority of HCAs appear in females taking oral contraceptives. Microscopically, the tumor consists of normal or near-normal hepatocytes arranged in cords or sheets with thin-walled vascular channels scattered throughout the lesion and scantly Kupffer cells. Bile ducts and portal areas are absent.

Hepatocellular adenoma may be an incidental finding or appear as an abdominal mass but most frequently patients seek attention for mild abdominal pain. Some 30%–50% of tumors present with hemorrhage either into the tumor or into the abdominal cavity, an unpredictable complication with a mortality of about 6% (Fig. 3).

There is strong evidence of a causal relationship between the use of oral contraceptives and the development of HCA, the risk increasing with the duration of use and the dose of hormones in the preparation [55]. Nevertheless, the pathogenetic mechanisms by which oral contraceptives induce the development and growth of HCA remain unknown. HCA has also been reported in a variety of conditions associated with high levels of exogenous or endogenous sex steroids, including long-term administration of noncontraceptive estrogens or anabolic steroids (mostly 17-alkylated androgens), hormone-secreting ovarian tumors, polycystic ovary, and partial androgen resistance. HCA is a common late complication of type 1 glycogenosis, in which hyperglucagonemia may play a role.

The term *liver adenomatosis* has recently been proposed for a syndrome consisting of multiple (arbitrarily >10) hepatic adenomas occurring in patients without a history of steroid use or glycogenosis and with frequent alterations in liver function tests [56]. Whether this syndrome is actually a separate entity or not awaits clarification.

The natural history of HCA is poorly understood since large series of patients followed up without resection are lacking. Withdrawal from oral contraceptives and dietary therapy for glycogenosis are likely to result in regression of most HCAs, but some tumors may grow and/or bleed despite discontinuation of oral contraceptive use. Pregnancy may induce HCAs to

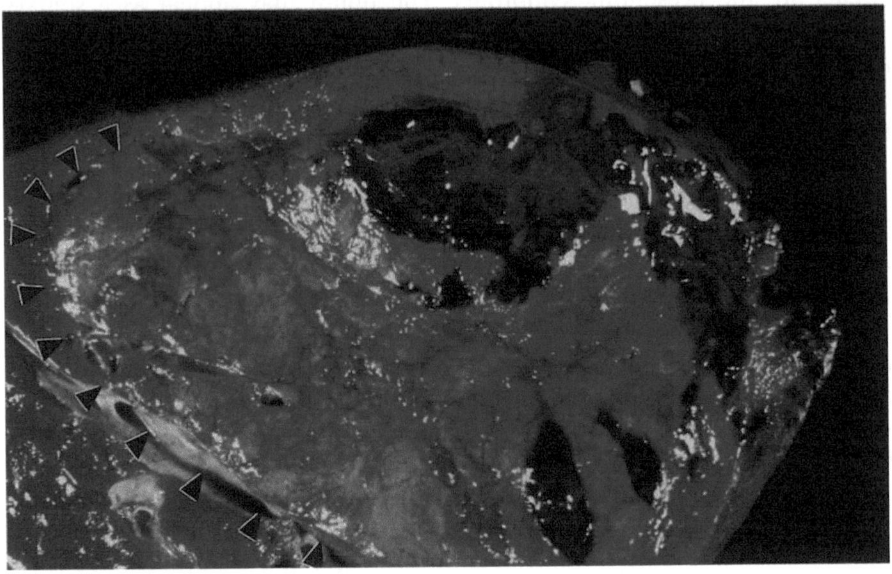

**Fig. 3.** Ruptured hepatocellular adenoma. *Arrowheads* indicate the internal limits of the lesion

grow, to become symptomatic, or to rupture. Regarding hemorrhage, most bleeding tumors are larger than 10 cm in diameter, but it should be taken into account that hemorrhage into the tumor may cause the size to be overestimated. Malignant transformation into hepatocellular carcinoma has been suggested to be an exceedingly rare complication of HCA, but conclusive evidence of such transformation is still lacking.

A confident preoperative diagnosis of HCA can be difficult to achieve. Anemia and/or abnormal liver function tests are almost exclusively found in bleeding tumors. HCA usually appears as a defect on $^{99m}$Tc scintigraphy, heterogeneous with a mixed echo pattern on US, hypodense with varying degrees of contrast enhancement on CT, heterogeneous and hyperintense on T2-weighted MRI, and hypervascular with frequent hypovascular areas on angiography. However, the detection of fresh blood on CT and MRI subsequent to acute hemorrhage is the only imaging feature highly suggestive of HCA. In many instances, imaging studies cannot reliably distinguish HCA from focal nodular hyperplasia or well-differentiated hepatocellular carcinoma. If the initial suspicion of HCA or focal nodular hyperplasia is strong, laparotomy should be preferred to needle biopsy because of its accuracy and safety.

The therapeutic approach to a patient with known or suspected HCA remains controversial. Avoidance of pregnancy and of the use of oral contraceptives is mandatory. The indication for surgery is clear in patients presenting with intraperitoneal hemorrhage. The reported high incidence of resectability and the low mortality and morbidity of elective resection make it appropriate to perform surgical resection of single, large, complicated or easily resectable tumors [57]. By contrast, for small, multiple, asymptomatic or anatomically unfavorable tumors, withdrawal of oral contraceptives and careful follow-up are likely to be a sensible policy, surgery being reserved for those tumors that fail to involute. Arterial embolization is an alternative to surgery for actively bleeding tumors and, in the case of large HCAs, may result in a preoperative reduction in tumor size.

## 2.2 Focal Nodular Hyperplasia

Focal nodular hyperplasia (FNH) is a rare entity that may appear in either sex at any age, although it has been more commonly reported in middle-aged females. FNH is usually a solitary, well-defined lesion with a characteristic central stellate scar (containing large arteries and bile ductular proliferation) (Fig. 4). Fibrous septa with mononuclear cell infiltration radiate from the central scar and surround nodules of normal-appearing hepatocytes. Unlike hepatocellular adenoma, FNH is usually a small lesion. Although its pathogenesis is still a matter of controversy, there is increasing evidence to suggest that a vascular malformation with secondarily altered sinusoidal blood flow is the primary event in the development of FNH [58]. Sex hormones do not seem to cause FNH but may eventually stimulate its growth.

Focal nodular hyperplasia is usually an incidental finding but a few patients may complain of abdominal pain or have a palpable mass or hepatomegaly. Reports of rupture and hemorrhage of FNH are exceedingly rare, and malignant transformation has not been demonstrated. A definite diagnosis nevertheless must be made because of the risk of mistaking FNH for hepatocellular adenoma or carcinoma. A variable proportion of cases of FNH (30%–70% in the available series) show normal or increased uptake on $^{99m}$Tc scintigraphy, a distinctive finding never so far reported in malignancies. FNH usually appears homogeneously hypo- or hyperechoic on US, hypodense on CT, homogeneous and isointense on T2-weighted MRI, and hypervascular on angiography. However, either US or CT may be normal in 15%–50% of cases. A central stellate scar is an uncommon but highly characteristic imaging feature that cannot be regarded as pathognomonic since it has also been reported in hepatocellular carcinoma. Although uncommon, the combination of a hypervascular lesion on angiography and normal or increased uptake on radioisotope imaging is nearly specific for FNH. Laparotomy is indicated if diagnosis remains uncertain after imaging procedures. Surgical resection is only warranted for symptomatic tumors.

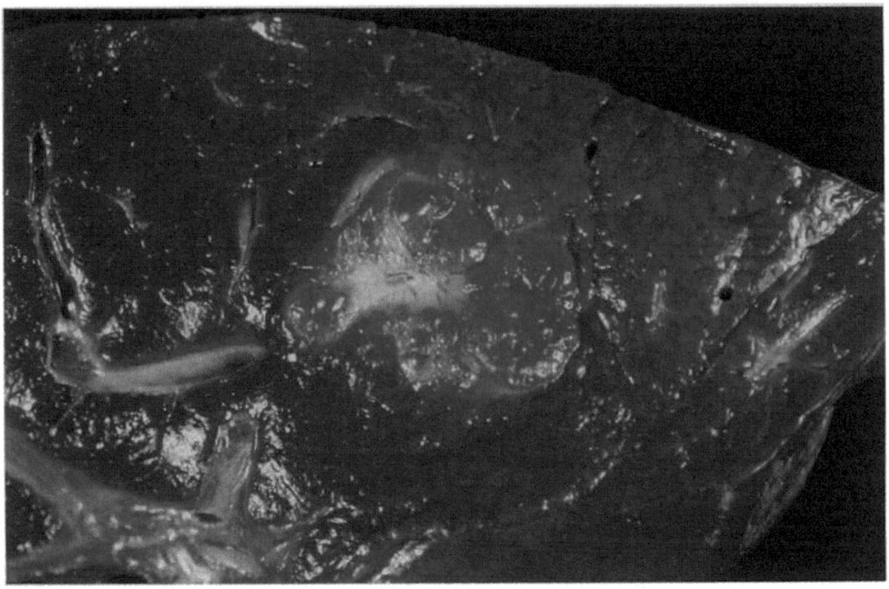

**Fig. 4.** Focal nodular hyperplasia with the characteristic central white scar

## 2.3 Nodular Regenerative Hyperplasia

Nodular regenerative hyperplasia (NRH) is an uncommon condition characterized by diffuse nodularity of the liver with little or no fibrosis. No age or sex predominance has been reported. There is a striking association between NRH and a wide variety of extrahepatic chronic diseases, especially myeloproliferative disorders (agnogenic myeloid metaplasia, polycythemia vera, primary thrombocytopenia, chronic myeloid leukemia), lymphoproliferative disorders (Hodgkin's and non-Hodgkin's lymphoma, chronic lymphocytic leukemia, Waldenström's disease, benign monoclonal gammapathy), immunologic diseases (rheumatoid arthritis, Felty's syndrome, progressive systemic systemic sclerosis, CRST syndrome, lupus erythematosus, lymphocytic thyroiditis, polyarteritis nodosa, cryoglobulinemia, myasthenia gravis, idiopathic thrombocytopenic purpura, Goodpasture's syndrome, polymyalgia rheumatica), and a miscellaneous group (toxic oil syndrome, massive metastatic carcinoma, bone marrow and renal transplant recipients usually receiving azathioprine) [59].

Two major theories have been proposed to explain the pathogenesis of NRH. The first regards NRH as a neoplastic process. The similarity between NRH and the nodules observed in experimental carcinogenesis in animals and the frequent history of drug therapy for the underlying disease (mainly corticosteroids and cytotoxic agents) suggest such a neoplastic nature. The second theory proposes a vascular origin of this lesion. A reduction in the number and size of portal vein branches has frequently been found in NRH. It has thus been theorized that decreased portal flow causes atrophy of the supplied acini, and that secondary hyperplasia of the intact acini will lead to nodule formation [59]. The primary event causing portal vein occlusion would be arteritis with secondary portal vein involvement in those cases associated with immune complex disorders or monoclonal gammapathy, and thrombosis in some hematologic diseases. According to this theory, portal hypertension would be the result of such occlusive venopathy rather than a consequence of the compression of the portal vein branches by the nodules themselves.

Sometimes NRH appears as an incidental finding at laparotomy or autopsy, but it may be associated with features of portal hypertension and subclinical cholestasis. The rupture of a nodule causing hemoperitoneum can be the first symptom of the disease.

Although NRH may be suspected from the appropriate clinical background, definite diagnosis relies on the demonstration of its characteristic pathologic features. The gross appearance of NRH is that of a finely nodular liver. The nodules are usually less than 1 cm in diameter, even though larger nodules resembling adenoma may be seen. Microscopically, they consist of normal or near-normal hepatocytes, often arranged in plates two or three cells thick. The hepatocytes between the nodules are atrophic and some degree of fibrosis may be observed in the portal areas; however, unlike in cirrhosis, nodularity always outweighs fibrosis. Nodularity is best disclosed by the reticulin stain and can be missed in small specimens. Hence, needle biopsy specimens may be misdiagnosed as either normal liver or micronodular cirrhosis. If needle biopsy is inconclusive, laparotomy and wedge biopsy are indicated.

Portocaval shunt is better tolerated than in cirrhosis and should be considered for symptomatic portal hypertension. Liver transplantation is rarely indicated because of the frequently associated systemic diseases.

### 2.4 Bile Duct Adenoma

Bile duct adenoma is an uncommon and usually solitary, small tumor. In most cases it appears as an unsuspected focal lesion incidentally detected during abdominal imaging or surgery for other indications or at necropsy. Its only clinical significance is the risk of confusion with a well-differentiated adenocarcinoma, although the absence of dysplasia and mitosis and the lack of desmoplastic fibrosis in the fibrous supporting stroma help to differentiate these entities.

## 2.5 Biliary Microhamartoma (Meyenburg Complex)

Meyenburg complexes are small, usually multiple lesions composed of dilated ductal structures embedded in connective tissue. Pathogenetically, they result from the arrest of development or wrong remodeling of the primitive ductal plate. Meyenburg complexes are regarded as a form of the adult-type fibropolycystic disease of the liver and may coexist with other features of such disease (e.g., Caroli's disease or congenital hepatic fibrosis) [60].

These lesions show no predilection for either sex, tend to be diagnosed in mid-adult life, and are almost always incidental findings upon laparotomy, abdominal imaging, or necropsy. However, they may be mistaken for metastatic disease to the liver, especially in the rare instances associated with abnormal liver function tests. In even rarer cases, Meyenburg complexes have been reported to result in portal hypertension or to display progression to carcinoma.

## 2.6 Biliary Cystadenoma

Biliary cystadenoma is a rare, cystic tumor of the liver or less frequently of the extrahepatic biliary system. It predominantly affects middle-aged females. Symptoms are the rule and depend on the size and location of the tumor, with abdominal pain and enlargement being the most frequent. Complications include biliary obstruction leading to jaundice or cholangitis, rupture, intracystic hemorrhage, and compression of adjacent organs.

Characteristically, the tumor is a large multilocular cyst, containing a clear to mucinous or gelatinous fluid. US and CT features do not allow differentiation from other benign cystic liver diseases or cystic metastases. Therefore, definite preoperative diagnosis may be difficult.

Biliary cystadenoma shows a high recurrence rate (nearly 100% for tumors not radically resected) and frequently undergoes malignant transformation [61]. Thus, an aggressive therapeutic attitude for this histologically benign tumor is warranted. Liver transplantation should be considered for unresectable tumors.

## 2.7 Biliary Papillomatosis

In biliary papillomatosis, of which less than 20 cases have been reported, multiple papillary adenomas (usually sessile) grow anywhere in the extra- or intrahepatic bile ducts and cause obstructive jaundice and secondary ascending infection and/or liver failure [62]. Occasionally, the tumors may transform into adenocarcinoma. Radical resection is efficacious when one single lobe is affected.

## 2.8 Hemangioma

Hemangioma is the most common benign hepatic tumor, with an estimated prevalence in the general population of 1%–5%. Hemangioma is more frequently found in adults and can be multiple in up to 20% of patients. Microscopically, it consists of vascular channels lined by endothelial cells and separated by a fibrous tissue. This tumor seems to grow by ectasia rather than by hyperplasia or hypertrophy.

Very little is known about the etiology of hemangioma. A possible role of steroid hormones in its pathogenesis is suggested by several observations, namely: (a) a consistent female predominance is found in the case of larger tumors; (b) tumor enlargement and recurrence after resection have been observed in hysterectomized women under estrogen replacement therapy and in patients who have continued to use oral contraceptives; (c) tumor enlargement has also been reported during pregnancy or after multiple pregnancies; (d) the association of hemangioma and focal nodular hyperplasia appears to be restricted to patients taking oral contraceptives. Nevertheless, sex hormones seem to favor tumor growth and complications rather than to play a causative role [63, 64, 65]. Hemangiomas are frequent among patients with tuberous sclerosis.

Symptoms rarely appear except in the case of so-called giant hemangioma (≥4 cm in diameter); they then consist of mild pain, hepatomegaly, or a palpable mass. Hemorrhage is life threatening but is an exceedingly uncommon complication.

An increasing number of hemangiomas are detected upon abdominal imaging for other indications and have to be differentiated from other asymptomatic focal hepatic diseases, especially occult malignancy. Thus, accurate, noninvasive diagnosis has become a major challenge. On US, hemangioma usually appears as a well-defined and homogeneously hyperechoic lesion, a pattern that is highly characteristic for tumors smaller than 3 cm. Dynamic CT usually shows contrast enhancement from the periphery of a hypodense lesion. Planar imaging or single-photon emission computed tomography (SPECT) using radiolabeled red blood cells may reveal the specific feature of slow filling and increased pool activity at 1–2 h. MRI findings are also highly characteristic when a hyperintense and homogeneous lesion is detected on heavily T2-weighted scans. Arteriographic features include nondilated arteries and delayed filling of the vascular lakes that gives a cotton wool appearance to the tumor.

In the workup of a focal lesion suspected to be a hemangioma, US diagnosis should be considered reliable when a single, small lesion is found in an otherwise healthy individual with normal liver function tests. For multiple or larger lesions or whenever any single study may be equivocal, the rational use of CT, MRI, and especially SPECT, either alone or in combination, can obviate the need for invasive procedures [66]. US follow-up is, however, sensible to confirm the diagnosis. Several reports have recently vindicated US-guided fine-needle aspiration biopsy of hemangioma as a safe procedure [67]. Unfortunately, the material obtained is usually too scanty to yield a definite diagnosis.

The natural history of hemangioma is still debated. The available reports on long-term follow-up of symptomless patients indicate that hemangioma seldom becomes symptomatic or grows. A conservative policy has thus been advocated for asymptomatic hemangioma, irrespective of its size. Surgery is restricted to complicated lesions and to cases in which the diagnosis is uncertain. Transcatheter arterial embolization is an alternative therapy for bleeding or symptomatic tumors, especially when surgery carries a high risk.

### 2.9 Lymphangiomatosis

Lymphangiomatosis is a rare congenital malformation of the lymphatic system that may affect the liver either alone or in combination with other organs, occasionally causing massive enlargement and liver failure. Liver transplantation has been carried out in one such case, with a favorable outcome [68].

### 2.10 Peliosis Hepatis

In peliosis hepatis, blood-filled cysts of various sizes appear scattered throughout the liver. The condition was first observed in patients with wasting diseases but in recent years it has increasingly been associated with a number of drug therapies, especially anabolic steroids. The pathogenesis is still unclear but focal hepatocellular necrosis, toxic endothelial injury, and obstruction of blood flow at the junction of sinusoids and centrilobular veins have all been proposed as possible primary events [46]. Peliosis hepatis frequently represents an incidental histologic finding but may become a clinically apparent disorder causing hepatomegaly, portal hypertension, hemoperitoneum, or liver failure.

### 2.11 Lipomatous Tumors

Lipomatous tumors of the liver include a number of rare benign neoplasms that contain fat in diverse combinations with other mesenchymal tissues such as hematopoietic tissue (*myelolipomas*), blood vessels alone (*angiolipomas*), or blood vessels together with smooth muscle (*angiomyolipomas*) or hematopoietic tissue (*angiomyelolipomas*) or both (*angiomyomyelolipomas*). They tend to be asymptomatic but mild elevations of liver function tests and pain derived from hemorrhage have been described. Sometimes they may appear as palpable masses. Lipomatous tumors are easily detectable by US and/or CT [69].

### 2.12 Other Mesenchymal or Mixed Tumors and Tumor-like Lesions

*Fibrous Mesotheliomas.* Fibromas grow attached to the surface of the liver and may reach a large size. Histologically, they consist of spindled fibroblast-like cells and collagen.

*Leiomyomas.* Benign smooth muscle tumors have been reported to arise in the liver.

*Benign Teratoma.* Tumors containing tissues derived from all three germ layers have also been described in the liver, sometimes coexisting with teratomas at other sites. They often present as a palpable mass.

*Inflammatory Pseudotumors.* A few tumor-like hepatic lesions histologically resembling inflammatory pseudotumors of other locations have been reported. Systemic symptoms such as fever, weight loss, and anemia are almost invariably present and may give rise to suspicion of an abscess [70]. The characteristic mesenchymal proliferation has caused some cases to be mistaken for sarcomas. Although different hypotheses have been proposed, the pathogenesis of inflammatory pseudotumors remains obscure.

*Miscellaneous.* Adrenal rest tumors and pancreatic heterotopia have presented as liver masses on rare occasions.

## 3 Liver Tumors of Childhood

Primary malignancies of the liver are rare in childhood. They account for 0.5%–2% of all pediatric tumors. The review by Weinberg and Finegold [71] of 1237 primary liver tumors in children showed that 43% (532 cases) were hapatoblastomas, 23% (284 cases) hepatocarcinomas, 13% (166 cases) benign vascular tumors, 6% (79 cases) sarcomas, 6% (75 cases) mesenchymal hamartomas, 2% (22 cases) adenomas, 2% (22 cases) focal nodular hyperplasia, and 5% (57 cases) other tumors. From this large series it is also evident that more than two-thirds of primary liver tumors in childhood are malignant. Most tumors cited above have already been described in this chapter. Because of their characteristic incidence in children, undifferentiated sarcoma, embryonal rhabdomyosarcoma, hepatoblastoma, mesenchymal hamartoma, and infantile hemangioendothelioma deserve special mention.

### 3.1 Undifferentiated Sarcoma

Primary undifferentiated sarcomas (also called embryonal sarcomas) are an exceptional form of hepatic tumor that in the vast majority of cases develop in children under 15 years of age. Common presenting symptoms and signs include abdominal pain and hepatomegaly, as well as unspecific general features such as fever, weight loss, and nausea. Liver function tests are normal or slightly altered. α-Fetoprotein is always normal [72]. Abdominal US and CT disclose the frequently mixed solid–cystic character of the tumor, which in most cases appears as a large and solitary hypovascular mass on arteriography. The right lobe of the liver is preferentially affected. Liver biopsy is essential for diagnosis [73].

Light microscopy shows poorly differentiated, irregularly shaped cells with eosinophilic, PAS-positive, diastase-resistant globules in the cytoplasm. Atypical mitoses are frequent [72].

There is no effective treatment and median survival is less than 1 year. A combination of surgery and polychemotherapy may improve survival [73].

### 3.2 Embryonal Rhabdomyosarcoma

Rhabdomyosarcoma of the biliary tree particularly affects children under 5 years old, with no sex predominance. Intermittent obstructive jaundice is the clinical presentation. Abdominal distention and fever are common symptoms, and the child is frequently diagnosed as having hepatitis. The obstructive nature of the jaundice is an important clue to the disease. Enlargement of the liver due to biliary obstruction is common. US and CT scans show a mass in the porta hepatis. An adequate combination of surgery, radiotherapy, and chemotherapy is essential to prolong survival [74].

### 3.3 Hepatoblastoma

Hepatoblastoma is the most common liver tumor of childhood, affecting children under 3 years of age. Males predominate in a ratio of 1.5:1. Frequently the child remains asymptomatic and is brought to the physician because of abdominal distention or hepatomegaly. Weight loss, anorexia, and fever are present in up to 20% of cases. An abdominal mass, most commonly in the right lobe of the liver, is the presenting finding [71]. Several clinical entities (corporeal hemihypertrophy, Meckel's diverticulum, Beckwith-Wiedemann syndrome, fetal alcohol syndrome, etc.) have been reported in association with the tumor.

Changes in liver function tests are non-specific, but high levels of serum α-fetoprotein are found in 80% of hepatoblastomas. Although of no prognostic value at the time of diagnosis, levels of α-fetoprotein correlate closely with the course of the tumor. Plain radiographs may show calcific densities in up to 15% of cases. US and CT disclose a hyperechoic, hyperdense single mass, which appears hypervascular on arteriograms. Pulmonary or skeletal metastases may be present.

Two histologic patterns have been recognized: epithelial and mixed epithelial and mesenchymal. Epithelial hepatoblastoma contains fetal and embryonic cells. Fetal cells are polyhedral, similar to normal hepatocytes but smaller in size, well defined, and showing an acidophilic cytoplasm. Mitoses are infrequent. Bile canaliculi may be seen between fetal-type cells. Extramedullary hematopoiesis in sinusoidal areas is consistently associated with this cell type. Embryonic cells are small, elongated, and hyperchromatic. They form tubular or rosette-like structures. Mitoses are more frequent. Mixed epithelial–mesenchymal hepatoblastoma shows, in addition to epithelial cells, spindle-shaped cells similar to young fibroblasts. Osteoid and cartilaginous foci are common [75].

Surgical resection, when possible, is the only hope for long-term survival or cure. At the time of diagnosis, 39%–70% of the tumors are unresectable, and preoperative chemotherapy may be used in order to reduce the size of the lesion and to permit resection [75, 76]. If surgery is not feasible, prognosis is poor because of rapidly progressive disease.

### 3.4 Mesenchymal Hamartoma

Mesenchymal hamartoma is a rare tumor-like lesion that probably represents an abnormal growth of mesenchymal tissue in and surrounding the portal vein areas with secondary cystic changes. Most cases appear in early childhood as an abdominal mass that grows due to fluid accumulation within the cystic component [77]. US and CT show a mixed but predominantly cystic mass that is occasionally unilocular. Mesenchymal hamartoma has not been reported to undergo malignant transformation. Cyst drainage or marsupialization should be considered whenever resection may have a high operative risk.

### 3.5 Infantile Hemangioendothelioma

Infantile hemangioendothelioma is a histologically benign tumor of early infancy (90% of cases are diagnosed in the first 6 months of life) with potentially fatal complications [78]. It can be single or multicentric and is easily detectable by US, CT, and angiography. Associated cutaneous hemangiomas are rather frequent. Symptoms are present in approximately half the patients and include hepatomegaly and/or abdominal mass, bleeding disorders, jaundice, and high-output congestive heart failure due to arteriovenous shunt through the tumor. The actual incidence of the latter is controversial (reports ranging from 8% to 65%), but it carries the poorest prognosis. As many as 70% of symptomatic patients may die from intractable heart failure, consumptive coagulopathy, tumor rupture, and hemorrhage or liver failure. In asymptomatic cases or when life-threatening complications can be avoided, spontaneous self-involution is the rule. Corticosteroids, arterial embolization, hepatic artery ligation, low-dose irradiation, and surgical resection have all been tried as alternative therapies with variable results.

## 4 Tumors of the Gallbladder

### 4.1 Primary Carcinoma of the Gallbladder

Gallbladder carcinoma (GBC) is the most frequent malignancy of the biliary tract. The incidence of GBC is highest in the 7th decade of life, and women outnumber men in a ratio of 3:1. In addition a higher incidence of GBC has been reported in a number of ethnic groups, i.e., American Indians, Swedish, Japanese, and Mexicans.

#### *Pathogenesis*

Gallstones are a very common finding among patients with GBC. Their prevalence ranges from 79% in postmortem studies to 92% in surgical series [79]. However, patients with gallstones are not likely to be at risk for this tumor. Thus, in a prospective cohort study on 2583 patients with gallstones followed for a median of 13.5 years, only five individuals developed GBC [80]. In addition, attempts to induce GBC in animals by means of introducing gallstones or a wide variety of foreign bodies inside the gallbladder have consistently failed. In contrast, a number of chemicals, including nitrosamines, are able to induce GBC in animal experimentation. Interestingly, nitrosamines are used in the manufacture of rubber and a high incidence of GBC has been reported in workers in the rubber industry [81].

A close association has been suggested between anomalous pancreatobiliary ductal union and GBC. Anomalous union at a distance greater than 15 mm from the papilla of Vater (normally <5 mm) occurred in 16.7% of 96 patients with GBC but in only 2.8% of 641 patients with various other hepatobiliary and pancreatic diseases [82]. Regurgitation of pancreatic juice into the bile duct has been regarded as a possible pathogenetic factor in this anomaly.

### *Pathology*

Most GBCs are adenocarcinomas. The remainder include anaplastic carcinoma, squamous carcinoma, and adenoacanthoma. Several classifications of GBC have been proposed. Microscopically, GBC can be divided into three types: tubular adenocarcinoma, papillary adenocarcinoma, and undifferentiated carcinoma. Tubular adenocarcinoma is the most common form. Papillary adenocarcinoma may have a lower association with gallstones and a somewhat more favorable prognosis [83].

Gallbladder carcinoma frequently infiltrates adjacent organs, especially the liver, extrahepatic bile ducts, and gastrointestinal tract (duodenum and colon). Lymphatic spreading occurs early in the natural history of the disease. Accordingly, regional lymph node involvement is detected in some 40%–50% of patients at the time of operation [79]. Hematogenous dissemination appears in end-stage disease, with peritoneum and lungs being the most common sites of distant metastases.

### *Presentation and Diagnosis*

Gallbladder carcinoma is rather commonly an unsuspected finding at cholecystectomy indicated for symptomatic cholelithiasis or cholecystitis. In large series, the most frequent presenting symptoms are pain (85%), anorexia and weight loss (66%), jaundice (50%), and fever (20%) [79]. A palpable mass is a common finding upon examination. Most patients have a history of chronic cholecystitis with recent changes in the pattern of pain [84]. Some others present with malaise, anorexia, weight loss, and pain in the right upper abdominal quadrant. Finally, a minority have a picture of acute cholecystitis or progressive jaundice.

Laboratory studies often show varying degrees of cholestasis; in particular, elevated serum alkaline phosphatase is frequently observed. Anemia is found in about 20% of patients. Imaging procedures hardly ever distinguish early malignant transformation from chronic calculous cholecystitis. In advanced tumors, US and CT may disclose a mass replacing the gallbladder. Percutaneous transhepatic or endoscopic retrograde cholangiography may show the features of malignant stricture in jaundiced patients, but they lack specificity. As a result of the paucity of specific symptoms and the relatively low sensitivity of the available diagnostic tools, early recognition of GBC is a more than difficult task. Indeed, preoperative diagnosis is correct in less than 30% of cases [85]. As a general rule. GBC should be suspected whenever pain becomes continuous in a patient with a history of chronic cholecystitis or cholelithiasis.

Inflammatory complications are common and include hydrops, empyema, cholangitis, and liver abscess. Free perforation into the abdominal cavity with secondary peritonitis occurs in 5%–10% of cases [79]. Fistulization to the duodenum or colon may also be observed.

*Therapy and Prognosis*

The prognosis of GBC is dismal. In a review of 4658 patients reported in the literature, only 32% were found to bear resectable tumors [79]. Furthermore, when those tumors incidentally detected after cholecystectomy were excluded from analysis, the resectability rate dropped to 10%.

Survival averages 4–6 months from the time of diagnosis. In a large series including nearly 6000 patients, 1- and 5-year survival rates were 11.8% and 4%, respectively [84]. Of those patients submitted to potentially curative resections, only 16% survived more than 5 years. Furthermore, of patients with GBC first diagnosed by microscopic examination of gallbladders removed for presumed benign disease, only 22% were alive 5 years after surgery and all of them had tumors that did not infiltrate beyond the muscularis mucosae [86]. Early recognition and radical surgery (including adjacent liver resection and regional lymph node dissection) may help to improve the outcome in patients with GBC.

The few available trials on radiotherapy and chemotherapy of GBC have not shown any conclusive benefit. It has been suggested, however, that radical irradiation may offer some palliation [87]. So that new, possibly more effective treatments can be evaluated, patients should be encouraged to enter controlled studies.

## 4.2 Benign Tumors of the Gallbladder

Benign changes of the gallbladder have been extensively reviewed by Christensen and Ishak [88]. True benign tumors may be epithelial (papillary and nonpapillary adenoma, benign mixed tumor) or mesenchymal (hemangioma, lipoma, leiomyoma, myoblastoma, neurofibroma, paraganglioma). Benign pseudotumors include a number of nonneoplastic changes that may appear grossly as a mass, namely: hyperplasia (adenomatous and adenomyomatous), heterotopia (gastric, enteric, pancreatic, hepatic, adrenal, thyroid), polyposis (cholesterol, inflammatory), and a miscellaneous group (xanthogranulomatous inflammation, parasitic infestations).

Adenoma accounts for 20% of all true benign tumors. they can be single or multiple and may be associated with gallstones (33%) and/or cholecystitis (59%) [88]. Adenomas are most commonly pedunculated (88%) but may be sessile.

Adenomyomatosis is the most frequent of all benign tumors and commonly coexists with gallstones and cholecystitis. It is usually asymptomatic but may cause a dyspeptic syndrome.

## References


1. Parkin DM, Stiernward J, Mujr CS (1984) Estimates of the worldwide frequency of the twelve major cancers. Bull WHO 62:163–182
2. Rustgi VK, Hoofnagle JH, Dusheiko GM, Lotze MT (1988) NIH Conference. Hepatocellular carcinoma. Ann Intern Med 108:390–401
3. Muñoz N, Bosch X (1987) Epidemiology of hepatocellular carcinoma. In: Okuda K, Ishak K (eds) Neoplasms of the liver. Springer, Berlin Heidelberg New York Tokyo, pp 3–19
4. Bosch X, Muñoz N (1988) Prospects for epidemiological studies on hepatocellular cancer as a model for assessing viral and chemical interactions. In: Bartsch H, Hemminki K, O'Neill IK (eds). Methods for detecting DNA damaging agents in humans: applications in cancer epidemiology and prevention. IARC Scientific Publications 89 IARC, Lyon, pp 427–438
5. The WHO Collaborative Study of Neoplasms and Steroid Contraceptives (1989) Combined oral contraceptives and liver cancer. Int J Cancer 43:254–259
6. Beasley RP (1988) Hepatitis B virus. The major etiology of hepatocellular carcinoma. In: Fortner CJ, Rhoads JE (eds) Accomplishment in cancer research. J.B. Lippincott, Philadelphia, p 80
7. Schröder CH, Zentgraf H (1990) Hepatitis B virus related hepatocellular carcinoma: chronicity of infection – the opening to different pathways of urobiquent transformations? Biochim Biophy Acte 1032:137–156
8. Tabor E (1989) Hepatocellular carcinoma: possible etiologies in patients without serologic evidence of hepatitis B infection. J Med Virol 27:1–6
9. Colombo M, Kuo G, Choo QL et al. (1989) Prevalence of antibodies to hepatitis C virus in Italian patients with hepatocellular carcinoma. Lancet II:1006–1008
10. Sherlock S (1988) Hepatocellular carcinoma. in: Sherlock S (ed) Diseases of the liver and biliary system. Blackwell Scientific, Oxford, p 584
11. Johnson PJ, Williams R (1987) Cirrhosis and etiology of hepatocellular carcinoma. J Hepatol 4:140–147
12. Liver Cancer Study Group of Japan (1988) The general rules for the clinical and pathological study of primary liver cancer. Jpn J Surg 19:98–129
13. Sheu JC, Sung JL, Chen DS et al. (1985) Early detection of hepatocellular carcinoma by real-time ultrasonography. Cancer 56:660–666
14. Ebara M, Ohto M, Shinagawa T et al. (1986) Natural history of minute hepatocellular carcinoma smaller than 3 centimeters complicating cirrhosis. Gastroenterology 90:289–298
15. Cottone M, Virdone R, Fusco G et al. (1989) Asymptomatic hepatocellular carcinoma in Child's A cirrhosis. Gastroenterology 96:1566–1571
16. Okuda K, Ohtsuky T, Obata H et al. (1985) Natural history of hepatocellular carcinoma and prognosis in relation to treatment. Cancer 56:918–928
17. Okuda K (1987) Early recognition of hepatocellular carcinoma. Hepatology 6:729–738
18. London WT, McMahon BJ (1990) Summary of a workshop on screening for hepatocellular carcinoma. MMWR 39:619–621
19. Franco D, Capussotti L, Smadja C et al. (1990) Resection of hepatocellular carcinoma. Results in 72 European patients with cirrhosis. Gastroenterology 98:733–738
20. Olthoff KM, Millis JM, Rosvoe MH, Goldstein LI, Ramming KP, Busuttil RW (1990) Is liver transplantation justified for the treatment of hepatic malignancies?. Arch Surg 125:1261–1268
21. Lai C, Wu P, Chang G et al. (1988) Doxorubicin versus no antitumor therapy in inoperable hepatocellular carcinoma. A prospective randomized trial. Cancer 62:479–483

22. Sugihara S, Kojiro M (1987) Pathology of cholangiocarcinoma. In: Okuda K, Ishak K (eds) Neoplasms of the liver. Springer, Berlin Heidelberg New York Tokyo, pp 143–158
23. Dayton MT, Longwire WP, Tompkins RK (1983) Caroli's disease: A premalignant condition? Am J Surg 145:41–48
24. Voravud N, Foster CS, Gilbertson JA, Sikora K, Waxman J (1989) Oncogene expression in cholangiocarcinoma and in normal hepatic development. Hum Pathol 20:1163–1168
25. Tada M, Omata M, Ohto M (1990) Analysis of *ras* gene mutations in human hepatic malignant tumors by polymerase chain reaction and direct sequencing. Cancer Res 50:1121–1124
26. Rabinowitz M, Zajko AB, Hassanein T et al. (1990) Diagnostic value of brush cytology in the diagnosis of bile duct carcinoma: a study in 65 patients with bile duct strictures. Hepatology 12:747–752
27. Scudera PL, Koizumi J, Jacobson IM (1990) Brush cytology evaluation of lesions encountered during ERCP. Gastrointest Endosc 36:281–284
28. Boerma EJ (1990) Research into the results of resection of hilar bile duct cancer. Surgery 108:572–580
29. Hadjis NS, Bleukharn JI, Alexander N, Benjamin IS, Blumgart LH (1990) Outcome of radical surgery in hilar cholangiocarcinoma. Surgery 107:597–604
30. Langer JC, Langer B, Taylor BR, Zeldin R, Cummings B (1985) Carcinoma of the extrahepatic bile ducts: results of an aggressive surgical approach. Surgery 98:752–757
31. O'Grady JG, Polson RJ, Rolles K, Calne RY, Williams R (1988) Liver transplantation for malignant disease. Ann Surg 207:373–379
32. Devier J, Baize M, de Toeuf J, Cremer M (1988) Long-term follow-up of patients with hilar malignant stricture treated by endoscopic internal biliary drainage. Gastrointest Endosc 34:95–101
33. Launois B, Campion JP, Brissot P, Gosselin M (1979) Carcinoma of the hepatic hilus. Surgical management and the case for resection. Ann Surg 190:151–157
34. Tomioka T, Tsunoda T, Harada N et al. (1987) Adenosquamous carcinoma of the liver. Am J Gastroenterol 82:1203–1206
35. Weiss SW, Enzinger FM (1982) Epithelioid hemangioendothelioma. A vascular tumor often mistaken for carcinoma. Cancer 50:970–981
36. Ishak KG, Sesterhenn IA, Goodman MD, Rabin L, Stromeyer FW (1984) Epithelioid hemangioendothelioma of the liver: a clinico-pathologic and follow-up study of 32 cases. Hum Pathol 15:839–852
37. Kelleher MB, Iwatsuki S, Sheahan DG (1989) Epithelioid hemangioendothelioma of the liver. Clinico-pathological correlation of 10 cases treated by orthotopic liver transplantation. Am J Surg Pathol 13:999–1008
38. Furui S, Itai Y, Ohtomo K et al. (1989) Hepatic epithelioid hemangioendothelioma: report of five cases. Radiology 171:63–68
39. Scoazec JY, Lamy P, Degott C, Reynes M, Feldmann G, Bismuth H, Benhamou JP (1988) Epithelioid hemangioendothelioma of the liver. Diagnostic features and role of liver transplantation. Gastroenterology 94:1447–1453
40. Falk H, Herbert J, Crowley S et al. (1981) Epidemiology of hepatic angiosarcoma in the United States: 1964–1974. Environ Health Perspect 41:107–113
41. Locker GY, Doroshow JH, Zwelling LA, Chabner BA (1979) The clinical features of hepatic angiosarcoma: a report of four cases and a review of the English literature. Medicine (Baltimore) 58:48–64
42. Ishak KG (1987) Malignant mesenchymal tumors of the liver. In: Okuda K, Ishak K (eds) Neoplasms of the liver. Springer, Berlin Heidelberg New York Tokyo, pp 160–176

43. Thomas LB, Popper H, Berk P, Selikoff I, Falk H (1975) Vinyl-chloride-induced liver disease. From idiopathic portal hypertension (Banti's syndrome) to angiosarcomas. N Engl J Med 292:17–22
44. Zafrani ES, Pinaudeau Y, Dhumeaux D (1983) Drug-induced vascular lesions of the liver. Arch Intern Med 143:495–502
45. Dannaher CL, Tamburro CH, Yam LT (1981) Occupational carcinogenesis: the Louisville experience with vinyl chloride-associated hepatic angiosarcomas. Am J Med 70:279–287
46. Zafrani ES (1989) Update on vascular tumors of the liver. J Hepatol 8:125–130
47. Palmer M, Braly LF, Schaffner F (1987) The liver in acquired immunodeficiency disease. Semin Liver Dis 7:192–202
48. Hassan F, Jeffers L, Welsh S, Reddy R, Schiff E (1989) Hepatic involvement as the primary manifestation of Kaposi's sarcoma in the acquired immunodeficiency syndrome. Am J Gastroenterol 84:1449–1451
49. Glasgow B, Anders K, Layfield J, Steinsapir K, Gitnic J, Lewin K (1985) Clinical and pathological findings of the liver in the acquired immunodeficiency syndrome (AIDS). Am J Clin Pathol 83:582–588
50. Schneiderman D, Arenson D, Cello J, Margaretten W, Weber T (1987) Hepatic disease in patients with the acquired immunodeficiency syndrome (AIDS). Hepatology 7:925–930
51. Luburich P, Bru C, Ayuso MC, Azon A, Condom E (1990) Hepatic Kaposi sarcoma in AIDS: US and CT findings. Radiology 175:172–174
52. Nakahama M, Takanashi R, Yamazaki I, Machinami R (1989) Primary fibrosarçoma of the liver. Immunohistochemical and electron microscopic studies. Acta Pathol Jpn 39:814–820
53. Katsuda S, Kawahara E, Matsui Y, Ohyama S, Nakanishi I (1988) Malignant fibrous histiocytoma of the liver: a case report and review of the literature. Am J Gastroenterol 83:1278–1282
54. Ryan J, Straus DJ, Lange C et al. (1988) Primary lymphoma of the liver. Cancer 61:370–375
55. Rooks JB, Ory HW, Ishak KG et al. (1979) Epidemiology of hepatocellular adenoma. The role of contraceptive use. JAMA 242:644–648
56. Flejou JF, Barge J, Menu Y, Degott C, Bismuth H, Potet F, Benhamou JP (1985) Liver adenomatosis. Gastroenterology 89:1132–1138
57. Leese T, Farges O, Bismuth H (1988) Liver cell adenomas. A 12-year surgical experience from a specialist hepatobiliary unit. Ann Surg 208:558–564
58. Wanless I, Mawdsley C, Adams R (1985) On the pathogenesis of focal nodular hyperplasia of the liver. Hepatology 5:1194–1200
59. Wanless IR (1990) Micronodular transformation (nodular regenerative hyperplasia) of the liver: a report of 64 cases among 2500 autopsies and a new classification of benign hepatocellular nodules. Hepatology 11:787–797
60. Summerfield J, Nagafuchi Y, Sherlock S, Cadafalch J, Scheuer PJ (1986) Hepatobiliary fibropolycystic diseases. A clinical and histological review of 51 patients. J Hepatol 2:141–156
61. Wheeler DA, Edmonson HA (1985) Cystadenoma with mesenchymal stroma in the liver and bile ducts. A clinicopathologic study of 17 cases, 4 with malignant change. Cancer 56:1434–1445
62. Gouma DJ, Mutum SS, Benjamin IS, Blumgart LH (1984) Intrahepatic biliary papillomatosis. Br J Surg 71:72–74
63. Conter RL, Longmire WP (1988) Recurrent Hepatic hemangiomas. Possible association with estrogen therapy. Ann Surg 207:115–119
64. Klatskin G (1977) Hepatic tumors: possible relationship to oral contraceptives. Gastroenterology 73:386–394
65. Mathieu D, Zafrani ES, Anglade MC, Dhumeaux D (1989) Association of focal nodular hyperplasia and hepatic hemangioma. Gastroenterology 97:154–157

66. Bennet W, Bova J (1990) Review of hepatic imaging and a problem-oriented approach to liver masses. Hepatology 12:761–775
67. Solbiati L, Livraghi T, De Pra L, <ierace T, Masciadri N, Ravetto C (1985) Fine-needle biopsy of hepatic hemangioma with sonographic guidance. AJR 144:471–474
68. Miller CH, Mazzaferro V, Makowka L et al. (1988) Orthotopic liver transplantation for massive hepatic lymphangiomatosis. Surgery 103:490–495
69. Roberts JL, Fishman EK, Hartman DS, Sanders R, Goodman Z, Siegelman SS (1986) Lipomatous tumors of the liver: evaluation with CT and US. Radiology 158:613–617
70. Kessler E, Turani H, Kayser S, Bar-Ziv J, Chainofff C (1988) Inflammatory pseudotumor of the liver. Liver 8:17–23
71. Weinberg AG, Finegold MJ (1983) Primary hepatic tumors of childhood. Hum Pathol 14:512–537
72. Stocker JT, Ishak KG (1978) Undifferentiated (embryonal) sarcoma of the liver. Report of 31 cases. Cancer 42:336–348
73. Vetter D, Bellocq JP, Amaral D et al. (1989) Sarcomes indifferenciees (ou embryonnaires) hepatiques. Problemes diagnostiques et therapeutiques a propos d'un rhabdomyosarcome botryoide. Gastroenterol Clin Biol 13:98–103
74. Ruymann FB, Raney RB, Crist WM et al. (1985) Rhabdomyosarcoma of the biliary tree in childhood. A report from the intergroup rhabdomyosarcoma study. Cancer 56:575–581
75. Stocker JT, Ishak KG (1987) Hepatoblastoma. In: Okuda K, Ishak K (eds) Neoplasms of the liver. Springer, Berlin Heidelberg New York Tokyo, pp 128–136
76. Weinblatt ME, Siegel SE, Siegel MM et al. (1982) Preoperative chemotherapy for unresectable primary hepatic malignancies in children. Cancer 50:1061–1064
77. Stocker JT, Ishak KG (1983) Mesenchymal hamartoma of the liver. Report of 30 cases and review of the literature. Pediatr Pathol 1:245–267
78. Dehner LP, Ishak KG (1971) Vascular tumors of the liver in infants and children. Arch Pathol 92:101–111
79. Vaittinen E (1970) Carcinoma of the gallbladder. A study of 390 cases diagnosed in Finland 1953–1967. Ann Chir Gynaecol Fenn [Suppl] 168:1–81
80. Maringhini A, Moreau JA, Melton LJ, Hench VS, Zinsmeister AR, DiMagno EP (1987) Gallstones, gallbladder cancer, and other gastrointestinal malignancies. An epidemiologic study in Rochester, Minnesota. Ann Intern Med 107:30–35
81. Mancuso TF, Brennan MJ (1970) Epidemiological considerations of cancer of the gallbladder, bile ducts and salivary glands in the rubber industry. J Occup Med 12:333–341
82. Kimura K, Ohto M, Saisho H et al. (1985) Association of gallbladder carcinoma and anomalous pancreatobiliary ductal union. Gastroenterology 89:1258–1265
83. Hisatomi K, Haratake J, Horie A, Ohsato K (1990) Relation of histopathological features to prognosis of gallbladder cancer. Am J Gastroenterol 85:567–572
84. Piehler JM, Crichlow RW (1978) Primary carcinoma of the gallbladder. Surg Gynecol Obstet 147:929–942
85. Litwin MS (1967) Primary carcinoma of the gallbladder: a review of 78 patients. Arch Surg 95:236–242
86. Bergdahl L (1980) Gallbladder carcinoma first diagnosed at microscopic examination of gallbladders removed for presumed benign disease. Ann Surg 191:19–22
87. Hanna SS, Rider WD (1978) Carcinoma of the gallbladder or extrahepatic bile ducts: the role of radiotherapy. Can Med Assoc J 118:59–61
88. Cristensen AH, Ishak KG (1970) Benign tumors and pseudotumors of the gallbladder. Arch Pathol 90:423–432

# 33 Liver Transplantation

E. ELIAS and P. BURRA

## 1 History of Liver Transplantation

Liver transplantation is now considered as standard treatment for end-stage chronic liver disease [1] and in some circumstances for acute hepatic failure. The first transplant was performed by STARZL in 1963 and led to pioneering programmes of liver transplantation in Denver, Colorado, and Cambridge, United Kingdom. Prior to 1980 transplants were performed only at Denver, Cambridge, and Hannover but since then the greatly improved survival rates have resulted in a rapid increase in both the number of patients undergoing transplantation and the number of centres involved, so that by 1990 the number of patients treated in this way worldwide had exceeded 10000.

## 2 Indications

The indications by diagnostic disease category for the patients who have undergone transplantation in the Birmingham programme are shown in Table 1. It can be seen that primary biliary cirrhosis (PBC) constitutes the commonest indication for transplantation in adults (Fig. 1). Experience has shown that age is not a major prognostic risk factor, and the patients in the Birmingham series have ranged from 3 months to 69 years old.

## 3 Selection of Patients

The selection of patients for the operation is crucial. Psychological assessment and education are essential in patient selection and all liver transplant programmes devote much time to preparing the patient and the patient's family for the ordeal. Hepatologists, transplant surgeons, and anaesthetists, together with nurses, chaplains, and social workers, are involved in preoperative counselling.

The final decision in our centre reflects the current indications and contraindications as well as the attitude of the patient and his or her family. Absolute contraindications include findings which render a successful outcome impossible (Table 2).

**Table 1.** Indications for liver transplantation in the Birmingham series, 1982–1990

| | |
|---|---|
| *Adults* | |
| Chronic liver disease | |
| – PBC | 35% |
| – PSC | 8% |
| – CAH | 4% |
| – Cryptogenic cirrhosis | 6% |
| – Alcoholic cirrhosis | 1% |
| Acute liver failure | 15% |
| Malignancy | 9% |
| – Primary | |
| – Secondary (e.g., carcinoid syndrome) | |
| Other | 10% |
| *Children* | |
| Inborn error of metabolism | 4% |
| – With intrinsic liver disease (e.g., $\alpha_1$-antitrypsin deficiency) | |
| – Without intrinsic liver disease (e.g., Crigler-Najjar syndrome) | |
| Cholestatic liver disease | |
| – Biliary atresia | 8% |

PBC, primary biliary cirrhosis; PSC, primary sclerosing cholangitis; CAH, chronic active hepatitis

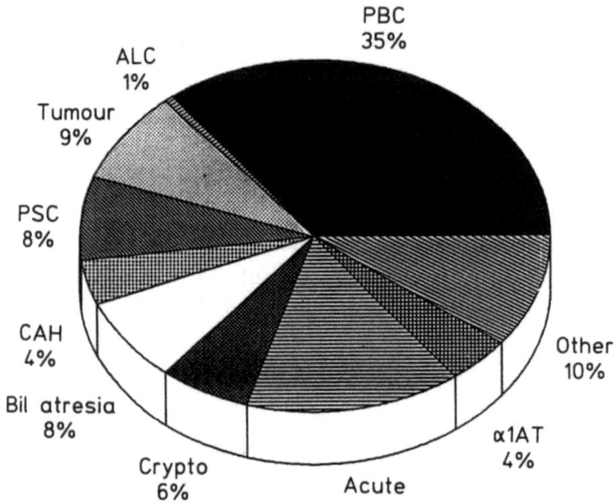


**Fig. 1.** Indications for liver transplantation in adults in the Birmingham programme. *PBC*, primary biliary cirrhosis; *αIAT*, $\alpha_1$-antitrypsin deficiency; *CAH*, chronic active hepatitis; *PSC*, primary sclerosing cholangitis; *ALC*, alcoholic hepatitis

The transplant operation should be delayed while the reversible abnormalities of hyponatraemia, spontaneous bacterial peritonitis, and post-sclerotherapy ulceration are corrected.

Hyponatraemia should be corrected so that the sodium concentration exceeds 125 mmol/litre, otherwise there is a risk of central pontine

**Table 2.** Absolute and relative contraindications to liver transplantation in the Birmingham series, 1982–1990

| |
|---|
| *Absolute* |
| Active sepsis outside the liver and biliary tree |
| HIV positivity |
| Metastatic hepatobiliary malignancy |
| *Relative* |
| Hyponatraemia |
| Impaired renal function |
| Muscle wasting |
| Hepatitis B or D |
| Pulmonary hypertension |
| Previous upper abdominal surgery |
| Active post-sclerotherapy ulceration |
| Bacteraemia |
| Spontaneous bacterial peritonitis |

myelinolysis [2]. Spontaneous bacterial peritonitis is diagnosed and treated on the sole criterion of finding more than 500 polymorphonuclear leucocytes per cc of ascites obtained by diagnostic aspiration. Active sepsis outside the liver is usually taken as an absolute contraindication, because postoperative immunosuppression may lead to overwhelming infection. There are circumstances, however, when infected patients may undergo transplantation. One example is the patient with biliary disease, such as primary sclerosing cholangitis or Caroli's syndrome, who may have localised biliary infection which is impossible to eradicate preoperatively but which will be removed along with the diseased liver [3].

Patients who have been treated by oesophageal sclerotherapy for bleeding varices and who have post-sclerotherapy ulceration at the time of their transplant may display ulcer perforation with mediastinal abscess formation some weeks after successful transplantation [4].

Many of the other factors which place patients in a high-risk category are indications that transplantation has been scheduled too late. Thus renal impairment, hypoalbuminaemia and gross muscle wasting are probably indications of a preterminal phase of the patient's chronic liver disease in which the optimal chance of surviving liver transplantation has been lost. Merely correcting the more apparent expression of this, e.g., a low serum albumin, does not remedy the situation. The Pittsburgh group identified renal impairment as the single most sinister independent variable in an analysis of pre-operative risk factors [5].

Previous upper abdominal surgery may also cause problems during the transplant surgery. In paediatric transplantation prior abdominal surgery does not affect mortality but does increase the number of red cell transfusions and infections, particularly abdominal infections [6]. In adults the risk of death within the 1st post-transplant month was initially reported by Starzl to be double that in patients without earlier operations. Though technical improvements have greatly diminished this hazard, surgery in the hepatobiliary area should be avoided prior to transplantation if possible.

Severe pulmonary hypertension, which occasionally complicates chronic liver disease, precludes liver replacement except in the exceedingly rare patient who is accepted for combined heart, lung, and liver transplantation. Only one patient in our series was successfully treated in this way. Arterial hypoxaemia due to intrapulmonary shunting may also be associated with cirrhosis but will tend to reverse following successful transplantation. Up to one-third of cirrhotics may experience mild to moderate arterial hypoxaemia in the absence of any apparent lung or heart disease [7–9].

### 3.1 Controversies in Selection of Patients

There is still no uniformity between centres in selection policies for patients with hepatocellular carcinoma, hepatitis B, alcoholic liver disease, and Budd-Chiari syndrome.

Patients presenting with a small (less than 2 cm diameter) *hepatocellular carcinoma* in a cirrhotic liver should be selected on the basis of Child-Pugh classification of the liver disease, tumour size and age. Partial hepatectomy carries a high risk in the presence of cirrhosis and cannot be performed in Child C subjects. Patients less than 55 years old with unresectable tumour may be considered for liver transplantation. However, a major consideration in this selection is the likelihood of recurrent disease after the operation. The assessment of the patient requires CT scan of chest and abdomen, bone scintigraphy and laparoscopy. Even then, the operation carries a reasonable prospect of long-term survival only when porta hepatis lymph nodes are shown to be free of tumour. Recurrence remains common despite the most stringent attempts to exclude extrahepatic spread prior to transplantation [10].

Liver transplantation in *hepatitis B virus* (HBV) infected patients may be indicated because of cirrhosis, hepatocellular carcinoma or fulminant hepatitis. The risk of recurrent HBV infection is very high in cirrhosis and lower in the case of hepatocellular carcinoma or fulminant hepatitis, when the virus does not replicate. In particular, serological positivity for HBe and/or HBV DNA at the time of transplantation is associated with almost certain recurrence. Attempts to prevent reinfection have been made with specific immunoglobulin for passive immunisation, active immunisation with vaccines and antiviral drugs such as interferon, but with generally poor results.

Attempts to prevent reinfection by the use of massive transfer of passive immunity with polyclonal or monoclonal antisera have generally proved very disappointing although reinfection of the graft is probably delayed. Anti-HBsAg monoclonal antibodies are currently in use but their long-term efficacy is unproven. Recurrence is due to the presence of a reservoir of the virus at the time of transplantation (leucocytes, spleen, pancreas).

A general reluctance to perform transplantation in patients with *alcoholic liver disease* can be due to several factors such as the fear of a return to alcohol (recidivism), the presence of social and behavioural problems (including poor compliance with medical advice, which is important following liver transplantation) and alcohol-related organic disorders such as nutritional deficiencies, subclinical cardiomyopathy, brain damage, chronic pancreatitis and infections.

There is no specific therapy of proven benefit for alcoholic liver disease other than removal of ethanol, correction of nutritional deficiencies and treatment of complications. Hepatic transplantation may be considered in patients who continue to deteriorate towards early death despite conventional management, and who appear committed to cease alcohol abuse [11]. The selection criteria for liver transplantation in patients with alcoholic cirrhosis should include poor quality of life due to persistent complications of portal hypertension and hepatic insufficiency despite maximum medical treatment during a minimum period of 6 months of abstinence before transplantation [12]. Alcoholic patients who manage to stop drinking generally fall into three categories: (a) the majority who will recover normal health though it may take 12 months or more for clinical evidence of liver disease to recede; (b) a small number who have lethargy, ascites and a poor quality of life despite abstinence of more than 12 months; (c) patients with severe acute alcoholic hepatitis, who may die within 6–8 weeks of their initial hospital admission. In category (c), if transplantation is successfully conducted the risk of recidivism is much greater.

Recent data from 73 alcoholics who underwent transplantation in Pittsburgh demonstrate that the survival rate and subsequent achievement of good health did not differ between alcoholic subjects and those transplanted for other causes. Thus, within the constraints of limited resources, including donor organ supply, orthotopic liver transplantation is a therapeutic option that may be considered for individuals with end-stage alcoholic liver disease who desire such therapy [13].

Transplantation is only rarely used in the management of patients with *Budd-Chiari syndrome*. Lesser treatments which can be offered to these patients consist in release of the obstruction with fibrinolysis, transcutaneous venoplasty, caval stenting or vena caval resection when a short length of stenosis is proved, mesocaval shunting or even meso-atrial shunts. Transplantation is usually reserved for those in whom the above measures are not successful or in whom they are judged to be insufficient because of severe irreversible liver lesions, including established cirrhosis.

## 4 Timing of Transplantation

It has been shown that the patient's pre-operative condition has a major influence on survival after transplantation. In view of this and because resources, including donor organs, are limited, transplant centres may be justified in adapting their selection policy to favour the better risk candidates.

Liver transplantation should ideally be performed as late in the course of the illness as is still compatible with an optimal chance of survival. Conversely, undue delay not only risks sudden death before transfer to the transplant centre, or death whilst waiting in hospital, but also diminishes the prospects of survival in those undergoing transplantation [14].

In practice, patients are monitored serially for signs of liver failure by simple analyses of the liver's metabolic, synthetic and excretory function. The parameters vary according to the type of liver disease involved and sometimes the decision is arrived at empirically on an individual case basis. For example, one of the most important aspects, which is not clearly quantifiable, is the patient's quality of life. The optimum is to define the criteria for timing liver transplantation within different diseases.
For *primary biliary cirrhosis* we consider the following features:

- Bilirubin >300 µmol/litre(should suffice even in the absence of any other indication)
- Bilirubin >100 µmol/litre and rising
- Diuretic-resistant ascites(with risk of hyponatraemia and hepatorenal syndrome)
- Spontaneous bacterial peritonitis
- Hepatic encephalopathy or grossly disabling lethargy
- Pain from osteoporotic bone disease
- Intractable pruritus
- Progressive muscle wasting
- Sclerotherapy-resisnant variceal bleeding

Patients selected for transplantation often have a combination of several of the above features.

For *cryptogenic cirrhosis* and *chronic active hepatitis* the commonest features indicating the appropriate time for transplantation are:

- Diuretic-resistant ascites
- Spontaneous bacterial peritonitis
- Hepatic encephalopathy or grossly disabling lethargy
- Low serum albumin (<26 g/litre)

For *primary hepatocellular carcinoma* the essential criterion is:

- Irresectable (by partial hepatectomy) tumour confined to the liver without spread to nodes at the porta hepatis.

Secondary malignancies are generally not accepted as an indication for transplantation, with the rare exception of massive deposits of slow growing, functioning tumours, e.g., carcinoids.

*Fulminant hepatic failure* has a high mortality which depends on the age of the patient, the aetiology of the liver disease, the rate of onset, and the depth and duration of encephalopathy. The interval from onset of the hepatic illness to development of encephalopathy in liver failure defines fulminant hepatitis (<8 weeks) and subacute hepatic necrosis (>8 weeks). Transplantation does improve the chance of survival in selected patients with fulminant hepatic failure, early referral and donor organ availability being important factors [15]. However, a notable feature of these series has been the failure of neurological recovery in a proportion of those in whom the grafted liver has functioned satisfactorily. Monitoring of intracerebral pressure and the development of reliable indices of cerebral viability are areas of intense activity and interest. We select the patients for transplantation on the basis of (a) factors which are most likely to carry a poor prognosis without transplantation, and (b) absence of adverse features for recovery following transplantation, e.g., neurological impairment secondary to cerebral oedema, or a psychiatric history of repeated suicide attempts.

In patients with fulminant hepatitis, O'Grady et al. [16] have shown that risk of death without transplantation correlates with aetiology, age, duration of jaundice before onset of encephalopathy and liver function (Table 3). Patients are placed on the emergency transplant list as soon as they have three of the risk factors.

In fulminant hepatitis due to paracetamol overdoes the poorest prognosis is indicated by acidosis, prolonged prothrombin time and renal impairment (Table 3).

In summary, in acute liver failure the early recognition of a severe prognosis and simultaneous transfer to a transplant centre are of prime importance. The decision to transplant needs to be taken sufficiently early to guarantee procurement of a donor organ, thus avoiding death prior to

**Table 3.** Factors associated with increased risk of death in fulminant hepatitis

| |
|---|
| *Non-paracetamol-induced* |
| Aetiology (non-A, non-B hepatitis and drug reactions, e.g., halothane, carry the worst prognosis) |
| Age <11 or >40 years |
| Duration of jaundice before onset of encephalopathy >7 days |
| Serum bilirubun >300 μmol/litre |
| Prothrombin time >50 s or factor V <20% (Paris criteria) |
| *Paracetamol overdose* |
| Arterial blood pH <7.30 |
| Prothrombin time >100 s |
| Serum creatinine >300 μmol/litre |

Modified from O'Grady JG et al. (1989) Gastroenterology 97:439–445 transplantation, and secondly to avoid fatalities due to cerebral oedema, which is apt to occur peri-operatively in the most advanced cases.

## 5 Operative and Postoperative Course

Intra-operative risk factors include severe bleeding, usually from a combination of adhesions, portal hypertension and coagulopathy, acute renal failure and, in fulminant hepatic failure, brain damage from cerebral oedema. Previous abdominal surgery may increase transfusion requirements and prolong the operation but is no longer a major contraindication to liver transplantation.

The new liver is inserted starting with the caval then the portal vein anastomosis. The liver is perfused through the portal vein with 5% dextrose to wash out any toxic metabolites prior to the completion of the portal vein anastomosis; it is then perfused with blood through the portal vein and the arterial anastomosis is completed. The biliary anastomosis is usually performed last.

Patients are ventilated postoperatively and usually extubation is achieved within 1–3 days. Abdominal drains and vascular access lines are removed within a few days and the intrabiliary T-tube is removed at 3 months. Oral intake is usually resumed in 2–3 days or nasogastric tube feeding is instituted. Daily liver function tests are performed. Most patients are well enough to leave hospital within a month of the operation [17].

## 6 Complications

Complications after liver transplantation can be classified into immediate, early and late (Table 4). Peri-operative complications include those instances in which the graft fails to function. The only recourse is retransplantation before cerebral oedema and brain stem herniation occur [18].

Early complications after surgery include cardiovascular instability, usually associated with intra-operative haemorrhage, primary non-function of the implanted liver and acute renal failure. One of the worst complications consists in early hepatic artery thrombosis which causes graft ischaemia with massive elevation of serum transaminases and is an indication for urgent regrafting. The hepatic artery is routinely imaged by Doppler ultrasonography and thrombosis confirmed angiographically. Infections (bacterial, viral, fungal) are other common causes of liver dysfunction or systemic disease.

Late complications are chronic rejection and recurrence of disease, such as hepatitis B and malignancies.

**Table 4.** Immediate, early and late complications after liver transplantation in the Birmingham series, 1982–1990

| | |
|---|---|
| *Immediate* | Haemorrhage<br>Renal failure<br>Primary graft failure |
| *Early* | |
| Day 0–3 | Hepatic artery thrombosis<br>Cerebral death (in acute liver failure) |
| Weeks 0–2 | Sepsis (pulmonary, abdominal, biliary)<br>Acute rejection (70%–80%)<br>Chronic rejection (rare) |
| Weeks 2–8 | Sepsis (perihepatic, biliary leaks or sludge in bile duct)<br>Acute rejection<br>Chronic rejection<br>Opportunistic infections (fungal, viral, e.g., CMV, herpesvirus)<br>Over-immunosuppression |
| *Late* | Chronic rejection (10–15%)<br>Acute rejection (rare)<br>Recurrent disease – HBV<br>– Malignancy<br>Biliary strictures |

Acute rejection is a very common finding associated with rising transaminases, bilirubin and alkaline phosphatase. Chronic rejection is associated with rising alkaline phosphatase and bilirubin, and clinical and histological findings confirm cholestatic features. Unfortunately, while increased immunosuppression is successful in overcoming most cases of acute rejection, chronic rejection is almost always irreversible and requires regrafting.

Disease has recurred in most patients who have undergone transplantation for hepatitis B despite attempts at its prevention with monoclonal antibodies or antiviral drugs.

Transplantation for hepatic malignancy leads to long-term survival in 20%–30%, recurrent disease being the major risk. In paediatric transplantations, primary or reactivation infection by herpesvirus, particularly cytomegalovirus, and Epstein-Barr virus can be an important cause of mortality [19]. Drug toxicity must also be considered a complication following liver transplantation during immunosuppressive therapy and can occur early or late (Table 5).

### 6.1 Rejection and Immunosuppression

Rejection is defined as graft damage arising from response of the recipient immune system to the transplanted liver. Although it has been suggested from animal studies that the liver is less susceptible to rejection than other organs, in humans there is little, if any, advantage [20]. Approximately 70%

**Table 5.** Drug toxicity following immunosuppressive therapy after transplantation

| |
|---|
| *Cyclosporine* |
| Nephrotoxicity |
| Hypertension |
| Hypertrichosis |
| Dyspepsia |
| Fine tremors, paraesthesia |
| *Azathioprine* |
| Myelotoxicity |
| Lymphoproliferative disorders |
| *Corticosteroids* |
| Cushing's syndrome |
| Psychotic manifestations |
| Osteoporosis |

of patients experience at least one episode of acute, reversible rejection and between 10% and 15% develop chronic rejection [21–24].

In cases of acute rejection, histology reveals a mixed inflammatory cell infiltrate concentrated around the bile ducts in the portal tract and the endothelium of the portal and hepatic vein radicles. Direction of the immune response to these cellular elements is thought to be due to the fact that, unlike hepatocytes, they normally express the major histocompatibility antigens (MHCs) of class I type, HLA-A, -B and -C, which makes them a potential target for CD8+ (cytotoxic) T cells. In rejection MHC class II (DR) antigens are expressed on biliary epithelial cells which can therefore act as antigen-presenting cells for CD4 (helper) T cells.

The cardinal feature of chronic rejection is the disappearance (sudden or gradual) of small intrahepatic bile ducts; the hepatic arterial lumen is occluded by foam cells and the parenchyma shows evidence of secondary cholestasis and ischaemia. The loss of bile ducts is described as the "vanishing bile duct syndrome"; its onset may be sudden or insidious with progressive deterioration in liver function [25].

Cyclosporine is the most commonly used maintenance drug [26]; it is usually employed in association with corticosteroids [27] and azathioprine [28] but regimens vary considerably between transplant centres. Our current protocol involves initial triple therapy with low dose prednisolone, 20 mg/day (reducing to zero at 3 months), azathioprine 2 mg/kg per day and cyclosporine 2 mg/kg per day i.v. continuing to 10 mg/kg per day orally and adjusted to maintain blood levels of 100–300 μg/litre.

Acute rejection is treated with methylprednisolone up to 1 g daily for 3 days. Patients who fail to respond to one or two courses of such a steroid bolus are treated for 10 days with the monoclonal antilymphocyte antibody OKT3.

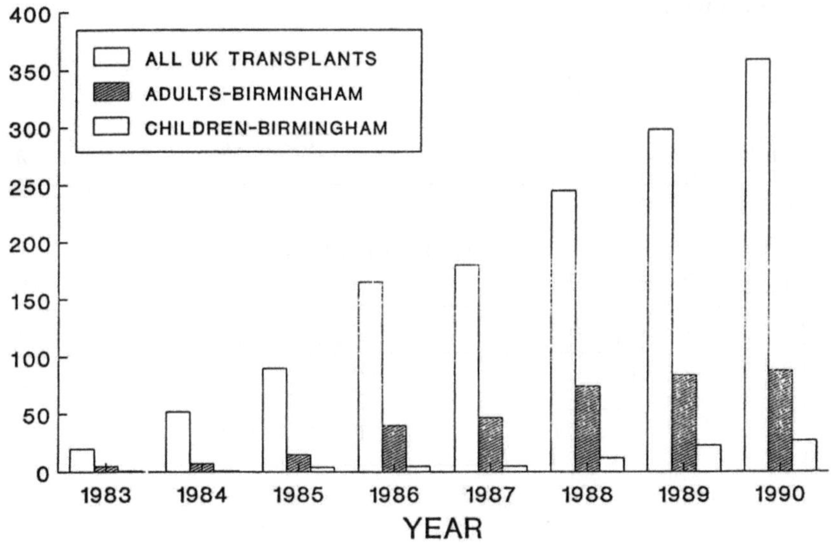


**Fig. 2.** Number of liver transplants in the United Kingdom and Birmingham by year

FK 506 is a powerful new immunosuppressant that has recently been demonstrated to successfully inhibit hepatic rejection in animal models. It is synergistic with cyclosporine but is usually substituted for it in clinical practise. FK 506 has been used following liver transplantation with promising early results from Pittsburgh [29, 30].

In post-transplant therapy it is crucial to balance the opposing constraints on immunosuppression so as to minimise both rejection and the risk of opportunistic infections. CMV infection is common after transplantation and CMV-negative donor livers are matched to CMV-negative recipients when possible; reduction of immunosuppression is sufficient to allow the patient to recover in most instances, but treatment with ganciclovir and hyperimmune globulin is instituted in severe cases.

## 7 Results

Between the start of the programme in January 1982 and May 1990, 370 transplants were performed in Birmingham in 317 patients, 268 adults and 49 children (Fig. 2).

Outcome depends on the timing of the transplant, selection of the patient, the severity of the disease and the extent of failure of other organ systems.

The actuarial survival at 1 year in the entire Birmingham series is more than 70% in PBC, more than 50% in other chronic liver disease and 40% in acute liver failure and malignancies (Fig. 3).

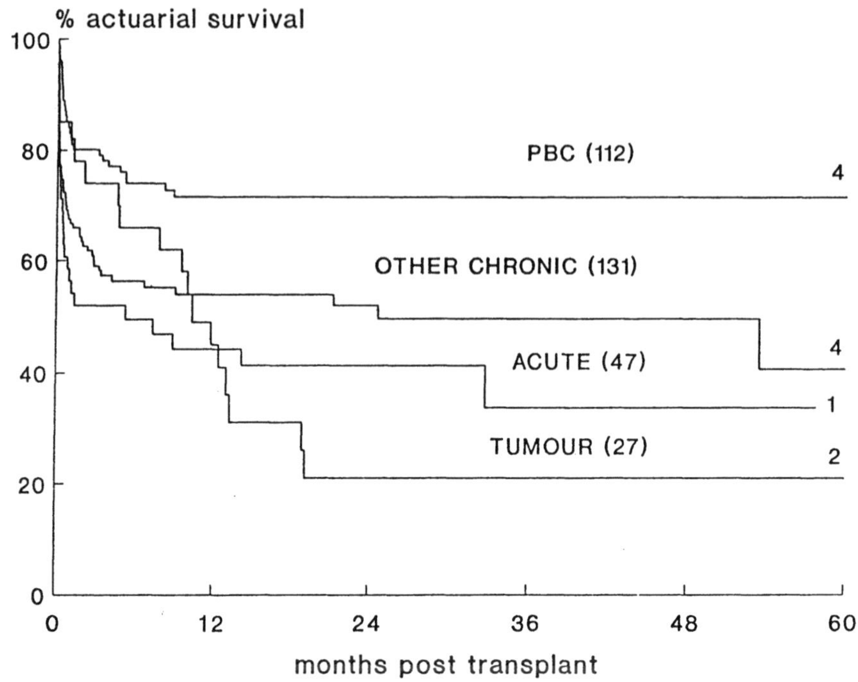


**Fig. 3.** Actuarial survival at 1 year in the entire Birmingham transplantation series, according to disease category. *PBC*, primary biliary cirrhosis

The results from Pittsburgh showed actuarial survival of 74% at 1 year and 64% at 5 years after transplantation.

Results are constantly improving, as can be seen from four consecutive series of 100 patients in our series in whom the actuarial survival at 1 year is likely to be respectively 51%, 55%, 73%, and 76% (Fig. 4). In these four series, 18, 13, 15 and 16 have undergone regrafting, receiving a total of 70 regrafts; the causes have been chronic rejection (22 cases), hepatic artery thrombosis (22), haemorrhagic necrosis (8), primary non-function (6), segmental infarction (6), non-A, non-B hepatitis (3), biliary complication (1), acute rejection (1) and portal vein thrombosis (1).

## 8 Conclusion

Improved results are likely to come with more stringent patient selection, opportune timing of liver replacement and more effective immunosuppression. Fatal delays occur due to late presentation and referral, rapidly progressive disease, difficulty in procuring organs and logistical difficulties in the transplant programme such as influx of more urgent cases which take priority. The patient should be offered the option of transplantation when the chances of success are still optimal (>70%). In acute liver failure, the

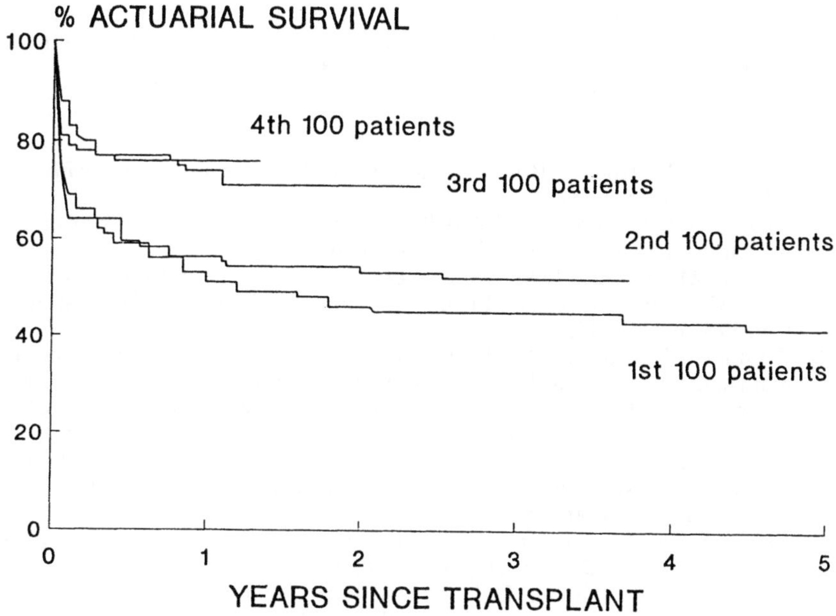


**Fig. 4.** Actuarial survival at 1 year in four consecutive series of 100 patients from the entire Birmingham transplantation programme

early recognition of a poor prognosis is of crucial importance. The decision to transplant needs to be taken sufficiently early to maximise the chances of procuring a donor organ and thus avoiding death due to cerebral oedema prior to transplantation.

The future of liver transplantation looks bright but contains many challenges [1]. "New and cheaper methods of monitoring and recognising rejection need to be developed: safer and less costly immunosuppressive agents need to be identified: better surgical techniques that result in fewer postoperative problems need to be developed" [31].

## References

1. National Institutes of Health Consensus Conference Development Statement (1984) Liver transplantation, June 20–23, 1983. Hepatology 4:13–45
2. Larner AJ, Vickers CR, Adu D et al. (1988) Correction of severe hyponatraemia by continuous arteriovenous haemofiltration before liver transplantation. Br Med J 297:1514–1515
3. Neuberger JM, Adams DH (1989) Liver transplantation. In: Davis M (ed) Clinical gastroenterology. Therapy of liver disease. Bailliere Tindall, London, p 231
4. Vickers CR, O'Connor HJ, Quintero GA et al. (1989) Delayed perforation of the esophagus after variceal sclerotherapy and hepatic transplantation. Gastrointest Endosc 35:459–461

5. Cuervas-Mons V, Millan I, Gavaler JS et al. (1986) Prognostic value of preoperatively obtained clinical and laboratory data in predicting survival following orthotopic liver transplantation. Hepatology 6:922–927
6. Cuervas-Mons V, Rimola A, Van Thiel D et al. (1986) Does previous abdominal surgery alter the outcome of pediatric patients subjected to orthotopic liver transplantation? Gastroenterology 90:853–857
7. Agusti AGN, Roca J, Bosch J et al. (1990) The lung in patients with cirrhosis. J Hepatol 10:251–257
8. Krowka MJ, Cortese DA (1985) Pulmonary aspects of chronic liver disease and liver transplantation. Mayo Clin Proc 60:407–418
9. Krowka MJ, Cortese DA (1987) Severe hypoxemia associated with liver disease: Mayo Clinic experience and the experimental use of almitrine bismesylate. Mayo Clin Proc 62:164–173
10. O'Grady JC, Polson RJ, Rolles K et al. (1988) Liver transplantation for malignant disease. Results in 93 consecutive patients. Ann Surg 207:373–379
11. Schenker S (1984) Alcoholic liver disease: evaluation of natural history and prognostic factors. Hepatology 4:365–435
12. Bird GLA, O'Grady JG, Harvey FAH et al. (1990) Liver transplantation in patients with alcoholic cirrhosis: selection criteria and rates of survival and relapse. Br Med J 301:15–17
13. Kumar S, Stauber RE, Gavaler JS et al. (1990) Orthotopic liver transplantation for alcoholic liver disease. Hepatology 11:159–164
14. Neuberger JM, Altman DG, Polson R et al. (1989) Prognosis after liver transplantation for primary biliary cirrhosis. Transplantation 48:444–447
15. Vickers C, Neuberger JM, Buckels JAC et al. (1988) Transplantation of the liver in adults and children with fulminant hepatic failure. J Hepatol 7:143–150
16. O'Grady JG, Alexander GJM, Hayllar KM et al. (1989) Early indicators of prognosis in fulminant hepatic failure. Gastroenterology 97:439–445
17. Buckels JAC (1989) Liver transplantation – techniques and results. In: Jewell DP, Snook JA (eds) Topics in gastroenterology. Blackwell Scientific, Oxford, p 93
18. Starzl TE, Demetris AJ, Van Thiel D (1989) Liver transplantation. N Engl J Med 321:1014–1022
19. Alonso EM, Fox AS, Franklin WA et al. (1990) Postnecrotic cirrhosis following varicella hepatitis A in a liver transplant patient. Transplantation 49:650–653
20. Starzl TE, Demetris AJ, Van Thiel DH (1989) Liver transplantation. N Engl J Med 321:1014–1022
21. Kirby RM, McMaster P, Clements D (1987) Orthotopic liver transplantation: post-operative complications and their management. Br J Surg 74:3–12
22. Snover DG, Freese DK, Sharp HL et al. (1987) Liver allograft rejection. An analysis of the use of biopsy in determining the outcome of rejection. Am J Surg Pathol 11:1–10
23. Ludwig J, Weisner RH, Batts KP et al. (1987) The acute vanishing bile duct syndrome (acute irreversible rejection) after orthotopic liver transplantation. Hepatology 7:476–483
24. Adams DH, Neuberger JM (1990) Patterns of graft rejection following liver transplantation. J Hepatol 10:113–119
25. Wight DGD, Portman B (1987) Pathology of rejection. In: Calne RY (ed) Liver transplantation, 2nd edn. Grune & Stratton, London, p 385
26. Calne RY, Rolles K, White DJ et al. (1979) Cyclosporine A initially as the only immunosuppressant in 34 recipients of cadaveric organs: 32 kidneys, 2 pancreases and 2 livers. Lancet II:1033–1036
27. Starzl TE, Weil R, Iwatsuki S et al. (1980) The use of cyclosporin A and prednisolone in cadaver kidney transplantation. Surg Gynecol Obstet 151:17–26
28. Gugenheim J, Samuel D, Saliba F et al. (1988) Use of cyclosporin A in combination with low-dose corticosteroids and azathioprine in liver transplantation. Transplant Proc 20 [Suppl]:366–368

29. Starzl TE, Makowka L, Todo S (1987) FK-506: a potential breakthrough in immunosuppression. Transplant Proc 19 [Suppl]:104
30. Hoffman AL, Makowka L, Banner B et al. (1990) The use of FK-506 for small intestine allotransplantation. Transplantation 49:483–490
31. Van Thiel DH, Tarter R, Gavaler JS et al. (1986) Liver transplantation in adults. An analysis of costs and benefits at the University of Pittsburgh. Gastroenterology 90:211–216

# 34 Gallstones

J.A. SUMMERFIELD

## 1 Gallstone Formation

Gallstones are common, affecting between 10% and 20% of the world's population. Gallstones are classified by their composition into two main groups: cholesterol stones and pigment stones. Cholesterol stones contain more than 70% cholesterol and usually have a dark central nucleus composed of a protein–pigment complex. Cholesterol stones are further classified into pure cholesterol stones, which are usually solitary, and mixed stones, which contain cholesterol in a matrix of calcium bilirubinate, calcium phosphate and protein. Mixed stones are usually multiple and faceted. Cholesterol gallstones account for about 70% of gallstones in Europe and the United States.

Pigment stones are also classified into two main groups. Brown pigment stones are soft and friable and consist of calcium bilirubinate, cholesterol and calcium soaps. Black pigment stones are hard and brittle and consist of an insoluble black pigment, calcium bilirubinate, calcium carbonate and phosphate, calcium salts of fatty acids and bile acids. Both types of pigment stone contain a large amount of mucoprotein matrix (up to 70%) and may contain up to 50% cholesterol.

### 1.1 Cholesterol Gallstones

Cholesterol gallstones result from the secretion of cholesterol-saturated bile by the liver. The cause of this cholesterol-saturated bile is unclear. Gallstone patients usually have a smaller bile acid pool than controls and it circulates more frequently. The small bile acid pool is probably not the most important factor in the production of saturated bile. This appears to be an elevated biliary cholesterol secretion rate. However, some normal subjects also have cholesterol-saturated bile intermittently, especially when fasting. Thus while cholesterol-saturated bile is a necessary prerequisite, it is not sufficient for gallstone formation. Other factors are important, such as the condition of the gallbladder, nucleation (seeding) factors in bile, race, age, sex, obesity, diet and drugs.

### 1.2 Bile Pigment Gallstones

Pigment stones are formed when bile contains excess unconjugated bilirubin which precipitates as calcium bilirubinate [1]. The solubility of unconjugated bilirubin is low so that it precipitates even when it constitutes only a small proportion of the total biliary bilirubin. Little is known of the factors causing pigment stone formation. The soft friable brown pigment stones are associated with bacterial infections of the biliary tract such as biliary strictures. Hydrolysis of conjugated bilirubin by bacterial β-glucuronidase increases the concentration of unconjugated bilirubin, which leads to its precipitation. The hard brittle black pigment stones develop in patients with cirrhosis, chronic haemolytic anaemias and malaria. The mechanism of stone production is unclear but increased unconjugated bilirubin in gallbladder bile in these patients is associated with increased enzymatic hydrolysis of bilirubin, probably due to β-glucuronidase secreted by the gallbladder or hepatocytes. Pigment gallstone formation is not related to cholesterol saturation of bile. Retained suture material may cause pigment stone formation in the bile duct.

## 2 Natural History of Gallstones

Most gallstones remain in the gallbladder (cholelithiasis) and are symptomless (silent gallstones), being discovered incidentally during investigation or at autopsy. Impaction of a gallstone in the neck of the gallbladder results in gallbladder inflammation and the symptoms and signs of acute or chronic cholecystitis. Acute cholecystitis will subside if the stone spontaneously disimpacts or may progress to gangrene and perforation or empyema of the gallbladder. Gallstones may pass through the cystic duct into the bile duct (choledocholithiasis), resulting in biliary obstruction and jaundice. Bacterial infection (cholangitis) commonly accompanies choledocholithiasis and can lead to liver abscess formation. Gallstones may perforate through the inflamed gallbladder wall to form an internal fistula (cholecystenteric fistula), usually to the small intestine or colon. A large gallstone passing into the small intestine may impact in the ileum, resulting in intestinal obstruction (gallstone ileus). Finally, surgical treatment for gallstones may result in a post-cholecystectomy syndrome or a benign stricture of the bile duct.

## 2.1 Acute Cholecystitis

### *Aetiology*

Acute cholecystitis is caused by gallstones in more than 90% of patients and follows the impaction of a stone in the cystic duct. Continued secretion by the gallbladder mucosa leads to a rise in gallbladder pressure. Inflammation of the gallbladder wall results from the toxic effects of the bile and bacterial infection by intestinal organisms, particularly anaerobes. In acute cholecystitis, gallbladder bile is usually turbid but may become frank pus (empyema of the gallbladder). Ischaemia of the distended gallbladder wall may result in infarction and perforation. Generalised peritonitis may follow but the leak is usually localised. Some patients appear to have repeated attacks of acute cholecystitis but these are usually recurrent bouts of chronic cholecystitis.

### *Symptoms and Signs*

The typical patient is an obese, middle-aged female, and the attack follows a large or fatty meal. However, there are many exceptions to this pattern. The principal symptom is severe pain, of sudden onset, which is continuous or minimally fluctuating, and localised to the epigastrium or right hypochondrium. The pain may radiate to the back. The constancy of the pain contrasts with the repeated bouts of biliary colic. In uncomplicated cases pain subsides over 12–18 h. Flatulence and nausea are common but persistent vomiting suggests the presence of a stone in the common bile duct.

Examination shows an ill, sweating patient with shallow respirations. Fever indicates a bacterial cholangitis. Jaundice is usually a sign of a stone in the bile duct. The abdomen moves poorly with respiration. Right hypochondrial tenderness is present and is exacerbated by inspiration (Murphy's sign). Muscle guarding and rebound tenderness are common. The gallbladder is usually impalpable but occasionally a tender mass of omentum and gallbladder may be felt under the liver.

### *Investigations*

A moderate polymorphonuclear leucocytosis ($12–15 \times 10^6$/litre) is common. Serum bilirubin concentrations between 17 and 68 µmol/litre may develop in uncomplicated acute cholecystitis but usually a raised bilirubin level indicates a stone in the bile duct. Modest rises in the serum alkaline phosphatase, aspartate aminotransferase and amylase may also develop. In about 10% of patients an abdominal x-ray will show calcified gallstones. Ultrasonography will reveal gallstones in the gallbladder (Fig. 1). Scintiscanning with $^{99m}$Tc-labelled dimethyl acetanilide iminodiacetic acid (HIDA) is also helpful. Entry of HIDA into the gallbladder usually rules out the

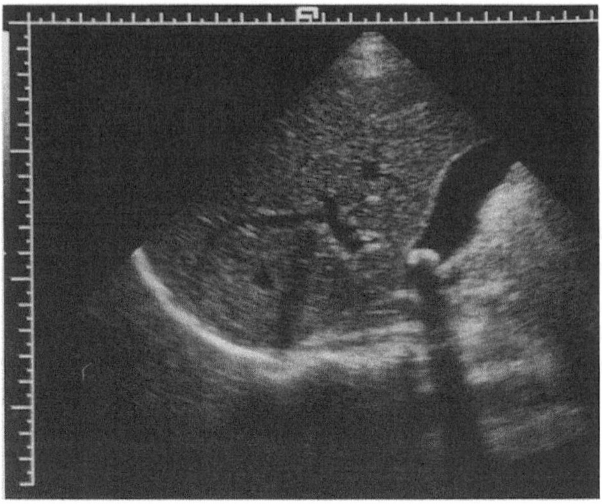

**Fig. 1.** Ultrasonography is a rapid and non-invasive method for detecting gallstones. Several stones can be seen in the gallbladder of this patient with acute cholecystitis. They are casting strong acoustic echoes

diagnosis and opacification of the bile duct without the gallbladder is evidence of blockage of the cystic duct. It is very important to establish the correct diagnosis before surgery is performed.

### *Differential Diagnosis*

Acute cholecystitis may be confused with other abdominal emergencies, including perforated peptic ulcer, acute pancreatitis, retrocaecal appendicitis, perforated carcinoma or diverticulum of the hepatic flexure of the colon and liver abscess. Cardiac infarction and pneumonia with right-sided pleurisy may give a similar clinical picture.

### *Complications*

*Gangrene of the Gallbladder.* Pain, tenderness and fever which increases progressively or persists for longer than 24–48 h are indications of gangrene of the gallbladder. The prognosis is poor if gallbladder perforation occurs. In elderly and obese patients perforation of the gallbladder may occur without definite signs. Perforation into an adjacent viscus produces a cholecystenteric fistula and may lead to gallstone ileus.

*Cholangitis.* Intermittent high temperatures sometimes accompanied by rigors indicate bacterial infection of the bile duct and usually indicate the passage of a gallstone into the bile duct.

## 2.2 Chronic Cholecystitis

Chronic cholecystitis is the commonest form of gallbladder disease caused by gallstones. Pathologically it is characterised by chronic inflammation and thickening of the gallbladder wall. In addition to stones, the gallbladder may contain a brown sediment (biliary mud). A proportion of patients with chronic cholecystitis have cholesterolosis of the gallbladder (strawberry gallbladder). This describes the deposition of yellow specks of cholesterol in the pink gallbladder wall and is a consequence of cholesterol-saturated bile. Cholesterolosis of the gallbladder is asymptomatic but about half the patients develop gallstones. Chronic cholecystitis usually develops insidiously but may follow an attack of acute cholecystitis.

### *Symptoms and Signs*

Many patients complain of bouts of constant right hypochondrial or epigastric pain. In some it is intermittent, the height of the pain being separated by 15 to 60-min intervals. The pain may last hours or be as brief as 15–20 min. It may radiate to the right shoulder or the back. More commonly symptoms are vague and include abdominal discomfort and distension, nausea, flatulence and intolerance of fatty foods. Unfortunately, many patients who do not have chronic cholecystitis complain of these symptoms. Examination of the abdomen may reveal tenderness of the gallbladder and a positive Murphy's sign. Laboratory investigations are usually unhelpful.

### *Imaging Techniques*

Ultrasonography should be the initial investigation to detect gallstones. Plain x-ray of the abdomen may reveal calcified stones (Fig. 2) or opacification of the gallbladder caused by high concentrations of calcium carbonate (limey bile). However, plain x-rays are rarely used now because of the low yield of this test. Oral cholecystography is only indicated if oral bile acid dissolution therapy is contemplated (see below). If these tests fail, ERCP should be performed in order to establish the diagnosis before cholecystectomy is performed (Fig. 3).

### *Differential Diagnosis*

Dyspepsia and fat intolerance are common symptoms that can be caused by many conditions, including peptic ulcers, hiatus hernia, chronic relapsing pancreatitis and tumours of the stomach, pancreas, colon or gallbladder. Functional disorders, such as irritable bowel syndrome, may also mimic chronic cholecystitis.

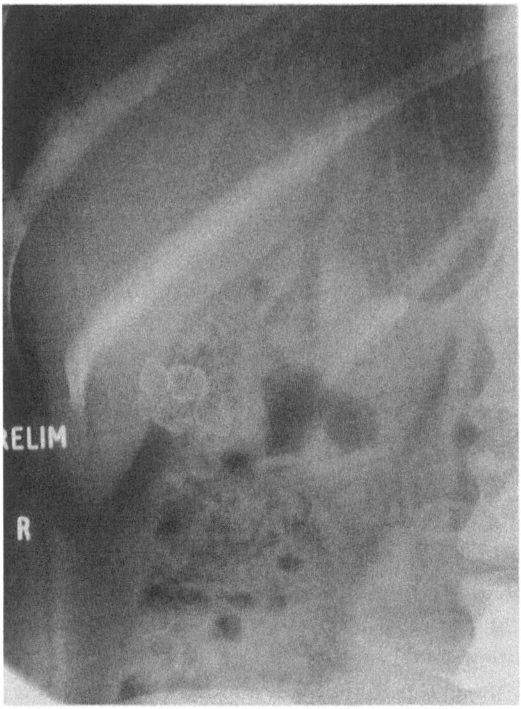


**Fig. 2.** Calcified gallstones. About 10% of gallstones contain sufficient calcium to be visible on a plain abdominal x-ray. CT scans will reveal calcification in a higher proportion. The calcium has been deposited as a peripheral ring

### *Complications*

Complications include acute exacerbations (acute cholecystitis), passage of stones into the bile duct (choledocholithiasis or Mirrizzi's syndrome), pancreatitis, cholecystenteric fistula and gallstone ileus. Carcinoma of the gallbladder is a very rare late complication. Occasionally the accumulation of the mucus and gallstones produces hydrops of the gallbladder, which presents as a tender mass.

## 2.3 Choledocholithiasis

Most stones in the common bile duct originate in the gallbladder. About 15% of patients with cholelithiasis will also have common duct stones. This proportion rises with age so that in the elderly nearly 50% of patients with cholelithiasis have common duct stones. Stones also develop in the bile duct in diseases causing chronic biliary obstruction, such as benign bile duct strictures and sclerosing cholangitis.

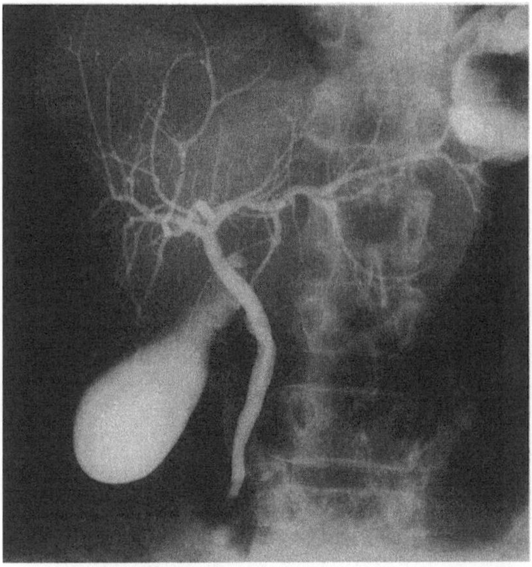

**Fig. 3.** ERCP is used to define accurately the state of the biliary tree. This jaundiced patient has a normal biliary tree. Jaundice was due to a drug

### *Clinical Features*

The classical triad of symptoms is right upper abdominal pain, jaundice and fever. The abdominal pain is typically colicky, severe and persists for hours. Pain is often associated with vomiting. Fever and rigors indicate cholangitis. The degree of jaundice is variable and may be intermittent. The urine is dark due to esterified bilirubin and the faeces are pale. The amount of pigment in the faeces may vary. Itching can be prominent. However, common bile duct stones may also be silent, especially in the elderly. Furthermore, only one of the triad of symptoms may be present, the patient presenting with jaundice, abdominal pain or cholangitis. The liver is moderately enlarged and there may be tenderness in the right upper quadrant. Prolonged biliary obstruction (lasting months or years) leads to biliary cirrhosis with portal venous hypertension and liver failure.

### *Laboratory Investigations*

Liver function tests show a cholestatic (biliary obstructive) pattern. Serum bilirubin level is raised, serum alkaline phosphatase and $\gamma$-glutamyltransferase activities are markedly elevated in contrast to a modest elevation of the serum aminotransferases. The prothrombin time may be prolonged due to inadequate absorption of vitamin K. The prothrombin time corrects after parenteral administration of vitamin K. A polymorphonuclear leucocytosis

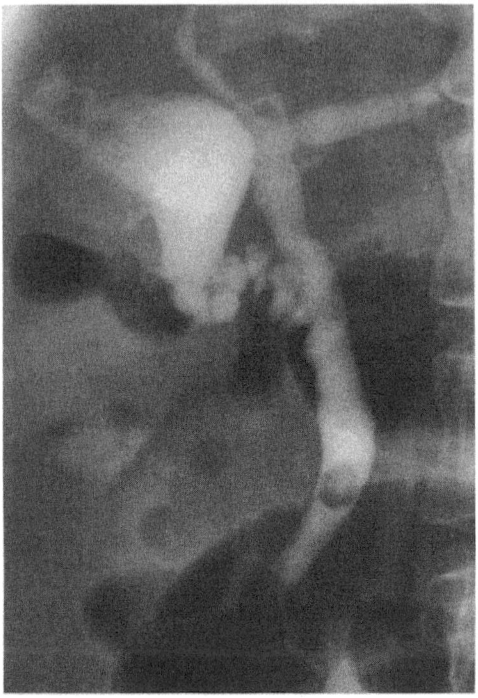

**Fig. 4.** Choledocholithiasis. ERCP in an elderly patient presenting with obstructive jaundice shows the common bile duct contains a gallstone. This was removed at ERCP by means of sphincterotomy

is common and indicates biliary infection. Blood cultures should be performed repeatedly during the fevers to isolate the organism and determine antibiotic sensitivities.

### *Imaging Techniques*

Ultrasonography is useful for demonstrating biliary dilatation and may reveal the gallstones. ERCP should then be performed to define the situation precisely. At ERCP the bile duct may be cleared of stones by sphincterotomy (Fig. 4).

### *Differential Diagnosis*

Gallstones are the most common cause of cholestatic (biliary obstructive) jaundice. Next in frequency are carcinomas of the head of the pancreas, ampulla of Vater and bile duct. Intrahepatic causes of cholestatic jaundice must also be considered. These include viral and alcoholic hepatitis, jaundice due to drugs and cholestasis of pregnancy.

# 3 Treatment of Gallstones

The mainstay of treatment for gallstones remains cholecystectomy. However, medical management can be used in selected patients. Treatment is obviously indicated for symptomatic gallstones and for their complications, but in patients with gallstones which are "silent" or give only minimal symptoms, treatment may be withheld. The problem revolves around the probability that these patients will develop serious complications in the future. It is appropriate to offer treatment of young patients (who, with many years ahead of them, will have a greater likelihood of developing the complications of gallstones) and to advise against treatment in the elderly with other major medical problems. However, in fit middle-aged patients with no or minimal symptoms it is reasonable to tell the patient of the finding and to withhold treatment until it is warranted by symptoms or complications.

There are now medical methods for removing gallstones from the gallbladder and bile ducts. The aim of these techniques is to avoid the discomfort, disability and risks of general anaesthesia and surgical exploration of the bile ducts. There are two types of medical method: chemical agents which dissolve gallstones and physical methods such as endoscopic sphincterotomy and extracorporeal shock wave lithotripsy (ESWL). The best success rates are obtained by the judicious combination of physical and chemical methods.

For practical purposes the agents used are all cholesterol solvents and will only dissolve stones containing a significant proportion of cholesterol. Pigment stones have proved very resistant to dissolution although some newer agents are claimed to be effective. There are two separate approaches to the dissolution of gallstones. In the first, agents are instilled topically through a percutaneous or nasobiliary catheter and in the second, agents are taken orally to alter the composition of bile so that it favours gallstone dissolution. Both approaches are used for stones in the gallbladder or in the bile ducts.

## 3.1 Silent and Minimally Symptomatic Gallbladder Stones

Apart from cholecystectomy there are two non-operative techniques for dissolving gallstones which may be used in selected patients, namely oral bile acid therapy and contact dissolution.

### *Oral Bile Acid Therapy*

Chenodeoxycholic acid (CDCA) was the first oral agent that was shown to dissolve cholesterol gallstones [2]. Calcified or pigment stones are not dissolved. In practical terms there need to be radiolucent stones in a functioning gallbladder (as judged by oral cholecystography) (Fig. 5). The stones

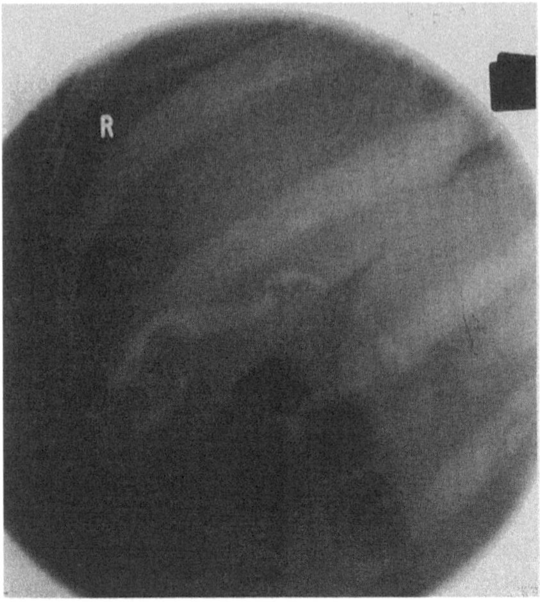


**Fig. 5.** Oral cholecystogram. This test is used in the assessment of patients for oral bile acid therapy. These radiolucent gallstones in a functioning gallbladder are composed of cholesterol. They were removed by ESWL and oral bile acid therapy

should not be larger than 15 mm in diameter and symptoms must be mild. The dose of CDCA is 15 mg/kg daily but obese patients require higher doses (20 mg/kg daily) to desaturate bile [3]. Unwanted effects include diarrhoea and modest elevations of serum aminotransferases and low density lipoprotein cholesterol. Gallstone dissolution is slow. While small stones may dissolve within 6 months, larger (15-mm) stones often require 2 years or more of continuous therapy. A low cholesterol diet and administration of CDCA as a single dose at bedtime aid gallstone dissolution [4]. The overall dissolution rate is unfortunately only about 40% [5] although the rate can be increased to about 75% by careful selection of compliant, non-obese patients and ensuring that a sufficient dose of CDCA is given to desaturate the bile. Some non-responders are patients with radiolucent pigment stones. Others have cholesterol stones containing surface salts (calcium phosphate, carbonate or bilirubinate) or an extensive mucoprotein matrix which inhibit cholesterol removal. In this latter group of patients, stones may be successfully dissolved after they have been shattered into small fragments by ESWL (see below).

Ursodeoxycholic acid (UDCA) is as effective as CDCA, is free from unwanted effects and a lower dose is required (8–13 mg/kg daily). However, UDCA is more expensive and is reported to cause calcification of some radiolucent stones [6]. The two bile acids differ in their mode of action.

CDCA dissolves cholesterol in micelles whereas UDCA promotes the removal of cholesterol as liquid crystals [7]. This difference in mode of action has prompted the use of combination therapy of 7 mg/kg daily of both bile acids. Combination therapy is now the preferred treatment [8].

There are three problems with oral bile acid therapy for gallstone dissolution. These are the small proportion of patients who are suitable, the slow pace of treatment and the tendency of gallstones to recur after they have been dissolved. About a quarter of patients re-form stones within 3 years and half the patients will re-form stones within 7 years [9]. Gallstone recurrence is not prevented by continuous low dose bile acid therapy or by high fibre or low refined carbohydrate diets. These factors limit the use of oral bile acid dissolution therapy and for most patients it is not a useful alternative to cholecystectomy.

### *Contact Dissolution of Gallstones*

Another approach to dissolving gallbladder stones is the direct instillation of an aliphatic ether into the gallbladder via a percutaneous catheter. Ethers are very effective cholesterol solvents but diethyl ether is too hazardous. However, a less volatile ether, methyl tertbutyl ether (MTBE), is effective at dissolving gallbladder cholesterol stones in situ [10].

Methyl tertbutyl ether is a foul-smelling, volatile, inflammable colourless liquid which, like diethyl ether, is anaesthetic at high concentrations. Unlike diethyl ether it is liquid at body temperature (boiling point 55°C). More than 90% of absorbed MTBE is eliminated intact by exhalation and the end-expiratory concentrations of MTBE are not explosive in air. MTBE dissolves cholesterol gallstones 50 times faster than mono-octanoin and in vitro dissolves stones containing only 40% cholesterol.

Suitable patients for MTBE therapy are those with radiolucent gallstones whose cystic duct is not occluded by fibrosis or a deeply impacted stone. Computed tomography is used to reveal gallstone calcium which is not dense enough to be seen on a plain abdominal x-ray. The number or size of the stones does not seem to matter. The gallbladder is catheterised by the transhepatic "skinny needle" technique entering it through the area of attachment of the gallbladder to the liver. This minimises the risk of leakage of bile, blood or MTBE. Location of the gallbladder is facilitated by prior opacification by oral cholecystography. Alternatively ultrasound guidance may be used. A thin (7 F, 1.7 mm) pigtail catheter is advanced into the gallbladder so that it loops on itself one or two times and is manipulated into the fundus away from the cystic duct. As many stones as possible are placed within the loops of the catheter as this is where optimal dissolution occurs. The volume of the gallbladder before overflow into the cystic duct is measured by injection of radio-opaque contrast medium. The volume of MTBE used is usually set at 5 ml less than gallbladder volume but not more than 10 ml is infused. MTBE is continually infused and aspirated with a glass syringe with the maximum vigour the patient will tolerate. Patient tolerance of the procedure is variable but many will require analgesia during the first hours of treatment. The gallbladder is aspirated completely to remove incoming bile and stone debris. To avoid cholesterol saturation of the solvent, fresh MTBE is used every 15 min. A note is kept of the volumes infused and aspirated to detect when solvent is being lost from the gallbladder by leakage. The cycles of MTBE infusion and aspiration are continued for 1–2 h after all radiological signs of the stones have disappeared. Typically this may take 5–7 h and may have to be repeated at another session. The procedure is normally performed manually but automated pumps are available.

The principal unwanted effects of MTBE therapy are sedation, burning upper abdominal pain, nausea and vomiting. Haemolysis and acute renal failure have been reported and appear to result from excessive escape of MTBE from the gallbladder. Latex (T-tubes and balloon catheters) and some plastics are dissolved by MTBE. Preliminary trials should be performed on the catheters that will be used.

Methyl tertbutyl ether is a rapid and effective method for dissolving cholesterol gallstones and is an option in patients with symptomatic cholesterol stones who are unsuitable for surgery. As with oral bile acid therapy, there is a possibility of gallstone recurrence after MTBE dissolution since the gallbladder remains intact.

Calcified gallstones and those with a high proportion of pigment or mucoprotein matrix will not dissolve with MTBE alone. One approach is to alternate MTBE with solvents for the non-cholesterol components of the stone. Calcified stones may be dissolved by alternating MTBE with a urea–EDTA (ethylenediamine tetra-acetic acid) solution which acts as a calcium chelator [11]. An alternative approach is first to shatter the calcified stone with lithotripsy (ESWL).

### *Combining Dissolution Therapy with Extracorporeal Shock Wave Lithotripsy*

Extracorporeal shock wave lithotripsy is a non-invasive and safe but expensive method which rapidly shatters gallstones into a coarse powder. Patients selected for ESWL have to satisfy similar criteria to those for oral bile acid therapy or MTBE, that is radiolucent stones in a functioning gallbladder with the added requirement that the gallbladder does not contain more than three stones. The limit on stone number relates to the technical difficulty of accurately focussing the shock waves on a number of small stones. Following stone fragmentation the debris is dissolved by combination therapy with CDCA and UDCA. Results in selected patients have been excellent [12]. Almost all cholesterol stones are shattered and after 18 months of adjuvant oral bile acid therapy more than 90% of stones up to 30 mm in diameter are completely cleared. Unwanted effects include biliary colic (in about 30%), skin petechiae and haematuria. The early machines required the patient to be submerged in a water bath and anaesthetised or heavily sedated. With the newer piezoceramic lithotriptors the patient lies on a bed for an hour or two and requires no sedation.

The combination of ESWL and oral bile acid therapy permits the non-operative removal of gallstones in the majority of patients with up to three radiolucent cholesterol gallstones. But such suitable patients are only a minority (about 10%) of all patients with gallstones.

Measures to increase the types of gallstones that can be treated include attacking calcified cholesterol stones by ESWL followed by oral bile acid therapy or MTBE. Here preliminary shattering of the stones allows the MTBE access to the cholesterol component and leaves an insoluble sludge which can be flushed out of the gallbladder. Solvents for non-cholesterol components of gallstones may also be used. Two limitations remain: the small number of stones that can be shattered and the tendency for the stones to recur.

#### *Current Status of Medical Therapy for Gallbladder Stones*

Currently only cholesterol stones are amenable to dissolution although agents that dissolve the non-cholesterol component of gallstones are being evaluated. Oral bile acid therapy is slow and unpredictable. MTBE therapy is invasive and the ether is unpleasant to use but dissolution is rapid. Calcified stones are resistant to dissolution by both methods. ESWL has provided an expensive but non-invasive and rapid treatment for cholesterol stones; it is usually used in conjunction with oral bile acid therapy. Combining ESWL with oral bile acid therapy or MTBE and non-cholesterol solvents also permits dissolution of some calcified stones.

These methods are only suitable for a minority of gallstones and there is a risk of gallstone recurrence. But they are realistic alternatives to cholecystectomy in suitable patients.

### 3.2 Cholecystitis

#### *Acute Cholecystitis*

Acute cholecystitis subsides in a few days with conservative treatment in most patients. Cholecystectomy is performed either a few days after the symptoms have settled or 2–3 months later. In the latter event, if the symptoms recur during the interval, cholecystectomy is performed without delay. Immediate surgery is mandatory if signs of gangrene or perforation develop.

*Conservative treatment.* Oral feeding is stopped. Intravenous fluids and analgesia with pentazocine or pethidine and atropine are administered.

Antibiotics are given to all but the most mild cases; tetracycline, ampicillin, a cephalosporin or ciprofloxacin is satisfactory. The patient should be observed frequently with abdominal examination and sequential leucocyte counts to detect signs of gangrene of the gallbladder or cholangitis.

*Surgical treatment.* Cholecystectomy is the operation of choice. About 10% of patients with acute cholecystitis will have common bile duct stones. Operative cholangiography is usually performed at the time of surgery to determine whether bile duct stones are present. Increasingly, operative cholangiography and exploration of the bile duct are avoided by performing preoperative ERCP and, if necessary, sphincterotomy. In poor-risk patients and when technical difficulties are encountered a cholecystotomy may be performed.

#### *Chronic Cholecystitis*

In established cases of chronic cholecystitis the treatment of choice is cholecystectomy. When the diagnosis is in doubt, especially when vague symptoms are associated with a functioning gallbladder containing stones, a conservative approach is worthwhile. This approach includes weight reduction and a low fat diet, especially if fatty food is associated with the symptoms. Treatment with CDCA or UDCA may also be considered. Chronic cholecystitis carries a good prognosis. Cholecystectomy is curative and should have a mortality well below 1%. However, if cholecystectomy is performed indiscriminately on patients with "dyspeptic" symptoms who happen to have incidental gallstones the results will be unpredictable and often unsatisfactory.

### 3.3 Choledocholithiasis

#### *Surgery and Endoscopic Sphincterotomy*

The options are surgery and endoscopic sphincterotomy. Both techniques clear the bile duct of stones in about 90% of patients. The mortality of surgery for stones in the common duct is of the order of 6%–8% [13, 14]. Postoperative complications such as wound infections, intra-abdominal sepsis, cholangitis, fistula and renal failure develop in about 46% of patients [15]. In contrast the mortality of endoscopic sphincterotomy is around 1.5% and the incidence of complications (haemorrhage, pancreatitis and perforation) around 10% [16].

Endoscopic sphincterotomy is the obvious choice in patients who have retained stones, are elderly, frail or very obese or have a pre-existing disease which precludes surgery. Endoscopic sphincterotomy is also the proper emergency treatment for patients with acute gallstone cholangitis and acute gallstone pancreatitis.

The question now is what should be done with younger patients with stones in the bile duct and a gallbladder in situ. Increasingly surgeons performing a cholecystectomy avoid exploring the bile duct and inserting T-tubes because retained stones can be removed later endoscopically. A related strategy is preoperative sphincterotomy to clear the bile ducts of stones before cholecystectomy. Preoperative sphincterotomy does reduce mean hospital stay [17]. Finally there is the option that bile duct stones are removed endoscopically and the gallbladder is then left in place. Current evidence indicates that very few patients treated in this way have further problems requiring cholecystectomy [18].

If sphincterotomy is adopted as the treatment of choice for bile duct stones, what can be done for the 10% of patients in whom sphincterotomy fails to clear the bile duct? Failure is due to stones that are too big to pass through the sphincterotomy or the presence of so many stones that the bile duct is packed solid. The dangers of haemorrhage and perforation are directly related to the size of the sphincterotomy. Help is at hand for these patients in the newer techniques including ESWL and medical treatments for the dissolution of bile duct stones.

If a T-tube is in place, the stones may be removed by a steerable basket-catheter manipulated down the T-tube track.

Preoperative preparation includes appropriate antibiotics for cholangitis, the correction of fluid and electrolyte balance, nutrition and anaemia, and if the prothrombin time is prolonged, parenteral vitamin K.

### *Oral Bile Acid Therapy*

Common bile duct stones are more serious clinical problems than gallbladder stones and require rapid removal. For this reason oral dissolution therapy, which is slow and uncertain, has found little place in their management. Nevertheless, there is limited clinical experience of the use of oral bile acid therapy for dissolving bile duct stones.

In a controlled study, administration of UDCA over 2 years dissolved gallstones in half the patients and also confirmed that common duct stones rarely disappear spontaneously [19]. The protracted nature of the treatment has led to the view that there are few circumstances in which oral dissolution therapy is appropriate for common bile duct stones. An exception is patients with gallstones complicating congenital biliary disease such as Caroli's syndrome. Here oral bile acid therapy may be tried when there are no alternatives for removing the stones.

### *Contact Dissolution of Common Bile Duct Stones*

Most stones in the common bile duct are either mixed cholesterol stones or bile pigment stones. The agents that are instilled into the bile duct to dissolve them are, in the main, cholesterol solvents. The solvents are instilled through T-tubes or nasobiliary tubes placed in the bile duct endoscopically. The aim is to dissolve the stones or to reduce their diameter so that the flushing action of the instillation will express the debris from the bile duct. Additionally endoscopic sphincterotomy and dormia baskets can remove or crush large stones that have been partially dissolved or softened by solvents. ESWL can be used to fragment large calcified calculi into fragments that the solvents can attack. Obviously contact dissolution does not work for bile pigment or calcified stones and because of the limited success rates obtained, contact dissolution has not established itself as a first-line treatment for common bile duct stones. The role of the available solvents is discussed below.

*Sodium Cholate.* Solutions of sodium cholate (100 mm) infused at 30 ml/h through a T-tube will dissolve some common bile duct stones. The treatment is protracted. Continuous infusion for up to 2 weeks may be necessary. Severe diarrhoea is common because of the load of bile acid reaching the gut. This can be alleviated by oral cholestyramine. In a collected series of 91 patients treated with sodium cholate stone disappearance was reported in only 60% [20]. Stone dissolution with sodium cholate has not become popular because of the limited success rate and the severe side-effects.

*Mono-octanoin.* Mono-octanoin (glyceryl-1-mono-octanoate) is a powerful cholesterol solvent. It is a viscous oil with a melting point of 20°C and samples are often solid. Mono-octanion is diluted with water (nine parts mono-octanoin: one part water) and filtered before use. The addition of water lowers the viscosity of mono-octanoin and markedly increases its cholesterol dissolution rate. Mono-octanoin is infused by gravity or an infusion pump with a manometer broken off at 15 cm between the infusion and the patient. This ensures that the infusion pressure does not exceed 15 cm $H_2O$. In an analysis of 343 patients treated with mono-octanoin [21], complete stone dissolution occurred in 26%. In a further 29% there was "some dissolution" which allowed bile duct clearance by endoscopic or percutaneous techniques. Thus mono-octanoin resulted in bile duct clearance in about half the patients. In 10% treatment had to be stopped because of side-effects. These included abdominal pain, nausea, vomiting and diarrhoea. Uncommon side-effects are acute cholangitis, septicaemia and acute pancreatitis. Treatment with mono-octanoin can last several weeks although the median treatment is 7 days. The modest success rate is probably because many bile duct calculi are brown pigment stones.

*Methyl Tertbutyl Ether.* The use of MTBE for contact dissolution of stones in the ballbladder has been discussed above. MTBE is less satisfactory for dissolving common bile duct stones probably because, as mentioned above, many of these stones are brown pigment calculi but it does work in some patients. MTBE is a very powerful cholesterol solvent and seems to be the preferred cholesterol solvent for common bile duct stones at present. MTBE is delivered to the bile duct through a nasobiliary tube. The principal problems are ensuring that the ether comes into contact with the stones and minimising losses of MTBE into the gut.

*Agents for Dissolving Pigment Stones.* A solution of EDTA and UDCA rapidly dissolves calcium bilirubinate stones in vitro [22]. Similar results are obtained using mixtures of EDTA, sodium cholate and UDCA. The dissolution rate of pigment stones is improved further if the bile acid/EDTA mixture is alternated with a modified mono-octanoin solution [23].

In clinical studies with these mixtures complete dissolution of bile duct stones has been achieved in 30% and partial dissolution in a further 30% over an average of 12 days' treatment [24] Side-effects are similar to those of mono-octanoin. Serum copper and zinc levels fall when EDTA solutions are instilled into the biliary tree and zinc supplements should be given during treatment. These regimens of bile acid/EDTA and mono-octanoin solutions are most successful with brown pigment stones. The hard black pigment stones contain calcium bilirubinate in a highly cross-linked network which makes them very resistant to dissolution.

### *Current Status of Medical Therapy*

Endoscopic sphincterotomy is the quickest and simplest way to clear the bile duct in most patients with common bile duct stones. However, sphincterotomy fails to clear the bile duct in about 10% of patients because the stones are either too large or too numerous. When sphincterotomy fails there are two options. The first is to shatter the stones by ESWL into fragments which will pass through the sphincterotomy. ESWL will clear the bile duct in about 80% of patients although most of these patients will require an additional endoscopic procedure to remove the fragments [25]. The second option is contact dissolution through a nasobiliary tube. ESWL seems to be the preferred method since it is quicker and has a higher success rate than contact dissolution. However, ESWL is expensive and not widely available. In these circumstances contact dissolution may be tried. MTBE is probably the agent of choice but there has been no formal comparison of efficacy with mono-octanoin. Because many common bile duct stones are bile pigment calculi, agents which dissolve calcium bilirubinate should be included. Alternating a bile acid/EDTA or a urea/EDTA mixture with MTBE may give much better results for common bile duct stones.

## References

1. Trotman BW, Soloway RD (1982) Pigment gallstone disease: summary of the National Institutes of Health-International Workshop. Hepatology 2:879–884

2. Danziger R, Hofmann AF, Schoenfield LJ, Thistle JL (1972) Dissolution of cholesterol gallstones by chenodeoxycholic acid. N Engl J Med 286:1–8
3. Iser JH, Maton PN, Murphy GM, Dowling RH (1978) Resistance to chenodeoxycholic acid (CDCA) treatment in obese patients with gallstones. Lancet I:1509–1512
4. Kupfer RM, Maudgal DP, Northfield TC (1987) Gallstone dissolution during chenic acid therapy. Effect of bedtime administration plus low cholesterol diet. Dig Dis Sci 27:1025–1029
5. Maton PN, Iser JH, Reuben A, Saxton HM, Murphy GM, Dowling RH (1982) Outcome of chenodeoxycholic acid (CDCA) treatment in 125 patients with radiolucent gallstones. Medicine (Baltimore) 61:85–96
6. Schoenfield LJ, Lachin JM (1981) Steering committee. Ann Intern Med 95:257–281
7. Fromm H (1986) Gallstone dissolution therapy. Current studies and future prospects. Gastroenterology 91:1560–1567
8. Podda M, Zuin M, Battezzati PM, Ghezzi C, de Fazio C, Dioguardi ML (1989) Efficacy and safety of a combination of chenodeoxycholic acid and ursodeoxycholic acid for gallstone dissolution: a comparison with ursodeoxycholic acid alone. Gastroenterology 96:222–229
9. Marks JW, Lan S-P (1984) The Steering Committee and the National Cooperative Gallstone groups. Low dose chendiol to prevent gallstone recurrence after dissolution therapy. Ann Intern Med 100:376–381
10. Thistle JL (1987) Direct contact dissolution of gallstones. Semin Liver Dis 7:311–316
11. Swobodnik W, Baumgaertel H, Janowitz P, Fuchs S, Ditschuneit H (1988) Dissolution of calcified gallbladder stones by treatment with methyl-hexyl ether and urea-EDTA. Lancet II:216
12. Paumgartner G (1987) Fragmentation of gallstones by extracorporeal shock waves. Semin Liver Dis 7:317–321
13. Doyle PJ, Ward-McQuaid JN, McEwen Smith A (1982) The value of routine per-operative cholangiography – a report of 4000 cholecystectomies. Br J Surg 69:617–619
14. Vellacott KD, Powell PH (1979) Exploration of the common bile duct: a comparative study. Br J Surg 66:389–391
15. Crumplin MKH, Jenkinson LR, Kassab JY, Whitaker CM, Al-Boutahi FH (1985) Management of gallstones in a district general hospital. Br J Surg 72:428–432
16. Cotton PB (1984) Endoscopic management of bile duct stones (apples and oranges). Gut 25:587–597
17. Neoptolemos JP, Carr-Locke DL, Fossard DP (1987) Prospective randomised study of preoperative endoscopic sphincterotomy versus surgery alone for common bile duct stones. Br Med J 294:470–474
18. Escourrou J, Cordova JA, Lazorthes F, Frexinos J, Ribet A (1984) Early and late complications after endoscopic sphincterotomy for biliary lithiasis with and without the gallbladder in situ. Gut 25:598–602
19. Salvioli G, Salati R, Lugli R, Zanni C (1983) Medical treatment of biliary duct stones: effect of ursodeoxycholic acid administration. Gut 24:609–614
20. Motson RW (1981) Dissolution of common bile duct stones. Br J Surg 68:203–208
21. Palmer KR, Hoffmann AF (1986) Intraductal mono-octanoin for the direct dissolution of bile duct stones: experience in 343 patients. Gut 27:196–202
22. Nakamura Y, Suzuki N, Takahashi W, Sato W (1982) A study on the dissolution and disintegration of calcium bilirubinate stones with special reference to effects of litholytic agents in human bile and to irrigation of bile duct in dogs. Tohoku J Exp Med 138:383–395

23. Leuschner U, Baumgartel H (1982) Gallstone dissolution in the biliary tract: in vitro investigations on inhibiting factors and special dissolution agents. Am J Gastroenterol 77:222–226
24. Leuschner U, Baumgartel H, David R, Kirchmeier CM, Sieratsic J (1984) Biochemical and morphological investigations on the toxicity of a Capmul preparation and a bile salt EDTA solution in patients with bile duct stones. Am J Gastroenterol 79:291–298
25. Sauerbruch T, Stern M (1989) Fragmentation of bile duct stones by extracorporeal shock waves. Gastroenterology 96:146–152

# Subject Index